Pharmacotherapeutics for Advanced Practice:
A Practical Approach

Second Edition

Virginia Poole Arcangelo, PhD, CRNP
Family Nurse Practitioner
Grove Family Medical Associates
Haddonfield, New Jersey
and
Clinical Associate Professor
College of Health Professions
Thomas Jefferson University
Philadelphia, Pennsylvania

Andrew M. Peterson, PharmD
Associate Professor of Clinical Pharmacy
Philadelphia College of Pharmacy
University of Sciences in Philadelphia
Philadelphia, Pennsylvania

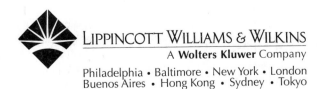

LIPPINCOTT WILLIAMS & WILKINS
A **Wolters Kluwer** Company
Philadelphia • Baltimore • New York • London
Buenos Aires • Hong Kong • Sydney • Tokyo

Acquisitions Editor: Margaret Zuccarini
Managing Editor: Helen Kogut
Senior Project Editor: Tom Gibbons
Senior Production Manager: Helen Ewan
Managing Editor/Production: Erika Kors
Creative Director: Doug Smock
Manufacturing Manager: William Alberti
Indexer: Ann Cassar
Compositor: Techbooks
Printer: Courier-Kendallville

2nd Edition

9 8 7 6 5 4 3 2 1

Library of Congress Cataloging-in-Publication Data

Pharmacotherapeutics for advanced practice : a practical approach/[edited by]
Virginia Poole Arcangelo, Andrew M. Peterson.—2nd ed.
    p. ; cm.
  Includes bibliographical references and index.
  ISBN 0-7817-5784-3 (pbk. : alk. paper)
    1. Chemotherapy. I. Arcangelo, Virginia Poole. II. Peterson, Andrew M.
  [DNLM: 1. Drug Therapy—methods. 2. Pharmaceutical Preparations—administration &
dosage. WB 330 P5354 2006]
  RM262.P4685 2006
  615.5'8—dc22   2005008048

Care has been taken to confirm the accuracy of the information presented and to describe generally accepted practices. However, the authors, editors, and publisher are not responsible for errors or omissions or for any consequences from application
of the information in this book and make no warranty, express or implied, with respect to the content of the publication.

The authors, editors, and publisher have exerted every effort to ensure that drug selectin and dosage set forth in this text
are in accordance with the current recommendations and practice at the time of publication. However, in view of ongoing
research, changes in government regulations, and the constant flow of information relating to drug therapy and drug reactions, the reader is urged to check the package insert for each drug for any change in indications and dosage and for added
warnings and precautions. This is particularly important when the recommended agent is a new or infrequently employed
drug.

Some drugs and medical devices presented in this publication have Food and Drug Administration (FDA) clearance for
limited use in restricted research settings. It is the responsibility of the health care provider to ascertain the FDA status of
each drug or device planned for use in his or her clinical practice.

LWW.com

Dedication

We would like to dedicate this book to our families, Roberta, Tony, David, Kristi, Hanna, Myrna, Maggie, Daniel and Sarah. This book is also dedicated to the memories of Bill and Midge, who are never far from our thoughts and always in our hearts.

CONTRIBUTORS

Edina Advic, PharmD, MBA
Specialty Resident in Infectious Diseases
Hospital of the University of Pennsylvania
Philadelphia, Pennsylvania
*Chapter 53: Opportunistic Infections in
Immunocompromised Patients*

Angela Allerman, PharmD, BCPS
Drug Information Specialist
DoD Pharmacoeconomic Center
Houston, Texas
Chapter 54: Coagulation Disturbances

Peter Anley, PharmD
Clinical Assistant Professor
Ernest Mario School of Pharmacy
Rutgers University
Piscataway, New Jersey
Chapter 4: Principles of Pharmacotherapy in Pediatrics

Robert W. Baran, PharmD
Outcomes Project Manager
Medical Outcomes Research and Economics
Roche Laboratories
Nutley, New Jersey
Chapter 41: Parkinson's Disease

Kelly Barringer, MSN, CRNP
Robert J. Maro Internal Medicine
Cherry Hill, New Jersey
Chapter 18: Hypertension
Chapter 55: Anemias

John Barron, BSPharm, PharmD
Senior Manager, Health Outcomes Research
HealthCore
Wilmington, Delaware
Chapter 19: Hyperlipidemia

Janis Bonat, MSN, CRNP
Family Practice Nurse Practitioner
Department of Family Medicine
Thomas Jefferson University
Philadelphia, Pennsylvania
*Chapter 29: Gastroesophageal Reflux Disease and
Peptic Ulcer Disease*
Chapter 49: Diabetes Mellitus

Mary Bowen, RN, DSN, CNAA
Assistant Professor, Nursing
College of Health Professions
Thomas Jefferson University
Philadelphia, Pennsylvania
Chapter 22: Dysrhythmias

Tim Briscoe, PharmD, CDE
Clinical Pharmacist Specialist–Primary Care
Department of Pharmacy and Drug Information
Grady Health Systems
Atlanta, Georgia
*Chapter 30: Constipation, Diarrhea and Irritable
Bowel Syndrome*

Angela Cafiero, PharmD, CGP
Assistant Professor of Clinical Pharmacy
Philadelphia College of Pharmacy
University of the Sciences in Philadelphia
Philadelphia, Pennsylvania
Chapter 41: Parkinson's Disease
Chapter 48: Alzheimer's Disease

Debra Carroll, MSN, CRNP
Adult/Gerontological Nurse Practitioner
Tri-Valley Primary Care
Telford, Pennsylvania
*Chapter 6: Principles of Pharmacotherapy
in Elderly Patients*

Tara Weikel Chapman, PharmD
Regulatory Project Associate
AstraZeneca LP
Wayne, Pennsylvania
Chapter 47: Attention-Deficit/Hyperactivity Disorder

Sandra Chase, BS, PharmD, FMPA
Clinical Pharmacy Specialist
Spectrum Health
Grand Rapids, Michigan
Chapter 21: Heart Failure

Anne Dellaira, BSN, MSN, PhD, RNCS
Consultant and School Nurse
Johnson's School, Cherry Hill School District
Cherry Hill, New Jersey
Chapter 45: Anxiety

Elyse L. Dishler, BA, MD
Family Physician
Cherry Hill Family Medical Associates
Cherry Hill, New Jersey
Chapter 42: Headaches

Quan V. Dong, PharmD
Project Manager
Health Process Management, Inc.
Owings Mills, Maryland
Chapter 3: Impact of Drug Interactions and Adverse Events on Therapeutics

Eileen Gleason Donnelly, BSN, RN, CCRN
Clinical Care Coordinator, Surgical Intensive Care Unit
Thomas Jefferson University
Philadelphia, Pennsylvania
Chapter 61: Weight Loss

Catherine J. Dragon, PharmD, BCPS
Director of Clinical Services
Office of Professional Programs
University of the Sciences in Philadelphia
Philadelphia, Pennsylvania
Chapter 29: Gastroesophageal Reflux Disease and Peptic Ulcer Disease

Mary Dressler-Carré, MSN, CRNP, CPNP
Director, Children's Clinic
North Penn Visiting Nurse Association
Lansdale, Pennsylvania
Chapter 15: Acne Vulgaris and Rosacea

Teena Eappen-Abraham, PharmD
Assistant Professor of Pharmacy Practice
Arnold and Marie Schwartz College of Pharmacy and Health Sciences
Long Island University
Brooklyn, New York
Clinical Coordinator of Pharmacy Services
New York Methodist Hospital
Brooklyn, New York
Chapter 26: Bronchitis and Pneumonia

Linda C. Foreman, MSN, FNP
Nurse Practitioner
Formerly of Amherst Family Physicians
Mount Holly, New Jersey
Chapter 13: Bacterial Infections of the Skin

Maria Foy, BS Pharm
Pharmacist
Doylestown Hospital
Doylestown, Pennsylvania
Chapter 13: Bacterial Infections of the Skin

Stephanie Gaber, PharmD
Clinical Coordinator
Methodist Hospital
Philadelphia, Pennsylvania
Chapter 5: Principles of Pharmacotherapy in Pregnancy and Lactation

Steven P. Gelone, PharmD
Associate Professor of Pharmacy, Department of Pharmacy Practice
Assistant Professor of Medicine, Section of Infectious Diseases
Temple University School of Pharmacy and Medicine
Philadelphia, Pennsylvania
Chapter 8: Principles of Antimicrobial Therapy

Ellen Boxer Goldfarb, CRNP
Outpatient Coordinator
Jefferson Antithrombic Services
Thomas Jefferson Internal Medicine Associates
Philadelphia, Pennsylvania
Chapter 54: Coagulation Disturbances

Gina M. Karcsh, PharmD
Philadelphia College of Pharmacy
University of the Sciences in Philadelphia
Philadelphia, Pennsylvania
Chapter 42: Headaches

Catherine Kirby, RN, MSN
Director of Quality Improvement
Jefferson Family Medicine
Thomas Jefferson University/Jefferson University Physicians
Philadelphia, Pennsylvania
Chapter 57: Immunizations

Jolynn Knoche, PharmD
Hematology/Oncology Clinical Pharmacist Specialist
Department of Pharmacy and Drug Information
Grady Health Systems
Atlanta, Georgia
Chapter 28: Nausea and Vomiting

Edward C. Li, PharmD
Assistant Professor
Department of Pharmacy Practice
Nesbitt School of Pharmacy
Wilkes University
Wilkes Barre, Pennsylvania
Chapter 56: Oncologic Disorders

Carol Gullo Mest, RN, PhD, CRNP
Director, Family Nurse Practitioner Program
Assistant Professor
DeSales University
Center Valley, Pennsylvania
Chapter 38: Ostoearthritis and Rheumatoid Arthritis

Janis Kubis Miller, CRNP, MS, CDE
Nurse Practitioner
Division of Internal Medicine
Thomas Jefferson University
Philadelphia, Pennsylvania
Chapter 27: Tuberculosis

Paul Miller, PharmD
Medical Information Manager
AstraZeneca LP
Wilmington, Delaware
*Chapter 7: Principles of Pharmacology
in Pain Management*

Samir K. Mistry, PharmD
Clinical Program Manager
Express Scripts, Inc.
Bloomington, Minnesota
Chapter 62: The Economics of Pharmacotherapeutics

Amy S. Morgan, PharmD, BCPS
Clinical Pharmacist
University of Pennsylvania Medical Center
Hospital of the University of Pennsylvania
Philadelphia, Pennsylvania
*Chapter 53: Opportunistic Infections in
Immunocompromised Patients*

Frank Natale, PharmD (Cand.), RPh, BS
Director of Pharmacy
Methodist Hospital Division
Thomas Jefferson University Hospital
Philadelphia, Pennsylvania
Chapter 44: Depressive Disorders

Anne Nichols, MSN, CRNP
Coordinator, Family Nurse Practitioner
Widener University
Chester, Pennsylvania
Chapter 33: Urinary Tract Infections

Judith A. O'Donnell, MD
Assistant Professor, Infectious Diseases
Drexel University College of Medicine
Philadelphia, Pennsylvania
Chapter 8: Principles of Antimicrobial Therapy

Tracy Offerdahl-McGowan, PharmD
Assistant Professor of Clinical Pharmacy
Philadelphia College of Pharmacy
University of the Sciences in Philadelphia
Philadelphia, Pennsylvania
Chapter 48: Alzheimer's Disease

Jessica O'Hara, PharmD
Medical Writer
Aston, Pennsylvania
Chapter 58: Smoking Cessation
Chapter 61: Weight Loss

Staci Pacetti, PharmD
Assistant Professor of Pharmacy
Temple University School of Pharmacy
Philadelphia, Pennsylvania
Chapter 8: Principles of Antimicrobial Therapy

Jeegisha Patel, PharmD
Assistant Professor of Clinical Pharmacy
Philadelphia College of Pharmacy
University of the Sciences in Philadelphia
Philadelphia, Pennsylvania
Chapter 58: Smoking Cessation

Kunjal Patel, PharmD
Centocor
Malvern, Pennsylvania
Chapter 43: Seizure Disorders

Louis R. Petrone, MD
Clinical Assistant Professor of Family Medicine
Jefferson Medical College
Philadelphia, Pennsylvania
Chapter 50: Thyroid Disorders

Silvana Poletajev, MSN, NP-C, CRNP
Family Nurse Practitioner
St. Francis Medical Center
Trenton, New Jersey
Chapter 23: Upper Respiratory Infections

Sherry Ratajczak, RN, MSN, CCRN, PhD (Cand.)
Assistant Professor of Nursing
DeSales University
Center Valley, Pennsylvania
Chapter 34: Prostatic Disorders and Erectile Dysfunction

Alicia Reese, PharmD, MS, BCPS
Assistant Professor of Clinical Pharmacy
Philadelphia College of Pharmacy
University of the Sciences in Philadelphia
Philadelphia, Pennsylvania
Chapter 20: Angina

Cynthia Sanoski, BS, PharmD
Associate Professor of Clinical Pharmacy
Philadelphia College of Pharmacy
University of the Sciences in Philadelphia
Philadelphia, Pennsylvania
Chapter 22: Dysrhythmias

Matthew Sarnes, PharmD
Clinical Consultant
Applied Health Outcomes
Tampa, Florida
*Chapter 3: Impact of Drug Interactions and Adverse
Events on Therapeutics*

Susan Schrand, RN, MSN, CRNP
Outpatient Intensivist
Renaissance Medical Management Co.
Wayne, Pennsylvania
Chapter 40: Fibromyalgia

Anita Siu, PharmD
Clinical Assistant Professor
Ernest Mario School of Pharmacy
Rutgers University
Piscataway, New Jersey
Neonatal/Pediatric Pharmacotherapy Specialist
Jersey Shore University Medical Center
Neptune, New Jersey
Chapter 4: Principles of Pharmacotherapy in Pediatrics

Anthony P. Sorrentino, BSc, PharmD
Director of Experiential Resources
Philadelphia College of Pharmacy
University of the Sciences in Philadelphia
Philadelphia, Pennsylvania
Chapter 51: Allergies and Allergic Reactions

Joshua J. Spooner, PharmD, MS
Director, Clinical Business Solutions
Advanced Concepts Institute
Philadelphia, Pennsylvania
Chapter 16: Ophthalmic Disorders
Chapter 42: Headaches
Chapter 62: The Economics of Pharmacotherapeutics

Linda M. Spooner, PharmD, BCPS
Clinical Assistant Professor
Ernest Mario School of Pharmacy
Rutgers University
Piscataway, New Jersey
Clinical Pharmacy Specialist in Infectious Diseases
Jersey Shore University Medical Center
Neptune, New Jersey
Chapter 52: Human Immunodeficiency Virus

Liza Takiya, PharmD
Associate Professor of Clinical Pharmacy
Philadelphia College of Pharmacy
University of the Sciences in Philadelphia
Philadelphia, Pennsylvania
Chapter 31: Inflammatory Bowel Disease

Nancy Tomaselli, RN, MSN, CRNP, CWOCN
Nurse Practitioner
Medical Center at Princeton
Continence Management Center
Princeton, New Jersey
President and CEO
Premier Health Solutions
Cherry Hill, New Jersey
Chapter 36: Sexually Transmitted Infections

Elena M. Umland, PharmD
Associate Professor of Clinical Pharmacy
Philadelphia College of Pharmacy
University of the Sciences in Philadelphia
Adjunct Clinical Assistant Professor of Family Medicine
Jefferson Medical College
Philadelphia, Pennsylvania
Chapter 60: Contraception

Denise Vanacore-Netz, MSN, CRNP
Coordinator, Adult NP Program
Graduate Nursing Division
Gwynedd Mercy College
Gwynedd Valley, Pennsylvania
Chapter 11: Fungal Infections of the Skin
Chapter 12: Viral Infections of the Skin
Chapter 14: Psoriasis

Samantha Venable, RN, MSN, FNP
Professor, Health Sciences and Human Services
Saddleback College
Mission Viejo, California
Chapter 32: Parasitic Infections

Eva Vivian, PharmD, CDE, BCPS
Associate Professor of Pharmacy Practice
College of Pharmacy
Western University of Health Sciences
Pomona, California
Chapter 18: Hypertension

Katherine Waltman, PharmD, BCPS
Medical Science Manager
Bristol-Meyers Squibb
Princeton, New Jersey
Chapter 48: Alzheimer's Disease

Veronica Wilbur, MSN, CRNP
Assistant Professor
Wilmington College
New Castle, Delaware
Chapter 30: Constipation, Diarrhea and Irritable Bowel Syndrome
Chapter 46: Insomnia and Sleep Disorders

Eric Wittbrodt, PharmD, BCPS, FCCM
Associate Professor of Clinical Pharmacy
Philadelphia College of Pharmacy
University of the Sciences in Philadelphia
Philadelphia, Pennsylvania
Chapter 26: Bronchitis and Pneumonia

Andrea Wolf, CRNP, MSN
Coordinator, Family Nurse Practitioner Program
Widener University School of Nursing
Chester, Pennsylvania
Family Practitioner
Lancaster, Pennsylvania
Chapter 37: Vaginitis

Nancy Youngblood, PhD, CRNP
Assistant Professor, Director, Adult Nurse Practitioner and
Family Nurse Practitioner
La Salle University, School of Nursing
Philadelphia, Pennsylvania
Chapter 20: Angina

Linda Zimmerman, MSN, FNP
Family Nurse Practitioner
Centro San Vicente Familiar de Salud
El Paso, Texas
Chapter 17: Otitis Media and Otitis Externa

REVIEWERS

Gary Arnold, MD
Associate Professor
College of Nursing and Allied Health Professions
University of Louisiana at Lafayette
Lafayette, Louisiana

Linda S. Baas, RN, PhD, ACNP
Professor and Director
Acute Care Graduate Program
University of Cincinnati
Cincinnati, Ohio

Steven L. Bents, MPAS, PA-C
Director, RMC PA Program
Rocky Mountain College
Billings, Montana

Donna G. Best, MN, ACNP
Associate Professor
Memorial University School of Nursing
St. John's, Newfoundland, Canada

Christine Bruce
Program Director, Physician Assistant Program
DeSales University
Center Valley, Pennsylvania

Susan A. Bruce, PhD(c), ANP
Clinical Associate Professor
University of Buffalo
Buffalo, New York

T. Joyce Bruce, RN, B, MSA, MSN-ANP
Faculty Primary Care Nurse
Nursing Division SIAST
Regina, Saskatchewan, Canada

Lucindra Campbell, MSN, RN
Adult Psychiatric Nurse Practitioner
Associate Professor
Houston Baptist University
Houston, Texas

Katherine Crabtree
Director of Nursing, Professor
Oregon Health and Science University
Portland, Oregon

Patsy E. Crihfield, MSN, RN, CCRN, FNP
Associate Professor of Nursing
Dyersburg State Community College
Dyersburg, Tennessee

Claire DeCristofaro, MD
Assistant Professor
College of Nursing and College of Health Professions
Medical University of South Carolina
Charleston, South Carolina

Glenn Donnelly, RN ENC, BscN, MN, PhD
Assistant Professor
College of Nursing, University of Saskatchewan
Regina, Saskatchewan, Canada

Dawn Lee Garzon, MSN, RN, CS, CPNP,
Clinical Assistant Professor
Barnes College of Nursing and Health Studies
University of Missouri—St. Louis
St. Louis, Missouri

Andy Grimone, PharmD
Clinical Pharmacy Specialist/Director
Pharmacy Residency Program
Saint Vincent Health Center
Erie, Pennsylvania

Brenda Halabisky, RN (EC), MSc, PHCNP, FNP-C
Curriculum Coordinator
University of Ottawa
Ottawa, Ontario, Canada

Margaret J. Halter, PhD, APRN
Professor of Nursing
Malone College
Canton, Ohio

Therese Jamison, MSN, RN, CS, ACNP
Assistant Professor
Madonna University
Farmington Hills, Michigan

Margaret C. Kydeman, RN, PhD, APRN, BC
Associate Professor
University of New Brunswick
Fredericton, Canada

Anisha Lakhani, BSc Pharm, PharmD
Drug Use Evaluation Coordinator, Clinical Pharmacist,
  Clinical Instructor
University of British Columbia
Surrey Memorial Hospital
Surrey, British Columbia, Canada

Mary Ann Lavin, ScD, RN, BC, ANP, FAAN
Associate Professor
St. Louis University School of Nursing
St. Louis, Missouri

David Miller, MD, FCCP
Adjunct Professor
College of Nursing and Health Sciences
Texas A&M University—Corpus Christi
Corpus Christi, Texas

Diane Montgomery, PhD, CPNP
Assistant Professor
Texas Woman's University College of Nursing
Houston, Texas

Patricia J. Neafsey, BS, MS, PhD
Professor
University of Connecticut School of Nursing
Stafford Springs, Connecticut

Dorothy Ochs, MSN, ARNP, BC
Assistant Professor
Fort Hays State University
Department of Nursing and Family
Hays, Kansas

Dale W. Quest, RN, PhD
Associate Professor
College of Nursing
University of Saskatchewan
Saskatoon, Saskatchewan, Canada

Elizabeth Sefcik, PhD, RNCS
Professor of Nursing
Texas A&M University—Corpus Christi
Corpus Christi, Texas

Beverly A. Sullivan, BS, PharmD
Director of Pharmacy Practice
Associate Professor
University of Wyoming School of Pharmacy
Laramie, Wyoming

Linda Tenofsky, PhD, APRN, BC
Professor and Basic Program Coordinator
Curry College
Milton, Massachusetts

Peggy Thweatt, RN, MSN
Nursing Faculty Development Coordinator
Coppin State College School of Nursing
Baltimore, Maryland

Deborah Williams, CRNP, PhD
Assistant Professor
DeSales University
Center Valley, Pennsylvania

PREFACE

INTRODUCTION

The origins of this text come from our combined experience in teaching nurse practitioners. As a nurse practitioner and educator herself, Virginia saw a need for practical exposure to the general principles of prescribing and monitoring drug therapy, particularly in the Family Practice arena. As a PharmD, Andrew saw a need to be able to teach new prescribers how to think about prescribing systematically, regardless of the disease state. We both found no suitable book that combined the practical with the systematic—most of the textbooks dedicated to this topic provided too much basic pharmacology with too little therapeutics. This book not only gives the basics on the pharmacology of the drugs, it also provides a process through which learners can begin to think pharmacotherapeutically—that is, learners will begin to identify a disease, review the drugs used to treat the disease, select treatment based on goals of therapy and special patient considerations, and learn how to adjust therapy if it fails to meet goals.

This is a book that meets the needs of both students and practitioners in a practical approach that is user friendly. It teaches the practitioner how to prescribe and manage drug therapy in primary care. The design of the book is based on input from both academicians and practitioners. Contributors were selected from academia and practice to provide a combination of evidence-based medicine and practical experience. The text considers disease- and patient-specific information. With each chapter, there are tables and algorithms that are practical and easy to read and that complement the text.

Additionally, the text guides the practitioner to a choice of second- and third-line therapy when the first line of therapy fails. Since new drugs are being marketed at all times, drug categories are discussed and information can be applied to the new drugs. Each chapter ends with case studies, and each case study asks the same questions. There are no answers to the questions since the authors believe the purpose of the case studies is to promote discussion, and that there may be more than one correct answer to each question, especially as new drugs are developed. What's more, the questions appear in the order in which they would be asked by a practitioner as he or she prescribes a medication.

ORGANIZATION OF THE BOOK

UNIT I—PRINCIPLES OF THERAPEUTICS

The first chapter introduces the prescribing process, including how to avoid medication errors. The next chapter provides the traditional, and necessary, information on the pharmacokinetics and pharmacodynamics of drugs. Using this foundation, the subsequent chapters apply this information to drug-drug and drug-food interactions, and discuss the changes in these parameters in pediatric, geriatric, and pregnant patients. The remaining chapters in the Principles unit give overviews of drugs that are used across many disease states: pain medications and antibiotics. These chapters discuss the principles of pain management and infectious disease therapy, so that the reader can learn how these concepts are applied to the disorders discussed in the following units. A full chapter on Complementary and Alternative Medicine (CAM) has been added to this section, recognizing the increased used of these modalities and attempting to meet the ever-growing need for information related to this aspect of patient care.

UNITS II THROUGH XII—DISORDERS

This section of the book, consisting of 47 chapters, reviews commonly seen disorders in the primary care setting. Although not all-inclusive, the array of disorders allows the reader to gain an understanding of how to approach the pharmacotherapeutic treatment of any disorder. The chapters are designed to give a brief overview of the disease process, including the causes and pathophysiology, with an emphasis placed on how drug therapy can alter the pathologic state. Diagnostic Criteria and Goals of Therapy are discussed and underlie the basic principles of treating patients with drugs.

In this second edition, several chapters have been condensed, such as Peptic Ulcer Disease and Gastroesophogeal Reflux Disease, and Irritable Bowel Syndrome and Constipation and Diarrhea, to avoid duplication. Other chapters have been expanded, such as Headaches to include all headaches and not just migraines, and Sleep Disorders to include restless leg syndrome and narcolepsy. The

Ophthalmic Disorders chapter also has been expanded. Chapters on Anemia and Cancer Chemotherapy have been added.

The drug sections review the agents' uses, mechanism of action, contraindications and drug interactions, adverse effects, and monitoring parameters. This discussion is organized primarily by drug class, with notation to specific drugs within the text and the tables. The tables provide the reader with a quick access to generic and trade names and dosages, adverse events, contraindications, and special considerations. Used together, the text and tables provide any reader with sufficient information to begin to choose a drug therapy for a patient.

The section on Selecting the Most Appropriate Agent aids the reader in deciding which agent to choose for a given patient. This section contains information on first-line, second-line and third-line therapies, with rationales for why agents are classified in these categories. Accompanying this section is an algorithm outlining the thought process by which clinicians select an initial drug therapy. Again, the text organization and the illustrative algorithms provide readers with a means of thinking through the process of selecting drugs for patients. In the second edition, we have kept the Recommended Order of Treatment tables and updated them, along with the algorithms and drug tables, to reflect current knowledge. Each chapter has been updated to reflect the most current guidelines available at the time of writing. However, medicine and pharmacotherapy are constantly changing, and it remains the clinician's responsibility to determine the most current information. To assist in this, we encourage you to access the companion website, http://connection.lww.com, which contains quarterly updated drug information from content published by Facts and Comparisons.

Included in each chapter is a section on monitoring a patient's response. This encompasses clinical and laboratory parameters, times when these items should be monitored, and actions to take in case the parameters do not meet the specified goals of therapy. In addition, special patient populations are discussed when appropriate. These discussions include pediatric and geriatric patients, but may also include ethnic- or sex-related considerations. Lastly, this unit includes a discussion of patient education material relevant to the disease and drugs chosen. In each chapter we have expanded the patient education section to include information on CAM related to that disorder; we have also added sections for patients and practitioners on sources of information external to the text.

Each of the case studies has been reviewed and updated as appropriate. The case study questions have been updated to reflect new content in the chapters. However, the pedagogical style of reasoning remains the same. Answers to these case studies are not supplied since the purpose is to promote discussion and evoke a thought process. Also, as time changes, so do therapies. Lastly, multiple "right" answers can be developed, and it is the responsibility of the instructor to help the student work through the process. In the last chapter, Integrative Approach, we do offer potential answers to the cases. These may not be the only answers, but indicate some of the thought processes that go into the decision-making process in pharmacologic management of a problem.

UNIT XIII—PHARMACOTHERAPY IN HEALTH PROMOTION

This unit discusses several areas of interest for promoting health or maintaining a healthy lifestyle using medications, including smoking cessation, immunizations, weight management, and contraception.

UNIT XIV—INTEGRATIVE APPROACH TO PATIENT CARE

This is a new section in the second edition. Chapter 62, The Economics of Pharmacotherapeutics, was moved here from Unit I to emphasize the need to balance clinical need with economic reality. This chapter discusses the economics of therapeutics, including formularies, co-pays, prior-authorizations, and managed care as it applies to prescribing medications.

The last chapter, Integrative Approaches to Pharmacotherapy, is an attempt to examine real-life, complex cases. Each case addresses the nine questions posed in the individual chapter case studies, but now provides the reader with examples of how to approach the case studies and examines issues to consider when presented with more than one diagnosis.

The book offers a consistent approach throughout each disorder chapter. The chapter format begins with the background and pathophysiology of the disorder, followed by a discussion of the relevant classes of drugs. These broad categories are then integrated in the section on Selecting the Most Appropriate Agent.

Drug overview tables are also organized consistently, giving the reader much information on each drug, including the usual dose, contraindications and side effects, and any special consideration a prescriber should be aware of during therapy. All of this information is supported by the significant text.

Algorithms provide the reader with a visual cue on how to approach treating a patient.

Recommended order of treatment tables provide the reader with basic drug therapy selection, from first-line to third-line therapies for each disorder. These, coupled with the algorithms and the drug tables, are the core of the text.

A **case study** is provided for each disorder discussed. These short cases are designed to stimulate discussion among students and with instructors. The nine questions at the end of each case are tailored to each disorder, but remain similar across all cases to reinforce the process of thinking pharmacotherapeutically.

This book is intended to provide primary care students with a reasoned approach to learning pharmacotherapeutics and to serve as a reference for the seasoned practitioner. As current instructors and practitioners, we are dedicated to providing you with a textbook that will meet your needs.

Virginia Poole Arcangelo
Andrew M. Peterson

ACKNOWLEDGMENTS

We would like to thank the people at Lippincott Williams & Wilkins, including Margaret Zuccarini, Joe Morita, Tom Gibbons, and Helen Kogut. We are also forever indebted to the contributors and reviewers who spent countless hours working on this project. Without them, this would never have become a reality.

TABLE OF CONTENTS

I

Principles of Therapeutics

ISSUES FOR THE PRACTITIONER IN DRUG THERAPY

■ VIRGINIA P. ARCANGELO

Drug therapy is often the mainstay of treatment of acute and chronic diseases. An important role of health care practitioners is to develop a treatment plan with the patient, and an integral part of treatment of disease and health promotion is drug therapy. In 2002, approximately 3.34 billion drugs were prescribed, up 4% from 2001 (Voczek, 2003). A nurse practitioner writes about 11 to 15 prescriptions a day.

In developing a treatment plan that includes drug therapy, the prescribing practitioner considers many issues in achieving the goal of safe, appropriate, and effective therapy. Among them are drug safety and product safeguards, the practitioner's role and responsibilities, the step-by-step process of prescribing therapy and writing the prescription, and follow-up measures; particularly important are promoting adherence to the therapeutic regimen and keeping up to date with the latest developments in drug therapy.

DRUG SAFETY AND MARKET SAFEGUARDS

In the United States drug safety is ensured in many ways, but primarily by the U.S. Food and Drug Administration (FDA), which is the federal agency charged with conducting and monitoring clinical trials, approving new drugs for market and manufacture, and ensuring safe drugs for public consumption. Although the federal government provides guidelines for a pure and safe drug product, guidelines for prescribers of drug therapy are dictated both by state and federal governments and licensing bodies in each state.

Clinical Trials

Various legislated mechanisms are in place to ensure pure and safe drug products. One of these mechanisms is the clinical trial process by which new drug development is carefully monitored by the FDA. Every new drug must successfully pass through several stages of development. The first stage is preclinical trials, which involve testing in animals and monitoring efficacy, toxic effects, and untoward reactions. Application to the FDA for investigational use of a drug is made only after this portion of research is completed.

Clinical trials, which begin only after the FDA grants approval for investigation, consist of four phases and may last up to 9 years before a drug is approved for general use. During clinical trials, performed on informed volunteers, data are gathered about the proposed drug's purity, bioavailability, potency, efficacy, safety, and toxicity.

Phase I of clinical trials is the initial evaluation of the drug. It involves supervised studies on 20 to 100 healthy people and focuses on absorption, distribution, metabolism (sometimes interchangeable with biotransformation), and elimination of the drug. In phase I, the most effective administration routes and dosage ranges are determined. During phase II, up to several hundred patients with the disease for which the drug is intended are subjects. The testing focus is the same as in phase I, except that drug effects are monitored on people with disease.

Phase III begins once the FDA determines that the drug causes no apparent serious adverse effects and that the dosage range is appropriate. Double-blind research methods (in which neither the study and control subjects nor the investigators know who is receiving the test drug and who is not) are used for data collection in this phase, and the proposed drug is compared with one already proven to be effective. Usually several thousand subjects are involved in this phase, which lasts several years and during which most risks of the proposed drug are discovered. At the completion of phase III, the FDA evaluates data presented and accepts or rejects the application for the new drug. Approval of the application means that the drug can be marketed—but only by the company seeking the approval.

Once on the market, the drug enters phase IV trials. Initially, the drug is released on a limited basis, then later on a more widespread basis. Everyone who takes the drug is monitored. Adverse drug reactions are reported and investigated. In late phase III and phase IV studies, the pharmaceutical companies have several objectives:

- To compare the drug with other drugs already available
- To monitor long-term effectiveness and impact on quality of life
- To determine cost effectiveness of the therapy in relation to other available therapies

Prevention of Harm and Misuse

Further safety promotion and harm prevention is ensured by the FDA's Controlled Substances Act of 1970, which establishes a schedule or ranking of drugs that have the potential for abuse or misuse. Drugs on the schedule are considered controlled substances. These drugs have the potential to induce dependency and addiction, either psychologically or physiologically. Box 1-1 defines the five categories of scheduled drugs, with Schedule 1 drugs having the greatest potential for abuse and Schedule 5 drugs the least.

Schedule drugs can be prescribed only by a practitioner who is registered and approved by the U.S. Drug Enforcement Agency (DEA). The DEA issues approved applicants a number, which must be written on the prescription for a

---

BOX 1–1. SCHEDULED DRUGS

Schedule 1 drugs have a high potential for abuse. There is no routine therapeutic use for these drugs and they are not available for regular use. They may be obtained for "investigational use only" by applying to the U.S. Drug Enforcement Agency. Examples include heroin and LSD.

Schedule 2 drugs have a valid medical use but a high potential for abuse, both psychological and physiologic. In an emergency, a Schedule 2 drug may be prescribed by telephone if a written prescription cannot be provided at the time. However, a written prescription must be provided within 72 hours with the words *authorization for emergency dispensing* written on the prescription. These prescriptions cannot be refilled. A new prescription must be written each time. Examples include certain amphetamines and barbiturates.

Schedule 3 drugs have a potential for abuse, but the potential is lower than for drugs on Schedule 2. These drugs contain a combination of controlled and noncontrolled substances. Use of these drugs can cause a moderate to low physiologic dependence and a higher psychological dependence. A verbal order can be given to the pharmacy and the prescription can be refilled up to five times within 6 months. Examples include certain narcotics (codeine) and nonbarbiturate sedatives.

Schedule 4 drugs have a low potential for abuse. They can cause psychological dependency but limited physiologic dependency. Examples include nonnarcotic analgesics and antianxiety agents, such as lorazepam (Ativan).

Schedule 5 drugs have the least potential for abuse. They contain a moderate amount of opioids and are used mainly as antitussives and antidiarrheals. Examples include antitussives and antidiarrheals with small amounts of narcotics.

---

controlled substance for the prescription to be valid. The prescriber's DEA number must also appear on a prescription that is being filled in another state.

Prescription Versus Nonprescription Drugs

Some drugs may be obtained without a prescription. Although they are commonly and legally obtained over the counter (OTC) without a prescription, these drugs also must have approval from the FDA for specific uses in specific doses. At one time, many of these drugs were available only by prescription. Currently, however, they are available in lower doses (ie, the lowest effective dose) without a prescription. These drugs carry user warnings on the labels. Many have the potential for interacting adversely with prescribed drugs or complicating existing disease. The self-prescribed use of OTC drugs may delay diagnosis and treatment of potentially serious problems. On the other hand, the use of OTC drugs can be beneficial for treatment of self-limiting disorders that are not serious.

Generic Drugs Versus Brand Name Drugs

Substituting a generic drug for a brand name drug is a common practice. When the patent on a brand name drug expires, other drug manufacturers can then produce the same drug formula under its generic name (the generic name and formula of a drug are always the same; only the brand names change). This practice not only benefits the manufacturer but decreases the cost to the consumer. To ensure safety, the FDA must grant approval for these drugs, and rigorous testing is again required to ensure that all generic drugs meet specifications for quality, purity, strength, and potency.

To obtain FDA approval, the generic drug is administered in a single dose to at least 18 healthy human subjects. Next, peak serum concentration and the area under the plasma concentration curve (AUC) are measured. The values obtained for the generic drug must be within 80% to 125% of those obtained for the brand name drug. Most generic drugs have a mean AUC within 3% of the brand name drug. There has been no reported therapeutic difference of a serious nature between brand name products and FDA-approved generic products. For more information, see Table 1-1, which presents FDA equivalency ratings for brand name and generic drugs.

Complementary and Alternative Medicine (CAM)

In the United States over the last 10 years the use of herbal preparations as treatments for disease and disease prevention has increased tremendously. Historically, herbs were the first healing system used. Herbal medicines are derived from plants and thought by many to be harmless because they are products of nature. Some prescription drugs in current use, however, such as digitalis, are also "natural," which is not synonymous with "harmless." Like synthetic products, natural substances may interact with

Table 1.1

FDA Therapeutic Equivalence Ratings

Rating Scale	Definition
A	*Therapeutically Equivalent*
AA	Products in conventional dosage forms not presenting bioequivalence problems
AB	Products meeting necessary bioequivalence requirements
AN	Solutions and powders for aerosolization
AO	Injectable oil solutions
AP	Injectable aqueous solutions and, in certain instances, intravenous nonaqueous solutions
AT	Topical products
B	*Not Therapeutically Equivalent*
BB	Drug products requiring further FDA investigation and review to determine therapeutic equivalence
BC	Extended-release dosage forms (capsules, injectables, and tablets)
BD	Active ingredients and dosage forms with documented bioequivalence problems
BE	Delayed-release oral dosage forms
BN	Products in aerosol–nebulizer drug delivery systems
BP	Active ingredients and dosage forms with potential bioequivalence problems
BR	Suppositories or enemas that deliver drugs for systemic absorption
BS	Products having drug standard deficiencies
BT	Topical products with bioequivalence issues
BX	Drug products for which the data are insufficient to determine therapeutic equivalence
AB	Potential equivalence problems have been resolved with adequate in vivo or in vitro evidence supporting bioequivalence

Compiled by Samir K. Mistry.

other drugs and may produce undesirable side effects as well.

Before 1962, herbal preparations were considered to be drugs, but now they are sold as foods or supplements and therefore do not require FDA approval as drugs. Hence, there are no legislated standards on purity or quantity of active ingredients in herbal preparations. The value of herbal therapy is usually measured by anecdotal reports and not verified by research.

The Dietary Supplement Health and Education Act (1994) requires labeling about the effect of herbal products on the body and requires the statement that the herbal product has not been reviewed by the FDA and is not intended to be used as a drug. CAM is discussed in Chapter 9.

PRACTITIONER'S ROLE AND RESPONSIBILITIES IN PRESCRIBING

Before prescribing therapy, the practitioner has a responsibility to gather data by taking a thorough history and performing a physical examination. Once the data are gathered and evaluated, one or more diagnoses are formulated and a treatment plan established. As noted, the most frequently used treatment modality is drug therapy, usually with a prescription drug.

If a drug is deemed necessary for therapy, it is essential for the practitioner to understand the responsibility involved in prescribing that drug or drugs and to consider seriously

which class of medication is most appropriate for the patient. The decision is reached based on a thorough knowledge of diagnosis and treatment.

Drug Selection

To determine which therapy is best for the patient, the practitioner conducts a risk–benefit analysis, evaluating the therapeutic value versus the risk associated with each drug to be prescribed. The practitioner then selects from a vast number of pharmacologic agents used for treating the specific medical problem. Factors to consider when selecting the drug or drugs are the subtle or significant differences in action, side effects, interactions, convenience, storage needs, route of administration, efficacy, and cost. Another factor in the decision may involve the patient pressuring the practitioner to prescribe a medication (because that is the expectation of many patients at the beginning of a health care encounter). Clearly, many responsibilities are inherent in prescribing a medication, and serious consequences may result if these responsibilities are not taken seriously and the prescription is prepared incorrectly.

Initial questions to ask when selecting drug therapy include "Is there a need for this drug in treating the presenting problem or disease?" and "Is this the best drug for the presenting problem or disease?" Additional questions are listed in Box 1-2.

BOX 1–2. QUESTIONS TO ADDRESS WHEN PRESCRIBING A MEDICATION

- Is there a need for the drug in treating the presenting problem?
- Is this the best drug for the presenting problem?
- Are there no contraindications to this drug with this patient?
- Is the dosage correct? Or is it too high or too low?
- Does the patient have allergies or sensitivities to the drug?
- What drug treatment modalities does the patient currently use, and will the potential new drug interact with the patient's other drugs or treatments?
- Is there a problem with storage of drug?
- Does the dosage regimen (schedule) interfere with the patient's lifestyle? For example, if a child is in school, a drug with a once- or twice-daily dosing schedule is more realistic than one with a four-times-daily schedule.
- Is the route of administration the most appropriate one?
- Is the proposed duration of treatment too short or too long?
- Can the patient take the prescribed drug?
- Has the patient been informed of possible side effects and what to do if they occur?

Concerns Related to Ethics and Practice

Certain ethical and practical issues must be considered as well. One overriding issue may be the lack of a clinical indication for using a medication. As mentioned, many patients visit a practitioner with the sole purpose of obtaining a prescription. In seeking medical attention, the ill patient expects the health care provider to promote relief from symptoms. In today's world, an abundance of information available in books, magazines, television, Web sites, and other media suggests that the health care provider can do this by prescribing a special medication. This expectation that a magic pill or potion—the prescription—is the ticket that will relieve reflux, kill germs, end pain, and restore health puts pressure on the practitioner to prescribe for the sake of prescribing. A common example of this involves the patient with a cold who seeks an antibiotic, such as penicillin. In such a situation, the practitioner has a responsibility to prescribe only medications that are necessary for the well-being of the patient and that will be effective in treating the problem. In the example of the patient with an uncomplicated head cold, an antibiotic would not be effective, and the responsible practitioner must be prepared to make an ethical and judicious decision and explain it to the patient.

Patient Education

An integral part of the practitioner's role and responsibility is educating the patient about drug therapy and its intended therapeutic effect, potential side effects, and strategies for dealing with possible adverse drug reactions. This may be explained verbally, with written instructions given, when appropriate. Instructions that are printed and handed to the patient must be readable and in a language that the patient can understand.

Medications can also have a placebo effect. Patients must believe that the drug will work for them to be committed to taking it as recommended. If that belief is not instilled in patients, the drug may not be perceived as effective and may not be taken as directed.

The practitioner may want to advise the patient to use only one pharmacy when filling prescriptions. The choice of only one pharmacy has several advantages, which include maintaining a record of all medications that the patient currently receives and serving as a double check for drug–drug interactions.

Prescriptive Authority

Prescribing practices of each practitioner are regulated by the state in which he or she practices. Each state determines practice parameters by statutes (laws enacted by the legislature) and rules and regulations (administrative policies determined by regulatory agencies). Each practitioner is responsible for knowing the laws and regulations in the state of practice. For instance, some states require a physician's signature on all prescriptions; other states require a physician's signature just on prescriptions for controlled substances.

Prescriptive authority is regulated by the State Board of Nursing, Board of Medicine, or Board of Pharmacy, depending on the state. States allow independent practice, collaborative practice, supervised practice, or delegated practice. Independent practice has no requirements for mandatory physician collaboration or supervision. Collaborative practice requires a formal agreement with a collaborating physician, ensuring a referral–consultant relationship. Supervised practice is overseen or directed by a supervisory physician. Delegated practice means that prescription writing is a delegated medical act.

Related to prescriptive authority issues is the issue of drug samples. Most drug companies engage in the promotional practice of distributing sample drugs to practitioners for use by patients. The Prescription Drug Marketing Act (PDMA), which was enacted in 1988 to protect the American consumer from ineffective drugs, also affects the receipt and dispensing of sample drugs. Prescription drugs can be distributed only to licensed practitioners (one licensed by the state to prescribe drugs) and health care entity pharmacies at the request of a licensed practitioner. PDMA protects the public in several ways. It forbids foreign countries to reimport prescription drugs; bans the sale, trade, and purchase of drug samples; prohibits resale of prescription drugs purchased by hospitals, health care entities, and charitable organizations; requests practitioners to ask for drug samples in writing; and regulates wholesale distributors of prescription drugs by requiring licensing in states where facilities are located. There are penalties for violation of the act. This act affects the distribution and use of pharmaceutical samples.

Because these samples are freely available, it might be assumed that they can be distributed by all practitioners, but this is not the case. The practitioner must be aware of the rules that govern requesting, receiving, and distributing these agents because the rules vary from state to state.

Specific procedures are required with drug samples. The pharmaceutical representative's Sample Request Form must be signed. It includes the name, strength, and quantity of the sample. The sample must be then recorded on the Record of Receipt of Drug Sample sheet. The samples must be stored away from other drug inventory and where unauthorized access is not allowed or in a locked cabinet or closet in a public area. Samples are to be inspected monthly for expiration dates, proper labeling and storage, presence of intact packaging and labeling, and appropriateness for the practice. If a sample has expired, it must be disposed in a manner that prevents accessibility to the general public. They cannot be disposed into the trash.

When distributing samples, each must be labeled with the patient's name, clear directions for use, and cautions. They are to be dispensed free of charge along with pertinent information. The medication is then documented in the patient's chart with dose, quantity, and directions.

Avoiding Errors

There are some common errors that can occur when prescribing drugs causing adverse drug events. A recent study in ambulatory care reported that 25% of 661 subjects reported an adverse drug event. Of these, 39% were avoidable and 6% were serious (Gandhi et al., 2003). Errors can be caused by a lack of drug knowledge, lack of patient information, poor communication, and failure to consider special populations (Doherty et al., 2004).

Lack of Drug Knowledge

There can be a lack of knowledge about indications and contraindications for drugs. This includes underuse, overuse, and misuse of drugs. An example of underuse is failure to prescribe an inhaled corticosteroid for an asthmatic who uses his albuterol daily. An example of overuse is prescribing an antibiotic for a cold or prescribing an antihypertensive drug for someone whose blood pressure is elevated because he is taking Sudafed. An example of misuse is prescribing hydrochlorothiazide to someone who is allergic to sulfa.

Dosing errors occur when a larger dose is prescribed than needed. Starting someone on 30 mg paroxetine instead of 20 mg may increase anxiety.

Lack of knowledge about drug–drug interactions can cause errors. For example, many drugs interfere with warfarin and cause increased bleeding if taken together.

Lack of Patient Information

A common error in prescribing is failure to obtain an adequate history from the patient. Often an adequate drug history is not obtained and the provider does not specifically inquire about OTC medications. Also information on allergies to medications is not always obtained. In addition to allergies, it is imperative to ascertain the reaction to the medication. Nausea is not considered an allergic reaction. An allergy history should be taken and documented at each visit before a new medication is prescribed.

Poor Communication

Poor communication can be a result of poor handwriting, incorrect abbreviations, misplaced decimals, and misunderstanding of verbal prescriptions. Poor communication also results when the prescriber fails to discuss potential side effects or ask about side effects at subsequent visits.

Special Population Considerations

Doses for children are usually based on weight in kilograms. The prescriber has a responsibility to calculate the dose and write the correct dose, rather than relying on the pharmacist to calculate the dose.

Elderly patients may have some difficulty hearing or reading small print. Additionally, they may be taking multiple prescription medications and OTC medications. The prescriber needs to be specific about when the patient should take each medication and if one drug cannot be taken with others. When the practitioner prescribes for the elderly, he or she one must consider renal function because some medications can cause toxicity, even in small doses, with decreased renal function.

STEPS OF THE PRESCRIBING PROCESS

At each visit, a medication history is obtained with the name of the drug, dosage, and frequency of administration. Information on any allergies should also be obtained. It is also helpful if the patient brings his or her actual drugs to the visit.

Multiple steps (Fig. 1-1) are involved in prescribing drugs and evaluating their effectiveness. Again, the first step is determining an accurate diagnosis based on the patient's history, physical examination, and pertinent test findings.

Next, in selecting the best agent, the practitioner thoroughly evaluates the patient's condition, taking into consideration the effect that various medications may have on the patient and the disorder, the expected outcomes of therapy, and other variables (Box 1-3). When prescribing any drug therapy, the practitioner must have a solid knowledge and background in the pathophysiology of disease, pharmacotherapeutics, pharmacokinetics, pharmacodynamics, and any interactions (see Chapter 3).

The practitioner needs to be knowledgeable about the best class of drugs for the diagnosed disorder or presenting problem, the recommended dosage, potential side effects, possible interactions with other drugs, and special prescribing considerations, such as required laboratory tests, contraindications, and patient instructions. To select the correct medication, the practitioner must thoroughly understand the pathophysiology of the condition being treated and the natural history of the disease. This information allows the practitioner to decide at which point in the disease process intervention

---

BOX 1–3. VARIABLES TO CONSIDER IN PRESCRIBING A MEDICATION

Age
Sex
Race
Weight
Culture
Allergies
Other diseases or conditions
Other therapies
   Prescription medications
   Over-the-counter medicines
   Alternative therapies
Previous therapies
   Effectiveness
   Adverse effects
   Adherence
Socioeconomic issues
   Insurance status
   Income level
   Daily schedule
   Living environment
   Support systems
Health beliefs

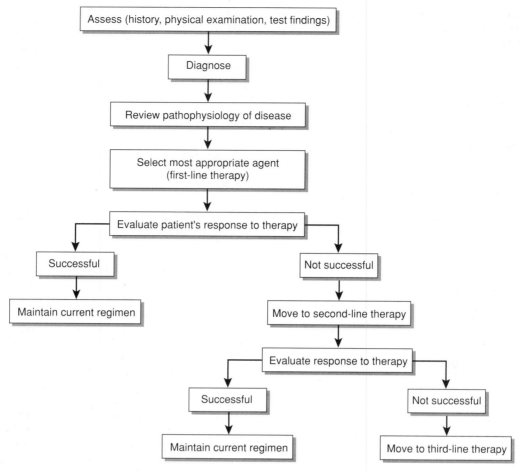

Figure 1-1   Process for prescribing.

with drug therapy is indicated because in many diseases or disorders, nonpharmacologic therapies are tried before drug therapy is initiated.

Next, the practitioner sets goals for therapy. Goals need to be realistic and outcomes measurable. All interventions, nonpharmacologic and pharmacologic, are initiated to meet these goals, and evaluation of the therapy's efficacy is based on these goals.

Lines of Therapy

For most disease entities, there is a recommended first-line therapy—that is, research shows certain agents to be more effective than others. Once initiated, the first-line therapy is evaluated and either continued or changed. If the desired goals are not achieved, or if an adverse reaction occurs, second-line therapy is initiated. The second-line therapy is then evaluated. If this therapy is not tolerated or efficacious, a third-line therapy is initiated, and so on. The practitioner continually evaluates the patient's response to therapy and maintains current therapy or changes it as indicated by the patient's response. For more information, see the case study outlining the prescribing process at the end of this chapter. Case studies such as this one are used throughout the text.

Consideration of Special Populations

Another step in prescribing drugs is considering specific concerns related to special populations, such as children, pregnant or breast-feeding women, and the elderly. Cultural beliefs are also considered to ensure that the drug regimen honors individual and family customs and preferences.

Identifying Outcomes

Expected outcomes can include improvement in clinical symptoms or pathologic signs or changes in biochemistry as determined by laboratory tests. To assess whether expected outcomes have been achieved, the practitioner reviews data collected on subsequent visits, evaluates the effectiveness of drug therapy, and investigates any adverse reactions.

The frequency of follow-up visits is determined by the disease and the patient's response to treatment. While outcomes are being assessed, the practitioner educates the patient about the outcomes of therapy as well. Topics for discussion include drug benefits, side effects, dosage adjustments, and monitoring parameters.

The patient as well as the practitioner must be informed about any undesirable outcomes of therapy with a prescription drug. Reactions that may be expected and must be discussed include side effects, drug or food interactions, and toxicity. Unexpected reactions include allergic reactions or intolerance to a drug. If a patient experiences a serious adverse drug reaction, the practitioner files a report with the FDA's MedWatch program on a special form obtainable from MedWatch (5600 Fishers Lane, Rockville, MD 20852-9787; see Chapter 4 for a sample of the MedWatch form). Similarly, adverse reactions to vaccines are reported through the Vaccine Adverse Event Reporting System. Adverse events are discussed in Chapter 4.

WRITING THE PRESCRIPTION

The prescription is a form of communication between the practitioner and the pharmacist. It is also the basis for written directions to patients, and it is a legal document. Each prescription should be clearly written to avoid errors of misinterpretation in filling the prescription. Although potentially serious errors occur infrequently, they are avoidable and should not occur at all.

An early step in the prescribing process involves ensuring that common but potentially serious errors are not made. The first is failure to identify a patient's allergies, particularly to a medication. In identifying a drug allergy, the practitioner should also investigate the kind of reaction experienced with the medication to differentiate between a true, life-threatening drug allergy and less serious drug sensitivity. Some cross-sensitivities must also be considered. Another error is failure to instruct the patient to stop a previously prescribed medication that treats the same condition. In some instances, an additional medication may be prescribed to increase the effect for the same problem, but the patient must be made aware of this. Otherwise, the original medication must be canceled. Failure to recognize the effect of a prescribed drug on other diseases or drugs can lead to potentially serious effects. There are now programs that can do multiple checks for interactions. One of these is Epocrates for PDAs and desktops.

Date, Name, Address, and Date of Birth

There are standard components of any prescription. One is the date and another is the full name, address, and date of birth of the patient. The name should be the patient's given name (the one on the medical record) and not a nickname. If a different name is used each time, the patient could have multiple records in pharmacy record-keeping systems. The address should be the current home address of the patient and not a work address or a post office box.

Prescriber's Name, Address, and Phone Number

The next components are the name, address and phone number of the prescriber and the collaborating physician if required by state law or regulations. This enables the pharmacist to contact the prescriber if there is a question about the prescription.

Name of Drug

Of course, the name of the drug is the most essential part of the prescription. Ideally, the generic name (with the trade or brand name in parentheses) is used. The name must be legible to avoid errors in filling the prescription correctly. For instance, some drugs have names that are commonly confused or misread, such as Norvasc and Navane, Prilosec and Prozac, carboplatin and cisplatin, and Levoxine and Lanoxin. Severe problems may result if the wrong drug is supplied erroneously. Adding the diagnosis to the prescription, although optional, can help the pharmacist avoid misinterpreting the prescribed drug.

Dose, Dosage Regimen, and Route of Administration

The drug dose is essential because many drugs are available in various strengths. The dose is written in numerals. If the dose is a fraction of 1, it is written in decimal form with a zero to the left of the decimal point (eg, 0.75). However, a whole number should not be followed by a decimal point (10.0 could be misinterpreted as 100). The numeric dose is followed by the correct metric specification such as milligram (mg), gram (g), milliliter (mL), or microgram (mcg). Many practitioners spell out *microgram* to avoid confusion with *milligram*. Some drugs are manufactured in units that should be specified, and the term *unit* should be written out (insulin 10 units, not 10 U). Usually, the strength of drugs that are combination products or that are manufactured only in one strength do not need to be included. The route of the drug is specified as well. (Routes of administration are discussed in Chapter 3.)

The prescription also specifies how frequently the drug is to be taken. A drug prescribed to be taken as needed is termed a *prn* drug. For example, dosage frequency can be written as "prn every 4 hours" (or another appropriate interval) for the problem for which the drug is prescribed (eg, "as needed for nausea"). It is good practice to write out the number (10–ten), especially with controlled substances. Any special instructions, such as "after meals," "at bedtime," or "with food," also should be specified. If the dose is once a day it is safer practice to write out daily than to write OD because this can be confused with every other day.

The prescription also includes the number of pills, vials, suppositories, or containers or amount in milliliters or ounces to be dispensed. Many prescription reimbursement or health care insurance programs allow only a 1-month supply to be dispensed at a time, so it is good practice to be knowledgeable about the rules of various prescription plans. The prescription indicates whether the prescription may be refilled and the number of refills permitted.

When prescribing a new drug for a patient, the practitioner may want to consider prescribing just a few doses or a 7-day supply initially. Alternatively, samples may be provided, if allowed by law or regulations, to determine if the patient can tolerate the drug and if it is effective. When deciding on the number of refills, the practitioner may decide when the patient should return for a follow-up visit

Sally Jones, FNP
111 High Street
Hometown, NH 00440
555-432-1111

Patient's Name ____________________ Date __________

Patient's Address ______________________________

____

Date of Birth __________

Drug ______________ Dosage ______________

Number ______________

Directions ____________________

Number of refills __________

Generic substitution yes _____ no _____

Signature ____________________

License Number ______________

DEA Number (if required) ____________

Sally Jones, FNP
111 High Street
Hometown, NH 00440
555-432-1111

Patient's Name John Smith Date 6/29/00

Patient's Address 13 Comstock Street

Newtown, NH 33300

Date of Birth 1/2/33

Enalapril (Vasotec) 5 mg

#30

Take one daily

Number of refills 5

Substitution yes X no

Signature *Sally Jones, FNP*

License Number RN0000033

DEA Number (if required) 012345-E

Figure 1–2 Example of a blank prescription form (*left*) and a completed form (*right*).

and allow just the number of refills that will take the patient until the next visit to ensure that the patient returns. Some drug prescriptions cannot be refilled. For all Schedule 2 drugs, for example, a new prescription must be written each time.

Allowable Substitutions

There are many generic equivalents for brand name drugs. Indication of whether a substitution is allowed is a part of the prescription. A generic drug substitute must have the same chemical composition and dosage as the brand name drug originally prescribed.

Prescriber's Signature and License Number

The signature of the prescriber is required. It should be legible and should be the person's legal signature. The license number of the prescriber or the collaborating physician is required on the prescription. In some instances, the DEA number of the prescriber is also required, especially when prescribing between states or prescribing a controlled substance. Figure 1-2 illustrates a blank prescription and a completed prescription. Each state has specific requirements for components on a printed prescription. The practitioner must be in compliance with state regulations and may prescribe only in the state in which he or she holds a license. Although the prescription may be filled in another state (if allowed by state regulations), a DEA number is usually required. If the practitioner is a federal employee, he or she may prescribe in any federal facility.

Any drug prescribed should be clearly documented in the medical record with date of order, dosage, amount prescribed, and number of refills. It is helpful to have a specific area in the record to record all drugs taken by the patient—prescription, OTC, and CAM—for ease of audit, reference, and communication among health care professionals.

BOX 1–4. FACTORS INFLUENCING THE PATIENT'S ADHERENCE TO A MEDICATION REGIMEN

- Approachability of the health care provider
- Perception of respect with which he or she is treated by the practitioner
- Belief that the therapy is beneficial
- Belief that the benefits of therapy outweigh the risks or side effects
- Degree to which the patient participates in developing the treatment regimen
- Cost of the regimen
- Simplicity of the regimen
- Understanding of the treatment regimen
- Degree to which the patient feels that expectations are being met
- Degree to which the patient perceives his or her concerns are important and being addressed
- Degree to which the practitioner motivates the patient to adhere to the regimen
- Degree to which the regimen is compatible with the patient's lifestyle

Table 1.2

Common Drug Reference Books

Reference	Features
American Hospital Formulary Service. Bethesda, MD: American Society of Hospital Pharmacists.	Drug entries are indexed by generic and brand names and organized by pharmacologic–therapeutic class.
Drug Facts and Comparisons St. Louis: Facts and Comparisons.	Drugs are indexed by generic and brand names and organized by major classes of drugs. Updates are issued monthly (in print and CD-ROM).
Physician's Desk Reference (PDR) Montvale, NJ: Medical Economics.	Drugs are indexed by manufacturer, brand name, generic name, and product category. Volume contains product identification section. Information replicates the official package insert from the drug manufacturer.

ADHERENCE ISSUES

A prescribed drug must be used correctly to produce optimal benefits. Patient nonadherence to a prescribed regimen leads to less-than-optimal outcomes, such as progression of the disease state and an increased incidence of hospitalizations. Studies demonstrate that the more complex the treatment regimen, the less likely the patient is to follow it. Platt, Tippy, and Turk (1994) reported that 30% to 40% of patients with epilepsy failed to take medications as prescribed, and only 7% of patients with insulin-dependent diabetes mellitus followed the prescribed regimen of care. Platt and colleagues also found that 50% of patients who begin antihypertensive therapy were no longer under medical care after 1 year. Stone (1979) reported that when patients were prescribed one medication, the rate of nonadherence was 15%. With two or three medications, the nonadherence rate was 25%. When more than five drugs were prescribed, the nonadherence rate rose to 35%. Inappropriate use of medications causes approximately 125,000 deaths per year. About 10% of all hospital admissions, 25% of hospital admissions of elderly, and 23% of nursing home admissions are a result of medication misuse and errors.

Several variables are associated with improved adherence to a drug regimen. These include variables associated with the patient's perception of the encounter and of the benefit of the treatment. If a patient is nonadherent to the prescribed regimen, it is important to document that in the chart. The risks of nonadherence are discussed and that discussion is documented. It is essential to ask why the patient is not following the prescribed treatment, and actions to rectify the problem should be taken. All of this is documented. One issue may be that the patient is unable to swallow the pill. The medicine may be available in liquid form or the pill may be split or crushed. The practitioner needs to review and understand the factors that affect adherence to a regimen (Box 1-4).

UPDATING DRUG INFORMATION

Many sources of drug information can be accessed by practitioners who must keep current on changes in drug therapy and continually update their fund of knowledge. Resources include reference books, pharmacists (who are expertly informed about drugs, interactions, dosages, etc), easy-to-carry drug handbooks and pocket guides for quick reference, and on-line databases and programs for PDAs (Tables 1-2 and 1-3).

Table 1.3

On-line Drug Reference Data

Reference	Address	Features
AHCPR Guidelines	www.ahrq.gov	Guidelines for clinical practice from the Agency for Health Care Policy and Research
Center Watch Clinical Trials	www.centerwatch.com	Lists clinical research trials and drug therapy newly approved by the U.S. FDA and the FDA New Drug Listing Service
Coreynahman	www.coreynahman.com	Pharmaceutical news and information Gives a choice of many sites for information
Epocrates	www.epocrates.com	Software for PDA with drug information, interactions, etc
Healthtouch Drug Information	www.healthtouch.com	Information for patient and provider
Mediconsult	www.mediconsult.com	Professional- and consumer-focused Detailed medical and drug information
Medscape	www.medscape.com	Drug search database Links to on-line journals
Pharmaceutical Information Network	www.pharminfo.com	Information about treatment and drug therapy Articles from clinical publications, symposium information and new drug information
RxList—The Internet Drug Index	www.rxlist.com	Cross-index of U.S. prescription products Links to full drug information and patient education materials

Bibliography

*Starred references are cited in the text.

DiPiro, J. T., Talbert, R. L., Hayes, P. E., et al. (Eds.). (1999). *Pharmacotherapy: A pathophysiologic approach* (4th ed.). East Norwalk, CT: Appleton & Lange.

*Doherty, K., Segal, A., & McKinney, P. (2004). The 10 most common prescribing errors: Tips on avoiding the pitfalls. *Consultant, 44*(2), 173–182.

*Gandhi, T. K., Weingart, S. N., Borus, J., et al. (2003). Adverse drug events in ambulatory care. *New England Journal of Medicine, 348,* 1556–1564.

*Platt, F. W., Tippy, P. K., & Turk, D. C. (1994). Helping patients adhere to the regimen. *Patient Care, 28*(17), 43–52, 57–58.

*Stone, G. C. (1979). Patient compliance and the role of the expert. *Journal of Social Issues, 35,* 34–59.

Tower, J. (2003). Nurse practitioner practice in 2003. *Journal of the American Academy of Nurse Practitioners, 15*(12).

*Voczek, D. (2003). Top drugs of 2002. *Pharmacy Times, 20* (April).

Wiltz, P., Zimer, P. A., & Scarcliff, K. J. (1999). NP authority to request, receive, and/or dispense drug samples: A state-by-state study. *American Journal for Nurse Practitioners, 3*(1), 7–24.

Visit the Connection web site for the most up-to-date drug information.

PHARMACOKINETIC BASIS OF THERAPEUTICS AND PHARMACODYNAMIC PRINCIPLES

■ ANDREW M. PETERSON

The art and science of clinical practice is based on understanding the relationship between the person and the disease and determining the most appropriate means for alleviating symptoms, curing disease, or preventing severe morbidity or even mortality. Very often, medications are prescribed to accomplish one or more of these goals.

Underpinning this treatment process is the intricate relationship between the body and the medication. Often, practitioners seek to understand the effect a drug has on the body (whether therapeutic or harmful) but neglect to consider the effect that the body has on the drug—even though one cannot be understood without the other. How the body acts on a drug and how the drug acts on the body are the subjects of this chapter.

Pharmacokinetics refers to movement of drug through the body—in essence, how the body affects the drug. This involves how the drug is administered, absorbed, distributed, and eventually eliminated from the body. *Pharmacodynamics* refers to how the drug affects the body—that is, how the drug initiates its therapeutic or toxic effect, both at the cellular level and systemically. Box 2-1 lists additional terms and definitions used in this chapter.

The purpose of pharmacokinetic processes is to get the drug to the site of action where it can produce its pharmacodynamic effect. There is a minimum amount of drug needed at the site of action to produce the desired effect. Although the amount of drug concentrated at the site of action is difficult to measure, the amount of drug in the blood can be measured. The relationship between the concentration of drug in the blood and the concentration at the site of action (ie, the drug receptor) is different for each drug and each person. Therefore, measuring blood concentrations is only a surrogate marker, an indication of concentration at the receptor (ie, the site of action). Figure 2-1 shows the relationship between pharmacokinetics and pharmacodynamics.

PHARMACOKINETICS

Using the surrogate marker of blood concentrations, the target drug concentration needed to produce desired effects can be determined. Assuming that the magnitude of the drug concentration at the site of action influences the drug effect, whether desired or undesired, it can be inferred that a range of drug levels produces a range of effects (Fig. 2-2). Below a specific level, or threshold, the drug exerts little to no therapeutic effect. Above this threshold, the concentration of drug in the blood is sufficient to produce a therapeutic effect at the site of action. However, as the drug concentration increases in the blood, so does the concentration at the site of action. Above a specific level, an increased therapeutic effect may no longer occur. Instead, an unacceptable toxicity may exist because the drug concentration is too high. Between these two levels—the minimally effective level and the toxic level—is the *therapeutic window*. The therapeutic window is the range of blood drug concentration that yields a sufficient therapeutic response without excessively toxic reactions. This range should not be considered absolute because it varies from individual to individual and therefore serves only as a guide to the practitioner.

Absorption

The first aspect of pharmacokinetics to consider is how drugs are administered, how they are absorbed into the body, and how they eventually reach the bloodstream. Merely introducing the drug into the body does not ensure that the compound will reach all tissues uniformly or even that the drug will reach the target site. Commonly recognized methods of absorption include enteral absorption (after the drug is administered by the oral or rectal route) and parenteral absorption (associated with drugs administered intramuscularly [IM], subcutaneously, or topically). The various administration routes and other factors affect a drug's ability to enter the bloodstream.

The extent to which the drug reaches the systemic circulation is referred to as *bioavailability*, or F, which is defined as the fraction or percentage of the drug that reaches the systemic circulation. Drugs administered intravenously are 100% bioavailable. Drugs administered by other routes (eg, oral, IM)

BOX 2–1. DEFINITIONS OF TERMS RELATED TO PHARMACOKINETICS AND PHARMACODYNAMICS

Affinity: The attraction between a drug and a receptor.

Allosteric site: A binding site for substrates not active in initiating a response; a substrate that binds to an allosteric site may induce a conformational change in the structure of the active site, rendering it more or less susceptible to response from a substrate.

Bioavailability (F): The fraction or percentage of a drug that reaches the systemic circulation.

Biotransformation: Metabolism or degradation of a drug from an active form to an inactive form.

Chirality: Special configuration or shape of a drug; most drugs exist in two shapes.

Clearance: Removal of a drug from the body.

Downregulation: Decreased availability of drug receptors.

Enantiomer (also called isomer): A mirror-image spatial arrangement, or shape, of a drug that suits it for binding with a drug receptor.

Enterohepatic recirculation: The process by which a drug excreted in the bile flows into the gastrointestinal tract, where it is reabsorbed and returned to the general circulation.

First-pass effect: The phenomenon by which a drug first passes through the liver for degradation before distribution to the tissues.

Half-life ($t_{1/2}$): The time required for half of a total drug amount to be eliminated from the body.

Hepatic extraction ratio: A comparison of the percentage of drug extracted and the percentage of drug remaining active after metabolism in the liver.

Pharmacodynamics: Processes through which drugs affect the body.

Pharmacokinetics: Processes through which the body affects drugs.

Prodrug: A drug that is transformed from an inactive parent drug into an active metabolite; in effect, a precursor to the active drug.

Receptor: The site of drug action.

Second messenger: A chemical produced intracellularly in response to a receptor signal; this second messenger initiates a change in the intracellular response.

Therapeutic window: The range of drug concentration in the blood between a minimally effective level and a toxic level.

Threshold: The level below which a drug exerts little to no therapeutic effect and above which a drug produces a therapeutic effect at the site of action.

Volume of distribution (V_d): The extent of distribution of a drug in the body.

---

may be 100% bioavailable, but more often they are less than 100% bioavailable. Therefore, bioavailability depends on the route of administration and, equally important, the drug's ability to pass through membranes or barriers in the body. Box 2-2 discusses oral bioavailability.

Factors Affecting Absorption

A variety of factors affect absorption, such as the presence or absence of food in the stomach, blood flow to the area for absorption, and the dosage form of the drug. The following sections discuss some of the major factors affecting absorption.

Movement Through Membranes and Drug Solubility

Throughout the body, biologic membranes act as barriers, blocking or permitting the passage of various substances. These membranes protect certain areas of the body from

Pharmacokinetics   Pharmacodynamics

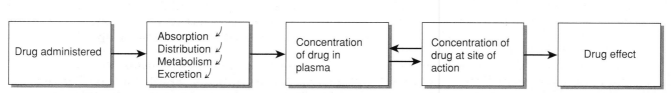

Figure 2–1   Relationship between pharmacokinetics and pharmacodynamics. Note the two-way relationship between the concentration of drug in the plasma and the concentration of drug at the site of action, depicting the interrelationship between pharmacokinetics and pharmacodynamics.

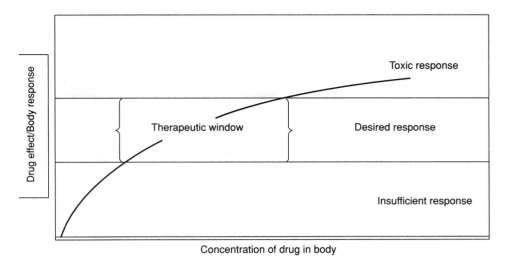

Figure 2–2 Therapeutic window: concentration versus response. The concentration of the drug in the body produces specific effects. A low concentration is considered subtherapeutic, producing an insufficient response. As the concentration increases, the desired effect is produced at a given drug level. A drug concentration that exceeds the upper limit of the desired response may produce a toxic reaction. The concentration range within which a desired response occurs is the therapeutic window.

BOX 2–2. ORAL BIOAVAILABILITY AND THE FIRST-PASS EFFECT

Drugs given by the oral route may be subject to the first-pass effect, by which drugs are metabolized by the liver before passing into circulation. After absorption from the alimentary canal, drugs go directly to the liver through the portal vein. In the liver, hepatic enzymes act on the drug, reducing the amount of active drug reaching the bloodstream and decreasing the amount available to the body. The fraction (or percentage) of medication reaching systemic circulation after the first pass through the liver is referred to as the drug's bioavailability (F).

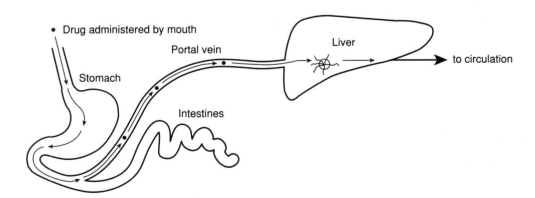

The first-pass effect is not the only factor contributing to the oral bioavailability of a drug. Poorly soluble drugs and drugs adversely affected by gastric pH or other presystemic factors can also have a low bioavailability.

Drugs not usually subject to the liver's first-pass effect are known as drugs with a low hepatic extraction ratio because the liver does not extract a large percentage of the drug before releasing it into the circulation. Usually, drugs with a low extraction ratio have high oral bioavailability. In contrast, drugs with a high extraction ratio have low oral bioavailability. For example, lidocaine has a hepatic extraction ratio of 0.7; that is, the liver metabolizes 70% of the drug before the drug reaches the circulation and, as such, only 30% remains available systemically. (This is one reason lidocaine is administered parenterally.) In other words, the first-pass effect for lidocaine is of such magnitude that an alternative route of administration is required. Giving large oral doses of a drug to compensate for the high extraction ratio is often an alternative to parenteral administration. For example, because of the high extraction ratio of propranolol, a l-mg dose administered intravenously is approximately equivalent to a 40-mg dose administered orally.

Examples of drugs with a high hepatic extraction ratio (70% or more) are imipramine (Tofranil), lidocaine (Xylocaine), and meperidine (Demerol); drugs with intermediate rankings are codeine, nortriptyline (Aventyl), and quinidine (Quinaglute); and some drugs with a low extraction ratio (30% or less) are barbiturates, diazepam (Valium), theophylline (Theo-Dur), tolbutamide (Orinase), and warfarin (Coumadin).

harmful chemicals and allow other areas to be accessed as needed.

Biologic membranes composed of cells serve as barriers primarily because of the structure and function of the cells that make up the membrane. Cell membranes are composed of lipids and proteins, creating a phospholipid bilayer. This bilayer acts as a barrier that is almost impermeable to water, other hydrophilic (water-loving) substances, and ionized substances. However, the bilayer does allow most lipid-soluble (hydrophobic) compounds to pass through readily. Interspersed throughout this bilayer are protein molecules and small openings, or pores. The proteins may act as carrier molecules, bringing molecules through the barrier. The pores allow hydrophilic molecules to pass through, if they are small enough. Therefore, drugs and other compounds that pass through membrane barriers can do so by passive and active means.

Passive Diffusion

Drugs can pass through membrane barriers by diffusion. In passive diffusion, molecules move from one side of a barrier to another without expending energy. In passing, the molecules move down a concentration gradient—that is, they move from an area of higher concentration to an area of lower concentration.

The rate of diffusion depends on the differences in concentrations, the relative strength of the barrier, the distance that the molecules must travel, and the size of the molecules. This relationship is known as Fick's law of diffusion. In essence, Fick's law states that the greater the distance and the larger the molecule, the slower the diffusion.

Another major barrier to the absorption of a drug is its solubility. To facilitate drug absorption, the solubility of the administered drug must match the cellular constituents of the absorption site. Lipid-soluble drugs can penetrate fatty cells; water-soluble drugs cannot. For example, a water-soluble drug such as penicillin cannot easily pass through the barrier between the blood and brain, whereas a highly lipid-soluble drug such as diazepam (Valium) can. The relative strength of the barrier is important because the barrier must be permeable to the diffusing substance. Drugs diffuse more readily through the lipid bilayer if they are in their neutral, non-ionized form. Most drugs are weak acids or weak bases, which have the potential for becoming positively or negatively charged. This potential is created through the pH of certain body fluids. In the plasma and in most other fluids, most drugs remain non-ionized. However, in the gastric acid of the stomach, weak bases become ionized and are more difficult to absorb. As this weak base progresses through the alkaline environment of the small intestines, it becomes non-ionized and therefore more easily absorbed. Similarly, weak acids remain non-ionized in the stomach and become ionized in the small intestines. The result is reduced absorption by the intestines.

Active Transport

In active transport, membrane proteins act as carrier molecules to transport substances across cell membranes. The role of active transport in moving drugs across cell membranes is limited. To be carried through by a protein, the drug must share molecular similarities with an endogenous substance the transport system routinely carriers. Cells can accomplish

this through the process of *endocytosis*. In this process, the cell forms a vesicle surrounding the molecule and subsequently invaginated in the cell. The vesicle is "pinched off" and the molecule is released into the cytoplasm of the cell.

Pharmaceutical Preparation

Drugs are formulated and administered in such a way as to produce either local or systemic effects. Local effects (eg, antiseptic, anti-inflammatory, and local anesthetic effects) are confined to one area of the body. Systemic effects occur when the drug is absorbed and delivered to body tissues by way of the circulatory system.

Depending on how a drug is formulated (eg, tablet or liquid), the means of drug delivery can target a site of action. Some drug formulations (dosage forms) deliver the drug into the gastrointestinal (GI) tract quickly (immediate release), whereas others release the drug slowly. This strategy for extending the activity of drugs in the body dampens the high and low swings of drug concentrations, thereby yielding a more constant blood level. Many medications are available in these controlled- or sustained-release dosage forms. The aims of sustained release are administration as infrequently as possible and, therefore, improved compliance and minimal hour-to-hour or day-to-day fluctuations in blood levels. The various release systems available are subject to physiologic and pathophysiologic changes in patient conditions.

Blood Flow

Blood flow ensures that the concentration across a gradient is continually in favor of passive diffusion—that is, as blood flows through an area, it continually removes drug from the area, thereby maintaining a positive concentration gradient. Many hydrophobic–lipophilic drugs can readily pass through membranes and be absorbed. However, if the blood flow to that area is limited, the extent of absorption is limited. Because of the minimal vascularization in the subcutaneous layer compared with the greater vascularity of the musculature, drugs injected subcutaneously may undergo limited absorption compared with drugs delivered by IM injection.

Gastrointestinal Motility

High-fat meals and solid foods affect GI transit time by delaying gastric emptying, which in turn delays initial drug delivery to intestinal absorption surfaces. The administration of agents that delay or slow intestinal motility (eg, anticholinergic agents) prolongs the contact time. This increased contact time secondary to prolonged intestinal transit time may increase total drug absorption. Conversely, laxatives and diarrhea can shorten an agent's contact time with the small intestine, which may decrease drug absorption.

Enteral Absorption

Enteral absorption, with the oral route of administration being the most common and probably the most preferred, occurs anywhere throughout the GI tract by passive or active transport of the drug through the cells of the GI tract.

Following Fick's law, low-molecular-weight, non-ionized drugs diffuse passively down a concentration gradient from the higher concentration (in the GI tract) to the lower concentration (in the blood). Active transport across the GI tract occurs more frequently with larger, usually ionized, molecules. These active mechanisms include binding of the drug to carrier molecules in the cell membrane. The molecules carry the drug across the lipid bilayer of the cells. However, most drugs are absorbed passively.

Oral Administration

The oral route of administration refers to any medication that is taken by mouth (*per os*, or PO). The ability to swallow is implicit in oral administration; however, many practitioners consider local action, in which absorption does not occur, also to be "oral" (eg, troches for fungal infections of the mouth). Common dosage forms administered by mouth include tablets, capsules, caplets, solutions, suspensions, troches, lozenges, and powders.

Absorption after oral administration usually occurs in the lower GI tract (small or large intestine), is usually slow, and depends on the patient's gastric emptying time, the presence or absence of food, and the gastric or intestinal pH. Variations in one or more of these factors can affect the stability of the drug, the contact time with the walls of the GI tract, or the blood flow to the GI tract and hence the ability of the drug to cross the epithelial lining of the GI tract. Most of the absorption occurs in the small intestine, where the large surface area enhances and controls drug entry into the body.

Drugs administered orally must be relatively lipid soluble to cross the GI mucosa into the bloodstream. The diffusion rate, a function of the lipid solubility of a drug across the GI mucosa, is a major factor in determining the rate of absorption of a drug. The acid pH of the stomach and the nearly neutral pH of the intestines can degrade some medications before they are absorbed. In addition, bacteria in various parts of the intestines secrete enzymes that also can break down drugs before absorption.

Although the GI tract is generally resistant to a variety of noxious agents, considerable irritation and discomfort can arise from certain medications in some people. Nausea, vomiting, diarrhea, and less often mucosal damage are common side effects of medications, and the practitioner should monitor all patients for these effects.

Sublingual Administration

Sublingual (SL, "under the tongue") drug administration relies on absorption through the oral mucosa into the veins that drain those vascular beds. These veins carry drug to the superior vena cava and eventually the heart. Drugs administered this way are not subject to the first-pass effect (see Box 2-2). This method of administration is limited by the amount of drug that can be placed sublingually and the drug's ability to pass through the oral mucosa into the venous system. Buccal administration, in which the drug is absorbed through the mucous membranes of the mouth, is similar to sublingual administration.

Rectal Administration

Drugs administered rectally (PR, *per rectum*) include suppositories and enemas. Primarily used in the treatment of local conditions (eg, hemorrhoids) and inflammatory bowel disease, this method is less effective than other enteral routes of administration because of the erratic absorption of most agents. Bowel irritation, early evacuation, and minimal surface area contribute to erratic absorption and poor tolerability of this route. Advantages, however, include the ability to administer a medication to an unconscious or nauseated patient.

Parenteral Absorption

All routes of administration not involving the GI tract are considered parenteral. Parenteral routes include inhalation, all forms of injection, and topical and transdermal administration.

Inhalation

Drugs that are gaseous or sprayable in small particles may be delivered by inhalation. The lungs provide a large surface area for absorption and quick entry into the bloodstream. Inhaled medications bypass the first-pass effect and therefore may have a high bioavailability. Examples of inhalants are anesthetic gases. Beta-adrenergic agonists used in treating asthma are also administered by inhalation. Conversely, agents such as inhaled corticosteroids are intended for local action in the lung tissue. Regardless of the intent of inhaled medications, the disadvantages include irritation to the alveolar space and the need for good coordination during self-administration, such as with metered-dose inhalers.

Intravenous Administration

The intravenous (IV) route provides rapid access to the circulatory system with a known quantity of drug. Bypassing the first-pass effect and any GI metabolism or degradation, drug absorption by this route is considered the gold standard with regard to bioavailability. IV bolus injections allow for large amounts of medication to be administered quickly for a high peak drug level and a rapid effect. However, adverse effects from these high levels of medications also occur with this form of administration. Repeated bolus doses of medications, at designated intervals, can produce large fluctuations in peak and trough (lowest concentration before next dose) levels. Although over time these peaks and troughs produce average desired concentrations, significant peak and trough fluctuations may not be desirable in some patients. Continuous administration by an infusion can minimize or eliminate these fluctuations and produce a consistent, steady-state concentration.

Like IV administration, intra-arterial administration produces a rapid effect. However, because the drug is directly instilled in an organ, this route is considered more dangerous than the IV route. Therefore, intra-arterial administration is usually reserved for a time when injection into a specific tissue is indicated (eg, anticancer treatment for a specific tumor).

Subcutaneous Administration

Subcutaneous (SC or SQ) administration produces a slower, more prolonged release of medication into the bloodstream. Injected directly beneath the skin, a drug must diffuse through layers of fat and muscle to encounter sufficient blood vessels for entry into the systemic circulation. This route is limited by the quantity of the liquid suitable for administration (usually 2 to 3 mL). Caution must also be taken because dermal irritation, or even necrosis, may occur. More recent technological advances allow the practitioner to implant drug-releasing mechanisms under the skin, providing a reservoir of drug for long-term absorption. Levonorgestrel (Norplant), a hormonal contraceptive, is administered in this manner.

Intramuscular Administration

Injecting medications into the highly vascularized skeletal muscle is a way of administering drugs quickly and avoiding the relatively large changes in plasma levels seen with IV administration. Local pain and muscle soreness are drawbacks to this method, as is the wide variability in the rate of absorption resulting from injections given in different muscles and in different patients. Blood flow to the area is the major factor in determining the rate of absorption. This is considered a safe way to administer irritating drugs, although not all IM injections are truly IM: in grossly obese patients, presumed IM injections may actually be intralipomatous, which decreases the rate of absorption because of the lower vascularity of fatty tissue.

Topical Administration

Topical drug administration involves applying drugs, in various vehicles (eg, liquids, powders), to the site of action, primarily the skin. Topical ointments, creams, drops, and gels typically produce a local effect. Ointments are occlusive, preventing water absorption or evaporation, and therefore have a hydrating effect and typically produce greater local effects than their cream counterparts. Creams are water soluble and therefore can be washed from the skin more readily than ointments. In hairy areas, creams are preferred over ointments because creams are hydrophilic and hence easier to apply and wash off. Gels, the most water-soluble topical dosage form, allow medication to be spread more easily over a larger area.

Transdermal Administration

Transdermal ("across the skin") administration refers to the systemic delivery of medication through the skin. Several transdermal drug delivery systems are available for a wide range of medications, including nitroglycerin (Transderm Nitro), estrogens (Estraderm), and fentanyl (Duragesic). In general, this method continuously delivers medication to achieve a constant blood level. The consistent delivery of drug throughout the dosing interval minimizes the peak-to-trough fluctuations seen with other forms of drug administration, thereby minimizing the toxicity associated with high blood levels while maintaining therapeutic concentrations.

Distribution

A discussion of the routes of administration offers the opportunity to consider the factors affecting drug absorption and bioavailability; once the medication is in the body, however, it must distribute to the site of action to be effective.

Distribution of an absorbed drug in the body depends on several factors: blood flow to an area, lipid or water solubility, and protein binding. For an absorbed drug to distribute from the blood to a specific site of action, there must be adequate blood flow to that area. In patients with compromised blood flow (eg, from shock), relying on the blood to deliver a drug to a site of action, such as the kidney, may be risky.

In addition, drug distribution may be affected by obesity, both immediately after absorption and after achieving an equilibrium or steady state in the body. Lipid-soluble drugs readily distribute into the fatty tissues, where they may be stored and even concentrated. Water-soluble drugs, however, tend to remain in the highly vascularized spaces of the skeletal muscle. Ideal body weight is usually considered the standard for determining drug dosage, which is often adjusted for obese or cachectic patients.

Protein Binding

After absorption into the blood (and lymph), a drug may circulate throughout the body bound to carrier proteins such as albumin or unbound (also called *free drug*). The extent of drug binding to carrier proteins depends on the affinity of the drug for the carrier protein and the concentrations of both the drug and the proteins. Acidic drugs commonly bind to albumin and basic drugs commonly bind to alpha$_1$-acid glycoprotein or lipoproteins.

Plasma protein binding is typically a reversible phenomenon, with binding and unbinding occurring within milliseconds. Therefore, the bound and unbound forms of the drug can be assumed to be at equilibrium at all times. As such, the degree of binding to plasma proteins can be expressed as a percentage of bound drug to total concentration (bound plus unbound). It is only the unbound or free drug that can exert a pharmacologic effect. If the drug becomes bound, it becomes inactive because it cannot leave the bloodstream or bind to an enzyme or receptor and exert its therapeutic action (Fig. 2-3).

Once free drug is eliminated from the body through metabolism or excretion, the bound drug can be released from the protein to become active. In essence, the bound drug may serve as a storage site or reservoir of drug. The percentage of free drug usually is constant for a single drug and varies among drugs. Patient-specific factors, such as nutritional status, renal function, and levels of circulating protein or albumin, can change the percentage of free drug.

Volume of Distribution

The amount of drug in the human body can never be directly measured. Observations are made of the concentration of

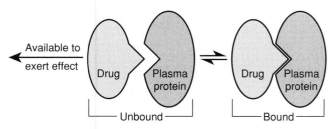

Figure 2–3   Relationship between bound and unbound drugs and plasma proteins.

BOX 2–3. CALCULATING THE APPARENT VOLUME OF DISTRIBUTION (V_d)

$$V_d = \frac{\text{Amount in body}}{\text{Plasma drug concentration}}$$

V_d is usually measured in liters (L); *amount in body* is usually measured in milligrams (mg); and *plasma drug concentration* is usually measured in milligrams per liter (mg/L).

The apparent volume of distribution is a theoretical parameter calculated by determining the amount of drug in the body (usually the dose administered) divided by the concentration of drug in the body taken at an appropriate time interval after administration.

drug in plasma or sometimes in blood. Over time, the concentration of drug in the plasma depends on the rate and extent of drug distribution to the tissues and on how rapidly the drug is eliminated. For most drugs, distribution occurs more rapidly than elimination. The resultant plasma concentration after distribution depends on the dose and the extent of distribution into the tissues. This extent of distribution can be determined by relating the concentration obtained with a known amount of administered drug.

For example, if 100 mg of an IV drug is administered to a person and remains only in the blood, and if that person's total blood volume measures 5 L, the resulting measured concentration of drug would be 20 mg/L [concentration = dose/volume: 100 mg/5 L]. However, in reality, few drugs distribute solely in the plasma, and many bind to plasma proteins. Drugs commonly bind not only to plasma proteins but also to tissue-binding sites on fat and muscle. In addition, drugs translocate into other "compartments" or spaces throughout the body. The apparent volume into which a drug distributes in the body at equilibrium is called the (apparent) volume of distribution (V_d). This volume does not refer to a real volume; rather, it is a mathematically calculated volume (Box 2-3). The V_d is a direct measure of the extent of distribution of a drug in the body and represents the apparent volume that a drug must distribute to contain the amount of drug homogenously.

Drugs that are highly water soluble or highly bound to plasma proteins remain in the blood compartment and do not distribute or bind to fatty tissue. These drugs have a low V_d, usually less than the volume of total body water (approximately 50 L, or 0.7 L/kg). Drugs with a low V_d usually circulate at high levels in the blood. In contrast, drugs that are not highly protein bound and are highly lipophilic have a high V_d (150 L, which is greater than the volume of total body water). These drugs distribute widely throughout the body and may even cross the blood–brain barrier.

Elimination

All drugs must eventually be eliminated from the body to terminate their effect. Drugs can be eliminated through metabo-

lism (or biotransformation) of the drug from an active form to an inactive form. Drugs can also be eliminated by excretion from the body. Therefore, elimination is a combination of the metabolism and excretion of drugs from the body. Important concepts in understanding drug elimination are half-life, steady state, and clearance. Knowledge of these phenomena in any given patient helps practitioners understand how long a drug will last in the body and how much should be given to maintain therapeutic levels and therefore helps in determining the appropriate dose and dosing intervals.

Metabolism

Metabolism is a function of the body designed to change substances into water-soluble, more readily excreted forms. The liver primarily performs the body's metabolic functions because of its high concentration of metabolic enzymes. This is why the first-pass effect is significant to the bioavailability of a drug administered orally.

Other organs, such as the kidneys and intestines, as well as circulating enzyme systems, also contribute to the metabolism of drugs. Metabolic processes are used to detoxify drugs and other foreign substances as well as endogenous substances. Drugs may be metabolized from active components into inactive or less active ones. Some drugs, however, may be biologically transformed from an inactive parent drug into an active metabolite. This type of drug is called a prodrug because it is a precursor to the active drug (Table 2-1). Not all drugs are metabolized to the same extent or by the same means. In fact, some drugs, such as the aminoglycosides (eg, gentamicin [Garamycin]), are not metabolized at all.

Enzyme actions are the primary means for metabolizing drugs, and these actions are broadly classified as phase 1 and phase 2 enzymatic processes. Phase 1 enzymatic processes involve oxidation, by which a drug is reduced to form a more polar or water-soluble compound. Phase 2 processes involve adding a conjugate (eg, a glucuronide) to the parent drug or the phase 1–metabolized drug to further increase water solubility and enhance excretion.

The oxidative process of phase 1 metabolism is catalyzed by a superfamily of more than 100 enzymes called the cytochrome P450 system (CYP). Three families and five isoforms of the CYP are important contributors to drug metabolism. The common feature of these enzymes is their lipid solubility. Most lipophilic drugs are substrates for one or more of the CYP enzymes (Table 2-2).

Some drugs can induce or stimulate the production of one or more isoforms of the enzymes by a process called enzyme induction, which increases the amount of enzyme available to metabolize drugs. The result of enzyme induction is an

Table 2.1

Selected Prodrugs and Metabolites

Parent Drug (Prodrug)	Active Metabolite
allopurinol	oxypurinol
codeine	morphine
enalapril	enalaprilat
prednisone	prednisolone
sulindac	sulindac sulfide

Table 2.2

Key Cytochrome P450 Families and Isoforms in Drug Metabolism

Family	Isoform	Example Drugs Metabolized
CYP1	CYP1A2	theophylline
CYP2	CYP2C	omeprazole
	CYP2D6	dextromethorphan
	CYP2E1	acetaminophen
CYP3	CYP3A4	quinidine

increased metabolism of other drugs, thereby decreasing the amount of drug circulating throughout the body.

Conversely, some drugs inhibit the production of CYP enzymes and thereby decrease the metabolism of drugs and increase circulating levels. This is known as enzyme inhibition. Both enzyme induction and inhibition are the basis of metabolically mediated drug–drug interactions. See Chapter 3 for further discussion of induction and inhibition and their role in drug–drug interactions.

Although the liver is regarded as the primary site of drug metabolism, other tissues also possess the enzymes necessary for metabolism. The kidneys, for example, have several enzymes needed for drug metabolism and can serve as the site of drug inactivation. The GI tract is also known to possess several of the CYP isoforms, contributing to the extrahepatic metabolism of drugs.

The nature, function, and amount of any drug-metabolizing enzymes can be different, resulting in differing drug disposition among patients. Disease-induced changes can affect drug metabolism as well. For example, alterations in liver function induced by long-standing cirrhotic changes can reduce the production of necessary enzymes, resulting in increased concentrations of drugs typically metabolized in the liver. Also, decreased blood flow to the liver, such as occurs in congestive heart failure, can decrease the delivery of drug to metabolic sites in the liver. Cigarette smoking, on the other hand, can increase the levels of enzymes responsible for drug metabolism, resulting in increased metabolic rates and the need for higher doses of drugs (eg, theophylline) in smokers than in nonsmokers.

Drug Excretion

Metabolism eliminates a drug from the body by changing the drug molecule into something else, but drugs also can be eliminated from the body by excretion. Excretory organs include the kidneys, lower GI tract, lungs, and skin. Other structures, such as the sweat, salivary, and mammary glands, are active in excretion as well. Drugs may also be removed forcibly by dialysis.

The primary route of excretion is the kidney. After the drug is metabolized, the resultant metabolite may be filtered by the glomerulus. As the drug continues through the proximal tubule, loop of Henle, and distal tubule, several things may occur: the drug may exert action (as in the case of diuretics), be reabsorbed into the bloodstream, or remain in the nephron, eventually reaching the collecting ducts, from which it ultimately leaves the body in the patient's urine. This filtration works well for hydrophilic, ionized compounds and is a common route of elimination. Conversely,

active secretion of drugs occurs in the proximal tubule. Two different systems exist, one for organic acids (eg, uric acid) and one for organic bases (eg, histamine). Once ionized by the acidic pH of the urine, organic bases are not reabsorbed back into the bloodstream. If the pH rises, then more of the organic base becomes non-ionized and becomes more readily reabsorbed. Similarly, changes in urine pH can alter the reabsorption of organic acids, increasing or decreasing the circulating levels as the pH changes. Drugs such as penicillin are excreted by the organic acid system.

Drugs are excreted by the liver into the gallbladder, resulting in biliary elimination. Biliary elimination can sometimes result in drug reabsorption. For example, if a drug is excreted in the bile, it goes into the GI tract, where it may be reabsorbed and returned to the general circulation. This is called *enterohepatic recirculation* (Fig. 2-4). The result of significant enterohepatic recirculation is a measurable increase in the plasma concentration of a drug and a delay in its elimination from the body.

Half-Life

The time required for a drug to be eliminated from the body varies according to the drug and the individual. However, useful generalizations can be made that help practitioners estimate how long a drug will remain in the body. The first generalization has to do with the elimination half-life ($t_{1/2}$), which is the time required for half of the total drug amount to be eliminated from the body. Assuming 100% of a drug exists in the body at time X, then one half-life later, 50% of the original amount would remain in the body. An additional half-life later, 25% would remain. For example, theophylline (Theo-Dur) has a $t_{1/2}$ of approximately 8 hours in nonsmokers. If the theophylline concentration in a patient's body is 15 mg/L, then it would take 8 hours to decline to 7.5 mg/L,

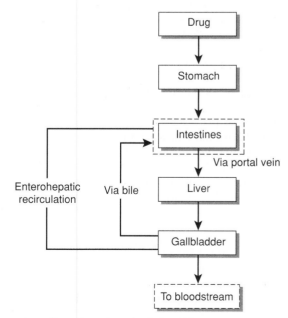

Figure 2–4 Enterohepatic recirculation. When a drug is absorbed from the intestine, travels to the liver and gallbladder, and into the bile unchanged, it has the potential for being reintroduced into the intestine and therefore reabsorbed. This is known as enterohepatic recirculation.

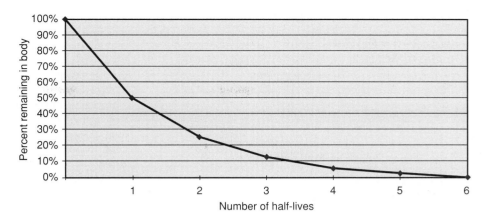

Figure 2–5 Drug elimination based on half-life (t$_{1/2}$).

another 8 hours (16 hours total) to fall to 3.75 mg/L, and so on. The actual rate of elimination of a drug remains constant, but as can be seen in Figure 2-5, the actual amount of drug eliminated is proportional to the concentration of the drug—that is, the more drug there is, the faster it is eliminated. This phenomenon, known as first-order kinetics, applies to most drugs. Rate processes can also be independent of concentration, and fixed amounts of drugs, rather than a fractional proportion, are eliminated at a constant rate. This phenomenon is called zero-order kinetics. Alcohol undergoes zero-order elimination.

After five half-lives, according to first-order kinetics, approximately 97% (96.875%) of the drug is eliminated from the body. Even after three half-lives, nearly 90% (87.5%) of the drug is eliminated. In most cases, after three to five half-lives, the amount of drug remaining is too low to exert any pharmacologic effect, and the drug is considered essentially eliminated. Understanding this concept is useful for practitioners in many situations. For example, if a drug reaches a toxic level, the practitioner knows that it will take three to five half-lives for the drug to be essentially eliminated from the body. The practitioner also can estimate when the drug level will approach a minimally effective concentration and can then calculate when to administer another dose of medication to reach a therapeutic drug level.

Steady State

In reality, patients take medications on a consistent basis, usually somewhere between one and four times daily. By doing so, they are absorbing and eliminating the drug throughout the

day. Because the rate of elimination is proportional to the concentration, at some point equilibrium is reached. Figure 2-6 demonstrates how doses of a drug with a half-life of 8 hours produce this equilibrium. Note that after approximately three to five half-lives, the curve levels off. This demonstrates equilibrium between the amount of drug entering the body and the amount leaving the body. This point, which is called *steady state*, reflects a constant mean concentration of drug in the body. At steady state, even though the blood levels of a drug fluctuate above and below this mean concentration and the drug level tends to have peaks and troughs during dosing intervals, the fluctuations remain within a constant range.

For some drugs, the time required to achieve steady state may be very long. For example, digoxin (Lanoxin) has a half-life of 39 hours (1.6 days), meaning that between 4.8 and 8 days are needed to achieve steady state. Clearly, when it is imperative to gain a therapeutic level quickly, waiting this long is unacceptable. Therefore, an initial loading dose of a drug is needed to reach the desired blood concentration quickly. The loading dose is based on the volume of distribution of the drug, independent of the half-life. The maintenance dose, however, is based on the half-life of the drug. Maintenance doses of the drug are given at scheduled intervals to replace the amount of drug eliminated.

Clearance

The concept of clearance, which refers to the removal of a drug from the body, is the final element in the process of elimination. Drugs with high clearances are removed from the body rapidly; those with low clearances are removed slowly.

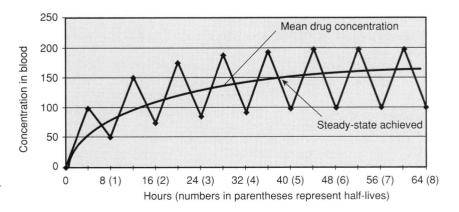

Figure 2–6 Steady state achieved with regular dosing (half-life = 8 hours).

BOX 2–4. RELATIONSHIP BETWEEN APPARENT VOLUME OF DISTRIBUTION, CLEARANCE, AND HALF-LIFE

$$\text{Clearance} = \frac{0.693 \times V_d}{t_{1/2}}$$

Clearance is usually expressed as L/hour; V_d is in L; $t_{1/2}$ is usually in hours.

Clearance of a drug from the body is directly dependent on the apparent volume of distribution and inversely related to the elimination half-life. The larger the V_d, the faster the clearance. Also, the smaller the $t_{1/2}$, the faster the clearance.

Drugs can be cleared by biliary, hepatic, and renal means. The following discussion highlights renal clearance.

Clearance is related to the volume of distribution and the half-life (Box 2-4). Clearance of a drug from the body depends directly on the apparent volume of distribution and is inversely related to the elimination half-life: the greater the volume of distribution and the shorter the half-life, the faster the clearance.

Because most drugs are "cleared" through the kidney, estimating the renal elimination rate or clearance can help the practitioner to understand how fast a drug is being eliminated in an individual patient. The kidney's ability to clear drugs is estimated through a surrogate substrate: creatinine. Creatinine, which is produced through the continual breakdown of muscle tissue and eliminated largely by glomerular filtration, is not significantly secreted or reabsorbed. Therefore, in estimating the creatinine clearance, the practitioner can also estimate the glomerular filtration rate. The level of creatinine is usually measured through a blood test (serum creatinine), with normal values ranging from 0.8 to 1.2 mg/dL. By combining this information with a patient's ideal body weight and age, the practitioner can use the formula of Cockroft and Gault to evaluate creatinine clearance and evaluate the kidney's ability to function and eliminate drugs (Box 2-5). For example, for a 40-year-old man of average height weighing 70 kg (154 lb)

BOX 2–5. COCKROFT AND GAULT FORMULA FOR ESTIMATING CREATININE CLEARANCE

$$CrCl_{est} = \frac{[140 - \text{age (y)}] \times IBW}{Scr \times 72}$$

Multiply $CrCl_{est}$ by 0.85 for women.

$CrCl_{est}$ = estimated creatinine clearance
Scr = serum creatinine (mg/dL)
IBW = ideal body weight in kilograms
    (kg; 2.2 lb = 1 kg)

and having a serum creatinine level of 1 mg/dL, the estimated creatinine clearance is 97 mL/minute. (This is only an estimate of this patient's creatinine clearance. The best method of determining the actual value is by a 24-hour urine specimen collection and measurement of excreted creatinine.)

Creatinine clearance values below 50 mL/minute suggest significant impairment of renal function and thus possible impairment of renal drug elimination. This may result in administered drugs having longer half-lives and higher steady-state concentrations, which may result in toxicity if the dose is not decreased or the length of time between doses is not increased.

Not every patient needs to have creatinine clearance estimated. Two rules of thumb are available for the practitioner: patients older than 65 years of age or those with a serum creatinine value greater than 1.5 mg/dL may be at risk for accumulating drug (and therefore toxicity) because of decreased renal function. In patients with either of these characteristics, a baseline and routine evaluation of renal function (eg, serum creatinine determination) should be performed.

PHARMACODYNAMICS

Pharmacodynamics refers to the set of processes by which drugs produce specific biochemical or physiologic changes in the body. Most often, pharmacodynamic effects occur because a drug interacts with a receptor. Receptors may be cell membrane proteins, extracellular enzymes, cytoplasmic enzymes, or intracellular proteins. A receptor is the component of the cell (or an enzyme) to which an endogenous substance binds, or attaches, initiating a chain of biochemical events. This chain of biochemical events culminates in a change in the physiologic function of the cell or activity of the enzyme. Like endogenous substances, drugs can initiate the biochemical chain of events. For example, a drug stimulating a receptor on the surface of an artery may ultimately cause vasoconstriction or vasodilation; or the drug's binding to a receptor may produce a change in cell wall permeability, thus allowing other substances to enter or leave a cell, such as occurs in nerve cells; or the drug attached to a receptor may initiate an increase or decrease in the production of an enzyme, thereby changing the amount of enzymatic activity for a given process.

Any chemical, endogenous or exogenous, that interacts with a receptor is called a *ligand*. Regardless of the ligand, or the actual interaction type, a substance can only alter or modify a cell or process, not impart a new function.

Drug Receptors

The capacity of a drug to bind to a receptor depends on the size and shape of the drug and the receptor. The drug acts as a "key" that fits into only a certain receptor or receptor type (Fig. 2-7). Once the drug fits into the receptor, it may act to "unlock" the activity of the receptor, thus initiating the biochemical chain of events, much like an ignition key initiates the chain of events that starts a car.

Drug receptors are commonly classified by the effect they produce. Some drugs interact with several receptors, causing multiple effects, whereas others interact with only a specific receptor, eliciting a single response. Epinephrine, for example, interacts with the alpha and beta receptors of the sympathetic

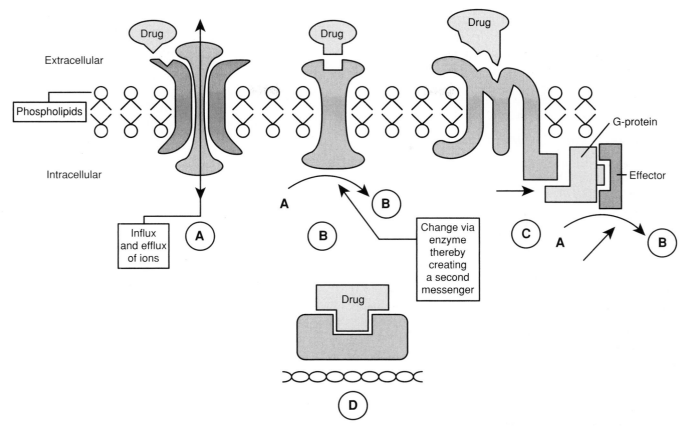

Figure 2–7 Drug and drug receptor interaction and signal transduction. The four primary receptors and their mechanisms of signal transduction include (A) gated ion channels; (B) transmembranous receptors; (C) G-protein-coupled receptors; and (D) intracellular receptors.

nervous system. As a result, epinephrine produces vasoconstriction (alpha receptor action) and an increase in heart rate (beta receptor action). Various molecules or enzymes can serve as drug receptors, such as ion channels (calcium channels), enzymes (angiotensin-converting enzyme [ACE]), and even receptors that generate intracellular second messengers (substances that interact with other intracellular components).

There are four known types of receptors: gated ion channels, transmembranous receptors, G-protein–coupled receptors, and intracellular receptors (see Fig. 2-7). Understanding these receptors and the signals they generate is central to understanding the actions of many drugs.

Gated Ion Channels

The function of gated ion channel receptors is to open or close channels to allow certain ions to pass through the cell membrane. Binding of ligands to these receptors produces a conformational change that widens or narrows the channel, thereby regulating the access of soluble ions. The nicotinic acetylcholine receptor is a good example. Its function is to translate the signal from acetylcholine into an electrical signal at the neuromuscular endplate. As such, when acetylcholine binds to this receptor, the channel opens, allowing sodium or potassium to enter the cell and cause cellular depolarization.

Other types of gated ion channel receptors are associated with the neurotransmitters. Gamma-aminobutyric acid

(GABA$_A$), the primary inhibitory neurotransmitter, opens a chloride channel in the cell, which minimizes the depolarization potential. Certain drugs, such as the benzodiazepines, bind to an allosteric site and enhance the activity of GABA$_A$ by increasing the opening of the chloride channel. There is no intrinsic activity at the allosteric site, and it serves only to enhance the primary action of the endogenous ligand. Other excitatory neurotransmitters, such as L-glutamate and L-aspartate, operate by this mechanism, called signal transduction, which transfers the signal quickly.

Transmembranous Receptors

A transmembranous receptor has its ligand-binding domain, the specific region to which ligands bind, on the cell's surface. The enzymatic portion of the receptor is in the cell cytoplasm. When a ligand binds to a transmembranous receptor, several things may occur. The receptor–ligand complex produces a conformational change in the receptor and triggers a response. Alternatively, the ligand–receptor complex can pass through the cell membrane and trigger an intracellular response directly. This intracellular response often is a change in enzymatic activity. A key feature of the transmembranous receptor response is the downregulation of the receptors, or a decrease in the number of receptors available for response. The opposite of this is upregulation, which does not occur as frequently. The nature of the signal depends on the specific ligand–receptor interaction, but it commonly results in the generation of second messengers. A second messenger is an intracellular chemical that interacts with other intracellular components. Ions such as calcium and potassium, along with cyclic adenosine monophosphate (cAMP), are common second messengers. Hormones and other endogenous substances, such as growth factors and insulin, often operate with this signaling mechanism.

G-Protein–Coupled Receptors

G-protein–coupled receptors are another family of receptors that generate intracellular second messengers. These receptors also exist as transmembranous receptors composed of an extracellular protein receptor and an intracellular type G protein. The interaction of a ligand and the receptor produces a conformational change in the receptor, bringing it in contact with the G protein. This contact results in activation of an enzyme or opening of an ion channel in the cell and, in turn, increased levels of the second messenger. It is the second messenger that triggers a change in the function of the cell. Alpha- and beta-adrenergic receptors, along with several hormone receptors, use G proteins to affect cell function.

Intracellular Receptors

Lipid-soluble drugs can traverse the lipid bilayer of the cell and enter the cytoplasm. Once inside, these drugs attach to intracellular receptors and initiate direct changes in the cell by affecting DNA transcription. Glucocorticoids and sex hormones are known to act by way of this signaling mechanism.

Drug–Receptor Interactions

The ability of a drug to bind to any receptor is dictated by factors such as the size and shape of the drug relative to the configuration of the binding site on the receptor. The electrostatic attraction between the drug and the receptor may also be important in determining the extent to which the drug binds to the receptor.

Affinity

A drug attracted to a receptor displays an *affinity* for that receptor. This affinity, the degree to which a drug is attracted to a receptor, is related to the concentration of drug required to occupy a receptor site. Drugs displaying a high affinity for a given receptor require only a small concentration in the circulation to elicit a response, whereas those with a low affinity require higher circulating concentrations. There exists equilibrium between the blood concentration of a drug, the concentration of drug at the site of action (ie, near the receptor), and the amount of drug bound to a receptor. The magnitude of a drug's effect can be explained by the receptor occupancy theory—that is, a response from a cell (or group of cells) depends on the fraction of receptors occupied by a drug or endogenous substance. Therefore, one can infer a relationship between the minimally and maximally effective concentrations needed at the site of action and the minimum and maximum blood concentrations.

Chirality

The shape of a drug can influence its interaction with a receptor. Most drugs display chirality—that is, they exist in two forms with mirror-image spatial arrangements called enantiomers, or isomers. Each enantiomer is distinguished from the other through its ability to rotate polarized light in pure solution to the right or left. This results in a dextrorotary, or *d*-enantiomer, and a levorotary, or *l*-companion.

A pair of entantiomers is like a left and a right hand. As such, enantiomeric pairs may not fit into a receptor equally well, just as a right hand does not fit well into a left-hand glove. This is called stereoselectivity; one enantiomer may fit better into a receptor than the other and, hence, be more active. For example, the drug dextromethorphan (Robitussin DM) is the *d*-isomer of a compound. This *d*-isomer is a common cough suppressant found in most over-the-counter medications. Its *l*-isomer counterpart, levorphanol (Levo-Dromoran), is an extremely potent narcotic analgesic. Although the *l*-isomer also possesses cough suppressant activity, the *d*-isomer is essentially devoid of analgesic activity at commonly used doses. This similarity coincident with dissimilarity illustrates the importance of isomers in pharmacodynamics.

Agonists and Antagonists

Not all drugs with an affinity for a receptor elicit a response. Drugs that display a degree of affinity for a receptor and stimulate a response are considered agonists. Others that display an affinity and do not elicit a response are called antagonists. Antagonists do not have intrinsic activity; they can only block the activity of the endogenous agonist. An antagonist may be viewed as a key that fits into the lock, but because of its different configuration cannot be turned. Because an antagonist can occupy, or fit into, a receptor, it competes with agonists for that receptor, thereby blocking the effect of the agonist. Antagonists with a high affinity for a receptor may be able to "bump" an agonist off the receptor and reverse the agonist activity. Antagonists usually are used to block the activity of an endogenous substance, but they also can be used to block the activity of exogenously administered drugs. For example, when naloxone (Narcan) is given to a patient taking opioid drugs, the analgesic (and adverse) effects of the opioid are reversed within 1 to 2 minutes. In most cases, naloxone has a higher affinity for the opioid receptor than the opioid itself. This rough explanation of drug–receptor interactions serves only as a basis for understanding the complexity of this interplay.

Dose–Response Relationships

For many drugs, the relationship between the dose and the response is obvious: lower doses produce smaller responses, whereas higher doses increase the response. This correlation is based on the amount of drug occupying specific receptors. As the amount of drug exceeds the number of available receptors, the response reaches a plateau, so that further increases in dose do not increase response. However, dose–response relationships such as these clearly depend on the affinity of a drug for a receptor: a drug with a high affinity for a receptor needs a significantly lower concentration

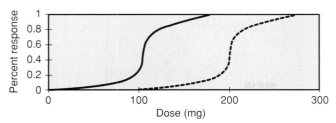

Figure 2–8   Two drugs with differing receptor affinities produce similar effects at different dosage ranges. The drug with the greater affinity (*solid line*) requires less drug to produce the same effect as a drug with less affinity (*dotted line*). This demonstrates the relationship between receptor affinity and drug potency.

to achieve the same effect compared with a drug with a lower affinity.

This difference in affinity accounts for the varying "potency" of drugs. For example, drugs such as hydromorphone (Dilaudid) and morphine produce the same effect: analgesia. However, hydromorphone is more potent than morphine and therefore requires a smaller concentration to elicit a similar level of analgesia. Figure 2-8 demonstrates a typical dose–response relationship.

FACTORS AFFECTING PHARMACOKINETICS AND PHARMACODYNAMICS

The goal of pharmacotherapeutics is to achieve a desired beneficial effect with minimal adverse effects. Once a medication has been selected for a patient, the practitioner must determine the dose that most closely achieves this goal. A rational approach to this objective combines the principles of pharmacokinetics with pharmacodynamics to clarify the dose–response relationship. Knowing the relationship between drug concentration and response allows the practitioner to take into account the various pathologic and physiologic features of a particular patient that make his or her response different from the average person's response to a drug.

Patient Variables

A host of variables affect the disposition of a drug in the body and the reaction the body has to the drug. People vary in their body type, weight, diet, ethnicity, and genetic makeup. These factors, individually and combined, contribute to significant variation in the response to drug therapy. For example, the genetic makeup of the people of Japan is known to affect the expression of certain hepatic enzymes involved in the metabolism of drugs. This suggests that, at least pharmacokinetically, some people of Japanese heritage respond differently to certain drugs. The same logic applies to people who are overweight and underweight, people of varying ages, people with various pathophysiologic problems, and even people with different diets and nutritional habits.

Genetics

Genetic differences are a major factor in determining the way that people metabolize specific compounds. Genetic variations

may result in abnormal or absent drug-metabolizing enzymes. The anomaly can be harmful or even fatal if the drug cannot be metabolized and therefore exerts a toxic effect from accumulation or prolonged pharmacologic activity. Some people, for example, lack the enzyme that breaks down acetylcholine. In these people, a drug such as succinylcholine (Anectine, an acetylcholine-like drug) is not degraded and therefore accumulates. The result is respiratory paralysis because the undegraded, accumulated succinylcholine has an increased half-life, causing it to remain active longer.

Age

The influence of age on pharmacokinetics and pharmacodynamics is well known. Developmental differences in the neonate, toddler, and young child, for instance, influence how drugs are handled by the GI tract, liver, and kidneys. Of equal importance is how these children respond to drugs in light of the presence or absence of receptors at different stages of development. For example, drug-metabolizing enzymes are deficient in the fetus and premature infant. The fetus can metabolize drugs early in its development, but its expression of drug-metabolizing enzymes differs from that of the adult and is usually less efficient.

Children can metabolize many drugs more rapidly than adults, and as children approach puberty, the rate of drug metabolism approaches that of adults. Similarly, older adults undergo physiologic changes that affect the absorption, distribution, and elimination of many agents. The pharmacodynamic changes imparted by age as well as accompanying diseases pose a greater challenge for the practitioner in understanding the impact a single agent has on a patient's health and well-being. Chapter 4 discusses pediatric considerations, and Chapter 6 discusses geriatric considerations in more depth.

Sex

The role of sex as a distinct patient variable is recognized by some but poorly understood by most. Most of the published clinical drug studies use male subjects as the primary study population, and clinicians then extrapolate the data to women. However, women in general have a higher percentage of body fat, which could ultimately alter the pharmacokinetic disposition of certain drugs. Similarly, the pharmacodynamic response of women may be different because of the presence or absence of hormones such as estrogen and testosterone.

Ethnicity

Ethnicity is a significant factor in both the pharmacokinetic and pharmacodynamic responses of patients. The genetic makeup of various ethnic populations governs the levels of hepatic enzymes expressed in these groups. Equally important are the habits and traditions of certain groups, such as diet or the use of home remedies.

Pharmacodynamically, ethnically based differences exist in the responses to agents. An example is the minimal response of African-American patients to monotherapy with some drugs, such as ACE inhibitors. African Americans produce a low level of renin, a key component in the renin–angiotensin–aldosterone system by which the ACE inhibitors work. This low level of renin makes this system untouchable by the ACE inhibitor, thereby negating its effect.

Diet and Nutrition

Diet affects the metabolism of and response to many drugs. Animal and human studies indicate that total caloric intake and the percentage of calories obtained from different sources (carbohydrates, proteins, and fats) influence drug pharmacokinetics. Specific dietary constituents, such as cruciferous vegetables and charcoal-broiled beef, can also alter drug metabolism. Fortunately, most food–drug interactions are not serious and do not alter the clinical effects of the drug. However, a few well-known food and drug combinations should be avoided because of their potentially serious interactions. For instance, certain tyramine-containing foods, such as fermented cheese and wine, should not be ingested with drugs that inhibit the monoamine oxidase enzyme (MAO inhibitors). Tyramine-rich foods stimulate the body to release catecholamines (norepinephrine, epinephrine). MAO-inhibiting drugs work by suppressing the destruction of catecholamines, thereby allowing higher levels of norepinephrine and epinephrine to accumulate. Consequently, when MAO inhibitors are taken with tyramine-containing foods, excessive catecholamine levels may develop and lead to a dangerous increase in blood pressure (hypertensive crisis). Practitioners should be aware of this and should be on the alert for other such interactions as new drugs arrive on the market.

Pathophysiology

Structural or functional damage to an organ or tissue responsible for drug metabolism or excretion presents an obvious problem in pharmacology. Diseases that initiate changes in tissue function or blood flow to specific organs can dramatically affect the elimination of various drugs. Certain diseases may also impair the absorption and distribution of the drug, complicating the problem of individualized response. The role of disease in affecting the patient's response is crucial because the response to the medication may be affected by the same pathologic process that the drug is being used to treat. For instance, renal excretion of antibiotics, such as the aminoglycosides, is altered radically in many types of bacterial infection, but these drugs are typically administered to treat the same infections that alter their own excretion. Consequently, great care must be taken to adjust the dosage accordingly when administering medications to patients with conditions in which drug elimination may be altered.

Bibliography

*Starred references are cited in the text.

Brody, T. M., Larner, J., & Minneman, K. (Eds.). (1998). *Human pharmacology: Molecular to clinical* (3rd ed.). St. Louis: Mosby–Year Book.

Goodman, L. S., Gilman, A., Hardman, J. G., Gilman, A. G., & Limbird, L. E. (Eds.). (1996). *Goodman and Gilman's the pharmacological basis of therapeutics* (9th ed.). New York: McGraw-Hill.

Gunaratna, C. (2000). Drug metabolism and pharmacokinetics in drug discovery: a primer for bioanalytical chemists, Part I. *Current Separations, 19*(1), 17–23.

Gunaratna, C. (2001). Drug metabolism and pharmacokinetics in drug discovery: a primer for bioanalytical chemists, Part II. *Current Separations, 19*(2), 87–92.

Katzung, B. G. (Ed.). (2001). *Basic and clinical pharmacology* (8th ed.). New York: McGraw-Hill.

Rowland, M., & Tozer, T. N. (Eds.). (1995). *Clinical pharmacokinetics: Concepts and applications* (3rd ed.). Philadelphia: J. B. Lippincott.

Smith, C. M., & Reynard, A. M. (Eds.). (1992). *Textbook of pharmacology*. Philadelphia: W. B. Saunders.

Williams, B. R., & Baer, C. L. (Eds.). (1998). *Essentials of clinical pharmacology in nursing* (3rd ed.). Spring House, PA: Springhouse Corp.

Visit the Connection web site for the most up-to-date drug information.

3

IMPACT OF DRUG INTERACTIONS AND ADVERSE EVENTS ON THERAPEUTICS

■ MATTHEW SARNES, QUAN V. DONG, AND ANDREW M. PETERSON

As the quantity and types of pharmacologic agents continue to expand, the likelihood of drug interactions and adverse reactions increases. Currently, more than 8000 drugs are available to treat various conditions. Each agent is designed to alter the homeostasis of the human body to some degree, and individual responses to these agents can be unpredictable.

In a meta-analysis, Lazarou, Pomeranz, and Corey (1998) found that 6.7% of hospitalizations were due to serious adverse drug reactions (ADRs), of which 0.32% resulted in death. Based on 1996 hospitalization rates, that accounts for approximately 100,000 deaths and more than 2 million serious ADRs (National Center for Health Statistics, 1996). Similarly, in hospitalized children, the overall incidence of ADRs was 9.5% and a rate of hospital admissions of 2.09% in this same age group (Impicciatore, et al., 2001). ADRs present an alarming problem that warrants significant attention from health care practitioners. Not only do ADRs affect morbidity and mortality, they also dramatically increase health care costs. Estimates suggest that an additional $1.56 to $4 billion is spent in direct hospital costs precipitated by ADRs (Bates, et al., 1997; Classen, et al., 1997).

Similarly, drug interactions are preventable ADRs posing a significant problem to the health care community. Therefore, a thorough understanding of how drug–drug interactions occur and how they relate to ADRs should help decrease the rate of occurrence and the associated morbidity/mortality. This chapter discusses the mechanisms of drug interactions and their potential consequences. For the purpose of this chapter, these interactions are broken down into three major categories: drug–drug interactions, drug–food interactions, and drug–disease interactions. Each of the interaction categories can affect the drug's pharmacokinetic or pharmacodynamic profile. The definition, identification, and management of ADRs are discussed at the end of the chapter.

DRUG–DRUG INTERACTIONS

When a person takes two or more medications concomitantly, the potential exists for one or more drugs to change the effect of other drugs. The drug whose effect is altered by another drug is termed the *object* or *target* drug. Although minor interactions between drugs probably occur frequently, these interactions may not be significant enough to alter the effect of either drug. However, it is important for the practitioner to understand the mechanisms behind these interactions to predict more accurately when significant (and potentially fatal) drug interactions may occur.

Pharmacokinetic Interactions

Absorption

Because most medications in the ambulatory care setting are administered orally, this route is the focus of discussion. For a drug to exert its effect, it must reach its site of action. Normally, this requires access to the bloodstream. As discussed in Chapter 2, drugs administered orally must be absorbed into the portal vein, through the intestinal wall, to reach the systemic circulation. The oral tablet must dissolve in the gastrointestinal (GI) tract before it can penetrate the intestinal wall.

Acidity (pH)

For some drugs, this process depends on the acidity in the GI tract. Therefore, if a drug that alters the gastric pH is administered concomitantly with a drug that depends on a normal gastric pH for dissolution, the absorption of the object drug will be affected. An example of this type of interaction is the concurrent administration of a histamine-2 (H_2) receptor antagonist (eg, ranitidine) and ketoconazole, an imidazole antifungal agent. Ketoconazole is the object drug that requires an acidic pH for absorption. When ranitidine is administered along with ketoconazole, the increase in gastric pH hinders the dissolution of ketoconazole and, therefore, decreases its absorption. Similarly, this change in pH can increase the absorption of other drugs. Similarly, the absorption is enhanced by an increased gastric pH secondary to H_2 antagonists.

Adsorption

Another mechanism of absorptive drug–drug interactions is adsorption. Adsorption occurs when one agent binds the other to its surface to form a complex. The most common agents associated with this type of interaction are divalent and trivalent cations (Mg^{2+}, Ca^{2+}, Al^{3+}, found in antacids) and anionic binding resins (colestipol, cholestyramine). This type of interaction occurs when certain medications such as tetracyclines or fluoroquinolones are given with antacids. The metal ions in the antacid chelate (form a complex with) the antibiotic, preventing absorption of both components (ion and antibiotic). Adsorbents can interact with a variety of drugs; therefore, appropriate intervals between doses of the interacting medications are warranted. In general, the agents known to interact in this manner should be administered at least 2 hours apart.

Gastrointestinal Motility and Rate of Absorption

Drugs that affect the motility of the GI tract produce a less common absorption-altering mechanism. These agents tend to affect the rate of absorption and not the amount of drug absorbed. Any agent—for example, metoclopramide—that stimulates peristalsis and increases gastric emptying time can increase the rate of absorption. This increase in rate of absorption occurs because the target drug reaches the duodenum faster, allowing absorption to occur sooner.

Conversely, anticholinergic agents and opiates decrease gastric motility, thereby decreasing the rate of absorption of object drugs. Because this type of interaction does not usually affect the amount of drug absorbed, it is usually clinically insignificant. Table 3-1 summarizes some of the major drug interactions that occur in the absorptive process.

Distribution

After drugs are absorbed into the bloodstream, most of them, to some degree, are bound to plasma protein such as albumin or α_1-acid glycoprotein. As described in Chapter 2, only an unbound drug is free to interact with its target receptor site and is therefore active. The percentage of drug that binds to plasma proteins depends on the affinity of that drug for the protein-binding site. If two drugs with high affinity for circulating proteins are administered together, they may compete for a single binding site on the protein. In fact, one drug may displace the other from the binding site with the result being an increase in the unbound (free) fraction of the displaced drug. This increase in free drug may trigger an exaggerated pharmacodynamic response or toxic reaction. However, because the excess unbound drug is now subject to elimination processes, the increases in both free drug fraction and the effects produced are usually transient.

Clinically significant drug displacement interactions normally occur only when drugs are more than 90% protein bound and have a narrow therapeutic index (Rolan, 1994). For example, warfarin is 99% protein bound, and therefore only 1% of the drug in the bloodstream is free to induce a pharmacodynamic response (inhibition of clotting factors). If a second drug is administered that displaces even 1% of the warfarin bound to albumin, the amount of free warfarin is doubled, to 2% free. This can result in a significant

---

Table 3.1

Drugs Affecting Absorption

	Mechanism of Action	Object Drug	Results
Absorption Inhibitors			
activated charcoal	Binding agent	digoxin	Decreased absorption
aluminum hydroxide	Unknown	allopurinol	Decreased absorption
antacids (Mg^{2+}, Ca^{2+}, Al^{3+})	Chelating agent	quinolones, tetracyclines, levodopa	Decreased absorption
anticholinergics	Decreases gastric emptying	acetaminophen, atenolol, levodopa	Decreased absorption rate
cholestyramine	Binding agent	acetaminophen, diclofenac, digoxin, glipizide, furosemide, iron, lorazepam, methotrexate, metronidazole, piroxicam	Decreased absorption
colestipol	Binding agent	carbamazepine, diclofenac, furosemide, tetracycline, thiazides	Decreased absorption
desipramine	Decreases GI motility	phenylbutazone	Decreased absorption
didanosine	Binding agent	ciprofloxacin	Decreased absorption
	Increases gastric pH	imidazole, antifungals	Decreased absorption
ferrous sulfate	Chelating agent	quinolones, tetracyclines, levodopa	Decreased absorption
histamine-2 receptor antagonists, omeprazole	Increases gastric pH	imidazole, antifungals, enoxacin	Decreased absorption
phenytoin	Unknown	furosemide	Decreased absorption
sucralfate	Binding agent	quinolones, tetracyclines, phenytoin	Decreased absorption
sulfasalazine	Unknown	digoxin	Decreased absorption
Absorption Enhancers			
cisapride	Increases gastric emptying	disopyramide	Increased absorption rate
histamine-2 receptor antagonists	Increases gastric pH	pravastatin, glipizide, dihydropyridine, calcium antagonists	Increased absorption
metoclopramide	Increases gastric motility	cyclosporine	Increased absorption rate
	Increases GI motility	acetaminophen, cefprozil, ethanol	Increased absorption rate

GI, gastrointestinal.

Table 3.2

Distribution Drug Interactions

Displacing Agent	Object Drug
aspirin	meclofenamate tolmetin
salicylates	methotrexate
TMP–SMZ	
sulfaphenazole	phenytoin
tolbutamide	
valproic acid	
halofenate	sulfonylureas
quinidine	digoxin
aspirin	warfarin
chloral hydrate	
diazoxide	
etodolac	
fenoprofen	
lovastatin	
nalidixic acid	
phenylbutazone	
phenytoin	
sulfapyrazone	

TMP-SMZ, Trimethophein–sulfamethoxazole

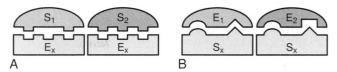

Figure 3–1 Substrate binding. **A.** Different substrates: Although Enzyme X (E_x) can bind to both Substrate 1 (S1) and Substrate 2 (S2), S2 has greater affinity for E_x than S1. Therefore E_x will bind to S2 most often. **B.** Different enzymes. Although Substrate X (S_x) can bind to both Enzyme 1 (E1) and Enzyme 2 (E2), E1 has a greater affinity for S_x than E2. Therefore S_x will bind to E1 most often.

increase in its pharmacodynamic action, leading to excessive bleeding. Table 3-2 lists examples of several displacement interactions.

Metabolism

Lipophilicity (fat solubility) enables drug molecules to be absorbed and reach their site of action. However, lipophilic drugs are difficult for the body to excrete. Therefore, they must be transformed by the body to more hydrophilic (water-soluble) molecules. This is accomplished primarily through phase I, or oxidation, reactions. The main sites of metabolism in the body are the liver (hepatocytes) and small intestine (enterocytes). Other tissues, such as the kidneys, lungs, and brain, play a minor role in the metabolism of drug molecules (Michalets, 1998). These sites of metabolism contain enzymes called cytochrome P450 isoenzymes. This group of isoenzymes has been identified as the major catalyst of phase I metabolic reactions in humans.

The nomenclature of the cytochrome P450 system classifies the isoenzymes (designated CYP) according to family (>36% homology in amino acid sequence), subfamily (77% homology), and individual gene (Brosen, 1990; Guengerich, 1994; Nebert, et al., 1987). For example, the isoenzyme CYP3A4 belongs to family 3, subfamily A, and gene 4. As one moves down the classification system from family to gene, the structures of the isoenzymes become more similar.

This enzyme system has evolved to form new isoenzymes that metabolize foreign substrates (ie, drugs) that are presented to the body. These enzymes are structured to recognize and bind to molecular entities on substrates. Many different substrates may have molecular structures that differ only slightly; therefore, an isoenzyme can bind to any one of these substrates. Although several different substrates may compete for the same enzyme receptor, the substrate with the highest affinity binds most often. The converse of this is also true. Two isoenzymes can bind to the same substrate (Fig. 3-1), but the substrate binds more often to the isoenzyme to which it has the most affinity. However, not every

drug molecule ("substrate") can be metabolized by every enzyme with which it binds; therefore, it is not a true substrate. These concepts form the backbone for the drug interactions that are expanded on later.

Six isoenzymes have been determined to be responsible for most metabolism-related drug interactions. They are the isoforms CYP1A2, CYP2C9, CYP2C19, CYP2D6, CYP2E1, and CYP3A4. The CYP3A4 isoform is responsible for 40% to 45% of drug metabolism, the CYP2D6 for the next 20% to 30%, CYP2C9 about 10%, and CYP2E1 and CYP1A2 each responsible for about 5% (Ingelman-Sundberg, 2004). The remaining 5% to 20% is accounted for by several lesser important isoforms. Because there are so few enzymes that transform a multitude of substrates, it is easy to see how there would be a great potential for interactions.

There are some genetic variations with respect to the distribution of the enzymes. For example, about 10% of Europeans lack the CYP2D6 enzyme and are therefore considered poor metabolizers of drugs using this pathway for biotransformation. These individuals, then, are at risk for ADRs related to drugs metabolized by the CYP2D6, or for underdosing of prodrugs requiring this enzyme for activation (eg, codeine). In contrast, about 5% of this population are considered ultra-metabolizers, have too rapid metabolism, and may show little to no response related to drugs metabolized by the CYP2D6 pathway (Ingelman-Sundberg, 2004). Similarly, there is variability within the CYP2C19 isoform, with about 15% of Asians being poor metabolizers and 2% to 4% of Africans, African Americans, or whites being poor metabolizers. At this time, there is no practical way of identifying poor metabolizers from others, but an unexpected response might be due to metabolic differences.

There are two types of metabolic drug interactions: drugs that inhibit the action of an enzyme and those that induce the activity of the enzyme.

Inhibition

Inhibition of drug metabolism occurs through competitive and noncompetitive inhibition. When two drugs, administered concurrently, are metabolized by the same isoenzyme, they are defined as competitive inhibitors of each other. In essence, they compete for the same binding site on an enzyme to be metabolized.

Noncompetitive inhibition also occurs when both drugs compete for the same binding site, but one drug is metabolized by that isoenzyme and the other drug is not. The best known example of a noncompetitive inhibitor is quinidine. Quinidine is metabolized by the CYP3A4 isoenzyme but can also bind to the CYP2D6 enzyme. Therefore, although

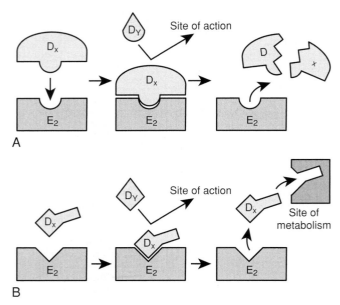

Figure 3-2 Inhibition. **A.** Competitive inhibition. Drug X (DX) and Drug Y (DY) are both metabolized by Enzyme 2 (E$_2$). **B.** Noncompetitive inhibition. Although DX and DY compete for the binding site on E$_2$, only DY is metabolized by E$_2$. Therefore DX noncompetitively inhibits DY.

quinidine does not compete for metabolism by the CYP2D6 isoenzyme, it does compete for the CYP2D6 isoenzyme binding site.

In both competitive and noncompetitive inhibition, the drug with the greatest affinity for the isoenzyme receptor is usually the inhibiting drug because it binds in the receptor site, preventing the other drug from being bound and metabolized (Fig. 3-2). The significance of the drug interaction depends on several characteristics of the inhibiting drug.

Affinity

The first characteristic, affinity, has already been mentioned. Many drugs may inhibit the same isoenzyme but not to the same extent. The greater the affinity of an inhibiting drug for an enzyme, the more it blocks binding of other drug molecules.

Half-Life

Along with affinity, the half-life (t½) of the inhibiting drug determines the duration of the interaction. The longer the half-life of the inhibiting drug, the longer the drug interaction lasts. For example, after a regimen of ketoconazole (t½ = 8 hours) is discontinued, its ability to inhibit the CYP3A4 enzyme lasts until it is eliminated, in three to five half-lives or approximately 1 day. However, the inhibiting effect of amiodarone, with a t½ of approximately 53 days, lasts for weeks to months after its discontinuation.

Concentration

The third major factor contributing to a drug's ability to inhibit hepatic enzymes is the concentration of the inhibiting

drug. A threshold concentration must be reached or exceeded to inhibit an enzyme. This is similar to the threshold concentration discussed in Chapter 2 regarding minimally effective concentrations and therapeutic responses. This minimally effective threshold concentration, or concentration-dependent inhibition, is exhibited by a variety of drugs. The dose yielding this concentration-dependent inhibition varies based on V$_d$, drug and receptor affinity, and characteristics of the individual patient. An example of a dose- or concentration-dependent inhibitor is cimetidine. In most patients, a dose of 400 mg/d results in only weak enzyme inhibition. However, at higher doses, it interacts significantly with both the CYP2D6 and CYP1A2 isoenzymes (Shinn, 1992).

Some enzyme inhibitors may affect one enzyme at a smaller concentration and more than one isoenzyme at higher concentrations. These enzyme inhibitors demonstrate that some isoenzymes have differing thresholds. For example, fluconazole at a dose of 200 mg/d significantly inhibits only the 2C9 isoenzyme, but as the dose increases above 400 mg/d, it also inhibits the 3A4 isoenzyme (Hansten, 1998; Kivisto, Neuvonen, & Koltz, 1994).

Toxic Potential

Another consideration with regard to inhibition interactions is the toxic potential of the object drug. For example, nonsedating antihistamines (ie, terfenadine and astemizole) are metabolized by the CYP3A4 isoenzyme to a nontoxic metabolite. The parent compound of both drugs is cardiotoxic. If a potent CYP3A4 inhibitor (eg, erythromycin) is administered concurrently with these agents, the parent compound accumulates in the body and causes a potentially fatal arrhythmia, such as torsades de pointes (Mathews, et al., 1991; Woosley, 1996). Because of their serious toxic potential, both terfenadine and astemizole have been removed from the market.

Not all inhibition reactions result in harmful effects, however. Some interactions may be inconsequential or even beneficial. For example, ketoconazole (a potent inhibitor of the CYP3A4 isoenzyme) can be given with cyclosporine. The consequent interaction enables practitioners to give less cyclosporine to achieve the same immunosuppressive response (Hansten & Horn, 1997).

The cytochrome P450 system is complex, but an understanding of the basic concepts of inhibitory interactions leads to the ability to anticipate which agents are likely to interact. The affinity, half-life, and drug concentration determine the potency of the inhibiting drug. A potent enzyme inhibitor inhibits most drugs metabolized by that enzyme. A clinically significant drug interaction also depends on the toxic potential of the drug being inhibited. Table 3-3 lists several enzyme inhibitors.

Induction

Drug–drug interactions can also result from the action of one drug (inducer) stimulating the metabolism of an object drug (substrate). This enhanced metabolism is thought to be produced by an increase in hepatic blood flow or an increase in the formation of hepatic enzymes. This process, known as *enzyme induction*, increases the amount of enzymes

Table 3.3

Drugs Affecting Metabolism Through Inhibition of Cytochrome P450 Isoenzymes

Inhibitors	Inducers	Substrates	Inhibitors	Inducers	Substrates
Isoenzyme 1A2			*Isoenzyme 3A4*		
cimetidine	carbamazepine	theophylline	amiodarone	carbamazepine	alprazolam
ciprofloxacin	phenobarbital		antifungals	dexamethasone	atorvastatin
clarithromycin	phenytoin	tricyclic antidepressants	clarithromycin	ethosuximide	calcium channel blockers
enoxacin	rifampin	benzodiazepines	erythromycin	phenobarbital	carbamazepine
erythromycin	ritonavir	warfarin	fluoxetine	phenytoin	clindamycin
norfloxacin	smoking		fluvoxamine	rifabutin	clomipramine
oral contraceptives	polycyclic		imidazole	rifampin	clonazepam
SSRIs	aromatic		nefazodone		cyclosporine
zileuton	hydrocarbons		norfloxacin		dapsone
			protease inhibitors		dexamethasone
Isoenzyme 2C (primarily 2C9, 2C19)			quinine		dextromethorphan
amiodarone	carbamazepine	amitriptyline	zafirlukast		disopyramide
cimetidine	phenobarbital	clomipramine			erythromycin
fluconazole	phenytoin	diazepam			oral contraceptives
fluoxetine	rifampin	imipramine			(estrogens)
fluvastatin		losartan			ethosuximide
fluvoxamine		phenytoin			fexofenadine
isoniazid		omeprazole			imipramine
metronidazole		tricyclic antidepressants			ketoconazole
omeprazole		warfarin			lidocaine
sertraline					lovastatin
zafirlukast					miconazole
					midazolam
Isoenzyme 2D6					nefazodone
amiodarone	carbamazepine				ondansetron
cimetidine	phenobarbital				pravastatin
clomipramine	phenytoin				prednisone
codeine	rifampin				protease inhibitors
desipramine					quinidine
haloperidol					quinine
perphenazine					rifampin
propafenone					sertraline
quinidine					tacrolimus
SSRIs					tamoxifen
thioridazine					temazepam
venlafaxine					triazolam
					verapamil
Isoenzyme 2E1					warfarin
disulfiram	ethanol	acetaminophen			zileuton
ritonavir	isoniazid	chloral hydrate			
		ethanol			
		isoniazid			
		ondansetron			
		tamoxifen			

SSRIs, selective serotonin reuptake inhibitors.

available to metabolize drug molecules, thereby decreasing the concentration and pharmacodynamic effect of the object drug.

Some of the more common enzyme inducers are rifampin, phenobarbital, phenytoin, and carbamazepine. Enzyme induction, like enzyme inhibition, is substrate dependent. Therefore, any drug that is a potent inducer of a cytochrome P450 system increases the metabolism of most drugs by that enzyme. Also, in a manner similar to that of enzyme inhibitors, inducers may affect more than one cytochrome P450 isoform; for example, phenobarbital is a potent inducer of the CYP3A4, CYP1A2, and CYP2C isoforms (Michalets, 1998).

Some enzyme inducers, such as carbamazepine, also increase their own metabolism. Over time, carbamazepine stimulates its own metabolism, thereby decreasing its half-

life and frequently resulting in an increased dose requirement to maintain the same therapeutic drug level (Hussar, 1995). This process is termed *autoinduction*.

The onset and duration/cessation of enzyme induction depend on both the half-life of the inducer and the half-life of the isoenzyme that is being stimulated. For example, rifampin (t½ = 3–4 hours) results in enzyme induction within 24 hours, whereas the enzyme induction capacity of phenobarbital (t½ = 53–140 hours) is not evident for approximately 7 days (Michalets, 1998; Spinler, Cheng, Kindwall, & Charland, 1995). The level of induction remains constant while the drugs are being administered. However, on discontinuation of the respective inducers, the inducing action of rifampin ends more rapidly because of its shorter half-life. This occurs because rifampin is removed from the body at a faster rate than phenobarbital and therefore is not available to inhibit hepatic enzymes for as long.

The initiation and duration of enzyme induction also depend on the half-life of the induced isoenzyme. It takes anywhere from 1 to 6 days for a cytochrome P450 enzyme to be degraded or produced (Cupp & Tracy, 1997). Therefore, even if a drug achieves a high enough concentration to produce induction of liver enzymes, the increase in metabolism of an object drug may not be evident until more liver enzymes have formed. The effect of rifampin on warfarin metabolism is a good example of this. Although induction begins within 24 hours of rifampin administration, its effect on warfarin metabolism is not evident for approximately 4 days (Harder & Thurmann, 1996). On discontinuation of rifampin, the remaining drug is metabolized to negligible levels before the effect on warfarin metabolism dissipates. This occurs because the half-life of the liver enzymes is greater than the half-life of rifampin, and therefore the enzymes remain to metabolize warfarin after rifampin is eliminated from the body.

These concepts are important to remember when monitoring laboratory values that demonstrate the effectiveness of the object medication. For example, the international normalized ratio (INR), which is a surrogate marker of warfarin levels, fluctuates significantly within a couple of days of the initiation or discontinuation of rifampin. However, no change in the INR is evident for approximately 1 week after administration of phenobarbital. This is also true when measuring levels of certain antibiotics and other agents that may be affected by inducers. Table 3-3 lists several enzyme inducers and the drugs they affect.

Excretion

Although most drugs are metabolized by the liver, the primary modes of elimination from the body are biliary and renal excretion. Drugs are removed from the bloodstream by the kidneys by filtration or by urinary secretion. However, reabsorption from the urine into the bloodstream may also occur.

Changes in these processes become important when they affect drugs that are unchanged or still active. Excretion of drug molecules can be affected in a number of ways; these include, but are not limited to, acidification or alkalinization of the urine and alteration of secretory or active transport pathways. Although they are not discussed here for various reasons, there are a select number of other mechanisms of renal drug interactions.

The ionization state of drug molecules plays a key role in the excretion process. The urine pH determines the ionization state of the excreted molecule. Because lipophilic membranes are less permeable to ionized molecules (hydrophilic), ionized molecules become "trapped" in the urine and are subsequently excreted. Drugs that are nonionized in the urine may be reabsorbed and then recirculated, effectively decreasing their elimination and increasing their half-lives.

Acidic drugs remain in their nonionized state in an acidic urine and become ionized in an alkaline urine. The opposite is true for basic drug molecules, which remain nonionized in an alkaline urine and are ionized in an acidic urine. When a drug is administered that alters the urine pH, it may promote an increased reabsorption or excretion of another drug. For example, the administration of bicarbonate can potentially increase the urine pH. This leads to the increased excretion of acidic drugs (eg, aspirin) and the increased reabsorption of basic drugs (eg, pseudoephedrine).

Although most drugs cross the membrane of the renal tubule by simple diffusion, some drugs are also secreted into the urine through active transport pathways. These pathways, however, have a limited capacity and can accommodate only a set amount of drug molecules. Therefore, if two different drugs using the same pathway are coadministered, the transport pathway may become saturated. This causes a "traffic jam" and the excretion of one or both of the drugs is inhibited.

These interactions can be beneficial or detrimental, depending on the agents that are administered. For example, when probenecid and penicillin are given together, they compete for secretion through an organic acid pathway in the renal tubule. The probenecid blocks the secretion of the penicillin, thereby increasing the therapeutic concentration of penicillin in the bloodstream. This is a prime example of drug interactions benefiting the patient. In contrast, digoxin and verapamil also share an active transport pathway. When they are administered concomitantly, their interaction leads to an increase in digoxin levels resulting in potential cardiotoxicity (eg, arrhythmia). Table 3-4 lists some other clinically important excretion interactions.

The other common pathway of excretion, the biliary tract, allows for the elimination of drugs and their metabolites into the feces. This route of excretion is involved in interactions with drugs that undergo enterohepatic recirculation. Drugs subject to this process are excreted into the GI tract through the biliary ducts and have the potential to be reabsorbed through the intestinal wall into the bloodstream. Some of these drugs depend on enterohepatic recirculation to achieve

Table 3.4

Drugs Affecting Excretion

Renal Elimination	Mechanism	Object Drug	Results
acetazolamide	Increases urine pH	salicylates	Increased elimination
losartan	Unknown	lithium	Decreased elimination
salicylates	Unknown	acetazolamide	Decreased elimination
acetazolamide	Increases urine pH	quinidine	Decreased elimination
triamterene	Unknown	amantadine	Decreased elimination
amiodarone	Unknown	digoxin	Decreased elimination
	Unknown	procainamide	Decreased renal and hepatic elimination
antacids	Increases urine pH	dextroamphetamine, quinidine, pseudoephedrine	Decreased elimination

therapeutic concentrations. An example of a drug class that undergoes enterohepatic recirculation is the oral contraceptive. After biliary excretion into the GI tract, estrogens in oral contraceptives are hydrolyzed by intestinal bacteria and then reabsorbed into the bloodstream. If an antibiotic is given with an oral contraceptive, the antibiotic may reduce the number of intestinal bacteria available to hydrolyze the oral contraceptive, thereby preventing reabsorption and decreasing the therapeutic concentration of the oral contraceptive in the bloodstream. Drugs that undergo enterohepatic recirculation are also greatly affected by binding agents because the drug has continued re-exposure to the binding agent in the GI tract.

Pharmacokinetic interactions make up a large part of the interactions that practitioners must contend with every day. These interactions are the most studied because they have an objective measurable outcome (eg, drug concentrations, enzyme concentrations). However, a drug's pharmacodynamic profile must also be considered when it is administered with other agents.

Pharmacodynamic Interactions

The responses or effects produced by a drug's actions are referred to as the drug's *pharmacodynamic profile*. Although drugs are administered to elicit a specific response or change in dynamics, an agent usually causes several changes in the body. When one or more drugs are coadministered, the entire pharmacodynamic profile of each drug must be considered because of the potential for their effects to interact. Drugs that have a similar characteristic in their pharmacodynamic profile may produce an exaggerated response. For example, when a benzodiazepine (eg, alprazolam) is administered with a muscle relaxant (eg, cyclobenzaprine), the sedative effects of both drugs combine to produce excessive drowsiness. A less obvious pharmacodynamic interaction occurs with the coadministration of angiotensin-converting enzyme inhibitors (eg, enalapril) and potassium-sparing diuretics (eg, triamterene). These agents individually can both produce an increase in the potassium (K^+) level. Unless the prescriber is aware of the pharmacodynamic profile of both drugs, the potential for an excessive increase in the potassium level may go unnoticed and arrhythmia may ensue.

In contrast, drugs may also produce opposing pharmacodynamic effects. This type of interaction may cause the expected drug response to be diminished or even abolished. Unfortunately, these interactions are often overlooked. Instead of the lack of response being interpreted as a pharmacodynamic drug interaction, it is suspected to be due to an ineffective dose or drug. This often leads to an increase in the amount of drug administered and consequent unwanted side effects or interactions. This type of interaction is illustrated by the concomitant administration of an antihypertensive agent (eg, a diuretic) and a nonsteroidal anti-inflammatory drug (NSAID). Thiazide diuretics produce their hypotensive effects by blocking sodium reabsorption in the distal tubule of the kidney, which leads to increased sodium and water excretion. If NSAIDs are administered concomitantly, the sodium and water retention effects of the NSAIDs may reduce or nullify the hypotensive action of the diuretic.

DRUG–FOOD INTERACTIONS

The interaction between food and drugs can affect both pharmacokinetic and pharmacodynamic parameters. The mechanism of these pharmacokinetic interactions is mediated by alteration of drug bioavailability, distribution, metabolism, or excretion, as seen with drug–drug interactions. The potential for pharmacodynamic drug–food interactions warrants concern about proper diet for patients on certain drugs. Although practicing clinicians often overlook drug–food interactions, these interactions can significantly affect efficacy of drug therapy. Awareness of significant drug–food interactions can reduce the incidence of these effects and optimize drug therapy.

Effect of Food on Drug Pharmacokinetics

Absorption

Food can affect the absorption of drugs in two ways: first, by altering the extent of drug absorption, and second, by changing the rate of drug absorption. Usually, changes in the rate of drug absorption have less significance if only the rate of absorption is delayed without affecting bioavailability. The underlying mechanisms that mediate these interactions are highly variable and depend on both the content of food and the properties of the drug involved.

Food can either increase or decrease the amount (extent) of drug absorption, potentially altering the bioavailability of a drug. One mechanism, similar to drug–drug interactions, is adsorption. For example, tetracycline and fluoroquinolone antibiotics (eg, ciprofloxacin, ofloxacin) can chelate with calcium cations found in milk or milk products, thus significantly limiting the drug's bioavailability (Deppermann & Lode, 1993).

A second type of drug–food interaction occurs when food serves as a physical barrier and prevents the absorption of orally administered drugs (Kirk, 1995). The absorptive capacity of the small intestine is related to the accessibility of a drug to the GI mucosal surfaces, the site where absorption occurs. When food is coadministered with a drug, access to the mucosa is reduced, resulting in delayed or decreased drug absorption. For example, the bioavailability of azithromycin is reduced by 43% when the drug is taken with food (Zithromax Package Insert, 2003). Similar types of interactions can be seen when erythromycin, isoniazid, penicillins, and zidovudine are given orally. To avoid such interactions, these drugs can be administered 2 hours apart from mealtime. Box 3-1 identifies some commonly prescribed drugs that should be taken on an empty stomach. Note, however, if patients cannot tolerate these medications on an empty stomach (because of GI side effects like diarrhea), coadministration with food may be advisable.

In contrast, food can also increase the absorption of some drugs. For example, a high-fat meal can significantly increase the absorption of lipophilic drugs like griseofulvin (Trovato, Nuhlicek, & Midtling, 1991). In another example, the concentration of a long-acting formulation of theophylline, such as Theo-24, can increase when taken with a high-fat meal (Jonkman, 1989). Conversely, only 40% of the Theo-Dur Sprinkle formulation is absorbed when given with meals. Because considerable variation can exist in the absorption of controlled-release

BOX 3–1. DRUGS TO BE TAKEN ON AN EMPTY STOMACH

azithromycin
captopril
erythromycin
fluoroquinolones (eg, ciprofloxacin, ofloxacin)
griseofulvin
isoniazid
oral penicillins
sucralfate
tetracycline
theophylline, timed release (eg, Theo-Dur Sprinkle,
    Theo-24, Uniphyl)
zidovudine

formulations of theophylline, the drug is recommended to be taken apart from meals (Hussar, 1995).

Metabolism

Food can also affect drug metabolism. Grapefruit juice, for example, can affect the metabolism of many drugs. Grapefruit juice specifically inhibits the 3A4 subset of intestinal cytochrome P450 enzymes and thus increases the serum concentration of drugs dependent on these enzymes for metabolism (Ameer & Weintraub, 1997; Huang et al., 2003).

The cytochrome enzymes are found in highest concentrations in the proximal two thirds of the small intestine. These enzymes are located at the distal portion of the villi that line the small intestine and are responsible for the extrahepatic metabolism of more than 20 drugs (Ameer & Weintraub, 1997; Huang et al., 2003). The component in grapefruit juice that is responsible for this interaction remains undetermined; however, the flavonoid naringin, found in high concentrations in grapefruit juice, is suspected. Increases in the bioavailability of verapamil and dihydropyridine calcium channel blockers such as felodipine, nisoldipine, nitrendipine, nifedipine, and amlodipine have been documented with the coadministration of grapefruit juice (Bailey, et al., 1993; Bailey, et al., 1992; Bailey, et al., 1991; Rashid, et al., 1993). The bioavailability of felodipine could be enhanced by as much as 2.8-fold by grapefruit juice (Bailey, et al., 1991). However, unlike verapamil and dihydropyridine, diltiazem does not demonstrate an increase in bioavailability with grapefruit juice. Because grapefruit juice appears to inhibit mostly intestinal CYP3A4 and not hepatic CYP3A4 enzymes, the metabolism of drugs administered intravenously is unlikely to be altered. Further, the data suggest that only those agents given at doses higher than usual or if the patients' liver is severely damaged, result in the intestinal CYP3A4 as the primary metabolic pathway (Huang et al., 2003). Box 3-2 identifies some drugs that may interact with grapefruit juice.

In contrast to the ability of grapefruit juice to inhibit drug metabolism, other components of food may induce drug metabolism and therefore decrease drug efficacy. For example, in the treatment of Parkinson disease, dopamine in the brain needs to be replenished. However, exogenous dopamine does not cross the blood-brain barrier, but its precursor, levodopa, does. Unfortunately, much of the levodopa is lost to metabolism when given orally and only approximately 1% of the administered amount enters the brain to be converted to dopamine (Trovato, et al., 1991). Concomitant administration with food containing pyridoxine (or vitamin B_6) can potentially further enhance the peripheral metabolism of levodopa, thus decreasing drug efficacy (Trovato, et al., 1991). Patients taking levodopa should therefore be educated about moderate intake of pyridoxine-rich foods, such as avocados, beans, bacon, beef, liver, peas, pork, sweet potatoes, and tuna. Similarly, charcoal-broiled meats can induce the activity of the CYP1A2 isoenzymes, thus increasing the metabolism of drugs such as theophylline (Kirk, 1995).

Excretion

Ingestion of certain fruit juices can alter the urinary pH and affect the elimination and reabsorption of drugs such as quinidine and amphetamine (Trovato, et al., 1991). Orange, tomato, and grapefruit juices are metabolized to an alkaline residue, which can increase the urinary pH. For drugs that are weak bases, making the urine more alkaline by raising the pH increases the proportion of nonionized drug and enhances the reabsorption of the drug systemically. (Recall that the ionization of drugs helps promote water solubility and ultimately enhances drug elimination into the urine.)

Effect of Food on Pharmacodynamics

Food affects the pharmacodynamics of drugs either by opposing or potentiating a drug's pharmacologic action. For example, warfarin exerts its anticoagulant effects by inhibiting synthesis of vitamin K-dependent clotting factors. Vitamin K is required for activation by several protein factors of the clotting cascade, namely, factors II, VII, IX, and X. When foods rich in vitamin K are ingested, they can significantly oppose the anticoagulatory efficacy of warfarin. Leafy green vegetables, such as collard greens, kale,

BOX 3–2. DRUGS THAT INTERACT WITH GRAPEFRUIT JUICE

benzodiazepines
    midazolam
    triazolam
cyclosporine
dihydropyridine calcium channel blockers
    amlodipine
    felodipine
    nifedipine
    nisoldipine
    nitrendipine
theophylline
verapamil
17β-estradiol

lettuce, spinach, mustard greens, and broccoli, are generally recognized to contain large quantities of vitamin K. Health care providers should educate patients who are taking warfarin about this interaction. More importantly, however, practitioners should stress maintaining a balanced diet without abruptly changing the intake of foods rich in vitamin K.

Another significant drug–food interaction occurs between monoamine oxidase inhibitors (MAOIs) and foods containing tyramine, an amino acid that is contained in many types of food. Tyramine can precipitate a hypertensive reaction in patients taking MAOIs, such as phenelzine, tranylcypromine, or isocarboxazid. Monoamine oxidases are enzymes located in the GI tract that inactivate tyramine in food. When patients are taking MAOIs, the breakdown of tyramine is prevented and therefore allows for more tyramine to be absorbed systemically. Because of the indirect sympathomimetic property of tyramine, this amino acid provokes the release of norepinephrine from sympathetic nerve endings and epinephrine from the adrenal glands, resulting in an excessive pressor effect. Clinically, patients may complain of diaphoresis, mydriasis, occipital or temporal headache, nuchal rigidity, palpitations, and elevated blood pressure. Common foods that contain tyramine are cheese and wine. Others are listed in Box 3-3.

Effect of Drugs on Food and Nutrients

Many of the aforementioned examples indicate that food can precipitate an interaction with a drug, but in some cases, a reciprocal relationship also holds true. First, some drugs can cause a depletion of nutrients or minerals found in food through various mechanisms. For example, drugs such as cholestyramine and colestipol, which were designed to bind

bile acid in the GI tract, could also potentially bind to fat-soluble vitamins (ie, vitamins A, D, E, K) and folic acid when taken with food, resulting in the decreased absorption of these vitamins. Similarly, the chronic use of mineral oil as a laxative acts as physical barrier and reduces the absorption of fat-soluble vitamins (Kirk, 1995).

Second, drug-induced malabsorption can occur in patients with pre-existing poor nutritional status. For example, long-term use of isoniazid can cause pyridoxine (vitamin B_6) deficiency. Pyridoxine supplementation is recommended for patients who are malnourished or predisposed to neuropathy (eg, patients with diabetes or alcoholism) when treated with isoniazid. In general, the clinical significance of these interactions depends on the baseline nutritional status of the patient. Patients with poor nutrition or inadequate dietary intake (eg, elderly or alcoholic patients) are potentially at greater risk for drug-induced vitamin and mineral depletion.

Third, drugs can change nutrient excretion as well. Both thiazide and loop diuretics can enhance the excretion of potassium, possibly leading to hypokalemia. Loop diuretics can increase urinary excretion of calcium, whereas thiazide diuretics can decrease it. In addition, ascorbic acid and potassium depletion can occur with high doses of long-term aspirin therapy (Trovato, et al., 1991).

DRUG–DISEASE INTERACTIONS

When drugs are used to treat diseases, another existing disease can cause unintended effects to occur. This is known as a drug–disease interaction. Certain diseases can change drug pharmacokinetic and pharmacodynamic parameters, leading to less-than-optimal drug therapeutic outcomes, greater risk for toxicity, physiologic changes, or exacerbation of existing diseases.

Effect of Disease on Drug Pharmacokinetics

Absorption

As already discussed, the absorption of drugs depends on the presence of other drugs and food in the GI tract. However, drug absorption also depends on the physiologic processes that maintain normal GI function. These processes can include enzyme secretion, acidity, gastric emptying, bile production, and transit time. Thus, any disease that alters the normal physiologic function of the GI system potentially alters drug absorption. For example, gastric emptying rate can be reduced in patients with duodenal or pyloric ulcers or hypothyroidism (Shargel & Yu, 1993). Also, diarrhea can pose a problem for oral absorption of drugs as well as food and nutrients in general.

Distribution

The distribution of drugs can be affected by certain disease states. Of significance are conditions that change plasma albumin levels and therefore can increase or decrease the concentration of drugs usually bound to albumin. Box 3-4 lists conditions that may change plasma albumin concentration.

BOX 3–3. FOODS HIGH IN TYRAMINE

Avocados (especially if over-ripe)
Bananas
Bean pods
Canned figs
Cheese (especially aged)
Chicken livers
Chocolate
Coffee
Cola beverages
Fermented meats (salami, pepperoni, summer sausage)
Herring (pickled or dry)
Raspberries
Soy sauce
Wines (especially red)
Yeast preparations
Yogurt

From May, R. J. (1993). Adverse drug reactions and interactions. In J. T. DiPiro, R. L. Talbert, P. E. Hayes, G. R. Matzke, & L. M. Posey (Eds.), *Pharmacotherapy: A pathophysiologic approach* (2nd ed., p. 71). Norwalk, CT, Appleton & Lange.

BOX 3–4. CONDITIONS THAT MAY CHANGE PLASMA ALBUMIN CONCENTRATIONS

Conditions That Decrease Plasma Albumin Level

Acute infection
Bone fractures
Burns
Cystic fibrosis
Inflammatory disease
Liver disease
Malnutrition
Myocardial infarction
Neoplastic disease
Nephrotic syndrome
Pregnancy
Renal disease
Surgical procedures

Conditions That Increase Plasma Albumin Level

Benign tumor
Gynecologic disorders
Myalgia
Schizophrenia

From Braun, L. D. (1997). Therapeutic drug monitoring. In L. Shargel, A. H. Mutnick, P. F. Souney, L. N. Swanson, & L. H. Black (Eds.), *Comprehensive pharmacy review* (3rd ed., pp. 586–597). Baltimore, Williams & Wilkins.

Metabolism

The metabolism of drugs can often be altered by diseases that affect the functions of the liver, such as liver cirrhosis. Failure of the liver (the primary organ responsible for drug metabolism) not only impairs drug metabolism, but can cause changes in liver blood flow and a reduction in albumin synthesis. Therefore, the clinical impact of liver failure includes a strong potential for interactions with drugs. Congestive heart failure is another disease that can cause direct reduction in the ability of the liver to metabolize drugs. In patients with congestive heart failure, however, decreased metabolic capacity of the liver is also caused by a decrease in blood flow to the liver owing to changes in cardiac output.

In some cases, normal liver function is needed to activate a drug rather than to inactivate it. Certain drugs like enalapril are called *prodrugs,* meaning the drug needs to be converted by the liver to its active form (enalaprilat) to achieve maximal therapeutic effect. Therefore, use of a prodrug in patients with liver dysfunction can potentially reduce the efficacy of the drug.

Excretion

Renal function can influence serum drug concentrations because most drugs are eliminated by the kidneys either as unchanged drug or as metabolites. Chronic renal diseases that compromise the function of the kidney to clear drugs can result in drug accumulation. Glomerulonephritis, interstitial nephritis, long-term and uncontrolled diabetes, and

hypertension are primary causes of declining renal function. In clinical practice, once the patient's estimated creatinine clearance has declined to less than 50 mL/min, dose adjustments usually are required for drugs that are primarily renally cleared. For example, drugs such as histamine (H_2) receptor antagonists and fluoroquinolone antibiotics commonly require dose adjustments for patients with renal insufficiency. In particular, the drug regimen of elderly patients or those with an elevated serum creatinine level above 1.5 mg/dL should be evaluated to detect any ADRs from possible drug accumulation secondary to declining renal clearance.

Effect of Disease on Pharmacodynamics

Drugs used to treat one medical condition can sometimes exacerbate the status of another comorbid disease. Practitioners, therefore, should be aware of potential drug–disease interactions that can affect pharmacodynamic parameters. A complete discussion of this topic is beyond the scope of this chapter; however, the use of β-adrenergic blockers in patients with diabetes mellitus is a good example to illustrate many important concepts. The β blockers in general are not considered the preferred antihypertensive agent for patients with diabetes mellitus, for several reasons. In patients with type 1 diabetes mellitus, β blockers can mask the symptoms of hypoglycemia, such as tachycardia, palpitation, tremor, and hunger, by opposing the compensatory effects of epinephrine. The β-blocking drugs can also prolong the hypoglycemic episode by preventing normal gluconeogenesis in the liver to occur in response to low blood glucose levels. By other mechanisms, β blockers can impair glucose tolerance and worsen diabetic control.

Although use of a β blocker as an antihypertensive agent is not absolutely contraindicated in patients with diabetes mellitus, it is best avoided because more appropriate, alternative agents are available.

PATIENT FACTORS INFLUENCING DRUG INTERACTIONS

The outcomes of drug interactions are highly variable from one person to another. Many patient factors can influence the propensity for an interaction to occur, such as genetics, diseases, environment, smoking, diet/nutrition, and alcohol (Hansten, 1998). An understanding of these factors can help to identify potential sources of drug interactions.

Heredity

The cytochrome P450 system can display genetic polymorphism (Ingelman-Sundberg, 2004; Hansten, 1998). That is, the variable metabolism of drugs by cytochrome P450 enzymes from one person to another in the population can be partly explained by genetic differences. Approximately 8% of Americans lack the gene to form the isoenzyme CYP2D6 and therefore are at greater risk for toxicity from psychotropic drugs and, potentially, other drugs that are metabolized by these isoenzymes (Hansten, 1998). The metabolism of isoniazid also demonstrates variation among different people; some acetylate isoniazid very rapidly, whereas others acetylate it slowly (Hussar, 1995).

Disease

Another important factor that influences drug interactions is the patient's existing disease state. Any disease affecting liver or kidney function can potentially predispose the patient to drug interactions and ADRs because these organs are primary sites of drug metabolism and elimination, respectively. Significant deterioration in drug metabolism or elimination can lead to increased serum drug concentrations and therefore increase the likelihood for drugs to interact. Consequently, elderly patients and those with a history of liver disease or renal insufficiency should be evaluated for dose adjustments of drugs significantly cleared by the liver and kidneys.

Environment

Environmental factors, such as DDT and other pesticides, can increase the activity of liver enzymes, potentially causing an increase in drug metabolism (Hussar, 1995). Although the general significance of the effect of environmental exposure on the clinical outcome of drug therapy has not been well studied, people working in occupations with prolonged exposure to toxins and chemicals should be more closely observed.

Smoking

Studies show that smoking can increase the liver's metabolism of certain drugs, including diazepam, propoxyphene, chlorpromazine, and amitriptyline (Hussar, 1995). For example, the polycyclic aromatic hydrocarbons in cigarettes can induce CYP1A2 metabolism, resulting in decreased theophylline serum concentrations (Schein, 1995).

Diet and Nutrition

The nutritional status and dietary intake of the patient can influence the importance of a drug–nutrient interaction. Drugs can deplete valuable vitamins and minerals from food; however, these interactions are often difficult to recognize and may go undetected. Patients with poor baseline nutrition (eg, alcoholics) may experience more pronounced effects mainly because of underlying nutritional deficiency. Practitioners should be aware of potential drug–nutrient interactions by identifying patients who have poor dietary intake and who concurrently take medications that can deplete vitamins and minerals.

Alcohol Intake

Alcohol can complicate drug therapy on many different levels. Alcohol has a variable effect on drug metabolism depending on acute or chronic intake. Acute alcohol ingestion can inhibit drug metabolism, thus increasing serum drug concentrations; it also can enhance the pharmacodynamic effect of drugs with properties of central nervous system depression. Patients concurrently taking narcotics, antihistamines, antidepressants, antipsychotics, and muscle relaxants with alcohol are at greatest risk for central nervous system depression and should be warned of this interaction (Trovato, et al., 1991).

In contrast, chronic alcohol intake tends to increase the synthesis of drug-metabolizing enzymes, leading to induction (Hansten, 1998). Enzyme induction causes decreases in serum drug levels. However, long-term abuse of alcohol leading to liver cirrhosis ultimately impairs drug metabolism by destruction of functional hepatocytes.

ADVERSE DRUG REACTIONS

An ADR can be defined as an undesirable clinical manifestation that is consequent to and caused by the administration of a particular drug. ADRs are basically drug-induced toxic reactions. The World Health Organization (WHO) defines an ADR as "a response to a medicine which is noxious and unintended, and which occurs at doses normally used in man."

There are two general types to consider.

The first type of ADR is an exaggeration of the principal pharmacologic action of the drug. The ADR is simply a more pronounced drug response than normal. These reactions usually are dose dependent and predictable. These are often referred to as type A reactions.

In the second type, type B reactions, the ADR is unrelated to the principal pharmacologic action of the drug itself (May, 1993; Plaa & Smith, 1995). These reactions are precipitated by the secondary pharmacologic actions of the drug, may be unpredictable, and may or may not be dose dependent. In either type, the ADR can result from overdosage of drug or administration of therapeutic doses to a patient hyperreactive to the drug, or as an indirect consequence of the primary action.

The term *ADR* implies a more severe reaction than a side effect. A side effect is also recognized as an undesirable pharmacologic effect that accompanies the primary drug action, but the effect is relatively mild compared with an ADR. A side effect usually occurs within the therapeutic dosing range (Plaa & Smith, 1995). Side effects, for example, are the dry mouth and blurred vision that occur from drugs with anticholinergic properties. In contrast, drug-induced liver damage (eg, increased hepatic enzymes on liver function test results) would not be considered as an undesirable side effect, but an ADR. Patients experiencing side effects from drugs do not necessarily require discontinuation of therapy; however, proper drug selection emphasizing agents with minimal side effect profiles may help improve patient acceptance of and compliance with the drug.

Tracking Drug Interactions and Adverse Drug Reactions

The initial source of documented ADRs comes primarily from the experience gained while using a drug during clinical trials. Usually, the number of people taking the drug in clinical trials, on the order of hundreds to several thousands, is too few to detect all the possible adverse reactions from the drug. However, after a drug is approved by the U.S. Food and Drug Administration (FDA), it becomes readily available for public use in hundreds of thousands to millions of people. The potential for drug interactions and ADRs then becomes much greater than during clinical trials. Therefore, practitioners should have a basic understanding of drug interactions and ADRs and report these events to the FDA when they occur.

MedWatch is a medical products reporting program conducted by the FDA (Fig. 3-3). The purpose of the MedWatch

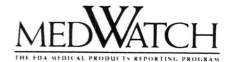

For **VOLUNTARY** reporting by health professionals of adverse events and product problems

THE FDA MEDICAL PRODUCTS REPORTING PROGRAM

Page _____ of _____

Form Approved OMB No. 0910-0291 Expires:12/31/94
Sen OMB statement on reverse

FDA Use Only **[DAVIS]**

Triage unit
sequence #

PLEASE TYPE OR USE BLACK INK

A. Patient information

1. **Patient identifier**

In confidence

2. **Age at time of event:**
or _____
Date of birth:

3. **Sex**
☐ female
☐ male

4. **Weight**
_____ lbs
or
_____ kgs

B. Adverse event or product problem

1. ☐ **Adverse event**   and/or   ☐ **Product problem** (e.g., defects/malfunctions)

2. **Outcomes attributed to adverse event**
(check all that apply)

☐ death _____ (mo day yr)
☐ life-threatening
☐ hospitalization − initial or prolonged

☐ disability
☐ congenital anomaly
☐ required intervention to prevent permanent impairment/damage
☐ other: _____

3. **Date of event** (mo day yr)

4. **Date of this report** (mo day yr)

5. **Describe event or problem**

6. **Relevant tests/laboratory data,** including dates

7. **Other relevant history, including preexisting medical conditions** (e.g., allergies, race, pregnancy, smoking and alcohol use, hepatic/renal dysfunction, etc.)

C. Suspect medication(s)

1. **Name** (give labeled strength & mfr/labeler, if known)
#1
#2

2. **Dose, frequency & route used**
#1
#2

3. **Therapy dates** (if unknown, give duration) from/to (or best estimate)
#1
#2

4. **Diagnosis for use** (indication)
#1
#2

5. **Event abated after use stopped or dose reduced**
#1 ☐ yes ☐ no ☐ doesn't apply
#2 ☐ yes ☐ no ☐ doesn't apply

6. **Lot #** (if known)
#1
#2

7. **Exp. date** (if known)
#1
#2

8. **Event reappeared after reintroduction**
#1 ☐ yes ☐ no ☐ doesn't apply
#2 ☐ yes ☐ no ☐ doesn't apply

9. **NDC #** (for product problems only)

10. **Concomitant medical products** and therapy dates (exclude treatment of event)

D. Suspect medical device

1. **Brand name**

2. **Type of device**

3. **Manufacturer name & address**

4. **Operator of device**
☐ health professional
☐ lay user/patient
☐ other: _____

5. **Expiration date** (mo day yr)

6.
model # _____
catalog # _____
serial # _____
lot # _____
other #

7. **If implanted, give date** (mo day yr)

8. **If explanted, give date** (mo day yr)

9. **Device available for evaluation?**   (Do not send to FDA)
☐ yes   ☐ no   ☐ returned to manufacturer on _____ (mo day yr)

10. **Concomitant medical products** and therapy dates (exclude treatment of event)

E. Reporter (see confidentiality section on back)

1. **Name, address & phone #**

2. **Health professional?**
☐ yes ☐ no

3. **Occupation**

4. **Also reported to**
☐ manufacturer
☐ user facility
☐ distributor

5. **If you do NOT want your identity disclosed to the manufacturer, place an " X " in this box.** ☐

Mail to: MEDWATCH
5600 Fishers Lane
Rockville, MD 20852-9787

or **FAX to:**
1-800-FDA-0178

FDA Form 3500 (6/93)   Submission of a report does not constitute an admission that medical personnel or the product caused or contributed to the event.

Figure 3–3   MedWatch form for reporting an adverse event or product problem to the U.S. Food and Drug Administration.

program is to enhance the effectiveness of surveillance of drugs and medical products after they are marketed and as they are used in clinical practice. The benefit to health care providers for reporting drug interactions and ADRs is to ensure that drug safety information is rapidly communicated to health care professionals, thus improving patient care. Health care providers should also be aware of programs in their own institutions that collect and report ADRs or drug interactions.

Bibliography

Starred references are cited in the text.

*Ameer, B., & Weintraub, R. A. (1997). Drug interactions with grapefruit juice. *Clinical Pharmacokinetics, 33*(2), 103–121.

*Bailey, D. C., Arnold, J. M. O., Strong, H. A., et al. (1993). Effect of grapefruit juice and naringin on nisoldipine pharmacokinetics. *Clinical Pharmacology and Therapeutics, 54*, 589–594.

*Bailey, D. G., Munoz, C., Arnold, J. M. O., et al. (1992). Grapefruit juice and naringin interaction with nitrendipine [Abstract]. *Clinical Pharmacology and Therapeutics, 51*, 156.

*Bailey, D. G., Spence, J. D., Munoz, C., et al. (1991). Interaction of citrus juices with felodipine and nifedipine. *Lancet, 337*, 268–269.

*Bates, D., Spell, N., Cullen, D., et al. (1997). The costs of adverse drug events in hospitalized patients. *Journal of the American Medical Association, 277*, 307–311.

*Brosen, K. (1990). Recent developments in hepatic drug oxidation: Implications for clinical pharmacokinetics. *Clinical Pharmacokinetics, 18*, 220–239.

*Classen, D. C., Pestonik, S. L., Evans, R. S., et al. (1997). Adverse drug events in hospitalized patients: Excess length of stay, extra costs, and attributable mortality. *Journal of the American Medical Association, 277*, 301–306.

*Cupp, M., & Tracy, T. (1997). Role of the cytochrome P450 3A subfamily in drug interactions. *US Pharmacist, 22*, HS9–HS21.

*Deppermann, K. M., & Lode, H. (1993). Fluoroquinolones: Interaction profile during enteral absorption. *Drugs, 45*(Suppl. 3), 65–72.

*Drew, R. H., & Gallis, H. A. (1992). Azithromycin—spectrum of activity, pharmacokinetics, and clinical applications. *Pharmacotherapy, 12*, 161–173.

*Fraser, A. G. (1997). Pharmacokinetic interactions between alcohol and other drugs. *Clinical Pharmacokinetics, 33*(2), 79–90.

*Guengerich, F. (1994). Catalytic selectivity of human cytochrome P450 enzymes: Relevance to drug metabolism and toxicity. *Toxicology Letters, 70*, 133–138.

*Hansten, P. D. (1998). Understanding drug–drug interactions. *Science and Medicine*, (Jan/Feb) 16–20.

*Hansten, P. D., & Horn, J. R. (1997). *Drug interactions: Analysis and management*. Vancouver, WA: Applied Therapeutics.

*Harder, S., & Thurmann, P. (1996). Clinically important drug interactions with anticoagulants: An update. *Clinical Pharmacokinetics, 30*, 416–444.

*Huang, S. M., Hall, S. D., Watkins P., et al. (2004). Drug interactions with herbal products and grapefruit juice: A conference report. *Clinical Pharmacology & Therapeutics, 75*, 1–12.

*Hussar, D. A. (1995). Drug interactions. *American Journal of Pharmacy, 167*, 1–39.

*Impicciatore P., Choonara I., Clarkson A., et al. (2001). Incidence of adverse drug reactions in paediatric in/out-patients: a systematic review and meta-analysis of prospective studies. *British Journal of Clinical Pharmacology, 52*, 77–83.

*Ingelman-Sundberg, M. (2004). Pharmacogenetics of cytochromes P450 and its applications in drug therapy; the past, present and future. *Trends in Pharmacological Sciences, 25*(4), 193–200.

Johnson, K. A., Strum, D. P., & Watkins, W. D. (1995). Pharmacology and the critical care patient. In P. L. Munson, R. A. Mueller, & G. R. Breese (Eds.), *Principles of pharmacology: Basic concepts and clinical application* (pp. 1673–1688). New York: Chapman & Hall.

*Jonkman, J. H. (1989). Food interactions with sustained-release theophylline preparations: A review. *Clinical Pharmacokinetics, 16*, 162–179.

Kirk, J. K. (1995). Significant drug-nutrient interactions. *American Family Physicians, 51*(5), 1175–1182.

*Kivisto, K., Neuvonen, P., & Koltz, U. (1994). Inhibition of terfenadine metabolism: Pharmacokinetic and pharmacodynamic consequences. *Clinical Pharmacokinetics, 27*, 1–5.

*Lazarou, J., Pomeranz, B., & Corey, P. (1998). Incidence of adverse drug reactions in hospitalized patients: A meta-analysis of prospective studies. *Journal of the American Medical Association, 279*, 1200–1205.

*Mathews, D., McNutt, B., Okerholam, R., et al. (1991). Torsades de pointes occurring in association with terfenadine use. *Journal of the American Medical Association, 266*, 2375–2376.

*May, R. J. (1993). Adverse drug reactions and interactions. In J. T. DiPiro, R. L. Talbert, P. E. Hayes, et al. (Eds.), *Pharmacotherapy: A pathophysiologic approach* (2nd ed., pp. 71–83). East Norwalk, CT: Appleton & Lange.

*Michalets, E. (1998). Update: Clinically significant cytochrome P-450 drug interactions. *Annals of Pharmacotherapy, 18*, 84–112.

*National Center for Health Statistics. (1996). *Vital and health statistics*. Series 13, No. 134 (FASTATS A to Z). [On-line; information updated 5/18/1999; retrieved 10/7/1999]. Available: http://www.cdc.gov/nchswww/gastats/hospital.htm

Nebert, D., Adesnich, M., Coon, M., et al. (1987). The P450 gene superfamily: Recommended nomenclature. *DNA, 6*, 1–11.

*Plaa, G. L., & Smith, R. P. (1995). General principles of toxicology. In P. L. Munson, R. A. Mueller, & G. R. Breese (Eds.), *Principles of pharmacology: Basic concepts and clinical application* (pp. 1537–1543). New York: Chapman & Hall.

*Rashid, J., McKinstry, C., Renwick, A. G., et al. (1993). Quercetin, an in vitro inhibitor of CYP3A, does not contribute to the interaction between nifedipine and grapefruit juice. *British Journal of Clinical Pharmacology, 36*, 460–463.

*Rolan, P. (1994). Plasma protein binding displacement interactions: Why are they still regarded as clinically important? *British Journal of Clinical Pharmacology, 37*, 125–128.

*Schein, J. R. (1995). Cigarette smoking and clinically significant drug interactions. *Annals of Pharmacotherapy, 29*, 1139–1147.

*Shargel, L., & Yu, A. B. C. (1993). *Applied biopharmaceutics and pharmacokinetics* (3rd ed.). East Norwalk, CT: Appleton & Lange.

*Shinn, A. F. (1992). Clinical relevance of cimetidine drug interactions. *Drug Safety, 7*, 245–267.

*Spinler, S., Cheng, J., Kindwall, K., & Charland, S. (1995). Possible inhibition of hepatic metabolism of quinidine by erythromycin. *Clinical Pharmacology and Therapeutics, 57*, 89–94.

*Trovato, A., Nuhlicek, D. N., & Midtling, J. E. (1991). Drug–nutrient interactions. *American Family Practitioner, 44*, 1651–1658.

*Woosley, R. (1996). Cardiac actions of antihistamines. *Annual Review of Pharmacology and Toxicology, 36*, 233–252.

PRINCIPLES OF PHARMACOTHERAPY IN PEDIATRICS

■ PETER ANLEY AND ANITA SIU

When treating pediatric patients, many health care practitioners use the terms *infant, child,* or even *kid* interchangeably. However, there are currently accepted terms that define the different age categories of pediatric patients (Table 4-1). These terms should be used for accuracy when describing young patients and especially when determining drug dosages. Safe and effective drug therapy in pediatric patients is based on a firm understanding of three concepts:

- Ongoing maturation and development in pediatric patients and their effect on a drug's absorption, distribution, metabolism, and excretion. Interpatient variabilities may be attributed to physiologic changes throughout childhood.
- Short- and long-term effects that the prescribed drug will have on a pediatric patient's growth and development
- Effects of underlying congenital, chronic, or current diseases on the prescribed drug, and vice versa

The popular concept that the pediatric patient is merely a "little or small adult," and therefore pediatric pharmacokinetics, drug dosing, and even adverse effects can be extrapolated from the results of adult clinical drug trials is a serious misconception. Although many drugs do exhibit similarities between the adult and pediatric populations, the assumption of resemblance should not be applied to all drugs. Several tragic drug misadventures in the 1960s and 1970s illustrate this. Extrapolated data from adult responses to chloramphenicol (Chloromycetin) led to its use in neonates in the 1960s. When given chloramphenicol, these neonates developed gray baby syndrome, hypotension, and hypoxemia, leading eventually to shock and death (Haile, 1977). This occurred because neonates, unlike adults, lack the enzyme needed to metabolize chloramphenicol. Another tragedy in the 1970s involved the topical antimicrobial cleanser hexachlorophene. Used routinely and safely in adults, hexachlorophene caused vacuolar encephalopathy of the brain stem in premature neonates after they were repeatedly bathed in a 3% solution (Anonymous, 1972).

The well-grounded fears that unforeseen adverse events may affect the growth or development of or may produce fatal outcomes in pediatric study subjects, combined with the difficulties associated with obtaining informed consent or blood samples, serve as major barriers to pharmaceutical manufacturers in conducting pediatric clinical trials. In turn, the lack of clinical trials in pediatric patients prevents the U.S. Food and Drug Administration (FDA) from approving drugs for use in the pediatric population. As such, the prescribing information commonly states "Pediatric Use: Safety and effectiveness in pediatric patients has not been established."

Without FDA approval or adequate documented information, many practitioners are uncertain how to use drugs in pediatrics. This leaves prescribers little choice but to use drugs in pediatric patients in an off-label capacity, based on adult data, uncontrolled pediatric studies, or personal experience.

In 1997, the FDA took the initiative to increase the quantity and quality of clinical drug trials in the pediatric population by proposing alternate ways to obtain FDA approval. The FDA would waive the need for well-controlled clinical drug trials if drug manufacturers provided other satisfactory data for drugs already approved for the same use in adults. These data could include the results of controlled or uncontrolled pediatric studies, pharmacodynamic studies, safety reports, and premarketing or postmarketing studies. Alternatively, the drug manufacturer could provide evidence demonstrating that the disease course and drug effects are sufficiently similar in adult and pediatric patients in order to support extrapolation of data from adult clinical trials. In addition, pediatric pharmacokinetic studies are necessary to provide data for an appropriate pediatric dosage recommendation, especially age-dependent dosing. An FDA regulation issued in December 1998 required manufacturers to provide additional information about the use of their drug products in pediatric patients. The nature of the studies required to support pediatric labeling will depend on the type of application, the condition being treated, and existing data about the product's safety and efficacy in pediatric patients. Manufacturers will be required to study the drug in all relevant pediatric age groups (U.S. FDA, 1998a).

PEDIATRIC PHARMACOKINETICS

Pediatric patients differ from adults, anatomically and physiologically. For safe use of drugs in pediatrics, prescribers and other caregivers need to recognize the potential for very different pharmacokinetics in pediatric patients as opposed

Table 4.1

Age Groups of Pediatric Population

Group	Age
Preterm or premature	Less than 36 wk gestational age
Neonate	Less than 30 d of age
Infant	1 mo until 1 y of age
Child	1 y until 12 y of age
Adolescent	12 y until 18 y of age

to adults. The differences are based on developing body tissues and organs, which affect a drug's absorption, distribution, metabolism, and excretion.

Changes in a pediatric patient's body proportions and composition and the relative size of the liver and kidneys can alter the pharmacokinetics of a drug. During the first several years of life, a child undergoes rapid changes in growth and development, most rapid during infancy. Growth is a quantitative change in the size of the body or any of its parts, and development is a qualitative change in skills or functions. Maturation, a genetically controlled development independent of the environment, is a slower process, lasting until late childhood. Table 4-2 summarizes pharmacokinetic differences in pediatric patients.

By the end of the first year of life, an infant's weight triples, whereas body surface area (BSA) and length double. Accompanying these changes in growth and development are changes in body composition, intracellular and extracellular body water, fat, and protein. Approximately 75% to 80% of a full-term neonate's body weight is total body water (Friis-Hansen, 1957). By 3 months of age, total body water constitutes approximately 65% of the patient's body weight. Extracellular water progressively declines and intracellular water increases faster than total body water, exceeding extracellular water (Friis-Hansen, 1957). The decreasing percentage of body weight from total body water is replaced by an increase in body fat during the first 5 months of life. In fact, the percentage of body weight from fat doubles in these 5 months.

The protein percentage increases during the second year of life as fat is lost, primarily because of ambulation. The liver and kidney reach their maximum size relative to body weight by 2 years of age, producing a "peak" in the child's metabolism and elimination. After 2 years of age, the child's liver and kidney size/body weight ratios steadily decrease until adult liver and kidney ratios are reached by adolescence.

Oral Absorption

The extent of a drug's absorption in a pediatric patient depends on a variety of factors: gastric pH, gastric and intestinal transit time, gastrointestinal surface area, enzymes, and microorganism flora, or any combination thereof.

Gastric pH

Basal and stimulated secretion of gastric acid controls the pH of the stomach. The stomach pH is alkaline at birth (>4) because of residual amniotic fluid and the immaturity of parietal cells. As gastric acid is produced, the pH falls. By the end of the first day of life, the basal and stimulated rates are equal, although lower than the rates in adults. An increased stomach pH (alkaline) adversely affects the absorption of weakly acidic drugs and improves the absorption of weakly basic drugs. This phenomenon results from increased ionization of the weakly acidic drug, producing more ionized (polar) drug, which moves poorly across the nonpolar gastric membrane—and vice versa for weakly basic drug. For example, the bioavailability of phenobarbital (a weak acid) is decreased in neonates, infants, and young children because their alkaline gastric pH produces more ionized phenobarbital, which crosses the gastric membrane poorly.

For weakly basic drugs, the alkaline stomach pH increases the non-ionized form of the drug, which then easily moves across the gastric membrane. By the second year of life, the child's gastric acid output on a per-kilogram body weight basis is similar to that observed in the adult (Deren, 1971). As a result, gastric pH affects the degree of drug ionization, thus changing the amount of drug absorbed.

Table 4.2

Age-Related Pharmacokinetic Differences in Children Compared With Adults

	Premature Neonate	Neonate	Infant	Child	Adolescent
Absorption					
Gastric acidity	↓	↓	↓	=	=
Gastric emptying time	↓	↓	=	=	=
GI motility	↓	↓	↓	=	=
Pancreatic enzyme activity	↓↓	↓	↓	=	=
GI surface area	↑	↑	↑	↑	=
Skin permeability	↑↑	↑	=	=	=
Distribution					
Body composition					=
Blood-brain barrier	↓	↓	=	=	=
Plasma proteins	↓↓	↓	=	=	=
Metabolism					
Liver	↓	↓	↓	=/↑	=
Elimination					
Renal blood flow	↓	↓	↓	=	=
Glomerular filtration	↓	↓	↓	=	=
Tubular function	↓	↓	↓	=	=

Gastric Emptying Time and Surface Area

The gastric emptying time is delayed in both preterm and full-term neonates during the first 24 hours of life. No studies have been conducted beyond the immediate neonatal period. The combination of delayed gastric emptying time and gastroesophageal reflux can result in the regurgitation of orally administered drugs, producing irregular drug absorption. In general, gastric emptying is more prolonged in neonates and infants than in children.

The characteristics of a drug's movement through the intestines can drastically affect the rate and extent of drug absorption because most drugs are absorbed in the duodenum. Both neonates and infants have irregular peristalsis, which can lead to enhanced absorption. In addition, the type of feeding an infant receives can affect intestinal transit time. For instance, the intestinal transit time in breast-fed infants is greater than in formula-fed infants (Cavell, 1981).

The relative size of the absorptive surface area in the duodenum can significantly influence the rate and extent of drug absorption. In the young, the greater relative size of the duodenum compared with adults enhances drug absorption.

Gastrointestinal Enzymes and Microorganisms

The absorption of drugs that are fat soluble or carried in fat vehicles depends on lipase. Premature neonates have low lipase concentrations and no alpha-amylase. The reduced activity of bile acids, lipase, alpha-amylase, and protease continues until approximately 4 months of age. Vitamin E absorption is decreased in neonates because of the diminished bile acid pool and biliary function; therefore, supplementation of this vitamin may be necessary.

The development of the intestinal microorganism flora depends more on diet than on age (Yaffe & Juchau, 1974), which may account for the more rapid development of flora in breast-fed infants than in formula-fed infants. The reduction of digoxin (Lanoxin) to inactive metabolites by anaerobic intestinal bacteria can be used as a marker for the development or changes in intestinal flora (Lindenbaum, Rund, Butler, et al., 1981). Digoxin metabolites are not detected in children until 16 months, and an adult-like reduction of digoxin does not occur until 9 years of age (Linday, Dobkin, Wang, et al., 1987).

Rectal Absorption

The rectal route of administration is seldom used; it usually is reserved for patients who cannot tolerate oral drugs or who lack intravenous access. In rectal administration, the drug is absorbed by the hemorrhoidal veins, which are not part of the portal circulation, therefore avoiding first-pass hepatic elimination. Unfortunately, most drugs administered by this route are erratically and incompletely absorbed. Feces in the rectum, frequent bowel movements in neonates and infants, and lack of anal sphincter muscle contribute to the poor absorption profile of drugs administered rectally.

Although rectal administration may not be appropriate for routine dosing of drugs, the rectal administration of diazepam (Valium), valproic acid (Depakote), or secobarbital (Seconal) has been used to control seizures when intravenous access could not be quickly established in infants or children with status epilepticus (Graves & Kriel, 1987).

Intramuscular and Subcutaneous Absorption

Both the characteristics of the patient and the properties of the drug influence the absorption of intramuscularly or subcutaneously administered drugs. Patient characteristics include blood flow to the muscle, muscle mass, tone, and activity. Important properties of the drug are its solubility, the pH of extracellular fluid, its ease in crossing capillary membranes, and the amount of drug administered at the injection site.

In pediatric patients, all the patient characteristics are highly variable. Neonates have decreased muscle mass, and their limited muscle activity decreases blood flow to and from the muscle. Collectively, these factors produce erratic and poor intramuscular drug absorption. On the contrary, infants possess a greater density of skeletal muscle capillaries than older children, allowing for more efficient drug absorption (Carry, Ringel, & Starcevich, 1986). Some drugs, such as erythromycin, can cause pain at the injection site and should not be administered intramuscularly. However, many drugs, such as the penicillins, reach concentrations in the serum with intramuscular administration that are comparable with those achieved after intravenous administration, with minimal adverse effects.

Percutaneous Absorption

Adverse effects resulting from the inadvertent systemic absorption of percutaneously administered hexachlorophene emulsion, salicylic acid ointment, and hydrocortisone creams in neonates have limited the use of this route of drug administration. The absorption of compounds is inversely related to the thickness of the stratum corneum and directly related to hydration of the skin (Morselli, Franco-Moselli, & Bossi, 1980). Relative to body mass, the BSA is greatest in the infant and young child compared with older children and adults. The decreased thickness of the skin with increased skin surface hydration relative to body weight produces much greater percutaneous drug absorption in neonates than in adults. The percutaneous administration of drugs in neonates does pose some risks of toxic effects. Neonatal skin is structurally immature, resulting in less subcutaneous fat and a thinner stratum corneum and epidermis (Rutter, 1987). Since a greater skin surface area/body weight ratio is observed during the neonatal period, percutaneous drug absorption is also superior. Both the advantages and subsequent disadvantages of enhanced percutaneous absorption disappear after infancy, however.

Pulmonary Absorption

Aerosolized drug delivery to the lungs continues to be a favorite technique in many respiratory disorders, such as asthma. Factors affecting drug deposition in the lungs include particle size, lipid solubility, protein binding, drug metabolism in the lungs, and mucociliary transport (American Academy of Pediatrics, 1997). Aerosol particle size and lipid solubility are factors in determining whether the drug is deposited in the upper or lower airways; smaller particle size and lipid-soluble drugs are more likely to be absorbed and deposited in the lower airways (Bond, 1993).

Besides drug considerations, pediatric characteristics also affect aerosol drug delivery. Infants and children have lower tidal volumes and increased respiratory rates (especially while crying), reducing drug delivery and absorption in the lungs (Dolovich, 1999). Studies have shown that less than 2% of aerosolized drugs are deposited in young infants and toddlers (Fok, Monkman, Dolovich, et al., 1996; Salmon, Wilson, & Silverman, 1990). Therefore, adult dosing may be necessary to counteract these effects.

Distribution

Six factors affect drug distribution in the pediatric population: vascular perfusion, body composition, tissue binding characteristics, physicochemical properties of the drug, plasma protein binding, and route of administration (Stewart & Hampton, 1987). During the neonatal period, most of these factors are significantly different from those in the adult population, while children and adolescents are very similar to or the same as adults.

Vascular Perfusion

Changes in vascular perfusion are common in neonates. For example, in neonatal respiratory distress syndrome and post-asphyxia, a right-to-left vascular shunt may occur and divert blood from the lungs to the tissues and organs.

Body Composition

Neonates have increased total body water (75% to 80%) with decreased fat compared with adults, resulting in a higher water-to-lipid ratio. After the neonatal period, fat increases and total body water decreases steadily until puberty, especially in girls. For instance, neonates and infants have increased total body and extracellular water, creating a larger volume of distribution and affecting the pharmacokinetics of some drugs, such as aminoglycoside. The larger volume, in turn, requires administering a larger milligram-per-kilogram dose of aminoglycoside to neonates and infants than to adults.

Tissue Binding Characteristics

The mass of tissue available for binding can affect drug distribution. Drugs extensively bound to tissues exhibit increased "free" blood levels when the mass of tissue is reduced by disease or degeneration or immaturity, as in pediatrics.

Physicochemical Properties

The physicochemical properties of a drug include lipid solubility (ionized vs. non-ionized) and molecular configuration. These properties affect the ability of a drug to move across membranes into target cells or tissues. Drugs that display favorable properties for absorption may pose a greater risk for toxicity in neonates, who have enhanced percutaneous drug absorption.

Plasma Protein Binding

Preterm neonates have lower circulating amounts of alpha$_1$-acid glycoprotein, which binds alkaline drugs, than full-term neonates, who have lower alpha$_1$-acid glycoprotein levels than adults. Neonates also have a reduced amount of circulating albumin compared with adults. Albumin is responsible for binding acidic drugs, fatty acids, and bilirubin. While the affinity of drugs for either of these plasma proteins is harder to determine, theoretically a neonate's affinity for protein binding is reduced, resulting in the likelihood of displacing drugs or bilirubin bound to albumin and leading to increased serum concentrations. All these factors produce a larger volume of distribution and increased free drug concentrations (eg, phenytoin [Dilantin]) in neonates than in adults.

Route of Administration

The route by which a drug is administered has a primary influence on the drug's distribution. If the drug is administered orally, the liver becomes the primary distribution site. However, if a drug is administered intravenously, the heart and lungs act as the primary distribution sites. This is important because when a drug passes through the liver before reaching its site of activity, it is subject to the first-pass effect of extensive hepatic metabolism, which typically reduces the amount of circulating active drug and thus limits its effects. Therefore, to achieve an equal effect, the dosage of a drug administered by the oral route usually needs to be higher than the dosage of a drug administered intravenously.

Metabolism

Clearance of many drugs is mainly reliant on hepatic metabolism. The two phases of drug metabolism in the liver are the oxidation, reduction, and hydrolysis reactions (phase I) and conjugation reactions (phase II). Age-related changes in metabolism affect how drugs are broken down or transformed in pediatric patients and how certain metabolic enzymes are activated (Table 4-3 summarizes developmental patterns in phase I oxidation reactions). Phase I and II reactions are delayed in neonates, infants, and young children, with consequential drug toxicities.

P450 cytochrome (CYP) is the most important component of phase I drug metabolism. Cytochromes in the CYP1, CYP2, and CYP3 families have been identified as important in human drug metabolism. Additional information suggests there is substantial genetic variability in the quantity and quality of P450 cytochromes in the human body (Kearns, 1995).

The metabolism of caffeine and theophylline, the prototypic substrate for CYP1A2, is reduced at birth; the drug concentration increases linearly over the first year of life and exceeds adult levels in older infants and children. To maintain therapeutic serum theophylline concentrations, smaller doses are prescribed and administered less frequently in neonates than in older infants and children.

In pediatrics, phase II reactions are less well studied than phase I reactions. In adults, acetaminophen (Tylenol) (a substrate for glucuronosyltransferase 1A6 and 1A9) is metabolized by a phase II glucuronidation reaction. In neonates and infants, however, this metabolic pathway is deficient. As a result, acetaminophen metabolism is shifted to sulfate conjugation, which results in a half-life for acetaminophen that is similar to its half-life in adults.

Table 4.3

Summary of Age-Related Changes in Metabolism

P450 Cytochromes	Reduced Activity Versus Adults	Increased Activity Versus Adults	Age at Which Adult Activity Is Reached
CYP 1A2	Until 4 mo of age	1–2 y of age	End of puberty
CYP 2C19	First week of life	3–4 y of age	End of puberty
CYP 2C9			
CYP 2D6	Until 3–5 y of age		3–5 y of age
CYP 3A4	First month of life	1–4 y of age	End of puberty
CYP 2E1	Unknown	Unknown	Unknown

(Based on data from Leader, J. S., & Kearns, G. L. [1997]. Pharmacogenetics in pediatrics: Implications for practice. *Pediatric Clinics of North America, 44*, 55–77.)

Elimination

Almost all drugs and their metabolites are excreted through the kidneys. The kidney eliminates drugs by glomerular filtration (passive diffusion) or tubular secretion (energy-dependent channels or pumps). The glomerular filtration rate (GFR) increases quickly during the first 2 weeks of postnatal life and does not approach adult rates until 2 years of age (Rubin, Bruck, & Rapoport, 1949); tubular secretion and reabsorption rates do not reach adult values until 5 to 7 months of age. The proximal tubules are characterized by an inability to concentrate urine or reabsorb various filtered compounds and a reduced ability to secrete organic acids. This immaturity of the renal system in neonates and infants results from restricted blood flow and a resultant decrease in cardiac output to the kidneys, combined with incomplete glomerular and tubular development. As a result, plasma clearance of many drugs via the kidneys is altered. For example, during infancy the response to thiazide diuretics, which require a GFR greater than 30 mL/minute to be effective, is diminished. Often, a larger dosage of a thiazide diuretic or substitution by a loop diuretic is required to produce adequate diuresis. Because the elimination of aminoglycosides is directly related to the GFR, aminoglycosides have a longer half-life in neonates and infants, thus requiring a longer dosing interval than in adults. In addition, decreased tubular secretion in neonates and infants can lengthen the elimination half-life of other antibiotics, such as the penicillins and sulfonamides. Selecting the appropriate dosing regimen based on age, weight, and kidney maturation and identifying concomitant agents renally eliminated are important factors to prevent toxicity. In general, renal excretion of many drugs is directly proportional to age.

DRUG SELECTION

Various factors are considered when prescribing a drug for a pediatric patient. Among them are the benefits of the drug in relation to the risks of administration, the long-term effects, the dosage form, and the route and frequency of administration (Fig. 4-1).

Risks and Benefits

Relatively few studies have been conducted to assess the risks versus the benefits of drug therapy in the pediatric population. Such studies can provide objective data that caregivers can use in choosing certain drugs to treat specific diseases. Risk data often encompass both short- and long-term risks of the disease and its treatment (including morbidity and mortality), adverse drug effects, cost, or negative quality-of-life issues; benefit data often include pertinent information about the natural history of the disease, drug safety profile, or positive quality-of-life issues.

For example, Redmond (1997) reviewed the risk–benefit data on ciprofloxacin (Cipro) for childhood infections. The major limiting factor to using any fluoroquinolone in pediatrics

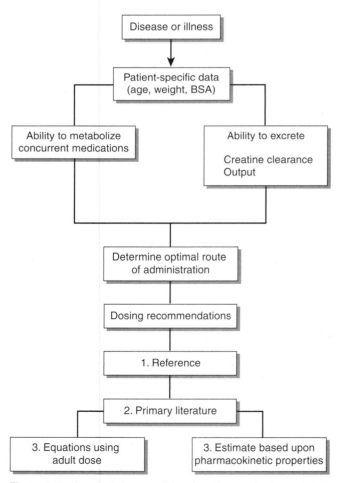

Figure 4–1   Approach to prescribing drug therapy for the pediatric patient.

is the risk of severe degenerative arthropathy, which was reported in studies of ciprofloxacin use in animals (Schluter, 1987). After 10 years of experience with ciprofloxacin in the United Kingdom, little risk of permanent joint damage was identified (Redmond, 1997). Therefore, ciprofloxacin can be used whenever the potential benefit of ciprofloxacin clearly outweighs the risk.

Long-Term Effects

Drugs administered to pediatric patients may take a longer time to produce adverse effects than in adults. Certain adverse effects may not be detected until decades after treatment. For example, secondary cancers, growth retardation, hypogonadism, and sterility have all been reported as late adverse effects associated with certain antineoplastic therapies. Inhaled and intranasal corticosteroids may decrease growth velocity, which is a means of comparing growth rates among children of the same age. Studies with inhaled steroids showed approximately a 1-cm/year reduction in growth velocity. The FDA suggests that the reduction is related to dose and how long the child takes the drug (U.S. FDA, 1998b). More recently, Lone and Pederson (2000) evaluated the long-term effect on growth of inhaled or intranasal budesonide in pediatric asthma patients. At the end of this 10-year study, the researchers concluded that normal adult height was achieved in patients receiving these corticosteroids.

Dosage Formulation

Commercially available dosage formulations often limit the drugs that can be prescribed to children. Many drugs are available only as an oral tablet, capsule, or intravenous dilution in adult dosage strengths. Prescribing a drug as a tablet or capsule for a pediatric patient has several drawbacks. He or she may have difficulty swallowing a whole or intact tablet or capsule, and attempting to break a tablet into smaller pieces or emptying part of a capsule to provide an appropriate dose leads to questionable accuracy of the administered dose. It is important to provide a dosage form that can be administered easily, accurately, and safely to a pediatric patient. A method to improve administration is via extemporaneous formulations, especially if a product is not commercially available as an elixir, solution, suspension, or syrup. Other alternatives to oral liquid formulations include tablet dispersion, powdered papers, and repacked capsules.

Ideally, a practitioner who is prescribing a dosage formulation not commercially available for a pediatric patient ought to work with a pharmacist who is willing and able to compound accurate pediatric drug dosages and formulas. Practitioners can familiarize themselves with additional drugs that can be extemporaneously compounded for use in pediatrics by a pharmacist in such publications as *Handbook on Extemporaneous Formulations* (Dice & Zenk, 1987); *Pediatric Drug Formulations* (Nahata & Hipple, 2000); *Teddy Bear Book: Pediatric Injectable Drugs* (Phelps, 2002); *Pediatric Dosage Handbook* (Taketomo, Hodding, & Kraus, 2003); or *The Children's Hospital of Philadelphia Extemporaneous Formulations* (Jew et al., 2003). A Medline search should be conducted for drugs not contained in these publications. Box 4-1 gives recommendations to assist healthcare professionals in reducing medication errors.

BOX 4–1. AMERICAN ASSOCIATION OF PEDIATRICS (AAP) RECOMMENDATIONS FOR REDUCING MEDICATION ERRORS

- Maintain an up-to-date patient allergy profile.
- Confirm the validity of a patient's weight for medications that are dosed by body weight (or body surface area [BSA] for medications dosed by BSA).
- State specific dosage strengths or formulation.
- Do not use abbreviations for drug names or patient instructions.
- Avoid using abbreviations for dosage units.
- Use a zero before a decimal point.
- Avoid a zero after a decimal point.

Dosage

In adult drug therapy, one standard dose of a drug can be used for almost all adults, but the opposite is true in pediatric drug therapy: a pediatric drug dose changes for different illnesses or as the patient grows or develops and requires age-dependent adjustments. Many drugs currently in use in pediatrics have established dosing recommendations based on body weight, BSA, concurrent drug therapy, and stage of development or physiologic function (age).

Body weight–based dosing is the most common method for pediatric dosing. A total daily dose, milligrams per kilogram per day (mg/kg/day), is divided by the dosing interval to calculate each individual dose. Analgesics, antipyretics, and emergency drugs are often administered on a dose-by-dose method; as such, the recommended pediatric dose is reported as milligrams per kilogram per dose (mg/kg/dose). The starting or maximum doses for pediatric intravenous infusions are usually reported as micrograms per kilogram per minute (mcg/kg/minute) or micrograms per kilogram per hour (mcg/kg/hour). Drug dosages based on a patient's BSA are usually reserved for antineoplastic agents or critically ill patients. Dosages of several drugs, including syrup of ipecac and kaolin (Kaopectate), are based on age.

General pediatric drug references such as the *Pediatric Dosage Handbook* (Taketomo et al., 2003) and Micro Medex (Drugdex, 2003) provide comprehensive drug monographs, including dosage formulations, adverse events, pharmacology, and pharmacokinetics. *The Harriet Lane Handbook* (Gunn & Nechyba, 2002) provides drug monographs based on the Johns Hopkins Hospital formulary and special drug topics. A specialty pediatric reference such as the *Red Book* (Pickering, 2003) covers only antimicrobial agents and vaccines; *Neofax '03* (Young & Mangum, 2003) and the *Neonatal Drug Formulary Book 2002* (Bhatt, Bruggman, Thayer-Thomas, et al., 2002) provide information about drug dosing in neonates.

In the absence of pediatric dosing recommendations, the traditional method for calculating dosage involves using the usual adult drug dosage adjusted by weight, BSA, or age. Body weight–based pediatric dosage calculation adjustment methods include Augsberger's and Clark's rules. One BSA-based

Table 4.4

Formulas for Calculating an Approximate Pediatric Dose Based on an Adult Dose

Formulas Based on Body Surface Area of the Pediatric Patient

Clarke's Body Area Rule

$$\frac{(\text{Body surface area in meters}^2) \times \text{adult dose}}{1.73}$$

Formulas Based on Body Weight of the Pediatric Patient

Augsberger's Rule

$$1.5 \times \text{Weight in kg} + 10 = \% \text{ of adult dose}$$

Clark's Rule

$$\frac{\text{Weight in pounds} \times \text{adult dose}}{150}$$

Formulas Based on Age of the Pediatric Patient

Augsberger's Rule

$$4 \times \text{Age in years} + 20 = \% \text{ of adult dose}$$

Bastedo's Rule

$$\frac{(\text{Age in years} + 3) \times \text{adult dose}}{30}$$

Cowling's Rule

$$\frac{(\text{Age at next birthday in years}) \times \text{adult dose}}{24}$$

Dilling's Rule

$$\frac{(\text{Age in years}) \times \text{adult dose}}{20}$$

Fried's Rule for Infants

$$\frac{(\text{Age in months}) \times \text{adult dose}}{150} = \text{infant dose}$$

Young's Rule

$$\frac{(\text{Age in years}) \times \text{adult dose}}{\text{Age in years} + 12}$$

dosage calculation method is Clarke's Body Area Rule, which helps approximate pediatric dosages. Age-based dosage calculations include Augsberger's Rule, Bastedo's Rule, Cowling's Rule, Fried's Rule for Infants, and Young's Rule (Table 4-4). Unfortunately, systematic comparative studies of dosages based on these formulas and dosages based on pediatric pharmacokinetic or clinical studies have not been conducted. An assumption is made that body mass and weight are linear, but growth and development are not linear processes.

BSA does correlate closely with many factors that influence drug elimination, including cardiac output, respiratory metabolism, blood volume, extracellular water volume, GFR, and renal blood flow. Therefore, the use of the Clarke's Body Area Rule is the preferred way to calculate a pediatric dose when the dose cannot be determined from published pediatric pharmacokinetic or clinical studies. However, before administering a dose calculated from Clarke's Body Area Rule, the caregiver should make sure that the dose is appropriate or reasonable based on his or her knowledge of pediatric pharmacokinetics.

Routes of Administration

Oral

When prescribing or administering oral drugs for pediatric patients, the caregiver needs to consider not only the drug's flavor and ease of delivery but the frequency of administration, dosage form, and "inactive" ingredients, such as alcohol and sugar. A liquid dosage form is preferred for most pediatric patients.

To ensure the accuracy of each dose administered, the drug should be measured and then administered with an oral syringe or a calibrated drug cup, with the base of the menis-cus viewed at eye level. If the drug is available only in tablet form, and the tablet can be broken, the tablet may be crushed and mixed in compatible syrup. However, mixing a crushed or whole tablet with food should be done cautiously because many foods interfere with drug absorption.

If the patient is an infant, the head should be raised to prevent aspiration of the drug. Applying gentle downward pressure on the chin with a thumb helps open the patient's mouth. If a syringe is used, the tip of the syringe should be placed in the pocket between the patient's cheek and gum and the drug administered slowly and steadily to reduce the risk of aspiration.

For bottle-fed infants, the drug can be placed in a nipple and the infant allowed to suck the contents. However, a drug should never be mixed with the contents of a baby's bottle because the correct dose will not be received if the infant does not consume the full contents of the bottle. In addition, a drug–nutrient interaction may occur if a drug is mixed with formula. A classic example of a drug–nutrient interaction is the significant reduction of oral phenytoin absorption after concurrent administration with an enteral feeding formula (Sacks & Brown, 1994).

Rectal

Toddlers being toilet trained, especially children experiencing stress or difficulty, often resist the rectal administration of drugs. Older children may perceive the procedure as an invasion of privacy and may react with embarrassment or anger and hostility. The best approach to reducing anxiety and increasing cooperation is to spend time explaining the procedure and to reassure the child that giving drugs by this route will not hurt. It may be necessary, after placing a suppository, to hold the child's buttocks together for a few minutes to prevent expulsion of the drug.

Parenteral

The use of topical anesthetics can minimize the pain associated with injections. EMLA cream (eutectic mixture of local anesthetics) has been used safely in infants as young as 6 months for venipuncture and intramuscular injections (Taddio, Nulman, Reid, et al., 1992).

The optimal site for intramuscular administration depends on the patient's age. In children younger than 3 years of age, the vastus lateralis (outer thigh) is the preferred site, whereas the gluteus (buttock) or ventrogluteal (hip) area is preferred in older children. Needle size depends on age, muscle mass, and drug viscosity. The patient should be told that the intramuscular injection will hurt but reassured that the drug will help. However, restraining or holding the patient still may be necessary. The patient should be comforted after the injection.

Subcutaneous administration of drugs (narcotics, insulin, heparin, vaccine) is performed similarly to intramuscular administration, but shorter needles are used and the injected volume is limited to less than 2 mL.

When administering an intravenous drug, it is important to check the compatibility of the drug with all other drugs administered through the same catheter or intravenous tubing. The concentration of the drug in solution can be adjusted to minimize vascular irritation by diluting the drug and adjusting the infusion time. The diameter and length of the intravenous tubing can affect the time it takes for a drug to be delivered to the patient.

Pulmonary

Nebulizers, metered-dose inhalers (MDIs), and dry powder inhalers (DPIs) can be used to deliver bronchodilators, aminoglycosides, and corticosteroids in the treatment of asthma or cystic fibrosis. Nebulized drugs require connecting an air or oxygen tube to the nebulizer machine and are often used in infants and young children. MDIs require coordination between actuation and inhalation; this is difficult in any age group, so a tube spacer is recommended for children less than 8 years old and a spacer connected to a face mask for children less than 4 years old (Tiddens, 2004). Spacer devices have expanded the use of MDIs even to the neonatal population. A DPI such as budesonide powder (Pulmicort Turbohaler) involves coordination with the patient's inspiratory flow; therefore, the delivery mechanism is not recommended in children less than 7 years of age.

Frequency

If adherence to a drug regimen is poor, the efficacy of treatment will be compromised. Both the drug administration frequency and the duration of treatment (the dosage) affect adherence to a drug regimen. The frequency of dosing depends primarily on the drug's pharmacokinetic profile (ie, a longer half-life results in less frequent dosing intervals). However, preparing the drug in different immediate- and delayed-release dosage formulations can also alter the dosing frequency.

To improve adherence to a drug regimen, especially in pediatric patients, the drug should be administered once or twice daily at most. There is an inverse relationship between adherence and the number of drugs, doses, and frequency in one day, as well as the duration of therapy. In response to the concerns about early cessation and improving the adherence of antimicrobial therapy for acute otitis media, Kozyrskyj and colleagues (Kozyrskyj, Hildes-Ripstein, Longstaffe, et al., 1998) reviewed the literature on short-course antibiotics. This meta-analysis supported shortening the course of antimicrobial therapy for acute otitis media from the traditional 7 to 10 days to 5 days. Other strategies for treating acute otitis media include the use of once-a-day antibiotics (Mandel, Casselbrant, Kurs-Lasky, & Bluestone, 1996) or one-time intramuscular injections (Bauchner, Adams, Barnett, & Klein, 1996). These changes in antimicrobial therapy may improve adherence, contain costs, and reduce the development of drug-resistant bacteria.

Some logistical and psychological implications are associated with the frequency of administering drugs to school-aged children, particularly during the school day. Most schools require notification by the prescriber that a drug needs to be administered during the school day and expect a separate supply of the drug to be kept at the school. To facilitate adherence to drug therapy and satisfy school requirements, the prescriber and pharmacy need to collaborate. The pharmacist can split the prescription based on the number of doses administered at home or school. With regard to psychological or emotional considerations, the prescriber needs to recognize that a student visiting the school nurse to receive the drug can create tension or a feeling of being different from his or her classmates.

For many years, the FDA has encouraged more well-controlled trials on drug efficacy and safety in pediatrics. The Food and Drug Administration Modernization Act of 1997 and the Best Pharmaceuticals for Children Act of 2002 offered support for the pharmaceutical industries to conduct and submit pediatric clinical trials. The Pediatric Research Equity Act of 2003 mandated that drugs used in pediatrics require literature or clinical trials supporting their use. Ensuring effective and safe delivery of drugs in pediatrics involves understanding the physiologic changes that occur throughout childhood. As a result, pediatric pharmacotherapy will evolve with additional clinical trials.

Bibliography

Starred references are cited in the text.

*American Academy of Pediatrics. (1997). Alternative routes of drug administration—advantages and disadvantages (subject review). *Pediatrics, 100,* 143–152.

*Anonymous. (1972). American Academy of Pediatrics committee on fetus and newborn: hexachlorophene and skin care of newborn infants. *Pediatrics, 49,* 625–626.

*Bauchner, H., Adams W., Barnett, E., & Klein, J. (1996). Therapy for acute otitis media. *Archives of Pediatric and Adolescent Medicine, 150,* 396–399.

Benitz, W. E., & Tatro, D. S. (1995). *The pediatric drug handbook* (3rd ed.). St. Louis: Mosby–Year Book.

*Bhatt, D. R., Bruggman, D. S., Thayer-Thomas, J. C., et al. (2002). *Neonatal drug formulary 2002* (5th ed.). Fontana, CA: N.D.F. Los Angeles.

*Bond, J. A. (1993). Metabolism and elimination of inhaled drugs and airborne chemicals from the lungs. *Pharmacology and Toxicology, 72,* 23–47.

*Carry, M. R., Ringel, S. P., & Starcevich, J. M. (1986). Distribution of capillaries in normal and diseased human skeletal muscle. *Muscle Nerve, 9,* 445–454.

*Cavell, B. (1981). Gastric emptying in infants fed human milk or infant formula. *Acta Paediatrica Scandinavica, 70,* 639–641.

Committee on Drugs/Committee on Hospital Care. (1998). Prevention of medication errors in the pediatric inpatient setting. *Pediatrics, 102,* 428–430.

*Deren, J. S. (1971). Development of structure and function of the fetal and newborn stomach. *American Journal of Clinical Nutrition, 24,* 144–159.

*Dice, J. E., & Zenk, K. E. (1987). *Handbook on extemporaneous formulations.* Bethesda, MD: American Society of Hospital Pharmacy.

*Dolovich, M. (1999). Aerosol delivery to children: what to use, how to choose. *Pediatric Pulmonology, 18* (Suppl.), 79–82.

*Drugdex. Micromedex Inc. Vol 117. 1975–2003.

*Fok, T. F., Monkman, S., Dolovich, M., et al. (1996). Efficacy of aerosol medication delivery from a metered-dose inhaler versus jet nebulizer in infants with bronchopulmonary dysphasia. *Pediatric Pulmonology, 21,* 301–309.

*Friis-Hansen, B. (1957). Changes in body water compartment during growth. *Acta Paediatrica, 46* (Suppl. 110), 1–68.

Grand, R. J., Ramakrishna, J., & Calenda, K. A. (1995). Inflammatory bowel disease in the pediatric patient. *Gastroenterology Clinics of North America, 24,* 613–632.

*Graves, N. M., & Kriel, R. L. (1987). Rectal administration of antiepileptic drugs in children. *Pediatric Neurology, 3,* 321–326.

*Gunn, V. L., & Nechyba, C. (2002) *The Harriet Lane handbook* (17th ed.). St. Louis: Mosby–Year Book.

*Haile, C. A. (1977). Chloramphenicol toxicity. *Southern Medical Journal, 70,* 479–480.

*Jew, R. K., Mullen, R. J., & Soo-Hoo, W. (2003). *Extemporaneous formulations* (1st ed.). Bethesda, MD: American Society of Hospital Pharmacists.

*Kearns, G. L. (1995). Pharmacogenetics and development: Are infants and children at increased risk for adverse outcomes? *Current Opinion in Pediatrics, 7,* 220–233.

*Kozyrskjy, A. L., Hildes-Ripstein, G. E., Longstaffe, S. E. A., et al. (1998). Treatment of acute otitis media with a shortened course of antibiotics: A meta-analysis. *Journal of the American Medical Association, 279,* 1736–1742.

Leeder, J. S., & Kearns, G. L. (1997). Pharmacogenetics in pediatrics: Implications for practice. *Pediatric Clinics of North America, 44,* 55–77.

*Linday, L., Dobkin, J. F., Wang, T. C., et al. (1987). Digoxin inactivation by the gut flora in infancy and childhood. *Pediatrics, 79,* 544–548.

*Lindenbaum, J., Rund, D. G., Butler, V. P., et al. (1981). Inactivation of digoxin by gut flora; reversal by antibiotic therapy. *New England Journal of Medicine, 305,* 789–794.

*Lone, A., & Pederson, S. (2000). Effect of long-term treatment with inhaled budesonide on adult height in children with asthma. *New England Journal of Medicine, 343,* 1064–1069.

*Mandel, E. M., Casselbrant, M. L., Kurs-Lasky, M., & Bluestone, C. D. (1996). Efficacy of ceftibuten compared with amoxicillin for otitis media with effusion in infants and children. *Pediatric Infectious Disease Journal, 15,* 409–414.

McEvoy, G. K. (Ed.). (2004). *AHFS drug information 2004.* Bethesda, MD: American Society of Health-System Pharmacists.

McGillis Bindler, R., & Berner Howry, L. (1997). *Pediatric drugs and nursing implications* (2nd ed.). Stamford, CT: Appleton & Lange.

*Morselli, P. L., Franco-Morselli, R., & Bossi, L. (1980). Clinical pharmacokinetics in newborns and infants: Age-related differences and therapeutic implications. *Clinical Pharmacokinetics, 5,* 485–527.

*Nahata, M. C., & Hipple, T. F. (2000). *Pediatric drug formulations* (4th ed.). Cincinnati, OH: Harvey Whitney.

*Phelps, S. J. (2002). *Teddy bear book: Pediatric injectable drugs* (6th ed.). Bethesda, MD: American Society of Hospital Pharmacists.

*Pickering, L. K. (Ed). *2003 Red book: Report of the Committee on Infectious Diseases* (26th ed.). Elk Grove Village, IL: American Academy of Pediatrics.

*Redmond, A. O. (1997). Risk-benefit experience of ciprofloxacin use in pediatric patients in the United Kingdom. *Pediatric Infectious Disease Journal, 16,* 147–149.

*Rubin, M. I., Bruck, E., & Rapoport, M. J. (1949). Maturation of renal function in childhood: Clearance studies. *Journal of Clinical Investigation, 28,* 1144–1162.

*Rutter, N. (1987). Percutaneous drug absorption in the newborn: Hazards and uses. *Clinical Perinatology, 14,* 911–930.

*Sacks, G. S., & Brown, R. O. (1994). Drug-nutrient interactions in patients receiving nutritional support. *Drug Therapy, 24,* 35–42.

*Salmon, B., Wilson, N. M., & Silverman, M. (1990). How much aerosol reaches the lungs of wheezy infants and toddlers? *Archives of Disease in Childhood, 65,* 401–404.

*Schluter, G. (1987). Ciprofloxacin: Review of potential toxicological effects. *American Journal of Medicine, 82*(Suppl. 4A), 91–93.

*Stewart, C. F., & Hampton, E. M. (1987). Effect of maturation on drug disposition in pediatric patients. *Clinical Pharmacy, 6,* 548–564.

*Taddio, A., Nulman, I., Reid, E., et al. (1992). Effect of lidocaine-prilocaine cream (EMLA) on pain of intramuscular Fluzone injection. *Canadian Journal of Hospital Pharmacy, 45,* 227–230.

*Taketomo, C. K., Hodding, J. H., & Kraus, D. M. (2003). *Pediatric dosage handbook* (10th ed.). Hudson, OH: Lexi-Comp.

*Tiddens, H. (2004) Matching the device to the patient. *Pediatric Pulmonology, 26* (Suppl.), 26–29.

*U.S. Food and Drug Administration. (1998a). Rules and regulations. *Federal Register, 63*(231), 66631–66672.

*U.S. Food and Drug Administration. (1998b). *FDA talk paper.* Rockville, MD: Author.

*Yaffe, S. J., & Juchau, M. R. (1974). Perinatal pharmacology. *Annual Review of Pharmacology, 14,* 219–238.

*Young, T. E., & Mangum, O. B. (2003). *Neofax '03: A manual of drugs used in neonatal care* (16th ed.). Raleigh, NC: Acorn Publishing.

Visit the Connection web site for the most up-to-date drug information.

PRINCIPLES OF PHARMACOTHERAPY IN PREGNANCY AND LACTATION

■ STEPHANIE GABER

Although very little is known about the effects of medications on the fetus, many women ingest drugs during their pregnancy. The World Health Organization states "there can be no doubt that at present some drugs are more widely used in pregnancy than is justified by the knowledge available." Although considerable attention has been given recently to illegal drug use during pregnancy, the use of legal drugs, both prescription and over-the-counter, for treating known maternal medical conditions, continues to be a controversial topic (Briggs et al., 2002).

ISSUES IN MEDICATION USE DURING PREGNANCY

Studies have determined that anywhere from 35% to 80% of all pregnant women will consume at least one medication during their pregnancy (McElhatton, 2003). As the number of medications being prescribed during pregnancy increases, the practitioner needs a solid understanding of the physiologic changes that occur during pregnancy and the effects that these changes have on medication use. The practitioner must also balance the need to treat the mother against the potential risk to the fetus. Because there are few studies available discussing the pharmacokinetic changes that occur during pregnancy, appropriate dosing of medications may be difficult. Understanding these changes will assist the practitioner in making recommendations during drug therapies. The maternal and fetal response to medications ingested during pregnancy may be influenced by two factors:

- Changes in the absorption, distribution, and elimination of the drug in the mother, which are altered by physiologic changes (Yankowitz & Niebyl, 2001)
- The placental–fetal unit, which affects the amount of drug that crosses the placental membrane, the amount of drug metabolized by the placenta, and the distribution and elimination of the drug by the fetus (Loebstein et al., 1997)

Pregnancy-Induced Maternal Physiologic Changes

Women undergo many physiologic changes during pregnancy (Table 5-1). These changes affect the way a medication exerts its effects on both the mother and fetus.

Absorption

Drug absorption into maternal bloodstream can occur by different processes, including the gastrointestinal (GI) tract, skin, or lungs, or the drug maybe directly placed into the bloodstream via intravenous administration.

Gastrointestinal Absorption

Pregnancy-induced maternal physiologic changes may affect GI function, and therefore the absorption of some drugs may be altered. Of the many factors that can affect GI absorption of drugs, one is the decrease in GI tract motility, especially during labor. It is believed that an increase in plasma progesterone levels causes this decrease in motility, which may delay the absorption of orally administered drugs (Fredericksen, 2001; Kraemer et al., 1997; Loebstein et al., 1997).

In addition, pregnant women experience a reduction in gastric acid secretions (up to 40% less than in nonpregnant women) as well as an increase in gastric mucous secretion (Fredericksen, 2001; Loebstein et al., 1997). Together, this may lead to an increase in gastric pH and a decrease in the absorption of medications that need an acidic pH for appropriate absorption.

Another reason for decreased GI absorption may be the nausea and vomiting that is common during the first trimester of pregnancy and that is thought to be associated with increased progesterone levels. Therefore, pregnant women may be well advised to take their medications at times when nausea is minimal (Loebstein et al., 1997).

Table 5.1

Physiologic Changes in Pregnancy

Organ System Dynamic	Change During Pregnancy
Cardiovascular	
Blood volume	Increased by 30%-50%
Cardiac output	Increased by 30%-50%
Systemic vascular resistance	Decreased
Gastrointestinal	
pH of intestinal secretions	Increased
Gastric emptying time	Increased
Gastric acid secretions	Decreased
Intestinal motility	Decreased
Kidney	
Renal blood flow rate	Increased
Glomerular filtration rate	Increased
Gynecologic	
Uterine blood flow	Increased

(Adapted from Kraemer, K. [1997]. Placental transfer of drugs. *Neonatal Network, 16* [2], 65–67.)

Lung Absorption

Physiologic changes in pregnancy favor the absorption of medications administered through the inhalation route. Both cardiac and tidal volumes are increased by approximately 50% in pregnancy; this results in hyperventilation and increased pulmonary blood flow (Loebstein et al., 1997). These alterations aid in the transfer of medications through the alveoli into the maternal bloodstream (Loebstein et al., 1997).

Transdermal Absorption

An increase in the absorption of medications through the skin is evident during pregnancy. The increase in peripheral vasodilation and increase in blood flow to the skin (Kraemer et al., 1997) enhance this increase in absorption. Because of an increase in total body water, there is increased water content in the skin, therefore favoring an increased rate and extent of absorption to water soluble medications like lidocaine, which is used as a topical anesthetic during pregnancy (Yankowitz & Niebyl, 2001).

Distribution

Maternal blood volume increases significantly during pregnancy. The 30% to 50% increase in blood volume (Guyton & Hall, 1996; Loebstein et al., 1997) is characteristically distributed to various organ systems serving the needs of the growing fetus. The full increase in total body water during pregnancy is 8 L, with 60% distributed to the placenta, fetus, and amniotic fluid and 40% going to maternal tissues (Loebstein et al., 1997). It is these increases that cause the volume of distribution of medications to increase, resulting in a decrease (dilutional effect) in drug concentrations. Studies show that serum levels of water-soluble drugs decrease because of the increased volume of distribution (Simone et al., 1994). Conversely, drug distribution is affected by an increase in maternal fat deposits. Medications that are highly lipophilic distribute to maternal fat deposits, also resulting in decreased serum drug levels. Body fat increases during pregnancy by 3 to 4 kg, and

may act as a reservoir for medications that favor a fat-soluble environment (Yankowitz & Niebyl, 2001). Another factor that may affect medication distribution is the concentration of albumin the maternal blood. The concentration of plasma albumin decreases during pregnancy (Fredericksen, 2001). This decrease is believed to be caused by a reduction in the rate of albumin synthesis or an increase in its rate of catabolism (Fredericksen, 2001). Medications that are highly bound to plasma albumin (eg, anticonvulsants) may have an increased drug concentration due to decreased albumin binding.

Elimination

Hormonal changes that normally occur during pregnancy can affect the elimination of various medications. The normal increase in progesterone levels can stimulate hepatic microsomal enzyme systems, thereby increasing the elimination of some hepatically eliminated medications (eg, phenytoin [Dilantin]). Progesterone may also decrease the elimination of some medications (eg, theophylline [Theo-Dur]) by inhibiting specific microsomal enzyme systems. Therefore, depending on the elimination pathway of a specific medication, the elimination rate cannot be predicted. The extent of these physiologic changes is difficult to quantify, and it is unknown whether changes in dosages are required.

As plasma volumes increase, so does renal blood flow (Fredericksen, 2001; Guyton & Hall, 1996; Loebstein et al., 1997). With the increase in renal blood flow by 50% (Loebstein et al., 1997) and increased glomerular filtration rate, drugs excreted primarily by the kidney show increased elimination. Again, the size of these increases in elimination is not known and therefore dosage adjustment may not be required.

Factors in Placental–Fetal Physiology

Until the 1960s, it was widely believed that the uterus provided a secure and protected environment for the developing fetus. Very little thought was given to the potential harm posed to the fetus from maternal drug use. After the thalidomide tragedy in the 1960s, the government required testing of drugs before human use. It is now known that by the fifth week of fetal development, virtually every drug has the ability to cross the placenta (Kraemer et al., 1997).

The treatment of medical conditions is complicated during pregnancy by various factors that must be considered before initiating drug therapy. A key factor is whether the drug will cross the placenta and potentially cause fetal harm.

Placental Transfer of Medications

The following factors affect a drug's ability to cross the placenta:

- Lipid-soluble drugs can cross the placenta more freely than water-soluble drugs because the outer layers of most cell membranes are made up of lipids. Many antibiotics and opiate compounds are highly soluble in lipids and can therefore easily cross the placental membrane (Kraemer et al., 1997).

Table 5.2

Effect of Molecular Weight on Placental Transfer of Drugs

Molecular Weight	Drug Example	Rate of Placental Transfer
<500 g/mole	acetaminophen, caffeine, cocaine, labetalol, morphine, penicillins, theophylline	Readily crosses the placenta
600-1000 g/mole	digoxin	Crosses placenta at a slower rate
>1000 g/mole	heparin, insulins	Transfer across placenta severely impeded

- The ionization status of the drug affects placental transfer. Drugs with high lipid solubility tend to remain in a nonionized state; therefore, placental transfer is increased. Heparin, for example, is a highly ionized drug, and therefore it does not readily cross the placental membrane (Kraemer et al., 1997).
- The molecular weight of the drug can determine the ease of placental transfer (Kraemer et al., 1997; Loebstein et al., 1997). The lower the molecular weight or the smaller the drug molecule, the more readily the drug crosses the placenta (Table 5-2).
- Only drugs that are not bound to a protein (eg, albumin) can cross the placenta. Albumin is the most abundant protein in the human body. During pregnancy, the concentration of albumin decreases, and therefore fewer proteins are present, allowing for more unbound or "free" drug to cross the placental membrane (Kraemer et al., 1997).

Placental and Fetal Metabolism

Evidence exists to support the theory that the human placenta and fetus are capable of metabolizing medications. Research findings suggest that liver enzyme systems are present in fetal livers as early as 7 to 8 weeks' gestation (Juchau & Choa, 1983). Although these enzyme systems are present, they are immature and any drug elimination that occurs is a result of drug diffusing back into maternal blood.

Fetal Physiology

Not all drugs that cross the placental barrier cause fetal harm. Therefore, the practitioner needs to ask whether a specific drug will cross the placenta and cause fetal harm. Fetal factors to be considered in answering the question include the gestational age at the time of exposure to the drug, which is important because some drugs can exert their effects on the fetus throughout gestation. On the other hand, some drugs exert their effects on the fetus at different stages of gestation. For example, angiotensin-converting enzyme (ACE) inhibitors, such as captopril (Capoten), quinapril (Accupril), and enalapril (Vasotec), are considered absolutely contraindicated in early pregnancy, being in category C in the second trimester and category D in the third trimester. In other words, they become less safe as the pregnancy advances.

Within the first 14 days after conception, the embryo is protected from exogenous toxicity (Kraemer et al., 1997; Rayburn, 1997). The cells at this time are totipotential, meaning that if one cell is damaged or killed, another cell can perform the dead cell's function, and the embryo remains unharmed (Dicke, 1989). After this point, the developing fetus is susceptible to the effects of drugs. The first 3 months of gestation are the most crucial in terms of abnormalities and malformations (Briggs et al., 2002). Some medications that may be relatively safe during the middle trimester of pregnancy may not be safe in the last trimester or during delivery. For example, aspirin use late in pregnancy is associated with increased bleeding at the time of delivery. Moreover, the effect that aspirin has on prostaglandins may delay labor.

Fetal total body water and fat deposition are associated with gestational age and they affect the absorption and distribution of drugs. As the fetus matures, total body water decreases and fat deposition increases, and the fetus is more likely to be affected by medications that are highly lipophilic (eg, opiates) than by medications that are water soluble (eg, ampicillin [Principen]).

Fetal circulatory patterns can alter the amount of drug distributed to the fetus. In early gestation, a disproportionately large percentage of the fetal cardiac output is presented to the brain, and consequently the concentration of drug in the fetal circulation is increased (Kraemer et al., 1997).

Teratogenicity of Medications

The word *teratogenicity* is derived from the Greek root *teras*, meaning "monster." Teratogenicity is the ability of an exogenous agent to cause the dysgenesis of fetal organs as evidenced either structurally or functionally (Koren et al., 1998; Kraemer et al., 1997).

The risk of fetal abnormality depends on many factors, including not only the gestational age of the fetus at the time of exposure but the agent or medications the fetus is exposed to and the length of exposure.

The health care provider must therefore balance the risk of exposing the fetus to the drug with the benefit of treatment to the mother. If it is determined that the drug is necessary, the drug with the safest profile should be used at the lowest effective dose. The practitioner always keeps in mind that the mother is not the only recipient of the drug—the fetus is as well. It is estimated that approximately 2% or 3% of all malformations and abnormalities in the developing fetus result from drug ingestion (Oakley, 1986).

To help prevent drug-induced abnormalities in the fetus, the U.S. Food and Drug Administration (FDA) has categorized drugs according to fetal risks. The categories are based on the presence or absence of controlled studies in women to determine the level of fetal risk (Table 5-3). Health care providers use these categories to determine the appropriate drug therapy that will effectively treat the mother but carries the least potential for fetal harm. In pregnant women, balancing the risk–benefit ratio is of great concern for the health care provider. Any illnesses or chronic medical conditions that go untreated during pregnancy could potentially cause harm to the mother and fetus, even though treating the illness or condition may be potentially harmful to the fetus. Therefore, weighing the benefit of drug therapy to the mother

Table 5.3

FDA Pregnancy Risk Categories

Category	Risk Summary	Example
A	Controlled studies in women fail to demonstrate a risk to the fetus in the first trimester (and there is no evidence of a risk in later trimesters), and the possibility of fetal harm appears remote.	folic acid, thyroid hormone
B	Either animal reproduction studies have not demonstrated a fetal risk but there are no controlled studies in pregnant women, or animal reproduction studies have shown an adverse effect (other than decrease in fertility) that was not confirmed in controlled studies in women in the first trimester (and there is no evidence of a risk in later trimesters).	erythromycin, penicillin
C	Either studies in animals have revealed adverse effects on the fetus and there are no controlled studies in women, or studies in women and animals are not available. Drugs should be given only if the potential benefit justifies the potential risk.	labetalol, nifedipine, ACE inhibitors
D	There is positive evidence of human fetal risk, but benefits from the use in pregnancy may be acceptable despite the risk.	glyburide, diazepam, aspirin, ACE inhibitors
X	Studies in animals or human beings have demonstrated fetal abnormalities, or there is evidence of fetal risk based on human experience, or both, and the risk of the use of the drug in pregnant women clearly outweighs any possible benefit. The drug is contraindicated in women who are or may become pregnant.	oral contraceptives, lovastatin, isotretinoin

with the risk of drug therapy to the fetus needs to be as balanced as possible.

DRUG THERAPY IN THE BREAST-FEEDING MOTHER

With the number of women who choose to breast-feed their infants increasing yearly, the number of questions presented to health care practitioners concerning the safety of medication use while breast-feeding is also increasing. Recommendations to discontinue or interrupt breast-feeding while taking medication are far too common. Health care practitioners are reluctant to recommend medication use while the mother is breast-feeding because of the potential adverse effects on the infant. Most research on lactation has been conducted in small groups or on animal models. The American Academy of Pediatrics has published lists of medications that are safe for use while breast-feeding (Boxes 5-1 and 5-2).

Human Breast Milk as a Drug Delivery System

Human breast milk is complex, nutrient-enriched fluid. Containing approximately 80% water, breast milk also has immunologic properties and proteins, fats, carbohydrates, minerals, and vitamins needed for normal development. The availability of the drug to be distributed into breast milk depends on many factors. For a drug to be distributed into breast milk, it must first be absorbed into the maternal circulation. The concentration or level of the drug in the mother's plasma influences the amount and degree of drug distributed into breast milk. Once drug is available for distribution into breast milk, several other factors need to be considered. These factors are similar to those determining whether a drug will cross the placental membrane, and include (Dillon et al., 1997):

- Blood flow to the breast—the greater the blood flow to the breast, the greater the drug level in breast milk.

- Plasma pH (7.45) and milk pH (7.08)—the medication will stay in the maternal plasma if the medication favors a higher pH.
- Mammary tissue composition—high adipose or fat content of the breast tissue causes lipophilic medications to be distributed into the breast tissue and then into breast milk.
- Breast milk composition—breast milk contains proteins, fat, water, and vitamins. Any medication that has a high affinity for any component will have an increased distribution into breast milk.
- Physicochemical properties (ie, lipophilicity, molecular weight, ionization of medication in plasma and breast milk) of the drug—drug characteristics that favor transfer of medication into breast milk are low molecular weight, low ionization in plasma, low protein binding, and high lipophilicity.
- Extent of drug protein binding in plasma and breast milk—medications that are highly protein bound in the plasma are less likely to be distributed into the breast milk.
- The rate of breast milk production—the more breast milk produced, the more diluted the medication will be in the breast milk.

When considering these factors, it can easily be appreciated that different medications distribute into breast milk at different rates and to different extents. That is one factor that makes prescribing medications to the breast-feeding woman problematic at best. Health care providers need to ask themselves many questions before selecting drug therapy.

First, is there a need to treat the maternal condition? Many prescriptions are written for conditions that do not need to be treated. Second, what medication can be prescribed that is least likely to be secreted into the breast milk, and for which there is the greatest information about its use in breast-feeding mothers?

Answers to these questions are often difficult or elusive. Referring to the FDA guidelines for medication use in pregnancy and lactation is helpful. Consulting the known pharmacokinetic parameters of medications can also be

BOX 5–1. SAFE MEDICATIONS TO USE IN BREAST-FEEDING

Analgesics
  acetaminophen
  propoxyphene
Narcotic analgesics
  codeine
  morphine
Anticoagulants
  warfarin
Anticonvulsants
  carbamazepine
  ethosuximide
  magnesium sulfate
  valproic acid
Antidepressants
  Consult health care provider
Antihistamines
  brompheniramine
  diphenhydramine
  triprolidine
Antihypertensives
  captopril
  clonidine
  hydralazine
  methyldopa
Anti-infectives
  cephalosporins
  penicillins
  macrolides
  tetracyclines
Nonsteroidal anti-inflammatory drugs
  ibuprofen
  mefenamic acid
  naproxen
Sedatives–hypnotics
  chloral hydrate
  secobarbital
Vitamins

BOX 5–2. MEDICATIONS CONTRAINDICATED IN BREAST-FEEDING

Antidepressant
  lithium
Chemotherapeutic agents
  methotrexate
  cyclophosphamide
  cisplatin
Radioactive isotopes
Recreational drugs
  alcohol
  amphetamines
  cocaine
  heroin, methadone
  marijuana
  lysergic acid diethylamide (LSD)
  nicotine
Thyroid agents
  thiouracil
  methimazole

discard the milk. Doing so relieves engorgement and promotes continued milk production and flow.

Balancing Benefits and Risks

Although the health benefits of breast-feeding are established, there remain a few medications that are unsafe to use during breast-feeding. As with medication use during pregnancy, the risk–benefit ratio needs to be assessed. Choice of the best medication to treat the maternal condition needs to be balanced against the risk of adverse effects to the infant.

Bibliography

Starred references are cited in the text.
*Briggs, C. G., Freeman, R. K., & Yaffe, S. J. (2001). *Drugs in pregnancy and lactation* (6th ed.). Baltimore: Williams & Wilkins.
Cordero, J. F., & Oakley, G. P. (1983). Drug exposure during pregnancy: Some epidemiological considerations. *Clinical Obstetrics and Gynecology, 26,* 418–428.
Dawes M., & Chowienczyk, P. J. (2001) Drugs in pregnancy. Pharmacokinetics in pregnancy. *Best Practice & Research in Clinical Obstetrics and Gynaecology, 15*(6), 819–826.
*Dicke, J. M. (1989). Teratology: Principles and practice. *Medical Clinics of North America, 73,* 567–582.
*Dillon, A. E., et al. (1997). Drug therapy in the nursing mother. *Obstetrics and Gynecology Clinics, 24,* 676–697.
*Fredericksen, M. C. (2001). Physiologic changes in pregnancy and their effect on drug disposition. *Seminars in Perinatology, 25*(3), 120–123.
*Guyton, A. C., & Hall, J. C. (1996). *Human physiology and mechanisms of disease* (6th ed.). Philadelphia: Saunders.
*Juchau, M. R., & Choa, S. T. (1983). Drug metabolism by the human fetus. In M. Gibaldi & L. Prescott (Eds.), *Handbook of clinical pharmacokinetics* (pp. 58–78). New York: Adis.
*Koren, G., et al. (1998). Drugs in pregnancy. *New England Journal of Medicine, 338,* 1128–1137.

helpful in prescribing medications. Selected drugs should have short half-lives, and the use of sustained-release products should be discouraged. Dosing schedules also help in minimizing the amount of drug reaching the infant. Scheduling the mother to take the medication immediately after breast-feeding minimizes the dose to the infant by circumventing peak breast milk levels (Dillon et al., 1997).

Patients with chronic conditions, such as hypertension, epilepsy, or diabetes, need to consult their health care practitioners about continuing treatment and minimizing risk to the infant. Without other options, patients with short-term illnesses can temporarily interrupt breast-feeding for the duration of treatment and resume breast-feeding a few days after therapy is completed. By this time, no residual drug should be concentrated in the breast milk. During the interruption, however, the mother must pump the breast and

*Kraemer, K., et al. (1997). Placental transfer of drugs. *Neonatal Network, 16*(2), 65–67.

*Loebstein, R., et al. (1997). Pharmacokinetic changes during pregnancy and their clinical relevance. *Clinical Pharmacokinetics, 33*, 328–343.

*McElhatton, P. R. (2003). General principles of drug use in pregnancy. *The Pharmaceutical Journal, 270*, 232–234.

*Oakley, G. P. (1986). Frequency of human congenital malformations. *Clinics in Perinatology, 13*, 545–554.

*Rayburn, W. F. (1997). Chronic medical disorders during pregnancy. *Journal of Reproductive Medicine, 42*, 1–24.

Scott, J. R., DiSaia, P. J., Hammond, C. B., & Spellacy, W. N. (Eds.). (1999). *Danforth's obstetrics and gynecology* (8th ed.). Philadelphia: Lippincott Williams & Wilkins.

*Simone, G., Derewlany, L., & Koren, G. (1994). Drug transfer across the placenta. *Clinics in Perinatology, 21*, 463–482.

Wyska E., & Jusko W. J. (2001). Approaches top pharmacokinetic/pharmacodynamic modeling during pregnancy. *Seminars in Perinatology, 25*, 124–32.

*Yankowitz, J., & Niebyl, J. R. (2001). *Drug therapy in pregnancy* (3rd ed.). Philadelphia: Lippincott, Williams & Wilkins.

Visit the Connection web site for the most up-to-date drug information.

PRINCIPLES OF PHARMACOTHERAPY IN ELDERLY PATIENTS

■ DEBRA CARROLL

The medical and pharmacologic management of the geriatric patient presents a challenge to the practitioner that warrants an understanding of aging and its effects on the body. In prescribing drug therapy for elderly patients, the practitioner must have a sound understanding of the physiologic and social issues that are unique to older adults and that may affect the safety and efficacy of prescribing practices. As the elderly population grows, the health care community must be prepared for the challenges ahead.

Indeed, the elderly population is the fastest growing of any age group, with people older than 85 years of age comprising the fastest-growing subset of that age group. By the year 2020, the "baby boomers" will reach seniority and continue to live longer than any prior generation. Modern technology has dramatically increased longevity, turning once fatal conditions, such as heart disease, into chronic illnesses (Guralnik & Havlik, 2000).

Aging leads to multiple chronic diseases affecting the elderly with disability, declining function, and frailty (Kasper & Burton, 2003). Treating multiple problems with prescription as well as over-the-counter (OTC) medications can result in adverse drug reactions (ADRs) and interactions related to changes produced by aging. Problems of polypharmacy (the use of multiple medications to treat a host of medical conditions), improper dosing for an older adult, and a lack of understanding by patients about medications can lead to complications and even death (Cusack & Vestal, 2000). This chapter discusses basic physiologic changes of aging, proper prescribing principles, and social concepts pertaining to safe medication use for the geriatric patient.

BODY CHANGES AND AGING

Every body system is affected by the aging process somewhat, although homeostasis is often maintained despite less-than-optimal functioning of organ systems. Certain systems are more vitally affected by aging and play significant roles in the pharmacokinetic and pharmacodynamic changes in drug effects. Box 6-1 summarizes the impact of aging on the pharmacokinetics of drugs.

Absorption

With aging, physiologic changes in the gastrointestinal (GI) tract may play a role in drug absorption and availability. Stomach pH may increase, blood flow may decrease, and gastric motility may be delayed. The significance of these changes for drug metabolism is controversial. Despite these changes, it is believed that the prolonged transit time in the GI tract still allows for adequate drug absorption (Cusack & Vestel, 2000).

Distribution

Body size decreases with age. Muscle that makes up lean body tissue decreases, shifting to increased fat stores, and body water content decreases by 10% to 15% by 80 years of age. Aging results in some reduction in serum albumin (by approximately 20%), leading to an increase in free drug concentration of drugs such as warfarin (Coumadin) and phenytoin (Dilantin) (Miller, 2004).

There are two important plasma-binding proteins in drug metabolism: albumin and α_1-acid glycoprotein. Albumin has an affinity for acid compounds or drugs such as warfarin, whereas α_1-acid glycoprotein binds more readily with lipophilic and alkaline drugs such as propranolol (Inderal) (Semla & Rochon, 2003). The effects of chronic disease, nutritional deficits, immobility, and age-related liver changes contribute to the changes in serum proteins. The significance of decreased serum proteins is realized when highly protein-bound drugs compete for decreased protein-binding sites. The result can be greater levels of free or unbound circulating drug and, therefore, potential toxicity (Miller, 2004).

Body mass changes may lead to changes in total body content of drugs in elderly patients. A water-soluble drug (low volume of distribution [V_d]) is taken up more readily by lean tissue or muscle and attains higher serum concentrations in patients with less body water or lean tissue. Conversely, a lipid-soluble (high V_d) drug is retained in body fat, resulting in a higher V_d for some drugs. Coupled with a decrease or no change in total body clearance, this increase in V_d can lead to increased half-lives and drug accumulation in elderly patients. For example, diazepam (Valium) has a half-life (t½) of approximately 20 hours in a young adult, but the t½ can exceed 70 hours in the older adult. In addition, some drugs, such as tricyclic antidepressants (TCAs) and long-acting benzodiazepines, pass more readily through the blood–brain barrier, causing more pronounced central nervous system (CNS) effects (Semla & Rochon, 2003). Elderly patients who are treated for depression and anxiety may experience fatigue and confusion from drug therapy because antidepressant and antianxiety agents more readily cross their blood–brain barrier.

Elimination

The liver is the major organ of drug metabolism in the body. With aging comes a decrease in blood flow and liver size. However, in the absence of disease, function is maintained. Decreased size and hepatic blood flow may slow the clearance of certain drugs, and reduced dosages may be required. This is particularly important for drugs with high hepatic extraction ratios. Phase I metabolism, particularly oxidation, is affected by aging. The result is decreased oxidation of drugs, which in turn results in a decreased total body clearance (Box 6-2). The phase II metabolism of drugs by conjugation, which promotes drug elimination by breaking the drug into water-soluble components, is not affected by age (Cusack & Vestal, 2000).

After the liver, the kidneys are the most important organs for drug metabolism and excretion. After 40 years of age, renal blood flow declines and the glomerular filtration rate (GFR) drops approximately 1% a year and accelerates with advancing age. Function is usually maintained despite decreased filtration unless illness or disease overstresses the kidney (Kelleher & Lindeman, 2003). In elderly patients, drugs excreted primarily by the kidney are given in smaller doses, or the time between doses is extended.

A serum creatinine level alone cannot be used to estimate renal function in the aging person because reductions in lean body mass result in decreased rates of creatinine formation. This, coupled with the decreased GFR, makes the serum creatinine appear normal. It cannot be assumed that the GFR is normal from a normal serum creatinine value. The most accurate means of measuring renal function is a 24-hour urine test for creatinine clearance; however, this is not standard procedure before ordering a medication. When there is a need to determine a drug choice in the setting of a potential reduction in creatinine clearance, the Cockcroft and Gault formula (see Chapter 2) provides an estimate based on age, weight, and serum creatinine level with an adjustment for sex (Semla & Rochon, 2003). Table 6-1 lists drugs eliminated by the kidney and recommended dosage adjustments based on estimated creatinine clearance.

PHARMACODYNAMIC CHANGES IN THE ELDERLY

Many of the changes that occur due to aging affect major organ systems and therefore affect the pharmacokinetic disposition of the drug. However, the clinician also must consider the impact drugs have on the aging body (or the pharmacodynamic effect). Although few data are available regarding age-related pharmacodynamic changes in elderly adults, it is known that the elderly may be more sensitive to drug–receptor interactions, either because of increased sensitivity of the receptor to the drug or decreased capacity to respond to drug-induced innervation of receptors. In addition, the number or affinity of receptors may be reduced (Cussack & Vestel, 2000). Nevertheless, it is commonly accepted that the CNS effects of drugs appear to be exaggerated in the elderly patient. Particularly egregious are the agents with anticholinergic affects, such as the TCAs, antihistamines, and

Table 6.1

Examples of Dose Adjustments Based on Estimated Creatinine Clearance

Drug	Usual Oral Dose (Nonrenally Impaired)	Dose Based on Estimated CrCl*		
		CrCl >50 mL/min	CrCl 10–50 mL/min	CrCL <10 mL/min
amantadine	100 mg q12h	Usual dose	Increase interval to q24–72h	Increase interval to q7 days
amoxicillin	250–500 mg q8h	Usual dose	Increase interval to q12h	Increase interval to q24h
cefaclor	250 mg tid	Usual dose	Decrease dose to 50%–100% of usual	Decrease dose to 50% of usual
ciprofloxacin	250–750 mg q12h	Usual dose	Reduce dose to 50% of usual	Reduce dose to 33% of usual or extend to q24h
codeine	30–60 mg q4–6h	Usual dose	Reduce dose to 75% of usual	Reduce dose to 50% of usual
digoxin[†]	0.125–0.5 mg q24h	Usual dose	Reduce dose to 25%–75% of usual OR increase interval to q48h	Reduce dose to 10%–25% of usual
enalapril	5–10 mg q12h	Usual dose	Reduce dose to 75% of usual	Reduce dose to 50% of usual
gabapentin[†]	400 mg tid (for CrCl >60)	300 mg bid (for CrCl 30–60 mL/min)	300 mg qd (for CrCl 15–30 mL/min)	300 mg qod (for CrCl <15 mL/min)
nadolol	80–120 mg/d	Usual dose	Reduce dose to 50% of usual	Reduce dose to 25% of usual
procainamide[‡]	350–400 mg q3–4h	Usual dose	Increase interval to 6–12h	Increase interval to q8–24h
ranitidine	150 mg q12h or 300 mg qhs	Usual dose	Decrease dose to 50% of usual OR increase interval to q24h	Decrease dose to 25% of usual OR increase interval to q48h

*Dose adjustments based on actual creatinine clearance or creatinine clearance estimated by the Cockroft and Gault formula (see Chapter 2).
[†]These drugs are best monitored using actual drug levels, and dose adjustments should be made based on these results.
[‡]Based on manufacturer's information.
(From Bennet, W. M., et al., [1991]. *Drug prescribing in renal failure: Dosing guidelines for adults* [2nd ed.]. Philadelphia: American College of Physicians; and *Physicians desk reference* [1998]. Medical Economics.)

antispasmodics. The anticholinergic effect induced by these agents can lead to excessive dry mouth, blurred vision, constipation, and even an exacerbation of benign prostatic hyperplasia. Caution should be used if these agents are prescribed at all.

Similarly, the sedative effects of agents may be intensified in elderly patients. The benzodiazepines and potent analgesic agents are examples of drugs for which older patients are particularly susceptible to this adverse effect. Overprescribing, or typical prescribing without considering the potential for exaggerated effect, can lead to oversedation and a greater risk of falls and fractures.

The cardiovascular system also can be affected by changes due to aging. Orthostatic hypotension is more common in the elderly because of a loss of the baroreceptor reflex and changes in cerebral blood flow. Moreover, drugs that lower blood pressure or decrease cardiac output put the elderly patient at risk for a syncopal episode.

POLYPHARMACY

Polypharmacy is a significant factor in the morbidity and mortality of elderly patients. Increasing age puts the person at risk for multiple chronic illnesses, many of which require drug therapy (Fig. 6-1). For example, the most common chronic disease in the United States, osteoarthritis, affects 40 million people, the majority being older adults. The costs in terms of morbidity are staggering. Chronic stiffness and pain from arthritis have an impact on function, prompting the routine use of nonsteroidal anti-inflammatory drugs (NSAIDs) and aspirin products (Luggen, 2003). Long-term use of NSAIDs lowers the prostaglandin level in the GI tract, which may result in esophagitis, peptic ulcerations, GI hemorrhage, and GI perforation (Chutka et al., 2004). In a geriatric patient, treatment with histamine-2 (H$_2$) blockers

or proton pump inhibitors to relieve the side effects of aspirin or other NSAIDs may cause additional side effects, such as confusion and mental status changes, in turn requiring more treatment. This demonstrates how easily adverse events occur and snowball in an elderly patient. These adverse events are detrimental to physical outcomes, causing approximately 1 death per 1000 hospitalized patients. Up to 30% of hospital admissions are due to ADRs, the result of improperly taking a prescribed medication, lack of instruction, interactions or allergic reactions, and other misfortunes (Horowitz, 2000).

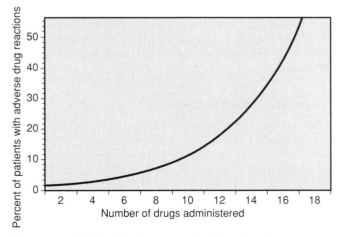

Figure 6–1 Relationship between probability of an adverse reaction and the number of medications taken. (Reproduced with permission from Smith, J. W., Seidl, L. G., & Cluff, L. E. [1966]. Studies on the epidemiology of adverse drug reactions: V. Clinical factors influencing susceptibility. *Annals of Internal Medicine 65*, 629.)

Several factors contribute to polypharmacy. Among them are the varied symptoms and complaints associated with multiple chronic illnesses. In addition, patients often believe that a "pill" will fix what ails them, and the health care provider feels pressured to "prescribe something" to satisfy the patients' expectations of a prescription for medication. When a particular medication regimen is unsuccessful, the health care provider typically prescribes another drug. Many elderly patients stockpile their discontinued medications in case they may be needed again—primarily because of the cost of prescription drugs (Rollason & Vogt, 2003).

Many providers who visit elderly patients in their homes have seen evidence of stockpiled medications. Some elderly patients keep a drawer or cabinet full of old prescription drug bottles. Some contain the same medication, differing only in brand name. Some patients may place a current medication (prescription or OTC) in a labeled prescription bottle that was used for another drug. In addition, the stockpile may reveal prescription bottles for other family members. Patients may be sharing medications or may have received medications from others who believed that the drug that helped them would help the patient (Peterson & Dragon, 1998).

Other sources of polypharmacy are "poly-providers." Many geriatric patients see multiple specialists for various chronic diseases. Medications prescribed without the provider carefully reviewing the patient's other medications can lead to drug overuse and complications. Without a primary care provider overseeing the care of the geriatric patient seeing multiple specialists, ADRs are sure to occur.

The health care provider sometimes creates a polypharmacy situation because multiple drugs are used to treat several chronic illnesses. The provider who is not astute in the principles of safe geriatric prescribing practices may create avoidable side effects and complications. In addition, the patient, who may be a great consumer of OTC medications, often self-prescribes without knowing the consequences of mixing OTC medications with current prescription drugs.

Drug Interactions in the Elderly

Because of normal, age-related physiologic changes, the geriatric patient is at greater risk for complications from medications. Complications related to drug–disease, drug–drug, and drug–food interaction are all commonly encountered. (For more information on drug–drug interactions, see Chapter 3.)

Adverse Drug Reactions

Although age itself creates a risk for ADRs, polypharmacy and the multiplicity of drugs taken by elderly patients present the greater risk. The geriatric patient with multiple chronic illnesses and medications must be identified as a potential candidate for ADRs (Fick et al., 2003). Older women in particular are at great risk for ADRs because they often receive more prescription drugs and have a more significant loss of muscle mass than older men.

There is a paucity of information on safety and efficacy of drugs for the elderly patient. Most research and clinical trials are performed with younger subjects. It often is difficult or impossible to predict the consequences of a medication for its intended use on an older adult because few data may be available. In an effort to better understand the effects of drugs on elderly patients, the FDA published guidelines in 1997 recommending older adults be included in clinical trials of drugs specifically being developed to treat prevalent diseases affecting older adults (Murray & Callahan, 2003).

Contributing Lifestyle Factors

Being unaware of potential drug interactions, elderly patients commonly take OTC medications with prescription drugs. Additional combinations of foods or nutritional supplements can slow absorption, prolonging the time for medications to reach peak levels (see Chapter 3). Fatty foods, in particular, can increase intestinal drug absorption because of the longer time required to digest a fatty meal. This, in turn, potentially leads to increased drug levels or toxicity.

Alcohol and Other Drugs

The ingestion of alcohol and other drugs can alter the metabolism of many medications in elderly patients. CNS effects such as lethargy and confusion occur, as does hypotension, when alcohol is combined with nitrates and some cardiovascular drugs. Alcohol can be found in many OTC products such as cough and cold syrups and mouthwashes (Miller, 2004).

Alcohol abuse may be overlooked as a potential problem in the elderly, but abuse among community-dwelling (non-institutionalized) people aged 65 years and older has a prevalence of 14% for men and 1.5% for women. High numbers of elderly alcoholics are treated in emergency departments and medical offices or are hospitalized for medical or psychiatric admissions (Lantz, 2002). Depression, which is more prevalent in the elderly, often coexists with alcohol abuse. Moderate to heavy drinkers older than 65 are 16 times more likely to die of suicide (National Institute on Alcohol Abuse and Alcoholism, 1998). Practitioners need to be more aware of the potential for alcohol abuse in elderly patients. Although alcohol use and abuse decline with age, approximately 50% of older adults use alcohol, with between 2% and 4% meeting the *Diagnostic and Statistical Manual* (American Psychiatric Association, 1994) criteria for alcohol abuse/dependency (Oslin, 2003). Life stressors such as retirement, loss of loved ones, dependency, and chronic illness are contributors to potential alcohol abuse.

Caffeine and Nicotine Use

Caffeine and nicotine are commonly used products that have the potential to interact with certain drugs, thereby altering efficacy and therapeutic drug levels. Besides its presence in coffee, tea, and some sodas, caffeine is found in many OTC drug products. The interaction of caffeine and certain medications may alter drug absorption, cause CNS effects, or decrease drug effectiveness (Miller, 2004). Table 6-2 summarizes selected caffeine–medication interactions.

Many elderly patients have lifelong smoking addictions and are unsuccessful in stopping. Patients and providers alike are frequently unaware of the effects of nicotine and medications. Nicotine alters the metabolism of many drugs, causes CNS effects, and interferes with platelet activity (Miller, 2004). Table 6-3 reviews nicotine–medication effects and interactions.

Table 6.2

Medication–Caffeine Interactions

Type of Interaction	Example of Interaction Effect
Caffeine-induced increase in gastric acid secretion	Decreased absorption of iron
Caffeine-induced gastrointestinal irritation	Decreased effectiveness of cimetidine; increased gastrointestinal irritation from corticosteroids, alcohol, and analgesics
Altered caffeine metabolism	Prolonged effect of caffeine when combined with ciprofloxacin, estrogen, or cimetidine
Caffeine-induced cardiac arrhythmic effect	Decreased effectiveness of antiarrhythmic medications
Caffeine-induced hypokalemia	Exacerbated hypokalemic effect of diuretics
Caffeine-induced stimulation of the central nervous system	Increased stimulation effects from amantadine, decongestants, fluoxetine, and theophylline
Caffeine-induced increase in excretion of lithium	Decreased effectiveness of lithium

ADHERENCE ISSUES

One reason elderly patients have problems with their medications is failure to adhere to the medication regimen. In many cases, prescription drugs are not taken as prescribed; up to 40% of elderly patients take their medications improperly (Cussack & Vestel, 2000). Studies have shown as the complexity of the medication regime increases, improper drug usage rises proportionately (Rollason & Vogt, 2003). In some cases, they may not take enough of the medication, either because they think that they will save money by making the prescription last longer or because they believe that the medicine is not needed daily. In other situations, a medication may not be taken if it interferes with the patient's lifestyle, for example, not taking a diuretic for fear of incontinence.

Table 6.3

Medication–Nicotine Interactions

Type of Interaction	Example of Interaction Effect
Nicotine-induced alteration in metabolism	Decreased efficacy of analgesics, lorazepam, theophylline, aminophylline, β blockers, and calcium channel blockers
Nicotine-induced vasoconstriction	Increased peripheral ischemic effect of β blockers
Nicotine-induced central nervous system stimulation	Decreased drowsiness from benzodiazepines and phenothiazines
Nicotine-induced stimulation of antidiuretic hormone secretion	Fluid retention, decreased effectiveness of diuretics
Nicotine-induced increase in platelet activity	Decreased anticoagulant effectiveness (heparin, warfarin); increased risk of thrombosis with estrogen use
Nicotine-induced increase in gastric acid	Decreased or negated effects of H_2 antagonists (cimetidine, famotidine, nizatidine, ranitidine)

Cost Factors

The cost of medications today is high. Unfortunately, many elderly patients do not have health insurance plans that cover prescription medications, or they quickly reach a capitated benefit with managed care plans when treated with several medications for multiple chronic illnesses. Many older adults on fixed incomes must make choices between buying food; paying rent, taxes, and utilities; or purchasing medications. In some cases, medication purchases become a low priority. The passage of the Medicare Prescription Drug Improvement and Modernization Act of 2003 promises to provide some relief for prescription drugs as it is phased in over several years (Herrick, 2004).

Side Effects

Other reasons for nonadherence to drug treatments include the unpleasant or inconvenient side effects accompanying some medications. Dry mouth, change in taste sensations, fatigue, or frequent urination are reported as reasons for stopping a medication. The form of the medication and ease of administration are reasons as well. Large tablets and capsules may be difficult to swallow. Swallowing problems may be compounded by insufficient fluid being taken with medications. Taking several oral medications at one dosing time with too little fluid may result in the medications "getting stuck," leading to chronic esophageal irritation. Presbyesophagus (the slowing of esophageal motility with advancing age) makes it difficult and frustrating to swallow multiple medications, and it can also lead to choking or aspiration.

Physical and Mental Changes

Functional deficits, especially those affecting the senses, can also challenge adherence to the medication regimen. Poor vision leads to difficulty reading labels and consequently taking the wrong pills or too many of the same pills. Arthritic hands and safety caps can make opening prescription bottles difficult and frustrating for an older adult.

The prevalence of dementia, which manifests in symptoms of cognitive impairment and poor short-term memory and recall, slowly progresses with age, affecting a substantial percentage of those residing in the community (Eslami & Espinoza, 2003). The condition may be unrecognized by the family because the patient may remain seemingly independent and functional despite mental deficits. The family may be fooled into believing the loved one is fine until the condition affects the person's ability to manage basic, daily routines. Unfortunately, the affected person is often responsible for taking his or her own medications. Poor memory results in not taking medication properly, forgetting doses, or taking too many doses of the same drug. Five to 28% of geriatric hospitalizations are estimated to be the result of ADRs (Semla & Rochon, 2003). Improperly taking digoxin, a drug with a narrow therapeutic range, is associated with drug toxicity in the elderly (Juurlink et al., 2003).

Self-Medication Issues

The use of OTC drugs is a significant issue. Noninstitutionalized elderly adults consume between 40% and 50% of all

OTC medications sold. Of more concern is the fact that 70% of those OTC medications were consumed without the patient consulting the health care provider (Meiner, 1997). Approximately 20% of ADRs in the elderly are due to OTC medications (Chutka et al., 2004). On average, the elderly take two OTC medications with 3.8 to 6.7 prescription drugs (Logue, 2002). Many OTC medications are taken without the medical provider's awareness to treat symptoms they do not want to report. Family members and friends often borrow medications believed to treat a particular ailment, again without consultation with their medical provider (Rollason & Vogt, 2003).

Many OTC medications are products that were once available only by prescription. Now, despite their decreased strength, these medications that once required medical supervision and monitoring present a potential hazard for side effects.

The most common OTC medications used by the geriatric patient include analgesics, vitamins and minerals, antacids, and laxatives (Rollason & Vogt, 2003). Cough and cold products and sleeping aids such as Tylenol PM are frequently used by older adults. Combining these products may result in confusion, change in mental status, fluid and electrolyte imbalances, dysrhythmias, and nervousness. Cold medications may worsen hypertension without the patient's knowledge or worsen glucose control in a patient with diabetes.

The geriatric patient must be educated to use OTC drugs safely and to do so only after consulting with the health care provider or pharmacist. If an alternative to drug use is feasible, such as initiating sleep hygiene practices versus taking a sleeping pill, the patient should be encouraged to try these measures first.

SPECIAL CONSIDERATIONS IN LONG-TERM CARE

Advanced age coupled with years of multiple illnesses and mental decline result in frailty and disability. Placement in a long-term care facility most often occurs when the older adult requires assistance with daily functions, such as bathing and dressing, shows cognitive impairment, or becomes incontinent. The national percentage of older adults in nursing homes is about 5%, rising to 20% for age 85 and older (Kasper & Burton, 2003). With a wide array of physical, psychiatric, neurologic, and behavioral problems, the long-term care resident is the most complex of all patients (Katz & Karuza, 2003). Consequently, the complexity of prescribing medications for the nursing home resident can be challenging and frustrating.

Falls and Medication

One of the most serious problems in long-term care facilities is falls. Approximately half of nursing home residents fall annually, sustaining fractures and soft tissue and other injuries (van Doorn Gruber-Baldini et al., 2003). Among the multiple causes of falls are medications, in particular psychotropic agents (eg, sedatives, hypnotics, antidepressants, and neuroleptics). These medications are useful for treating the depression, anxiety, and behavioral problems that are not unusual in the long-term care resident. However, their use presents an ongoing treatment challenge.

The practitioner is often pressured by family members and nursing staff to "do something" when the elderly patient's behavior becomes difficult and unmanageable. At one time, psychotropics such as haloperidol (Haldol) were used to control behavior chemically. In 1987, the Omnibus Budget Reconciliation Act (OBRA) was enacted. Strict regulations were introduced to prevent inappropriate psychotropic drug use in long-term care, and compliance with the regulations is strictly monitored (Katz & Karuza, 2003).

Antipsychotics

Psychotropic drugs, such as the antipsychotics, are appropriately intended to treat schizophrenia, hallucinations, and violent behaviors that pose the potential for physical harm. Environmental and organic causes of aberrant behavior need to be ruled out before prescribing an antipsychotic, and all nonpharmacologic means should be explored *before therapy begins* (American Geriatric Society & American Association for Geriatric Psychiatry, 2003). Consulting with a geropsychiatrist regarding psychotropic management is recommended. In addition, monthly chart reviews are performed to evaluate side effects and the necessity of using psychotropic drugs. Long-term care facilities are subject to citation and loss of licensure for inappropriate use of psychotropic or chemical restraints.

The host of side effects of psychotropic agents makes monitoring the elderly resident receiving psychotropic therapy imperative. Extrapyramidal symptoms (EPSs), tardive dyskinesia, dystonic reactions, and anticholinergic effects can be severe. Older drugs, such as haloperidol, fluphenazine (Prolixin), and trifluoperazine (Stelazine), have a greater propensity to cause EPSs.

The newer, atypical antipsychotic agents (ie, serotonin–dopamine antagonists) are better tolerated and are associated with fewer side effects than the older agents. Advantages include less tardive dyskinesia and fewer EPSs, although risperidone (Risperdal) has a greater dose-related response for EPSs. Increased weight gain and the potential for metabolic changes are common with the atypical antipsychotics. Somnolence, which usually subsides, may occur with initial titration of risperidone and olanzapine (Zyprexa). Frail elderly patients may experience more sedation with quetiapine (Seroquel). Risperidone should be avoided or used cautiously with patients who have Parkinson disease because of their greater potential for EPSs.

One of the newest atypical antipsychotics for the treatment of psychosis in patients with Alzheimer disease is aripiprazole (Abilify), a partial dopamine agonist. Somnolence, the most common side effect, is dose related (Jeste Schneider et al., 2003).

For patients exhibiting hyperactivity, aggression, increased motor activity, and excitability and inability to tolerate the usual antipsychotics, the anticonvulsants divalproex (Depakote), carbamazepine (Tegretol), oxcarbazepine (Trileptal), and lamotrigine (Lamictal) are being used with greater frequency. Hyponatremia or syndrome of inappropriate antidiuretic hormone (SIADH) has been associated with carbamazepine and oxcarbazepine. Caution should be used with divalproex in patients with hepatic impairment (Espinoza & Eslami, 2004). Lamotrigine has been associated with serious and life-threatening rashes (toxic epidermal necrolysis or

Stevens-Johnson syndrome) in 0.3% of adults, usually within 2 to 8 weeks of treatment initiation (Burdick & Goldberg, 2002; Espinoza & Eslami, 2004).

Anxiolytics

Anxiety is a problem frequently confronted in the nursing home setting. It may be precipitated by physical causes such as pain, infection, or chronic illness. Other stressors that contribute to anxiety include fatigue and change, such as a change in a daily routine or change of caregiver. An overly stimulating environment or expectations of staff members hurrying the elderly resident through daily routines may evoke anxiety. Initially, nonpharmacologic measures should be used to assess and ameliorate anxiety; prescribing a medication to relieve anxiety should be a last choice.

Several nonpharmacologic antianxiety treatments may be beneficial. They include establishing daily routines in a structured environment, consistently providing the same caregiver for bathing and hygiene assistance, avoiding overstimulation from activities, limiting social visits, and scheduling quiet time with rest or nap periods (Flint, 2001).

When anxiolytic drugs are prescribed, the benzodiazepines are often chosen for patients 65 years of age and older. Unfortunately, side effects are prevalent, among which are the discomforts of discontinuing the therapy. The patient may experience increased agitation, anxiety, and insomnia. More serious symptoms include tremors, tachycardia, diaphoresis, nausea, vomiting, and alterations in perception, anterograde amnesia, and seizures. The benzodiazepines have a propensity for dependence by accumulating in the elderly body. For this reason they should be prescribed for short courses of up to 2 weeks at most (Pontillo et al., 2002).

The elderly patient receiving benzodiazepine therapy often experiences significant daytime sedation, dizziness, and subsequent falls. Studies indicate the "oldest old," those older than 85 years of age, have a 15-fold increased risk of falls with benzodiazepine use. When a benzodiazepine with a long half-life is prescribed, the fall rate is 10-fold greater than when a benzodiazepine with a short to moderate half-life is prescribed (Caramel et al., 1998). Benzodiazepines with a long half-life include diazepam and flurazepam (Dalmane); benzodiazepines with a shorter half-life include lorazepam (Ativan), alprazolam (Xanax), and oxazepam (Serax). When a benzodiazepine is prescribed, it should have a short half-life, be for short-term use, and be given in the lowest dose possible.

The selective serotonin reuptake inhibitors (SSRIs), which treat depression, general anxiety, and panic and obsessive–compulsive disorders are now considered the better choice for treating anxiety in the frail elderly due to their favorable side effect profile (Sheikh & Cassidy, 2003). There is often comorbid depression with anxiety, so an SSRI may treat both conditions, such as paroxetine (Paxil) for panic and depression (Pontillo et al., 2002).

An alternative anxiolytic is buspirone (BuSpar). It is nonsedating, has minimal drug interactions and a slow onset of action, 2-3 weeks. For that reason it is not indicated for acute anxiety but works well as an add-on drug (Flint, 2001). Caution must be used with buspirone in patients with Parkinson disease because EPS symptoms can occur. For anxiety with underlying depression and insomnia, trazodone (Desyrel) is an alternative. Because of its sedating properties, it promotes sleep and treats underlying depression that may exacerbate anxiety (Pontillo et al., 2002).

Antidepressants

The prevalence of depression increases with age, as evidenced by a 25% to 30% rate of depression among residents in long-term care. In such settings, elderly patients with depression should be treated because antidepressant treatment usually improves nutrition and function and decreases symptoms of pain and insomnia (Lantz, 2001). Better choices for antidepressants include the SSRIs (eg, paroxetine, fluoxetine [Prozac], sertraline [Zoloft], citalopram [Celexa]) and escitalopram [Lexapro]. The SSRIs have the advantage of daily dosing and fewer side effects than TCAs, which were used frequently before the advent of SSRIs. Although the TCAs are still used, they are associated with many side effects that can lead to cognitive impairment and falls. Cardiovascular effects include hypotension, arrhythmias, and sudden death. Other troublesome side effects include sedation, dry mouth, urinary retention, and dizziness from anticholinergic properties.

Significant drug interactions and toxicity may occur with SSRI use because these drugs inhibit oxidative metabolism. Drugs that may be affected by SSRIs include warfarin, phenytoin, and class 1C antiarrhythmics (Lavretsky, 2001). Studies indicate that older adults taking SSRIs have a greater risk of falls than older adults not taking antidepressants (Leipzig et al., 1999). Hyponatremia has been increasingly noted to occur in elderly patients on SSRIs. On withdrawal of the SSRI, sodium levels return to normal within days to weeks (Kirby & Ames, 2001). The prescriber needs to be aware of early signs of hyponatremia: lethargy, fatigue, muscle cramps, anorexia, and nausea.

Other Disorders and Drug Therapies

Pain medications such as narcotic analgesics should be avoided to reduce the risk of confusion, delirium, and falls. Acetaminophen (Tylenol) is often sufficient to reduce pain and discomfort. Propoxyphene (Darvon), which is frequently overused, causes many central nervous system effects and should be avoided in the nursing home (Caracci, 2002).

The chronic pain of degenerative joint disease unrelieved by acetaminophen can be treated with an NSAID. Long-term treatment with NSAIDs can result in GI bleeding, anemia, and renal insufficiency. The cyclooxygenase 2 (COX-2) inhibitors, celecoxib (Celebrex), and valdecoxib (Bextra) are nontraditional anti-inflammatory drugs developed to prevent GI bleeding by not affecting platelet aggregation and bleeding. Although the risk of bleeding with COX-2 inhibitors may be lower than traditional NSAIDs such as naproxen or ibuprofen, it can still occur (Luggen, 2003). Cardiovascular safety concerns about rofecoxib (Vioxx) led to its removal from the market. The other two COX-2 inhibitors are being reevaluated for safety as well.

Other commonly encountered drug-related problems in long-term care are urinary incontinence and recurrent urinary tract infections, evidenced by confusion and mental status changes. Respiratory infections such as bronchitis and pneumonia quickly spread through a facility because of the compromised immune state of frail residents. Thus, antibiotic use is called on more frequently than for the community-residing adult. The frail elderly patient with pneumonia may not have typical signs of illness. For example, the patient may not have a cough or a fever. Moreover, the frail elderly patient becomes ill more quickly and decompensates rapidly if untreated. Dehydration, sepsis, or even death may result.

Constipation is another concern, and sometimes an obsession, of elderly patients. In many instances, they think they need medications to promote bowel movements. However, alternate methods of treating this problem may be judicious, including increasing physical activity and consumption of fluids, fiber, and fruit. One or two tablespoons of a mixture of prune juice, unprocessed bran, and applesauce taken daily are an alternative to stool softeners and laxatives. When assessing constipation, a review of current medications may yield clues to drug use that contributes to the constipation. For example, anticholinergics, such as oxybutynin (Ditropan) used for urinary incontinence; antidepressants, such as the TCAs; and calcium channel blockers may all cause constipation in the frail elderly patient.

In summary, the elderly resident in long-term care is usually the frailest and at greatest risk for complications related to improper drug administration. The health care provider should attempt to keep medications at a minimum with the lowest dosage possible. A monthly or bimonthly review of all medications should be done to review medical necessity. A pharmacist from within the facility or from the company supplying the facility with medications should routinely review charts and write recommendations to decrease or stop medications. The suggestions should be evaluated by the health care provider and acted on if appropriate to reduce polypharmacy, side effects, and costs for the resident.

GUIDELINES FOR SAFE PRESCRIBING

The goal of prescribing for patients in long-term care should be to prevent adverse events, falls, and injuries that will further degrade the patient's function, both physical and mental. The provider must prescribe cautiously and keep the patient's safety in mind while promoting his or her comfort and dignity. Providers in long-term care need to familiarize themselves with the Beers criteria, a consensus-based document listing potentially inappropriate medications for use in elderly patients and guidelines for safe prescribing practices. This extensive list of medication guidelines was created by a consensus panel of nationally recognized experts in geriatrics and updated in 2002 (Fick et al., 2003).

Exploring Alternatives to Medication

The health care provider must evaluate new problems and determine if a medication is necessary as part of the treatment plan. If there are alternatives to medications, such as diet, exercise, and weight loss for borderline hypertension,

or antiembolism stockings instead of a diuretic for pedal edema, these options should be explored. Only after non-pharmacologic treatments fail should a medication be initiated. In knowing the patient's overall situation—physically, mentally, and socially—the provider has a baseline from which to consider the risks and benefits of medication therapy. Table 6-4 lists 20 medications that should not be prescribed to any elderly patient (General Accounting Office, 1995). All of the drugs in this table are also present in the 2002 Beers Criteria (Fick et al., 2003) except for phenylbutazone, which is no longer marketed.

Choosing Drugs Efficiently

When deciding on a medication for an older adult, a drug that treats two coexisting conditions should be considered. For example, a calcium channel blocker might be selected for the patient with angina and hypertension. An elderly man with hyperplasia of the prostate and hypertension may benefit from an α-adrenergic blocking agent such as terazosin (Hytrin). Treating two conditions with one medication reduces cost, cuts down on dosing schedules, and improves adherence and patient satisfaction.

Simplifying the Regimen

Simplifying the medication plan is a key to therapeutic adherence and safety. Drugs are started at the lowest dose possible and the dosage increased as needed (Routledge et al., 2003). Lower doses are often effective and reduce the risk of toxicity. Dosing schedules must be easy to follow and remember. If two drugs are equally suitable to treat the same condition, it is desirable to prescribe the one that requires the least frequent dosing.

Another important concern is cost of the drug, especially if the drug is for long-term use. Many elderly patients are on fixed incomes and find the cost of prescription drugs unaffordable. If the most suitable medication for the condition is expensive, this is explained to the patient before purchase to prevent "sticker shock" or the embarrassment of not having enough money to pay for the prescription. A generic drug should be prescribed whenever possible.

Educating Patients and Caregivers

Potential side effects of new medications need to be discussed in a nonthreatening way so that the patient is not frightened by anticipating a side effect that may not occur. The media are powerful in alarming patients about potentially undesirable or dangerous adverse effects, proven or not. Many older patients stop taking essential medications after reading or hearing something in the media pertaining to that particular drug.

Reviewing Medications

The provider working with a geriatric population should have the patient bring in all of his or her medications to each office visit or review a current medication card if the patient carries one. The current medications taken by the patient are recorded at each office visit as part of the progress note. This review alerts the provider to improper dosing and drug administration,

Table 6.4

Twenty Drugs to Avoid in Elderly Patients

Prescription Drug	Use	Reason for Avoiding
amitriptyline	To treat depression	Other antidepressant medications cause fewer side effects.
carisoprodol	To relieve severe pain caused by sprains and back pain	Minimally effective while causing toxicity. Potential for toxic reaction is greater than potential benefit.
chlordiazepoxide	To tranquilize or to relieve anxiety	Shorter-acting benzodiazepines are safer alternatives.
chlorpropamide	To treat diabetes	Other oral hypoglycemic medications have shorter half-lives and do not cause inappropriate antidiuretic hormone secretion.
cyclandelate	To improve blood circulation	Effectiveness is in doubt. This drug is no longer available in the United States.
cyclobenzaprine	To relieve severe pain caused by sprains and back pain	Minimally effective while causing toxicity. Potential for toxic reaction is greater than potential benefit.
diazepam	To tranquilize or to relieve anxiety	Shorter-acting benzodiazepines are safer alternatives.
dipyridamole	To reduce blood clot formation	Effectiveness at low dosage is in doubt. Toxic reaction is high at higher dosages. Safer alternatives exist.
flurazepam	To induce sleep	Shorter-acting benzodiazepines are safer alternatives.
indomethacin	To relieve the pain and inflammation of rheumatoid arthritis	Other nonsteroidal anti-inflammatory drugs cause fewer toxic reactions.
isoxsuprine	To improve blood circulation	Effectiveness is in doubt.
meprobamate	To tranquilize	Shorter-acting benzodiazepines are safer alternatives.
methocarbamol	To relieve severe pain caused by sprains and back pain	Minimally effective while causing toxicity. Potential for toxic reaction is greater than potential benefit.
orphenadrine	To relieve severe pain caused by sprains and back pain	Minimally effective while causing toxicity. Potential for toxic reaction is greater than potential benefit.
pentazocine	To relieve moderate to severe pain	Other narcotic medications are safer and more effective.
pentobarbital	To induce sleep and reduce anxiety	Safer sedative–hypnotics are available.
phenylbutazone	To relieve the pain and inflammation of rheumatoid arthritis	Other nonsteroidal anti-inflammatory drugs cause fewer toxic reactions.
propoxyphene	To relieve mild to moderate pain	Other analgesic medications are more effective and safer.
secobarbital	To induce sleep and reduce anxiety	Safer sedative–hypnotics are available.
trimethobenzamide	To relieve nausea and vomiting	Least effective of the available antiemetics.

(From General Accounting Office. [1995]. *Prescription drugs and the elderly: Many still receive potentially harmful drugs despite recent improvements* [HEHS-95–152]. Washington, DC: Author.)

misunderstanding of medications, and changes made by specialists and other professionals. The specialist is not always aware of all the medications or OTC drugs the patient takes and may prescribe a drug that places the patient at risk for interactions. As part of the review, the health care provider should ask about topical creams, vitamins, eye drops, and OTC products that may interact with prescription drugs. Patients do not always view these products as medications.

The provider should review all drugs periodically to determine if the dosage can be reduced or the drug discontinued. The goal should always be to use as little medication as possible to treat the multiple illnesses that challenge the older adult.

At the end of each office visit, the provider needs to give the medication list to the patient. Doses and times to take the medications and any special instructions need to be clearly stated and communicated in writing as appropriate. New medications should be listed by brand and generic name so there is no confusion. Clear writing with large lettering should be used, particularly if the patient has common vision impairments, such as cataracts, glaucoma, or macular degeneration.

The caps of the medication bottles that the patient brings to the office can be labeled with the reason for the drug (eg, "blood pressure," "water pill," or "diabetes"). This helps to ensure that the patient has a basic understanding of the importance of each drug. If the caregiver of an older patient is available, the provider should explain any new medication changes or special instructions, especially for the patient with cognitive impairment or other changes in mental status.

THERAPEUTIC MONITORING

When memory problems are an issue, a medication planner helps. Labeled with the days of the week and four dosing times per day, the planner is a useful device for preparing medications for a week. A patient who fails to take the medications despite visual cues and careful labeling may be sending a signal that the family or other responsible caregivers need to investigate additional interventions, home care services, or future placement in assisted living or long-term care facilities.

It is important routinely to schedule and monitor the results of laboratory tests when the patient is taking medications that may result in fluctuating drug blood levels. For example, elderly patients taking such drugs as warfarin, theophylline (Theo-Dur), digoxin, and quinidine (Quinaglute) need careful monitoring, as do patients taking anticonvulsant medications, such as phenytoin, carbamazepine (Tegretol), and valproic acid (Depakote), for seizure disorders.

Patients taking diuretics or angiotensin-converting enzyme (ACE) inhibitors require periodic evaluation with a renal profile to detect electrolyte imbalances, as well as renal insufficiency (as evidenced by rising blood urea nitrogen [BUN] and creatinine levels). Patients starting ACE inhibitor therapy should have a baseline BUN/creatinine level documented with a follow-up test in 2 weeks to alert for renal artery stenosis (evidenced by a rise in the BUN/creatinine levels). Because of the potential for elevations in serum potassium concentration with ACE inhibitor therapy, the elderly need routine renal profiles to detect such changes, especially when

BOX 6–3. GUIDELINES FOR SAFE PRESCRIBING FOR ELDERLY PATIENTS

- Schedule routine follow-up examinations for the patient who has multiple chronic illnesses and who takes multiple medications.
- Review the risks and benefits of adding a medication. Explore nonpharmacologic options first.
- If possible, choose one medication that treats two coexisting problems.
- Always start with the lowest dose possible and titrate up slowly. "Start low; go slow."
- Choose a drug with the fewest daily required doses (ie, daily vs. twice daily).
- Remember to consider the cost of the brand name drug and consider generic equivalents if cost issues will deter compliance.
- Reduce dosages or discontinue medications if possible to avoid polypharmacy.
- Advise patients to bring all medications (prescription or over-the-counter) to each office visit for review.
- Write down all current medications and dosages on the progress note for each office visit.
- Review medications added by other practitioners and specialists. Inform these professionals of changes made by the primary health care provider.
- Give a written list to the patient after each office visit of the medications to be taken.
- Write written medication instructions and changes in large print.
- Explain and write both the generic and brand name of the prescribed drug to avoid confusing the patient.
- Review medications and changes in the regimen with the caregivers of patients with cognitive impairments.
- Recommend or provide medication planners or weekly/daily dosage containers to improve compliance and promote safe medication administration.
- Schedule blood tests regularly to monitor levels of such medications as diuretics, ACE inhibitors, antiseizure medications, anticoagulants, antiarrhythmics, and digitalis.

drug therapy also includes diuretics and digoxin (Lanoxin). Box 6-3 presents guidelines for prescribing drugs safely for elderly patients.)

Bibliography

Starred references are cited in the text.

*American Psychiatric Association. (1994). *Diagnostic and statistical manual of mental disorders* (4th ed.). Washington, DC: Author.

*American Geriatric Society & American Association for Geriatric Psychiatry. (2003). Consensus statement on improving the quality of mental health care in U.S. nursing homes: Management of depression and behavioral symptoms associated with dementia. *Journal of the American Geriatric Society, 51*(9), 1287–1298.

*Bennett, W. M., Aranoff, G. R., Golper, T. A., et al. (1991). *Drug prescribing in renal failure: Dosing guidelines for adults* (2nd ed.). Philadelphia: American College of Physicians.

*Burdick, K., & Goldberg, J. (2002). Cognitive advantages of new anticonvulsants in treating a geriatric population. *Clinical Geriatrics, 10* (10), 25–36.

*Caracci, G. (2003). The use of opioid analgesics in the elderly. *Clinical Geriatrics, 11*(11), 18–21.

*Caramel, V., Remarque, E., Knook, D., et al. (1998). Benzodiazepine users aged 85 and older fall more often. *Journal of the American Geriatric Society, 46*(9), 1178–1179.

*Chutka, D., Takahashi, P., & Hoel, R. (2004). Inappropriate medications for elderly patients. *Mayo Clinic Proceedings, 79*(1), 122–139.

*Cooke, C., & Proveaux, W. (2003). A retrospective review of the effect of COX-2 inhibitors on blood pressure change. *American Journal of Therapeutics, 10*(5), 311–317.

*Cusack, B., & Vestel, R. (2000). Clinical pharmacology. In M. Beers & R. Berkow (Eds.), *The Merck manual of geriatrics* (3rd ed., pp. 54–74). Whitehouse Station, NJ: Merck Research Laboratories.

*Eslami, M., & Espinoza, R. (2003). Update on treatment for Alzheimer's disease-Part 1: Primary treatments. *Clinical Geriatrics, 11*(12), 42–49.

*Espinoza, R., & Eslami, M. (2004). Update on treatment for Alzheimer's disease-Part II: Management of noncognitive, psychiatric, and behavioral complications. *Clinical Geriatrics, 12*(1), 45–53.

*Fick, D., Cooper, J., Wade, W., et al. (2003). Updating the Beers criteria for potentially inappropriate medication use in older adults. *Archives of Internal Medicine, 163*, 2716–2724.

*Flint, A. (2001). Anxiety disorders. *Clinical Geriatrics, 9*(11), 21–30.

*General Accounting Office. (1995). *Prescription drugs and the elderly: Many still receive potentially harmful drugs despite recent improvements* (HEHS-95-152). Washington, DC: Author.

*Guralnik, J., & Havlik, R. (2000). Demographics. In M. Beers & R. Berkow (Eds.), *The Merck manual of geriatrics* (3rd ed., pp. 9–21). Whitehouse Station, NJ: Merck Research Laboratories.

*Herrick, T. (2004). The long-awaited Medicare overhaul: The prescription drug benefit. *Clinician News, 8*(2), 25.

*Horowitz, M. (2000). Aging and the gastrointestinal tract. In M. Beers & R. Berkow (Eds), *The Merck manual of geriatrics* (3rd ed., pp. 1000–1052). Whitehouse Station, NJ: Merck Research Laboratories.

*Jeste, D., Schneider, L., De Deyn, P., et al. (2003). Atypical antipsychotics for the management of patients with dementia and psychotic symptoms. *Clinical Geriatrics & Annals of Long-Term Care* (Suppl.), December.

*Juurlink, D., Mamdani, M., Kopp, A., et al. (2003). Drug-drug interactions among elderly patients hospitalized for drug toxicity. *Journal of the American Medical Association, 289*(13), 1652–1658.

*Kasper, J., & Burton, L. (2003). Demography. In E. Flaherty, T. Fulmer, & M. Mezey (Eds), *Geriatric nursing review syllabus* (pp. 7–12). New York: American Geriatric Society.

*Katz, P., & Karuza, J. (2003). Nursing-home care. In E. Flaherty, T. Fulmer, & M Mezey (Eds.), *Geriatric nursing review syllabus* (pp. 97–102). New York: American Geriatric Society.

*Kelleher, C., & Lindeman, R. (2003). Renal diseases and disorders. In E. Flaherty, T. Fulmer, & M. Mezey (Eds.), *Geriatric *nursing review syllabus* (pp. 357–365). New York: American Geriatric Society.

*Kirby, D., & Ames, D. (2001). Hyponatremia and selective serotonin re-uptake inhibitors in elderly patients. *International Journal of Geriatric Psychiatry, 16*(5), 484–493.

*Lantz, M. (2001). Depression in the elderly: Recognition and treatment. *Clinical Geriatrics, 10*(10), 18–24.

*Lantz, M. (2002). Alcohol abuse in the older adult. *Clinical Geriatrics, 10*(2), 40–42.

*Lavretsky, H. (2001). Choosing appropriate treatment for geriatric depression. *Clinical Geriatrics, 9*(5), 30–46.

*Leipzig, R., Cumming, R., & Tinetti, M. (1999). Drugs and falls in older people: A systematic review and meta-analysis: Psychotropic drugs. *Journal of the American Geriatric Society, 47*(1), 30–39.

*Logue, R. (2002). The impact of advanced practice nursing on improving medication adherence in the elderly: An educational intervention. *American Journal for Nurse Practitioners, 6*(5), 9–15.

*Luggen, A. (2003). Arthritis in older adults. *Advance for Nurse Practitioners, 11*(3), 26–35.

*Meiner, S. (1997). Polypharmacy in the elderly. *Advance for Nurse Practitioners, 5*(7), 26–34.

*Miller, C. (2004) *Nursing for wellness in older adults: Theory and practice* (4th ed., pp. 503–537). Philadelphia: Lippincott Williams & Wilkins.

Murray, M., & Callahan, C. (2003). Improving medication use for older adults: An integrated research agenda. *Annals of Internal Medicine, 139*(5), 425–428.

*National Institute on Alcohol Abuse and Alcoholism. (1998). Alcohol and aging. *Alcohol Alert No. 40.* Bethesda, MD.

*Oslin, D. (2003). Substance abuse. In E. Flaherty, T. Fulmer, & M. Mezey, (Eds.), *Geriatric nursing review syllabus* (pp. 234–239). New York: American Geriatric Society.

*Peterson, A. M., & Dragon, C. J. (1998). Improving medication compliance in patients receiving home care. *Home HealthCare Consultant, 5*(9), 25–27.

Physicians desk reference. (1998). Montvail, NJ: Medical Economics.

*Pontillo, D., Lang, A., & Stein, M. (2002). Management and treatment of anxiety disorders in the older patient. *Clinical Geriatrics, 10*(10), 38–49.

*Rollason, V., & Vogt, N. (2003). Reduction of polypharmacy in the elderly. *Drugs & Aging, 20*(11), 817–832.

*Routledge, P., Mahony, M., & Woodhouse, K. (2003). Adverse drug reactions in elderly patients. *British Journal of Clinical Pharmacology, 57*(2), 121–126.

*Semla, T., & Rochon, P. (2003). Pharmacotherapy. In E. Flaherty, T. Fulmer, & M. Mezey (Eds.), *Geriatric nursing review syllabus* (pp. 35–42). New York: American Geriatric Society.

*Sheikh, J., & Cassidy, E. (2003). Anxiety disorders. In E. Flaherty, T. Fulmer, & M. Mezey (Eds). *Geriatric nursing review syllabus* (pp. 220–223). New York: American Geriatric Society.

*van Doorn, C., Gruber-Baldini, A., Zimmerman, S., et al. (2003). Dementia as a risk factor for fall and fall injuries among nursing home residents. *Journal of the American Geriatric Society, 51*(9), 1213–1218.

Visit the Connection web site for the most up-to-date drug information.

PRINCIPLES OF PHARMACOLOGY IN PAIN MANAGEMENT

■ ANDREW M. PETERSON AND PAUL MILLER

One of the most widely encountered clinical situations is the patient in pain. It is also one of the most difficult aspects of care. Pain is a subjective response to noxious stimuli and its intensity varies from patient to patient, day to day. The clinician has a large array of medications available to assist patients in relieving their pain, and this chapter describes the principles of pain management and introduces the student to the many types and classes of drugs available for the practicing nurse.

Analgesics represent one of the most frequently prescribed and administered classes of medications. Managing pain in the acutely or chronically ill patient requires both a sound comprehension of the clinical pharmacology of analgesics and a clear understanding of the patient's perception of pain. Clinicians caring for chronically ill patients not only find themselves assisting the patient in dealing with the physical component of pain, but often are confronted by the patient's psychological, spiritual, and social perceptions of pain and pain medication.

Age is often a major consideration in achieving pain relief. For example, elderly patients are less likely to complain about pain and therefore request fewer analgesics to alleviate pain. A corollary exists in pediatric patients, whose inability to express adequately their suffering led some clinicians to believe that children could not feel pain. Clinicians, however, now realize that pediatric patients experience as much pain as adults. Because of the identified communication barrier, clinicians need to use special techniques to assess and understand children's pain.

TYPES OF PAIN

Pain can be classified into two categories, which first helps to identify the derivation of pain and then provides a framework for treatment. The two types of pain based on onset and duration are acute and chronic. Pain can also be classified and subsequently treated based on specific symptoms.

Acute Pain

Acute pain has a sudden onset, usually subsides in a short period of time and is characterized by sharp, localized sensation with an identifiable cause. Surgical intervention and trauma are commonly identified sources of pain. Often, acute pain is a natural physiologic response to injury, useful in warning individuals of diseases or harmful situations. This process is often seen as a signal that the body is invoking critical immunologic and physiologic responses to cellular or tissue damage. Concomitant physiologic responses include excessive sympathetic nervous system activity, such as tachycardia, diaphoresis, and increased respiratory rate. When acute pain responses become unremitting, constant, or undertreated, these biologic responses outlive their usefulness and lead to additional undesired consequences such as anxiety or depression. Avoiding the progression to a chronic state of pain is an underlying goal of acute pain management. However, the primary goal is an amelioration of the pain.

Chronic Pain

Chronic pain is arbitrarily defined as pain lasting longer than 3 to 6 months, although some argue that chronic pain begins sooner than after 3 months of continuous pain. Further classification of chronic pain is based on the taxonomy of malignancy. *Chronic nonmalignant pain* comes in a variety of forms, including, but not limited to, rheumatoid arthritis and osteoarthritis, pain originating in nerve tissue, or reflex sympathetic dystrophy. *Chronic malignant pain* is associated with a cancer, where the pain may be due to the cancer tissue itself or damage to secondary tissue. The pain is often found in alternative sites (eg, bone pain).

It is important to differentiate between these different types of pain through careful history of the location, quality, and nature of the pain because treatment is dictated by the cause and type of pain. In any case, the primary goal of therapy in chronic pain is to decrease the pain to a tolerable level so the patient may function in daily life.

Chronic Nonmalignant Pain

In the past, chronic nonmalignant pain was called *chronic benign pain*, a name that belies its dangerous effects. Most pain syndromes can be classified into several categories:

BOX 7–1. CLASSIFICATION OF CHRONIC PAIN

Nociceptive Pain
Arthropathies (eg, rheumatoid arthritis, osteoarthritis, gout)
Ischemic disorders
Myalgia (eg, myofacial pain syndromes)
Nonarticular inflammatory disorders (eg, polymyalgia rheumatica)
Skin and mucosal ulcerations
Visceral pain

Neuropathic Pain
Painful diabetic polyneuropathy
Postherpetic neuralgia
Poststroke pain (central pain)
Trigeminal neuralgia

Mixed or Undetermined Pathophysiology
Chronic recurrent headaches
Painful vasculitis

nociceptive pain, neuropathic pain, and mixed or undetermined pain. This classification system, with examples, is shown in Box 7-1. Nociceptive pain may be visceral (arising from internal organs) or somatic (arising from skin, bones, joints, muscles) and is most often derived from stimulation of pain receptors. Nociceptive pain may arise from tissue inflammation, mechanical deformation, ongoing injury, or destruction. Nociceptive mechanisms usually respond well to traditional approaches to pain management, including common analgesic medications and nonpharmacologic strategies. Neuropathic pain is described by patients as radiating, burning, or tingling, which is due to abnormal processing of sensory input by the nervous system. Neuropathic pain is often resistant to opioid therapy; therefore, alternative treatment choices including anticonvulsants and tricyclic antidepressants (TCAs) may need to be considered.

Chronic Malignant Pain

The causes of cancer pain can include pain induced by the disease and pain secondary to treatment. The disease-induced pain includes pain secondary to direct tumor involvement of bone, nerves, viscera, or soft tissue. In addition, muscle spasm, muscle imbalance, or other body structure/function changes secondary to the tumor are considered disease induced. Commonly, treating cancer using techniques such as surgery, chemotherapy, radiation therapy, or immunotherapy can induce significant and long-lasting chronic pain.

Cancer and its treatment may activate peripheral nociceptors, causing somatic and visceral nociceptive pain. Cancer and its treatment can also induce neuropathic pain that may involve the sympathetic nervous system, thereby maintaining the perception of pain.

PAIN TRANSMISSION

Several theories exist as to how pain is registered in the brain as an occurrence. The signal transmission can occur through one or more of the proposed mechanisms described.

Gate Theory

The most widely accepted hypothesis about the nature of pain is known as the gate theory. In essence, the gate theory of pain suggests that a combination of neurons in the dorsal horn regulates the transmission of pain signals to the brain. Small pain-conducting fibers transmit the signal of injury (extreme heat, cold, mechanical injury) to areas of the higher brain centers such as the thalamus and limbic system. The transmission conducted by these fibers is regulated by larger *mechanofibers*; if these fibers are stimulated (through pressure, electrical stimulation, or other counterirritant), the original perception of pain is diminished. In a sense, these fibers close the pain gateway (Fig. 7-1).

Chemical Mediators

Coupled with the neuronal component of pain is the release of chemical mediators initiating or continuing the stimulation of small pain-conducting fibers. These chemical mediators include the neurotransmitters acetylcholine and histamine, and polypeptides such as bradykinin, prostaglandins (PGs), and substance P. These substances play a role in the pain pathway as neurotransmitters or neuromodulators. Blocking the production of these substances, particularly inhibiting the production of PG with aspirin or similar compounds, minimizes the pain signal, hence the perception of pain. Regardless of their role, these chemicals are sources of pain transmission and are targets for many of the drugs used to treat pain.

Pain-Modulating Receptors

Tolerance for pain varies widely and may be due to individual production of endogenous pain-relieving substances such as enkephalins and endorphins. Today, β-endorphin is considered the most important of these endogenous analgesics. Secondary to a painful stimulus or stressor, β-endorphin is released by the pituitary gland into the bloodstream or by specific neurons containing high concentrations of the substance.

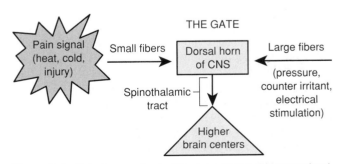

Figure 7–1 Gate theory of pain. When a pain signal is transmitted to the dorsal horn, small pain-conducting fibers carry this signal to higher brain centers. This signal transmission can be attenuated through stimulation of the large fibers, closing the gate to the pain signal and transmitting the large-fiber signal.

Once released, β-endorphin stimulates inhibitory neuronal receptors known as the opioid receptors. Stimulation of these receptors, particularly the *mu* (μ) receptor, inhibits the transmission of pain signals to and from the higher brain centers. These receptors are also stimulated by morphine-like drugs (opiates) and therefore account for a great deal of the pain relief associated with opioid analgesics.

In contrast, neuropathic pain syndromes do not respond to conventional analgesic therapy as predictably as nociceptive pain. However, they have been noted to respond to unconventional analgesic drugs such as TCAs, anticonvulsants, or antiarrhythmic agents. Mixed or unspecified pain is often regarded as having mixed or unknown mechanisms. Response to treatment of these syndromes is more unpredictable and may require various trials of different or combined approaches.

GENERAL PRINCIPLES OF PAIN MANAGEMENT

Treatment of pain in today's society rests on two major principles: appropriate assessment of the severity and intensity of the pain and selection of the most appropriate agent to relieve pain with minimal side effects.

Pain Assessment

The assessment of each patient's pain is extremely important for determining proper treatments as well as determining their effectiveness over time. According to the National Institutes for Health, self-reporting by patients is "the most reliable indicator of the existence and intensity of pain." Along with self-reporting, it may also be helpful to involve a patient's caregiver in assessing pain, especially for the very young or older patients when other factors may affect communication. The self-report should include a description of the pain; its location, intensity/severity, and aggravating and relieving factors; and the patient's cognitive response to pain. It is best to work with brief, easy-to-use assessment tools that reliably document pain intensity and pain relief and to relate these to other dimensions of pain, such as mood. One routine clinical approach to pain assessment and management is summarized by the mnemonic ABCDE (Box 7-2). It is also important to note that assessment tools should be used both initially to obtain a baseline as well as throughout therapy to monitor progress.

Because pain is very subjective and is not easily quantifiable, several tools are available to determine the quantity and quality of a patient's pain. The various pain scales can be classified as single or multidimensional and self-report or observational. Common single-dimension tools include the visual analog scale (VAS), numeric rating scales (NRSs), and verbal description scales (VDSs; Fig. 7-2). The single-dimension scales evaluate only one aspect of pain, which is intensity, whereas multidimensional scales also consider location, pattern, and affective effects. Examples of multidimensional scales include the Brief Pain Inventory and the McGill Pain Questionnaire.

The information gleaned, particularly from the numeric and visual analog scales, can be used in determining treatment and drug selection. Both the Agency for Health Care Policy and Research (AHCPR) and the World Health Organization

(WHO) have published guidelines on the appropriate evaluation and treatment of acute and chronic pain. Both organizations suggest using a 10-point scale to assess a patient's current level of pain. A "0" defines a pain-free state, and a "10" describes the most severe pain ever experienced by the patient. The WHO defines pain rated at 1 to 4 as mild; 5 to 6 as moderate; and 7 to 10 as severe.

Subsequent assessments should evaluate the effectiveness of the treatment plan and, if pain is unrelieved, determine whether the cause is related to the progression of disease, a new cause of pain, or the cancer treatment. The assessment of the patient's pain and the efficacy of the treatment plan should be ongoing, and the pain reports should be documented. Continued use of the same pain scale is crucial to the continued assessment of treatment progress and communication between health care providers.

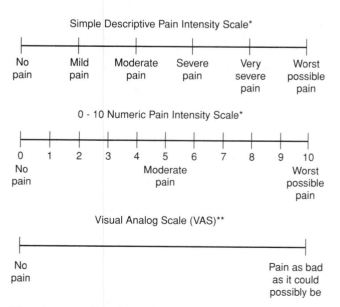

Figure 7–2 Visual analog scales used for ranking pain.

BOX 7–3. PAIN CONTROL OPTIONS

Cognitive–Behavioral Therapy
Relaxation
Imagery

Physical Agents
Massage
Heat or cold applications

Transcutaneous Electrical Nerve Stimulation (TENS)

Medications
Nonnarcotic Agents
Acetaminophen
NSAIDs
Local anesthetics

Narcotic Agents
Systemic administration
Patient-controlled analgesia
Spinal analgesia

Pain Management

The options available to control pain are listed in Box 7-3. These options include nonpharmacologic and pharmacologic treatment. Often, a combination of treatments is necessary to reduce the pain to a tolerable level or eliminate it completely. The goals of any pain therapy include relieving pain, maintaining patient function, and maximizing the patient's quality of life. All of these should be accomplished with a minimum of side effects.

An essential principle in using medications to manage chronic pain is to individualize drug regimens according to the type and severity of pain. When at all possible, however, the oral route should be considered as first-line therapy because this is the least invasive pain management modality.

For mild to moderate pain, acetaminophen (Tylenol), aspirin, or a nonsteroidal anti-inflammatory drug (NSAID) is usually considered initial therapy. Acetaminophen is used for mild pain across all age groups, mainly due to its favorable side effect profile. NSAIDs are among the most widely prescribed drugs in the world. Newer agents known as cyclooxygenase-2 (COX-2) inhibitors (celecoxib, rofecoxib, and valdecoxib) are commonly prescribed they have fewer gastrointestinal (GI) side effects.

For pain that persists or increases, an opioid, such as codeine or hydrocodone (Vicodin), can be added to the regimen. Pain management for moderate to severe pain begins with a more potent opioid, such as morphine, hydromorphone (Dilaudid), or fentanyl (Duragesic), and can be administered with acetaminophen or an NSAID. The concurrent use of opioids and an NSAID or acetaminophen often provides more analgesia than either of the drug classes alone.

When developing a treatment plan, members of the health care team should pay particular attention to the preferences and needs of patients whose education or cultural traditions may impede effective communication. Certain cultures have strong beliefs about pain and its management, and members of these cultures may hesitate to report unrelieved pain or may have specific preferences for pain-relieving measures. When developing a treatment plan, clinicians should be aware of the unique needs and circumstances of patients from different age groups or various ethnic and cultural backgrounds.

Certainly, pharmacologic treatment is the most common modality in pain control; however, nonpharmacologic options have been evaluated. Behavioral therapy, including systematic approaches to coping strategies, has been used to help control pain. Other, nonpharmacologic, approaches include the use of physical therapies such as heat, massage, and muscle stretching. Transcutaneous electrical nerve stimulation (TENS) therapy has also been used to help control certain types of pain.

Drug Therapy by Type of Pain

The AHCPR suggests that mild to moderate pain be treated with step 1 drugs (Table 7-1). Examples of step 1 drugs include acetaminophen, aspirin, and NSAIDs. Maximal doses of these drugs should be used before proceeding to opioid analgesics.

Step 2 drugs, such as codeine, hydrocodone, oxycodone, and propoxyphene, are commonly used to treat moderate pain. These drugs are restricted to this use because their side effects are dose limiting or they are usually prepared in combination with nonopioid analgesics (eg, oxycodone/acetaminophen or hydrocodone/acetaminophen).

Severe pain is most commonly treated with step 3 drugs, of which morphine is the classic example. When used in equivalent doses, most pure opioids can be used as step 3 drugs. These include morphine, oxycodone, hydromorphone, fentanyl, and meperidine. Morphine is considered the gold standard and it should be considered as the first step 3 drug for use in all patients, including elderly patients.

In all cases, pain medications should be administered around the clock, and as-needed medications used to treat "breakthrough" pain. This recommendation is based on the finding that regularly scheduled medications maintain a constant level of drug in the body and help prevent a recurrence of pain.

Table 7.1

Recommended Order of Treatment for Pain

Kind of Pain	Agent(s)	Comments
Mild to moderate	acetaminophen, aspirin, NSAIDs	Maximum doses should be used before proceeding to opioid analgesics.
Moderate to severe	codeine, hydrocodone, oxycodone, propoxyphene	Usually prepared in combination with nonopioid analgesics. Side effects are dose limiting.
Severe	morphine, oxycodone, hydromorphone, fentanyl, meperidine	Morphine is the gold standard and the first step 3 drug in all patients, including the elderly

An essential principle in using medications to manage chronic pain is to individualize drug regimens according to the type and severity of pain. When at all possible, however, the oral route should be considered as first-line therapy. In most cases, this is the least invasive pain management modality. For mild to moderate pain, acetaminophen, aspirin, or an NSAID is usually considered initial therapy. For pain that persists or increases, an opioid, such as codeine or hydrocodone, should be added. Management for moderate to severe pain should begin with a more potent opioid, such as morphine, hydromorphone, or fentanyl, which can be administered with acetaminophen or an NSAID. The concurrent use of opioids and an NSAID or acetaminophen often provides more analgesia than either of the drug classes alone (Table 7-2).

Acute Pain

Acetaminophen is the drug of choice for treating minor, non-inflammatory pain, especially in patients prone to gastric damage. In addition, NSAIDs are effective as monotherapy in mild to moderate pain and are often used in combination with opioids in treating severe pain.

The opioids as a class generally exhibit equal analgesic effects when given at equipotent doses (adjusted for route of administration and duration of action). Although propoxyphene possesses analgesic activity, it has been shown to be no more effective than codeine or aspirin. Pentazocine is effective in relieving moderate pain but is less effective than morphine in relieving severe pain. Oxycodone is a mild analgesic, and the combination of oxycodone and acetaminophen or aspirin has no advantage over the combination of codeine with acetaminophen or aspirin.

Chronic Pain

Nonmalignant

The NSAIDs and salicylates, including aspirin, are effective for chronic inflammatory conditions, such as arthritis, and musculoskeletal conditions. Efficacy of NSAID treatment varies greatly among patients. Those who do not respond to one NSAID in one class may respond to an NSAID from the same or a different class. The opioids should be considered as an alternative or an addition to NSAID therapy in chronic nonmalignant pain. Administration of a lower-potency opioid in conjunction with an NSAID is a beginning to therapy. Combination products (eg, Tylenol with codeine) should be avoided when opioids are used adjunctively with NSAIDs.

Although still controversial, the role of opioids in treating chronic nonmalignant pain is becoming increasingly accepted. However, they have little efficacy in neuropathic pain. Care should be taken when administering opioids to the elderly because of the chance of sedation, cognitive impairment, and constipation. Physical dependence and addiction should not be the overriding considerations when choosing a pain modality for elderly patients.

Malignant

The WHO outlines an approach to the management of cancer pain. The titration of therapy for cancer pain using this method has been effective in relieving pain for approximately 90% of patients with cancer pain (AHCPR, 1994; WHO, 1996). With this "ladder" approach, the first step is acetaminophen, aspirin, or NSAIDs. Patients with moderate to severe pain should be started at the second or third step of the ladder. If pain persists or increases, codeine or hydrocodone should be added to the regimen. As pain continues to increase or persist, substituting higher-potency opioids or increasing the dose is the next consideration. Levorphanol and methadone should not be used in treating chronic pain in elderly patients because their long half-lives and potency make dose titration difficult and frequently cause oversedation and toxicity.

DRUGS USED IN PAIN MANAGEMENT

The current pharmacotherapeutic options for pain management include the nonnarcotic (nonopioid) and the narcotic (opioid) agents. Nonnarcotic analgesics include agents such as acetaminophen, salicylates, and NSAIDs. The narcotic analgesics include opioids such as oxycodone, morphine, and fentanyl. Selection of which agent to use rests on an assessment of the patient's type and source of pain as well as the intensity level of the pain.

Nonopioid Analgesics

The nonnarcotic analgesics are considered first-line therapy in treating of mild and mild to moderate pain (Table 7-3). All are effective at decreasing pain, and many have the added benefit of anti-inflammatory action. These agents each have an onset of analgesia within 1 hour of oral administration, and drug effects last anywhere from 4 to 12 hours. The agents can be classified by their mechanism of action, inhibition of PG synthesis, and mediation of pain through opioid receptor activity. Aspirin, salicylates, and, to a lesser extent, acetaminophen are inhibitors of PG synthesis, and they mediate pain through this pathway.

Acetaminophen

Acetaminophen is one of the most commonly prescribed analgesic–antipyretic medications. It is an effective alternative to aspirin. Acetaminophen's antipyretic activity comes from its direct action on the hypothalamic heat-regulating center to increase the dissipation of heat through increased vasodilation and perspiration. The analgesic activity is mediated through PG inhibition in the central nervous system (CNS); however, its lack of peripheral PG inhibition makes it a weak anti-inflammatory agent and it is therefore not considered useful in treating inflammatory disorders such as rheumatoid arthritis.

Acetaminophen is almost completely absorbed from the GI tract and thus has an onset of action ranging from 30 to 45 minutes. Its extensive liver metabolism to inactive substances makes it a relatively nontoxic agent. However, a small portion (4%) of the drug is converted to a toxic metabolite, normally inactivated by glutathione pathways. If glutathione stores are depleted, as seen in cases of chronic ingestion or acute overdosage, the toxic metabolite can cause potentially fatal liver necrosis. Acetaminophen toxicity should be considered when a single ingestion exceeds

Table 7.2

Pharmacokinetic and Pharmacodynamic Properties of Narcotic Analgesics

Pain Type	Generic Name	Trade Name(s)	Onset of Analgesia (min)	Half-life (h)	Duration of Analgesia (h)	Route	Equinanalgesia Dose (mg)	Usual Starting Dose
Mild–moderate	codeine	various	15–30	2–4	4–6	IM, PO	130 / 200	60 mg q3–4h (PO)
	hydrocodone	Vicodin,* others	NA	4	4–8	PO	5–10	10 mg q4h
	propoxyphene	Darvon,† Darvocet, others	30–60	6–12	4–6	PO	130	
	pentazocine	Talwin	15–20	4–5	3	IM, SQ / PO	30–60 / 120–180	50 mg q6h (PO)
	butorphanol	Stadol	<10	2.5–4	3–4	IM	2	
	nalbuphine	Nubain	<15	2–5	3–6	IM	10	
	buprenorphine	Buprenex	15	2–3	6	IM	0.3–0.6	
	dezocine	Dalgan	15–30	2.4	2–4	IM	10	
Moderate–severe	oxycodone	Percocet,‡ Percodan,‖ others	15–30	3–4	4–5	PO	30	10 mg q4h
	oxymorphone	Numorphan	5–15	2–3	4–6	IM, SQ / PO	1 / 5	1 mg q4h (IM)
Severe	morphine	Various	15–60	2–4	3–7	IM, SQ / PO	10 / 30–60	10 mg q4h (IM) / 30 mg q4h (PO)
	hydromorphone	Dilaudid	15–30	2–3	4–5	IM, SQ / PO	1.5 / 7.5	1.5 mg q4h (IM) / 6 mg q4h (PO)
	levorphanol	Levo-Dromoran	30–90	12–16	6–8	IM, SQ / PO	2 / 4	2 mg q6–8h (IM) / 4 mg q6–8h (PO)
	methadone	Dolophine, others	30–60	15–40	4–5 (acute) / >8§ (chronic)	IM / PO	10 / 10–20	10 mg q6–8h (IM or PO)
	fentanyl	Duragesic	up to 24 h	1.5–6	48–72	Transdermal	100 µg/h = 60 mg PO morphine	25 µg patch q72h
	meperidine	Demerol, others	10–45	2–4	2–4	IM, SQ / PO	75 / 300	100 mg q3h (IM) / Oral not recommended

*Combination product, hydrocodone and acetaminophen.
†Combination product, propoxyphene and acetaminophen.
‡Combination product, oxycodone and acetaminophen.
§Due to accumulation.
‖Combination product, oxycodone and aspirin.

Table 7.3

Pharmacokinetic and Pharmacodynamic Properties of Nonnarcotic Analgesics

Generic Name	Trade Name(s)	Dosage Forms	Half-life (h)	Onset of Analgesia (h)	Duration of Analgesia (h)	Route	Usual Starting Dosage	Maximum Daily Dose
acetaminophen	Tylenol, others	Tablet, suspension, elixir, suppository	6–7	0.5–0.75	3–5	PO, PR	650 mg q4–6h	4000 mg
aspirin	Bayer, Excedrin, others	Tablet	0.25–0.33 (2–3 salicylic acid)	0.5–0.75	3–5	PO	650 mg q4–6h	4000 mg
tramadol	Ultram	Tablet	6–7	1	5–7	PO	50–100 mg q6h	400 mg
salsalate	Disalcid, others	Capsule/tablet	2–3	NA	NA	PO	750–1000 mg bid	
magnesium salicylate	Original Doan's, others	Capsule/tablet	2–3	NA	NA	PO	650 mg q4h	
choline magnesium salicylate	Trilisate	Tablet	2–12	NA	NA	PO	1000 mg bid	
diflunisal	Dolobid	Tablet	8–12	1	8–12	PO	1 g load, then 500 mg q8–12h	1500 mg

140 to 200 mg/kg or chronic use exceeds 10 days with usual doses. Generally, the maximum daily dose of acetaminophen should not exceed 4000 mg.

Nonsteroidal Anti-inflammatory Drugs

The NSAIDs are divided into a variety of chemical classes. Their physical and chemical properties determine their distribution in the body and, therefore, lead to different therapeutic responses. Despite the difference in chemical class, the NSAIDs as a group exert their action through the same mechanism. All NSAIDs have anti-inflammatory, analgesic, and antipyretic activity because of their ability to inhibit cyclooxygenase, an enzyme necessary for PG synthesis. Many NSAIDs inhibit both cyclooxygenase-1 (COX-1) and cyclooxygenase-2 (COX-2). Most NSAIDs including aspirin, ketoprofen, and indomethacin inhibit both enzymes but are mostly selective for COX-1. Ibuprofen and naproxen are considered slightly selective for COX-1, whereas others, including etodolac and nabumetone, may be considered slightly selective for COX-2. Newer agents, known as the COX-2 inhibitors, primarily block COX-2, and at therapeutic concentrations do not inhibit COX-1, therefore decreasing GI side effects. Similarly, acetaminophen inhibits cyclooxygenase, but does not act peripherally; it lacks anti-inflammatory activity. Aspirin irreversibly inhibits platelet cyclooxygenase; however, other salicylates (choline magnesium trisalicylate, choline salicylate, sodium salicylate, magnesium salicylate, and salsalate) reversibly inhibit platelet cyclooxygenase, like NSAIDs.

All NSAIDs are highly protein bound. Lower doses should be used in elderly patients to adjust for the decline in renal function due to aging. A significant analgesic effect is achieved within 1 hour of NSAID administration, with maximal effects within 2 or 3 hours.

Long-term use of NSAIDs at high doses (anti-inflammatory doses) can cause serious adverse effects. The most common, potentially serious side effects are those affecting the kidney and GI tract. The newer COX-2 inhibitors have less GI toxicity; however, risk for renal adverse events is similar to traditional NSAIDs. Indomethacin (Indocin) is associated with more CNS adverse effects than other NSAIDs. NSAID-induced anemia can occur although the incidence is very low. If anemia is suspected in patients on long-term therapy, the clinician needs to determine hemoglobin and hematocrit values and consider discontinuing therapy. Aspirin is associated with a high incidence of adverse GI effects. Aspirin and NSAIDs should be taken with food or milk to minimize GI distress. Unlike NSAIDs, acetaminophen, choline magnesium trisalicylate, and salsalate have minimal GI toxicity and no effect on platelet aggregation at usual doses. See Chapter 41 for more discussion of NSAIDs and acetaminophen.

Opioids

Opioids bind to one of the four opiate receptors: mu (μ), kappa (κ), sigma (σ), or delta (δ). An analgesic effect is associated with binding to μ and κ receptors. Full agonists, acting at μ, κ, and possibly δ receptors, include morphine, hydrocodone, hydromorphone, levorphanol (Levo-Dromoran), fentanyl, methadone (Dolophine), meperidine (Demerol), propoxyphene (Darvon), codeine, and oxycodone. Pentazocine (Talwin) is a partial agonist–antagonist of opioid receptors. Tramadol (Ultram) is a weak agonist of all opioid receptors, inhibiting norepinephrine reuptake and causing serotonin release.

Activation of the μ opioid receptor produces excellent analgesia as well as undesired effects, including respiratory depression, euphoria, mydriasis, and sedation. Morphine and other μ opioid receptor agonists provide excellent pain relief over a broad dosage range. At equianalgesic doses and appropriate dosing intervals, there is no appreciable difference in pain relief among all of the opioid agents. The described potency is only a reflection of the dose needed to achieve a desired level of analgesia; the more potent the agent, the fewer milligrams needed (Table 7-4).

All opioids are hepatically metabolized to active and inactive metabolite, which are eliminated in the urine. Meperidine is metabolized to an active metabolite, normeperidine,

Table 7.4

Pain Receptors and Their Biologic Effects

Receptor	Biologic Response to Stimulation
Mu (μ)	Respiratory depression, physical depression, tolerance, constipation, euphoria, miosis
Kappa (κ)	Spinal-level analgesia and sedation, without respiratory depression, miosis
Sigma (σ)	Vasomotor stimulation, psychotomimetic effects, miosis

which can accumulate and induce seizures with high doses or in patients with decreased renal function. Propoxyphene also is metabolized to an active metabolite, norpropoxyphene, which has a half-life of approximately 34 hours; metabolism is decreased in elderly patients, and accumulation of both propoxyphene and the active metabolite can occur.

The analgesic effects of opioids begin within 30 to 60 minutes and reach peak effect within 1 to 2 hours. Short-acting opioids include propoxyphene (2–3 hours) and meperidine (2–4 hours). Moderate-acting opioids, with duration of actions between 4 and 6 hours, include morphine, codeine, hydromorphone, levorphanol, and oxycodone. Methadone is considered a long-acting opioid with a duration of action of approximately 24 to 36 hours in elderly patients.

Morphine and Congeners

Morphine is a low-cost, readily available agent with well-characterized pharmacokinetic and pharmacodynamic properties. Morphine is absorbed erratically from the GI tract, and it undergoes significant first-pass hepatic metabolism when given by this route. Morphine is distributed throughout the body, and sufficient amounts cross the blood–brain barrier to account for most of its pharmacologic effects. Morphine has a plasma half-life of approximately 3 hours, which is due mainly to its nearly complete metabolism in the liver. Morphine crosses the placental barrier well and is excreted in maternal milk.

Morphine may be administered orally, rectally, by injection, intrathecally, or intraspinally. The agent is available in short-acting, immediate-release dosage forms (tablets and liquid) and sustained-release tablets, such as MS Contin. Single-dose studies suggest that the oral dose is six times the parenteral dose, but with multiple doses the oral dose is three times the parenteral dose. This is due to the accumulation of an active metabolite, 6-morphine glucuronide, which has a longer half-life than the parent drug.

Morphine effectively relieves severe pain, particularly dull, chronic pain, regardless of its cause or anatomic source. Analgesia is due to the drug's effects in the CNS and spinal cord. Morphine not only alleviates pain but alters the perception of pain, so that discomfort is less distressing or more tolerable.

Therapeutic doses of morphine can cause respiratory depression. Low doses mainly depress respiratory depth, whereas higher doses also depress rate. This effect is due both to the drug's actions on the brain's medullary respiratory control center and to the drug's ability to suppress the medulla's response to blood carbon dioxide levels. Tolerance develops to respiratory depression. A person in whom tolerance has developed may experience only slight effects after receiving doses that could cause serious or fatal respiratory depression in a nontolerant person.

Morphine also increases smooth muscle tone in various parts of the GI tract. Stimulation of intestinal κ receptors results in reduced peristalsis and increased tone of the rectal sphincter. The overall effect of increased smooth muscle tone is constipation.

Hydromorphone is considered more potent and more soluble than morphine; however, it has a similar pharmacologic profile. Hydromorphone is available in both tablet and injection forms.

Oxycodone is similar to morphine except that it is less potent. Although it may be used alone, it is more commonly used in combination with nonopioid analgesics, such as aspirin and acetaminophen, for the reduction of moderate pain. Oxycodone is also available as a sustained-release tablet that is used to treat severe chronic pain, such as the pain associated with cancer.

Codeine is usually administered orally either alone or in combination with nonopioid analgesics, such as aspirin or acetaminophen, for mild to moderate pain. It is also an effective antitussive agent. Codeine has more of a stimulant effect on the CNS than morphine. This stimulatory effect of codeine is due to the formation of the metabolite norcodeine.

Codeine salts are well absorbed orally and have a higher oral bioavailability than morphine; this is reflected by the fact that codeine has the lowest oral-to-parenteral dose ratio of all the injectable opioid analgesics. However, codeine has few advantages over morphine as an analgesic. The liability for drug dependence with this compound appears to be less than that of morphine, but at equianalgesic doses, codeine induces greater histamine release than morphine. This increases the risk of hypotension, cutaneous vasodilation, urticaria, and bronchoconstriction. Hydrocodone, which is a derivative of codeine, is often used in combination with nonnarcotic analgesics and has a similar profile to codeine.

Meperidine and Congeners

Meperidine and fentanyl are the most commonly used alternatives to morphine and its congeners. These agents offer low to no cross-allergenicity in patients hypersensitive to morphine-like drugs, yet, at equianalgesic doses, they offer similar pain relief. Other agents, such as sufentanil (Sufenta) and alfentanil (Alfenta), also fall in this class, but are used primarily for perioperative and postoperative pain relief and are available only in an injectable form.

Meperidine is a highly effective and commonly used synthetic analgesic that binds strongly to both μ and κ receptors. It is less potent than morphine. Most of the pharmacologic effects of this drug are similar to those of morphine sulfate, with the following exceptions: (1) high-dose meperidine may cause CNS excitation characterized by tremors and seizures, (2) it induces a lower incidence of constipation than morphine, and (3) the drug has little effect on the cough reflex.

Meperidine has an oral bioavailability of approximately 50% and distributes similarly to other opioids. Meperidine appears to be more rapidly acting than morphine, and one of its metabolites, normeperidine, is approximately one-half as active as an analgesic as the parent compound. The CNS excitation seen after large doses of meperidine can be attributed to the accumulation of the normeperidine metabolite.

The half-life of normeperidine ranges between 15 and 20 hours; the metabolite is almost completely renally eliminated. The possibility of accumulation of this metabolite leading to detrimental CNS effects makes meperidine almost contraindicated in patients with renal impairment.

Fentanyl is available in as an injectable agent for intramuscular administration (Sublimaze), a transdermal patch (Duragesic), and a lollipop (Actiq) for oral administration. The transdermal patch is not indicated for acute pain management because of the kinetic characteristics of the delivery system. The drug delivery system of the patch deposits a concentration of fentanyl in the upper skin layers, where the drug becomes available to the systemic circulation. The patches are designed to deliver a near-constant rate of drug to the skin at rates of 25, 50, 75, and 100 mg/h, although individual skin type and metabolism may vary. Peak systemic concentrations occur between 24 and 72 hours after initial application of the patch. The patch remains on the patient for 72 hours, after which it is exchanged for a fresh patch. After several sequential patches, the patient achieves a steady-state systemic concentration. After removal of the patch, serum concentrations fall by one half in 13 to 22 hours (average, 17 hours).

Methadone-Like Agents

Methadone and propoxyphene are in yet another chemical class and can therefore be used as alternatives to the morphine- and meperidine-like drugs in cases of hypersensitivity. However, the long half-life of methadone and the purported lack of efficacy of propoxyphene make these agents less favorable.

Methadone hydrochloride is effective both parenterally and orally and has an oral bioavailability exceeding 90%. It is more than 90% bound to plasma and tissue proteins and is extensively metabolized in the liver to inactive products. The drug, which has a long half-life, nearly 40 hours in some patients, accumulates on repeated administration. Patients with reduced renal or hepatic function should be monitored carefully for signs of drug accumulation or toxicity. The long biologic half-life probably accounts for the mild, but prolonged, withdrawal syndrome if drug use stops abruptly. Methadone is used in treating severe pain. In addition, it is indicated for detoxification of opioid-dependent people.

Mixed Opioid Agonists–Antagonists

The mixed agonist–antagonist agents include pentazocine, butorphanol (Stadol), buprenorphine (Buprenex), dezocine (Dalgan), and nalbuphine (Nubain). These are indicated for moderate to severe pain and apparently have a ceiling effect on respiratory depression. The pharmacology of the agents suggests that at therapeutic doses, there is an agonistic effect on the μ receptor, which produces analgesia. However, at higher doses, these agents create an antagonistic activity, diminishing the analgesic effect and, in some cases, potentially precipitating a withdrawal syndrome. These agents were once thought to have little to no addictive properties because of their antagonistic activity, However, a low abuse potential does exist. Nalbuphine and dezocine are not controlled substances, and butorphanol has recently been listed as a Schedule 4 drug.

The advantages of using these agents comprise the lower abuse potential and the lower risk of respiratory depression. The drawbacks include the psychotomimetic effects, the ceiling analgesic effect, and the withdrawal-like syndrome seen particularly in narcotic-dependent patients.

Opioid Antagonists

Naloxone (Narcan) and naltrexone (ReVia) are pure opioid antagonists that competitively bind to all opioid receptors without producing an analgesic response. Naloxone is inactivated when given orally and therefore is given only by injection. Naloxone is indicated for treating narcotic-induced respiratory depression (known or suspected), whereas naltrexone is indicated for the adjunct maintenance of opioid-free states in detoxified patients.

The half-life of naloxone ranges between 60 and 90 minutes in adults and up to 3 hours in neonates. However, the duration of drug action is approximately 45 minutes. In most cases, this duration is shorter than the offending narcotic action and the overdose effect from the offending narcotic usually returns, requiring readministration of naloxone.

Conversely, naltrexone is well absorbed after oral administration but undergoes extensive first-pass metabolism, resulting in only 5% to 20% of the administered agent reaching systemic circulation. Naltrexone is metabolized to an active metabolite, which also contributes to the pharmacologic activity. The half-life of the parent compound is approximately 4 hours and 13 hours for the active metabolite. A careful drug history and even a naloxone challenge should be administered to a patient under consideration for naltrexone therapy. The patient should be narcotic free for 7 to 10 days before naltrexone is administered. Baseline liver function tests should be obtained and values monitored frequently during therapy.

The side effects of naloxone include tachycardia and hypertension, ventricular fibrillation, and even cardiac arrest. Seizures have been reported, particularly in patients addicted to medications. Insomnia, anxiety, hepatotoxicity, and headache are common in patients taking naltrexone.

Central Analgesic Agents

Tramadol is a centrally acting, nonnarcotic agent that weakly and predominantly binds to the μ receptor. It is chemically unrelated to both the opiates and the NSAIDs. Overall, tramadol has an advantage over opioids for treating chronic pain, but it may be very useful for acute pain in patients for whom an opioid is not a viable option and an NSAID may introduce undue risk (eg, GI bleed). It has little propensity for abuse and tolerance and is indicated for moderate to moderately severe pain. Tramadol is rapidly absorbed, and peak serum levels, which are obtained within 2 hours, persist for 4 to 6 hours. Tramadol is metabolized in the liver to an active metabolite (O-dimethyl tramadol) and the elimination half-life is approximately 5 hours. Tramadol is also available in combination with acetaminophen as Ultracet.

Safety of Opioids

Side effects common to all opioids include sedation, euphoria, and GI disturbances. The GI disturbances are primarily constipation and nausea, presumably due to stimulation of the κ opioid receptors located in the GI tract, which, when stimulated, decrease peristalsis and lead to constipation. Although considered the most dangerous side effect, severe respiratory depression is rarely seen in patients without underlying pulmonary dysfunction. Other important contraindications related to respiratory depression include closed head injury or recent brain surgery. The increase in intracranial pressure, cerebral vasodilation, and hypotension associated with these conditions can decrease brain tissue oxygenation and exacerbate injury.

Opioid Dependence

Opioid tolerance develops when chronic use of opioids causes the need for increased doses to maintain analgesia. Tolerance and physical dependence on opioids can develop quickly. Even patients taking the medication as briefly as 2 or 3 days can experience mild withdrawal symptoms on discontinuation. These symptoms range from mild tremors to sweating and fever, and mimic flulike symptoms. Severe withdrawal, from chronic users or abusers, may consist of increased respiratory rate, perspiration, lacrimation, mydriasis, hot and cold flashes, and anorexia.

The drug-seeking behavior often seen in the patient with chronic pain may result from a worsening of the pain rather than a tolerance to the drug action. Apparent tolerance in a patient with chronic pain should not impede aggressive therapy.

Tolerance to the effects of opioids is not necessarily a sign of substance abuse or addiction. The concept of substance abuse with respect to opioids is an important consideration, but beyond the scope of this chapter.

Adjunctive Agents

Several medications have been evaluated for use either alone or in conjunction with other analgesics to treat many persistent pain conditions. This can include many types of pain; however, specific agents have been proven beneficial in neuropathic pain and postoperative pain. TCAs have been useful particularly in patients with diabetes or postherpetic neuropathy. The exact mechanism behind their effects in not fully understood; however, it is believed to be partially due to effects on serotonin and norepinephrine uptake. Several agents have beneficial effects in neuropathic pain, including amitriptyline, desipramine, imipramine, clomipramine, doxepin, and maprotiline. It is important to remember the anticholinergic side effects with TCAs, most commonly glaucoma, urinary retention, confusion, and sedation; these should be monitored especially in the elderly population.

Another group of agents commonly prescribed for diabetic neuropathy and postherpetic or trigeminal neuralgia includes the anticonvulsants. The most common agents used are carbamazepine, valproic acid, and phenytoin. Common side effects include sedation drowsiness and confusion and should be monitored closely. Recently the use of gabapentin has been increasing due to less adverse events. Gabapentin has been shown to be effective in diabetic neuropathy, postherpetic or trigeminal neuralgia, restless legs syndrome, phantom limb and stump pain, and pain after a stroke. Generally doses are started at 100 to 300 mg once daily and titrated up to 1800 to 3600 mg daily in three divided doses. To date, no evidence has indicated that gabapentin would be useful for acute musculoskeletal pain, chronic musculoskeletal strain, or tendinitis. The common side effects associated with gabapentin include dizziness, somnolence, and peripheral edema. Caution should be taken in patients also receiving morphine because CNS depression could occur due to increased gabapentin concentrations; thus, the dose of morphine may need to be reduced.

Skeletal Muscle Relaxants

Several drugs are used to relieve symptoms of acute musculoskeletal disorders such as whiplash, muscle sprains, or athletic injury. Many of these disorders are accompanied by spasm and pain. Most of the drugs used to treat these disorders are given orally and are indicated for short-term use adjunctively with bed rest and an individualized physical therapy plan. Many of the drugs are available in narcotic/nonnarcotic fixed-dose combinations to provide multiple drug actions. All these drugs cause CNS depression as a side effect, and their effects are potentiated by other CNS depressants, including alcohol.

Peripherally Acting Skeletal Muscle Relaxants

These drugs interfere with the transmission of cholinergic impulses between the somatic motor neurons and skeletal fibers at the neuromuscular junction. They usually produce paralysis of the skeletal muscles involved. Another term for these agents is neuromuscular-blocking agents. They are used principally as adjuncts to general anesthetics and in minor surgical procedures or shock therapy. These agents are not used in the acute or chronic treatment of pain. Examples of these agents include succinylcholine (Anectine) and vecuronium (Norcuron).

Centrally Acting Skeletal Muscle Relaxants

The aim of centrally acting skeletal muscle relaxants is to produce decreased muscle tone and involuntary movement without loss of voluntary motor function or consciousness. These drugs either act directly on the contractile mechanism of the skeletal musculature or on transmission in spinal cord motor reflex pathways, primarily to elicit varying degrees of skeletal muscle relaxation. They are used to afford a degree of relief from muscle spasms and hyperreflexia resulting from conditions such as inflammation, anxiety, stress, and other neurologic disorders.

Commonly used agents are described in Table 7-5. There are few differences in efficacy among these agents, and selection is usually based on past experience, cost, and formulary status. Carisoprodol (Soma) is a congener of meprobamate and has a similar onset of action (30 minutes) and a similar duration of action (4–6 hours). However, carisoprodol is available only in an oral form, compared with the oral and intravenous forms of methocarbamol (Robaxin).

Cyclobenzaprine (Flexeril) is structurally related to the TCAs. As such, it is contraindicated for use in patients taking monoamine oxidase inhibitors, in the acute recovery phase of a myocardial infarction, or with arrhythmias or significant heart block. The onset of action of cyclobenzaprine

Table 7.5

Overview of Selected Skeletal Muscle Relaxants

Generic (Trade) Name and Dosage	Selected Adverse Events	Contraindications	Special Considerations
cyclobenzaprine (Flexeril) Usual dose: 10 mg tid to a maximum of 60 mg/d	Anticholinergic effects, drowsiness	Use cautiously in glaucoma, hyperthyroidism, arrhythmias, congestive heart failure, acute recovery phase of myocardial infarction	Geriatric—not recommended Pediatric—safety and efficacy in children <15 y old is not established Unknown
carisoprodol (Soma) Usual dose: 350 mg tid	GI upset, drowsiness	Acute intermittent porphyria	Not recommended for use in children younger than 12 y
chlorzoxazone (Paraflex, Parafon Forte) Usual dose: 1 tablet 3–4 times/d May be increased to 750 mg 3–4 times/d	May impair mental and physical abilities; driving and operating machinery not recommended	Intolerance to chlorzoxazone	May cause GI irritation Decrease dosage as improvement occurs
methocarbamol (Robaxin) Usual dose: 1.5 g qid initially; reduce to 750 mg/d	May impair mental and physical abilities; driving and operating machinery not recommended	Contraindicated in patients with renal dysfunction	Pregnancy category B
metaxalone (Skelaxin) Usual dose: 800 mg 3–4 times/d	May impair mental and physical abilities; driving and operating machinery not recommended		Pregnancy category B Use cautiously in anemia, renal or hepatic impairment Liver function studies should be done regularly
tizanidine (Zanaflex) Usual dose: 4 mg q6–8h Do not exceed 36 mg in 24 h	Somnolence, dry mouth, dizziness	Hypersensitivity to tizanidine	Limited experience in long-term use or doses >8 mg

is approximately 1 hour and its effects can last up to 12 hours. However, the drug is often given three times daily to ensure efficacy during the day. When the drug is considered for use in elderly patients, its anticholinergic properties also must be taken into account, particularly dry mouth, drowsiness, dizziness, and constipation.

Tizanidine (Zanaflex) is a newer, centrally acting, α_2-adrenergic agonist, putatively reducing spasticity by increasing presynaptic inhibition of motor neuron excitation. The peak effect occurs within 1 to 2 hours of oral administration and lasts 3 to 5 hours. It has an oral bioavailability of approximately 40% because of first-pass metabolism. The half-life of the agent is approximately 2.5 hours, and clearance is delayed by a factor of four in elderly patients.

Diazepam (Valium) is also used as a centrally acting skeletal muscle relaxant. It is indicated for relief of skeletal muscle spasm caused by inflamed muscles or joints and upper motor neuron disorders such as cerebral palsy. Dosing is similar to that for anxiety. For more information, see Chapter 45.

Baclofen (Lioresal) is indicated for managing signs and symptoms of spasticity resulting from multiple sclerosis and for spinal cord injuries or diseases. It is available as an oral tablet. An injectable form for intrathecal administration is available for severe spasticity. Common side effects of the oral form include drowsiness, hypotension, weakness, nausea and vomiting, and headache. Intrathecal administration results in hypotension, somnolence, dizziness, constipation, and headache. Respiratory depression and difficulty with concentration or coordination are also seen with intrathecal administration.

Many CNS depressants (alcohol, barbiturates) elicit varying degrees of muscle relaxation but are of little use clinically because they also produce marked sedation and addiction. Attempts to dissociate this CNS depressant action from the muscle-relaxing effect by synthesis of various centrally acting muscle relaxants has met with limited success, and all currently useful muscle relaxants evoke a degree of sedation that makes their long-term use undesirable.

Their advantage over neuromuscular blockers is their oral efficacy; their disadvantages are the sedation and sensorimotor impairment that accompany their use.

Centrally acting muscle relaxants are similar in pharmacology and toxicology. No one drug possesses a significant therapeutic advantage over any other agent.

Bibliography

*Starred references are cited in the text.

*Agency for Health Care Policy and Research, United States Department of Health and Human Services, Public Health Service. (1994). *Management of cancer pain.* Rockville, MD: Author.

Amadio, P., Jr., Cummings, D. M., & Amadio, P. (1993). Nonsteroidal anti-inflammatory drugs: Tailoring therapy to achieve results and avoid toxicity. *Postgraduate Medicine, 93*(4), 73–76, 79–81, 85–86, 88, 93–97.

Ballantyne, J. C., & Mao J. (2003). Opioid therapy for chronic pain. *New England Journal of Medicine, 349*(20), 1943–1953.

Beers, M. H., & Berkow, R. (Eds.). (1999). *Merck manual of diagnosis and therapy* (17th ed.). Whitehouse Station, NJ: Merck.

Bushnell, T. G., & Justins, D. M. (1993). Choosing the right analgesic: A guide to selection. *Drugs, 46,* 394–408.

Carns, P., Stang, H., Kaye, C., et al. (2004). *Assessment and management of acute pain.* (4th ed.). Bloomington, MN: Institute for Clinical Systems Improvement.

Clive, D. M., & Stoff, J. S. (1984). Renal syndromes associated with nonsteroidal anti-inflammatory drugs. *New England Journal of Medicine, 310,* 563–572.

Cepeda M.S., et al. (2003). Side effects of opioids during short-term administration: Effect of age, gender, and race. *Pharmacodynamics and drug action,* 74(2), 102–112.

Cuny, C.J., et al. (1979). Pharmacokinetics of salicylate in elderly. *Gerontology, 25,* 49–55.

Ivey, K. J. (1983). Gastrointestinal effects of antipyretic analgesic. *American Journal of Medicine, 75,* 53–64.

Kane, F. J., & Pokorny, A. (1975). Mental and emotional disturbance with pentazocine (Talwin) use. *Southern Medical Journal, 68,* 808–811.

Lazarus, H., et al. (1990). A multi-investigator clinical evaluation of oral controlled-release morphine (MS Contin®) administered to cancer patients. *Hospice Journal, 6,* 1–15.

Levy, G. (1965). Pharmacokinetics of salicylate elimination in man. *Journal of Pharmaceutical Sciences, 54,* 959–967.

McEvoy, G. K., & Litvak, K. (Eds.). (2004). *AHFS drug information 04.* Bethesda, MD: American Society of Hospital Pharmacists.

Moreland, L. W., & St. Clair, E. W. (1999). The use of analgesics in the management of pain in rheumatic diseases. *Rheumatic Diseases Clinics of North America, 25,* 153–191.

Nikolaus, T., & Zeyfang, A. (2004). Pharmacological treatments for persistent non-malignant pain in older persons. *Drugs & Aging, 21,* 19–41.

Olin, B.R., et al. (Eds.). (2000). *Drug facts and comparisons.* St. Louis: Lippincott Williams & Wilkins.

Ortho-McNeil Pharmaceutical. (1997). *Product information: ULTRAM® (Tramadol hydrochloride tablets).* Raritan, NJ: Author.

Pasternak, G. W. (1987). Morphine 6-glucuronide, a potent mu agonist. *Life Science, 41,* 2845–2849.

Portenoy, R. K. (1996). Opioid therapy for chronic nonmalignant pain: A review of the critical issues. *Journal of Pain and Symptom Management, 11,* 203–217.

Ripamonti, C., & Dickerson, E. D. (2001). Strategies for the treatment of cancer pain in the new millennium. *Drugs, 61,* 955–977.

Vickers, M.D., et al. (1992). Tramadol: Pain relief by opioid without depression of respiration. *Anesthesia, 47,* 291–296.

Von Feldt, J. M., & Ehrlich, G. E. (1998). Pharmacologic therapies. *Physical Medicine and Rehabilitation Clinics of North America, 9,* 473–487.

Wall, R. T. (1990). Use of analgesics in the elderly. *Clinics in Geriatric Medicine, 6,* 345–364.

Wang, R. I. H., & Sandoval, R. G. (1971). The analgesic activity of propoxyphene napsylate with and without aspirin. *Journal of Clinical Pharmacology, 11,* 310–317.

Washington Department of Labor and Industries, Washington State Medical Association. (2002). *Guideline for the use of Neurontin in the management of neuropathic pain.* Seattle: Washington Department of Labor and Industries, Washington State Medical Association.

Willcox, S. M., Himmelstein, D. U., & Woolhandler, S. (1994). Inappropriate drug prescribing for the community-dwelling elderly. *Journal of the American Medical Association, 272,* 292–296.

World Health Organization (1990). Cancer pain relief and palliative care: Report of a WHO expert. *Committee Technical Report Series, No. 804.* Washington, DC: Author.

*World Health Organization (1996). *Cancer pain relief: With a guide to opioid availability* (2nd ed.). Washington, DC: Author.

Visit the Connection web site for the most up-to-date drug information.

PRINCIPLES OF ANTIMICROBIAL THERAPY

■ STEVEN P. GELONE, STACI PACETTI, AND JUDITH A. O'DONNELL

The selection of an appropriate antimicrobial agent to treat an infection is guided by a number of factors. Typically, empiric antimicrobial therapy is based on the epidemiology of the suspected infection, with therapy directed toward the most likely organisms. Laboratory studies, including Gram stain as well as culture and sensitivity testing, help to identify the pathogen and its susceptibility to a variety of antimicrobials. Although there may be several options, efficacy, toxicity, pharmacokinetic profile, and cost ultimately determine the agent of choice. The optimal dose and duration of the antimicrobial therapy are then determined by patient factors such as age, weight, and concurrent disease states as well as the site of infection.

This chapter presents the major antimicrobial classes, provides an overview of the agents' pharmacology and clinical uses, and outlines an approach to appropriate antibiotic selection. The classes are presented in alphabetical order for ease of reference.

FACTORS IN SELECTING AN ANTIMICROBIAL REGIMEN

Before initiating antibiotic therapy, a systematic approach to identify the source and site of infection must be undertaken. A complete medical history and physical examination should be conducted to identify signs and symptoms consistent with the presence of infection. Identifying underlying medical or social conditions such as diabetes, immunosuppression (cancer, human immunodeficiency virus [HIV] infection), past medications, or intravenous (IV) drug use may help in identifying a predisposition toward infection or the most likely pathogen causing disease. In addition, determining where the infection was acquired (in the community versus a nursing home or hospital setting) may also help limit the list of most likely pathogens.

Identifying the causative pathogen is the ultimate goal because it allows for optimal antibiotic selection and patient outcome. Specimens from the most likely body sites should be properly collected and sent to the microbiology laboratory. Depending on the body site involved, specimens will be stained (eg, Gram stain) to determine morphology and cell wall structure and to detect white blood cells (which indicate inflammation and infection). The gold standard of diagnosis in infectious diseases is to be able to grow the causative organism in culture and perform antibiotic susceptibility

testing to determine which agents are most likely to be effective in eradicating the pathogen.

Often, antibiotic therapy is initiated before culture and sensitivity testing is complete. Empiric antibiotic therapy is based on the premise of providing coverage for the most likely pathogens (Table 8-1). Table 8-2 outlines key pathogens and spectra of activity for the most commonly prescribed antibiotics. In general, the most likely organism is based on the body site of the infection, the setting in which the infection was located when laboratory data, such as cultures and sensitivities, become available. In addition, if the patient was being treated initially with a parenteral antibiotic, therapy should be switched to the oral route. This conversion should be based on the following criteria:

- The patient is responding to therapy, as evidenced by a return to normal of signs and symptoms of infection. Evidence includes a trend toward normal values in the patient's temperature and white blood cell counts.
- The patient can take oral medications and absorb them adequately.
- An oral equivalent to the parenteral regimen exists. Not all parenteral agents are available orally. In choosing the oral equivalent, the goal is to select an agent (or agents) that provides a similar spectrum of antimicrobial activity and possesses good oral bioavailability. This may necessitate the use of oral agents that are from a different class from the parenteral agent.

The patient's response to therapy should be monitored regularly. This includes monitoring both efficacy and toxicity. If the patient responds to the prescribed antibiotic regimen, the presenting signs and symptoms of the infection should resolve. Parameters to be considered for response regardless of the site of infection include vital signs, white blood cell count, and, if the culture proved positive for bacteria, subsequent cultures that prove negative. Other signs and symptoms are specific to the body site involved. Monitoring for adverse events is specific to the agents prescribed (review the drug overview sections for common adverse events). All patients should be taught how to recognize the most common adverse events, and they should be advised to notify their health care provider if an adverse reaction occurs.

Table 8.1

Infection and Most Likely Infecting Organism

Body Site (Infection)	Most Likely Organism
Heart (Endocarditis)	
Subacute	*viridans* streptococci
Acute	
Injection drug user	*Staphylococcus aureus*, gram-negative aerobic bacilli, *Enterococcus* spp.
Prosthetic valve	*Staphylococcus epidermidis*
Intra-abdominal tissues	*Escherichia coli, Enterococcus* spp., anaerobes (especially *Bacteroides fragilis*), other gram-negative aerobic bacilli
Brain (Meningitis)	
Children <2 mo	*E. coli*, group B streptococci, *Listeria monocytogenes*
Children 2 mo–12 y	*Streptococcus pneumoniae, Neisseria meningitidis, Haemophilus influenzae*
Adults (community acquired)	*S. pneumoniae, N. meningitides*
Adults (hospital acquired)	*S. pneumoniae, N. meningitides*, gram-negative aerobic bacilli
HIV co-infected	*Cryptococcus neoformans, S. pneumoniae*
Respiratory Tract	
Upper tract, community acquired	*S. pneumoniae, H. influenzae, Moraxella catarrhalis*, group A streptococci
Lower tract, community acquired	*S. pneumoniae, H. influenzae, M. catarrhalis, Klebsiella pneumoniae* *Mycoplasma pneumoniae, Chlamydia pneumoniae*, viruses
Aspiration pneumonia	Mouth flora (anaerobic and aerobic)
Lower tract, hospital acquired	*S. aureus, Pseudomonas aeruginosa*, other gram-negative aerobic bacilli
HIV co-infected	*Pneumocystis carinii, S. pneumoniae*
Skin and Soft Tissue	
Diabetic ulcer	*Staphylococcus* spp., *Streptococcus* spp., gram-negative aerobic bacilli, anaerobes
Urinary Tract	
Community acquired	*E. coli*, other gram-negative aerobic bacilli, *Enterococcus* spp., *Staphylococcus saprophyticus*
Hospital acquired	*E. coli*, other gram-negative aerobic bacilli, *Enterococcus* spp.

AMINOGLYCOSIDES

Despite the advent of many new antibiotics over the past several decades, the aminoglycosides remain an important therapeutic drug class. Their major drawback has been their potential for drug-related toxicities (nephrotoxicity and ototoxicity); because of these, their use or the length of therapy has been restricted. More recently, however, the introduction of a modified dosing regimen that uses once-daily (or extended-interval) dosing of these agents for a variety of infections has provided a way of maximizing their therapeutic effects while minimizing the risk of toxicity.

Pharmacokinetics and Pharmacodynamics

The aminoglycosides are poorly absorbed from the gastrointestinal (GI) tract, and parenteral administration is necessary to treat systemic infections. They are weakly bound to serum proteins (10%) and freely distribute into the extracellular fluid. The approximate volume of distribution is 0.25 L/kg, which may be significantly affected in intensive care patients and in disease states such as malnutrition, obesity, and ascites. The aminoglycosides are excreted unchanged via glomerular filtration. The half-life of aminoglycosides in an adult with normal renal function is approximately 2 to 3 hours. Dosage adjustments are necessary in patients with renal impairment, as substantial increases in the half-life are seen. Aminoglycosides can be removed by hemodialysis, peritoneal dialysis, and continuous hemofiltration/dialysis.

Because of a narrow range between efficacy and toxicity, renal function and serum levels are used to monitor therapy with aminoglycosides. Table 8-3 gives dosage guidelines.

Pharmacodynamically, the bactericidal effect of the aminoglycosides depends on the drug's concentration: the number of organisms decreases more rapidly when a higher peak concentration is achieved. In addition, the aminoglycosides exhibit a post-antibiotic effect for both gram-positive and gram-negative organisms.

Mechanism of Action and Spectrum of Activity

The aminoglycosides are actively taken up by bacteria and subsequently bind to the smaller 30S subunit of the bacterial ribosome, thus inhibiting bacterial protein synthesis. They are considered bactericidal.

The principal activity of the aminoglycosides is against aerobic gram-negative bacilli such as *Escherichia coli, Klebsiella* species, *Proteus mirabilis, Enterobacter* species, *Acinetobacter* species, and *Pseudomonas aeruginosa*. They are also generally active against gram-positive cocci, particularly *Staphylococcus* species, *Enterococcus* species, and *Streptococcus* species, but they must be used in combination with a cell wall-active agent such as ampicillin (Principen), nafcillin (Unipen), or vancomycin (Vancocin). Streptomycin is also active against *Francisella tularensis*.

Table 8.2

Sensitivity of Organisms to Specific Agents

Agent	Staphylococci and Streptococci	Enterococcus	Methicillin-Sensitive Staphylococcus aureus	Methicillin-Resistant S. aureus	Gram-Negative Aerobes	Pseudomonas	Gram-Negative Anaerobes (Bacteroides fragilis)	Chlamydia pneumoniae, Legionella pneumophila
Aminoglycosides								
gentamicin	++	++	++	++	+++	++	–	–
tobramycin	–	–	–	–	+++	+++	–	–
amikacin	–	–	–	–	+++	+++	–	–
Antianaerobic Agents								
clindamycin	+++	–	+++	–	–	–	+++	–
metronidazole	–	–	–	–	–	–	+++	–
Beta-Lactam/Beta-Lactamase Inhibitors								
piperacillin–tazobactam	+++	+++	+++	–	+++	+++	+++	–
amoxicillin–clavulanic acid	+++	+++	+++	–	++	–	+++	–
ampicillin–sulbactam	+++	+++	+++	–	++	–	+++	–
ticarcillin–clavulanic acid	+++	++	+++	–	+++	++	+++	–
Carbapenems								
ertapenem	+++	++	+++	–	+++	–	+++	–
imipenem	+++	++	+++	–	+++	++/+++	+++	–
meropenem	+++	++	+++	–	+++	++/+++	+++	–
First-Generation Cephalosporins								
cefazolin	+++	–	+++	–	++	–	–	–
cephalexin	+++	–	+++	–	++	–	–	–
cefadroxil	++	–	+++	–	++	–	–	–
Second-Generation Cephalosporins								
cefuroxime	+++	–	+++	–	++	–	++	–
cefoxitin	++	–	++	–	++	–	++/+++	–
cefotetan	++	–	++	–	++/+++	–	++	–
Third-Generation Cephalosporins								
ceftriaxone	+++	–	++	–	+++	+	+	–
cefotaxime	+++	–	++	–	+++	+	+/++	–
ceftazidime	++	–	+	–	+++	++	–	–
Fourth-Generation Cephalosporins								
cefepime	+++	–	++	–	+++	++	–	–
chloramphenicol	+/++	++	–	–	+	–	+++	–
Fluoroquinolones								
ciprofloxacin	+/++	++	+++	+	+++	+++	–	++
ofloxacin	++	+	+++	+	+++	++	–	++
norfloxacin	++*	++*	+++	+	+++*	+++*	–	–
levofloxacin	++/+++	+/++	++	+/++	+++*	++	–	+++
gatifloxacin	++/+++	++	++	+/++	++	–	+/++	+++
moxifloxacin	++/+++	++	+++	+/++	++	–	+/++	+++
sparfloxacin	+++	++	+++	++	++	–	–	+++
trovafloxacin	+++	++/+++	+++	++/+++	+++	+++	+++	+++

The following table lists antimicrobial agents by class with a spectrum-of-activity grid (8 data columns; column headers appear on the facing page).

Class / Agent								
Lipopeptides								
daptomycin	−	−	−	+++	+++	+++	++	+++
Macrolides								
erythromycin	+++	−	+/+++	−	++	−	+++	+++
clarithromycin	+++	−	++	−	++	−	+++	+++
azithromycin	++	−	++/+++	−	+	+++	++	++
dirithromycin	+++	−	+/++	−	++	−	+++	+++
telithromycin	+++	−	++	−	++	−	+++	+++
Monobactams								
aztreonam	−	++	++/+++	−	−	−	−	−
Oxazolidinediones								
linezolid	++	−	+	+++	+++	+++	+++	+++
Penicillins								
penicillin G	−	−	−	−	+	++	++	+++
penicillin V	−	−	−	−	+	++	++	+++
ampicillin	−	−	+/++	−	+	+++	+++	+++
amoxicillin	−	−	+/++	−	+	+++	+++	+++
nafcillin	−	−	−	−	++	−	+++	+++
dicloxacillin	−	−	−	−	++	−	+++	+++
carbenicillin	−	+++*	+++*	−	++	+++	+++	+++
ticarcillin	−	++	++	−	++	++	+++	+++
piperacillin	−	+++	++	−	++	+++	+++	+++
Rifampin								
rifampin	++	+	+	++	++	−	++	++/+++
Streptogramins								
quinupristin–dalfopristin	++	−	+	+++	+++	++	+++	+++
Sulfonamides								
trimethoprim–sulfamethoxazole	−	−	++/+++	++	++	−	++	++
Tetracyclines								
tetracycline	+++	−	+	+/++	++	++	++/+++	++/+++
doxycycline	+++	−	+/++	+/++	++	++	++/+++	++/+++
minocycline	++	−	+/++	++/+++	++	++	+++	+++
Vancomycin								
vancomycin	−	−	−	+++	+++	+++	+++	+++

Table 8.3

Aminoglycoside Dosages

Aminoglycoside	Dosages	Target Peak and Trough
Multiple Daily Dosing		
gentamicin, tobramycin	1.7 mg/kg IV q8h	Peak 6–8 μg/mL, trough <2 μg/mL
netilmicin	1.7–2 mg/kg IV q8h	Peak 6–8 μg/mL, trough <2 μg/mL
amikacin, kanamycin	5 mg/kg IV q8h or 7.5 mg/kg IV q12h	Peak 20–30 μg/mL, trough <8 μg/mL
streptomycin	0.5–2 g IV q24h	Peak 20–30 μg/mL, trough <8 μg/mL
Once-Daily Dosing*		
gentamicin, tobramycin	5–7 mg/kg IV q24h	Peak >15 μg/mL, trough <1 μg/mL
netilmicin	5–7 mg/kg IV q24h	Peak >15 μg/mL, trough <1 μg/mL
amikacin	15–20 mg/kg IV q24h	Peak >50 μg/mL, trough <5 μg/mL

Note: Dosage adjustment required for all above drugs administered to patients with renal impairment.
*Once-daily dosing of aminoglycosides is not recommended for enterococcal infections; during pregnancy; in instances of gram-positive synergy; for endocarditis, meningitis, or ascites.

Mechanism of Resistance

There are three mechanisms by which resistance to the aminoglycosides may arise:

- Decreased aminoglycoside uptake
- Enzymatic modification of the drug
- Alteration of the ribosomal binding site

The most common of these mechanisms is enzymatic modification of the aminoglycosides that renders them inactive. Resistance to aminoglycosides resulting from changes in the ribosomal binding site is a less common mechanism but may be seen in isolates resistant to streptomycin. The third mechanism is impaired aminoglycoside uptake due to decreased active uptake or membrane changes of the gram-negative organisms that reduce permeability of the drug. Resistance to the aminoglycosides, unlike the beta-lactams and quinolones, is relatively stable and slow to develop, particularly when they are used in combination with other antibiotics.

Clinical Uses

The aminoglycosides are primarily used in treating gram-negative infections. They have long been used in the empiric treatment of neutropenic fever and nosocomial infections because of their broad coverage of *P. aeruginosa* and Enterobacteriaceae. They are also frequently used with cell wall-active agents such as penicillins, cephalosporins, and vancomycin to achieve synergy in treating gram-positive infections, including staphylococcal and enterococcal infections. They are routinely used in combination with other agents in treating pneumonia, bacteremia, and skin and soft tissue infections. Monotherapy usually is not recommended, with the noted exception of patients with urinary tract infections. The aminoglycosides have been used in treating tuberculosis, with streptomycin having the greatest activity against *Mycobacterium tuberculosis*. Streptomycin is also the treatment of choice for tularemia, a potential agent of bioterrorism.

Adverse Events

In general, the aminoglycosides have been associated with a variety of adverse events (GI and central nervous system [CNS]), most of which are mild and transient. They rarely produce hypersensitivity reactions and are well tolerated at the sites of administration. Nephrotoxicity and ototoxicity are also associated with aminoglycoside use.

Nephrotoxicity results from accumulation of the drug in the proximal tubule cells of the kidney, causing nonoliguric renal failure. This renal failure is usually mild and reversible and rarely progresses to the need for dialysis; dosage changes are required. Factors that increase the risk of toxicity to the kidney include increased age, renal disease, increased trough levels, dehydration, and concomitant administration of nephrotoxic agents such as amphotericin B (Fungizone), cyclosporine (Sandimmune), and vancomycin. Blood urea nitrogen (BUN) and serum creatinine values are monitored in addition to serum levels to ensure safe and effective therapy.

Two forms of ototoxicity—auditory and vestibular—may occur alone or simultaneously. Auditory toxicity presents as hearing loss and tinnitus; vestibular toxicity is manifested by nausea, vomiting, and vertigo. Ototoxicity may be irreversible and has been associated with high serum trough levels. The risk of ototoxicity increases when the aminoglycosides are administered in combination with high-dose loop diuretics, high-dose macrolide antibiotics, or vancomycin.

The aminoglycosides have the potential to cause or prolong neuromuscular blockade, although this is uncommon. It is recommended that parenteral aminoglycosides be administered over a 30-minute interval. The risk of neuromuscular blockade increases in patients receiving concurrent neuromuscular blockers, general anesthetics, or calcium channel blockers, and in those with myasthenia gravis. Administration of calcium gluconate usually reverses the neuromuscular blockade.

ANTIANAEROBIC AGENTS

Clindamycin (Cleocin) has been used extensively in treating gram-positive and anaerobic bacterial infections. It was first used orally to treat streptococcal and staphylococcal infections, but it soon became the drug of choice for anaerobic infections. The combination of clindamycin and gentamicin (Garamycin) has become the standard of care in treating mixed aerobic and anaerobic infections.

Metronidazole (Flagyl) was first recognized for its antiprotozoal activity in treating *Trichomonas vaginalis* infections. Subsequently, its utility as an anti-anaerobic agent was used in treating *Bacteroides fragilis* infections. Metronidazole has become a treatment of choice for *Clostridium*

Table 8.4

Antianaerobic Agent Dosages

Drug	Adult Dosages	Pediatric Dosages
clindamycin	150–450 mg PO q6h 600 mg IV q8h	10–30 mg/kg/d PO q6–8h 25–40 mg/kg/d IV q6–8h
metronidazole	250–500 mg PO q6–8h 500 mg IV q6–12h	30 mg/kg/d q6h

Note: Dosage adjustment recommended for all above drugs for patients with liver dysfunction.

difficile colitis and is part of a number of regimens to eradicate *Helicobacter pylori*–associated duodenal ulcers.

Pharmacokinetics and Pharmacodynamics

Both clindamycin esters, palmitate and phosphate, are absorbed and converted to active forms in the blood. Clindamycin reaches most tissues and bone, but its distribution into the cerebrospinal fluid (CSF) is limited. The half-life is approximately 3 hours. Most of the drug is metabolized by the liver, necessitating dosage adjustment in patients with liver impairment (Table 8-4). Hemodialysis and peritoneal dialysis do not remove clindamycin to a significant extent.

Metronidazole is completely absorbed from the GI tract after oral administration. It penetrates well into most tissues, with an apparent volume of distribution of 0.6 to 0.9 L/kg. Its binding to plasma protein is minimal. Metronidazole is metabolized by the liver, and dosage adjustments are necessary in patients with hepatic impairment. The half-life is approximately 6 to 9 hours. Metronidazole is removed by hemodialysis and peritoneal dialysis.

Mechanism of Action and Spectrum of Activity

Clindamycin binds to the 50S subunit of the bacterial ribosome and inhibits protein synthesis. It acts at the same site as chloramphenicol (Chloromycetin) and the macrolides.

Metronidazole is reduced to a toxic product that interacts with DNA, causing strand breakage and resulting in protein synthesis inhibition.

The principal activity of clindamycin is against aerobic gram-positive cocci, gram-positive and gram-negative anaerobic organisms, including *Bacteroides*, and protozoa. It lacks significant coverage against aerobic gram-negative organisms.

Metronidazole has excellent activity against both gram-positive and gram-negative anaerobes, *H. pylori*, and protozoa, such as *T. vaginalis*.

Mechanism of Resistance

The primary mechanism of resistance to clindamycin occurs as a result of alterations of the binding site on the 50S ribosomal subunit. Metronidazole resistance is conferred by decreased enzymatic activity of reductases, resulting in less activation and uptake of the drug. Development of resistance to metronidazole is rare in anaerobes but common in *H. pylori*.

Clinical Uses

Clindamycin and metronidazole are typically included in regimens for their anaerobic coverage in mixed infections. In addition, metronidazole is the drug of choice for *C. difficile* diarrhea. Clindamycin is also used in treating gram-positive infections, toxoplasmosis, and *Pneumocystis carinii* pneumonia. In addition, it is frequently used to inhibit toxin production as part of the treatment for staphylococcal or streptococcal toxic shock. The Centers for Disease Control and Prevention recommendations include clindamycin in the treatment guidelines for pelvic inflammatory disease, whereas metronidazole is recommended as the treatment of choice for bacterial vaginosis and trichomoniasis.

Adverse Events

The major side effect associated with clindamycin is diarrhea and associated *C. difficile* colitis. This adverse event is unrelated to dose and may range from acute, self-limiting symptoms to life-threatening megacolon. Clindamycin use in combination with skeletal muscle relaxants has been reported to potentiate neuromuscular blockade in rare cases. Pain at the site of administration may occur.

Metronidazole is usually safe and well tolerated. GI side effects such as nausea, vomiting, abdominal pain, and a metallic taste are most common. More serious but rare effects include seizures, peripheral neuropathy, and pancreatitis. Seizures have been associated with high doses, whereas peripheral neuropathy has been documented in patients receiving prolonged courses of metronidazole.

Metronidazole enhances the anticoagulant effect of warfarin (Coumadin), resulting in a prolonged half-life of warfarin. A disulfiram-like reaction characterized by flushing, palpitations, nausea, and vomiting may occur when alcohol is consumed during metronidazole therapy. Phenobarbital (Luminal), phenytoin (Dilantin), and rifampin (Rifadin) increase the metabolism of metronidazole, which may result in treatment failure. Cimetidine (Tagamet), an enzyme inhibitor, decreases the metabolism of metronidazole.

BETA-LACTAM/BETA-LACTAMASE INHIBITOR COMBINATIONS

Resistance to penicillin develops when the drug is inactivated by the enzymes known as penicillinases or beta-lactamases produced by bacteria. After several attempts over the years to prevent penicillin degradation by this enzyme, clavulanic acid became the first beta-lactamase inhibitor introduced and commercially available in combination with a beta-lactam. The role of the beta-lactamase inhibitor is to prevent the breakdown of the beta-lactam by organisms that produce the enzyme, thereby enhancing the antibacterial activity. These combinations are suitable alternatives for infections caused by resistant organisms such as *S. aureus* and *Haemophilus influenzae*.

Pharmacokinetics and Pharmacodynamics

The beta-lactam/beta-lactamase inhibitors diffuse into most body tissues, with the exception of the brain and CSF. The half-life of both components in each combination is approximately 1 hour. Because these drugs are eliminated by glomerular filtration, renal dysfunction necessitates dosage changes (Table 8-5). The compounds are removed by hemodialysis and peritoneal dialysis.

Table 8.5

Beta-Lactam/Beta-Lactamase Inhibitor Dosages

Drug	Adult Dosages	Pediatric Dosages
amoxicillin–clavulanic acid	250–500 mg PO q8h 500–875 mg PO q12h	20–40 mg/kg/d q8–12h
ampicillin–sulbactam	1.5–3.0 g IV q6h	100–400 mg/kg/d q4–6h
piperacillin– tazobactam	4.5 g IV q6–8h or 3.375 g IV q4–6h	240 mg/kg/d q8h
ticarcillin–clavulanic acid	3.1g IVq4–6h	200–300 mg/kg/d q4–6h

Note: Dosage adjustment required for all above drugs administered to patients with renal impairment.

Mechanism of Action and Spectrum of Activity

The beta-lactam components of the combinations are cell wall-active agents. They interfere with bacterial cell wall synthesis by binding to and inactivating penicillin-binding proteins (PBPs). The beta-lactamase inhibitors irreversibly bind to most beta-lactamase enzymes, protecting the beta-lactam from degradation and improving their antibacterial activity. The beta-lactamase inhibitors alone lack significant antibacterial activity.

Mechanism of Resistance

Resistance to the beta-lactam/beta-lactamase inhibitor combinations occurs in two ways: either there is an overproduction of penicillinases not susceptible to the beta-lactamase inhibitors, or the beta-lactamases produced are less sensitive to the inhibitors. The latter can result in cross-resistance among all the combinations. In addition, as with all penicillins, a modification in the PBP can result in decreased activity.

Clinical Uses

Based on their broad spectrum of activity, the beta-lactam/beta-lactamase inhibitors are frequently used in treating polymicrobial infections. They are used extensively to treat intra-abdominal and gynecologic infections and skin and soft tissue infections, including human and animal bites, as well as foot infections in diabetic patients. Respiratory tract infections, including aspiration pneumonia, sinusitis, and lung abscesses, have been successfully treated with these combinations.

Adverse Events

The addition of the beta-lactamase inhibitor to the penicillins has not resulted in any new or major adverse events. The major effects associated with the beta-lactam/beta-lactamase inhibitor combinations are hypersensitivity reactions and GI side effects such as nausea and diarrhea associated with oral administration. Elevated aminotransferase levels have been documented for all agents.

The combinations are physically incompatible with parenteral aminoglycosides. Each of the penicillins in the combinations has been associated with the inactivation of aminoglycosides in vitro. The clinical significance of this interaction is unknown.

CARBAPENEMS

The carbapenems—ertapenem (Invanz), imipenem (Primaxin), and meropenem (Merrem)—are bicyclic beta-lactams with a common carbapenem nucleus (Table 8-6). Imipenem is extensively metabolized by renal dehydropeptidases, yielding only limited activity in the urine. Cilastatin, a competitive inhibitor of the dehydropeptidases, was introduced to overcome imipenem's degradation and is commercially available in combination with imipenem in a one-to-one ratio. Subsequently, ertapenem and meropenem were developed; they maintain stability against dehydropeptidase metabolism without the addition of a cilastatin-like agent. The carbapenems are the most broad-spectrum agents commercially available.

Pharmacokinetics and Pharmacodynamics

Carbapenems are not absorbed after oral administration. They exhibit linear pharmacokinetics; thus, peak serum levels increase proportionately as the dose is increased. They are widely distributed into most tissues, with an approximate volume of distribution of 0.25 L/kg. They are weakly bound to plasma proteins. Penetration into the CSF varies and depends on the degree of meningeal inflammation. The half-life of the carbapenems is approximately 1 hour. They are primarily eliminated by urinary excretion of unchanged drug. Both imipenem and meropenem are removed by hemodialysis and hemofiltration.

The carbapenems, like other beta-lactams, exhibit time-dependent bactericidal effects. Unlike other beta-lactams, they exhibit a significant post-antibiotic effect against gram-negative aerobes lasting at least 1 to 2 hours.

Mechanism of Action and Spectrum of Activity

Similar to the penicillins and cephalosporins, the carbapenems bind to the PBPs on the cell wall and interfere with bacterial cell wall synthesis. They have excellent stability against beta-lactamases and bind to a variety of PBPs.

Imipenem and meropenem possess the broadest spectrum of activity of any of the beta-lactam compounds. They have excellent activity against aerobic gram-positive organisms, including staphylococci and streptococci and gram-negative organisms such as Enterobacteriaceae, *P. aeruginosa*, and *Acinetobacter* species. They are also active against most gram-negative anaerobic organisms, including *B. fragilis*. Ertapenem has a similar spectrum of activity as the other carbapenems, with the noted exceptions of *P. aeruginosa*

Table 8.6

Carbapenem Dosages

Drug	Adult Dosages	Pediatric Dosages
ertapenem	1 g IV/IM daily	Not recommended
imipenem	250–1,000 mg IV q6h	40–60 mg/kg/d, individual doses q6h
meropenem	500 mg–1 g IV q6–8h	60–120 mg/kg/d, divided doses q8h

Note: Dosage adjustment required for all above drugs administered to patients with renal impairment.

and *Acinetobacter species*, for which ertapenem has no clinically significant activity.

Mechanism of Resistance

Decreased affinity for the PBPs on the cell wall is an important mechanism of resistance of gram-positive organisms. Alteration of membrane porins by Enterobacteriaceae and *P. aeruginosa* is a second mechanism that renders the membrane impermeable to the carbapenems. Methods to overcome resistance to carbapenems include combination therapy to achieve additive or synergistic effects and optimal drug dosing regimens.

Clinical Uses

Their broad spectrum of activity and stability to beta-lactamases make the carbapenems useful as single agents in treating polymicrobial infections. They have been used extensively in treating skin and soft tissue, bone and joint, intra-abdominal, and lower respiratory tract infections. In addition, meropenem is used in treating CNS infections because it has a lower risk than imipenem of causing seizures.

Adverse Events

Neurotoxicity, a well-known effect of the carbapenems, is characterized by seizure activity. Imipenem has been reported to lower the seizure threshold more frequently than meropenem. A difference in side chains may account for the lower incidence and risk with meropenem. Risk factors include impaired renal function, improper dosing, age, previous CNS disorder, and concomitant agents that lower the seizure threshold. Meropenem has therefore been the carbapenem of choice in patients with a seizure disorder or underlying risk factors, and it is the only carbapenem indicated in treating bacterial meningitis.

GI side effects such as nausea, vomiting, and diarrhea have also been reported. Decreasing the infusion rate may lessen their severity.

Concomitant administration of probenecid and meropenem results in decreased clearance of meropenem and a substantial increase in half-life, so the concurrent administration of these two agents is not recommended. A similar interaction with imipenem occurs, but to a lesser degree.

CEPHALOSPORINS

The cephalosporins, a beta-lactam group, are structurally similar to the penicillins. Substitutions on the parent compound, 7-aminocephalosporanic acid, produce compounds with different pharmacokinetic properties and spectra of activity. The cephalosporins are divided into "generations" based on their antimicrobial spectrum of activity. The progression from first to third generation in general reflects an increase in gram-negative coverage and a loss of gram-positive activity.

Pharmacokinetics and Pharmacodynamics

The cephalosporins are well absorbed from the GI tract. In some cases, food enhances absorption. They penetrate

Table 8.7

Cephalosporin Dosages

Drug	Adult Dosages	Pediatric Dosages
First Generation		
cefazolin	500 mg–1 g IV q8h	50–100 mg/kg/d q8h
cephalothin	0.5–2 g IV q6h	80–150 mg/kg/d
cephapirin	500 mg–1 g IV q6h	40–80 mg/kg/d q4–6h
cephalexin	250–500 mg PO q6h	25–100 mg/kg/d q6h
cephradine	250–500 mg PO q6–12h	25–100 mg/kg/d q6–12h
cefadroxil	500 mg–1 g PO q12h	30 mg/kg/d q12h
Second Generation		
cefotetan	1–2 g IV q12h	40–80 mg/kg/d q12h
cefoxitin	1–2 g IV q6–8h	80–160 mg/kg/d q4–8h
cefuroxime	750–1.5 g IV q8h	75–150 mg/kg/d q8h
cefuroxime axetil	250–500 mg PO q12h	20–30 mg/kg/d q12h
loracarbef	200–400 mg PO q12–24h	15–30 mg/kg/d q12h
cefaclor	250–500 mg PO q8h	20–40 mg/kg/d q8–12h
Third Generation		
cefoperazone†	1–2 g IV q12h	100–150 mg/kg/d q8–12h
cefotaxime	1–2 g IV q8h	100–300 mg/kg/d q6–6h
ceftazidime	1–2 g IV q8h	100–150 mg/kg/d q8h
ceftizoxime	1–2 g IV q8h	150–200 mg/kg/d q6–8h
ceftriaxone†	1–2 g IV q24h	50–100 mg/kg/d q12–24h
ceftibuten	400 mg PO q24h	9 mg/kg/d q24h
cefpodoxime proxetil	200–400 mg PO q12h	10 mg/kg/d q12h
cefprozil	250–500 mg PO q12h	15–30 mg/kg/d q12h
cefdinir	300 mg PO q12h or 600 mg q24h	7–14 mg/kg/d q12–24h
Fourth Generation		
cefepime	1–2 g IV q8–12h	50 mg/kg/d q8h

*Dosage adjustment necessary in patients with renal impairment.
†Dosage adjustment necessary in patients with liver dysfunction.

well into tissues and body fluids and achieve high concentrations in the urinary tract. Non-cephamycin second-generation agents and all third- and fourth-generation agents penetrate the CSF and play a role in treating bacterial meningitis. Most of the oral and parenteral cephalosporins are excreted by the kidney, with the exception of ceftriaxone (Rocephin) and cefoperazone (Cefobid), which are eliminated by the liver. The cephalosporins exhibit a time-dependent bactericidal effect and a prolonged post-antibiotic effect against staphylococci. Table 8-7 gives more information.

Mechanism of Action and Spectrum of Activity

Like other beta-lactams, the cephalosporins interfere with bacterial cell wall synthesis by binding to and inactivating the PBPs.

Mechanism of Resistance

One of the main mechanisms of cephalosporin resistance involves production of beta-lactamases that hydrolyze the beta-lactam ring and destroy the antibacterial activity. Other mechanisms that confer resistance are alterations in PBPs and changes in porin size, resulting in decreased entry of the drug.

Clinical Uses

The cephalosporins are used in treating a variety of infections. In general, the first-generation cephalosporins are used in treating gram-positive skin infections, pneumococcal respiratory infections, and urinary tract infections, and for surgical prophylaxis. The second-generation cephalosporins are used in treating community-acquired pneumonia, other respiratory tract infections, skin infections, and, in some settings, meningitis. Mixed aerobic and anaerobic infections may be treated with the second-generation cephamycins. In addition, treating community-acquired bacterial meningitis typically includes a third-generation cephalosporin such as ceftriaxone or cefotaxime (Claforan). Nosocomial infections are commonly treated with ceftazidime (Fortaz) or cefepime (Maxipime), whose broad spectrum of activity includes gram-negative organisms, especially *P. aeruginosa*.

Adverse Events

The cephalosporins are a safe class of antimicrobials with a favorable toxicity profile. With a few exceptions, the adverse events are similar across the generations. Hypersensitivity reactions, not unlike those with the penicillins, are characterized by maculopapular rash and urticaria. The cross-reactivity between penicillins and cephalosporins is 3% to 10%. The most common side effects with oral administration are nausea, vomiting, and diarrhea. GI effects are usually transient. Less common reactions include Coombs' positivity and rare hemolytic reactions.

CHLORAMPHENICOL

Chloramphenicol has a wide spectrum of activity against gram-positive, gram-negative, and anaerobic organisms. However, its use has been limited by its toxicity profile, which includes "gray baby" syndrome, optic neuritis, and fatal aplastic anemia. Nonetheless, in selected situations, chloramphenicol remains an important agent.

Pharmacokinetics and Pharmacodynamics

Specific parameters of chloramphenicol are determined by the form, dosage, and route of elimination (Table 8-8). Chloramphenicol is available in oral capsule form, palmitate suspension, and IV succinate ester. The ester formulations are hydrolyzed in the body to active drug. Chloramphenicol penetrates well into most tissues and bodily fluids, including the CSF. It is conjugated in the liver and excreted by the kidney in an inactive, nontoxic form. The serum half-life is 3 to 4 hours. Chloramphenicol is 25% to 50% bound to protein.

Serum levels are frequently monitored in high-risk patients. The therapeutic range of chloramphenicol is 5 to 25 mg/dL. Dose-related myelosuppression typically occurs at serum levels exceeding 25 mg/dL.

Mechanism of Action and Spectrum of Activity

Chloramphenicol reversibly binds to the larger 50S subunit of the ribosome, thereby inhibiting bacterial protein synthesis. It is variably bactericidal.

Table 8.8

Chloramphenicol Dosages

Patient Group	Dosage
Older children and adults	50 mg/kg/d PO/IV in 6-h intervals
Older children and adults with meningitis	100 mg/kg/d PO/IV in 6-h intervals

Chloramphenicol is active against gram-positive and gram-negative aerobes and anaerobes as well as atypical organisms, including spirochetes, chlamydiae, and rickettsiae. Its gram-negative activity includes *E. coli*, *Proteus* species, and *Salmonella* species but not *P. aeruginosa*.

Mechanism of Resistance

Organisms acquire resistance to chloramphenicol in two ways. First, the enzyme chloramphenicol acetyltransferase converts the drug into a product lacking antimicrobial activity. The second mechanism is based on the organism's loss of an outer membrane protein. Without the protein, chloramphenicol cannot penetrate the organism and exert its effects. This mechanism is characteristic of *E. coli*, *H. influenzae*, *P. aeruginosa*, and *Serratia marcescens*.

Clinical Uses

Newer agents have reduced the need to use chloramphenicol in treating infection. However, it can be used as an alternative in treating bacterial meningitis when a patient has a life-threatening penicillin allergy. It is also useful in treating rickettsial diseases such as Rocky Mountain spotted fever and typhus fever in patients allergic to tetracyclines, or in pregnant women. Chloramphenicol may be used in treating vancomycin-resistant enterococcal infections as well.

Adverse Events

The major adverse events associated with chloramphenicol are "gray baby" syndrome, blood dyscrasias, and optic neuritis. "Gray baby" syndrome typically occurs in neonates and is manifested by vomiting, lethargy, respiratory collapse, and death. It results from drug accumulation because neonates cannot conjugate chloramphenicol. Two forms of hematologic toxicity may occur with chloramphenicol administration. Dose-related bone marrow suppression has occurred in patients receiving more than four doses exceeding 4 g/day and at serum levels exceeding 25 mg/dL. It may present as a combination of anemia, leukopenia, and thrombocytopenia. Aplastic anemia is an idiosyncratic effect that is independent of dose and may occur weeks after therapy with chloramphenicol. It is more common with oral administration and often necessitates bone marrow transplantation. Optic neuritis is a major neurologic complication and is associated with long courses of chloramphenicol. The toxicity involves red-green color changes and loss of vision. It may be reversible or permanent. GI side effects have been associated with high doses of chloramphenicol.

Chloramphenicol is metabolized by the liver and is an inhibitor of the cytochrome P450 enzyme system. It prolongs the half-life of warfarin, phenytoin, and cyclosporine.

FLUOROQUINOLONES

Since 1990, the fluoroquinolones (FQs) have become a dominant class of antimicrobial agents. No other class of antimicrobial agents has grown so rapidly or been developed with such interest by pharmaceutical research companies. This drug class will likely double in size, with several approvals currently before the FDA. Since 1997, six new agents have been released into the U.S. market: levofloxacin (Levaquin), sparfloxacin (Zagam), trovafloxacin (Trovan), which has recently been limited to inpatient therapy, moxifloxacin (Avelox), and gatifloxacin (Tequin).

Pharmacokinetics and Pharmacodynamics

The FQs are bactericidal antibiotics. They display a concentration-dependent killing effect. Therefore, achieving a higher peak concentration of the FQs results in more rapid and complete killing of susceptible organisms (Table 8-9).

All FQs also exhibit a post-antibiotic effect, which also appears to be a concentration-dependent parameter. The newer compounds have been reported to have post-antibiotic effects of 1 to 6 hours, depending on the pathogen and drug studied.

Mechanism of Action and Spectrum of Activity

The quinolone antibiotics are strong inhibitors of DNA gyrase and topoisomerase IV. These enzymes are critical to the process of supercoiling DNA. Without such enzymatic activity, DNA cannot replicate.

Mechanism of Resistance

The selective pressure associated with widespread use of FQs has led to the emergence of quinolone-resistant bacteria. These microorganisms become resistant to FQs through two mechanisms: chromosomal mutations or alterations in their ability to permeate the bacterial cell wall. Mutational FQ resistance arises in a stepwise manner. Active efflux limits intracellular accumulation of antimicrobials and may lead to clinically significant quinolone resistance, warranting a change in therapy.

Table 8.9

Fluoroquinolone Dosages

Drug	Adult Dosage
norfloxacin	400 mg PO bid
ciprofloxacin	250–500 mg PO bid; 200–400 mg IV q12h
enoxacin	200–400 mg PO bid
ofloxacin	300–400 mg PO bid; 200–400 mg IV q12h
levofloxacin	250–500 mg PO/IV daily
sparfloxacin	400 mg on day 1, then 200 mg PO daily
gatifloxacin	200–400 mg PO/IV daily
moxifloxacin	400 mg PO/IV daily
lomefloxacin	400 mg PO daily at bedtime

Note: These drugs are not recommended for use in children younger than 16 years.

Table 8.10

Adverse Events Associated With Fluoroquinolones

Body System	Adverse Event
Cardiovascular	Hypotension, tachycardia, prolonged QTc interval
Central nervous system	Headache, dizziness, sleep disturbances, mood change, confusion, psychosis, tremor, seizures
Integumentary	Rash, pruritus, photosensitivity, leg pigmentation, urticaria
Hepatic	Transient increase in aminotransferases, cholestatic jaundice, hepatitis, hepatic failure
Musculoskeletal	Arthropathy, tendinitis, tendon rupture
Renal	Azotemia, crystalluria, hematuria, interstitial nephritis, nephropathy, renal failure
Other	Drug fever, chills, serum sickness–like reaction, anaphylaxis, angioedema, bronchospasm, vasculitis, hypo/hyperglycemia

Clinical Uses

The FQs have been shown to be effective in treating a variety of infections, including urinary tract infections (for which they are one of the agents of choice), sexually transmitted diseases, skin and soft tissue infections, GI infections (including traveler's diarrhea), and osteomyelitis. Their track record in treating respiratory tract infections has also been quite good, but there are some adverse events (Tables 8-10, 8-11, and 8-12). There are also some caveats. First, for hospital-acquired infection, ciprofloxacin (Cipro) is the preferred agent because it has the best activity against *P. aeruginosa*. For community-acquired infections, one of the newer agents (ie, levofloxacin, sparfloxacin, gatifloxacin, or moxifloxacin) is preferred because these agents have the greatest activity against *S. pneumoniae*. Last, ciprofloxacin is recommended for meningococcal prophylaxis as a single 500-mg oral dose.

LIPOPEPTIDES

Lipopeptides are large-molecular-weight antibacterial agents that have been under evaluation over the past several decades. Daptomycin is an antibacterial agent of a new class of antibiotics, the cyclic lipopeptides. Daptomycin is a natural product that has clinical utility in the treatment of infections caused by aerobic gram-positive bacteria.

Pharmacokinetics and Pharmacodynamics

Daptomycin pharmacokinetics are nearly linear and time independent at doses up to 6 mg/kg administered once daily for 7 days. Its half-life is approximately 8 hours. The apparent volume of distribution of daptomycin at steady state in healthy adults was approximately 0.09 L/kg. Daptomycin is excreted primarily by the kidney (approximately 78% of the administered dose). Because renal excretion is the primary route of elimination, dosage adjustment is necessary in patients with severe renal insufficiency (creatinine clearance less than 30 mL/min). The pharmacokinetics of daptomycin are not altered in subjects with moderate hepatic impairment. Daptomycin is reversibly bound to human plasma proteins, primarily to serum albumin, in a concentration-independent manner. The mean serum protein binding of

Table 8.11

Drug Interactions of the Newer Fluoroquinolones

	Gatifloxacin	Levofloxacin	Moxifloxacin	Trovafloxacin
Antacids	Yes	Yes	Yes	Yes
Vitamins/minerals	Yes	Yes	Yes	Yes
Theophylline	No	No	No	No
NSAIDs	No	Yes	No	No
Warfarin	No	No	No	Yes
Digoxin	No	No	No	No
Milk products	No	No	No	No
Morphine	No	No	No	Yes
Medications that prolong the QTc interval	No	No	Yes	No

daptomycin is approximately 92% in healthy adults after the administration of 4 or 6 mg/kg. Serum protein binding is not altered as a function of daptomycin concentration, dose, or number of doses received. Daptomycin does not inhibit or induce the activities of human cytochrome (CYP) P450 isoforms 1A2, 2A6, 2C9, 2C19, 2D6, 2E1, and 3A4.

Daptomycin exhibits rapid, concentration-dependent bactericidal activity against gram-positive organisms in vitro. This has been shown both by time-kill curves and by MBC/MIC ratios using broth dilution methodology.

Mechanism of Action and Spectrum of Activity

The mechanism of action of daptomycin is distinct from that of any other antibiotic. Daptomycin binds to bacterial membranes and causes a rapid depolarization of membrane potential. The loss of membrane potential leads to inhibition of protein, DNA, and RNA synthesis, which results in bacterial cell death.

The in vitro spectrum of activity of daptomycin encompasses most clinically relevant gram-positive pathogenic bacteria. Daptomycin retains potency against antibiotic-resistant gram-positive bacteria, including isolates resistant to methicillin, vancomycin, and linezolid.

Mechanism of Resistance

At present, no mechanism of resistance to daptomycin has been identified. There are no known transferable elements that confer resistance to daptomycin. Cross-resistance has not been observed with any other class of antibiotic.

Clinical Uses

Daptomycin is indicated for the treatment of complicated skin and skin structure infections caused by susceptible

strains of the following gram-positive microorganisms: *S. aureus* (including methicillin-resistant strains), *Streptococcus pyogenes*, *Streptococcus agalactiae*, *Streptococcus dysgalactiae* subspecies *equisimilis*, and *Enterococcus faecalis* (vancomycin-susceptible strains only). Combination therapy may be clinically indicated if the documented or presumed pathogens include gram-negative or anaerobic organisms. The dose for patients with normal renal function is 4 mg/kg IV administered daily. Daptomycin is not indicated for the treatment of pneumonia.

Adverse Events

Daptomycin may cause GI reactions such as constipation, nausea, diarrhea, and vomiting. Injection site reactions and headache may occur. Skeletal muscle toxicity manifested as muscle pain has been reported with daptomycin. This is accompanied by an increase in creatinine phosphokinase (CPK) levels. Caution should be used in patients concomitantly receiving an HMG-CoA reductase inhibitor, as these agents can also cause myopathy.

MACROLIDES

Erythromycin (E-Mycin), the prototypical macrolide, has been used in treating a variety of infections over the years. However, its use has been diminished by its GI side effects. This toxicity has even been used as a means of treating patients with diabetic gastroparesis. Newer agents have been developed with improved GI tolerance and longer half-lives.

Pharmacokinetics and Pharmacodynamics

The macrolides are usually administered orally and are absorbed from the GI tract if not inactivated by gastric acid. They have good tissue penetration and achieve high intracellular concentrations. The macrolides are excreted in both the liver and the urine. Half-lives vary throughout the class. Azithromycin (Zithromax) has the longest half-life, approximately 50 hours. Dosage adjustment in patients with renal failure is necessary with clarithromycin (Biaxin) and erythromycin (Table 8-13).

Table 8.12

Agent-Specific Issues With Fluoroquinolones

Drug	Adverse Event
sparfloxacin (Zagam)	Phototoxicity, prolonged QTc interval
trovafloxacin (Trovan)	Liver toxicity
moxifloxacin (Avelox)	Prolonged QTc interval
lomefloxacin (Maxaquin)	Phototoxicity

Table 8.13

Macrolide Antibiotic Dosages

Drug	Adult Dosage	Pediatric Dosages
azithromycin	250–500 mg IV/PO daily	5–12 mg/kg/d
clarithromycin*	250–500 mg PO q12h	15 mg/kg/d q12h
dirithromycin	250–500 mg PO daily	
erythromycin*	250 mg–1 g PO q6h	
	0.5–1 g IV q6–8h	15–50 mg/kg/d q6h
ethyl succinate base		30–50 mg/kg/d q6–8h
estolate		20–50 mg/kg/d q6–12h
stearate		20–40 mg/kg/d q6h
injection		15–50 mg/kg/d q6h
telithromycin	800 mg PO daily	Not recommended

*Dosage adjustment necessary in patients with renal impairment.

Mechanism of Action and Spectrum of Activity

The mechanism of action of the macrolides is inhibition of bacterial protein synthesis by binding to the 50S ribosomal subunit. The spectrum of activity of the macrolides includes gram-positive and gram-negative aerobes and atypical organisms, including chlamydiae, mycoplasma, legionellae, rickettsiae, and spirochetes.

Mechanism of Resistance

Resistance may occur as a result of alterations in the macrolide binding site on the ribosomal subunit, modification of the drug, or altered transport of the macrolides.

Clinical Uses

The macrolides are used in a variety of settings. Their broad spectrum of activity makes them useful in treating skin, soft tissue, and respiratory tract infections, sexually transmitted diseases, HIV-related *Mycobacterium avium-intracellulare* complex infection, and other infections caused by atypical organisms such as chlamydiae, rickettsiae, and legionellae.

Adverse Events

The macrolides are in general considered safe agents. GI effects such as abdominal pain, nausea, and vomiting are the most common side effects. The newer macrolides cause fewer GI effects. Hepatotoxicity related to the macrolides is rare but serious; it also is less frequent with the newer agents. Extremely high doses of IV erythromycin and oral clarithromycin have been associated with ototoxicity. Phlebitis may occur with IV administration.

The macrolides are separated into groups based on the clinical significance of drug interactions. It is postulated that structural features of the compounds contribute to the interacting potential. Group 1 includes erythromycin and troleandomycin (TAO), inhibitors of the cytochrome P450 enzyme system with documented interactions. They have been shown to prolong the half-life of an extensive list of agents, including cyclosporine, theophylline (Theo-Dur), rifampin, and the HMG-CoA reductase inhibitors. These interactions also are likely to occur in group 2, which includes clarithromycin. The newer macrolides in group 3,

azithromycin (Zithromax) and dirithromycin (Dynabac), do not form cytochrome P450 complexes, so the possibility of similar interactions is low.

Macrolides have the potential to increase the QTc interval, so caution should be used in patients receiving concomitant medications that can prolong the QTc interval.

MONOBACTAMS

The monobactams are a unique class of beta-lactams with a four-membered ring but lacking a fifth or sixth member, like other beta-lactams. Because aztreonam (Azactam) is the only agent of its class commercially available, most of the information relates specifically to that agent. With primary activity against gram-negative organisms, including *Pseudomonas*, aztreonam is considered a safer version of the aminoglycosides, with a similar spectrum of activity.

Pharmacokinetics and Pharmacodynamics

Aztreonam distributes well into most tissue, with a volume of distribution of 0.16 L/kg. Penetration into the CSF is increased in the presence of inflamed meninges. Aztreonam is not extensively bound to proteins. The approximate half-life is 2 hours, and dosages are typically calculated according to the severity of disease (Table 8-14). Aztreonam is excreted unchanged by glomerular filtration, so dosage adjustments are necessary in patients with renal insufficiency. Aztreonam is cleared by hemodialysis and peritoneal dialysis.

Mechanism of Action and Spectrum of Activity

Aztreonam, like other beta-lactams, interferes with bacterial cell wall synthesis by binding to and inactivating PBPs. The principal activity of aztreonam is against most aerobic gram-negative organisms, including *P. aeruginosa, S. marcescens,* and *Citrobacter* species. It has virtually no activity against gram-positive organisms. Its gram-negative coverage is similar to that of the aminoglycosides and third-generation cephalosporins. Aztreonam is not active against anaerobic organisms.

Mechanism of Resistance

Resistance to aztreonam occurs when the outer membrane of the gram-negative organism (ie, *P. aeruginosa*) becomes partially or wholly impermeable to the agent. Although aztreonam is relatively stable to hydrolysis by beta-lactamases, this mechanism of resistance is becoming more prevalent in hospital-acquired infections as well.

Table 8.14

Aztreonam Dosages

Severity of Infection	Adult Dosages	Pediatric Dosages
Mild	500 mg IV q8–12h	90–120 mg/kg/d q6–8h
Moderate	1–2 g IV q8–12h	
Severe	2 g IV q6–8h	

Note: Dosage adjustment required in patients with impaired renal function.

Clinical Uses

Aztreonam is commonly used in treating both complicated and uncomplicated urinary tract infections and respiratory tract infections such as pneumonia and bronchitis when aerobic gram-negative coverage is necessary. It usually is used in combination with an agent with gram-positive activity to broaden coverage. It is a reasonable substitute for the aminoglycosides in treating gram-negative infections in patients at high risk of toxicity.

Adverse Events

Aztreonam has a relatively safe toxicity profile. Most of the adverse events associated with aztreonam are local reactions and GI symptoms. Elevated aminotransferase levels have also been documented. Despite its beta-lactam structure, patients allergic to penicillins and cephalosporins usually do not manifest an allergic reaction to aztreonam. A cross-allergy specifically with ceftazidime has been reported and linked to an identical side chain on both compounds. No clinically significant drug interactions have been documented with aztreonam.

OXAZOLIDINONES

The oxazolidinones are a totally synthetic antibiotic class first investigated in the late 1980s as antidepressant agents. Serendipitously, these agents were discovered to have excellent antibacterial activity. The main reason for their clinical development has been the development and spread of resistance in gram-positive pathogens. The first agent in this class, linezolid (Zyvox), was approved by the FDA on April 18, 2000.

Pharmacokinetics and Pharmacodynamics

The oxazolidinones are well absorbed from the GI tract. Peak levels are achieved within 1 to 2 hours, and levels increase linearly as the dose is increased. The absolute bioavailability is approximately 100%. The oral formulation may be administered without regard to meals. Linezolid is predominantly eliminated by nonrenal mechanisms. Its metabolism does not involve the cytochrome P450 enzyme system. Two inactive metabolites are the major byproducts of this conversion to more water-soluble products that are excreted by the kidney. Dosage (adult, oral or IV: 200 to 600 mg twice daily) adjustment is not required for age or weight or in patients with altered renal or hepatic function.

Pharmacodynamically, this class most commonly produces a bacteriostatic effect. The most important parameter for predicting efficacy appears to be the time during which concentrations are maintained above the minimum inhibitory concentration. A post-antibiotic effect of 3 to 6 hours has been reported, but this has little clinical significance.

Mechanism of Action and Spectrum of Activity

The oxazolidinones are protein synthesis–inhibiting compounds. They bind to the 50S ribosome at a unique binding site and disrupt protein synthesis. To date, neither cross-resistance nor synergy or additivity has been described with other antibiotic classes. Antagonism has been described with chloramphenicol and clindamycin.

The principal activity of linezolid is against gram-positive aerobic organisms, including staphylococci, streptococci, and enterococci. In particular, activity against resistant pathogens, including methicillin-resistant staphylococci, penicillin-resistant streptococci, and vancomycin-resistant enterococci, is excellent.

Mechanism of Resistance

Resistance has been reported in 15 patients, all of them infected with an enterococcal species. The mechanism is a mutation at the binding site for linezolid at the 50S ribosome.

Clinical Uses

Linezolid has been approved by the FDA for the treatment of community- and hospital-acquired pneumonia, skin and skin structure infections, and vancomycin-resistant *Enterococcus faecium* infections. For the foreseeable future, this agent will likely be used specifically to treat multiply resistant gram-positive infections caused by methicillin-resistant staphylococci, penicillin-resistant *Streptococcus pneumoniae*, and vancomycin-resistant *E. faecium*.

Adverse Events

In general, linezolid is well tolerated. The most common adverse events include diarrhea, nausea, taste perversion, and vomiting. As mentioned earlier, this class of agents was initially investigated for its antidepressant activity. Thrombocytopenia has been reported on average in 3% to 4% of patients in studies, so caution should be used in patients at risk for this adverse reaction. These agents possess weak monoamine oxidase inhibitory activity. There is a potential for drug interactions with sympathomimetic agents, such as pseudoephedrine (Sudafed), or foods rich in tyramine.

PENICILLINS

First isolated in 1928, the penicillins were used successfully to treat streptococcal and staphylococcal infections. Since then, many synthetic penicillins have been developed to address the emerging problem of resistance. Despite resistance, the penicillins remain an important class of antimicrobials. They are classified based on their spectra of activity.

Pharmacokinetics and Pharmacodynamics

Most of the penicillins are unstable in the acid environment of the stomach and must be administered parenterally. Those that are acid stable are given orally (Table 8-15). They are widely distributed in the body and penetrate the CSF in the presence of inflammation. Most of the penicillins are excreted by the kidneys, and renal impairment necessitates dosage adjustment. The half-life of the penicillins in general is 30 to 60 minutes. The penicillins are removed by hemodialysis, with the exception of nafcillin (Unipen) and oxacillin (Bactocill). The penicillins exhibit

Table 8.15

Penicillin Dosages

Drug	Adult Dosages	Pediatric Dosages
Natural		
penicillin G	2–4 million units q4–6h IV	100,000–400,000 units/kg/d IV q4–6h
penicillin G benzathine	1.2–2.4 million units IM at specified intervals	300,000–2.4 million units IM
penicillin G procaine	0.6–4.8 million units IM in divided doses q12–24h at specified intervals	25,000–50,000 units/kg/d IM
penicillin VK	250–500 mg PO q6h	25,000–50,000 units/kg/d q6–8h
Aminopenicillins		
ampicillin	1–2 g q4–6h IV	
amoxicillin–ampicillin	250–500 mg PO q8h	100–400 mg/kg/d IV q4–6h
	400–800 mg PO q12h	50–100 mg/kg/d q6–8h PO
Carboxypenicillins		
carbenicillin indanyl	382–764 mg PO q6h	30–50 mg/kg/d q6h PO
ticarcillin sodium	3 g q4–6h IV	200–300 mg/kg/d q4–6h
Penicillinase Resistant		
cloxacillin	250–500 mg PO q6h	50–100 mg/kg/d q6h PO
dicloxacillin	250–500 mg PO q6h	25–100 mg/kg/d q6h PO
nafcillin	500 mg–1 g IV q4–6h	50–200 mg/kg/d q4–6h PO/IV
oxacillin	250–500 mg PO q4–6h	100–200 mg/kg/d q4–6h IV
	1–2 g q4–6h	
Ureidopenicillins		
mezlocillin	3–4 g IV q4–6h	200–450 mg/kg/d q4–6h
piperacillin	3–4 g IV q4–6h	200–300 mg/kg/d q4–6h

Note: Dosage adjustment of all above drugs required in patients with impaired renal function, with the exception of penicillinase-resistant penicillins.

time-dependent bactericidal activity and a post-antibiotic effect against most gram-positive organisms.

Mechanism of Action and Spectrum of Activity

The mechanism of action of the penicillins is inhibition of bacterial cell growth by interference with cell wall synthesis.

Mechanism of Resistance

Resistance to the penicillins occurs primarily through inactivation of the beta-lactam ring by the beta-lactamase enzymes. Other mechanisms include alteration in porin size and PBP target site, which result in decreased penetration of the penicillins.

Clinical Uses

The penicillins are effective in a variety of infections, including those of the upper and lower respiratory tract, urinary tract, and CNS, as well as sexually transmitted diseases. They are the agents of choice for treating gram-positive infections such as endocarditis caused by susceptible organisms. Both the carboxypenicillins and ureidopenicillins are useful in treating infections caused by *P. aeruginosa*.

Adverse Events

There is a low incidence of adverse reactions with penicillin administration. Hypersensitivity reactions characterized by maculopapular rash and urticaria are most common. GI side effects are most common with oral administration. In the presence of severe renal dysfunction, high-dose penicillins have been associated with seizures and encephalopathy. Thrombophlebitis has occurred with IV administration. The Jarisch-Herxheimer reaction, characterized by fevers, chills, sweating, and flushing, may occur when penicillin is used in treating spirochetal infections, in particular syphilis. Release of toxic particles from the organism precipitates the reaction.

Drug interactions involving penicillins are rare. Probenecid has been shown to increase the half-life of the penicillins by inhibiting the tubular secretion of penicillins. Both the carboxypenicillins and ureidopenicillins have been shown to inactivate the aminoglycosides, and these agents should not be mixed in the same IV solution. Also, the parenteral carboxypenicillins have a high sodium content. Caution should be used in patients with fluid or sodium restrictions.

RIFAMPIN

Rifampin is a macrocyclic antibiotic used in a variety of settings; it has become a first-line agent in treating tuberculosis. It is typically combined with vancomycin in treating methicillin-resistant *S. aureus* (MRSA) infections.

Pharmacokinetics and Pharmacodynamics

Rifampin is completely absorbed after oral administration. It distributes into most tissues and fluids, including the CSF. Oral adult dosage is 600 to 1,200 mg daily; parenteral dosage is 10 to 20 mg/kg IV daily. The half-life of rifampin is approximately 3 hours. It is metabolized by the liver and is not removed by hemodialysis or peritoneal dialysis. Rifampin exhibits a post-antibiotic effect against mycobacteria.

Mechanism of Action and Spectrum of Activity

Rifampin inhibits bacterial RNA synthesis by binding to the beta subunit of DNA-dependent RNA polymerase, blocking RNA transcription.

Rifampin is extremely active against gram-positive cocci. It has moderate activity against aerobic gram-negative bacilli. *Neisseria meningitidis*, *Neisseria gonorrhoeae*, and *H. influenzae* are the most sensitive gram-negative organisms. It is also active against *Legionella*. Rifampin maintains its activity against *M. tuberculosis*.

Mechanism of Resistance

Resistance to rifampin is conferred by modification of the beta subunit, resulting in decreased binding affinity of the drug. Multiple agents are used to delay emergence of resistance in treating tuberculosis.

Clinical Uses

Rifampin is commonly used in combination with a cell wall-active agent to treat serious, gram-positive infections that fail to respond to other courses of therapy. It is the drug of choice for postexposure meningitis prophylaxis against *N. meningitidis* and *H. influenzae* type B. Rifampin is a first-line agent in the treatment of *M. tuberculosis* infection, and it is used to treat nontuberculous mycobacterial infections as well.

Adverse Events

The most common side effects associated with rifampin are GI distress (nausea, vomiting, and diarrhea), headache, and fever. Although not a true adverse effect, rifampin changes bodily fluids such as sweat, saliva, and tears to a red-orange color. Hepatotoxicity is rare, but the risk increases when it is administered in combination with isoniazid (Laniazid). Anemia or thrombocytopenia also has been reported. Uveitis, an inflammation of the eye, is a rare but dose-related side effect.

Rifampin is a potent inducer of hepatic cytochrome P450 drug metabolism and precipitates many drug interactions. Rifampin increases the clearance of agents such as antiarrhythmics, azole antifungals, clarithromycin, warfarin, and protease inhibitors.

STREPTOGRAMINS

The streptogramin antibiotics are naturally occurring products that have been used clinically in Europe for more than 30 years as oral agents to treat mild to moderate infections. A parenteral formulation has recently become available. A semisynthetic derivative, quinupristin/dalfopristin (Synercid), is the first injectable streptogramin antibiotic.

Pharmacokinetics and Pharmacodynamics

Synercid is not absorbed from the GI tract. After IV administration, both quinupristin and dalfopristin have a serum half-life of approximately 1 hour. Clearance of both agents is through the liver. Conjugation with glutathione or cysteine results in at least two active metabolites from each of the parent compounds. Although the cytochrome P450 enzyme system is not involved in the metabolism of Synercid, cytochrome P450 3A4 (responsible for the metabolism of many drugs) is significantly inhibited by Synercid. Close clinical or serum level monitoring of agents such as cyclosporine is recommended.

Pharmacodynamically, Synercid is a bactericidal agent against most organisms, with the noted exception of vancomycin-resistant *E. faecium*. The parameter that appears to be most predictive of efficacy is the ratio of the area under the concentration curve over the minimum inhibitory concentration. Synercid possesses a post-antibiotic effect ranging from 8 to 18 hours. The dosage for adults and children is 7.5 mg/kg every 8 to 12 hours.

Mechanism of Action and Spectrum of Activity

The streptogramins inhibit protein synthesis by binding to the 50S ribosome. The interaction of quinupristin and dalfopristin is synergistic. Either compound alone is bacteriostatic, whereas the combination results in a bactericidal effect. Additivity or synergy has been described with vancomycin, ampicillin, cefotaxime, and doxycycline (Vibramycin).

The principal activity of Synercid is against gram-positive aerobic organisms, including staphylococci, streptococci, and enterococci. In particular, its activity against resistant pathogens, including methicillin-resistant staphylococci, penicillin-resistant streptococci, and vancomycin-resistant *E. faecium*, is excellent. Synercid is not active against *Enterococcus faecalis*, however.

Mechanism of Resistance

Several mechanisms of resistance to the streptogramins have been identified. The most clinically important mechanism is a result of a change in the binding site for quinupristin. This resistance trait is known as the MLSB form of resistance. To date, this mechanism has not resulted in an organism becoming nonsusceptible to Synercid. The clinical relevance of this characteristic is controversial, and it will likely play a larger role because this trait is widespread in a variety of organisms. The other mechanisms include enzymatic modification of the streptogramins and active efflux of the drugs out of the bacterium. The clinical significance and prevalence of these mechanisms are unknown.

Clinical Uses

Synercid is approved by the FDA for treating skin and skin structure infections and vancomycin-resistant *E. faecium* infections. For the foreseeable future, this agent will likely be used specifically to treat multiply resistant gram-positive infections caused by methicillin-resistant staphylococci, penicillin-resistant *S. pneumoniae*, and vancomycin-resistant *E. faecium*.

Adverse Events

The most common adverse reactions are infusion related. Infusion site reactions, including pain, inflammation, edema, and thrombophlebitis, have been reported in as many as 75% of patients who have received Synercid through a peripheral IV catheter. Arthralgias and myalgias have also been reported. They may be severe and result in discontinuation of therapy.

Table 8.16

Sulfonamide Dosages

Drug	Adult Dosages	Pediatric Dosages
sulfadiazine	4–8 g PO in divided doses	120–200 mg/kg/d q6h
sulfamethoxazole	1 g PO q8h	50–60 mg/kg/d q12h
sulfisoxazole	4–8 g PO in divided doses	120–150 mg/kg/d q4–6h
trimethoprim	100 mg PO q12h	4–6 mg/kg/d q12h
trimethoprim– sulfamethoxazole	160/800 mg PO q12h 10–20 mg/kg/d IV in divided doses	6–20 mg/kg/d q6–12h

Note: Dosage adjustment necessary in patients with renal impairment.

They usually occur after several days of therapy. After discontinuation of therapy, these reactions are uniformly reversible. The most common laboratory abnormality is an increased level of conjugated bilirubin.

SULFONAMIDES

In 1932, the dye prontosil rubrum was found to be effective in treating streptococcal infections. Subsequent studies found that one of its byproducts was sulfanilamide. Manipulation of this byproduct created the class of antimicrobials known as the sulfonamides.

Pharmacokinetics and Pharmacodynamics

Oral sulfonamides are readily absorbed from the GI tract. They are distributed through all body tissues and enter the CSF, pleural fluid, and synovial fluid. They are eliminated from the body by glomerular filtration and metabolism. The half-lives of the sulfonamides vary from hours to days; sulfadoxine (Fansidar), at 5 to 10 days, has the longest half-life. Table 8-16 gives dosing information.

Mechanism of Action and Spectrum of Activity

The sulfonamides work by inhibiting the incorporation of para-aminobenzoic acid (PABA) into DNA, thereby inhibiting folic acid production and bacterial cell growth.

Trimethoprim (Primsol) inhibits the enzyme dihydrofolate reductase, synergistically inhibiting folic acid formation at another step in the pathway.

The sulfonamides are active against a wide range of gram-positive and gram-negative organisms, with the exception of *Pseudomonas* species and group A streptococci. In combination with other folate antagonists, they also demonstrate activity against *P. carinii* and *Toxoplasma gondii*.

Mechanism of Resistance

Resistance to the sulfonamides occurs as a result of overproduction of PABA or structural changes in enzymes so there is less affinity for the sulfonamide substrate.

Clinical Uses

The sulfonamides are frequently used in treating a number of infections. Poorly absorbed, sulfasalazine (Azulfidine) is used in the management of ulcerative colitis. Because of their limited spectrum of activity and increasing resistance, the sulfonamides are typically used in combination with other agents to increase efficacy or expand coverage. Trimethoprim–sulfamethoxazole (Bactrim) is the combination of choice in treating urinary tract infections, *P. carinii* pneumonia, toxoplasmosis, and some resistant gram-negative infections.

Adverse Events

A variety of side effects are reported for sulfonamides. The most common are rash, fever, and GI side effects. The rash occurs within 1 to 2 weeks of initiating therapy. Severe dermatologic reactions, such as Stevens-Johnson syndrome and vasculitis, are uncommon and associated more with the longer-acting preparations. Hemolytic anemia can occur in patients with glucose-6-phosphate dehydrogenase deficiency.

The sulfonamides potentiate the effects of warfarin, phenytoin, hypoglycemic agents, and methotrexate (MTX) as a result of drug displacement or decreased liver metabolism.

TETRACYCLINES

The tetracyclines possess activity against gram-positive, gram-negative, and atypical organisms, including rickettsiae, chlamydiae, mycobacteria, and spirochetes. They are separated into short-, intermediate-, and long-acting agents. Doxycycline and minocycline (Minocin) are considered the most active of the class. The tetracyclines became the first class of antimicrobials to be labeled "broad spectrum," and they remain a frequently used class of antimicrobials.

Pharmacokinetics and Pharmacodynamics

Absorption from the GI tract varies among agents, along with protein binding. The long-acting agents have the highest absorption and are bound to protein to the greatest extent. With the exception of the long-acting agents, absorption of the agents is improved with administration on an empty stomach. The tetracyclines have excellent tissue distribution. The primary route of elimination is through the kidney by glomerular filtration, with the exception of doxycycline. In general, the short-acting agents have a half-life of 8 hours, and the long-acting agents, 16 to 18 hours. The tetracyclines are removed to a small degree by hemodialysis, but it does not warrant a dosage adjustment. Table 8-17 gives dosing information.

Table 8.17

Tetracycline Dosages*

Drug	Adult Dosages
demeclocycline	150 mg PO q6h
	300 mg PO q12h
doxycycline	100 mg IV/PO q12h
minocycline	100 mg PO q12h
oxytetracycline	1–2 g/d PO in divided doses
	300 mg/d PO in divided doses
tetracycline	1–2 g/d PO in divided doses

*The tetracyclines are not recommended for use in children.
Note: Dosage adjustment for all above drugs necessary in patients with renal impairment, with the exception of doxycycline.

Mechanism of Action and Spectrum of Activity

The tetracyclines inhibit bacterial protein synthesis by binding to the 30S subunit of the ribosome. The tetracyclines are active against gram-positive and gram-negative bacteria and atypical organisms, including spirochetes, rickettsiae, chlamydiae, mycoplasma, and legionellae. They typically are bacteriostatic agents.

Mechanism of Resistance

The most common mechanism of resistance to the tetracyclines is decreased entry of drug into the cell or an increased ability of the organism to export antibiotic. A second mechanism, not clearly understood, is inactivation of tetracycline by resistant organisms. Development of resistance to one agent typically confers resistance to the entire class.

Clinical Uses

Because of their broad spectrum of activity, the tetracyclines are used extensively in a variety of settings. They are typically used as alternatives when beta-lactams are not an option. They are frequently used in treating rickettsial, chlamydial, and gram-negative infections, in addition to acne vulgaris and pelvic inflammatory disease. Doxycycline is the drug of choice for the treatment of early Lyme disease. Demeclocycline (Declomycin) is commonly used to treat the syndrome of inappropriate antidiuretic hormone secretion.

Adverse Events

The most frequent side effects associated with the tetracyclines are anorexia, nausea, vomiting, and epigastric distress. These are typically lessened if the agents are administered with food. Thrombophlebitis is associated with IV administration, and it is recommended that the tetracycline be administered in a large volume of fluid and at rotated sites. Hepatotoxicity is a rare but fatal toxicity. The risk of hepatotoxicity increases if the patient is concurrently receiving other hepatotoxic agents. The Fanconi syndrome, characterized by nausea, vomiting, polydipsia, and acidosis, may develop if outdated tetracyclines are ingested. The toxic effects have been associated with citric acid in the formulation, which has been removed from current products. Gray-brown discoloration of the teeth can be a permanent effect of the tetracyclines. It results from stable tetracycline/calcium complexes in bone and teeth and is related to dose and duration of therapy. Patients receiving tetracyclines are more sensitive to the effects of the sun because of accumulation of the drug in the skin. Minocycline has been associated with dose-related vertigo.

There are multiple drug interactions involving the tetracyclines. The absorption of the tetracyclines is affected by a number of agents. Tetracyclines form chelating complexes with divalent and trivalent cations, decreasing the absorption of the tetracycline. It is recommended that the administration of tetracyclines and antacids, iron, and sucralfate (Carafate) be separated. Likewise, food decreases the absorption of most tetracyclines, with the exception of doxycycline. Milk and dairy products also impair their absorption. Phenytoin and carbamazepine (Tegretol), enzyme inducers, decrease the half-life of doxycycline. Concomitant administration of tetracyclines and oral contraceptives results in decreased levels of the oral contraceptive, so an additional form of contraception is recommended. The tetracyclines potentiate the effect of warfarin by impairing vitamin K production by intestinal flora.

VANCOMYCIN

Vancomycin is a glycopeptide antibiotic with a narrow spectrum of activity directed toward gram-positive organisms. Its potential for drug-related toxicities has limited its use as a first-line agent. Emergence of resistant gram-positive pathogens such as MRSA has made vancomycin an important agent in treating these serious infections.

Pharmacokinetics and Pharmacodynamics

Vancomycin is poorly absorbed from the GI tract except in patients with pseudomembranous colitis and concomitant renal insufficiency. Oral administration of vancomycin achieves concentrations in the stool sufficiently high to treat *C. difficile* colitis. The volume of distribution ranges from 0.6 to 0.9 L/kg, with good penetration into most bodily fluids and tissues. Unpredictable levels are attained in the CSF and bone. Vancomycin is almost completely excreted by the kidney through glomerular filtration. Monitoring renal function is important in determining proper dosing. Dosage adjustment is necessary in patients with renal insufficiency. The half-life in adults with normal renal function is 5 to 11 hours. Vancomycin is not cleared to a significant extent by hemodialysis or peritoneal dialysis. Many clinicians advocate the use of therapeutic drug monitoring to maximize efficacy and minimize toxicity. In general, the target trough concentration ranges between 5 to 10 mg/mL, and the peak concentration is 20 to 40 mg/mL. Vancomycin exhibits time-dependent bactericidal activity. Table 8-18 gives dosing information.

Mechanism of Action and Spectrum of Activity

Vancomycin is a cell wall–active agent that inhibits the second stage of bacterial cell wall synthesis by binding to the D-alanyl D-alanine portion of the cell wall precursor. It also alters membrane permeability and RNA synthesis.

The principal activity of vancomycin is limited to gram-positive aerobic and anaerobic bacteria such as methicillin-

Table 8.18

Vancomycin Dosages

Estimated Creatinine Clearance (mL/min)	Dosing Interval		
	40–55 kg, 500 mg*	55–75 kg, 750 mg*	75–100 kg, 1,000 mg*
>80	q8h	q12h	q12h
54–80	q12h	q18h	q18h
40–53	q18h	q24h	q24h
27–39	q24h	q36h	q36h
21–26	q36h	q48h	q48h
16–20	q48h		

Note: These recommendations represent one of several nomograms used in the empiric dosing of vancomycin. Some prescribers use pharmacokinetic calculations and monitor serum trough levels to evaluate the efficacy and toxicity of a particular regimen. Therapeutic trough levels are typically maintained between 5 and 10 μg/mL.
*Patient's body weight and IV dose of vancomycin.

sensitive and methicillin-resistant staphylococci and *Clostridium* species.

Mechanism of Resistance

As a result of increased use of vancomycin, resistance to the glycopeptides has developed. Resistance to vancomycin is mediated by enzymatic alteration of vancomycin's binding site so the drug cannot work effectively.

Clinical Uses

Vancomycin is used to treat a variety of infections. It is frequently used to treat serious gram-positive infections in patients allergic to or unable to tolerate beta-lactams, and it is the drug of choice for MRSA and other resistant gram-positive infections. Neutropenic fever, endocarditis, and meningitis are commonly treated with vancomycin. Oral vancomycin is used in treating *C. difficile* colitis that has failed to respond to metronidazole.

Adverse Events

The most common side effects associated with vancomycin administration are fever and chills, phlebitis, and "red man" syndrome. "Red man" syndrome is a histamine-mediated phenomenon associated with the rate of vancomycin infusion. The typical syndrome consists of pruritus; flushing of the head, neck, and face; and hypotension; it usually resolves on discontinuation of the drug. Vancomycin has been classified as an ototoxic and nephrotoxic agent. Although rare, ototoxicity has occurred in patients receiving high-dose therapy or concurrent other relatively toxic agents (eg, aminoglycosides).

Nephrotoxicity as a result of vancomycin alone is uncommon. Typically, a combination of variables and risk factors precipitates renal insufficiency. Risk factors include age, pre-existing renal disease, and the use of other nephrotoxic agents such as aminoglycosides, amphotericin B, acyclovir, and cyclosporine. Hematologic effects such as thrombocytopenia and neutropenia are rare.

IV vancomycin is incompatible with a variety of agents in solution, such as corticosteroids, aminophylline, and barbiturates.

Bibliography

Buckley, M. M., Brogden, R. N., Barradell, L. B., & Goa, K. L. (1992). Imipenem-cilastatin: a reappraisal of its antibacterial activity, pharmacokinetic properties, and therapeutic efficacy. *Drugs, 44*, 408.

Carpenter, C. F., & Chambers, H. F. (2004) Daptomycin: another novel agent for treating infections due to drug-resistant gram-positive pathogens. *Clinical Infectious Diseases, 38*, 994–1000.

Gelone, S. P., & Lorber, B. (1998). Clindamycin. *Antibiotics for the Clinician, 2*, 1–9.

Gilbert, D. N. (1991). Once-daily aminoglycoside therapy. *Antimicrobial Agents and Chemotherapy, 35*, 399–405.

Gilbert, D. N. (1995). Aminoglycosides. In G. L. Mandell, J. E. Bennett, & R. Dolin (Eds.), *Principles and practice of infectious diseases* (p. 281). New York: Churchill Livingstone.

Hellinger, W. C., & Brewer, N. S. (1999). Carbapenems and monobactams: imipenem, meropenem, and aztreonam. *Mayo Clinic Proceedings, 74*, 420.

Kasten, M. J. (1999). Clindamycin, metronidazole, and chloramphenicol. *Mayo Clinic Proceedings, 74*, 825.

Mayer, K. H. (1996). Sulfonamides and trimethoprim. In V. T. Andriole (Ed.), *Current infectious disease drugs* (p. 164). Philadelphia: Current Medicine.

McKinnon, P. S., Freeman, C., & Sougakoff, W. (1999). Beta-lactam and beta-lactamase inhibitor combinations. In V. L. Yu, T. C. Merrigan, Jr., & S. L. Barriere (Eds.), *Antimicrobial therapy and vaccines* (p. 676). Baltimore: Williams & Wilkins.

Morris, A. B., Kanyok, T. P., Scott, J., et al. (1999). Rifamycins. In V. L. Yu, T. C. Merrigan, Jr., & S. L. Barriere (Eds.), *Antimicrobial therapy and vaccines* (pp. 901–962). Baltimore: Williams & Wilkins.

Myers, B. R., Gurtman, A. C., & Farrington, J. M. (1996). Cephalosporins. In V. T. Andriole (Ed.), *Current infectious disease drugs* (p. 13). Philadelphia: Current Medicine.

Neu, H. C. (1992). Quinolones antimicrobial agents. *Annual Review of Medicine, 43*, 465.

O'Donnell, J. A., & Gelone, S. P. (2000). Fluoroquinolones. *Infectious Disease Clinics of North America, 14*, 489–513.

O'Donnell, J. A., & Gelone, S. P. (2004). The newer fluoroquinolones. *Infectious Disease Clinics of North America, 18*, 691–716.

Saxon, A., Beall, G. N., Rohr, A. F., et al. (1987). Immediate hypersensitivity reactions to beta-lactam antibiotics. *Annals of Internal Medicine, 107*, 204.

Smilack, J. D. (1999). The tetracyclines. *Mayo Clinic Proceedings, 74*, 727.

Spiers, K. M., & Zervos, M. J. (2004) Telithromycin. *Expert Review Anti-Infective Therapy, 2*, 685–693.

Westley-Horton, E., & Koestner, J. A. (1991). Aztreonam: a review of the first monobactam. *American Journal of Medical Science, 302*, 46.

Wilhelm, M. P., & Estes, L. (1999). Vancomycin. *Mayo Clinic Proceedings, 74*, 928.

Williams, J. D., & Sefton, A. M. (1993). Comparison of macrolide antibiotics. *Journal of Antimicrobial Chemotherapy, 31*(Suppl. C), 11.

Wrighet, A. J. (1999). The penicillins. *Mayo Clinic Proceedings, 74*, 290.

Visit the Connection web site for the most up-to-date drug information.

COMPLEMENTARY AND ALTERNATIVE MEDICINE (CAM)

■ VIRGINIA P. ARCANGELO

There has been a tremendous growth in the use of complementary and alternative medicine (CAM) in the United States in recent years. *Complementary medicine* is defined as that used together with conventional medicine. *Alternative medicine* is that used in place of conventional medicine. Users of CAM are mostly between 30 and 49 years of age. Women use CAM more frequently than men. People use CAM because they want more control over their medical care, they feel an affinity for a holistic or "natural" approach, they are dissatisfied with the attitudes of their health care providers, or conventional medicine fails to meet their needs (Box 9-1). *Integrative medicine*, a combination of mainstream medical treatment and CAM, appears to have more scientific evidence regarding safety and efficacy. This chapter will focus on the agents that are in the mainstream of Western society, such as herbal or dietary supplements.

In 1995, the National Institute of Health's Office of Alternative Medicine (OAM) defined CAM as the "broad domain of healing resources that encompasses all health systems, modalities, and practices and their accompanying theories and beliefs other than those intrinsic to the politically dominant health system of a particular society or culture in a given historical period. CAM includes all such practices and ideas self-defined by their users as preventing or treating illness or promoting health and well-being. Boundaries within CAM and between CAM and domains of the dominant system are not sharp or fixed" (Panel on Definition and Description, CAM Research Methodology Conference, 1995).

DOMAINS OF CAM

There are five domains of CAM (Box 9-2): alternative medicine system, mind/body interventions, biologically based therapy, manipulation and body-based methods, and energy therapies. Alternative medicine systems are based on complete systems of theory and practice. Mind/body interventions incorporate a variety of techniques to enhance the mind's capacity to affect bodily function; a common practice is biofeedback. Biologically based therapy is treatment with substances found in nature. Manipulation and body-based methods are based on manipulation or movement of body parts; an example is chiropractic manipulation.

Energy therapies involve the use of energy fields such as magnets.

NATIONAL CENTER FOR COMPLEMENTARY AND ALTERNATIVE MEDICINE

The National Center for Complementary and Alternative Medicine (NCCAM) was established in 1998 by congressional mandate. It is dedicated to exploring complementary and alternative healing practices in the context of rigorous science. Its purpose is to train CAM researchers and disseminate authoritative information to the public and professionals. It serves as an information clearinghouse and facilitates research and training programs, which are funded by the federal government. NCCAM has four areas of focus: research, research training and career development, outreach, and integration.

NCCAM identifies CAM practitioners. It also publishes alerts and advisories for specific products and practices, lists clinical trials of CAM, and provides treatment information.

REGULATION

Over 100 million Americans use dietary supplements, which are defined as products taken orally that contain a "dietary product" intended to supplement the diet. These may include vitamins, minerals, herbs, amino acids, other botanicals, or substances such as enzymes, organ tissues, and metabolites. The products may be in the form of powder, capsules, tablets, gelcaps, or liquids. The increasing use of dietary supplements reflects the increased interest in "natural" medicine, fitness, health, and disease prevention. Also, consumers want to avoid the high cost of traditional drugs and the side effects of these drugs.

More than 500 herbs are marketed in the United States; indeed, about 25% of the current pharmacopoeia is derived from botanicals. The cardiac glycoside digoxin comes from the foxglove plant. Aspirin comes from willow bark, oral contraceptives from Mexican yam, warfarin from sweet clover, and capsaicin from the red pepper plant.

BOX 9–1. REASONS TO USE CAM

- Advertising
- Desire to have control over treatment
- Desperation
- Dissatisfaction with prescription drugs
- Perceived effectiveness
- Perceived safety
- Rejection of established medical practices

In March 2003, the FDA published new guidelines for dietary supplements that would prevent contamination with other herbs, pesticides, heavy metals, or prescription drugs. Manufacturers do not have to prove the supplement's quality but must meet certain FDA standards. The FDA can take action only if it finds that a product is unsafe once it is on the market. Each product must have a label accurately listing the product's ingredients. Box 9-3 lists label requirements for herbal preparations.

Products also have a "Supplemental Facts" panel that lists the appropriate serving size. Natural remedies cannot be

---

BOX 9–2. DOMAINS OF COMPLEMENTARY AND ALTERNATIVE MEDICINE

Alternative Medicine Systems — These are built upon complete systems of theory and practice and have often evolved apart from and earlier than the conventional medical approach popular in the United States. Examples are homeopathic and naturopathic medicine and traditional Chinese medicine.

Mind-Body Interventions — This incorporates a variety of techniques designed to enhance the mind's capacity to affect bodily function and symptoms. This includes biofeedback, meditation, dance therapy, and art therapy.

Biologically Based Therapy — This is treatment with substances found in nature, including dietary supplements, herbal supplements, and "natural" but scientifically unproved treatment.

Manipulation and Body-Based Methods — These are based on manipulation or movement of body parts. Examples include chiropractic manipulation and massage therapy.

Energy Therapies — This is the use of energy fields. Biofield therapy affects the energy fields that purportedly surround and penetrate the human body and includes Reiki and Therapeutic Touch. Bioelectromagnetic therapy is based on treatment involving the unconventional use of electromagnetic fields. An example is magnet therapy.

BOX 9–3. LABEL REQUIREMENTS FOR HERBAL PREPARATIONS

- Name
- Quantity of contents
- Ingredients and amounts
- Disclaimer: "This statement has not been evaluated by the FDA. This product is not intended to diagnose, treat, cure or prevent disease."
- Supplemental facts panel
  - Serving size
  - Amount
  - Active ingredients
- Other ingredients such as herbs for which no daily values exist
- Name and address of manufacturer, packer, or distributor

---

patented, so the manufacturer does not need to take the time and money to conduct necessary tests.

Nutrition Labeling and Education Act (NLEA)

NLEA was enacted by Congress in 1990 to provide a clear relationship of nutrition to disease. The purpose of the act was to educate consumers. Information required on the label includes nutritional information, in an easy-to-read format, with the amount of ingredient per serving, the percentage of daily values of the ingredients, and the standard serving size. The act also established that disease-related health claims could be used on labeling of nutritional products, provided there is agreement among qualified scientists that the claim is valid. A sample of a dietary supplement label is shown in Box 9-4.

Dietary Supplement Health and Education Act

DSHEA, passed in 1994, restricted the FDA's control over dietary supplements. It defined herbal products as dietary

---

BOX 9–4. SAMPLE OF LABEL FOR HERBAL PRODUCT

Supplemental Facts

Serving size 1 capsule	Amount per	%Daily
Chromium	serving	value
Other ingredients: flour, rice, gelatin	500 mg	400%
Supports glucose and fat metabolism		

supplements, which are considered foods. Before this, products had to be proven safe by the FDA; those introduced after the act's passage had to be proven safe by the manufacturer. The manufacturer of an herbal preparation is responsible for the truthfulness of the claims made on a label and must have evidence supporting the claims; however, there is no standard for this evidence, nor does the manufacturer need to submit it to the FDA. The manufacturer may claim that the product affects the structure or function of the body as long as there is no claim of effectiveness in the prevention or treatment of a specific disease. A disclaimer must be provided stating that the FDA has not evaluated the product. Since health claims are not pre-approved, the statement "This statement has not been evaluated by the Food and Drug Administration. This product is not intended to diagnose, treat, cure or prevent any disease" must be on the label. Information regarding therapeutic claims for herbal products can be disseminated as long as the information is not misleading or product-specific, is physically separated from the product, and has no product stickers affixed to it.

In 2000, the FDA allowed "structure and function" statements to be made. For example, cranberry products could say that the product supports urinary health, but not that it treats urinary tract infections. It allowed for claims that do not relate to disease but are health maintenance claims ("maintains a healthy circulatory system"), non-disease claims ("helps you relax"), and claims for minor symptoms associated with life stages ("for common symptoms of PMS"). Anything that uses words such as "prevents," "treats," "cures," "mitigates," or "diagnoses disease" is subject to drug requirements.

This act led to enormous growth in the dietary supplement industry, which today grosses over $18 billion annually.

RISKS

Many herbs and alternative medicines have not been studied adequately and may in fact be toxic. The fact that plants are "natural" does not make the use of agents from that plant free of risks! Adverse reactions can result from direct exposure to the component of the plant or from poor manufacturing process. The law does not require that adverse events resulting from the use of dietary supplements be reported to the FDA. Research studies of safety in people are not required because, as noted above, these agents are considered dietary supplements, not drugs. There is inappropriate dissemination of information and weak regulation in the industry. Box 9-5 lists the dangers of herbal preparations.

One example of an adverse reaction that has brought about governmental action is ephedra. Ephedra, a common ingredient in weight-loss products, can cause an increase in blood pressure, tremors, arrhythmia, seizures, strokes, myocardial infarction, and death. In April 2004 the FDA banned its sale.

There is no check on the ingredients in a preparation. Analyses of herbal supplements have found differences between what is on the label and what is actually in the bottle. There may be less or more of the supplement than the label indicates.

Herbal medicines can be purchased and consumed by anyone. They are less expensive than prescription drugs but can still be costly.

BOX 9–5. DANGERS OF HERBAL PRODUCTS

- Many herbs and alternative medicines have not been studied adequately and may be toxic.
- Research studies of safety in people are not required.
- Natural remedies cannot be patented, so the manufacturer does not take the time and money to conduct necessary tests.
- There is inappropriate dissemination of information and weak regulation in the industry.
- Herbal supplements can be bought by anyone.
- There can be herb–drug interactions.

HERB/DRUG INTERACTIONS

Interactions between dietary supplements and drugs can be pharmacokinetic or pharmacodynamic. Pharmacokinetic interactions can be a change in the amount of active compounds available and are the consequence of alteration in absorption, distribution, metabolism, or excretion. For example, senna, a common ingredient in weight-loss products, has a laxative effect that can affect drug transit time and reduce absorption. Zinc lozenges, often used to relieve cold symptoms, may chelate fluoroquinolones and tetracyclines, decreasing serum levels of these antibiotics.

Pharmacodynamic interactions occur at the site of action and may be additive or antagonistic to prescribed drugs or other herbal preparations. Vitamin E doses of greater than 1,000 units per day can increase the anticoagulant effect of warfarin. Ephedra has additive effects with caffeine and at high doses can cause death.

There can be an effect on drug metabolism. Herbal products can affect cytochrome P-450 isoenzymes. For example, St. John's wort is a potent herbal inducer of cytochrome P-450 3A4.

PATIENT EDUCATION

Patients must be aware that herbal preparations have pharmacologic properties. There are interactions with many prescription and over-the-counter medications. All products should be purchased from a reliable source. The more ambitious the claim, the more suspicious the consumer should be of the product.

The consumer can request professional health information from the company such as the nature of the company, testing procedures, quality control standards, and so forth.

Consumers should avoid excessive dosing. Taking higher than the recommended dosage can increase the possibility of adverse effects. All supplements should be discontinued during pregnancy and lactation and avoided in children under 12.

Dietary supplements should not be used for serious health conditions without the advice and supervision of a qualified health professional. Most dietary supplements are meant to treat mild, short-term disorders.

Combination products should be avoided. Combining more than two or three ingredients in one product is not good because it is impossible to tell which ingredient is causing side effects if they develop. Multivitamins are the exception.

All side effects should be reported to a health professional. The side effects may be due to the dietary supplement or from interaction with a prescribed drug.

Consumers can obtain information about CAM from many websites (Box 9-6).

COMMONLY USED HERBS

The following section reviews some commonly used dietary supplements (herbs). Table 9-1 lists them by use for various organ systems.

Acidophilus

Action and Proof of Efficacy

Acidophilus is a nonpathologic bacteria that resides in the gastrointestinal (GI) tract. It helps maintain a balance of bacterial diversity. It binds enterocytes within the GI tract and prevents harmful bacteria from attaching to these cells. Clinical trials have not yielded many positive results.

Uses and Dosage

Acidophilus is commonly used to restore normal oral, GI, and vaginal flora. This is potentially useful in patients taking antibiotics because the normal flora may be disturbed by the bactericidal or bacteriostatic activity of the drug. Further, patients with *Candida* and bacterial infections may have an imbalance of normal flora. The dosage of acidophilus ranges from 1 to 10 billion viable organisms a day in three or four divided doses.

Adverse Reactions

Adverse reactions are GI-related, primarily flatulence. Warfarin's efficacy may be reduced because acidophilus may enhance the intestinal absorption of vitamin K.

Black Cohosh

Action and Proof of Efficacy

Black cohosh has vascular and estrogenic activity. Some studies have shown that black cohosh binds to estrogen receptors.

Uses and Dosage

The action of estrogen-receptor binding is thought to mimic natural estrogen activity. Therefore, black cohosh is used for dysmenorrhea and vasomotor menopausal symptoms. The recommended dosage is 40 to 200 mg daily.

Adverse Reactions and Drug Interactions

Black cohosh can cause nausea, dizziness, increased perspiration, and bradycardia. It interacts with several classes of drugs, such as anesthetics and sedatives. It may increase the hypotensive effect of many antihypertensive agents. It also may increase the effects of estrogen supplements. Black cohosh is contraindicated in patients with estrogen-dependent tumors.

Echinacea

Action and Proof of Efficacy

Echinacea stimulates phagocytosis and increases respiratory cellular activity and mobility of leukocytes. A review of 19 German controlled studies in treatment of the common cold showed that there may be some effect on the immune system, but a recent study showed no effect on children ages 2 to 11.

Uses and Dosage

Echinacea is used to help heal abscesses, burns, eczema, and skin wounds and to treat the common cold. The recommended dosage is 1 g three times a day for capsules; 6 to 9 mL per day for expressed juice; or 0.75 to 1.5 mL two to five times a day as a tincture. It can also be ingested as a tea, using 2 teaspoonfuls of the herb simmered in 1 cup of boiling water for 10 minutes. It should be taken for no more than 8 weeks.

Adverse Reactions and Drug Interactions

Echinacea may cause a rash. It should not be taken by immunocompromised patients. Long-term use may suppress T cells. There are no reported drug interactions.

Garlic

Action and Proof of Efficacy

Garlic has lipid-lowering and antithrombotic properties. Results from clinical studies are varied. Cholesterol-lowering effects, if any, have been shown to be small.

Table 9.1

Common Herbal Preparations

Suggested System	Name/Dosage	Use	Selected Adverse Events	Contraindications/ Interactions	Special Considerations
Gastrointestinal (GI)	Acidophilus 1–10 billion viable organisms daily in 3 or 4 doses orally	Restore normal oral, GI, and vaginal flora altered by antibiotics or *Candida* and bacterial infections	Flatulence	Warfarin — may decrease efficacy	
Health promotion	Black cohosh 40–200 PO mg/day	Relief of menstrual and menopausal symptoms	Increased perspiration, dizziness, nausea/ vomiting, visual disturbances, reduced pulse	Anesthetics, antihypertensives, sedatives — may increase hypotensive effect. Not for use in patients with estrogen-dependent tumors	May increase effects of estrogen supplements
Respiratory disorders	Echinacea Capsule, 1 g PO TID; expressed juice, 6–9 mL daily; tea, 2 tsp herb simmered in boiling water for 10 min; tincture, 0.75–1.5 mL 2–5 times a day	Shorten duration of symptoms of URI, wound healing	Nausea, rash	Those who are immunocompromised (may suppress T cells). Human immunodeficiency virus. Tuberculosis. Multiple sclerosis	Only taken for 8 weeks
Cardiovascular disorders	Garlic 600–900 mg/day 1 clove of garlic daily	Lower cholesterol, prevent clot formation	Dizziness, irritation of mouth and esophagus, nausea, flatulence, malodorous breath and body, sweating	Warfarin (increased risk of bleeding)	The preparation must contain allicin, the active ingredient in garlic.
Neurologic/psychological	Gingko biloba 120–240 PO mg/day in 2 or 3 divided doses	Peripheral vascular insufficiency, memory loss	Headache, dizziness, heart palpitations	Aspirin (increased risk of bleeding). Nifedipine (elevated nifedipine levels). Trazodone (increased sedation). Warfarin (increased risk of bleeding). Hypoglycemic agents (facilitates clearance to elevate blood sugar). Thiazide diuretics (increases blood pressure when combined)	
Musculoskeletal	Glucosamine 500 mg PO TID	Antiarthritic	Potential to alter blood glucose levels, heartburn, diarrhea, nausea, abdominal pain	Sulfa allergy	
Neurologic/psycho-logical	Kava kava	Depression	Headaches, disturbance in visual accomodation	Alcohol (increases activity). Alprazolam (may induce coma). CNS depressants (additive sedative effects). Levodopa (increases parkinsonian symptoms)	
Neurologic/psycho-logical	Melatonin 5 mg PO HS Jet lag: 5 mg/day for 3 days before departure and ending 3 days after departure	Insomnia Jet lag	Headache, depression, drowsiness, confusion, hypothermia	Nifedipine (interferes with antihypertensive effect). Increased anxiolytic action with benzodiazipines	Drowsiness may occur within 30 minutes, so avoid operating machinery.

Table 9.1

Common Herbal Preparations (*Continued*)

Suggested System	Name/Dosage	Use	Selected Adverse Events	Contraindications/ Interactions	Special Considerations
Neurologic/ psychological	St. John's wort 320 mg PO daily	Depression, anxiety, neuralgic pain	Dizziness, restlessness, sleep disturbances, dry mouth, constipation, GI distress, photosensitivity	Oral contraceptives (decreased efficacy) Cyclosporine (decreased levels) Digoxin (decreased levels) Nifedipine (decreased levels) TCA (decreased levels) SSRIs (increased sedative effects and serotonin syndrome) Simvastatin (decreased cholesterol-lowering effect) Theophylline (decreased levels) Warfarin (decreased anticoagulant effect) Alcohol MAO inhibitors	Considered an MAO inhibitor
Neurologic/psycho- logical	Valerian 200–500 mg PO HS for insomnia 200–300 mg PO BID for anxiety	Sleep disorders, anxiety	Excitability Blurred vision, nausea	Additive effects with alcohol and CNS depressants	
Respiratory	Zinc	Cold symptoms, wound healing	Nausea, bad taste, diarrhea, vomiting, mouth irritation		
Genitourinary disorders	Saw palmetto 320 mg/day PO	BPH	GI side effects, decreased libido, headache, back pain	Warfarin (increased risk of bleeding)	

Uses and Dosage

Garlic is used to treat hyperlipidemia and to prevent clot formation. The dosage is 600 to 900 mg/day. The product must contain allicin, the active ingredient in garlic. Fresh garlic is the most effective (one clove a day).

Adverse Reactions and Drug Interactions

Garlic can cause dizziness, irritation of the mouth and esophagus, nausea, flatulence, malodorous breath and body odor, and sweating. Garlic increases the risk of bleeding when taking with anticoagulants. Garlic oil can reduce CYP2E1 activity by almost 40%, causing elevated serum levels of drugs whose major metabolic pathway includes CYP2E1, such as alcohol.

Gingko Biloba

Action and Proof of Efficacy

Gingko biloba promotes arterial and venous vascular changes that increase tissue perfusion and cerebral blood flow. It is also considered an antioxidant. Results from clinical trials are varied. Cholesterol-lowering effects, if any, have been shown to be small.

Uses and Dosage

Gingko biloba is used to treat peripheral vascular insufficiency and dementia. The dosage is 120 to 240 mg/day in two or three divided doses.

Adverse Reactions and Drug Interactions

Gingko biloba can cause headache, diarrhea, flatulence, nausea, and dermatitis. It interacts with anticoagulants and antiplatelets by affecting platelet activity. When taken with insulin and oral hypoglycemic agents, it causes increased clearance of insulin and oral hypoglycemic agents, resulting in elevated blood glucose levels. When taken with thiazide diuretics, it increases blood pressure.

Glucosamine

Action and Proof of Efficacy

Glucosamine stimulates the production of cartilage components and allow rebuilding of damaged cartilage. Studies have proven its safety and effectiveness in the treatment of osteoarthritis.

Uses and Dosage

Glucosamine is used for osteoarthritis and other joint diseases. The recommended dosage is 500 mg three times a day. It may take 2 weeks to realize the positive effect.

Adverse Reactions and Drug Interactions

Glucosamine can cause drowsiness, headache, abdominal pain, constipation, diarrhea, epigastric discomfort, and nausea. There are no known drug interactions.

Kava

Action and Proof of Efficacy

Kava inhibits the limbic system, suppressing emotional excitability and mood enhancement. Randomized, controlled clinical trails of kava use with anxiety provide some reasonable support for its use, but there are no clinical comparison trials with existing anxiolytics.

Uses and Dosage

Kava has been used to treat anxiety disorders. Dosage is based on the kavapyrone content. The recommended content is 70 to 240 mg kavopyrone in three divided doses.

Adverse Reactions and Drug Interactions

Kava can cause headaches, dizziness, and disturbances in visual accommodation. Alcohol can increase kava's activity. Central nervous system (CNS) depressants can cause an additive sedative effect. Taken together, levodopa and kava can cause an increase in parkinsonian symptoms. Absorption of kava is increased if it is taken with food.

Melatonin

Action and Proof of Efficacy

Melatonin release corresponds to periods of sleep. Studies have proven melatonin to be safe and effective for the short-term prevention of jet lag.

Uses and Dosage

Melatonin is used to prevent and treat jet lag and sleeping disturbances. The recommended dosage for sleeping disturbances is 5 mg at bedtime. The recommended dosage for jet lag is 5 mg/day for 3 days before departure and ending 3 days after departure.

Adverse Reactions and Interactions

Melatonin can cause altered sleep patterns, confusion, headache, hypothermia, sedation, tachycardia, hypertension, hyperglycemia, and pruritus. Interactions include increased anxiolytic action when taken with benzodiazepines.

Saw Palmetto

Action and Proof of Efficacy

Saw palmetto inhibits the production of enzymes responsible for converting testosterone to more reactive dihydrotestosterone (DHT). Saw palmetto blocks the binding of DHT to prostate cells, inhibiting enlargement. Studies have shown a decrease in symptoms in patients with noncancerous enlargement of the prostate. Saw palmetto also increases urine flow and improves emptying of the bladder.

Uses and Dosage

Saw palmetto is used to treat benign prostatic hyperplasia (BPH) (see Chapter 34 for more information on BPH). The recommended dosage is 320 mg daily.

Adverse Reactions and Drug Interactions

Adverse reactions include headache, hypertension, constipation, diarrhea, decreased libido, and back pain. There are no known drug interactions.

St. John's Wort

Actions and Proof of Efficacy

St. John's Wort is a monoamine oxidase (MAO) inhibitor. It inhibits reuptake of serotonin, noradrenaline, adrenaline, and dopamine. Numerous studies of St. John's Wort in patients with depressive disorders have shown that it is more effective than placebo and as effective as antidepressants; however, these studies had many flaws, and more studies need to be done.

Uses and Dosage

St. John's Wort is used to treat depression, anxiety, and neuralgic pain. The recommended dosage is 320 mg daily.

Adverse Reactions and Drug Interactions

St. John's Wort can cause dizziness, restlessness, sleep disturbances, dry mouth, constipation, GI distress, and photosensitivity. Drug interactions include an increase in MAO inhibition activity when taken with alcohol, MAO inhibitors, narcotics, and over-the-counter cold and flu medicines. There is a decrease in levels of digoxin and cyclosporine. Serotonin syndrome may develop when used concurrently with amphetamines, selective serotonin reuptake inhibitors, trazodone, and tricyclic antidepressants.

Valerian

Actions and Proof of Efficacy

Valerian binds to GABA alpha-receptor sites in the brain and CNS. It acts in a competitive action with any benzodiazepine. In nine randomized, placebo-controlled, double-blind studies in which valerian was used a treatment for sleep disorders, some studies showed effectiveness but others showed none.

Uses and Dosage

Valerian is used for insomnia, anxiety, and stress. The recommended dosages are 200 to 500 mg at bedtime for insomnia and 200 to 300 mg two times a day for anxiety.

Adverse Reactions and Drug Interactions

Valerian can cause excitability, blurred vision, and nausea. There are additive effects with alcohol and CNS depressants.

INCREASING AWARENESS

Since the use of CAM is increasing, health care providers must be aware of the different modalities. At each visit, the patient should be asked about the use of over-the-counter medications, vitamins, and supplements. The health care provider should check whether there are any interactions between medications and supplements.

Patients who choose to use CAM can be directed to reliable providers and reliable dietary supplements. NCCAM is an excellent source of information for both the patient and provider and can be accessed on the Internet (*www.nccam.nih.gov*) or by phone (1-888-644-6226).

Bibliography

Starred references are cited in the text.

Austin, J. A. (1998). Why patients use alternative medicines: results of a national study. *JAMA, 279*(19), 1548–1553.

Bernstein, N. J. (2000). Discussing complementary therapies with cancer patients: what we should be talking about. *Journal of Clinical Oncology, 18*, 2501–2504.

DerMarderosian, A., & Beutler, J. A. (Eds.) (2002). *The review of natural products* (3rd ed.). Missouri: Facts and Comparisons.

DeSmet, P. (2002). Herbal remedies. *New England Journal of Medicine, 347*, 2046–2056.

Fetrow, C. W., & Avila, J. R. (2004). *Professional's handbook of complementary and alternative medicines.* Philadelphia: Lippincott Williams & Wilkins.

*Panel on Definition and Description. CAM Research Methodology Conference (1995). Defining and describing CAM. *Alternative Therapy, 3*(2), 49–57.

Pappas, S., & Perlman, A. (2002). Complementary and alternative medicine: the importance of doctor-patient communication. *Medical Clinics of North America, 86*(1), 1–10.

Steiger, T. E. (2002). Complementary and alternative medicine: a primer. *Family Practice Management, 8*(3), 37–42

Visit the Connection web site for the most up-to-date drug information.

II

Pharmacotherapy for Skin Disorders

10

CONTACT DERMATITIS

■ VIRGINIA P. ARCANGELO

Dermatitis is an alteration in skin reactivity caused by exposure to an external agent. It is a combination of genetic and environmental factors. It can occur after a single exposure or multiple exposures to an agent or in response to an allergen. The resulting dermatitis usually appears as an inflammatory process. According to the American Academy of Dermatology, contact dermatitis is a common problem and results in approximately 5.7 million visits to health care providers each year. Almost any substance can be a potential irritant. Diaper dermatitis (sometimes called *diaper rash*) is the most common form of irritant contact dermatitis in childhood.

CAUSES

Two types of contact dermatitis are irritant and allergic dermatitis. *Irritant* contact dermatitis results from exposure to any agent that has a toxic effect on the skin. *Allergic* contact dermatitis results from exposure to an antigen that causes an immunologic response. Atopic dermatitis (eczema), a form of allergic dermatitis characterized as a pruritic, chronic inflammatory condition, affects between 5% and 10% of the population in the United States (Goodheart, 1999). It most often begins in childhood.

PATHOPHYSIOLOGY

Irritant contact dermatitis is not an allergic response. It is a result of damage to the water–protein–lipid matrix of the outer layer of skin. It appears as an erythematous, scaly eruption resulting from friction, exposure to a chemical, or a thermal injury (Fig. 10-1). The severity of the reaction depends on the condition of the skin, the concentration and the toxicity of the irritant, and the length of exposure. The reaction appears only in the area exposed to the irritant.

Allergic contact dermatitis (eg, poison ivy) is an immunologically mediated response to an allergen (antigen). The allergen penetrates the skin and is processed by cutaneous macrophages, which present the antigen to the T lymphocytes that proliferate and circulate throughout the lymph system. This is the beginning of sensitization. In a complex process, the lymph system "remembers" the allergen. Then, 5 to 7 days after sensitization, there is visual evidence of the response. On subsequent exposures, however, dermatitis may develop within 6 to 18 hours (Fig. 10-2). Hypersensitivity can occur after one exposure or after years of repeated exposures. Contact dermatitis may spread extensively beyond the area of contact.

In atopic dermatitis, there are high concentrations of serum immunoglobulin E (IgE), decreased numbers of immunoregulatory T cells, defective antibody-dependent cellular cytotoxicity, and decreased cell-mediated immunity.

DIAGNOSTIC CRITERIA

Irritant contact dermatitis and allergic contact dermatitis appear as linear streaks of papules, vesicles, and blisters that are very pruritic. In irritant contact dermatitis, the lesions are found only in the area of exposure to the irritant. In allergic contact dermatitis, the lesions are usually more diffuse, and they may present over an underlying area of edema.

Atopic dermatitis is characterized by a strong family or patient history of atopy. Lesions include papules, erythema, excoriations, and lichenification. In infants, the face, chest, legs, and arms are the most commonly involved areas; lesions are scaly and red and may be crusted patches and plaques. In children, the most common sites are the antecubital and popliteal fossae, the neck, wrists, ankles, eyelids, scalp, and behind the ears. Lesions are usually lichenified because of constant scratching. In adults, the neck, antecubital and popliteal fossae, face, wrist, and forearms are the most commonly involved areas. Lesions may appear as poorly defined, pruritic, erythematous papules and plaques.

INITIATING DRUG THERAPY

The most effective form of treatment for contact dermatitis is prevention. The patient must become aware of the causes or triggers and plan ways to avoid them. Before initiating therapy, the practitioner first needs to determine the severity of the problem. If the symptoms are mild, cool compresses may offer relief, and baths with colloidal oatmeal may offer relief from pruritus. Compresses of Burow's solution are effective for drying the vesicles and bullae that may be associated with contact dermatitis. If these treatments fail or if the dermatitis is more extensive, drug therapy is initiated.

Before initiating drug therapy, delivery of the drug to the skin, protection/barrier function, and cosmetic acceptability must be considered. Ointment and gels offer the best delivery

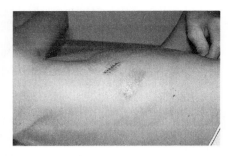

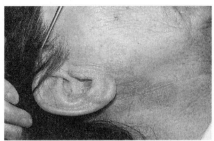

Figure 10–1   Examples of irritant contact dermatitis from **(A)** an adhesive bandage and **(B)** from contact with hair dye. (From Goodheart, H.P. [1999]. *A photoguide of common skin disorders: Diagnosis and management* [pp. 42, 44]. Baltimore: Williams & Wilkins.)

and protection barrier. Creams are less greasy but less effective. Lotions are dilute creams. Solutions are alcohol-based liquids and are useful for treating the scalp because they do not coat the hair.

Goals of Drug Therapy

The goals of drug therapy for dermatitis are:

- Restoration of a normal epidermal barrier
- Treatment of inflammation of skin
- Control of itching

The mainstays of therapy for contact dermatitis are topical corticosteroids and oral antihistamines. There are also topical immunosuppressives available. Systemic corticosteroids are recommended for widespread symptoms and antihistamines are used for relieving intense pruritus.

Topical Corticosteroids

Topical steroidal therapy is safer than systemic steroidal therapy. Steroidal agents are effective for smaller outbreaks.

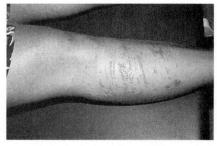

Figure 10–2   Example of the rash characteristic of allergic contact dermatitis—in this case from contact with poison ivy. (From Goodheart, H.P. [1999]. *A photoguide of common skin disorders: Diagnosis and management* [p. 42]. Baltimore: Williams & Wilkins.)

Because of their anti-inflammatory and antimitotic actions, they reduce inflammation and the buildup of scale.

Topical corticosteroids are classified according to potency (Table 10-1), with the fluorinated agents being more potent. Ideally, the least potent topical corticosteroid should be used for the shortest possible time in treating dermatitis. Topical corticosteroids should be avoided if there are additional bacterial, viral, or fungal skin infections, and they are not recommended for prophylaxis.

Dosage

Treatment may be initiated with an intermediate- or high-potency topical corticosteroid. A lower-potency corticosteroid may be used after the symptoms subside. As a rule, short-term therapy with more potent topical corticosteroids is preferred to longer-term therapy with less potent corticosteroids. Low-potency corticosteroids should be used in the facial and intertriginous regions because fluorinated and high-potency corticosteroids applied to the face may cause atrophy of the tissue or trigger steroidal rosacea. If it is necessary to use either type of agent, use should be limited to a very brief time. The maximum recommended length of treatment with topical corticosteroids is 2 weeks for adults and 1 week for children.

Preparations

Topical corticosteroids are available in creams, ointments, lotions, gels, solutions, or sprays. Creams are the most desirable because they are not as obvious when applied. They are, however, water based, which causes more skin drying. Ointments and gels are the most potent and the most lubricating, and have occlusive properties. In areas with large amounts of hair or widespread dermatitis, lotions, gels, spray products, and solutions are easiest to apply. Occlusion by a dressing of an area of a topical corticosteroid application increases hydration and hence penetration, thereby enhancing efficacy.

Correct Usage

Tolerance to a topical corticosteroid is common. To prevent this, chronic use is not recommended. Using the topical corticosteroid preparation only in the case of recurrence of contact dermatitis, and not prophylactically, or prescribing intermittent dosing (eg, every 4 days) may be effective methods of controlling tolerance.

Application

Penetration of a topical corticosteroid is enhanced when the skin is hydrated. This can be accomplished by moistening the skin before application or by using an occlusive dressing constructed from a material such as a plastic shower cap (for the scalp), gloves (for hands), or plastic wrap or a sock (on other extremities).

Adverse Events

Although topical corticosteroids are relatively safe to use, some adverse events may occur. The prolonged use of fluorinated corticosteroids on the face can cause atrophy and acne-like eruptions. This usually is seen after therapy stops,

Table 10.1

Classification of Topical Corticosteroids by Potency

Low Potency	Intermediate Potency	High Potency	Very High Potency
aclometasone dipropionate 0.05% (Aclovate—c, o)	desonide 0.05% (DesOwen—c, l, o Tridesilon—c, o)	amcinonide 0.1% (Cyclocort—c, l, o)	betamethasone dipropionate augmented 0.05% (Diprolene—o, g)
fluocinolone acetonide 0.01% (Synalar—s)	desoximetasone 0.05% (Topicort LP—emollient cream)	betamethasone dipropionate augmented 0.05% (Diprolene AF—emollient cream Diprolene—lotion)	cobetasol propionate 0.05% (Temovate—c, g, o, scalp preparation Temovate-E—emollient cream)
hydrocortisone base or acetate 0.5% (Cortisporin—c Mantadil—c)	diflorasone diacetate 0.05% (Florone—c Florone—emollient cream)	desoximetasone 0.05% (Topicort—g) desoximetasone 0.25% (Topicort—emollient cream, o)	diflorasone diacetate 0.05% (Psorcon—o)
hydrocortisone base or acetate 1% (Cortisporin—o Hytone (1% or 2.5%)—c, l, o Proctocort—c Vytone—c)	fluocinolone acetonide 0.025% (Synalar—c, o)	fluocinonide 0.05% (Lidex—c, g, o, s Lidex-E—emollient cream)	halobetasol propionate 0.05% (Ultravate—c, o)
triamcinolone acetonide 0.025% (Aristocort—c Aristocort A—c Kenalog—c, l, o)	flurandrenolide 0.025% or 0.05% (Cordran-SP—c Cordran—o)	diflorasone diacetate 0.05% (Florone—o Psorcon—c)	
	fluticasone propionate 0.005% or 0.05% (Cutivate—o 0.005%, c 0.05%)	halcinonide 0.1% (Halog—c, o, s Halog-E—emollient cream)	
	hydrocortisone buteprate 0.1% (Pandel—c)	triamcinolone acetonide 0.5% (Aristocort—c, o Aristocort A—c Kenalog—c)	
	hydrocortisone butyrate 0.1% (Locoid—c, o, s)		
	hydrocortisone valerate 0.2% (Westcort—c, o)		
	mometasone furoate 0.1% (Elocon—c, o, l)		
	prednicarbate 0.1% (Dermatop—emollient cream)		
	triamcinolone acetonide 0.1% (Aristocort—c, o Aristocort A—c, o Kenalog—c, o)		
	triamcinolone acetonide 0.2% (Kenalog—aerosol)		

c, cream; l, lotion; o, ointment; g, gel; s, solution.

and may last for several months. With prolonged use, ecchymoses may develop on the arms in elderly patients. Moreover, epidermal atrophy, manifested by striae, shiny, thin skin, or telangiectases, can occur with prolonged use, or a hypersensitivity reaction may occur, usually in response to the vehicle in which the medication is delivered. Topical corticosteroids can potentiate or cause cataract formation or glaucoma when used around the eyes for prolonged periods.

Systemic Corticosteroids

If the dermatitis is widespread or resistant to treatment with topical steroidal preparations, oral corticosteroids may be used. Systemic corticosteroids inhibit cytokine and mediator release, attenuate mucus secretion, upregulate beta-adrenergic receptors, inhibit IgE synthesis, decrease microvascular permeability, and suppress the influx of inflammatory cells and the inflammatory process.

Systemic corticosteroids are prescribed in a tapering dose schedule. The starting dose of 1 mg/kg is decreased by 5 mg every 2 days for at least 2 weeks. Medications should be taken in the morning or early afternoon to minimize sleep disturbances. Taking the corticosteroids for less than 2 weeks may cause rebound dermatitis, especially with poison ivy. If dermatitis flares up during the tapering, the dosage can be increased and tapered again.

Although these medications are readily absorbed when taken orally, peak plasma concentrations are not achieved for 1 to 2 hours. For more information about systemic corticosteroids, refer to Chapter 24.

Contraindications

Because they suppress the immune response, systemic corticosteroids are contraindicated in patients with systemic mycoses and in patients receiving a vaccination. These drugs also should be used cautiously in people with tuberculosis, hypothyroidism, cirrhosis, renal insufficiency, hypertension, osteoporosis, and diabetes mellitus.

Adverse Events

Systemic corticosteroids mask infection. In short-term use, they may cause gastrointestinal upset. Mood changes (hyperactivity, anxiety, depression) may be evident and sleep disturbances may occur, especially if medication is taken late in the day. The effects of systemic corticosteroids may be decreased if they are administered with barbiturates, hydantoins, or rifampin.

Topical Immunosuppressives

Topical immunosuppressives act on T cells by suppressing cytokine transcription. These agents are used in patients with moderate to severe atopic dermatitis who cannot tolerate topical steroids or are not responsive to other treatments, or where there is a concern for topical steroid-induced atrophy.

Tacrolimus and pimecrolimus are the preparations currently available. They are applied twice a day until the lesions clear and then for an additional 7 days. The skin is dried before application.

Table 10.2

Overview of Topical Corticosteroids Used for Contact Dermatitis

Generic (Trade) Name & Dosage	Selected Adverse Events	Special Considerations
Low Potency		
aclometasone dipropionate 0.05% (Aclovate—c, o)	Skin irritation Acneiform lesions Striae Skin atrophy	Applying to moist skin and covering with occlusive dressing increases efficacy.
fluocinolone acetonide 0.01% (Synalar—s)	Same as above	Same as above
hydrocortisone base or acetate 0.5% (Cortisporin—c Mantadil—c) hydrocortisone base or acetate 1% (Cortisporin—o Hytone [1% or 2.5%]—c, l, o Proctocort—c Vytone—c)	Same as above	Same as above
triamcinolone acetonide 0.025% (Aristicort—c Aristicort A—c Kenalog—c, l, o)	Same as above	Same as above
Intermediate Potency		
desonide 0.05% (DesOwen—c, l, o Tridesilon—c, o)	Same as above	Same as above
desoximetasone 0.05% (Topicort LP—emollient cream)	Same as above	Same as above
diflorasone diacetate 0.05% (Florone—c Florone—emollient cream)	Same as above	Same as above
fluocinolone acetonide 0.025% (Synalar—c, o)	Same as above	Same as above
flurandrenolide 0.025% or 0.05% (Cordran-SP—c Cordran—o)	Same as above	Same as above
fluticasone propionate 0.005% or 0.05% (Cutivate—o 0.005%, c 0.05%)	Same as above	Same as above
hydrocortisone buteprate 0.1% (Pandel—c)	Same as above	Same as above
hydrocortisone butyrate 0.1% (Locoid—c, o, s)	Same as above	Same as above
hydrocortisone valerate 0.2% (Westcort—c, o)	Same as above	Same as above
mometasone furoate 0.1% (Elocon—c, o, l)	Same as above	Same as above
prednicarbate 0.1% (Dermatop—emollient cream)	Same as above	Same as above
triamcinolone acetonide 0.1% (Aristicort—c, o Aristicort A—c, o Kenalog—c, o)	Same as above	Same as above
triamcinolone acetonide 0.2% (Kenalog—aerosol)		
High Potency		
amcinonide 0.1% (Cyclocort—c, l, o)	Same as above	Same as above
betamethasone dipropionate augmented 0.05% (Diprolene AF—emollient cream Diprolene—l)	Same as above	Same as above
desoximetasone 0.05% (Topicort—g)	Same as above	Same as above
desoximetasone 0.25% (Topicort—emollient cream, o)		
diflorasone diacetate 0.05% (Florone—o Psorcon—c)	Same as above	Same as above
fluocinonide 0.05% (Lidex—c, g, o, s Lidex-E—emollient cream)	Same as above	Same as above
halcinonide 0.1% (Halog—c, o, s Halog-E—emollient cream)	Same as above	Same as above
triamcinolone acetonide 0.5% (Aristicort—c, o Aristicort A—c Kenalog—c)	Same as above	Same as above
Very High Potency		
betamethasone dipropionate augmented 0.05% (Diprolene—o, g)	Same as above	Do not apply under or around eyes. Avoid using occlusive dressing.
cobetasol propionate 0.05% (Temovate—c, g, o, scalp preparation Temovate-E—emollient cream)	Same as above	Same as above
diflorasone diacetate 0.05% (Psorcon—o)	Same as above	Same as above
halobetasol propionate 0.05% (Ultravate—c, o)	Same as above	Same as above
Topical Steroids		
See Table 10-1 for listing	Burning Irritation Pruritus Erythema Folliculitis	Can cause or intensify cataracts or glaucoma if used near eyes Use lowest potency on thin/atrophic skin and children. Pregnancy category C
Topical Immunosuppressants		
pimecrolimus (Elidel) 1% tacrolimus topical (Protopic) 0.03%, 0.1% Apply light layer bid For use for 2 years and over	Skin burning Pruritus Flu-like symptoms Erythema Alcohol intolerance Folliculitis	Do not use with occlusive dressing. Apply for 1 week after clearing. Pregnancy category C Not recommended for under 2 years old

c, cream; o, ointment; g, gel; s, solution; l, lotion.

Contraindications

Care should be used when administering these drugs with drugs in the CYP3A family. The drugs should not be used under occlusive dressings.

Adverse Effects

There can be transient burning and pruritus, which disappear with continued use. The concomitant ingestion of alcohol can cause redness and flushing. Sun protection is recommended.

Antihistamines

Antihistamines are used to relieve pruritus associated with contact dermatitis. One side effect is drowsiness. Antihistamines are discussed in Chapter 51.

Selecting the Most Appropriate Agent

In contact and atopic dermatitis, topical corticosteroids are the first line of therapy (Table 10-2). These agents are for short-term use. The recommended treatment order is listed in Table 10-3.

First-Line Therapy

A topical corticosteroid preparation with low to intermediate potency applied twice a day is the appropriate first-line therapy. If improvement does not occur, a higher-potency topical corticosteroid may be tried rather than increasing the time of administration of the lower-potency agent. Occlusive dressings and application to moist skin may be efficacious in treating the acute phase. Low-potency topical corticosteroids are used on the face and intertriginous areas. Oral antihistamines are used to relieve pruritus and reduce the response to the cause.

Second-Line Therapy

Second-line therapy calls for a more potent topical corticosteroid. Topical immunosuppressants are another consideration for second-line therapy.

Third-Line Therapy

Systemic corticosteroids are useful for treating widespread dermatitis. They are given on a tapered-dose schedule. The recommended dose is 1 mg/kg, with the dose decreased every 2 days for at least 2 weeks and up to 3 weeks. If a flare-up occurs during the tapering, the dosage can be increased again. When treating severe poison ivy, for example, oral corticosteroids are continued for 2 to 3 weeks to prevent rebound dermatitis, which may occur if therapy is discontinued before that time.

Figure 10-3 provides an algorithm of contact dermatitis treatment.

Special Populations

Pediatric

Topical corticosteroids should be used for only 7 days in children younger than 6 years of age, and at the lowest

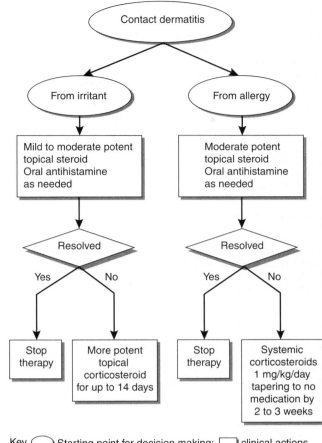

Figure 10–3 Treatment algorithm for contact dermatitis.

potency. Topical corticosteroids can cause atrophy of the skin. Topical immunosuppressants are considered only for those 2 and older. Topical immunosuppressants will not cause atrophy of the skin.

Geriatric

The most common causes of contact dermatitis in elderly patients are topical medications (eg, neomycin [Myciguent]) and the bases of other topical medications. The adhesives on adhesive patches may also cause contact dermatitis. The

---

Table 10.3

Recommended Order of Treatment for Contact Dermatitis

Order	Agent	Comments
First line	Apply low-potency topical corticosteroid two times a day. Take oral antihistamine for relief of symptoms.	Occlusive dressing is helpful. Apply to moist skin surface. Use only for 14 d in adult and 7 d in child.
Second line	Increase potency of topical corticosteroid.	Avoid using moderate- or high-potency topical corticosteroid on face or intertriginous areas.
Third Line	Prescribe oral corticosteroid on tapered dosage regimen.	Common dosage: 1 mg/kg decreased by 5 mg every 2 d. Continue therapy for at least 2 wk. Consider increasing dose if dermatitis flares up; then taper as above.

rash of contact dermatitis does not present in a classic pattern in the elderly. Instead of vesicles or inflammation, the area exposed to the irritant may simply become scaly. Topical corticosteroids can cause atrophy of the skin in elderly people, which is a problem because their skin is already friable.

MONITORING PATIENT RESPONSE

The response to therapy is monitored by visual examination of the affected parts of the anatomy and the reported resolution of symptoms. The patient should return for follow-up evaluation within 2 or 3 days of initiation of therapy. If a bacterial infection recurs secondary to contact dermatitis, it may be treated as discussed in Chapter 13.

PATIENT EDUCATION

Drug Information

Education includes teaching patients to avoid the causative substance. Using mild soaps without perfume is an important preventive measure. As appropriate, the practitioner can demonstrate how to apply topical preparations to moist skin and apply an occlusive dressing to increase the efficacy of topical corticosteroids. Penetration of topical steroids is enhanced 10- to 100-fold by hydrating (moistening) the area before applying the medication. An easy-to-make occlusive dressing consists of plastic wrap applied over the medicated area and held in place by a sock or tape. On the hands, a glove can act as an occlusive dressing. On the head area, a shower cap can be used.

Occlusive dressings should not be used with topical immunosuppressives. The patient should avoid alcohol and should use sunscreen.

Complementary and Alternative Medicine

Some supplements are thought to be helpful in atopic dermatitis. Gingko biloba antagonizes platelet-aggregating factors, a key chemical mediator in atopic dermatitis. Zinc can be used at a dosage of 50 mg/day until the condition clears. Use of fish oil supplements incorporates omega-3 fatty acids into the membrane phospholipid pools.

Recommendations for supplements are as follows:

- Vitamin A 50,000 IU daily
- Vitamin E 400 IU daily
- Zinc 50 mg daily, to be decreased as the condition clears
- EPA 540 mg and DHA 360 mg daily or flaxseed oil 10 g daily
- Evening primrose oil 3,000 mg daily

■ Case Study

J.F., a 15-year-old boy who weighs 110 pounds, is seeking treatment for a very itchy rash consisting of linear streaks of papules, vesicles, and blisters on his arms, legs, and face. He tells you he was hiking in the woods 2 days ago along trails lined with patches of shiny weeds with three leaves. He tried using calamine lotion and over-the-counter hydrocortisone cream but has had no relief from the itching.

Diagnosis: Contact dermatitis (poison ivy)

1. List specific goals of treatment for J.F.

2. What drug therapy would you prescribe? Why?

3. What are the parameters for monitoring the success of the therapy?

4. Discuss specific patient education based on the prescribed therapy.

5. List one or two adverse reactions for the selected agent that would cause you to change therapy.

6. What would be the choice for second-line therapy?

7. What over-the-counter and alternative medications would be appropriate for J.F.?

8. What lifestyle changes would you recommend to J.F.?

9. Describe one or two drug/drug or drug/food interactions for the selected agent.

Bibliography

*Starred references are cited in the text.

Beltranic, V. S. (2002). Clinical features of atopic dermatitis. *Immunology and Allergy Clinics of North America, 22*(1), 25–42.

Fitzpatrick, S. D., & Elsner, P. (1997). Clinical irritant contact dermatitis syndromes. *Immunology and Allergy Clinics of North America, 17*, 367–375.

Friedlander, S. F. (1998). Contact dermatitis. *Pediatrics in Review, 19*, 166–171.

*Goodheart, H. P. (1999). *A photoguide of common skin disorders: diagnosis and management*. Philadelphia: Williams & Wilkins.

Kennedy, M. (1999). Evaluation of chronic eczema and urticaria and angioedema. *Immunology and Allergy Clinics of North America, 17,* 19–33.

Larsen, F. S., & Hanifen, J. M. (2002). Epidemiology of atopic dermatitis. *Immunology and Allergy Clinics of North America, 22*(1), 1–24.

Murray, M. T., & Pizzorno, J. E. (1999). Atopic dermatitis-eczema. In *Pizzorno's textbook of natural medicine* (2d ed.). New York: Churchill Livingstone.

Schauder, L. C. (2002). New treatment for atopic dermatitis. *Immunology and Allergy Clinics of North America, 22*(1), 141–152.

Shaw, J. C. (1996). Differential diagnosis of allergic disease: masquerades of allergy. *Immunology and Allergy Clinics of North America, 16*, 119–135.

Webster, G. (2001). Topical medications: a focus on antifungals and topical steroids, *Clinical Cornerstone, 4*(1), 33–36.

Visit the Connection web site for the most up-to-date drug information.

FUNGAL INFECTIONS OF THE SKIN

■ VIRGINIA P. ARCANGELO AND DENISE VANACORE-NETZ

Fungi live in the dead, horny outer layer of the skin. The organisms penetrate only the stratum corneum—the surface layer of the skin—and infect the skin, hair, and nails. They cause tinea, tinea versicolor, and candidiasis.

TINEA

Dermatophytes are a group of fungi that infect nonviable keratinized cutaneous tissues. Dermatophytosis, more commonly called *tinea*, is a condition caused by dermatophytes. Tinea is further classified by the location of the infection (Box 11-1).

Tinea capitis primarily affects children 3 to 9 years of age. This age group may also be infected with tinea corporis. *Tinea pedis* most commonly affects the adolescent population and young adults. Immunocompromised patients have an increased incidence and more intractable dermatophytosis. *Tinea unguium*, infection of the nails, is also called *onychomycosis*. It is caused by various yeast, fungi, and molds.

CAUSES

General factors that predispose to fungal infections include warm, moist, occluded environments, family history, and a compromised immune system. Infection is spread from person to person by animals, especially cats and dogs, and by inanimate objects.

PATHOPHYSIOLOGY

Dermatophytes grow only on or within keratinized structures. Most infections result from five specific species of fungus: *Trichophyton rubrum, Trichophyton tonsurans, Trichophyton mentagrophytes, Microsporum canis,* and *Epidermophyton floccosum*. These can be found on humans, animals, and in the soil. They produce enzymes (keratinases) that allow them to digest keratin, causing epidermal scale; thickened, crumbly nails; or hair loss.

DIAGNOSTIC CRITERIA

General symptoms of fungal infections in hair and skin include pruritus, burning, and stinging of the scalp or skin. An inflammatory dermal reaction may cause erythema and vesicles. Diagnosis is confirmed by several mechanisms. One mechanism is microscopic evaluation of the stratum corneum with 10% potassium hydroxide (KOH) preparation. At the margin of the lesion, scale is scraped with a No. 15 knife blade and placed on a slide. KOH is then added and the slide inspected under the microscope. Fungi appear as rod-shaped filaments with branching.

Another mechanism for diagnosis is the fungal culture. A specimen of infected tissue is applied to a dermatophyte test medium on an agar plate. If the infecting organism is a fungus, the plate will change color—from yellow to pink or red—in approximately 2 weeks.

A third diagnostic method involves using a Wood's lamp, which produces a bright green fluorescence in the presence of a tinea infection caused by *Microsporum* species. A major disadvantage of this test is that other fungal infections may be undiagnosed because the Wood's lamp test identifies only *Microsporum*.

Tinea can affect various areas of the body. The condition is named based on the area effected. Box 11-1 lists the names for the different areas effected.

Tinea Capitis

Presentation of tinea capitis varies widely. There may be generalized, diffuse seborrheic dermatitis-like scalp scaling, although more common signs and symptoms include impetigo-like lesions with crusting and redness, areas of hair loss with broken hairs, and possibly inflammatory nodules. Although often impressive, cervical lymphadenitis does not correlate with the extent of scalp inflammation. Finally, approximately 15% of patients have a cross-infection with tinea corporis. Most cases of tinea capitis are found in prepubertal children, with a disproportionate amount in African Americans. It is very contagious.

Most cases (90%) are caused by *T. tonsurans. Microsporum audouinii*, spread from human to human, and *M. cania*, spread from animals, are other organisms.

Tinea capitis presents in several ways:

- Inflamed, scaly, alopecic patches, especially in infants
- Diffuse scaling with multiple round areas with alopecia secondary to broken hair shafts, leaving residual black stumps

Tinea infections are identified by their location on the body as follows:

- Head: tinea capitis
- Body: tinea corporis
- Hand: tinea manus
- Foot: tinea pedis
- Groin: tinea cruris
- Nails: tinea unguium (onychomycosis)

- "Gray patch" type with round, scaly plaques of alopecia in which the hair shaft is broken off close to the surface
- Tender pustular nodules

Tinea Corporis

Tinea corporis is called "ringworm" when it affects the face, limbs, or trunk, but not the groin, hands, or feet. The typical presentation of tinea corporis is a ring-shaped lesion with well-demarcated margins, central clearing, and a scaly, erythematous border. It is caused by contact with infected animals, human-to-human transmission, and from infected mats in wrestling. The organisms responsible are *M. canis,* *T. rubrum,* and *T. mentagrophytes.*

Tinea Cruris

Tinea cruris is often referred to as *jock itch.* A fungal infection of the groin and inguinal folds, tinea cruris spares the scrotum. The most common causes are *T. rubrum* or *E. floccosum.* Typically, the lesion borders are well demarcated and peripherally spreading. The lesions are large, erythematous, and macular, with a central clearing. A hallmark of tinea cruris is pruritus or a burning sensation. There is often an accompanying fungal infection of the feet.

Tinea Pedis

Interdigital tinea pedis, commonly called *athlete's foot,* is characterized by scaling and itching in the web spaces between the toes and sometimes denudation and sodden maceration of the skin. Another variation is inflammatory tinea pedis, which presents with vesicles involving the toes or instep. A third variety is the moccasin style, which presents with itching, chronic noninflammatory scaling, and thickness and cracking of the epidermis on the sole, heel, and often up the side of the foot. This is a common problem in young men.

Most cases are caused by *T. rubrum,* which evokes a minimal inflammatory response. The *T. mentagrophytes* organism produces vesicles and bullae.

There are three types of tinea pedis:

- Interdigital, which presents as scaling, maceration, and fissures between the toes

- Plantar, which presents as diffuse scaling of the soles, usually on the entire plantar surface
- Acute vesicular, which presents as vesicles and bullae on the sole of the foot, the great toe, and the instep

Tinea Manus

Tinea manus is a dermatophyte infection of the hand. This is always associated with tinea pedis and is usually unilateral. The lesions are marked by mild, diffuse scaling of the palmar skin, and vesicles may be grouped on the palms or fingernails involved.

Tinea Unguium

Tinea unguium (onychomycosis) is a fungal infection of the nail. Typically affected are the toenails, which become thick and scaly with subungual debris. Onycholysis, a separation of the nail from the nail bed, may be seen. The infection usually begins distally at the tip of the toe and moves proximally and through the nail plate, producing a yellowish discoloration and striations in the actual nail. Under the nail, a hyperkeratotic substance accumulates that lifts the nail up. If untreated, the nail thickens and turns yellowish brown. Onychomycosis is usually asymptomatic but can act as a portal of entry for a more serious bacterial infection.

Organisms causing onychomycosis include dermatophytes, *E. floccosum, T. rubrum, T. mentagrophytes, Candida albicans, Aspergillus, Fusarium,* and *Scopulariopsis.*

Some health insurance plans refuse to reimburse for drug therapy without confirmation of the diagnosis. Tests that verify the diagnosis include the KOH test and culture.

INITIATING DRUG THERAPY

Fungal infections can be prevented by applying powder containing miconazole (Monistat) or tolnaftate (Tinactin) to areas prone to fungal infections after bathing. The areas can be dried completely with a hair dryer on low heat.

Goals of Drug Therapy

Pharmacologic therapy is directed against the offending fungus and the site of infection. Therapy is topical or systemic, depending on the location of the lesion. Topical therapy is used for most skin infections. The exceptions are tinea capitis and tinea unguium (onychomycosis).

Topical Azole Antifungals

Topical azoles (Table 11-1) impair the synthesis of ergosterol, the main sterol of fungal cell membranes. This allows for increased permeability and leakage of cellular components and results in cell death. Topical azoles are fungicides that are effective against tinea corporis, tinea cruris, and tinea pedis as well as cutaneous candidiasis. They should be applied once or twice a day for 2 to 4 weeks. Therapy should continue for 1 week after the lesions clear. However, therapy is not recommended during pregnancy or lactation and is administered cautiously in hepatocellular failure. Ketoconazole (Nizoral), in particular, should be avoided in patients with sulfite sensitivity. Adverse effects include pruritus, irritation, and stinging.

Table 11.1

Overview of Antifungal Medications

Generic (Trade) Name and Dosage	Selected Adverse Events	Contraindications	Special Considerations
Topical Agents			
clotrimazole ointment (Lotrimin), powder (Desenex) Gently massage ointment into affected and surrounding skin areas bid × 4 wk; powder as needed	Erythema, irritation, stinging, pruritus	Pregnancy or lactation Use cautiously in patients with hepatocellular failure	May be purchased OTC
miconazole (Micatin, Monostat Derm) Cover affected areas with cream lotion, or powder bid for 2–4 wk	Irritation, maceration	Pregnancy or lactation	Avoid applying near eyes
ketoconazole (Nizoral) Apply to affected and surrounding areas once daily for 2–4 wk	Irritation, stinging, pruritus	Asthma Not administered to people who are sensitive to sulfites Pregnancy or lactation	Not recommended in children
oxiconazole (Oxistat) Apply to affected and surrounding areas 1–2 times daily for 2–4 wk	Pruritus, burning	Pregnancy or lactation	Avoid applying near eyes or mucous membranes
sulconazole (Exelderm) Apply to affected and surrounding areas bid × 4 wk	Pruritus, burning sensation, erythema	Pregnancy or lactation	Not recommended in children Avoid contact with eyes
ciclopirox (Loprox) Apply to affected area bid × 4 wk	Pruritus, burning sensation		Not recommended in children younger than 10 y Lotion formulation good for nails Avoid occlusive dressing
naftitine (Naftin) Apply to affected area once daily × 4 wk	Burning, stinging, dryness, erythema, itching		Not recommended in children Avoid occlusive dressings Avoid contact with mucous membranes
terbinafine (Lamisil) Apply to affected area bid × 4 wk	Burning, irritation, skin exfoliation, dryness		Not recommended in children Avoid occlusive dressings Avoid contact with mucous membranes
tolnaftate (Tinactin) Apply small amount bid × 4 wk	Stinging, burning, irritation		Not recommended in children younger than 2 y
selenium sulfide (Selsun) 1% (OTC); 2.5% Massage into affected area, rest 15 min, rinse thoroughly	Irritation, hair loss		
nystatin (Mycostatin) 100,000 units/mL Infants: 1 mL each side of mouth Adults: 2–3 mL each side of mouth	GI upset, oral irritation		Continue use for at least 48 h after clinical cure Keep in mouth as long as possible before swallowing
Oral Agents			
griseofulvin (Grifulvin V) Microsize: Adult 500–1000 mg Child 10–15 mg/kg/d Ultramicrosize: Adult 330–660 mg Child 10 g/kg/d	Headaches, nausea, vomiting, diarrhea, photosensitivity	Pregnancy Patients with porphyria or hepatic failure	Ultramicrosize particle increases absorption Prescribe with caution to patients who are sensitive to penicillin Drug is most effective when taken with a high-fat meal. Drug is well tolerated in young children. Monitor complete blood count and LFT with long-term use. Drug use may aggravate lupus erythematosus. Use with alcohol produces Antabuse-like effects. Drug interactions: antagonizes oral contraceptives and warfarin, and is antagonized by barbiturates
ketoconazole (Nizoral) 200 mg/d	Nausea, vomiting, abdominal pain, urticaria, pruritus	Do not use with other drugs metabolized by CYP3A	Not recommended in children

Table 11.1

Overview of Antifungal Medications (*continued*)

Generic (Trade) Name and Dosage	Selected Adverse Events	Contraindications	Special Considerations
itraconazole (Sporanox) 200 mg/d	GI upset, rash, fatigue, headache, dizziness, edema	Do not use with other drugs metabolized by CYP3A	Not recommended in children May use pulse dosing Remains in nails for 4–5 mo Ingestion of food increases absorption
terbinafine (Lamisil) 62.5–250 mg/d	GI disturbance, LFT abnormalities, urticaria, pruritus	Liver or renal disease	Not recommended in children
fluconazole (Diflucan) Adults: 100–200 mg/d Children: 3–6 mg/kg/d	GI disturbance, headache, rash, hepatotoxicity		Decrease dose if creatinine clearance <50 mL/min Drug interactions: potentiates warfarin, theophylline, oral hypoglycemics May increase serum levels of phenytoin, cyclosporine Thiazides increase fluconazole levels May decrease effect of oral contraceptives

CYP3A, cytochrome P450 enzyme 3A; GI, gastrointestinal; LFT, liver function tests; OTC, over the counter.

Topical Allylamine Antifungals

These agents are effective against dermatophyte infections but have limited effectiveness against yeast. Patients treated with these agents may undergo a shorter treatment period with less likelihood of relapse. Topical allylamines are applied twice daily. Potential side effects include burning and irritation.

Griseofulvin

Mechanism of Action

Griseofulvin in a fungistatic that deposits in keratin precursor cells, increasing new keratin resistance to fungal invasion.

Adverse Events

Adverse effects include nausea, vomiting, diarrhea, headache, or photosensitivity. Evaluation of renal, hepatic, and hematopoietic systems is recommended before initiating therapy, particularly because this drug may aggravate lupus erythematosus.

Interactions

Griseofulvin increases levels of warfarin (Coumadin) and decreases levels of barbiturates and cyclosporine (Sandimmune). It may decrease the efficacy of oral contraceptives and may cause a serious and unpleasant reaction with alcohol. Patients should be advised not to drink beverages or any other preparation containing alcohol while taking the drug.

Systemic Allylamine Antifungals

Terbinafine (Lamisil) is a synthetic allylamine derivative that inhibits squalene epoxidase, a key enzyme in fungal biosynthesis. This causes a deficiency of ergosterol causing fungal cell death. It is used in the treatment of onychomycosis.

Dose

For fingernail onychomycosis the dose is 250 mg/d for 6 weeks; toenail onychomycosis requires 250 mg/d for 12 weeks.

Adverse Events

Adverse events include diarrhea, dyspepsia, rash, increase in liver enzymes, and headache. Evaluation of alanine aminotransferase (ALT) and aspartate aminotransferase (AST) levels is recommended before starting therapy and at 6 to 8 weeks into therapy if it is long-term because it can cause liver failure, although this is rare.

Interactions

Terbinafine is potentiated by cimetidine (Tagamet) and antagonized by rifampin (Rifadin). Cyclosporine levels should be monitored when the patient is taking both cyclosporine and terbinafine.

Systemic Azole Antifungals

Systemic azoles inhibit cytochrome P450 (CYP) enzymes and fungal 14-α-demethylase, inhibiting synthesis of ergosterol. Systemic therapy is required for tinea capitis and tinea unguium. Itraconazole (Sporanox), a systemic azole, has a high affinity for keratin and is lipophilic, which causes high levels to accumulate in the hair and nail. It has a long half-life, so pulse dosing, in which periods of drug therapy are alternated with periods without therapy, is feasible.

Dosage

The dosage of itraconazole is 200 mg once daily for 12 weeks for toenail infection. For fingernail infection, the dose is 200 mg twice daily for 1 week, then 3 weeks off, and repeat dosing with 200 mg twice daily for 1 week. The drug is not recommended for children, and ingestion of food increases absorption.

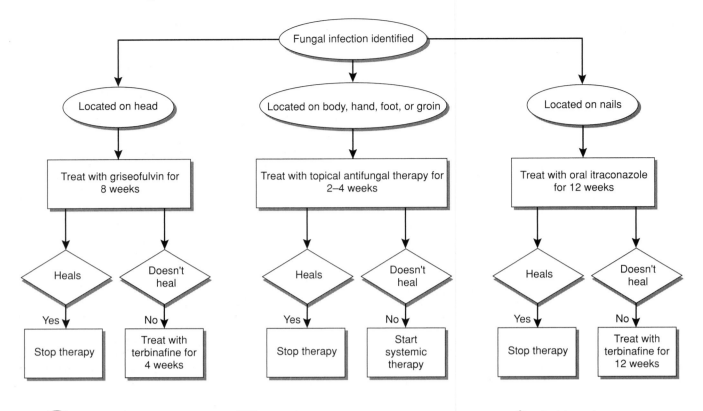

Figure 11–1 Treatment options for fungal skin infections.

The dosage of fluconazole usually 200 mg on the first day then 100 mg each day for at least 2 weeks. For children it is 6 mg/kg/d on day 1, then 3 mg/kg/d.

Contraindications

A systemic azole should not to be given with drugs metabolized by the CYP3A enzyme, including β-hydroxy-β-methylglutaryl coenzyme A (HMG-CoA) reductase inhibitors such as quinidine (Quinidex) or others. The azole antifungals should not be used in pregnancy.

Adverse Events

Adverse effects associated with systemic azole therapy include gastrointestinal (GI) upset, rash, fatigue, hepatic dysfunction, edema, and hypokalemia.

Interactions

Severe hypoglycemia may occur with hypoglycemic drugs. In addition, systemic azole therapy may potentiate triazolam (Halcion), midazolam (Versed), and warfarin. Fluconazole (Diflucan) levels are increased with use of hydrochlorothiazide (HydroDIURIL). Anticholinergics, histamine-2 (H₂) blockers, and antacids should be avoided within 2 hours of taking an oral azole so that absorption is not compromised.

Selecting the Most Appropriate Agent

Topical agents work well for most tineas but not for tinea capitis and tinea unguium. If the tinea capitis is especially severe

and painful in a child, prednisone (Deltasone) 1 mg/kg/d can be given for 3 to 4 days as adjunct therapy. To be effective, all therapy must be adequate in dose and duration. If a pet carries the fungus, the pet must be treated. For more information, see Figure 11-1.

When selecting an oral agent to treat onychomycosis, consideration must be given to cost of the agent, patient motivation and compliance, the age and health of the patient, and drug interactions and side effects of the medications.

First-Line Therapy

Topical therapy is recommended for cases of tinea corporis, pedis, cruris, or manus when the infection affects a limited area. The topical antifungal is applied 3 cm beyond the margin of the lesion. Therapy should continue for at least 2 weeks and for 1 week after the lesion clears (Table 11-2).

Table 11.2

Recommended Order of Treatment for Tinea Capitis

Order	Agent	Comments
First line	griseofulvin (Grifulvin V)	Treatment lasts a minimum of 8 wk
		Take medication with a high-fat meal
Second line	terbinafine (Lamisil) or itraconazole (Sporonax)	Treatment lasts 4 wk

Table 11.3

Recommended Order of Treatment for Tinea Corporis, Tinea Cruris, and Tinea Pedis

Order	Agent	Comments
First line	Topical azole antifungals for 2–4 wk (1 wk past clinical cure)	Use medications for 2 wk even after the rash is gone
Second line	Systemic therapy: terbinafine (Lamisil) or fluconazole (Diflucan)	

First-line therapy for tinea capitis is microsize griseofulvin (Table 11-3) administered with milk or food to promote absorption. Treatment is for 8 weeks. The adult dose is 500 mg/d, and the pediatric dose ranges between 10 and 20 mg/kg/d. Children may attend school during therapy.

First-line therapy for tinea unguium (onychomycosis) consists of systemic agents. Topical preparations are not effective because they penetrate the nails poorly. Itraconazole is given by pulse dosing, 200 mg twice daily with a full meal for 7 days of each month. Treatment for fingernails lasts 3 months and for toenails, 4 months. Also effective for toenails is 200 mg itraconazole per day for 12 weeks (Table 11-4). Pulse dosing has less impact on the liver and is more popular than continuous dosing. Fluconazole can be given at a dose of 150 to 400 mg/d for 1 to 4 weeks or 150 mg once a week for 9 to 10 months. Treatment for onychomycosis is only 40% to 50% effective.

Second-Line Therapy

Second-line therapy for tinea corporis, pedis, cruris, or manus is needed if the infection fails to respond to topical therapy, if there are multiple lesions, or if treatment areas are repeatedly shaved. Second-line therapy consists of terbinafine 250 mg/d for 2 to 6 weeks or fluconazole 150 mg/wk for 2 to 4 weeks.

Second-line therapy for tinea capitis involves using itraconazole, terbinafine, or fluconazole if treatment failure occurs with griseofulvin despite adequate dosage and time.

MONITORING PATIENT RESPONSE

When patients use terbinafine or itraconazole, the AST/ALT levels and white blood cell counts need to be monitored at 6 to 8 weeks. Follow-up evaluations need to monitor both the effectiveness of the therapy and results of liver, kidney, and hematopoietic diagnostic studies. If tests disclose elevated liver function or if creatinine clearance exceeds 40 mL/min, drug therapy should be discontinued.

Table 11.4

Recommended Order of Treatment for Onychomycosis

Order	Agent	Comments
First line	itraconazole (Sporonax) or terbinafine (Lamisil)	Take with food Treatment lasts 12 wk Not recommended for children

PATIENT EDUCATION

An important role of the practitioner is to teach the patient about hygiene and ways to avoid transferring fungal infection to others. Patients should be instructed to complete the full course of treatment and not to stop treatment when symptoms subside. Parents and other caregivers also need to know that children can attend school while being treated.

Vinegar soaks and Vicks VapoRub can be used for onychomycosis. Vinegar is mixed with 1 part vinegar to 2 parts warm water. Feet are soaked for 15 to 20 minutes daily. It should not be used long-term. Vicks VapoRub can be applied to the toenails and socks put over the feet. Neither of these remedies have been thoroughly researched. Areas with fungal infections should be carefully dried. Antifungal powders and sprays can be used for prophylaxis.

TINEA VERSICOLOR

Tinea versicolor, also called pityriasis versicolor, is an opportunistic superficial yeast infection. It is a chronic, asymptomatic infection characterized by well-demarcated, scaling patches of varied coloration, from whitish to pink, tan, or brown.

CAUSES

An overgrowth of the hyphal form of *Pityrosporum ovale* causes tinea versicolor, which is most common in young adults (>15 years). The fungal infection occurs mostly in subtropical and tropical areas. In temperate zones, it is more common in the summer months but is seen in physically active people year round. Moist skin surfaces predispose to tinea versicolor. The infection rarely causes symptoms other than discoloration, and patients usually seek treatment for cosmetic purposes.

PATHOPHYSIOLOGY

P. ovale has an enzyme that oxidizes fatty acids in the skin surface lipids, forming dicarboxylic acids, which inhibit tyrosinase in epidermal melanocytes and cause hypomelanosis (loss of pigmentation).

DIAGNOSTIC CRITERIA

Skin lesions of tinea versicolor are well-defined, round or oval macules with an overlay of scales that may coalesce to form larger patches. They most often form on the trunk, upper arms, and neck. There may be mild itching. The diagnosis is confirmed by positive KOH test findings, which reveal budding yeast and hyphae.

INITIATING DRUG THERAPY

Topical agents for treating tinea versicolor include selenium sulfide lotion or shampoo and azole creams. The treatment may be repeated in 3 to 4 weeks and before the next warm season or travel to a tropical area. For widespread or stubborn disease systemic itraconazole or fluconazole may be prescribed for 7 to 10 days.

Table 11.5

Recommended Order of Treatment for Tinea Versicolor

Order	Agent	Comments
First line	selenium sulfide solution 1% or 2.5% topical azole cream or spray	Topical therapy is used for localized lesions. Use if lesions are resistant or widespread.
Second line	itraconazole (Sporonax)	

Goals of Therapy

The goal of therapy for tinea versicolor is resolution of lesions. Therapy lasts for 3 to 4 weeks. Because the lesions may recur in warm weather, prophylaxis consists of applying selenium sulfide lotion or shampoo twice a month.

Selenium Sulfide

Selenium sulfide, the drug of choice for tinea versicolor, has antifungal properties (Table 11-5). It is applied once a day to the affected skin for 15 minutes and then rinsed off. Contraindicated during pregnancy and lactation, it can be used with caution in instances of acute inflammation or exudation. Skin folds and genitalia are carefully rinsed. Selenium sulfide must be kept away from eyes. Potential adverse effects include irritation and increased hair loss.

Selecting the Most Appropriate Agent

Lesions may reappear because the infection is a result of microorganisms that normally inhabit the skin, so twice-monthly application of selenium sulfide is suggested as prophylaxis.

First-Line Therapy

Selenium sulfide solution (2.5%) as a lotion or shampoo (Selsun) is applied once a day. Pyrithione zinc (Head and Shoulders shampoo) can also be used. An antifungal topical agent is used. Choices include terbinafine cream or spray, ketoconazole, or sulconazole (Exelderm) nitrate for 3 to 4 weeks. The treatment can be repeated before the next warm season.

Second-Line Therapy

For resistant or widespread tinea versicolor, systemic therapy with itraconazole (200 mg for 5 days) may be prescribed.

PATIENT EDUCATION

It may take several months for the discoloration to disappear. Prophylactic application of ketoconazole cream or shampoo 1 to 2 times a week can prevent recurrence. The treatment can be repeated before the next exposure to warm weather.

CANDIDIASIS

Cutaneous candidiasis is a superficial fungal infection of the skin and mucous membranes. It is commonly found in the diaper area, oral cavity, intertriginous areas, nails, vagina,

---

BOX 11–2. VARIETIES OF CANDIDIASIS

Candidal infections are identified by their location on the body as follows:

- Axillae, under pendulous breasts, groin, intergluteal folds: intertrigo
- Glans penis: balanitis
- Follicular pustules: candidal folliculitis
- Nail folds: candidal paronychia
- Mouth and tongue: oral candidiasis (thrush)
- area included under diaper—diaper dermatitis

---

and male genitalia. It can occur at any age and in both sexes. It is classified by its location on the body (Box 11-2).

CAUSES

Cutaneous candidiasis, which is caused by *Candida albicans*, a yeast-like fungus, occurs on moist cutaneous sites. Predisposing factors include infection, diabetes, use of systemic and topical corticosteroids, and immunosuppression. It is commonly found in people who immerse their hands in water. It thrives in occluded sites.

Pathophysiology

Normally found on the skin and mucous membranes, *C. albicans* invades the epidermis when warm, moist conditions prevail or when there is a break in the skin that allows overgrowth.

DIAGNOSTIC CRITERIA

Candidiasis has several classifications. Intertrigo presents as red, moist papules or pustules. It is found in the axillae, inframammary areas, groin, and between fingers and toes.

Diaper dermatitis presents as erythema and edema with papular and pustular lesions, erosion, and oozing. Scaling may be evident at the margin of the lesions.

Interdigital candidiasis is an erythematous eroded area with surrounding maceration between the fingers and toes, whereas balanitis presents as multiple discrete pustules on the glans penis and preputial sac. Balanitis that involves the scrotum can be painful. It is most common in uncircumcised men.

Paronychia and onychia present as redness and swelling of the nail folds. Swelling lifts the wall from the nail plate, causing purulent infection.

Follicular candidiasis appears as small, discrete pustules in the ostia of hair follicles, and oral candidiasis (thrush) presents as white plaques on an erythematous base. It is found mostly in infants and immunocompromised patients. The tongue is usually involved.

INITIATING DRUG THERAPY

Candidiasis can be prevented by keeping intertriginous areas dry when possible. Also, washing with benzoyl peroxide and applying powder containing miconazole may be beneficial.

Table 11.6

Recommended Order of Treatment for Candidiasis

Order	Cutaneous Agent	Oral Agent	Comments
First line	Cool soaks with Burow's solution Topical azole	oral nystatin (Mycostatin)	Burow's solution is used in macerated areas. Topical azole is used for 10 days. Systemic therapy is used if no response to topical therapy.
Second line	itraconazole (Sporonax) or fluconazole (Diflucan)	itraconazole or fluconazole	NA

Goals of Therapy

The goal of therapy is restoration of the mucous membranes to normal.

Nystatin

Nystatin (Mycostatin) is a fungicide that binds to sterols in the cell membrane of the fungus, causing a change in the membrane's permeability. This allows intracellular components to leak, thereby causing cell death.

Used to treat thrush in infants and adults, nystatin is placed in each side of the mouth 3 times daily (see Table 11-1). The solution is kept in the mouth as long as possible, then swallowed. Therapy continues for 10 to 14 days and at least 48 hours after clinical clearing. Adverse effects include GI upset and oral irritation.

Selecting the Most Appropriate Agent

First-Line Therapy

For cutaneous candidiasis, cool wet soaks with Burow's solution can be applied 2 to 3 times daily in macerated areas. Intertriginous areas are kept dry by powdering (eg, with Zeasorb A-F Powder), exposing them to air, or by drying with a hair dryer after bathing. Antifungal creams (clotrimazole [Lotrimin], ketoconazole) can be applied once or twice a day for 10 days (Table 11-6).

For oral candidiasis, oral nystatin is used for 10 to 14 days, or one clotrimazole troche is given orally 5 times a day for 2 weeks.

Second-Line Therapy

For failure to respond to treatment, patients have the option of second-line therapy. Systemic itraconazole may be prescribed to adults only for cutaneous or oral candidiasis. For children and adults, oral fluconazole may be prescribed.

MONITORING PATIENT RESPONSE

Response to therapy should be evaluated in 2 weeks. Follow-up for patients receiving long-term systemic therapy (2 weeks; not necessary for pulse therapy) is recommended every month to monitor liver function. Patients undergoing pulse therapy do not need monitoring as regularly. Human immunodeficiency virus infection and diabetes mellitus should be ruled out in patients who have recurring problems with candidiasis.

■ Case Study

M. B. is a 42-year-old diabetic woman who presents with thickened, yellow toenails that are painful when she wears dress shoes. Her blood sugar level is well controlled. She is taking the following medications: metformin 500 mg tid, cimetidine 300 mg qid, Accupril 10 mg daily. A toenail culture comes back positive for fungus.

→ 1. List specific goals for treatment for M. B.

→ 2. What drug therapy would you prescribe? Why?

→ 3. What are the parameters for monitoring success of the therapy?

→ 4. Discuss specific patient education based on the prescribed therapy.

→ 5. List one or two adverse reactions for the selected agent that would cause you to change therapy.

→ 6. What would be the choice for second-line therapy?

→ 7. What over-the-counter and/or alternative medications would be appropriate for M. B.?

→ 8. What lifestyle changes would you recommend to M. B?

→ 9. Describe one or two drug–drug or drug–food interaction for the selected agent.

PATIENT EDUCATION

Education of the patient regarding hygiene and preventing or decreasing the transfer of the organism to others is important. It is equally important to stress air drying or drying with a hair dryer after bathing to ensure complete drying. Antifungal powder can be applied to areas predisposed to fungal infections.

Bibliography

*Starred references are cited in the text.

Daniel, C. R., Gupta, A. K., Joseph, W. S., et al. (2004). Onychomycosis disease management. *Medical Crossfire, 5*(5), 3–17.

Fitzpatrick, T. R., Johnson, R. A., Wolff, K., et al. (1997). *Color atlas and synopsis of clinical dermatology: Common and serious diseases* (3rd ed.). New York: McGraw-Hill.

Goodheart, H. P. (2003). *A photoguide of common skin disorders* (2nd ed.). Philadelphia: Lippincott Williams & Wilkins.

Habif, T. P. (2004). *Clinical dermatology: A color guide to diagnosis and therapy* (4th ed., Chap. 13). Philadelphia: Mosby.

Kelechi, T. J., & Stroud, S. (2004). The four 'Vs' for foot care. *Advances for Nurse Practitioners, 12*(6), 67–70, 84.

VanderStraden, M. R., Hossain, M. A., & Ghannoum, M. A. (2003). Cutaneous infections: Dermatophytosis, onychomycosis and tinea versicolor. *Infectious Disease Clinics of North America, 17*, 87–112.

Visit the Connection web site for the most up-to-date drug information.

VIRAL INFECTIONS OF THE SKIN

■ VIRGINIA P. ARCANGELO AND DENISE VANACORE-NETZ

Viruses producing skin lesions may be categorized into three groups: herpes viruses, papilloma viruses, and pox viruses. Herpes and papilloma viruses each affect approximately 20% of the adult population in the United States, with an even distribution between the sexes (Dambro, 2004).

Viruses are further classified by family—either the ribonucleic acid (RNA) family or the deoxyribonucleic acid (DNA) family. Herpes viruses, papilloma viruses, and pox viruses are members of the DNA family.

Viruses are obligate intracellular parasites that consist of a nucleic acid core surrounded by one or more proteins. A host cell is required for viral replication. Several mechanisms exist for viral replication, and different DNA viruses replicate by their own specific mechanism. Pox viruses replicate entirely in the cytoplasm. Herpes viruses replicate their own polymerase, along with several of their own enzymes. Papilloma virus proteins contribute to the initiation of DNA replication.

HERPES VIRUS INFECTIONS

CAUSES

Seven types of herpes viruses are associated with human illness: herpes simplex type 1 (HSV-1), herpes simplex type 2 (HSV-2), varicella-zoster virus (VZV), Epstein-Barr virus, cytomegalovirus, human herpes virus type 6 (HHV-6), and human herpes virus type 8 (HHV-8).

HSV-1 infection usually involves the face and skin above the waist. HSV-2 is most commonly associated with the genitalia and the skin below the waist. A life-threatening neonatal infection is associated with HSV-2 in a baby whose mother is infected with the virus; the infection is transmitted during vaginal birth. Herpes zoster (shingles) and varicella (chickenpox) are the result of VZV infection. Infectious mononucleosis is a result of Epstein-Barr virus infection. HHV-6 is associated with a mild childhood illness called roseola. HHV-8 is associated with Kaposi's sarcoma, especially in patients with HIV infection. HSV-1 and VZV are discussed in this chapter; HSV-2 is discussed in Chapter 36.

PATHOPHYSIOLOGY

Herpes viruses replicate their own polymerase along with several of their own enzymes. HSV is highly contagious. It is spread by direct contact with skin or mucous membrane. After the primary infection, the virus retreats to the dorsal root ganglion, where it remains latent until it is reactivated by triggers such as stress, viral infections, or sunlight.

DIAGNOSTIC CRITERIA

Infection with HSV-1 and HSV-2 causes vesicular eruptions that are painful and often recurrent. The common incubation period of 4 to 10 days is followed by the eruption of clustered vesicles on an erythematous base. Distribution of the virus into autonomic and sensory nerve endings allows the virus to remain latent.

Typically, HSV-1 causes oral or facial infections, with the most common sites being the mouth, pharynx, lips, or face. Primary occurrences usually have intense symptoms. Prodromal symptoms include burning, tingling, or itching; these symptoms may accompany recurrent infection as well. Recurrence of the infection is thought to be precipitated by fatigue, stress, trauma, fever, or ultraviolet radiation. The lesion presents as a single vesicle or group of vesicles that overlie an erythematous base. They become pustules and become crusted or erode. Lesions recur at the site innervated by the dorsal root ganglion inhabited by the virus.

The two different diseases caused by VZV (primary varicella infection, known as *chickenpox*, and herpes zoster, known as *shingles*) have similar symptoms. After an incubation period of 10 to 20 days, chickenpox (primary varicella) manifests with fever and malaise followed by the outbreak of itchy, vesicular lesions on an erythematous base. The outbreak usually begins on the trunk and progresses to the extremities and face. Primary varicella occurs most often in children. Adults infected with primary varicella tend to have more systemic effects, especially if they have pre-existing medical conditions.

A reactivation of VZV in the nerve root ganglion is referred to as herpes zoster or shingles. The infection characteristically begins with neuralgia in the affected dermatome, followed by an outbreak of grouped vesicles on an erythematous base, clustered in a unilateral pattern of the dermatome. In two thirds of infections, the lesions are on the trunk. Additional symptoms include fever, myalgia, and increasing localized pain. The most common presentation of herpes virus infection in the elderly is VZV in the form of herpes zoster. Three fourths of all cases of shingles occur in patients older than 50 years. A significant complication of herpes zoster is postherpetic neuralgia, pain in the dermatome site that lasts longer than 6 weeks after resolution of the infection.

INITIATING DRUG THERAPY

Although nonpharmacologic interventions, such as soaks with Burow's solution, help to relieve symptoms, HSV-1 infection is treated primarily with other topical agents. In the case of severe infection in an immunocompromised patient, treatment may be with systemic drug therapy, which shortens the duration of symptoms; however, there is no treatment to prevent recurrence.

For oral HSV-1 infections (oral herpes), symptoms may or may not respond to viscous lidocaine (Xylocaine) 2% applied to the lesion. A solution of diphenhydramine (Benadryl) elixir and aluminum hydroxide/magnesium hydroxide (Maalox) mixed in a 1:1 proportion can be used as an oral rinse four times a day. Sucking on Popsicles also can provide temporary relief.

For primary VZV infections that manifest as chickenpox, systemic therapy is used only in special cases and is not recommended for uncomplicated disease. The only approved pharmacologic agent for primary VZV is acyclovir (Zovirax).

Dosing is significantly higher than for HSV infections. For VZV infections that manifest as herpes zoster, or shingles, antiviral agents may help relieve symptoms. Patients should be treated if the rash has been present for fewer than 72 hours or if new lesions are still developing. If therapy starts within 72 hours of the appearance of the lesion, systemic therapy decreases the duration of the rash and the acute pain associated with herpes zoster. In addition, any patient who is older than 50 years who is immunocompromised should be treated with antiviral agents. The use of antiviral therapy in herpes zoster decreases the symptoms of postherpetic neuralgia from 62 days with placebo to 20 days with acyclovir.

Goals of Drug Therapy

In herpes virus infections, the goal of therapy is to reduce the duration of symptoms and suppress pain.

Topical Antiviral Agents

Two topical agents—acyclovir 5% and penciclovir (Denavir)—are available to treat herpes infections. These agents work by inhibiting viral DNA synthesis (Table 12-1).

Patients usually apply topical acyclovir every 3 hours, six times per day, for 7 days. Penciclovir is applied every 2 hours,

Table 12.1

Overview of Antiviral Agents for Herpes Virus Infections

Generic (Trade) Name and Dosage	Selected Adverse Events	Contraindications	Special Considerations
Topical Therapy			
acyclovir 5% (Zovirax) Apply every 3 h, 6 times per day for 7 d	Pruritus, pain on application	Do not use on mucous membranes or near eyes.	Must use glove or finger cot for application
penciclovir 1% (Denavir) Apply every 2 h for 4 d while awake	Headache, mild skin irritation	Renal impairment	Begin using drug at earliest sign or symptom.
Systemic Therapy			

acyclovir (Zovirax)
  For HSV-1
    200 mg five times per day for 10 d for initial outbreak;
    200 mg five times a day for 5 d for recurrence
  For VZV infection
    Children: 20 mg/kg qid for 5 d
    Adults: 800 mg five times a day for 7 d
	Nausea, vomiting, headache, CNS disturbance, rash, malaise	Renal impairment	Do not exceed maximum dose.

famciclovir (Famvir)
  For HSV-1
    250 mg tid for 10 d for initial outbreak; 125 mg tid for recurrence
  For VZV infection
    500 mg tid for 7 d
	Headache, GI disturbance, paresthesias	Renal dysfunction	May be affected by drugs metabolized by aldehyde oxidase

valacyclovir (Valtrex)
  For HSV-1
    1 g bid for 10 d
  For VZV infection
    1 g tid for 7 d
  For recurrent HSV
    2000 mg bid for 1 d
	GI upset, headache, dizziness, abdominal pain	Renal impairment	Be alert for renal or CNS toxicity with nephrotoxic drugs.

HSV, herpes simplex; virus; VZV, varicella-zoster virus.

during waking hours, for 4 days. Adverse effects include mild skin irritation and pruritus.

Systemic Antiviral Agents

The three first-line systemic agents are acyclovir (Zovirax), famciclovir (Famvir), and valacyclovir (Valtrex). Systemic antivirals are highly effective against herpes virus. In general, antiviral therapy is recommended for adolescents, adults, and high-risk patients, but not usually for healthy children below the age of 12 years (see Table 12-1).

Contraindications

Caution should be used in patients with renal disease because antivirals are excreted by the renal system. They are also contraindicated in patients with congestive heart failure and in lactation. Dosage adjustments are made for patients with a creatinine clearance rate less than 25 mL/minute.

Adverse Events

Adverse effects include headaches, vertigo, depression, and tremors. Patients may also experience gastrointestinal symptoms and rashes.

Interactions

The effect of antiviral agents is increased in patients taking probenecid, and patients taking zidovudine (Retrovir) may experience drowsiness.

Acyclovir

The prototypical antiviral agent acyclovir acts by inhibiting viral DNA replication. The drug works only in cells infected by HSV. A disadvantage of oral acyclovir is its low bioavailability of 10% to 20%.

The recommended acyclovir dosage for an initial episode of HSV disease in an immunocompetent host is 200 mg orally five times per day for 10 days (see Table 12-1). The recommended dosage for recurrent episodes is 200 mg five times per day for 5 days. For patients with recurrent infections, treatment prophylaxis is recommended with 400 mg twice daily. For an immunocompromised patient, the recommended treatment is 400 mg five times per day for 7 to 10 days. For suppression therapy, 400 mg twice a day is the dosage. The children's dosage of acyclovir is 5 mg/kg/day in five divided doses for 7 days.

The recommended dosage for treating VZV infections in children is 20 mg/kg four times per day for 5 days. Adult dosing is 800 mg five times per day for 7 to 10 days.

Famciclovir

Famciclovir is the diacetyl ester prodrug of penciclovir. It is an acyclic guanosine analog. After first-pass metabolism, it is well absorbed and converted to penciclovir. The oral bioavailability of famciclovir ranges from 5% to 75%.

The dosage of famciclovir is 250 mg three times per day for 10 days for an initial episode of illness; for recurrent episodes, the dose is 125 mg twice daily for 5 days and 200 mg twice a day for suppression therapy.

Valacyclovir

Valacyclovir is a prodrug of acyclovir and is converted rapidly. First-pass metabolism converts valacyclovir to acyclovir with 50% bioavailability.

The dosage of valacyclovir is 500 mg twice a day for 10 days for initial infection, 500 mg five times a day for recurrent infections, and 200 mg twice a day for suppression therapy. For cold sores 2,000 mg can be given twice a day for 1 day (two doses).

Selecting the Most Appropriate Agent

Of the various antiviral agents available, which is most effective for which disorder? Which agents are used when the first choice fails?

First-Line Therapy: Herpes Simplex Virus Type 1

First-line therapy for HSV-1 is topical acyclovir 5% every 3 hours six times a day for 7 days or penciclovir cream 1% every 2 hours during waking hours for 4 days in immunocompetent patients. Acyclovir is usually the first choice because it is less expensive than valacyclovir or famciclovir.

Immunocompromised patients may need oral acyclovir 200 mg five times a day for 7 days, valacyclovir 500 mg twice a day for 5 days, or famciclovir 500 mg twice a day for 7 days (Fig. 12-1 and Table 12-2).

First-Line Therapy: Varicella-Zoster Virus

Systemic therapy is used only in patients with complicated disease or in children with pulmonary disease or taking steroids, and not for uncomplicated disease. It is prescribed only if the rash has been present for less than 24 hours. Acyclovir is used at a dosage of 20 mg/kg four times a day for 5 days (Fig. 12-2 and Table 12-3).

First-Line Therapy: Herpes Zoster

Systemic antiviral therapy can be started if the herpes zoster outbreak is less than 72 hours in duration or longer than 72 hours but with new lesions appearing, the patient is older than 50 years of age, or the patient is immunosuppressed. Therapy consists of valacyclovir 1 g three times a day or famciclovir 500 mg three times a day for 7 days (Fig. 12-3). Cost is a driving force in prescribing valacyclovir before famciclovir because it is less expensive.

Table 12.2

Recommended Order of Treatment for HSV-1 Infection

Order	Agent	Comments
First line	Topical therapy with acyclovir 5% (Zovirax) or penciclovir 1% (Denavir)	Begin treatment at earliest sign of outbreak.
Second line	Systemic therapy with acyclovir (Zovirax), famciclovir (Famvir), or valacyclovir (Valtrex)	

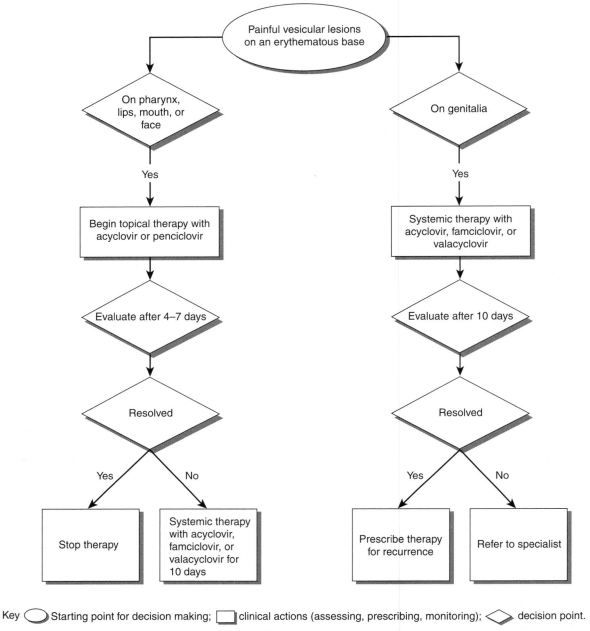

Key ⬭ Starting point for decision making; ▭ clinical actions (assessing, prescribing, monitoring); ◇ decision point.

Figure 12–1   Treatment recommendations (left) for outbreaks of herpes simplex virus type 1 (HSV-1) and (right) for HSV-2.

Table 12.3

Recommended Order of Treatment for Varicella-Zoster Virus Infection

Order	Agents	Comments
First line	acyclovir (Zovirax), famciclovir (Famvir), valacyclovir (Valtrex)	For children the maximum dose is 800 mg qid. Acyclovir is the only approved agent for primary varicella. Antiviral therapy for primary varicella is recommended for adolescents, adults, and high-risk patients, but not for healthy children.

MONITORING PATIENT RESPONSE

Follow-up evaluation of HSV infection is not required if the symptoms resolve. For patients with herpes zoster, follow-up is recommended at 3 days after starting therapy, then at 1 week.

PATIENT EDUCATION

Lifestyle Changes

Educating the patient about hygiene, precipitating factors, and prevention is imperative. For patients with the HSV-2 infection manifested as genital herpes, education regarding sexual activity, recurrence, and the unpredictable course of the

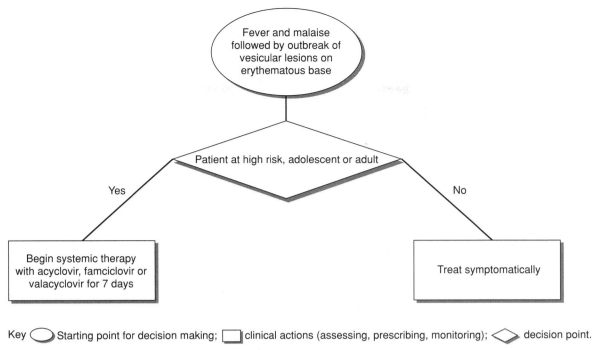

Figure 12–2 Treatment algorithm for the varicella zoster virus infection manifested as chickenpox.

disease is necessary. Moreover, these patients should be screened for other sexually transmitted diseases (see Chapter 36 for more information). In patients with more than five recurrences per year, prophylactic treatment is recommended.

In patients with herpes zoster, follow-up monitoring for postherpetic neuralgia is important. Patients with postherpetic neuralgia should understand that pain management is the goal of therapy.

Because herpes virus is spread by skin contact, patients need to recognize the importance of wearing gloves when applying medications and of thorough, careful hand washing. Skin-to-skin contact is avoided. Patients with herpes zoster can transmit the virus as chickenpox to anyone who has not been infected with the virus.

Complementary and Alternative Medicine

Capsaicin is used for pain control in herpes zoster. It is most effective when applied three or four times a day. Tea tree oil has reported antiseptic properties and is used in herpes simplex.

WARTS (VERRUCAE)

Warts are caused by the human papilloma virus (HPV). There are more than 80 types of HPV. They are transferred by skin-to-skin contact. The common viruses can be classified as those causing anogenital infections and non-anogenital infections. Anogenital infections are discussed in Chapter 36. The most common non-anogenital infections present as warts. These are very common, especially in children: at some time in their life, approximately 20% of school-aged children have one or more warts, which usually regress spontaneously. Categories of warts include plantar, filiform, flat, and common.

CAUSES

Plantar warts result from HPV-1 and commonly occur on the soles of the feet and the palms of the hands. Verruca vulgaris—common warts—is an infection with HPV-2. These

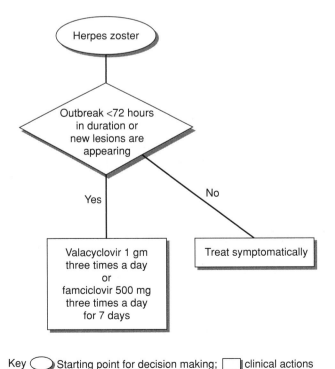

Figure 12–3 Treatment algorithm for the varicella herpes zoster virus infection manifested as shingles.

present on the fingers or toes or at sites of trauma. They are flesh-colored to brown, hyperkeratotic papules. HPV-3 produces flat warts, which are located on the face, neck, and chest or flexor regions of the forearms and legs.

Factors that predispose to HPV include:

- Infection with HIV
- Intake of drugs that decrease cell-mediated immunity (prednisone, cyclosporin)
- Chemotherapeutic agents
- Pregnancy (may cause proliferation)
- Handling raw meat, fish, or other animal matter

PATHOPHYSIOLOGY

Papilloma virus proteins contribute to the initiation of DNA replication.

DIAGNOSTIC CRITERIA

Warts are papillomatous, corrugated, hyperkeratotic growths found only on the epidermis, especially in areas subjected to repeated trauma. They can be solitary, multiple, or clustered. Warts are named based on their clinical appearance, location, or both.

Filiform warts are found primarily on the face and neck and present as tan, finger-like projections. Plantar warts (verruca plantaris) are found on the metatarsal areas, heels, and toes. Common warts (verruca vulgaris) occur most often on the hands and fingers, knees, and elbows and have an asymmetric distribution. Flat warts (verruca plana) are found mostly on the forehead, chin, cheeks, arms, and dorsa of the hands. They are flat and well defined and may be flesh-colored or darker brown. Flat warts can be spread by shaving and are found in the beard area in men and on the legs in women. These HPV infections are rarely associated with malignancy. Typically, the incubation period is 2 to 6 months.

INITIATING DRUG THERAPY

The natural history of cutaneous HPV infection is spontaneous resolution in months or a few years, so aggressive therapy may not be needed unless the patient reports pain. If treatment is initiated, the choice of medication depends on age of the patient, whether pain is involved, and the location of the wart. Filiform and flat warts are removed by a dermatologist. Topical treatment with salicylic acid (DuoFilm) is usually the starting point for all other warts. It is easier to treat small verrucae rather than waiting until they are large.

Goals of Therapy

The goal of therapy is eradication of the virus and lesion, although there is no way to actually kill HPV.

Salicylic Acid

Salicylic acid is a keratolytic (peeling) agent. It is available in a variety of strengths for specific types or sites of verrucae. It comes in liquid, gel, and patches. Usually, 17% salicylic acid is used to treat small lesions. Mediplast is a patch

product that is 40% salicylic acid plaster; it is useful for large lesions and can be cut to fit the wart.

Dosage

The solution is left on overnight. The patch is applied and left on for 5 to 6 days. Treatment continues for up to 12 weeks. The patient is instructed to soak the area in water for 5 minutes and dry the area before applying the topical preparation.

Contraindications

Topical therapy is contraindicated in patients with diabetes mellitus or impaired circulation and on moles, birthmarks, or unusual warts with hair growth. The most common adverse effect is skin irritation.

Selecting the Most Appropriate Agent

Since the immune system seems to play the most important role in HPV, treatment stimulates the immune system to deal more effectively with the virus. Most warts cure themselves over time, especially in the immunocompetent host.

First-Line Therapy

Filiform or flat warts are removed by a dermatologist. For common warts, topical salicylic acid in a 17% concentration is used; it is applied at bedtime for approximately 8 weeks or until the wart is gone. For plantar warts, a 40% salicylic

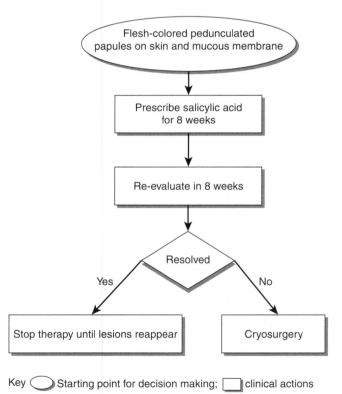

Key ⬭ Starting point for decision making; ▭ clinical actions (assessing, prescribing, monitoring); ◇ decision point.

Figure 12–4 Treatment algorithm for nonanogenital human papilloma virus infection.

Table 12.4

Recommended Order of Treatment for Non-anogenital Infection with Human Papilloma Virus

Order	Agents	Comments
First line	salicylic acid	Used as first-line agent to treat all types of verrucae
Second line	cryosurgery, electrosurgery, or CO_2 laser surgery	Refer patient to specialist.

acid preparation is used in plaster or patch form that is cut to the size of the wart and applied at bedtime. The preparation remains in place for 24 to 48 hours. When removed, the area is rubbed with a pumice stone to remove dead white keratin. This is repeated for approximately 8 weeks or until the wart is gone (Fig. 12-4 and Table 12-4).

Second-Line Therapy

If patient-applied therapy fails, cryosurgery, electrotherapy, or CO_2 laser surgery can be performed.

MONITORING PATIENT RESPONSE

In non-anogenital HPV infections, multiple treatments may be necessary. Patients should understand the importance of follow-up beyond the initial wart removal, because the virus may remain. Patients may need weekly treatment until the wart is eradicated.

PATIENT EDUCATION

Patients need to be informed that viral warts may recur.

■ Case Study

B.H. is a 72-year-old man who presents for evaluation of several painful red bumps on his left side. The pain radiates around to his chest. The rash resembles blisters that are just forming. He noticed them yesterday, and more are forming. His wife is receiving chemotherapy for breast cancer. His laboratory results are all normal, and his creatinine is 1.2.

Diagnosis: Herpes zoster

1. List specific treatment goals for B.H.
2. What, if any, drug therapy would you prescribe? Why?
3. What are the parameters for monitoring the success of the therapy?
4. Discuss specific patient education based on his history and the therapy.
5. List one or two adverse effects he may get from the prescribed therapy.
6. What over-the-counter and/or alternative therapy might you recommend?
7. What lifestyle changes might you recommend for B.H.?
8. Describe one or two drug/drug or drug/food interaction for the selected agent.

Bibliography

Starred references are cited in the text.

Brown, T. J. (2001). Antiviral agents. *Dermatological Clinics, 19*(1), 23–34.

Dambro, M. R. (2004). *Griffith's 5-minute clinical consult 2004.* Philadelphia: Lippincott Williams & Wilkins.

Emmert, D. H. (2000). Treatment of common cutaneous herpes simplex virus infection. *American Family Physician, 61*(1), 1697–1706.

Fitzpatrick, T. B., Johnson, R. A., Wolff, K., Polano, M. K., & Suurmond, D. (1997). *Color atlas of clinical dermatology* (3rd ed.). New York: McGraw-Hill.

Goodheart, H. P. (2003). *A photoguide of common skin disorders* (2nd ed.). Baltimore: Lippincott Williams & Wilkins.

Stankus, S. J. (2000). Management of herpes zoster (shingles) and postherpetic neuralgia. *American Family Physician, 61*(8), 2437–2448.

Traton, E. (2002). Visceral zoster as a presenting feature of disseminated herpes zoster. *Journal of the American Academy of Dermatology, 46*(5), 834–839.

Visit the Connection web site for the most up-to-date drug information.

BACTERIAL INFECTIONS OF THE SKIN

■ MARIA FOY AND LINDA C. FOREMAN

Bacterial skin infections range from those that are minor and heal without consequence to those that are more severe and may be disfiguring or even life-threatening. Minor infections are quite common and are often self-treated by patients without formal medical care. For the most part, wounds seen in health care practice are easily managed with appropriate wound care and antibiotic therapy, if indicated.

Common primary skin infections resulting from bacteria include impetigo, bullous impetigo, folliculitis, felons, paronychias, and cellulitis (see Box 13-1 for information about associated problems). These are discussed in this chapter, along with the less common infections erysipelas, ecthyma, furuncles, and carbuncles. This chapter also contains a brief discussion of necrotizing fasciitis, a very serious infection treated in an inpatient setting by specialists. See the accompanying color plates for an illustration of some of these infections.

CAUSES

The bacterial organisms most commonly responsible for causing skin infections are *Streptococcus pyogenes* (group A *Streptococcus*, or GAS) and *Staphylococcus aureus* (Tables 13-1 and 13-2).

Impetigo and Ecthyma

In the past, superficial skin infections, such as impetigo, a common infection characterized by scattered vesicular lesions, were caused by GAS. However, a shift in normal skin flora has occurred in the United States, and now impetigo is due primarily to *S. aureus* alone or less commonly in combination with GAS. Bullous impetigo, a variation of impetigo, is caused primarily by *S. aureus*.

Ecthyma is a chronic form of impetigo that affects deeper layers of the skin. Usually the causes are the same as those of impetigo. However, gram-negative organisms, such as *Pseudomonas*, or fungal organisms may play a role, especially in diabetic or immunocompromised patients. Ecthyma can develop from minor wounds, scabies, insect bites, or any condition that causes itching, scratching, and excoriation.

Impetigo is more common among children but is also seen in adults. It most often occurs during hot, humid weather. Both impetigo and ecthyma are contagious and can be spread through person-to-person contact, often in schools or day care centers. Poor hygiene and crowded living conditions are other factors that can contribute to the development of these infections (Gorbach, 2004).

Cellulitis and Erysipelas

Cellulitis is an infection involving the skin and subcutaneous layers. It has the potential to spread systemically and cause serious illness. It can develop in any type of wound, ranging from a minor break in the skin to more serious laceration, puncture, or burn. Other common precipitants include stasis dermatitis, stasis ulcers, edema of the lower extremity, venous insufficiency, and obesity (Odell, 2003). In intravenous drug users, cellulitis typically develops at injection sites. The characteristics of infection depend on many factors, including the type of wound, the organisms involved, and the patient.

Most cases of cellulitis result from GAS and *S. aureus* infection, though patients with predisposing factors may acquire cellulitis from any organism, including *Escherichia coli*, *Pseudomonas*, and *Klebsiella* (see Table 13-2) (Goldstein & Shellow, 1995). A *Pasteurella* species often causes cellulitis related to animal bites and scratches. Table 13-2 lists additional causes.

Erysipelas, predominantly caused by *S. pyogenes*, is a superficial form of cellulitis and is seen more often in children, especially infants, and the elderly. Also known as St. Anthony's fire, it is an acute condition that can spread rapidly through the skin and lymphatics, causing significant mortality (up to 5%) if left untreated.

Pustular Infections

Pustular infections include folliculitis, furunculosis, and carbunculosis. Folliculitis is a common superficial infection associated with *S. aureus*. However, patients who have been taking prolonged antibiotic therapy for acne may acquire folliculitis from gram-negative organisms such as *Klebsiella*, *Enterobacter*, or *Proteus*. These lesions are usually found on the cheek or chin, under the nose, or on the central facial areas (Trent et al., 2001). *Pseudomonas* may cause folliculitis in those who frequently use hot tubs, usually due to inadequate chlorination.

BOX 13–1. DANGER: BITES AND OTHER PUNCTURE WOUNDS

Human and animal bites and puncture wounds of other sorts are infections waiting to develop. Because these wounds are associated with such a high risk for infection, antibiotic prophylaxis with a broad-spectrum penicillin or quinolone usually begins with the patient's request for health care. Tetanus is also an important consideration in puncture wounds and bites, and patients should be immunized as needed.

If the wound was created by a clean object and is in an area that is well vascularized, treatment, in addition to antibiotic prophylaxis, may consist simply of washing thoroughly; soaking in warm, soapy water several times a day; and observing the site for a few days.

If the wound was made by an object contaminated with fecal material, soil, or other debris, or if the patient is diabetic or has a compromised circulation, broad-spectrum antibiotic prophylaxis is required with amoxicillin-clavulanate potassium or ciprofloxacin based on probable causative organism.

Care for bite wounds depends on several factors, including whether the biter was a human or an animal, the location of the wound, and whether the wound is primarily a puncture or a laceration. All bite wounds should be cleaned thoroughly with soap and water. Puncture bites should be irrigated with normal saline solution. Extensive wounds may require surgical débridement, tendon repair, or suturing. If the bite is located on an extremity elcoation of the extremity will help prevent swelling.

All human bites that break the skin should be treated with broad-spectrum antibiotic prophylaxis. Appropriate, choices include amoxicillin-clavulanate, or ampicillin–sulbactam of intravenous treatment needed. Oral doxycycline can be used for patients who are allergic to penicillin. Treatment should be given for a full 7 to 10 days.

Minor animal bites may not require antibiotic prophylaxis unless the wound is on the hand, foot, or face. However, the infection rate in animal bites can range from 2% to 20%, and it may be prudent to treat the wound with a course of antibiotic prophylaxis. The possibility of rabies must also be addressed. The same agents used for human bites are also appropriate for animal bites.

Although most puncture wounds heal without incident, patients should be instructed to observe for signs of infection, including inflammation, persistent pain, swelling, or purulent drainage. If a puncture wound becomes infected, further systemic antibiotic therapy is required and should be based on culture and Gram stain results. A follow-up visit should be scheduled within days to ensure that the wound is healing without further infection.

Furunculosis (furuncles) and carbunculosis (carbuncles) are pustular infections usually caused by *S. aureus*. Both conditions can develop from an unresolved case of folliculitis (Bisno et al., 1997).

Irritation from shaving, plucking, and waxing of hair may contribute to folliculitis. Other predisposing factors include humid conditions, tight clothing, diabetes, occlusion of the hair follicles from cosmetics or sunscreens, poor hygiene, and occupational exposure to heavy grease or solvents.

Other common skin infections, such as paronychia (an infection surrounding a nail bed) and a felon (an infection affecting the tip of a digit) are usually caused by *S. aureus*, *S. pyogenes*, or *Pseudomonas*, and occasionally gram-negative bacilli. *Candida* may also contribute, especially in diabetic patients.

Necrotizing Fasciitis

Necrotizing fasciitis, an extremely serious infection of the subcutaneous tissues, is life-threatening if not diagnosed early and treated appropriately. It is most likely to occur in middle-aged, elderly, or seriously debilitated patients (Sadick, 1997). The mortality rate is 20% to 30%; it approaches 50% in patients

Table 13.1

Selected Organisms That Cause Skin Infections

	Impetigo and Ecthyma	Bullous Impetigo	Erysipelas	Folliculitis, Furuncles, and Carbuncles	Paronychias
Gram-Positive Organisms					
Staphylococcus aureus	X	X	X (very few)	X	X
Group A *Streptococcus*	X		X		X
Group B *Streptococcus*	X (newborn impetigo)		X (newborn)		
Gram-Negative Organisms					
Proteus				X (facial) (folliculitis)	
Pseudomonas	X (occasionally ecthyma)			X (hot tub folliculitis)	X
Klebsiella				X (folliculitis)	
Enterobacter				X (occasionally folliculitis)	

Table 13.2

Organisms That Cause Cellulitis

Organism	Condition
Staphylococcus aureus	Common
Group A *Streptococcus*	Common
Haemophilus influenzae B	Children (periorbital cellulitis*)
Pneumococcus	Children
Escherichia coli	Opportunistic in compromised patients
Pseudomonas	
Klebsiella	
Enterobacter	
Pasteurella multocida	Animal bites and scratches
Anaerobic organisms	Diabetes, ulcers, trauma, crush wounds
Erysipelothrix rhusiopathiae	Fish handlers, usually on the hand
Aeromonas hydrophila	Fresh water-related injury, immunosuppressed patients
Vibrio species	Sea water-related injuries

*Uncommon now because of use of HIB vaccine.

BOX 13–2. PREDISPOSING FACTORS IN SKIN INFECTIONS

Chronic carriers of *Staphylococcus aureus*
Diabetes mellitus
Peripheral vascular disease
Venous stasis
Alcoholism (malnutrition)
Immune deficiency
Corticosteroid therapy
Obesity
Trauma or burns
Poor hygiene
Warm, humid conditions
Topical irritants
Tight clothing

---

with underlying vascular disease. Often, the initial lesion is minor, such as an insect bite or boil; it is rarely associated with Bartholin's gland or perianal abscesses (Gorbach, 2004). However, 20% of cases have no visible lesions (Gorbach, 2004). Patients with diabetes and alcoholism may have no evidence of trauma (Odell, 2003).

Necrotizing fasciitis can be either monomicrobial from β-hemolytic *S. pyogenes, S. aureus,* or anaerobic streptococcus, or polymicrobial, often involving 1 to 15 organisms. Varicella infections can also be a risk factor for invasive infections (Wilhelm et al., 2001).

Patients with necrotizing fasciitis are very ill and require intensive care. Usually, treatment by surgeons and infectious disease specialists is indicated. Patients who are elderly or debilitated or who have predisposing medical conditions, such as diabetes, advanced atherosclerotic disease, and lesions starting in an extremity and progressing into the back, chest wall, or buttock muscles, have a poor prognosis (Gorbach, 2004).

PATHOPHYSIOLOGY

The skin is composed of three layers. The outer layer is the epidermis, the first line of defense against infection. Nail tissue is part of the epidermis. Underneath is the dermis, which contains connective tissue, blood vessels, nerves, hair follicles, sweat glands, and sebaceous glands. The innermost layer is composed of subcutaneous tissue. Skin infections may be classified according to the depth of penetration and the layer and skin structure affected.

Under normal circumstances, bacteria present on the skin as normal flora cause no harm. However, a break in the skin can allow these organisms to penetrate and proliferate, resulting in a skin infection. Some people are persistent carriers of *S. aureus* in the nasal, perineal, or axillary areas. These people may be more prone to development of skin infections and more likely to experience recurrences.

Patients with predisposing medical conditions (Box 13-2), such as diabetes, immune system disorders, and malnutrition from alcoholism or other causes, are more prone to skin infection because of poor wound healing ability. Also at a higher risk for skin infection are those with circulatory com-

promise of the arterial, venous, or lymphatic systems. Wound infections in patients with these conditions have the potential to become more serious and invasive, requiring intravenous antibiotic therapy, hospitalization, or referral to a specialist. Wound infections can also become more serious when treatment is delayed. The practitioner must be alert for these situations and act promptly.

In addition, any organism, not just GAS or *S. aureus,* may become opportunistic in these patients and cause infection. Some common opportunistic organisms include *E. coli, Klebsiella,* and *Pseudomonas aeruginosa*. Opportunistic infections are more difficult to treat. They require a wider variety of antibiotic agents and tend to be chronic.

DIAGNOSTIC CRITERIA

Impetigo and Ecthyma

Impetigo, a highly contagious, common primary skin infection in children, is most frequently found on the face, scalp, or extremities. Impetigo in adults is not as contagious as in children. Impetigo begins as scattered, discrete macules that itch and are spread by scratching. These macules then develop into vesicles and pustules on an erythematous base that eventually rupture, oozing a purulent liquid. Once dried, the lesions appear thick, with a characteristic honey-colored crust on the surface. Once healed, scarring is rare. Regional lymphadenopathy may be present and lesions may itch; however, fever or other systemic complaints are uncommon. The infection is diagnosed clinically by the appearance of hallmark honey-colored crusts; a Gram stain of the vesicular fluid can confirm the diagnosis if there is any doubt.

Bullous impetigo is a variation of impetigo. Found on the face, scalp, extremities, trunk, and intertriginous areas, it affects primarily newborns and children between the ages of 3 and 5 (Wilhelm et al., 2001). Bullous impetigo is characterized by the formation of superficial, flaccid bullae on the skin. The brownish-gray lesions are sometimes crusted or have an erythematous halo. They also appear smooth and shiny, as if they were coated with lacquer.

In its most severe form, bullous impetigo denudes large areas of skin in what is referred to as "scalded skin" syndrome. This is most common in infants but can occur in those who are immunosuppressed. It is thought to occur in patients who are sensitive to toxins produced by staphylococcal organisms (Barg et al., 1998). Such cases carry a greater risk for more invasive infection because of the loss of large amounts of the skin, which is the body's protective barrier.

Ecthyma occurs when a case of impetigo worsens and spreads deeply to the dermis. Much less common than impetigo, ecthyma usually affects debilitated individuals and the elderly (Odell, 2003). Signs of ecthyma are usually found on the lower extremities, beginning with the formation of vesicles that then develop into shallow ulcerations. The ulcerations enlarge over several days and are surrounded by an erythematous halo. Because the infection affects the deeper layers of the skin, scarring is often seen after ulcerations heal (Wilhelm et al., 2001). Lesions are usually painful and may persist for weeks to months.

Cellulitis and Erysipelas

Cellulitis is a potentially serious infection involving the skin and subcutaneous tissue. In adults, it most commonly affects the lower extremities and may begin with a skin break due to local trauma, but this area of trauma may not be apparent. In children, cellulitis usually results from an insect bite or a wound. The disease causes spreading and painful erythema, with the affected area warm and tender to the touch. Pitting edema is often present. The skin may also be shiny and have an "orange peel" appearance. The margins of cellulitis are diffuse, not sharply demarcated, and the affected area is flat and usually edematous. In open wounds, purulent drainage and necrosis may be present. Red streaks may develop proximal to the area of infection, indicating lymphatic spread. Crepitus may be present, suggesting involvement of anaerobic organisms.

Systemic symptoms of fever, chills, and malaise and regional adenitis are common and can indicate impending bacteremia. In fact, these symptoms may be present before cellulitis is clearly evident.

Erysipelas, a type of cellulitis limited to the superficial layers of the skin, is most common in children, especially infants and the elderly, but it can occur in healthy individuals who have sustained only minor wounds. Others patients who are at risk include those with venous insufficiency or underlying skin ulcers, diabetics, alcoholics, or those with nephritic syndrome. Erysipelas is most commonly found on the lower extremities but can be also found on the face and scalp. Erysipelas begins as an area of sharply demarcated erythema that spreads rapidly over a period of minutes to hours. The affected area is slightly raised, firm, warm, and tender to the touch. Erythema spreads along local lymphatic channels, which gives the skin a typical "orange peel" appearance due to lymphatic obstruction.

Common systemic symptoms include pain, malaise, chills and fever. In more serious cases, patients may appear seriously ill. Erysipelas occurring on the face often follows a respiratory infection; this can be very serious due to the occurrence of cavernous sinus thrombosis (Odell, 2003). Erysipelas can recur, usually in the same area as a previous infection, especially in patients with venous insufficiency or lymphedema (Wilhelm et al., 2001).

Pustular Infections

Folliculitis, a noninfectious pustular infection of the hair follicles, is usually superficial and can occur in any hairy area, especially the bearded parts of the face and the intertriginous areas. Early lesions appear as erythematous papules; they turn into small pustules within approximately 48 hours. The lesions may itch initially, then rupture and form crusts. It is common to see various lesions at different stages of development. Folliculitis often recurs over months or even years.

A furuncle, which develops from folliculitis, is a painful, pus-filled nodule that develops around a hair follicle. The condition is most commonly found in adolescents or in those with predisposing conditions such as diabetes, immunodeficiency, or poor hygiene. A carbuncle is a confluence of several furuncles that form deep within the dermis. They are often found on the upper back or the thick skin at the back of the neck, especially in men over 40.

Furuncles and carbuncles are found in hairy areas or in areas of friction. Common sites are the neck, face, axillae, forearms, upper back, groin, buttocks, and thighs. A lesion begins with pruritus and tenderness. It becomes fluctuant in several days as the collection of pus enlarges. Ranging in size from 0.5 to 3 cm, it appears as a pointed, yellow lesion on the skin. As the lesion enlarges, tenderness increases and the lesion often ruptures spontaneously. Systemic manifestations are not usually seen with furuncles, but carbuncles are frequently accompanied by systemic signs such as fever, malaise, and headache.

A paronychia is infection of the tissue surrounding a nail bed. It is associated with nail biting, hangnails, or finger sucking; it may occur in people who have their hands in water frequently. Diabetic patients are also at a higher risk. A paronychia involving the toenail most often results from an ingrown nail. The infected area appears red and swollen and is painful. Pus, which may accumulate, may sometimes be expressed with gentle pressure; this usually relieves the discomfort. Systemic symptoms are uncommon.

A felon, which may follow a fingertip wound, is an infection that involves the pulp space in the tip of a digit. It is potentially more serious than a paronychia because it is confined in a closed space. The affected digit is erythematous, edematous, and exquisitely tender. The edema has the potential to compromise the arterial supply of the digit. If left untreated, abscess and tissue necrosis can occur. An additional danger is the possibility of bony or joint involvement, which can lead to loss of function.

Necrotizing Fasciitis

Necrotizing fasciitis should be suspected in any case of presumed cellulitis that does not respond to the usual treatment. Patients with this condition are extremely ill and require intensive care and treatment by specialists. Necrotizing fasciitis initially appears similar to cellulitis, with severe pain, erythema, and edema. The infection can be differentiated from cellulitis by its rapid spread, tissue destruction, and lack of response to usual antibiotic therapy. The subcutaneous tissue will have a wooden-hard feel, as compared to cellulitis and erysipelas, where this tissue is yielding and can be palpated. Other symptoms that distinguish necrotizing fasciitis from cellulitis are high fever (102°F to 105°F), intense pain and tenderness at the site, and swelling of the affected extremity. As tissue destruction spreads, pain is replaced by anesthesia. Drainage is usually present and is described as "dishwater pus" (Sadick, 1997). As toxicity increases, abnormal renal function ensues and patients become confused.

INITIATING DRUG THERAPY

An increasing challenge in treating skin infections is the problem of antibiotic-resistant organisms. Choosing the appropriate agent is not as simple as it once was, and prescribers must be aware of this fact, as well as of regional variations in infecting organisms.

Because warm, humid conditions and poor hygiene may play a role in skin infections, especially impetigo, treatment begins with good hygiene (Box 13-3), avoidance of irritants, and meticulous wound care as appropriate. For some very minor infections, these measures along with a topical agent may be sufficient. Adjunctive treatment for all skin infections (bullous impetigo and erysipelas, for example) includes warm soaks and elevation of the affected area if it involves an extremity. However, most bacterial skin infections require treatment with systemic antibiotic therapy.

Most infections are treated on an outpatient basis with oral antibiotic agents. Patients with more serious infections may require hospitalization and intravenous medication or referral to a specialist. Treatment decisions are based on the practitioner's knowledge of the patient and predisposing conditions, the patient's present state of health, the type of infection, and the stage of infection.

In many cases of skin infection, systemic antibiotic therapy (Table 13-3) is prescribed empirically based on knowledge of the organisms commonly responsible for specific infections, such as S. aureus and GAS. With potentially serious infections such as a felon or cellulitis, a specimen of wound drainage should be obtained for culture and sensitivity testing. Empiric therapy will be initiated pending the results.

In the case of puncture or bite wounds that are not initially infected, antibiotics are prescribed as prophylaxis because of the high risk of infection associated with these wounds.

Topical medications might be used as primary treatment or adjunctively with systemic agents. Topical agents include mupirocin (Bactroban) and gentamicin (Garamycin) solutions. In some patients thought to be chronic carriers of S. aureus, infections may be recurrent. Topical mupirocin ointment applied to the nares or perineal or axillary areas may be used as a prophylactic agent to eliminate this chronic carrier state (Fitzpatrick et al., 1997).

Several adjunctive measures may also be used with drug therapy. Besides warm soaks, incision and drainage may help resolve pustular lesions. Sterile saline dressings and cool Burow's compresses may be used to decrease the pain associated with cellulitis (Rose, 2004). Patients with a paronychia may need to have the nail bed decompressed to relieve the pressure, and deeper and more invasive infections almost always require incision and drainage.

Goals of Drug Therapy

The goals in treating bacterial skin infections are to cure the infection, prevent worsening, minimize scarring, and prevent recurrence. Many minor infections resolve within 10 to 14 days. If resolution does not occur, alternative agents may be prescribed. The prescriber must decide when it is appropriate to initiate treatment with an alternative agent or whether a referral to a specialist for more definitive diagnosis and treatment is indicated.

Antibiotics

Several classes of antibiotic agents are useful for treating bacterial skin infections. For information on specific agents, refer to Table 13-3. Antibiotic agents are bactericidal to specific microorganisms. Agents may be administered topically, orally, intramuscularly, or intravenously, depending on the specific infection and the condition of the patient.

The most common adverse effects occurring with most antibiotics are nausea, vomiting, diarrhea, rashes, allergic reactions, and urticaria. Also, patients taking antibiotic therapy, especially prolonged therapy, sometimes acquire fungal infections such as vaginal candidiasis or thrush.

A less common but potentially life-threatening adverse effect of antibiotic therapy is pseudomembranous colitis. This causes severe diarrhea and is usually a result of overgrowth of the bacterium Clostridium difficile. Anaphylaxis and seizures (especially when high doses of antibiotics are used) may also occur. To minimize the risk of these events, a thorough patient history is essential before prescribing these drugs. There are also many interactions between antibiotics and other medications a patient might be taking. For information on selected drug interactions, see Table 13-3.

Broad-Spectrum Penicillins

Most skin infections are caused by GAS and S. aureus. In the past, simple penicillin was usually effective in treating these

---

BOX 13–3. STRATEGIES TO PREVENT SKIN INFECTIONS

Wash hands frequently to prevent spread of infecting organisms.
Clean skin twice daily with soap and water or antibacterial soap (eg, Hibiclens, Lever 2000).
Avoid scratching.
Use warm soaks to promote drainage of pustular matter.
Avoid irritants, including tight clothing, shaving, sunscreens, and occlusive cosmetics and deodorants.

Table 13.3

Overview of Selected Antibiotics for Skin Infections

Generic (Trade) Name and Dosage	Selected Adverse Events	Contraindications	Special Considerations
Broad-Spectrum Penicillins			
amoxicillin–clavulanate (Augmentin) Adults: 500–875 mg q12h or 250–500 mg q8h PO Children: 22.5 mg/kg q12h PO or 13.3 mg/kg q8h PO	Nausea, vomiting, diarrhea, rash, allergic reactions, fungal infection **Serious:** pseudomembranous colitis, seizures (high doses)	Allergy to penicillin or clavulanate, serious allergy to imipenem, or cephalosporins Use with caution in severe renal disease, less severe allergy to cephalosporins.	Take with or without food. Food may decrease GI symptoms. Interactions: warfarin, oral contraceptives Probenecid decreases renal excretion. Increased risk of rash with allopurinol Safe for young children
dicloxacillin (Dynapen) Adults: 125–250 mg 6h PO Children: 3.125–6.25 mg/kg q6h PO	Same as amoxicillin–clavulanate Drug-induced hepatitis	Penicillin allergy Use with caution in severe renal or hepatic disease, pregnancy, lactation.	Take on empty stomach for best absorption. Interactions: probenecid, warfarin
First-Generation Cephalosporins			
cephalexin (Keflex) Adults: 500 mg q12h PO Children: 12.5–25 mg/kg q12h PO	Nausea, vomiting, diarrhea, rash, allergic reactions, fungal infections **Serious:** pseudomembranous colitis, seizures (high doses) Stevens-Johnson syndrome, hemolytic anemia	Serious penicillin allergy, allergy to cephalosporins Use with caution in renal disease, pregnancy, lactation.	Take with or without food. Food may decrease GI symptoms. Probenecid decreases renal excretion.
cefadroxil (Duricef) Adults: 500 mg q12h PO or 1 g q24h PO Children: 15 mg/kg q12h or 30 mg/kg q24h PO	Same as cephalexin	Same as cephalexin	Same as cephalexin
Second-Generation Cephalosporins			
cefaclor (Ceclor) Adults: 250–500 mg q8h or 375–500 mg q12h PO (extended release) Children: 6.7–13.3 mg/kg q8h Not to exceed 1 g/day	Same as cephalexin	Same as cephalexin	Same as cephalexin
cefuroxime (Ceftin, Zinacef) Adults: 250–500 mg q12h PO Children: 15 mg/kg q12h PO	Same as cephalexin	Same as cephalexin	Same as cephalexin; swallow whole because of bitter taste
cefprozil (Cefzil) Adults: 250–500 mg q12h PO or 500 mg q24h PO Children: 20 mg/kg q24h	Same as cephalexin	Same as cephalexin	Same as cephalexin
Third-Generation Cephalosporins			
cefpodoxime (Vantin) Adults: 400 mg q12h PO	Same as cephalexin	Same as cephalexin	Same as cephalexin
ceftriaxone (Rocephin) Adults: 0.5–1.0 g q12h IM or IV or 1–2 g q24h IM or IV Children: 50–75 mg/kg q24h IM or IV not to exceed 2 g	Same as cephalexin and also pseudolithiasis	Same as cephalexin	No known interactions IM: dilute with lidocaine to reduce pain at injection site.
Macrolides			
erythromycin base (E-Mycin, Erytab) Adults: 250–500 mg q6h PO Children: 5–12.5 mg/kg q6h PO	Nausea, vomiting, diarrhea, rash, allergic reactions, fungal infection, hepatitis, ototoxicity **Serious:** pseudomembranous colitis	Allergy to erythromycin or macrolide Caution in hepatic disease	Better absorbed on an empty stomach 1 h before or 2 h after a meal. Enteric-coated form can be taken with or without food. Interactions include warfarin, theophylline, digoxin. Consult other sources (see Chapter 8).
azithromycin (Zithromax) Adults: 500 mg on day 1, then 250 mg once daily × 4 d PO Children: 10 mg/kg on day 1, then 5 mg/kg once daily × 4 d PO	Nausea, diarrhea, abdominal pain, rash, photosensitivity, allergic reaction, fungal infection, dizziness, fatigue, headache, palpitations **Serious:** pseudomembranous colitis	Allergy to macrolides. Use with caution in hepatic disease, patients with prolonged QT interval. Safety not established in pregnancy, lactation, and children younger than 2 y.	Take on empty stomach. Antacids with aluminum or magnesium decrease serum levels. Interactions: warfarin, pimozide, carbamazepine. Consult other sources (see Chapter 8).
clarithromycin (Biaxin) Adults: 250 mg q12h PO Children: 7.5 mg/kg q12h PO	Nausea, vomiting, diarrhea, dyspepsia, abnormal taste, allergic reactions, fungal infection **Serious:** pseudomembranous colitis	Allergy to macrolides Pregnancy and lactation Use with caution in severe hepatic or renal disease.	Take with or without food. Interactions: warfarin, digoxin, carbamazepine, theophylline. Consult other sources (see Chapter 8).

(continued)

Table 13.3

Overview of Selected Antibiotics for Skin Infections (*Continued*)

Generic (Trade) Name and Dosage	Selected Adverse Events	Contraindications	Special Considerations
Fluoroquinolones			
ciprofloxacin (Cipro) Adults: 500–750 mg q12h PO Children: not approved	Nausea, diarrhea, altered taste, dizziness, drowsiness, headache, insomnia, agitation, confusion **Serious:** pseudomembranous colitis, Stevens-Johnson syndrome	Allergy to fluoroquinolone. Children younger than 18 y, pregnancy. Use with caution in renal disease, CNS disease, elderly, lactation (safety not established).	Food slows absorption Interactions: antacids, zinc, sucralfat, iron, theophylline, warfarin, probenecid, foscarnet, glucocorticoids, didanosine.
Levofloxacin (Levagium) Adults: 500–750 mg qd PO Children: not approved	Same as ciprofloxacin		
Moxifloxacin (Avelox) Adults: 400 mg qd PO	Same as ciprofloxacin		
Miscellaneous			
clindamycin (Cleocin) Adults: 150–450 mg q6h PO Children: 2–5 mg/kg q6h PO or 2.7–6.7 mg/kg q8h	Nausea, vomiting, diarrhea, rash, allergic reaction, fungal infections **Serious:** pseudomembranous colitis	Allergy, previous pseudomembranous colitis, severe hepatic disease. Use with caution in pregnancy and lactation.	Take with or without food with full glass of water. Interactions include kaolin (decreases absorption).

infections. With the growing problem of antibiotic resistance, it is now necessary to choose a broad-spectrum penicillin to overcome organism resistance. Also, many strains of *S. aureus* produce the enzyme penicillinase, which can inactivate penicillin. The provider should choose an agent that is penicillinase-resistant. Useful agents in this class for treating specific skin infections include amoxicillin–clavulanate (Augmentin) or dicloxacillin (Dynapen).

Amoxicillin–clavulanate has bactericidal action against many organisms, including streptococci, pneumococci, *Haemophilus influenzae, E. coli*, and *Proteus mirabilis*. The clavulanate portion of the drug can also resist the action of beta-lactamase, an enzyme that can also inactivate penicillin. Amoxicillin–clavulanate is well absorbed orally and is more resistant to acid inactivation than other penicillins.

Common side effects are nausea, vomiting, diarrhea, rash, and urticaria. Fungal infections may also occur. Patients who are allergic to penicillin should not be given this agent. It should be used with caution in patients with severe renal impairment.

Dicloxacillin has bactericidal activity against penicillinase-producing strains of *S. aureus*. It is active against most gram-positive aerobic cocci but is not as effective as plain penicillin. Dicloxacillin is given by the oral route. The adverse effect profile is similar to that of amoxicillin–clavulanate. In addition, dicloxacillin should be used with caution in patients with severe renal and hepatic impairment (see Table 13-3).

First-Generation Cephalosporins

In this class, commonly used drugs for treating skin infections are cephalexin (Keflex) and cefadroxil (Duricef). They have bactericidal activity against many organisms, including GAS and penicillinase-producing *S. aureus*. They have limited activity against *Klebsiella pneumoniae, P. mirabilis*, and *E. coli*.

Both agents are well absorbed orally. Their adverse effect profiles are similar to that of the broad-spectrum penicillins.

These drugs should not be used in patients with a severe penicillin allergy. Care should be used in the presence of severe renal disease (see Table 13-3).

Second-Generation Cephalosporins

Second-generation cephalosporins that are useful for skin infections include cefaclor (Ceclor), cefuroxime (Ceftin, Zinacef), and cefprozil (Cefzil). They are effective against the same organisms as first-generation cephalosporins but are much more effective against certain gram-negative organisms, including *H. influenzae, E. coli, K. pneumoniae*, and *Proteus* organisms. These agents are all well absorbed orally. Their adverse effect profile is similar to that of the first-generation cephalosporins. They should not be given to patients who have a severe allergy to penicillin or an allergy to other cephalosporins. Care should be used in patients with severe renal disease (see Table 13-3).

Third-Generation Cephalosporins

Useful third-generation cephalosporins for treating skin infections include cefpodoxime (Vantin), ceftriaxone (Rocephin), and ceftazidime (Fortaz). These drugs are usually reserved for more serious infections and are not typically chosen as first-line agents. In addition, ceftriaxone and ceftazidime are not available as oral agents. Ceftriaxone is administered either intramuscularly or intravenously, with ceftazidime administered intravenously only. Cefpodoxime is available only as an oral agent.

These agents' spectrum of antibacterial activity is similar to that of the second-generation cephalosporins. However, they are less effective against *S. aureus* and more effective against certain gram-negative organisms, including *Enterobacter, H. influenzae, E. coli, K. pneumoniae*, and *Proteus*. Ceftazidime would be recommended for infections caused by *Pseudomonas*. Ceftriaxone is absorbed intramuscularly, but this route of administration may be painful. Cefpodoxime is well absorbed orally.

The adverse effect profile for these agents is similar to that of the other cephalosporins. Care should be taken in prescribing them in the presence of severe renal and hepatic impairment. Rarely, ceftriaxone causes pseudolithiasis (see Table 13-3).

Macrolides

Among the macrolide antibiotics used for treating skin infections are erythromycin (E-Mycin, Ery-Tab), azithromycin (Zithromax), and clarithromycin (Biaxin). These drugs are often used in patients allergic to penicillin. Topical erythromycin may be useful for treatment of some skin infections.

These agents have bactericidal activity against streptococcal and staphylococcal organisms. Erythromycin is also active against several gram-negative organisms, although not the ones usually responsible for skin infections. Azithromycin and clarithromycin also are effective against gram-negative organisms, including *H. influenzae*, which does play a role in certain skin infections. These agents are well absorbed orally.

The adverse effect profile of erythromycin is similar to that of the penicillins and the cephalosporins. Gastrointestinal adverse reactions are common with oral erythromycin. Azithromycin and clarithromycin may cause abdominal pain and other gastrointestinal side effects, but the incidence is less than with erythromycin. Clarithromycin may also cause an abnormal metallic taste in the mouth and taste disturbances. Both drugs are contraindicated in patients allergic to any other macrolide. Caution should be used in patients with liver disease, and clarithromycin should not be used during pregnancy or lactation or in patients with severe renal impairment (see Table 13-3).

Fluoroquinolones

Levofloxacin (Levaquin), moxifloxacin (Avelox), and ciprofloxacin (Cipro) are the fluoroquinolone antibiotics used in the treatment of skin and skin structure infections. They are useful for serious infections, for infections in which the causative organisms are unknown, in patients with penicillin allergies, or for infections from gram-negative organisms. They have a broad spectrum of activity against many organisms, including *S. aureus, Staphylococcus epidermidis, E. coli, Klebsiella, Enterobacter, P. aeruginosa*, and many other organisms. Levofloxacin and moxifloxacin may offer slightly better coverage against gram-positive organisms than ciprofloxacin. They are all well absorbed orally.

Common adverse effects are diarrhea, nausea, abdominal pain, dizziness, drowsiness, headache, and insomnia. Uncommon but severe events include Stevens-Johnson syndrome, seizures, Achilles tendon rupture, and pseudomembranous colitis. These drugs are associated with a variety of drug interactions (see Table 13-3).

Fluoroquinolone antibiotics are contraindicated in children younger than 18 years of age and during pregnancy and lactation. They are also contraindicated in patients allergic to other fluoroquinolones. These medications should be used cautiously in elderly patients and patients with central nervous system diseases, seizure disorders, or renal impairment.

Topical Agents

Topical agents may be used as first-line treatment or adjunctively in bacterial skin infections. Mupirocin ointment is effective against *S. aureus* and some streptococcal infections. It is also used over the long term to eliminate nasal, axillary, or groin carriage of *S. aureus*, which is thought to contribute to recurrent infections in some patients.

Mupirocin ointment is minimally absorbed systemically. It is metabolized by the skin and usually well tolerated. Adverse effects are few but include headache, cough, rhinitis, pharyngitis, upper respiratory tract congestion, and taste perversion with nasal use. Burning, stinging, rash, erythema, or itching can occur when applied topically. Mupirocin should not be used in patients with an allergy to the drug and should not be used with other nasal products. It should be used with caution in patients with impaired renal function due to possible absorption of polyethylene glycol through an open wound (Drug Facts and Comparisons, 2004).

The topical preparation of gentamicin is available in a cream or an ointment. It is a powerful topical agent and is effective against many organisms, including GAS, *S. aureus*, and *Pseudomonas* species. Topical gentamicin can be used for a variety of primary and secondary skin infections. It is safe for children older than 12 months. It is usually well tolerated, although irritation may occur. Occasionally, fungal infection or overgrowth of nonsusceptible bacteria may occur at the site of use.

Selecting the Most Appropriate Agent

Most bacterial skin conditions are treated empirically based on the prescriber's knowledge of the organisms most likely to cause a particular infection (Table 13-4). When the organism is not known, the potential for serious infection is present, or the patient is already extremely ill, the prescriber needs to confirm the diagnosis and organism either by skin biopsy or wound culture. In such cases, empiric treatment begins with a broad-spectrum agent until organism susceptibility is available and a diagnosis is made.

Other important factors in choosing an antibiotic agent include patient allergies, pregnancy status, renal and hepatic function, and age. Practical concerns that affect compliance include the taste of the medication (especially in treating children), its adverse effect profile, how frequently it must be taken, and how much it costs. An antibiotic agent may be changed if the condition does not improve or if intolerable effects impede compliance or pose a danger to the patient. Figures 13-1 and 13-2 give an overview of the drug selection process.

First-Line Therapy: Impetigo and Ecthyma

For minor cases of impetigo, topical mupirocin ointment applied three times daily for 7 to 10 days may be sufficient treatment (Fitzpatrick et al., 1997). Some practitioners advocate debriding the crusts to promote topical absorption, but debridement is painful and often unnecessary. Mupirocin is less effective in the bullous form of impetigo (Gorbach, 2004).

In most cases, an oral antibiotic is prescribed for 7 to 10 days. A broad-spectrum penicillin (eg, amoxicillin–clavulanate or dicloxacillin) is a good first choice.

Table 13.4

Recommended Order of Treatment for Bacterial Skin Infections

Infection	First-Line Therapy	Second-Line Therapy	Third-Line Therapy
Impetigo, bullous impetigo, and ecthyma	Oral antibiotic for 7–10 d	Alternate oral antibiotic for 7–10 d or refer	
Cellulitis	Oral antibiotic for 7–10 d	Admit for intravenous antibiotic treatment or refer	
Erysipelas	Oral antibiotic for 7–10 d	Admit for intravenous antibiotic treatment or refer	
Furuncles and carbuncles	Oral antibiotic for 7–10 d or refer	Alternate oral antibiotic for 7–10 d or refer	
Paronychias	Tetanus prophylaxis, as appropriate, and oral antibiotic for 7–10 d	Alternate oral antibiotic for 7–10 d or refer	
Felon and puncture wound	Tetanus prophylaxis, as appropriate, and oral antibiotic for 7–10 d	Continue oral antibiotic if infection continues	Alternate oral antibiotic for 7–10 d or refer

Cephalosporins (eg, cephalexin) are also effective. In cases of penicillin allergy, erythromycin is an alternative, but in many communities, *S. aureus* and GAS have become resistant to this agent. In this case, another macrolide such as azithromycin or clarithromycin may be acceptable. In patients suspected of being chronic carriers of *S. aureus*, the

nostrils may be treated with topical mupirocin ointment to eradicate the organisms and prevent recurrence (Fitzpatrick et al., 1997).

Oral agents, such as dicloxacillin or cephalexin, are usually required for the treatment of ecthyma. Because of the chronicity of this condition, antibiotics are often given for a 2- to

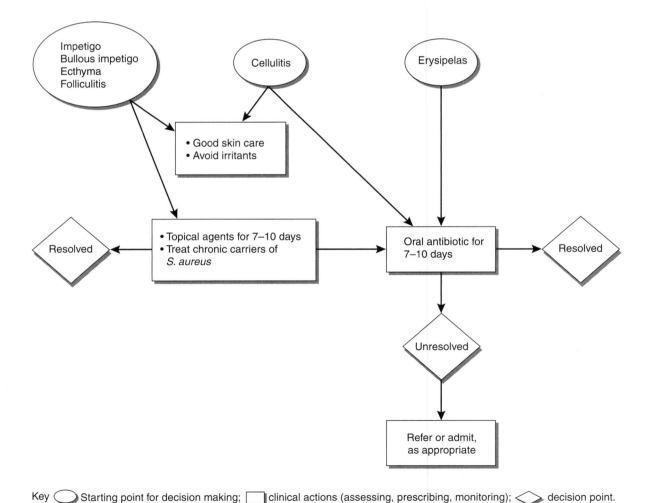

Key ⬭ Starting point for decision making; ▭ clinical actions (assessing, prescribing, monitoring); ◇ decision point.

Figure 13–1   Treatment algorithm for impetigo, cellulitis, erysipelas, and other bacterial skin infections. *Note:* if patient has necrotizing fasciitis, admit to hospital and refer to specialist.

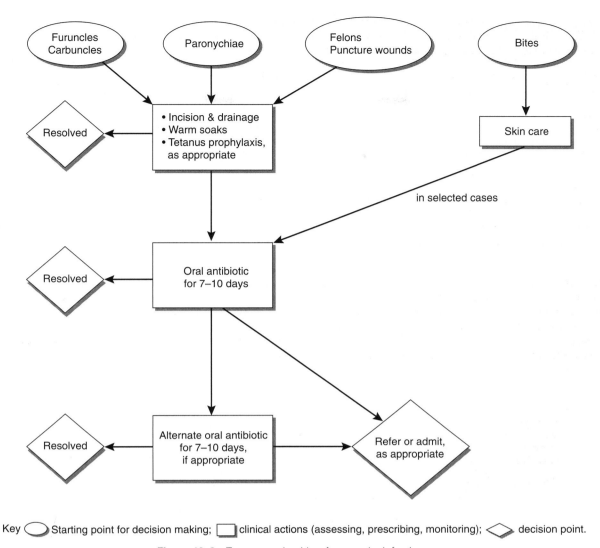

Figure 13–2 Treatment algorithm for pustular infections.

Key ⬭ Starting point for decision making; ▭ clinical actions (assessing, prescribing, monitoring); ◇ decision point.

3-week period; intravenous antibiotics may be required (Swartz, 2000). The same agents used to treat impetigo are effective for ecthyma unless the practitioner suspects a pseudomonal infection. In these cases, a medication that provides gram-negative coverage, such as ciprofloxacin, may be prescribed. Because of the depth of ulceration and chronic nature of ecthyma, healing may take weeks to months, and scarring is probable (Fitzpatrick et al., 1997). Debridement is not recommended due to the increased chance of bacteremia.

Second-Line Therapy: Impetigo and Ecthyma

Although bullous impetigo is treated initially with the same agents used for impetigo (see Table 13-4), severe cases, or cases of scalded skin syndrome, may need to be treated intravenously with a drug such as nafcillin (Swartz, 2000).

First-Line Therapy: Cellulitis and Erysipelas

Treatment for mild cellulitis should begin promptly and usually on an outpatient basis with oral antibiotic therapy. Those who are more seriously ill require parenteral therapy and pos-

sibly hospitalization. Systemic treatment is always required for cellulitis.

After culturing any drainage, the prescriber may select empiric treatment with a broad-spectrum penicillin such as amoxicillin–clavulanate or dicloxacillin. Alternative agents include cephalexin or a macrolide such as erythromycin or clarithromycin. In patients with predisposing conditions that encourage opportunistic organisms, drug selection is based on coverage for these conditions, and the course of therapy is at least 10 to 14 days, continuing until the infection resolves.

Erysipelas is treated aggressively because it has the potential to spread so rapidly. A good first choice is an oral agent such as oral penicillin V or amoxicillin–clavulanate or a cephalosporin such as cephalexin. In patients who are seriously ill, hospitalization and intravenous antibiotic therapy are required. Even in serious cases, improvement usually occurs rapidly within the first 48 hours.

Second-Line Therapy: Cellulitis and Erysipelas

If the infection does not respond to the initial course of treatment, patients should be promptly referred or admitted for intravenous therapy. Wounds that become secondarily infected may require debridement, with frequent cleansing and dressing changes. Surgical debridement may be necessary.

First-Line Therapy: Pustular Infections

Systemic therapy may not be needed for folliculitis; warm compresses can be used to facilitate drainage. Topical treatments may be helpful and include mupirocin, gentamicin, or bacitracin. However, if folliculitis is deep, with extensive involvement, systemic therapy may be started empirically with an oral antistaphylococcal agent. *Pseudomonas* folliculitis may be treated with an antipseudomonal quinolone if it is persistent or severe (Rose, 2004).

Moist heat applications are usually adequate for the treatment of mild furunculosis. However, if drainage is performed, if the furuncle is located above midface, or if the furuncle is surrounded by an area of cellulitis, oral antistaphylococcal antibiotics (dicloxacillin, clindamycin, erythromycin) may be indicated. Treatment is continued for up to 2 weeks until the area of acute inflammation has improved. Intravenous antibiotics may be indicated in patients who are systemically ill.

For patients with a paronychia, systemic antibiotics are necessary if the infection does not resolve on its own or after surgical drainage. Topical preparations do not penetrate the nail bed well and generally are not indicated for treatment (Hacker & Roaten, 1999). Effective agents include amoxicillin–clavulanate, cephalexin, dicloxacillin, or erythromycin. This condition is often recurrent.

After surgical drainage, a felon is treated with antibiotic therapy based on culture and Gram stain results. Tetanus prophylaxis is given as needed.

Second-Line Therapy: Pustular Infections

Folliculitis and furuncles may recur in patients who are chronic carriers of *S. aureus*. Treatment applied to the nostrils, perineum, or axillae with topical mupirocin may be needed to eradicate the organism and prevent recurrence. Very severe cases of furunculosis or carbunculosis may require parenteral therapy.

First-Line Therapy: Necrotizing Fasciitis

Aggressive surgical intervention is usually needed for the treatment of necrotizing fasciitis. Empiric antibiotic therapy usually includes combination therapy with ampicillin, gentamicin, and metronidazole; ampicillin, gentamicin, and clindamycin; ampicillin–sulbactam and gentamicin; or imipenem and metronidazole. Vancomycin can be used in place of ampicillin in penicillin-allergic patients or in patients suspected of having resistant organisms. Once culture and biopsy results are available, therapy can be tailored appropriately.

SPECIAL CONSIDERATIONS

When choosing topical or systemic therapy in a pregnant patient, a drug in category B should be chosen over a drug in category C whenever possible. Below is a list of commonly used medications for skin and skin structure infections and their associated categories:

Augmentin: category B
Dicloxacillin: category B
Cephalexin and other cephalosporins: category B
Erythromycin and azithromycin: category B
Clarithromycin: category C
Fluoroquinolones: category C
Clindamycin: category B
Mupirocin: category C
Gentamicin topical: category C

MONITORING PATIENT RESPONSE

The therapy for bacterial skin conditions is monitored by follow-up visits (see Figs. 13-1 and 13-2). Most cases of impetigo heal rapidly without scarring or other adverse effects. These patients may not need to be seen again unless the condition does not resolve. However, untreated lesions may last for weeks and develop into ecthyma, which is the more chronic and severe form of impetigo. These patients do require follow-up. Folliculitis, although not serious, is often recurrent or chronic. Emphasis should be placed on controlling aggravating factors and promoting good hygiene measures. Follow-up or referral is required if the condition spreads or does not resolve.

Secondary infection such as osteomyelitis or endocarditis is a risk in carbunculosis. For this reason, systemic antibiotics are always given after lesions are drained. These patients also may require parenteral therapy. In recurrent cases of carbunculosis, the patient should be tested for HIV. Close follow-up is important.

Patients with cellulitis and erysipelas should be followed closely because of the potential for a serious systemic infection. It is sometimes necessary to change antibiotic agents or increase the duration of treatment if the patient fails to improve. Follow-up or referral may be necessary for paronychia, which often recurs.

PATIENT EDUCATION
Drug Information

Patients treated with systemic antibiotic therapy must be taught to take their medication around the clock to sustain the proper blood level. They also must understand the importance of taking the medication for the prescribed length of time and not to discontinue their medication even if they feel their infection is resolved.

There are common side effects with most antibiotics, such as nausea, vomiting, diarrhea, and rash. Some medications must be taken with or without food. These instructions should be emphasized to the patient. Some medications may cause dizziness, drowsiness, or photosensitivity, and patients should be advised accordingly.

Antibiotics can predispose a patient to fungal infections such as vaginal candidiasis or oral thrush. Patients should be told to report these symptoms so that appropriate treatment can be implemented. Some antibiotics may cause a decreased effectiveness of oral contraceptives, so patients should be told to use an alternate form of contraception while on their medication until their next menstrual cycle. They should also be told if their medication is not safe to use during pregnancy or lactation if applicable. Alternate medication should be prescribed in those cases or if there is any uncertainty about their pregnancy status.

Patients should be told to report signs of allergic reaction, fever, or severe diarrhea, especially if it contains blood, mucus, or pus. Unusual bleeding or bruising should also be reported. These adverse effects may be signs of a serious medication reaction.

Most topical medications are relatively well tolerated. However, some are in an alcohol base and are flammable if exposed to flames. Patients should avoid smoking while and shortly after applying their medication. Other topical agents, such as clindamycin, may be absorbed systemically even when used in the topical form, putting the patient at risk for adverse effects.

Nutrition/Lifestyle Changes

Patients need to learn proper methods of hygiene (see Box 13-3) to prevent the spread of infection, secondary infection, or recurrence. Patients with paronychia must be instructed to keep their hands dry as much as possible. An antifungal cream may be useful when indicated to prevent superinfection.

In cases where there are open wounds, wound care instruction is essential. Some infections, such as impetigo, present a risk to others. Patients with impetigo should avoid contact with infants, small children, the elderly, or those who are debilitated due to the highly contagious nature of the illness.

Although most bacterial skin infections are self-limiting and resolve quickly with treatment, some have the potential to become much more serious. Patients should be taught to report symptoms such as fever, increased erythema or streaking, chills, or malaise that may indicate a worsening of their condition. Also, the chronic nature of some skin infections, such as folliculitis, should be emphasized so that patients understand that treatment may be long term and recurrent.

Complementary and Alternative Medicine

Topical magnesium and iodine topical solutions are likely to be effective for the treatment of skin infections. Magnesium can speed the healing of wounds in patients with skin ulcers, boils, and carbuncles. However, if treatment is prolonged, damage can occur to the skin around the area of treatment (Natural Medicines Comprehensive Database, 2004). Iodine is an effective antiseptic agent; a 2% solution is recommended. Skin irritation, stains, and sensitization have been associated with its use.

Topical trypsin is possibly effective for wound cleansing and wound healing. Trypsin is contained in some FDA-approved products for wound debridement such as Granulex and Dermuspray (Natural Medicines Comprehensive Database, 2004). Pain and burning may occur with its use.

Other complementary therapies have been tried for wound healing, but there are insufficient data about their effectiveness. Some of these therapies include aloe, gota kula, hyaluronic acid, goldenseal, bee propolis, and cartilage.

■ Case Study

M.R. is a 66-year-old woman with diabetes mellitus. She is obese and has difficulty seeing and caring for herself. She presents with an oozing erythematous area on her left lower leg that began 2 weeks ago as an insect bite. The area was itchy but not painful. She has had an intermittent, low-grade fever for the past week but otherwise feels well. She states that the redness has gotten worse and the lesion began oozing purulent fluid approximately 1 week ago. She also notes mild swelling in her lower leg near the lesion. Her only medication is insulin, and she has no allergies.

Diagnosis: Cellulitis

1. List two specific goals of treatment for M.R.

2. What drug therapy would you prescribe, and for how long? Why?

3. What would you monitor to determine the success or failure of this regimen? When would you monitor them?

4. What would you tell M.R. about the drugs you prescribed?

5. What over-the-counter or alternative medications would be appropriate for this patient?

6. What dietary and lifestyle changes should be recommended for this patient?

7. Describe one or two drug/drug or drug/food interactions for the selected agent.

8. List one or two adverse reactions for the selected agent that would cause you to change therapy.

9. If one of these adverse reactions occurred, what would your second-line therapy be?

Bibliography

Starred references are cited in the text.

Abyad, A. (2004). Cellulitis. In M. R. Dambro (Ed.). *Griffith 5-minute clinical consult* (12th ed.). New York: Lippincott Williams & Wilkins. Web site: http://online.statref.com. Retrieved Aug. 1, 2004.

*Barg, N., Gantz, N., Jarvis, W., & Talarico, L. D. (1998). Common and potentially fatal *Staph* infections. *Patient Care, 32*(6), 26–49.

Billica, W. H. (2004). Impetigo. In M. R. Dambro (Ed.). *Griffith 5-minute clinical consult* (12th ed.). New York: Lippincott Williams & Wilkins. Web site: http://online.statref.com. Retrieved Aug. 1, 2004.

Drug Facts and Comparisons. (2004). St. Louis, MO: Facts and Comparisons.

*Fitzpatrick, T. B., Johnson, R. A., Wolff, K., Polano, M. K., & Suurmond, D. (1997). Cutaneous bacterial infections. In: *Color atlas and synopsis of clinical dermatology: Common and serious diseases* (3rd ed., pp. 604–621). New York: McGraw-Hill.

*Gorbach, S. L. (2004). Skin and soft tissue infections. In S. L. Gorbach, J. Q. Bartlett, & N. R. Blacklow (Eds.). *Infectious disease* (3rd ed.). New York: Lippincott Williams & Wilkins.

Hacker, S. M., & Roaten, S. P. (1999). Strategies for managing bacterial skin infections. *Patient Care, 33*(2), 53–71.

Kincaid, S. A. (2004). Erysipelas. In M. R. Dambro (Ed.). *Griffith 5-minute clinical consult* (12th ed). New York: Lippincott Williams & Wilkins. Web site: http://online.statref.com. Retrieved August 1, 2004.

Kravetz, J. D., & Federman, D. G. (2004). Treatment of mammalian bites. In J. D. Kravetz, editorial consultant. ACP's PIER: The Physicians' Information and Education Resource. Philadelphia: American College of Physicians. Web site: http://online.statref.com. Retrieved August 1, 2004.

Mancini, A. J. (2002). Skin infections and exanthems. In A. M. Rudolph & C. D. Rudolph (Eds.). *Rudolph's pediatrics* (21st ed.). New York: McGraw-Hill Medical Publishing Division. Web site: http://online.statref.com. Retrieved August 1, 2004.

Micromedex Healthcare Series: Thomson Micromedex, Greenwood Village, Colorado Edition expires September 2004.

Millikan, L. (2004). Paronychia. In M. R. Dambro (Ed.). *Griffith 5-minute clinical consult* (12th ed.). New York: Lippincott Williams & Wilkins. Web site: http://online.statref.com. Retrieved August 1, 2004.

*Natural Medicines Comprehensive Database on line. Retrieved August 6, 2004, through Doylestown Hospital's web site. (http://www.naturaldatabase.com).

*Odell, M. L. (2003). Skin infections and infestations. In A. K. David, T. A. Johnson, M. Phillips, & J. E. Scherger (Eds.). *Family medicine: Principles and practice* (6th ed.). New York: Springer-Verlag. Web site: http://online.statref.com. Retrieved August 1, 2004.

Pierce, N. F. (1995). Bacterial infections of the skin. In L. R. Barker, J. R. Burton, & P. D. Zieve (Eds.), *Principles of ambulatory medicine* (4th ed., pp. 300–306). Baltimore: Williams & Wilkins.

*Rose, L. C. (2004). Folliculitis. In M. R. Dambro (Ed.). *Griffith 5-minute clinical consult* (12th ed.). New York: Lippincott Williams & Wilkins. Web site: http://online.statref.com. Retrieved August 1, 2004.

*Sadick, N. S. (1997). Current aspects of bacterial infections of the skin. *Dermatology Clinics, 15*, 341–349.

Stevens, D. L. (2004). In: D. L. Stevens, editorial consultant. ACP's PIER: The Physicians' Information and Education Resource. Cellulitis and Soft Tissue Infections. Philadelphia: American College of Physicians. Web site: http://online.statref.com. Retrieved August 1, 2004.

*Swartz, M. (2000). Cellulitis and subcutaneous tissue infections. In G. L. Mandell, J. E. Bennett, & R. Dolin (Eds.). *Mandell, Douglas, and Bennett's principles and practices in infectious disease* (5th ed.). New York: Churchill Livingstone.

The Natural Pharmacist, Consumer Edition on-line. Retrieved August 9, 2004, through Gadsden Regional Medical Center's web site: http://www.gadsdenregional.com.

*Trent, J. T., Federman, D., & Kirsner, R. S. (2001). Common bacterial skin infections. *Ostomy Wound Management, 47*(8), 30–34.

*Wilhelm, M. P., & Edson, R. S. (2001). Clinical syndromes 13: Skin and soft tissue infections. In W. R. Wilson & M. A. Sande (Eds.). *Current diagnosis and treatment of infectious diseases, section II.* New York: Lange Medical Books/McGraw-Hill Medical Publishing Division, 2001. Web site: http://online.statref.com. Retrieved August 1, 2004.

Visit the Connection web site for the most up-to-date drug information.

14

PSORIASIS

■ VIRGINIA P. ARCANGELO AND DENISE VANACORE-NETZ

Psoriasis is a debilitating disease characterized by recurrent exacerbations and remissions. It affects between 2% and 3% of the U.S. population, with a higher incidence in whites and an equal distribution between the sexes. Approximately 36% of patients with psoriasis have a positive family history. The cost of outpatient treatment for psoriasis averages $1.6 to $3.2 billion annually.

There appear to be two peak ages of onset: between 16 and 22 years, and between 57 and 60 years. Psoriasis has an element of physical discomfort, with pain, itching, stinging, cracking, and bleeding of the lesions. In approximately 10% of patients with psoriasis, the disease develops into psoriatic arthritis.

Psoriasis affects almost all aspects of life, including sexual relationships and emotional well-being. In addition, patients with psoriasis spend 1 or more hours a day caring for their skin (Fleischer, Feldman, Rapp, et al., 1996). Of a survey group of patients with psoriasis, up to 25% felt at some point in their life that they would rather be dead than alive with psoriasis (Rapp, Exum, Reboussin, et al., 1997).

CAUSES

A definitive cause for psoriasis is unknown, although there are several possible etiologic factors: abnormal epidermal cell cycle, hereditary factors, and trigger factors, including trauma, infection, endocrine imbalance, climate, and emotional stress.

Physical trauma, such as rubbing, scratching, or sunburn, is a major exacerbating factor in psoriasis, and this is referred to as *Koebner's phenomenon*. A precipitating event in some cases of guttate psoriasis is a streptococcal infection. Stress plays a role in as many as 40% of psoriasis flares in adults and children. Exacerbations of psoriasis may develop from the use of certain drugs (Box 14-1).

PATHOPHYSIOLOGY

In psoriasis, there is an alteration of the cell kinetics of keratinocytes. The normal epidermal cell turnover is 14 days. In psoriasis, this cell turnover drops to 2 days, resulting in 28 times the normal production of epidermal cells. Immunologic phenomena are a major factor in the pathogenesis of psoriasis. Normal T cells help protect the body against infection and disease. In psoriasis, T cells are put into action by mistake and become so active that they trigger other immune responses. There is inflammation and a rapid turnover of skin cells. In some cases, use of immunosuppressive drugs causes remission.

Additionally, tumor necrosis factor (TNF) causes inflammation, leading to the formation of painful, disfiguring psoriasis plaques. TNF is found in high levels in psoriatic plaques and plays a critical role in their formation and inflammation.

DIAGNOSTIC CRITERIA

Psoriasis is diagnosed by observation of characteristic, well-demarcated, erythematous papules or plaques surrounded by silvery or whitish scales. The lesions are symmetric and usually found on the face, extensor joints, anogenital area, palms and soles, intertriginous areas, trunk, scalp, ears, and nails.

The varieties of psoriatic disease include plaque, guttate, erythrodermic, and pustular. The plaque type is the most common form. The guttate type is characterized by small, scattered, teardrop-shaped papules and plaques. In many cases, psoriasis begins as the guttate form. The erythrodermic form is characterized by generalized intense erythema and shedding of scales. Finally, the pustular type has three additional forms: generalized, localized, and hand and foot. All share a similar characteristic: 2- to 3-mm pustules on specific body regions.

Clinical presentation of the plaque type of psoriasis consists of sharply demarcated, erythematous papules and plaques with marked silvery-white scales. Bleeding may follow removal of the scales (Auspitz sign). The elbows, knees, and scalp are the most common areas for psoriatic plaques. Pitting and discoloration of the nails also characterizes psoriasis. In some cases, the nail may separate from the nailbed.

INITIATING DRUG THERAPY

Before beginning drug therapy, the patient is usually counseled to avoid precipitating factors. Then, to select the most appropriate treatment, the prescriber must determine whether the patient has localized or generalized psoriasis. Patients with 10% or less of body involvement can usually

BOX 14–1. DRUGS KNOWN TO EXACERBATE PSORIASIS

Systemic corticosteroids (when dose is decreased or stopped)
Lithium carbonate
Antimalarials
Beta blockers
Systemic interferon
Alcohol

be successfully treated in a primary care setting with topical agents, whereas those with greater body surface area (BSA) involvement usually require treatment by a dermatologist with phototherapy or systemic therapy. In estimating BSA involvement, the prescriber keeps in mind that the palm represents 1% BSA; this can be used as a tool to estimate total BSA involvement.

Goals of Drug Therapy

The goals of therapy are to:

- Decrease the size and thickness of the plaques
- Decrease pruritus
- Improve emotional well-being and quality of life
- Remission
- Minimal side effects from treatment

It is imperative to use a management strategy that has the least possible toxicity and that is acceptable to the patient. Sequential therapy is thought to be effective because psoriasis is a chronic disease requiring long-term maintenance therapy and treatment of exacerbations. The three phases of sequential therapy are the clearing, transitional, and maintenance phases. Table 14-1 identifies topical and systemic preparations used in psoriasis treatment.

Emollients

Emollients are useful for all cases of psoriasis as an adjunct therapy. These agents hydrate the stratum corneum, decrease water evaporation, and soften the scales of the plaques. They are available in lotions, creams, and ointments. The thicker the preparation, the more effective it is. Commercially available agents include Eucerin cream/lotion, Lubriderm, and Moisturel. In addition to preserving moisture, emollients have a mild antipruritic effect.

Topical Corticosteroids

The foundation of topical treatment is topical corticosteroids. They play an important role in treating psoriasis by decreasing erythema, pruritus, and scaling. They promote vasoconstriction. They are fast-acting but not intended for long-term use. Topical corticosteroids are classified into several categories based on potency and vasoconstrictive properties.

Low-potency corticosteroids are safer for long-term use and for use at thin-skinned sites such as the face and groin. For moderate psoriatic disease, a potent or superpotent agent is used with occlusive dressings. A less potent agent is used once improvement occurs.

Topical corticosteroids may be used for longer periods on thicker skin because thicker skin does not absorb medication as well as thinner skin. Topical corticosteroids have a rapid onset of action. They decrease erythema, inflammation, and pruritus. For more information on topical corticosteroids, see Chapter 10. See also the color plates of skin disorders.

Topical Immunosuppressives

Topical immunosuppressives act on T cells by suppressing cytokine transcription. These agents are used for patients with moderate to severe atopic dermatitis who cannot tolerate topical steroids or are not responsive to other treatments, or where there is a concern for topical steroid-induced atrophy. Tacrolimus and pimecrolimus are the preparations currently available. They are applied twice a day until the lesions clear and then for an additional 7 days. The skin is dried before application. These agents are discussed in detail in Chapter 10.

A study using tacrolimus ointment for treatment of psoriasis on the face and intertriginous area showed that 81% of the patients experienced complete clearance of the lesions; it was a very small study, however (N = 21) (Freeman et al., 2003).

Coal Tars

Coal tar (Zetar) contains polycyclic hydrocarbon compounds formed from bituminous coal. It depresses DNA synthesis and has anti-inflammatory and antipruritic properties. Several preparations are available, including an ointment, a gel preparation, a bath preparation, and shampoo. Coal tar can be used as an initial therapy, usually with adjunct topical corticosteroids.

Coal tar is applied overnight and at home because of the offensive odor. The emulsion is dissolved in bath water (15 to 25 mL) and the patient immerses the affected area in the water for 10 to 20 minutes. It is used for 30 to 45 days, three to seven times a week. The shampoo preparation is massaged into a wet scalp and rinsed. It is applied a second time and left on the scalp for 5 minutes.

Efficacy of the ointment or gel is based on the amount of time that the medication is on the body. There is a slow response to coal tar therapy, and it is not used for acute exacerbations or on open or infected lesions.

Some disadvantages of coal tar include the unpleasant odor, staining of clothes and skin (even with the clear preparation), and photosensitivity. These disadvantages tend to lead to poor compliance. In addition, folliculitis commonly occurs, especially in areas with dense hair follicles. This requires discontinuing the medication.

Anthralin

Anthralin (Drithocreme, Micanol) is another topical treatment for psoriasis. It is a coal tar derivative.

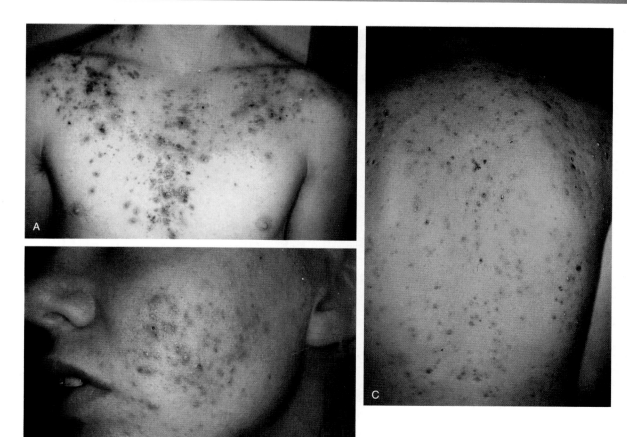

Color Plate 1. A. Acne vulgaris: Chest, B. Acne vulgaris: Face, C. Acne vulgaris: Back

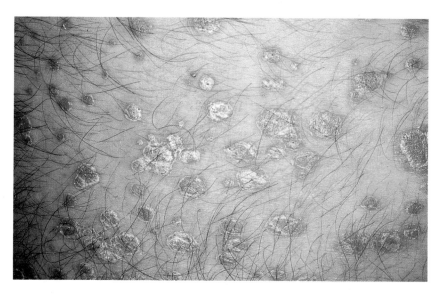

Color Plate 2. Psoriasis

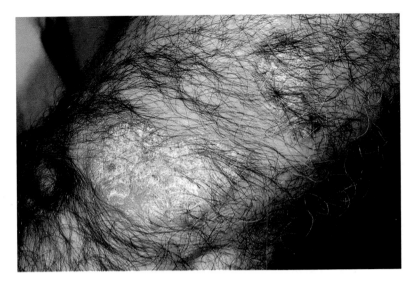

Color Plate 3. Plaque psoriasis

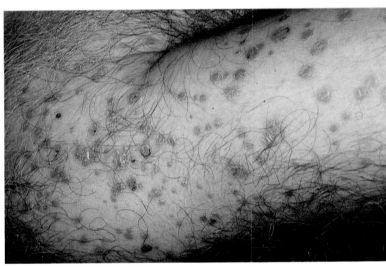

Color Plate 4. Guttate psoriasis

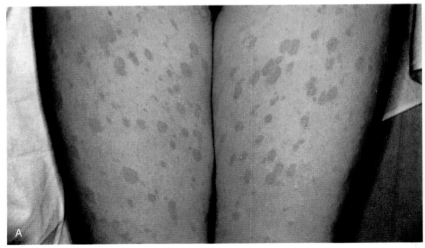

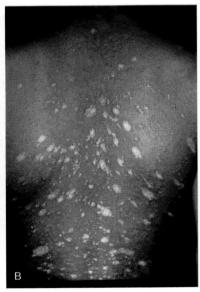

Color Plate 5. A. Pityriasis rosea: Thighs, B. Pityriasis rosea on the back of an African American male

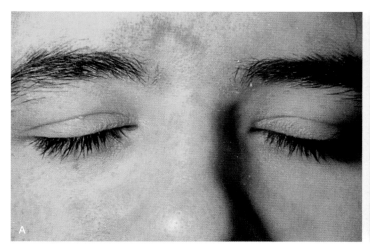
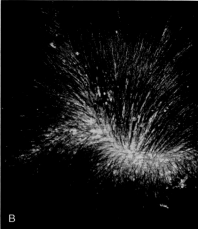

Color Plate 6. A. Seborrheic dermatitis: Eyes and nose, B. Seborrheic dermatitis

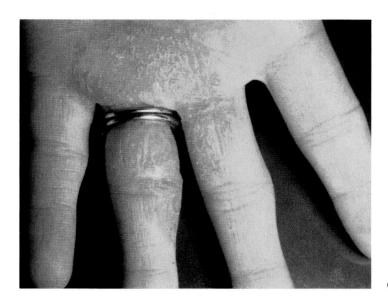

Color Plate 7. Contact dermatitis from soap under rings

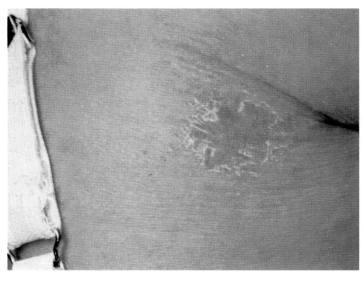

Color Plate 8. Contact dermatitis

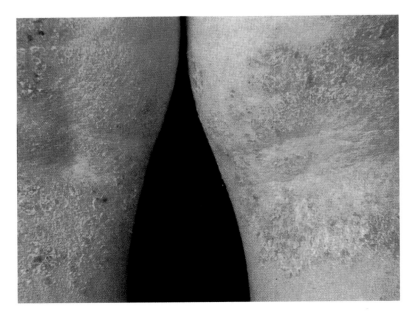

Color Plate 9. Atopic dermatitis

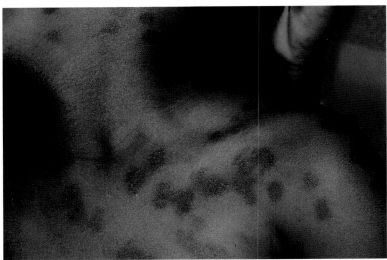

Color Plate 10. Tinea corporis

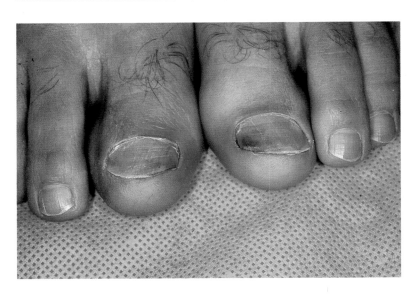

Color Plate 11. Tine ungium

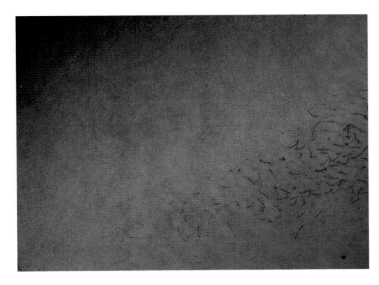

Color Plate 12. Tinea versicolor

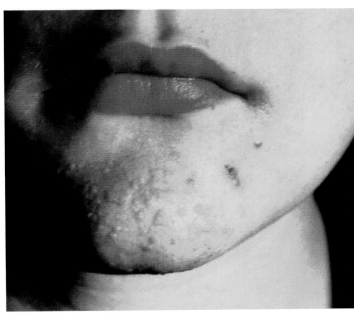

Color Plate 13. Herpes simplex

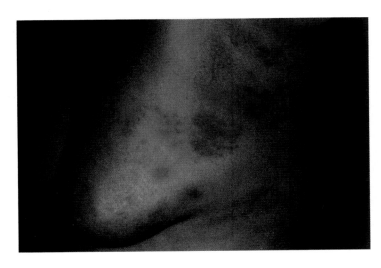

Color Plate 14. Herpes zoster

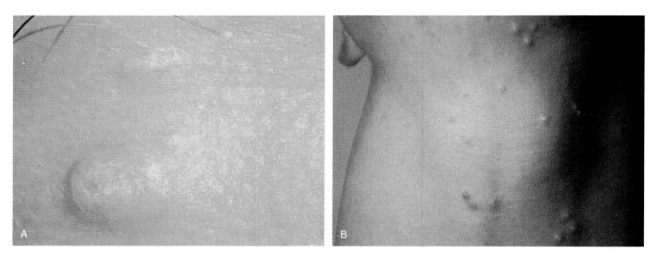

Color Plate 15. A. Molluscum contagiosum up close, B. Molluscum contagiosum: Neck

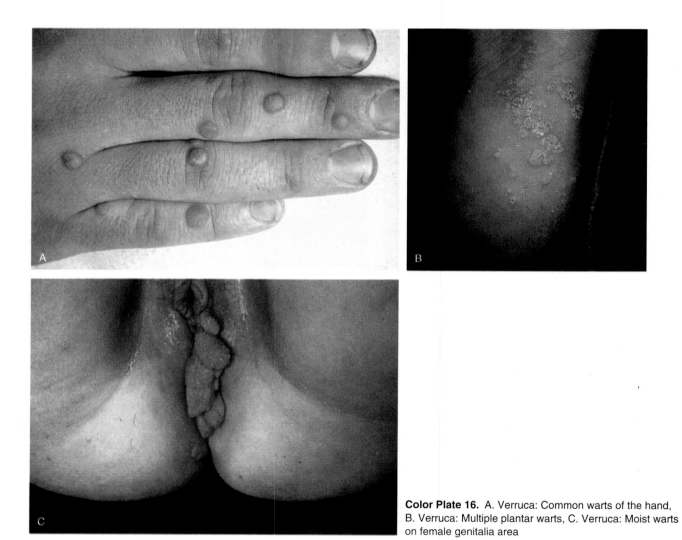

Color Plate 16. A. Verruca: Common warts of the hand, B. Verruca: Multiple plantar warts, C. Verruca: Moist warts on female genitalia area

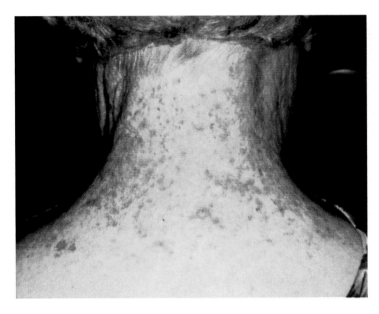

Color Plate 17. Actinic keratoses

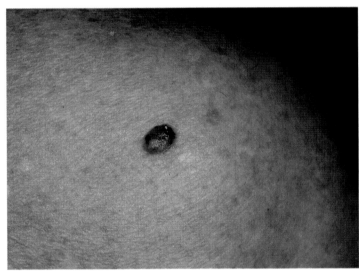

Color Plate 18. Basal cell carcinoma

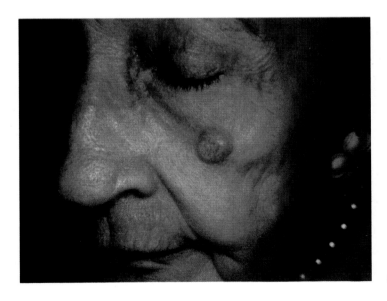

Color Plate 19. Squamous cell carcinoma on cheek

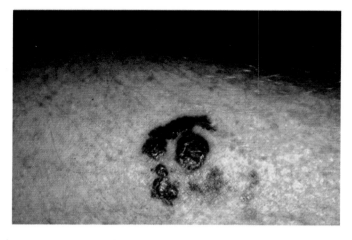

Color Plate 20. Malignant melanoma

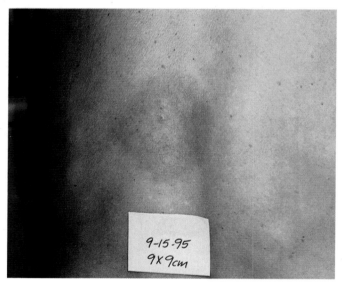

9-15-95
9 X 9 cm

Color Plate 21. Classic erythema migrans rash

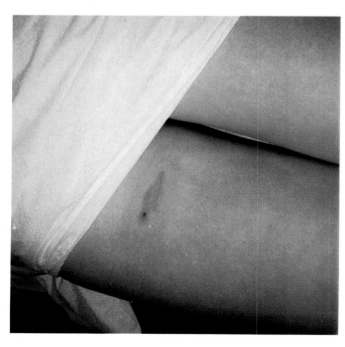

Color Plate 22. Brown recluse spider bite

Table 14.1

Overview of Selected Agents for Psoriasis

Generic (Trade) Name and Dosage	Selected Adverse Events	Contraindications	Special Considerations
Topical Agents			
emollients (Eucerin, Lubriderm, Moisturel) Apply to affected skin three or four times daily.	Folliculitis, maceration, miliaria		Avoid applying near eyes.
TAR PREPARATIONS coal tar (Zetar) Apply at bedtime and allow to remain on skin. Emulsion: 15–25 mL dissolved in bath water Shampoo	Irritation, photoreactions, unpleasant odor, folliculitis	Open or infected lesions	Preparation may stain skin and clothing. With emulsion, immerse affected area for 10 to 20 minutes three to seven times a week. Shampoo should be massaged into wet scalp and rinsed, then applied a second time and left on for 5 min.
ANTIPSORIATICS anthralin (Drithocreme, Micanol) Apply for 30–60 minutes, then remove.	Irritation	Renal disease, acute psoriasis	Preparation may stain skin, towels, sinks, and tubs. Avoid applying near eyes and mucous membranes. Irritation can be avoided by applying emollients to unaffected skin.
VITAMIN D ANALOGS calcipotriene (Dovonex) Apply bid.	Burning and stinging, skin peeling, rash	Hypercalcemia, vitamin D toxicity	Do not use on face.
VITAMIN A DERIVATIVE tazarotene (Tazorac) Once a day at bedtime	Pruritus, erythema		Avoid vitamin A.
TOPICAL CORTICOSTEROIDS hydrocortisone (Cortisporin)	Burning, folliculitis, hypothalamic–pituitary–adrenal axis suppression	Primary bacterial infections or fungal infections	Use lowest effective dose. Avoid prolonged use. Use occlusive dressing.
TOPICAL IMMUNOSUPPRESSIVES tacrolimus (Protopic) Pimecrolimus (Elidal)	Transient burning; alcohol use can chase redness & flushing	Not under occlusive dressing	Use suncause screen.
Systemic Agents etretinate (Acitretin) 25–50 mg daily	Elevation in lipid levels, abnormal liver function, alopecia, rash, dry skin, pruritus	Alcohol use, pregnancy and lactation	Perform pretreatment lipid and liver function tests. Advise female patients not to become pregnant while taking this medication. Take with meals.
methotrexate (MTX, Rheumatrex) 10–25 mg/kg/wk	Headache, blurred vision, fatigue, malaise, GI distress, gingivitis, hepatotoxicity, chills, bone marrow depression, rash alopecia, fever	Pregnancy and lactation; caution in patients with renal and hepatic compromise, leukopenia	Drug decreases the level of digoxin. Increased risk of toxicity with salicylates, phenytoin, sulfonamides
cyclosporine (Cyclosporine A, Sandimmune) maximum dose 5 mg/kg/d	Tremor, gingival hyperplasia GI upset, hypertension, renal dysfunction, acne	Pregnancy and lactation; caution in impaired renal and hepatic function	Increased risk of digoxin toxicity Interacts with lovastatin, diltiazem, ketoconazole Decreased therapeutic effect with use of hydantoins, rifampin, sulfonamides
Etanercept (Enbrel) 50 mg twice a week for 3 months, then 50 mg weekly by subcutaneous injection	Infection, injection site pain, localized erythema, rash, upper respiratory infection, abdominal pain, vomiting	Concurrent live vaccine, active infection; caution in pregnancy, impaired renal function, asthma, blood dyscrasia, CNS demyelinating disease, history of recurrent infections	A maximum of 25 mg can be given in each site, requiring two injections. It is given subcutaneously.

Mechanism of Action

There are two possible mechanisms of action: inhibition of DNA synthesis, and a decrease in epidermal proliferation. Anthralin is a good therapy if the patient has a limited number of lesions, but its use is time-consuming.

Dosage

Anthralin is applied for 30 minutes to 1 hour and then removed. It should be applied only to the lesion, not to unaffected skin. Treatment starts with a low strength that is gradually increased. Staining of the psoriasis plaques signifies that treatment is decreasing cellular proliferation. Treatment is time-consuming but short term.

Time Frame for Response

There is a slow onset of action, and response is slow as well.

Contraindications

Anthralin therapy is contraindicated in acute psoriasis and inflammation.

Adverse Events

Anthralin therapy may be limited by irritation of the unaffected skin. Irritation can be prevented by applying emollients to the normal skin. The medication stains clothing a brownish-purple and permanently stains towels, tubs, and sinks.

Vitamin D Analogs

Calcipotriene (Dovonex) is a vitamin D analog for treating mild to moderate psoriasis.

Mechanism of Action

Its mechanism of action is a reduction of cell proliferation by binding to receptors in epidermal keratinocytes. The drug is also thought to have an anti-inflammatory effect. It is effective for long-term use and maintenance therapy and is often used as rotational therapy with topical steroids.

Dosage

A thin layer is applied twice a day to affected skin for 6 to 8 weeks. It is also used as rotational therapy or by pulse dosing (off-and-on therapy), in which the patient follows the therapeutic regimen for 2 weeks, followed by 1 week off. Use with a potent topical corticosteroid is most effective. The patient must be cautioned not to use more than 100 g per week.

Time Frame for Response

Some improvement is usually seen in 2 to 4 weeks, although therapy is recommended for 6 to 8 weeks. An advantage of calcipotriene is its similar efficacy to that of medium- to high-potency topical corticosteroids. Unlike corticosteroids, however, calcipotriene does not cause skin atrophy or hypothalamic–pituitary–adrenal axis suppression. However, it is an irritant and therefore should not be used on the face. It is contraindicated in patients with hypercalcemia and vitamin D toxicity.

Adverse Events

The most common adverse effects of calcipotriene are mild and include dry skin, peeling, and rash. Hypercalcemia may be caused by vitamin D ingestion but is rare if the patient uses less than 100 g of calcipotriene per week.

Retinoid (Vitamin A Derivative)

Tazarotene (Tazorac) is a topical retinoid used for mild to moderate psoriasis.

Mechanism of Action

This drug normalizes epidermal differentiation, decreases hyperproliferation, and diminishes inflammation of the cells in the skin. Use of tazarotene promotes longer remission of psoriasis.

Dosage

It comes in a clear, nonstaining gel (0.05% and 0.1%) and is applied in a thin layer once a day at bedtime. Skin must be air dried and the area left unoccluded. The preparation can be used for the body, scalp, hairline, and face, but not on the genitalia or intertriginous areas or around the eyes.

Time Frame for Response

After 1 week of therapy, diminished scaling is noted. Clearing is seen in approximately 8 weeks.

Contraindications

Tazarotene can cause fetal harm, so it is started in menstruating women during menses; these women should ensure that they do not become pregnant during therapy.

Adverse Events

Adverse effects of tazarotene include pruritus, erythema of the skin, and mild to moderate burning. The use of topical corticosteroids counteracts these effects. The patient must be warned that the psoriasis may get worse before it improves.

Interactions

Vitamin A ingestion is to be avoided, and tazarotene is used with caution with other photosensitizers such as tetracyclines and with other topical irritants such as abrasives, depilatories, or permanent wave solutions.

Systemic Retinoids

Acitretin (Soriatane) is a systemic retinoid used for long-term psoriasis therapy.

Mechanism of Action

Acitretin normalizes epidermal differentiation and diminishes hyperproliferation and inflammation of cells in the skin.

Dosage

A 25- to 50-mg dose is given once a day with the main meal until the lesions clear, which occurs gradually.

Contraindications

Acitretin is contraindicated in pregnancy and lactation and with the use of alcohol. It cannot be used in patients with severe renal impairment and increased lipid levels. The patient cannot donate blood for 3 years after therapy. Caution is used if there is a history of depression, obesity, or alcohol abuse.

Adverse Events

Adverse effects include lipid elevations, abnormal liver function, alopecia, skin peeling, pruritus, dry skin, dry mouth, epistaxis, paresthesia, paronychia, and pseudotumor cerebri.

Interactions

Drug interactions occur with methotrexate (MTX, Rheumatrex), alcohol, and progestin-only contraceptives. Women must not ingest alcohol during therapy or for 2 months afterward because alcohol prolongs the teratogenic potential of the drug.

Methotrexate

Methotrexate is used to treat generalized psoriasis.

Mechanism of Action

Methotrexate inhibits folic acid reductase, resulting in the inhibition of cellular replication and selection of the most rapidly dividing cells.

Dosage

The dose is 10 to 25 mg/kg per week orally in a single weekly dose, or 2.5 mg/kg per day for 5 days followed by at least 2 days off. With improvement in the disease, the dose is reduced and other agents are used.

Contraindications

Methotrexate is contraindicated in pregnancy and lactation, and the drug is used with caution in patients with renal and hepatic disorders and leukopenia.

Adverse Events

Common adverse effects include headache, blurred vision, fatigue, malaise, gastrointestinal distress, gingivitis, hepatic toxicity, bone marrow depression, rash, alopecia, and chills and fevers.

Interactions

There is an increased risk of toxicity if the patient is taking other medications, such as salicylates, phenytoin (Dilantin), and sulfonamides. Use of methotrexate also decreases the serum level of digoxin (Lanoxin).

Cyclosporine

Mechanism of Action

Cyclosporine (Cyclosporin A, Sandimmune) inhibits T-helper and T-suppressor cells and inhibits the production of cytokines.

Dosage

The maximum dose for use in psoriasis is 5 mg/kg per day.

Contraindications

Cyclosporine is contraindicated in pregnancy and lactation and must be used cautiously in patients with impaired renal function and malabsorption.

Adverse Events

Adverse effects include tremor, gingival hyperplasia, gastrointestinal upset, hypertension, renal dysfunction, and acne.

Interactions

Cyclosporine use increases the risk for nephrotoxicity if the patient uses other nephrotoxic agents, and also increases the risk for digoxin toxicity. Cyclosporine interacts with lovastatin (Mevacor), diltiazem (Cardizem), and ketoconazole (Nizoral), and its therapeutic effect is decreased with concomitant hydantoin (Dilantin), rifampin (Rifadin), and sulfonamide use.

Etanercept

Etanercept (Enbrel) is a human TNF receptor.

Mechanism of Action

It binds TNF cytokines that help regulate the body's immune response to infection and inflammation. It is used in moderate to severe psoriasis.

Dose

The dose of etanercept in psoriasis is 50 mg subcutaneously twice a week initially for 3 months. Maintenance dose is 50 mg sq weekly, with a maximum of 25 mg given at one site. It requires two injections in separate sites. A PPD test must be negative before treatment starts.

Contraindications

Contraindications include a concurrent live vaccine and an active infection. Caution is recommended in pregnant patients (although it is a category B drug) and patients with impaired renal function, asthma, a history of blood dyscrasias, CNS demyelinating disease, and a history of chronic recurrent infections.

Adverse Events

Adverse events include infection, injection site pain, localized erythema, rash, upper respiratory infections, abdominal pain, and vomiting.

Interactions

There is an increased chance of infection with immunosuppressants. Live vaccines should be given 2 weeks before or 3 months after therapy to ensure adequate immunization.

Selecting the Most Appropriate Agent

Selection of therapy depends on the patient's age, type of lesion, site and involvement, and previous treatments. Mild to relatively moderate psoriasis (<10% BSA) can be treated by a primary care provider. Topical treatment of psoriasis is the first step and is usually effective for mild disease. Patients with more generalized disease are referred to a dermatologist for treatment and phototherapy, and systemic agents are used (Table 14-2 and Fig. 14-1).

It appears that combination therapy with systemic agents and other modalities has synergistic value. In combination therapy, the dose can often be reduced, causing less toxicity from the drugs. Systemic therapy with phototherapy is also effective.

First-Line Therapy

First-line therapy includes moisturizers and topical steroids. For 2 weeks, a high-potency or very–high-potency topical steroid is applied twice a day and covered by an occlusive dressing of plastic wrap. A low-potency preparation is used on the face and intertriginous areas. An ointment is recommended because it provides the most moisture. An emollient also is used to keep the area moist.

Second-Line Therapy

If the patient's response to first-line therapy is not optimal, several second-line choices are available. If the patient had a good response to first-line therapy, therapy may consist of a 1-week rest from the topical corticosteroids and then another 2 weeks of therapy with the same agent for two more times. If the psoriasis goes into remission, applying the topical steroids once or twice a week may maintain the remission.

Another option is to taper the high-potency topical corticosteroid use to once or twice a week and add a vitamin D analog twice a day to the regimen. This produces a better result than either drug used alone. The topical corticosteroid helps clear the plaques and reduces irritation from the vitamin D preparation.

Third-Line Therapy

If first- and second-line treatments fail, a patient is referred to a dermatologist, who may use ultraviolet B light treatments, antimetabolites, etanercept or psoralens plus ultraviolet A light therapy (PUVA).

MONITORING PATIENT RESPONSE

The goal of chronic topical corticosteroid therapy is to use the lowest effective potency to control symptoms. Follow-up initially may need to be monthly, then may progress to every 2 to 3 months. In addition, referral for counseling, if desired, may help address related emotional issues.

PATIENT EDUCATION

Drug Information

In patients with psoriasis, education regarding stress monitoring and control is important, as is education regarding the disease process and treatment goals. The patient should understand that psoriasis is not contagious.

Patients may also benefit from information and support from groups such as the National Psoriasis Foundation (1-800-723-9166, www.psoriasis.org).

Showing the patient how to apply topical steroids is an important aspect of care, particularly if the medications are to be used only twice a day and applied lightly on moist skin.

Table 14.2

Recommended Order of Treatment for Psoriasis

Order	Therapy	Comments
First line	High-potency to very–high-potency topical corticosteroids applied to moist skin and use of occlusive dressing twice a day for 2 wk. Use emollients as adjunct therapy.	Use when less than 10% of body surface area is affected.
Second line	If the patient responded well to first-line therapy, provide a 1-wk rest from the topical corticosteroids and initiate another 2 wk of therapy with the same agent for two more times. OR Taper the high-potency topical corticosteroid to once or twice a week and add a vitamin D analog twice a day.	If there is remission, applying the topical steroids once or twice a week may maintain remission.
Third line	Refer to dermatologist for systemic therapy.	For use with greater than 20% body surface area, PUVA is used with coal tar or anthralin; PUVB is used with psoralens.

PUVA (B), psoralens with ultraviolet A (B).

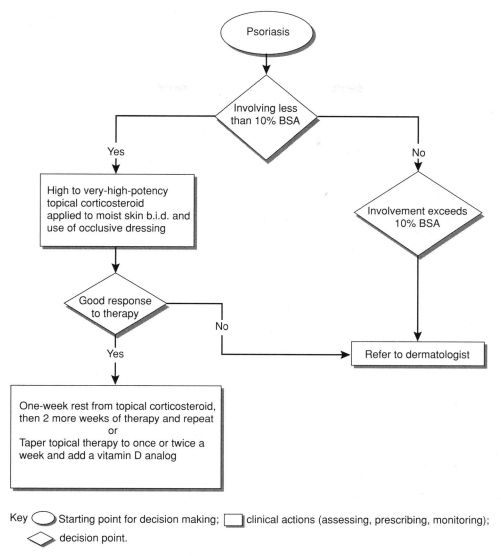

Figure 14–1 Treatment algorithm for psoriasis.

Lifestyle Changes

Symptom control, rather than cure, is the goal of therapy. Patients may help control symptoms by exposing their skin to the sun. This should be accomplished by gradually increasing the length of exposure. Emphasis should be placed on the importance of using sunscreen and avoiding sunburn. To prevent infection, patients must take care not to cut the lesions when shaving (if there are lesions in the area).

Psoriasis can be triggered by infections, stress, and changes in climate that can dry skin. These should be avoided when possible.

Complementary and Alternative Medicine

Fish oil is thought to alter the immune response and in small quantities can relieve itching and scaling. It has shown effect in chronic plaque psoriasis in doses of 6 to 15 g daily. An alternative is to eat fish three times a week. Aloe vera was shown to be effective in treatment of psoriasis. In a 16-week study, there was 82.8% clearing of psoriatic plaque using 0.5% hydrophilic aloe vera cream three times a day. Glucosamine has been shown to relieve some of the pain of arthritis from psoriasis.

■ Case Study

P.B. is a 58-year-old woman with a history of hypertension. She seeks treatment for small, scattered papules and plaques with a silvery-white scale on her elbows, forearms, and knees. The BSA affected is approximately 8%. She is very self-conscious about the lesions: "I just want them to go away." Her medications include propranolol 40 mg TID and furosemide 40 mg daily. She has a positive family history of psoriasis and reports high levels of stress in her job and life.

Diagnosis: Psoriasis

1. List specific goals for treatment for P.B.
2. What drug therapy would you prescribe? Why?
3. What are the parameters for monitoring the success of the therapy?
4. Discuss specific patient education based on the prescribed therapy.
5. List one or two adverse reactions for the selected agent that would cause you to change therapy.
6. What would be the choice for second-line therapy?
7. What OTC or alternative medications would be appropriate for P.B.?
8. What lifestyle changes would you recommend to P.B.?
9. Describe one or two drug/drug or drug/food interactions for the selected agent.

Bibliography

Starred references are cited in the text.

Bowcoch, A. M., & Barker, J. N. (2003). Genetics of psoriasis: the potential impact on new therapies. *Journal of the American Association of Dermatology, 49*(2 Suppl), S51–56.

Calan, J. P., Krueger, G. G., Lobwohl, M., et al. (2003). AAD consensus statement on psoriasis therapy. *Journal of the American Association of Dermatology, 49*(5), 897–899.

Choi, J., & Koo, Y. M. (2003). Quality of life issues in psoriasis. *Journal of the American Association of Dermatology, 49*(2 Suppl), S57–61.

*Fleischer, A. B., Feldman, S. R., Rapp, S. R., et al. (1996). Alternative therapies commonly used within a population of patients with psoriasis. *Cutis, 58,* 216–220.

*Freeman, A. K., Lenowske, B. S., Brady, C., et al. (2003). Tacrolimus ointment for treatment of psoriasis in the face and intertriginous areas. *Journal of the American Association of Dermatology, 48*(4), 564–568.

Guyette, J. R., & Rygwelski, J. M. (2002). Complementary of alternative medicine: therapies for common dermatological conditions: atopic dermatitis, psoriasis, and acne. *Clinics in Family Practice, 4*(4), 947–950.

Lohwahl, M. (2003). Combining the new biologic agents with our current psoriasis armamentarium. *Journal of the American Association of Dermatology, 49*(2 Suppl), S118–124.

Naldi, L., Peli, F., Parazzini, F., & Carrel, C. F. (2001). Family history of psoriasis, stressful life events and recent infectious disease are risk factors for the first episode of acute guttate psoriasis: results of case-control study. *Journal of the American Association of Dermatology, 44*(3), 433–438.

*Rapp, S. R., Exum, M. I., Reboussin, D. M., et al. (1997). The physical, psychological and social impact of psoriasis. *Journal of Health Psychology, 2,* 525–537.

Weinstein, G. D., Koo, J. Y. M., & Krueger, G. G. (2003). Tazarotene cream in the treatment of psoriasis: two multi-center, double-blinded, randomized, vehicle-controlled studies of the safety and efficacy of tazarotene cream 0.05% and 0.1% applied once a day for 12 weeks. *Journal of the American Association of Dermatology, 48*(5), 760–767.

Yamauci, P. S., Rizk, D., & Kormeili, G. G. (2003). Current systemic therapy for psoriasis: where are we now? *Journal of the American Association of Dermatology, 49*(2 Suppl), S66–77.

Visit the Connection web site for the most up-to-date drug information.

ACNE VULGARIS AND ROSACEA

■ MARY DRESSLER-CARRÉ

ACNE VULGARIS

Acne vulgaris is viewed by many as a rite of passage during the adolescent years. Up to 90% of all teenagers report having some form of acne. Adults suffer from the effects of acne as well: between 30% and 50% of adult women report experiencing acne. Consumers spend millions of dollars annually on prescription and over-the-counter (OTC) acne preparations.

The psychosocial costs of acne are great. Adolescents are particularly affected by physical defects, no matter how minor they appear to others. The health care practitioner must be particularly sensitive to the perceived seriousness of the acne in addition to the clinical picture. What may seem inconsequential to the practitioner may be devastating to the patient. No matter how minor the acne may appear to the provider, it is important to ask patients if they are concerned about their acne and whether they would like treatment (see the color plates in this book for more information).

CAUSES

Historically, numerous theories of the cause of acne vulgaris have been proposed, yet the exact cause remains unknown. Foods, stress, and dirt, although not causative, may exacerbate existing acne, which is why it is important to obtain a complete health history to ascertain precipitating factors. For example, a variety of drugs, physical occlusants, and conditions may exacerbate acne. Certain drugs used to treat tuberculosis, seizure disorders, or steroid-dependent chronic illness or depression may cause a drug-induced acneiform rash (Table 15-1). Drug-induced acne should be suspected when all lesions are in the same stage (eg, the lesions are uniformly all pustules or all open comedones), covering the face, chest, trunk, arms, and legs.

Acne may be exacerbated in teenagers and adults whose skin is exposed to oily agents, such as makeup, oil-based sunscreen, and oil-based hair products that come in contact with the forehead and temporal regions of the face (referred to as *pomade acne*). Friction acne from tight-fitting clothes, such as football helmets and hatbands, is found over the skin rubbed by the clothes. Exposure to animal-, vegetable-, and petroleum-based oils used in workplaces such as fast-food restaurants and automotive garages may also exacerbate acne. Thus, although eating French fries may not cause acne, cooking them may make the acne worse. Emotional stress may contribute to acne exacerbations in persons prone to breakouts, but studies have not consistently proven the correlation.

Women with a history of menstrual irregularities, hirsutism, and treatment-resistant acne should be evaluated for androgen excess associated with polycystic ovarian disease.

PATHOPHYSIOLOGY

Acne usually begins 1 to 2 years before the onset of puberty, when androgen production increases. Excess androgen causes increased sebum production. For unknown reasons, abnormal keratinization causes retention of sebum in the pilosebaceous follicle. This produces open comedones (blackheads) and closed comedones (whiteheads) (see Color Plate 1).

When closed comedones continue to produce keratin and sebum, the pilosebaceous follicle ruptures and inflames the surrounding tissue. If the inflammation is close to the surface, a papule forms. If it is deeper in the dermis, a larger papule or nodule forms. These deeper, nodular acne cysts cause permanent scars.

Although *Propionibacterium acnes*, an anaerobic gram-positive bacterium, is present as normal flora in the pilosebaceous follicle, acne vulgaris is not an infectious entity. Rather, it is believed that *P. acnes* produces lipolytic enzymes that in turn produce biologically active extracellular products. These in turn attract polymorphonuclear leukocytes and monocytes, which increase inflammation.

DIAGNOSTIC CRITERIA

Acne vulgaris is diagnosed from the clinical presentation of the patient's skin. It is classified and subsequently treated depending on its severity.

The mildest form of acne is comedonal. Both open and closed comedones may be present. Mild inflammatory acne is manifested by papules. Moderate inflammatory acne consists of pustules and some cysts. Severe cystic acne consists of cysts, nodules, and scarring (Table 15-2).

Table 15.1

Medications That Cause Acneiform Rash

Medication	Underlying Condition
Isoniazid	Tuberculosis
Phenytoin	Seizure disorder
Trimethadione	Seizure disorder
Lithium	Depression
Corticosteroids	Chronic inflammatory conditions

INITIATING DRUG THERAPY

Skin care is the most important nonpharmacologic tool in the management of acne vulgaris. The patient should be instructed to wash the face gently two or three times a day with a mild soap such as Basis, Cetaphil, Neutrogena, or Purpose. Care should be taken to avoid harsh, drying cleansers. Washing should be gentle because scrubbing the skin may exacerbate the acne. Comedo removal, although therapeutic, should be undertaken only by someone skilled in the proper technique. Picking or popping pimples may increase tissue damage and infection. The health care provider should advise the patient to avoid manipulating the acne with the fingers.

In general, use of personal care products should be minimized. Moisturizers and cosmetics should be water-based, noncomedogenic, and fragrance-free. If hair preparations are used, they should also be water-based. The patient should be instructed to apply hair products so that they do not come in contact with facial skin.

The practitioner also needs to stress that ingestion of specific foods, such as chocolate, greasy foods, colas, and iodide-containing foods, does not cause acne. Elimination diets are not considered therapeutic unless the patient reports an exacerbation associated with a certain food. In that case, the food must be avoided for 4 to 6 weeks and then gradually reintroduced to see what effect that food has on the acne.

Goals of Drug Therapy

The goal of pharmacotherapy is to minimize the number and severity of new lesions. Patients must be counseled that improvement of acne vulgaris takes time—usually 4 to 6 weeks. There is no cure for acne. Some form of therapy will probably need to be continued throughout adolescence and even into young adulthood.

Pharmacotherapy choices are based on the severity of the acne. Currently, successful therapy usually relies on a combination of medications. The synergistic effect of two or more drugs from different classes produces the best results. See Table 15-3 for a summary of acne medications.

Table 15.2

Classification of Acne Vulgaris

Classification	Physical Findings
Comedonal acne	Open comedones (blackheads), closed comedones (whiteheads)
Mild inflammatory acne	Papules
Moderate inflammatory acne	Pustules, cysts
Severe cystic acne	Cysts, nodules, "ice-pick" scarring

Comedolytics

Retinoic Acid (Tretinoin)

Marketed under the trade names Retin-A and Avita, retinoic acid is the acid form of vitamin A. When applied topically, retinoic acid acts on the epidermis with little systemic absorption to decrease cohesion between epidermal cells and increase epidermal cell turnover. The result is expulsion of open comedones and the conversion of closed comedones to open ones.

When used properly, retinoic acid causes mild erythema and peeling of the skin. Some patients cannot tolerate daily use or prolonged contact at the initiation of therapy. For example, fair-skinned patients should be advised to start out using the product every other day. Alternatively, the patient may be instructed to apply retinoic acid to the face for 15 to 30 minutes each night and then wash off the medication. Gradually, the length of time the medication remains on the face is increased until it can be tolerated overnight. It is best to apply the medication on clean, thoroughly dry skin to avoid excessive irritation. Side effects of retinoic acid include erythema, local skin irritation, and photosensitivity. Patients should be advised to avoid prolonged exposure to the sun or to wear a noncomedogenic sunscreen formulated specifically for use on the face.

Retinoic acid is available in cream (0.025%, 0.05%, 0.1%), gel (0.01%, 0.025%), liquid (0.05%), and microsphere (0.04% and 0.1%) formulations. The microsphere formulation encapsulates the active ingredient in microspheres, which act as a reservoir that slowly releases the retinoic acid. Although the microsphere product contains a higher percentage of medication, the slow-release formulation produces less irritation, making it one of the mildest dosage forms.

Adapalene Gel

Adapalene (Differin), a topical medication for treating non-inflammatory acne, is a derivative of naphthoic acid, which binds to retinoid receptors. It is considered less irritating than retinoic acid. Up to 40% of patients report irritation, but it subsides during the first month of treatment. Adapalene is applied in the same way as retinoic acid. A small amount is applied either every other day or for short periods in the evening until the drug can be tolerated overnight. Side effects of adapalene include hyperpigmentation and photosensitivity.

Comedolytic Bactericidals

Benzoyl Peroxide

Benzoyl peroxide is both a comedolytic and bactericidal agent specific to *P. acnes*. It has a role in inflammatory acne because of its antibacterial qualities. By decreasing *P. acnes* levels, it decreases the inflammation caused by leukocytic and monocytic attraction to the pilosebaceous follicle.

The major side effect of benzoyl peroxide is irritation. Like all comedolytics, benzoyl peroxide is applied initially in a low-percentage formulation in a nonirritating base. The patient increases the dosage strength and frequency. Because benzoyl peroxide may bleach colored items, the patient should be instructed not to let the product

Table 15.3

Overview of Topical and Oral Acne Preparations

Generic (Trade) Name and Dosage	Selected Adverse Events	Contraindications	Special Considerations
Topical Medications			
retinoic acid (Retin-A, Avita) 0.025%, 0.05% cream, gel 0.04%, 0.1% microspheres Apply once daily; increase strength as tolerated.	Erythema, local skin irritation, photosensitivity	Eczema, sunburn	Apply to dry skin for short periods or on alternate nights until better tolerated. Avoid products with high concentrations of alcohol, astringents, spices, lime. Pregnancy category C
adapalene (Differin) 0.1% gel, cream, liquid Apply once daily.	Hyperpigmentation, photosensitivity		Same as above
benzoyl peroxide (many) 2.5%–5.0% once a day; increase to two or three times daily	Irritation	Sunscreens containing para-aminobenzoic acid (PABA) may cause transient skin discoloration.	Product may bleach fabrics. Apply at different time from other topical medications.
azelaic acid (Azelex) 20% cream Apply twice a day.	Pruritus, irritation		Darker-pigmented people may have hypopigmentation. Exacerbation of asthma.
clindamycin (Cleocin T) Apply to skin twice a day.	Burning; stinging of eyes; possibly pseudomembranous colitis		Discontinue use if diarrhea develops. Pseudomembranous colitis may develop. Drug may potentiate neuromuscular blocking agents.
erythromycin (many) 2%–3% topical Apply twice daily.	Irritation	Allergy to erythromycin	None
tazarolene (Tazorac) 0.05%, 0.1% gel, cream Apply once daily.	Irritation, photosensitivity	Pregnancy category X	Obtain negative pregnancy test and use reliable contraception during medication use.
Oral Medications			
tetracycline (many) 500–1,000 mg daily divided bid/qid Taper to 250 mg/d after improvement; attempt to discontinue after 4–6 months of therapy.	Photosensitivity, gastric irritation, decreased effectiveness of oral contraceptives	Age younger than 12 years Pregnancy category D	Drug may increase serum digoxin levels. Drug absorption is reduced if taken with antacids, iron, zinc, dairy products. Drug use may increase blood urea nitrogen values if renal system is impaired.
erythromycin (many) 500–1,000 mg/d divided bid/qid	Nausea, vomiting, diarrhea, rash, allergic reactions, fungal infection, hepatitis, ototoxicity	Allergy to erythromycin or macrolide Not recommended for children younger than 2 months of age	Take on an empty stomach for better absorption 1 h before or 2 h after a meal. Enteric-coated form can be taken with or without food. Interactions: warfarin, theophylline, cisapride, digoxin, and others
isotretinoin (Accutane, generic) 0.5–1.0 mg/kg bid	Increased cholesterol and triglyceride levels; dry skin and mucous membranes; depression; aggressive, violent behaviors; back pain; arthralgias in pediatric patients	Adolescents before cessation of growth Pregnancy category X	Prescriber must be registered in SMART program. Female patients of childbearing age must have 2 negative pregnancy tests prior to therapy initiation, monthly negative pregnancy test while on therapy. Monitor cholesterol and triglyceride levels, CBC, liver function tests before therapy, at 4 weeks, and as indicated
ethinyl estradiol with norgestrate (Ortho Tri-Cyclen, Tri-Spiritec) 1 tablet daily		Premenarchal girls, male patients	Women who smoke should avoid use of oral contraceptives.

come in contact with brightly colored towels, pillowcases, or clothing. If used with retinoic acid, benzoyl peroxide should be applied in the morning and retinoic acid before bedtime.

Benzoyl peroxide is available in various strengths and bases, both OTC and by prescription. Gel formulations, which are considered more effective, are available in 2.5%, 4%, 5%, 10%, and 20% strengths. Lotions (5%, 10%, and 20%) and creams (5% and 10%) are also available.

Before using prescription-strength benzoyl peroxide, the patient should be instructed to discontinue any washes or lotions containing benzoyl peroxide that he or she may already be using. Inadvertent use of the two products may increase irritation.

Azelaic Acid

Azelaic acid (Azelex) is believed to interfere with the DNA synthesis of acne-causing bacteria. The drug is considered as effective as topical macrolide antibiotics in treating papulopustular acne. Azelaic acid is supplied as a 20% cream and is applied topically twice a day. In dark-pigmented people, hypopigmentation may develop from use.

Topical Antibiotics

Topical antibiotics may be prescribed when comedolytic antibacterials are either not effective or not tolerated and systemic antibiotics are not desired. Topical antibiotics inhibit the growth of *P. acnes* and decrease the number of comedones, papules, and pustules. Clindamycin 2% (Cleocin T) or erythromycin 2% or 3% (many brands) is supplied in solutions, saturated pads, lotions, and gels. Rarely, topical clindamycin has been implicated in pseudomembranous colitis and regional enteritis. The practitioner should advise patients to discontinue therapy if diarrhea develops.

Oral Antibiotics

When improvement cannot be achieved with topical therapy, oral antibiotics may be considered. Oral antibiotics are indicated for inflammatory acne because they suppress *P. acnes* as well as inhibit bacterial lipases, neutrophil chemotaxis, and follicular inflammation. There is no indication for their use in noninflammatory acne.

Tetracycline

Tetracycline is the most commonly used oral antibiotic for treating inflammatory acne. Doses begin at 500 to 1,000 mg/day and are tapered to 250 mg/day after improvement occurs. Clinical improvement takes at least 3 to 4 weeks.

Tetracycline permanently stains the teeth in children, so it should not be prescribed for patients younger than 12 years of age. Moreover, the drug is a teratogen. It may also decrease the effectiveness of oral contraceptives. Therefore, caution should be used when prescribing it for sexually active female patients. Patient education should include directions to avoid concurrent ingestion of milk products, iron preparations, and antacids, which decrease absorption. Ideally, the medication should be taken on an empty stomach.

Side effects of tetracycline include photosensitivity, gastric irritation, blood dyscrasias, and pseudotumor cerebri (benign intracranial hypertension). Caution should be used in treating patients who have renal failure or who are concurrently taking digoxin because tetracycline may increase serum digoxin levels.

Other Systemic Drugs

Given in doses between 500 and 1,000 mg/day, erythromycin is as effective as tetracycline. It is helpful in treating people with tetracycline allergy. Minocycline and doxycycline have also been used, but there is no advantage over tetracycline or erythromycin. Minocycline is considerably more expensive.

Retinoic Acid Derivatives: Isotretinoin

Isotretinoin (Accutane) has changed the management of acne therapy. It is reserved for patients with severe nodulocystic acne when other treatments fail. Isotretinoin is a retinoic acid derivative. Although the exact mechanism is unknown, it decreases sebum production, follicular obstruction, and the number of skin bacteria. It also has an anti-inflammatory action.

Dosage

Isotretinoin is given at a dose of 0.5 to 1 mg/kg/day. Therapy continues for 15 to 20 weeks unless significant improvement occurs sooner. If therapy needs to be repeated, 2 months should elapse before restarting the drug.

Contraindications

Because isotretinoin, a teratogen, is associated with serious birth defects, only prescribers registered in the SMART (System to Manage Accutane-Related Teratogenicity) Program (Roche Laboratory) may prescribe Accutane. Similar programs are in place for generic isotretinoin. The SMART program requires prescribers to study Roche's Guide to Best Practices and sign and return a letter of understanding that details the risks of pregnancy while on Accutane. The letter of understanding is an agreement to follow the recommendations of the SMART program, which includes obtaining two negative pregnancy tests prior to initiation of the drug and obtaining monthly pregnancy tests during therapy for all female patients. A yellow self-adhesive Accutane qualification sticker is to be placed on every prescription written, regardless of the gender of the patient. Only 30 days of drug can be prescribed at one time. Female patients able to bear children should be counseled to use two forms of contraception (Roche Laboratories, 2002).

In spite of this program, initiated in 2002, 120 pregnancies were reported the following year, in comparison to 127 pregnancies in the previous year. In 2004 the FDA's Drug Safety and Risk Management Advisory Committee and Dermatologic and Ophthalmic Drugs Advisory Committee proposed adopting a more restrictive risk management program. It will most likely entail a national registry of all persons receiving isotretinoin and the ability to track negative pregnancy tests. This program would be based on those currently used for clozapine and thalidomide (Mechcatie, 2004).

Before initiating therapy, a baseline complete blood count and chemistry profile and fasting triglyceride and cholesterol levels should be obtained. A complete blood count and a chemistry profile should then be obtained 1 month after the start of therapy. Pregnancy should be avoided for 1 month after therapy is discontinued.

Adverse Events

The most significant adverse effect of isotretinoin is teratogenicity. A 25-fold increase in fetal abnormalities has been documented. Even without external abnormalities, approximately 50% of children exposed to isotretinoin in utero have subnormal intelligence.

Approximately 25% of patients experience cholesterol and triglyceride elevations. Pseudomotor cerebri has been reported when isotretinoin therapy is combined with tetracycline. Almost all patients report dry skin and mucous membranes, including cheilitis, severe dry skin, and difficulty wearing contact lenses. Other side effects include musculoskeletal aches and corneal opacities. Therapy should not be initiated in adolescents who have not finished growing because the drug may cause premature closure of the epiphyses.

A "black box" warning was added in 2002, warning of an increase in aggressive or violent behaviors in patients as well as back pain in children: 29% of children developed back pain and 22% experienced arthralgias (FDA MedWatch October, 2002).

Other Medications

Topical Antibiotic–Benzoyl Peroxide Combinations

Marketed as Benzamycin, the combination of erythromycin 3% and benzoyl peroxide 5% in a gel base may increase compliance when a topical antibiotic is needed in addition to one or more other topical medications. The gel is applied once or twice a day. Although the product requires refrigeration, small quantities may be transferred to another container for up to 10 days, which tends to promote therapeutic adherence. Benzamycin is also marketed in pouches (Benzamycin Pak) that are mixed by the patient and therefore do not require refrigeration. The pack holds the two active ingredients in separate chambers, and they can be mixed as needed.

Similarly, a combination of clindamycin 1% and benzoyl peroxide 5% gel (Benzaclin Gel, Duac Gel) is available. Unlike Benzamycin, these products have a shelf life of 3 months at room temperature and do not require refrigeration.

Ethinyl Estradiol With Norgestimate

Oral contraceptives (OCs) that contain ethinyl estradiol and norgestimate (Ortho Tri-Cyclen, Tri-Spritec) have been approved by the FDA for the treatment of acne. Relative to other therapies, OCs are inexpensive. They reduce both comedonal and inflammatory acne and are worth considering for women who are already taking or considering taking systemic contraceptives.

Tazarotene Gel

A retinoid pro-drug, tazarotene gel (Tazorac) is effective against both comedonal and inflammatory acne as well as psoriasis. Despite being a topical drug, tazarotene is considered teratogenic (pregnancy category X) and should be used only by women who take systemic contraceptives and who have a negative pregnancy test.

Care should be taken when using the medication with tetracycline because it potentiates the photosensitivity reaction. Other side effects include dry skin, erythema, and pruritus.

Selecting the Most Appropriate Agent

The most important consideration in selecting a therapeutic regimen is matching the severity of the acne to the appropriate pharmacologic agent (Fig. 15-1 and Table 15-4).

First-Line Therapy

The first line of therapy for comedonal acne is topical medication. Topical comedolytics encourage faster turnover of the surface skin. The addition of bactericidals or topical antibiotics enhances results for patients with closed comedones and pustules.

Second-Line Therapy

Patients whose acne does not respond to topical therapy may need oral medications. The practitioner may initiate treatment with oral antibiotics in addition to topical medications for more severe papulocystic acne. Oral contraceptives are a useful and cost-effective alternative for sexually active women.

Third-Line Therapy

Isotretinoin is reserved for the most severe forms of nodulocystic acne. Special care must be taken when prescribing this agent for women who can become pregnant. Practitioners who are not registered with the SMART program or who cannot comply with the necessary monitoring and follow-up may feel more comfortable referring the patient to a dermatologist for evaluation and treatment.

SPECIAL POPULATION CONSIDERATIONS

Pediatric

Because of the risk of dental enamel defects and bone growth retardation, the use of tetracycline is contraindicated in children younger than 12 years of age. Growth retardation in children who have not reached adult height is associated with isotretinoin use. Children may also experience increased arthralgias and back pain with the use of isotretinoin.

Women of Childbearing Age

Women of childbearing age who are using isotretinoin or tazarotene gel must not become pregnant because of the teratogenicity of the products. Practitioners may suggest that a long-acting contraceptive, such as Depo-Provera, be used. If pregnancy occurs, the patient must be counseled accordingly. Tetracycline, also considered teratogenic, may decrease the effectiveness of oral contraceptives. Women taking this antibiotic should rely on a long-acting contraceptive or a barrier method to prevent pregnancy. Retinoic acid is labeled pregnancy category C and is not recommended for use in pregnant women or nursing mothers.

Table 15.4

Recommended Order of Treatment for Acne

Order	Agent	Comments
First line	Topical therapy	Improvement takes approximately 6 weeks.
Second line	Oral medications	Monitor in 6 weeks.
Third line	Isotretinoin or refer to dermatologist	Prescribe with caution to women of childbearing age. Pregnancy category X.

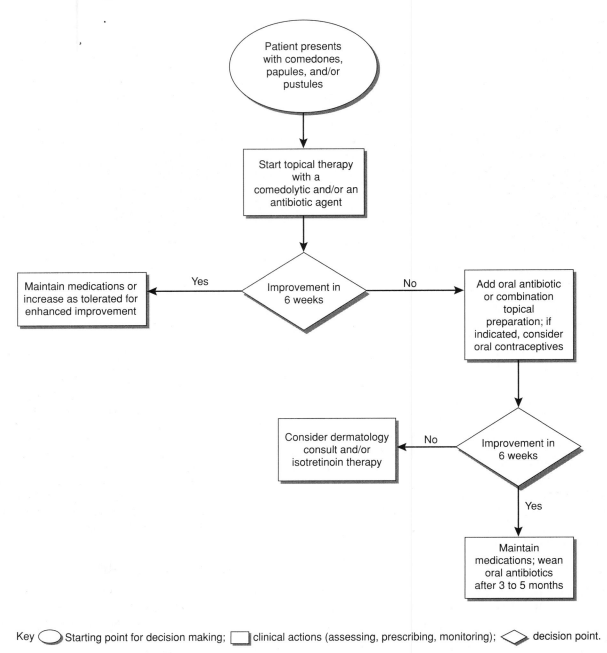

Key ⬭ Starting point for decision making; ▭ clinical actions (assessing, prescribing, monitoring); ◇ decision point.

Figure 15–1 Treatment algorithm for acne.

Ethnic

Azelaic acid may cause hypopigmentation in patients with dark skin.

MONITORING PATIENT RESPONSE

Follow-up should be scheduled monthly to monitor the patient's response to therapy, provide reassurance, and encourage adherence to therapy. Monthly visits provide the opportunity to adjust medications and dosages as the patient's acne responds to treatment. The ideal management is long-term topical therapy. If isotretinoin is prescribed, laboratory tests should be obtained before therapy and 1 month into therapy, as described previously.

PATIENT EDUCATION

Drug Information

The practitioner may show the patient how to apply topical preparations correctly to prevent excessive irritation (Box 15-1). An important consideration in prescribing topical therapy is that many gels and solutions contain significant amounts of alcohol. If a patient is sensitive to alcohol-based preparations or is experiencing significant dryness despite low concentrations of active ingredients, the practitioner may consider switching to a preparation that does not contain alcohol, such as a cream or aqueous gel.

Patients should be cautioned to avoid using excessive amounts of topical medications in the hope that it will speed

> **BOX 15–1. GENERAL PRINCIPLES FOR APPLYING TOPICAL ACNE PREPARATIONS**
>
> - Initiate therapy with a lower concentration of active ingredient, then work up to a higher concentration as tolerated.
> - Choose a product with a lower percentage of alcohol for people with sensitive skin.
> - Apply the product to clean, dry skin. Allow at least 20 minutes to elapse between washing the face and applying the medication.
> - Use the smallest amount of medication necessary for coverage.
> - Apply in "dots" over the desired area, then rub into skin.
> - Apply one drying agent in the morning, another in the evening to avoid excessive irritation.

improvement. Instead, irritation will most likely be the result, and that may discourage continuation of therapy.

Patience is the key to resolution of acne. Adolescents looking for a quick cure may be disappointed. All forms of acne therapy require a minimum of 4 to 6 weeks before results are seen. It is important to provide appropriate follow-up and encouragement and to have the patient return for evaluation and refinement of the treatment program.

Patient-Oriented Information Sources

The websites www.acne.org and www.nih.gov/medlineplus/acne.html (a site from the National Institutes of Health) provide information about acne and treatment.

ROSACEA

Occasionally mistaken for acne vulgaris, rosacea is an acneiform disorder that begins in midlife (30 to 50 years of age). The rash is symmetric and limited to the central part of the face. Fair-skinned people with a tendency to blush are more often affected. Although rosacea is more likely to develop in women, men who are affected may have a more severe form of the disorder.

CAUSES

Rosacea does not have a clear cause. Various theories suggest bacterial infection, fungal infection, hair follicle mite (*Demodex folliculorum*) infestation, menopausal changes, and, more recently, *Helicobacter pylori* infection. Alcohol and stress exacerbate but do not cause rosacea.

PATHOPHYSIOLOGY

Early vascular rosacea consists of simple erythema in response to cold exposure. Extravascular fluid accumulates as a result of various factors (exposure to cold, ingestion of hot or spicy food, intake of alcohol, local irritants). As a result, blood flow to the superficial dermis increases. Persistent telangiectasia occurs late in the vascular stage of the disorder. During this period, ocular involvement may develop, consisting of mild conjunctivitis, dry eyes, burning, blepharitis, and occasionally keratitis and corneal ulceration.

The second stage of rosacea represents lymphatic failure. It results in epidermal epithelial hyperplasia and pilosebaceous gland hyperplasia with fibrosis, inflammation, and telangiectasia. Clinical changes include persistent erythema, telangiectases, papules, and pustules. Rhinophyma, the characteristic deep inflammation and connective tissue hypertrophy of the nose, may begin to develop during this stage. Rhinophyma is almost exclusively seen in men older than 40 years of age and is treatable only by surgery.

Late-stage rosacea is recognized by persistent deep erythema, dense telangiectases, papules, pustules, nodules, and persistent edema of the central part of the face.

DIAGNOSTIC CRITERIA

The diagnosis of rosacea is based on the history and clinical presentation. Fixed telangiectasia is the hallmark of this disorder. In patients younger than 30 years of age, acne should be ruled out. In patients with systemic symptoms, systemic lupus erythematosus should be ruled out. Bacterial cultures should be performed to rule out *Staphylococcus aureus* folliculitis and gram-negative folliculitis. Patients who do not respond to systemic antibiotics should be evaluated for *D. folliculorum* infestation.

Approximately 50% of patients report ocular involvement, so any ocular symptoms should be investigated. Referral to an ophthalmologist should be considered if the practitioner suspects corneal ulceration or keratitis.

INITIATING DRUG THERAPY

The goal of therapy is to minimize the disfiguring effects of rosacea and prevent further tissue damage. As with acne, the patient's concerns with regard to appearance must be considered. Patients with rosacea may feel stigmatized. Treatment during the early phase (vasodilation) is difficult. Patients may not respond to treatment until the condition progresses to the inflammatory stage.

Topical Antibacterials

Metronidazole

Topical metronidazole (MetroGel, Noritate) has anti-inflammatory properties (Table 15-5). It is available in 0.75% and 1% strengths and is applied twice a day in a thin layer on the face, avoiding the eyes. Adverse events include burning, skin irritation, transient erythema, mild dryness, and pruritus. Metronidazole is available in cream, gel, and lotion. Initial results should be seen in approximately 3 weeks and the full effect in approximately 9 weeks. Patients are then maintained on the agent indefinitely. Patients who receive concurrent anticoagulant therapy should be monitored closely for an enhanced anticoagulation effect.

Table 15.5

Overview of Topical Agents for Rosacea

Generic (Trade) Name and Dosage	Selected Adverse Events	Contraindications	Special Considerations
metronizadole 0.75% gel, cream, lotion (MetroGel, etc.) 1.0% cream (Noritate)	Burning sensation, irritation, erythema (transient), mild dryness, pruritus	Children Breast-feeding mothers	Avoid eyes. With anticoagulant therapy, monitor closely for enhanced anticoagulation.
sodium sulfacetamide 10% with sulfa 5% (Sulfacet-R, Novalcet) sodium sulfacetamid 10% with sulfa 5% and urea 10% (Rosula) One to three times a day in thin layer	Local irritation, allergic dermatitis	Kidney disease Breast-feeding mothers Sulfa allergy	Avoid eyes and denuded skin. Pregnancy category C
Azelaic Acid 15% (Finacea) Apply thin film two times daily.	Burning, stinging, pruritus	Children	Hypopigmentation in patients with dark complexions

Combination Medications

Sodium sulfacetamide 10% with sulfur 5% (Sulfacet-R, Novalcet, Clenia) also has anti-inflammatory properties when used to treat rosacea. It is applied one to three times a day. It is contraindicated in patients with kidney disease and in those sensitive to sulfa drugs. Application to eyes and areas of denuded skin is to be avoided. Adverse events include local irritation and allergic dermatitis.

Rosula is a combination of sulfacetamide 10%, sulfur 5%, and urea 10%. The addition of urea helps to soothe and relieve redness and inflammation.

Azelaic Acid

Azelaic acid (Finacea), also indicated for acne, has been shown to be effective in treating papules and pustules associated with rosacea. Supplied as a 15% gel, it is indicated for the topical treatment of inflammatory papules and pustules of mild to moderate rosacea. Patients with dark complexions may experience hypopigmentation.

Oral Antibiotics

When topical agents have not improved the patient's condition, oral antibiotic agents may be considered. Antibiotics are used for their anti-inflammatory effect rather than their antibiotic properties. Oral antibiotics are indicated for patients with ocular symptoms.

Tetracycline

Tetracycline is the antibiotic of choice for treating rosacea. Tetracycline is prescribed in doses of 500 mg twice a day to initiate remission. After 2 weeks, the dose can be lowered to 250 mg twice a day for an additional 4 weeks. If no inflammatory lesions are present at 6 weeks, the dose may be lowered to 250 mg once a day. After 3 to 5 months, the practitioner may consider discontinuing the oral antibacterial while continuing topical metronidazole therapy.

Doxycycline

Doxycycline (Vibramycin, Monodox, Doryx), a tetracycline derivative, is sometimes more effective than tetracycline. It is given in doses of 100 mg twice daily, then tapered after 2 weeks to 50 mg twice daily. After improvement occurs, the dose may be lowered to 50 mg/day, then stopped after 3 to 5 months while maintaining metronidazole cream. Patients should be cautioned to avoid sun exposure while taking doxycycline.

Erythromycin

Erythromycin (E-mycin, Ery-Tab) is a useful agent when tetracycline is contraindicated. Dosages and tapering regimens are identical to those used for tetracycline.

Isotretinoin

Isotretinoin (Accutane) may be prescribed for patients who do not respond to oral and topical antibiotics. It is given in doses of 0.5 to 1.0 mg/kg/day for up to 8 months. Precautions and laboratory follow-up as described in the section on acne should be maintained.

Selecting the Most Appropriate Agent

Initial drug therapy choices should include a topical agent. Cases that involve ocular symptoms should be treated with oral antibiotics.

First-Line Therapy

The first-line treatment of rosacea consists of topical therapy. If no improvement is seen after 6 weeks, second-line therapy begins.

Table 15.6

Recommended Order of Treatment for Rosacea

Order	Agent	Comments
First line	Topical medication	Improvement takes 6 weeks.
Second line	Oral antibiotics	Improvement takes 6 weeks.
Third line	Oral isotretinoin; consider referral to dermatologist.	Pregnancy category X

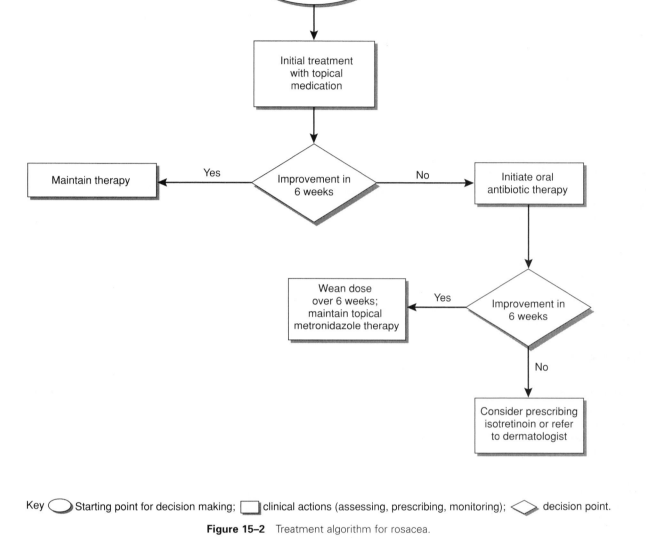

Figure 15–2 Treatment algorithm for rosacea.

Second-Line Therapy

Second-line treatment consists of adding an oral antibiotic. After 2 weeks, the dose is reduced by 50%; then, after 6 weeks, the oral antibiotic is discontinued altogether and the topical treatment continues indefinitely.

Third-Line Therapy

Third-line treatment consists of oral isotretinoin or referral to a dermatologist. Table 15-6 lists the lines of therapy for rosacea, and Figure 15-2 outlines rosacea treatment.

MONITORING PATIENT RESPONSE

As discussed throughout this chapter, the patient's response is monitored regularly by observation and follow-up visits to adjust medications and provide support and encouragement during therapy.

PATIENT EDUCATION

Patients with rosacea need to recognize what triggers the condition. The goal of management is to avoid flare-ups. Although each patient responds differently to triggers, common triggers are sun exposure, strong winds, cold weather, warm environment, strenuous exercise, alcoholic beverages, spicy foods, hot foods and beverages, and stress.

Patients may be advised to avoid harsh cleansers, rough washcloths, and pulling or tugging at the skin. Cosmetic foundations with a green tint may camouflage redness. Additional information and consumer education may be obtained through the National Rosacea Society (1-888-NO BLUSH, http://www.Rosacea.org).

■ Case Study

Jane, age 16, comes to your office for a routine physical examination. You notice that she has facial acne that she is hiding with heavy makeup. She has tried Clearasil inconsistently without relief. She works at a fast-food restaurant as a cook after school and on the weekends. Her mother has made her stop eating chocolates and greasy foods, but that has not seemed to help her. She is concerned because her prom is in 6 weeks and she wants her face clear. On physical examination, there are open and closed comedones as well as papules on her face and back. No scarring is evident. Jane confides that she has recently become sexually active.

Diagnosis: Acne vulgaris

1. List specific treatment goals for Jane.
2. What drug therapy would you prescribe? Why?
3. What are the parameters for monitoring the success of the therapy?
4. Describe specific patient education based on the prescribed therapy.
5. List one or two adverse reactions for the selected agent that would cause you to change therapy.
6. What would be the choice for second-line therapy?
7. What dietary and lifestyle changes should be recommended for Jane?
8. Describe one or two drug/drug or drug/food interactions for the selected agent.

Bibliography

*Starred references are cited in the text.

Blount, B. W., and Pelletier, A. L. (2002). Rosacea: a common, yet commonly overlooked, condition. *American Family Physician, 66*(3), 435–442.

Callender, V. D. (2004). Acne in ethnic skin: special considerations for therapy. *Dermatologic Therapy, 17*(2), 184.

Del Rosso, J. Q. (2004). Medical treatment of rosacea with emphasis on topical therapies. *Expert Opinion on Pharmacotherapy, 5*(1), 5–13.

Fitzpatrick, T. B., Johnson, R. A., Wolff, K., et al. (2000). *Color atlas and synopsis of clinical dermatology* (3rd ed.). New York: McGraw-Hill.

Goldsmith, L. A., Bolognia, J. L., Callen, J. P., et al. (2004). American Academy of Dermatology Consensus Conference on the safe and optimal use of isotretinoin: summary and recommendations. *Journal of the American Academy of Dermatology, 50*(6), 900–906.

*Mechcatie, E. (2004). Pregnancies lead to more isotretinoin restrictions. *Pediatric News, 38*(4), 5.

*Roche Laboratories. (2002). Accutane (isotretinoin) capsules complete product information. Nutley, NJ: Author.

Thiboutot, D. M. (2002). Acne and rosacea: new and emerging therapies. *Dermatologic Clinics, 18*, 63–71.

U.S. Food and Drug Administration. (2002). Accutane risk management program strengthened. *FDA Consumer Magazine, 36*(1). Rockville, MD: Author. [on-line: retrieved August 29, 2004]. Available: http://www.fda.gov/fdac/features/2002/102_acne.html.

*U.S. Food and Drug Administration. (2002). MedWatch 2002 Safety Alert – Accutane (isotretinoin) Dear Accutane Prescriber letter. Rockville, MD: Author [on-line: retrieved September 6, 2004]. Available: http://www.fda.gov/medwatch/SAFETY/2002/accutane_deardoc_10-2002.htm.

Weston, W. W., Lane, A., & Morelli, J. (2002). *Color textbook of pediatric dermatology*. St. Louis: Mosby.

Wilkin, J., Dahl, M., Detmar, M., et al. (2002). Standard classification of rosacea: report of the National Rosacea Society Expert Committee on the Classification and Staging of Rosacea. *Journal of the American Academy of Dermatology, 46*(4), 584–587.

Visit the Connection web site for the most up-to-date drug information.

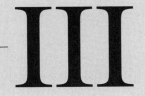

Pharmacotherapy for Eye and Ear Disorders

OPHTHALMIC DISORDERS

■ JOSHUA J. SPOONER

There are many conditions and disorders of the eye, but only a few, such as blepharitis and conjunctivitis, should be treated by a primary care provider. The remaining conditions are usually treated by eye care specialists. Nonetheless, prescribers should be familiar with drug therapy for the more common ophthalmic conditions (glaucoma, keratoconjunctivitis sicca) because they may encounter patients being treated for these disorders.

EYELID MARGIN INFECTIONS: BLEPHARITIS

The eye is well protected externally by the eyebrow, eyelashes, and eyelids. If these protective mechanisms are compromised, the eye becomes predisposed to disease. Externally, the eyelid structures are composed of skin with a high degree of elasticity, muscles that elevate the upper eyelid and close the eyelids, and the tarsal plate, which contains the meibomian glands. Through frequent blinking, the eyelids maintain an even flow of tears over the cornea. Internally, the eyelid structure is lined by the palpebral conjunctiva, which folds upon itself and then covers the sclera of the eyeball up to the corneoscleral junction. Located at the lid margins are the openings to the long sebaceous meibomian glands; these glands secrete the oily film that prevents tears from evaporating. At the base of the eyelash hair follicles are the superficial modified sebaceous glands of Zeiss and the sweat glands of Moll. Any of these glands may become functionally disrupted.

Blepharitis is an inflammation of the eyelid margin. Although it is a common eye disorder in the United States, epidemiologic information on its incidence or prevalence is lacking.

CAUSES

Blepharitis can be caused by a bacterial infection (staphylococcal blepharitis), inflammation or hypersecretion of the sebaceous glands (seborrheic blepharitis), meibomian gland dysfunction (MGD blepharitis), or a combination of these (American Academy of Ophthalmology [AAO], 2003a). Staphylococcal and seborrheic blepharitis involve the anterior eyelid; both have been referred to as anterior blepharitis.

PATHOPHYSIOLOGY

Alhough the gram-positive organisms *Staphylococcus epidermidis* and *Staphylococcus aureus* are found in a high proportion of both normal subjects and patients with blepharitis, *S. aureus* is isolated with greater frequency from the eyelids of patients with staphylococcal blepharitis. Both *S. epidermidis* and *S. aureus* are thought to play a role in the development of staphylococcal blepharitis, but the mechanism of disease production is poorly understood. Toxin production, immunologic mechanisms, and antigen-induced inflammatory reactions have all been reported with blepharitis (AAO, 2003a; Song et al., 2001).

Seborrheic blepharitis typically occurs as part of the more comprehensive condition of seborrheic dermatitis, with dandruff of the scalp, eyebrows, eyelashes, nasolabial folds, and external ears. In one study, 95% of patients with seborrheic blepharitis also had seborrheic dermatitis (McCulley et al., 1982). Seborrheic blepharitis is more commonly found in the geriatric population because of its association with rosacea.

Eyelid manifestations of MGD include prominent blood vessels crossing the mucocutaneous junction, thickening of the eyelid margin, plugging of the meibomian orifices, and formation of chalazia (painless firm lumps on the eyelid). These changes may lead to atrophy of the meibomian glands (AAO, 2003a). Compared to healthy patients, meibomian gland secretions are more turbid among patients with MGD blepharitis. These secretions block the gland orifices and become a growth medium for bacteria. Patients with MGD blepharitis frequently have coexisting rosacea or seborrheic dermatitis.

DIAGNOSTIC CRITERIA

There are no specific diagnostic tests for blepharitis. Patients with blepharitis frequently present with irritated red eyes and report a burning sensation. Increases in tearing, blinking, and photophobia are frequently reported, as is eyelid sticking and contact lens intolerance. Upon close inspection, the eyelid margins appear red, greasy, and crusted, with eyelid deposits that cling to the eyelashes. The eyelid margins may be ulcerated and thickened, and eyelashes may be missing.

Although the clinical features of staphylococcal, seborrheic, and MGD blepharitis are similar, there are differences that can aid in the differential diagnosis of these conditions. Eyelash loss and eyelash misdirection frequently occur in staphylococcal blepharitis but are rare in seborrheic blepharitis. The eyelid deposits are matted and scaly in staphylococcal blepharitis, oily or greasy in seborrheic blepharitis, and fatty and possibly foamy in MGD blepharitis. Chalazia are most likely to occur in MGD blepharitis.

INITIATING DRUG THERAPY

The underlying cause of the blepharitis must be treated, particularly if it is due to seborrheic dermatitis or rosacea. Treatment for all types of blepharitis includes strict eyelid hygiene and warm compresses. The use of warm compresses with a clean washcloth can soften adherent encrustations; once-daily use of compresses is generally sufficient, although some patients report benefit from using warm compresses two to four times a day (AAO, 2003a). Patients with MGD blepharitis often benefit from eyelid massage following warm compress use to remove excess oil (Shovlin & DePaolis, 2002). Following warm compress use, eyelid cleaning is performed by having the patient rub the base of the eyelashes with a commercially available eyelid cleaner (EyeScrub, OcuSoft) or a 1:1 mixture of baby shampoo (eg, Johnson & Johnson) and water on a cotton swab, cotton ball, or gauze pad (Shields, 2000). Performing eyelid hygiene daily or several times a week often blunts the symptoms of chronic blepharitis (AAO, 2003a). Patients with seborrheic or MGD blepharitis should be advised that eyelid hygiene may be required for life.

Patients suspected of having a new case of seborrheic or MGD blepharitis should be referred to an eye care specialist for a workup. Patients with staphylococcal blepharitis need a topical antibiotic.

Goals of Drug Therapy

The goals of drug therapy are to eradicate the pathogens causing the blepharitis and to reduce the signs and symptoms of blepharitis.

Topical Ophthalmic Antimicrobials

Topical ophthalmic antimicrobials are used for the treatment of and prophylaxis against external bacterial infections (Table 16-1). They kill the offending pathogen and other susceptible organisms.

Selecting the Most Appropriate Agent

Topical antimicrobials that are effective against staphylococci are listed in Table 16-2.

First-Line Therapy

Topical antibiotics such as bacitracin ointment or erythromycin 0.5% ophthalmic ointment are used. Therapy selection is based on allergies and patient preference for ointment or solution (drops). Ointments tend to cause a greater degree of

blurry vision than the solutions; if a patient prefers a solution, one of the newer fluoroquinolones (gatifloxacin, levofloxacin, or moxifloxacin) would be suitable. The AAO (2003a) recommends that the frequency and duration of treatment should be guided by the severity of the blepharitis.

Second-Line Therapy

If the blepharitis fails to respond to the first-line therapy after several weeks or the condition appears to worsen at any time (including any vision loss or corneal involvement), the patient should be referred to an ophthalmologist for a complete evaluation.

PATIENT EDUCATION

Patients should be educated about the chronic nature of blepharitis. While chronic blepharitis can rarely be eliminated, improved eyelid hygiene, warm massages, and occasional antibiotic use (for staphylococcal blepharitis) can improve symptoms. Contact lens wearers should refrain from wearing contact lenses during an acute case of blepharitis, especially if antibiotic therapy has been initiated. Contact lens wearers with chronic blepharitis should consult with their eye care professional to determine whether contact lens use is safe.

EXTERNAL SURFACE OCULAR INFECTIONS: CONJUNCTIVITIS

Conjunctivitis is the most common cause of a red, painful eye in the United States (Horton, 1998). Conjunctivitis is an inflammation of the bulbar or palpebral conjunctiva, the clear membrane that covers the white part of the eye and lines the inner surfaces of the eyelids. Conjunctivitis is commonly referred to as *pink eye*.

CAUSES

Approximately 15% of conjunctivitis cases in adults are bacterial in origin. The most common organisms seen in acute bacterial conjunctivitis are the gram-positive *Staphylococcus* and *Streptococcus* species and the gram-negative *Pneumococcus*, *Moraxella*, and *Haemophilus* species; less common organisms include *Neisseria gonorrhoeae* and *Chlamydia trachomatis* (Silverman & Bessman, 2003). In children, up to 50% of conjunctivitis cases are of bacterial origin. The most common pathogens in neonates are *N. gonorrhoeae* and *C. trachomatis*, while *H. influenzae*, *S. pneumoniae*, and *M. catarrhalis* are the most commonly isolated organisms in children with bacterial conjunctivitis (Silverman & Bessman, 2003; Teoh & Reynolds, 2003).

Viruses account for the majority of conjunctivitis cases in adults. The most common viral etiology is adenovirus infection (Horton, 1998); conjunctivitis due to an adenovirus is highly contagious (Shields, 2000; Teoh & Reynolds, 2003). Other viruses associated with conjunctivitis include the herpes simplex virus and molluscum contagiosum (AAO, 2003b).

Table 16.1

Overview of Antimicrobial Ophthalmic Agents

Generic (Trade) Name and Dosage	Selected Adverse Events	Contraindications	Special Considerations
Single-Agent Products			
sulfacetamide sodium 10% solution or ointment (AK-Sulf, Bleph-10, Sodium Sulfamyd, Cetamide) Dosing Solution: 1–2 drops every 1–4 hours initially according to the severity of infection Ointment: ½ inch 3 or 4 times a day and at bedtime Dosing may be tapered as the condition responds. Usual duration of therapy is 7–10 days.	Local irritation, itching, stinging, burning, periorbital edema	Allergy to sulfa drugs Do not use in infants < 2 years of age.	A significant percentage of *Staphylococcus* species are resistant to sulfa drugs. Ointments may blur vision and retard corneal wound healing. Do not use in patients with purulent exudates.
bacitracin 500 units/g ointment (AK-Tracin)	Blurred vision, redness, burning, eyelid edema		Ointments may blur vision and retard corneal wound healing.
erythromycin 0.5% ointment (Ilotycin)			Ointments may blur vision and retard corneal wound healing.
gentamicin 0.3% solution or ointment (Garamycin, Genoptic, Gentak) Dosing Solution: 1–2 drops in the affected eye(s) every 4 hours Ointment: ½ inch to the affected eye 2 or 3 times a day	Ocular burning and irritation, nonspecific conjunctivitis, conjunctival epithelial defects, conjunctival hyperemia, bacterial and fungal corneal ulcers		In severe infections, dosage of the solution may be increased to as much as 2 drops every 2 hours. Ointments may blur vision and retard corneal wound healing.
tobramycin 0.3% solution or ointment (Tobrex, AKTob) Dosing Solution: 1–2 drops into the infected eye every 4 hours Ointment: 1 inch every 8–12 hours	Lid itching, lid swelling, conjunctival hyperemia, nonspecific conjunctivitis, bacterial and fungal corneal ulcers		Ointments may blur vision and retard corneal wound healing. For more severe infections, the initial dose may be increased to 2 drops every 30–60 minutes initially (solution) or 1 inch every 3–4 hours (ointment).
ciprofloxacin 0.3% solution or ointment (Ciloxan) Dosing Solution: 1–2 drops every 2 hours while awake for 2 days, then 1–2 drops every 4 hours while awake for 5 days Ointment: ½ inch three times a day for 2 days, then ½ inch twice a day for 5 days	Local burning and discomfort, white crystalline precipitate formation, conjunctival hyperemia, altered taste		Ointments may blur vision and retard corneal wound healing. This is the only ophthalmic fluoroquinolone available as an ointment.
gatifloxacin 0.3% solution (Zymar) Dosing: One drop in the affected eye every 2 hours while awake for 2 days, then 1 drop in the affected eye up to 4 times daily while awake	Conjunctival irritation, tearing, papillary conjunctivitis, eyelid edema, ocular itching, dry eye		
levofloxacin 0.5% solution (Quixin) Dosing: One drop in the affected eye every 2 hours while awake for 2 days, then 1 drop in the affected eye up to 4 times daily while awake	Temporarily decreased or blurred vision, eye irritation, itching, dry eye		A higher-dose levofloxacin product is available (Iquix) for use in bacterial corneal ulcer.
moxifloxacin 0.5% solution (Vigamox) Dosing: One drop in the affected eye 3 times a day for 7 days	Decreased visual acuity, dry eye, ocular itching and discomfort, ocular hyperemia		

(continued)

Table 16.1

Overview of Antimicrobial Ophthalmic Agents (*Continued*)

Generic (Trade) Name and Dosage	Selected Adverse Events	Contraindications	Special Considerations
norfloxacin 0.3% solution (Chibroxin) Dosing: 1–2 drops in the affected eye 4 times a day for up to 7 days; first-day dosing may be increased to 1–2 drops every 2 hours while awake for severe infections	Local burning and discomfort, conjunctival hyperemia, photophobia, altered taste		
ofloxacin 0.3% solution (Oculfox) Dosing: 1–2 drops in the affected eye every 2–4 hours for 2 days, then 1–2 drops 4 times a day	Ocular burning and stinging, itching, redness, edema, blurred vision, photophobia		Rare reports of dizziness and nausea with use
Combination Products polymixin B sulfate, bacitracin ointment or solution (Polytrim, Polysporin) Dosing Solution: 1 drop in the affected eye(s) every 3 hours (maximum 6 doses a day) for 7–10 days Ointment: Apply every 3–4 hours for 7–10 days, depending upon the severity of infection.	Local irritation (burning, stinging, itching, redness), lid edema, tearing, rash		Ointments may blur vision and retard corneal wound healing.
polymixin B sulfate, bacitracin zinc, neomycin ointment and solution (Neosporin) Dosing Solution: 1–2 drops into the affected eye(s) every 4 hours for 7–10 days Ointment: Apply every 3–4 hours for 7–10 days, depending upon the severity of infection	Itching, swelling, conjunctival erythema, local irritation		Ointments may blur vision and retard corneal wound healing. Dosage of the solution may be increased to as much as 2 drops every hour for severe infections.

Allergic conjunctivitis is fairly common and is frequently mistaken for bacterial conjunctivitis. There are three types of allergic conjunctivitis: hay fever conjunctivitis, due to seasonal release of plant allergens; vernal conjunctivitis, which is of unknown origin but is thought to be due to seasonal airborne antigens; and atopic conjunctivitis, which occurs in people with atopic dermatitis or asthma.

Conjunctivitis can also be caused by mechanical or chemical irritants. A foreign body on the eye (typically a contact lens) can lead to giant papillary conjunctivitis.

Table 16.2

Recommended Order of Treatment for Blepharitis

Order	Agent	Comments
First line	Erythromycin 0.5% ophthalmic ointment *or* Bacitracin 500 units/g ointment *or* An ophthalmic fluoroquinolone solution (gatifloxacin, levofloxacin, or moxifloxacin)	Ointments tend to cause a greater degree of blurry vision than solutions. Erythromycin and bacitracin are available as inexpensive generic products. The remaining ophthalmic fluoroquinolones do not provide good staphylococcal coverage.
Second line	Referral to an ophthalmologist	

PATHOPHYSIOLOGY

General mechanisms of infection are at work in bacterial and viral conjunctivitis. In bacterial conjunctivitis, the infecting organism is obtained via contact with an infected individual and transmitted to the eye by fingertips. Neonates with conjunctivitis may have become inoculated during childbirth by their infected mother (AAO, 2003b). Transmission of viral conjunctivitis is usually through direct contact with infected persons, contact with contaminated medical instruments, or contaminated swimming pool water (Morrow & Abbott, 1998). In both bacterial and viral conjunctivitis, the infectious agent causes the inflammation of the conjunctiva. Mechanical and chemical irritants that cause conjunctivitis operate in the same manner.

In hay fever conjunctivitis, symptoms are caused by the IgE-mediated release of mast cells in the conjunctiva (Horton, 1998).

DIAGNOSTIC CRITERIA

In addition to the hallmark red or pink eye, classic patient complaints that occur in conjunctivitis include itching or burning sensations of the eyes, ocular discharge ("leaky eye"), eyelids that are stuck together in the morning, and a sensation that a foreign body is lodged in the eye. Patients may also report a feeling of fullness around the eye. Moderate to severe pain and light sensitivity are not typical features of a primary conjunctival inflammatory process (Morrow & Abbott, 1998). If these symptoms are present, or if the patient reports blurred vision that does not improve with blinking, the patient should be referred to an eye care professional, as a more serious ocular disease process (such as keratoconjunctivitis) may be occurring (Morrow & Abbott, 1998). Neonates with signs of conjunctivitis should be referred to an eye care professional for immediate examination, as bacterial conjunctivitis due to *C. trachomatis* or *N. gonorrhoeae* can lead to serious eye damage.

Although many symptoms of conjunctivitis are nonspecific (tearing, irritation, stinging, burning, and conjunctival swelling), inspection and patient history can help determine the cause of illness. Patients who report that their eyelids were stuck together upon awakening most likely have bacterial conjunctivitis (Morrow & Abbott, 1998); this sticking is caused by a purulent ocular discharge. Because gonococcal conjunctivitis produces a copiously purulent discharge, the cause of any copiously purulent conjunctivitis should be suspected as *N. gonorrhoeae* until Gram-stain testing proves otherwise. Bacterial conjunctivitis usually starts in one eye and can become bilateral a few days later.

Viral conjunctivitis produces a profuse watery discharge. Similar to bacterial conjunctivitis, viral conjunctivitis usually starts in one eye and can become bilateral within a few days. While unlikely, photophobia and a foreign-body sensation may be reported. Examination may reveal a tender preauricular node.

In allergic conjunctivitis, itching is the hallmark symptom; it can be mild to severe and may manifest as excessive blinking. A history of recurrent itching or a personal or family history of hay fever, asthma, atopic dermatitis, or allergic rhinitis is suggestive of allergic conjunctivitis. In general, a patient with conjunctivitis who does not report an itchy eye does not have allergic conjunctivitis. Unlike bacterial or viral conjunctivitis, allergic conjunctivitis usually presents with bilateral symptoms. An ocular discharge may or may not be present; if present, it may be watery or mucoid. Aggressive forms of allergic conjunctivitis are vernal conjunctivitis in children and atopic conjunctivitis in adults. Vernal conjunctivitis is associated with shield corneal ulcers and perilimbal accumulation of eosinophils (Horner-Trantas dots) (Silverman & Bessman, 2003). Atopic conjunctivitis is associated with eyelid thickening and scarring, blepharitis, and corneal scarring (AAO, 2003b).

Giant papillary conjunctivitis occurs mainly in contact lens wearers. These patients report excessive itching, mucus production and discharge, and increasing intolerance to contact lens use. Giant papillae form on the upper palpebral conjunctiva and can be seen upon lid eversion (AAO, 2003b; Silverman & Bessman, 2003).

INITIATING DRUG THERAPY

Before drug therapy is prescribed, both the patient and the practitioner should be aware that bacterial and viral conjunctivitis are highly contagious and are spread by contact. Therefore, good hand-washing and instrument-cleansing techniques are imperative. The etiology of illness should be determined, as treatment is different for bacterial, viral, and allergic conjunctivitis.

Goals of Drug Therapy

The goals of drug therapy are to eradicate the offending organism (for bacterial conjunctivitis) and to relieve symptoms (for all types of conjunctivitis). A patient with bacterial conjunctivitis should experience improvement in symptoms a few days after the start of antibiotic therapy; the organisms remain active (and contagious) for 24 to 48 hours after therapy begins. With viral conjunctivitis, the disease is contagious for at least 7 days after symptoms appear; it may be contagious for up to 14 days.

Antibiotics

Although bacterial conjunctivitis caused by typical pathogens (*Staphylococcus*, *Streptococcus*, *Pneumococcus*, *Moraxella*, and *Haemophilus* species) is usually self-limiting, antibiotic therapy is justified because it can shorten the course of the disease, which reduces person-to-person spread, and lowers the risk of sight-threatening complications. The choice of antibiotic is usually empirical. Although no single topical antibiotic covers all potential conjunctival pathogens, selection of agents with good gram-positive coverage (especially good staphylococcal coverage) is essential (Morrow & Abbott, 1998). Five to 7 days of therapy with agents such as erythromycin ointment or bacitracin-polymyxin B ointment or solution is usually effective. While well tolerated, sulfacetamide has weak to moderate activity against many gram-positive and gram-negative organisms. The aminoglycosides have good gram-negative coverage but incomplete coverage of *Streptococcus* and *Staphylococcus* species and a relatively high incidence of corneal toxicity. The fluoroquinolones also have good gram-negative coverage; the older fluoroquinolones (ciprofloxacin, norfloxacin, and ofloxacin) have poor coverage of *Streptococcus* species, while the newer fluoroquinolones (gatifloxacin, levofloxacin, and moxifloxacin) offer improved gram-positive coverage.

Because gonococcal infection is serious, immediate treatment of conjunctivitis due to *N. gonorrhoeae* with a 1-g IM injection of ceftriaxone (Rocephin) is recommended for adults and children who weight at least 45 kg. For cephalosporin-allergic patients, alternatives include single doses of ciprofloxacin 500 mg, ofloxacin 400 mg, or IM spectinomycin 2 g. Children who weigh less than 45 kg should receive a single 125-mg IM injection of ceftriaxone, while 25 to 50 mg/kg of ceftriaxone IV or IM (not to exceed 125 mg) is the appropriate dose for neonates. Topical antibiotic therapy is not necessary, but topical bacitracin or erythromycin ointment is often initiated to prevent secondary infection (AAO, 2003b).

As *C. trachomatis* is now the most common cause of conjunctivitis in neonates in the United States, the long-time standard prophylactic agent for neonates, topical 1% silver nitrate solution, is no longer recommended or commercially available in America. Topical erythromycin or tetracycline ointments are now used for prophylaxis, but their effectiveness in preventing neonatal chlamydial conjunctivitis is questionable (American Academy of Pediatrics, 2000; Chen, 1992). In adults and children at least 8 years old, *C. trachomatis* infection is treated with a single 1-g dose of azithromycin or 7 days of therapy with doxycycline 100 mg twice daily (AAO, 2003b). Children who weigh at least 45 kg but are less than 8 years old should receive the single dose of azithromycin 1 g. Neonates and children who weigh less than 45 kg should receive 50 mg/kg/day of erythromycin base or erythromycin ethylsuccinate, divided into four doses a day for 10 to 14 days (AAO, 2003b). Identification of either *Chlamydia* or *N. gonorrhoeae* conjunctivitis requires that the patient's sexual partner also be treated.

Antihistamines

The ophthalmic antihistamines (emedastine, levocabastine) prevent the histamine response in blood vessels by preventing histamine from binding with its receptor site. They are useful in reducing the symptoms of allergic conjunctivitis. Ocular adverse events include transient stinging or burning upon instillation, eye pain, dry eyes, red eyes, visual disturbances, watery ocular discharge, and eyelid edema. Oral antihistamines can also help to relieve symptoms in many patients. Table 16-3 gives details on these agents.

Mast Cell Stabilizers

The mast cell stabilizers (cromolyn, lodoxamide, nedocromil, and pemirolast) inhibit hypersensitivity reactions and prevent the increase in cutaneous vascular permeability that accompanies allergic reactions. These agents may be helpful for patients with allergic conjunctivitis. Ocular adverse events include transient burning, stinging or discomfort, pruritus, blurred vision, dry eyes, taste alteration, and foreign body sensation (see Table 16-3).

Antihistamine/Mast Cell Stabilizer

Several new products (azelastine, epinastine, ketotifen, and olopatadine) have the combined properties of an antihista-

mine and a mast cell stabilizer, providing immediate relief of itching and long-term suppression of histamine release. These agents are given two or three times a day and have a side effect profile similar to the antihistamines and mast cell stabilizers (see Table 16-3).

Nonsteroidal Anti-inflammatory Ophthalmic Drugs

The ophthalmic nonsteroidal anti-inflammatory (NSAID) ketorolac may be useful for treating the itch associated with allergic conjunctivitis. The NSAIDs inhibit the biosynthesis of prostaglandin by decreasing the activity of the enzyme cyclooxygenase. Ketorolac is administered 1 drop four times a day into the affected eye. It is contraindicated in patients who wear soft contact lenses. It should be used with caution in patients with aspirin sensitivities and patients who have bleeding disorders or are receiving anticoagulant therapy, as ophthalmic NSAIDs are absorbed systemically. Adverse events include transient stinging and burning, irritation and inflammation, corneal edema, and iritis (see Table 16-3).

Vasoconstrictors

Vasoconstrictor eye drops (naphazoline, oxymetazoline, phenylephrine, and tetrahydrozoline) may offer relief to patients with allergic conjunctivitis. With the exception of the higher-strength (0.1%) naphazoline solution, these agents are available without a prescription. Side effects include stinging, blurred vision, mydriasis, and increased redness; punctate keratitis and increased intraocular pressure (IOP) may also occur. These agents are contraindicated in patients with narrow-angle glaucoma or a narrow angle without glaucoma. Rebound congestion may occur with frequent or extended use of these agents; use should be limited to a maximum of 72 hours (see Table 16-3).

Topical Corticosteroids

Topical corticosteroids have been shown to reduce inflammation in allergic conjunctivitis. Low-dose corticosteroid therapy can be used at infrequent intervals for short-term periods (1 to 2 weeks) (AAO, 2003b). If a topical corticosteroid fails to improve inflammation or pain within 48 hours, therapy should be discontinued. Long-term use of topical corticosteroids is associated with severe side effects, including ocular hypertension, cataract formation, glaucoma, and infection (Calonge, 2001) (see Table 16-3).

Selecting the Most Appropriate Agent

Treatment of bacterial conjunctivitis is aimed at eradicating the offending organism. Cultures are not indicated unless the infection does not resolve with first-line therapy (Table 16-4 and Fig. 16-1). A variety of treatments can be used to maintain eye comfort of patients with allergic conjunctivitis. Viral conjunctivitis is self-limiting and is treated with cool compresses; giant papillary conjunctivitis is often treated by changes in contact lens use or discontinuation and symptomatic therapy.

There is conflicting information about the use of soft contact lenses while taking ophthalmic medications that

Table 16.3

Overview of Antiallergy Ophthalmic Agents

Generic (Trade) Name and Dosage	Selected Adverse Events	Contraindications	Special Considerations
Antihistamines			
emedastine 0.05% solution (Emadine) Dosing: 1 drop in the affected eye up to 4 times a day	Blurred vision, burning and stinging, dry eyes, foreign body sensation, hyperemia, itching		Labeling: Wait 10 minutes following administration before inserting contact lenses.
levocabastine 0.05% suspension (Livostin) Dosing: 1 drop in the affected eyes 4 times a day	Burning and stinging, headache, visual disturbances, dry mouth, fatigue, eye pain, dry eye, eyelid edema		Indicated use limited to 2 weeks. Labeling: Do not administer while wearing contact lenses.
Mast Cell Stabilizers			
cromolyn 4% solution (Crolom) Dosing: 1–2 drops in each eye 4–6 times a day at regular intervals	Burning and stinging, conjunctival injection, watery eyes, itching, dry eye, styes		Labeling: Refrain from contact lens use while under treatment.
lodoxamide 0.1% solution (Alomide) Dosing: 1–2 drops in each eye 4 times a day	Burning and stinging, ocular itching, blurred vision, dry eye, tearing, hyperemia, foreign body sensation		Labeling: Refrain from contact lens use while under treatment.
nedocromil 2% solution (Alocril) Dosing: 1–2 drops in each eye twice a day	Ocular burning and stinging, unpleasant taste, redness, photophobia		Labeling: Refrain from contact lens use while exhibiting the signs and symptoms of allergic conjunctivitis.
pemirolast 0.1% solution (Alamast) Dosing: 1–2 drops in each affected eye 4 times daily	Burning, dry eye, foreign body sensation, ocular discomfort		Pemirolast contains lauralkonium chloride, not benzalkonium chloride. Labeling: Wait 10 minutes following administration before inserting contact lenses.
Antihistamine / Mast Cell Stabilizer			
azelastine 0.05% solution (Optivar) Dosing: One drop into each affected eye twice daily	Ocular burning and stinging, headache, bitter taste, eye pain, blurred vision		Labeling: Wait 10 minutes following administration before inserting contact lenses.
epinastine 0.05% solution (Elestat) Dosing: One drop in each eye twice a day	Burning sensation, folliculosis (hair follicle inflammation), hyperemia, itching		Labeling: Wait 10 minutes following administration before inserting contact lenses.
ketotifen 0.025% solution (Zatidor) Dosing: 1 drop in the affected eye(s) every 8–12 hours	Conjunctival injection, burning and stinging, conjunctivitis, dry eye, itching, photophobia		Labeling: Wait 10 minutes following administration before inserting contact lenses.
olopatadine 0.1% solution (Patanol) Dosing: 1–2 drops in each affected eye twice daily at an interval of 6–8 hours	Ocular burning and stinging, dry eye, foreign body sensation, hyperemia, lid edema, itching		Labeling: Wait 10 minutes following administration before inserting contact lenses.
Nonsteroidal Anti-inflammatory Drugs			
ketorolac 0.5% solution (Acular) Dosing: 1 drop 4 times a day	Stinging and burning, corneal edema, iritis, ocular irritation or inflammation		Use with caution in patients with aspirin sensitivities and patients with bleeding disorders or those receiving anticoagulant therapy. Labeling: Do not administer while wearing contact lenses.
Decongestants			
naphazoline 0.012%, 0.02%, or 0.03% solutions (Clear Eyes, Naphcon, Vasoclear), and 0.1% solution (Vasocon, Naphcon Forte, Albalon, AK-Con)	Stinging, blurred vision, mydriasis, redness, punctate keratitis, increased IOP	Narrow-angle glaucoma Narrow-angle without glaucoma	Use should be limited to 72 hours. Contains benzalkonium chloride; use with contact lenses not addressed in labeling

(continued)

Table 16.3

Overview of Antiallergy Ophthalmic Agents (*Continued*)

Generic (Trade) Name and Dosage	Selected Adverse Events	Contraindications	Special Considerations
Dosing: 1–2 drops in the affected eye(s) every 3–4 hours, up to 4 times a day			
oxymetazoline 0.025% solution (OcuClear, Visine L.R.) Dosing: 1–2 drops in the affected eye(s) every 6 hours	Stinging, blurred vision, mydriasis, redness, punctate keratitis, increased IOP	Narrow-angle glaucoma Narrow-angle without glaucoma	Use should be limited to 72 hours. Contains benzalkonium chloride; use with contact lenses not addressed in labeling
phenylephrine 0.12% solution (Relief, Prefrin Liquifilm) Dosing: 1–2 drops up to 4 times a day as needed	Stinging, blurred vision, mydriasis, redness, punctate keratitis, increased IOP	Narrow-angle glaucoma Narrow-angle without glaucoma	May cause rebound miosis and decreased mydriatic response in older persons Use should be limited to 72 hours. Contains benzalkonium chloride; use with contact lenses not addressed in labeling 2.5% and 10% solutions are available for pupil dilation for diagnostic procedures.
tetrahydrozoline 0.05% solution (Visine, Murine Plus, Collyrium Fresh) Dosing: 1–2 drops up to 4 times a day	Stinging, blurred vision, mydriasis, redness, punctate keratitis, increased IOP	Narrow-angle glaucoma Narrow-angle without glaucoma	Use should be limited to 72 hours. Contains benzalkonium chloride; use with contact lenses not addressed in labeling
Topical Corticosteroids medrysone 1% suspension (HMS) Dosing: 1 drop every 4 hours	IOP elevation, loss of visual acuity, cataract formation, stinging and burning	Acute superficial herpes simplex Fungal disease Viral disease of the cornea and conjunctiva Ocular tuberculosis Iritis or uveitis	Not recommended for use in iritis and uveitis Labeling: Wait 15 minutes following administration before inserting contact lenses.
prednisolone 0.12%, 0.125%, or 1% suspension (Pred Mild, Econopred, Pred Forte) or 0.125% or 1% solution (AK-Pred, Inflamase) Dosing Solution: 1–2 drops every hour during the day and every 2 hours at night initially, reduced to 1 drop every 3–4 times a day with favorable response Suspension: 1–2 drops 2–4 times a day; dose may be increased during the initial 24–48 hours	IOP elevation, cataract formation, delayed wound healing, secondary ocular infection, acute uveitis, globe perforation, stinging and burning, conjunctivitis	Dendritic keratitis Fungal disease Viral disease of the cornea and conjunctiva Mycobacterial eye infection Acute, purulent, untreated eye infections	Labeling: Wait 15 minutes following administration before inserting contact lenses.
dexamethasone 0.1% solution (AK-Dex, Decadron) or 0.1% suspension (Maxidex) or 0.05% ointment (Decardon) Dosing Solution: 1–2 drops every hour during the day and every 2 hours at night initially, reduced to 1 drop every 4 hours with favorable response Suspension: 1–2 drops <4–6 times a day in mild disease; hourly in severe disease Ointment: Apply a thin coating of ointment 3 or 4 times a day	IOP elevation, loss of visual acuity, cataract formation, secondary ocular infection, globe perforation, stinging and burning	Dendritic keratitis Fungal disease Viral disease of the cornea and conjunctiva Mycobacterial eye infection	Labeling: Wait 15 minutes following administration before inserting contact lenses.

(continued)

Table 16.3

Overview of Antiallergy Ophthalmic Agents (*Continued*)

Generic (Trade) Name and Dosage	Selected Adverse Events	Contraindications	Special Considerations
loteprednol 0.2% or 0.5% suspension (Alrex, Lotemax) Dosing 0.2% solution: 1 drop in the affected eye(s) 4 times a day 0.5% solution: 1–2 drops in the affected eye(s) 4 times a day	IOP elevation, loss of visual acuity, cataract formation, secondary ocular infection, globe perforation, stinging and burning, dry eye, itching, photophobia	Dendritic keratitis Fungal disease Viral disease of the cornea and conjunctiva Mycobacterial eye infection	If needed, dosing of the 0.5% solution can be increased to 1 drop every hour during the first week of therapy. Labeling: Wait 10 minutes following administration before inserting contact lenses.

contain the preservative benzalkonium chloride (BAK). This preservative, which is in all of the ophthalmic antihistamines, mast cell stabilizers, NSAIDs, vasoconstrictors, and topical steroids reviewed in this section (except for pemirolast), may be absorbed by contact lenses. While no products identify contact lens use as an absolute contraindication to therapy, some (eg, cromolyn, lodoxamide, and nedocromil) have warnings advising against the use of contact lenses during therapy; others advise patients to wait 10 to 15 minutes after administering the medication before reinserting contact lenses (see Table 16-3). Regardless of the etiology, contact lens wearers should refrain from wearing contact lenses during an acute case of conjunctivitis.

Bacterial Conjunctivitis

The treatment of bacterial conjunctivitis is aimed at the organisms *S. aureus*, *S. pneumoniae*, and *H. influenzae*. First-line treatments include 7 to 10 days of therapy with erythromycin ointment (two or three times a day) or polymyxin B–trimethoprim solution (1 drop every 3 to 4 hours). Therapy selection can be based on patient preference for ointment or solution. If bacterial conjunctivitis does not resolve with first-line therapy, the patient should be referred to an eye care professional so that cultures may be taken to rule out *C. trachomatis*. The ophthalmic fluoroquinolones with improved gram-positive organism coverage (gatifloxacin, levofloxacin, or moxifloxacin) can be used as second-line therapy.

Gonococcal infection requires immediate treatment. Ceftriaxone is recommended for adults and children who weigh at least 45 kg; alternatives include ciprofloxacin, ofloxacin, and spectinomycin. Children who weigh less than 45 kg and neonates should receive a reduced dose of ceftriaxone. In adults and children at least 8 years old, *C. trachomatis* infection is treated with azithromycin or doxycycline. Azithromycin should be used in children who weigh at least 45 kg but are less than 8 years old, while neonates and children who weigh less than 45 kg should receive erythromycin base or erythromycin ethylsuccinate.

Seasonal Allergic Conjunctivitis

An ophthalmic antihistamine (emedastine, levocabastine) can be used as first-line therapy for mild seasonal allergic conjunctivitis. If symptom control is inadequate, a brief course

(1 to 2 weeks) of a low-potency topical corticosteroid can be added to the regimen. If the condition is persistent, a mast cell stabilizer or, preferably, an agent with antihistamine and mast cell stabilizer properties (azelastine, epinastine, ketotifen, or olopatadine) can be used. The ophthalmic NSAID ketorolac should be reserved for third-line therapy.

Vernal/Atopic Conjunctivitis

Topical antihistamines (emedastine, levocabastine), oral antihistamines, or mast cell stabilizers (cromolyn, lodoxamide, nedocromil, or pemirolast) can be used as first-line agents for the treatment of vernal or atopic conjunctivitis. For patients with acute exacerbations, a topical corticosteroid can be added to the first-line agent for control of severe symptoms.

Viral Conjunctivitis

There is no effective treatment for viral conjunctivitis; patients should be informed of the risk of spreading the infection to the other eye (in unilateral infection) or to other people. Topical antihistamines, artificial tears, or cool compresses can be used to relieve symptoms. In severe cases of adenoviral keratoconjunctivitis with marked chemosis or lid swelling, epithelial sloughing, or membranous conjunctivitis, topical corticosteroids can be helpful in preventing scarring.

Giant Papillary Conjunctivitis

Treatment of giant papillary conjunctivitis centers around modifying the causative entity. Treatment of mild giant papillary conjunctivitis due to contact lens use can consist of one or more of the following: more frequent replacement of contact lenses, decrease in contact lens wearing time, increase in the frequency of enzyme treatment, use of preservative-free lens care systems, switching to disposable lenses, administration of a mast cell stabilizer, and change of the contact lens polymer. In moderate or severe giant papillary conjunctivitis due to contact lens use, discontinuation of contact lens use for several days or weeks or a brief course of topical corticosteroid therapy may be necessary.

MONITORING PATIENT RESPONSE

If symptoms begin to improve within 48 hours, no follow-up is needed. If there is no improvement, the patient should be referred to an eye care professional for evaluation.

Table 16.4

Recommended Order of Treatment for Conjunctivitis

Order	Agent	Comments
Bacterial Conjunctivitis (non-gonococcal, non-chlamydial)		
First line	Erythromycin ointment *or* Bacitracin-polymyxin B ointment or solution	Ointments tend to cause a greater degree of blurry vision than solutions.
Second line	Ophthalmic fluoroquinolones (gatifloxacin, levofloxacin, or moxifloxacin)	The remaining ophthalmic fluoroquinolones do not provide good staphylococcal coverage.
Seasonal Allergic Conjunctivitis		
First line	Ophthalmic antihistamine	
Second line	Addition of a brief course of low-potency topical corticosteroid to the first-line agent *or* For recurrent or persistent disease: a product with antihistamine/ mast cell stabilizer properties	Use of the topical corticosteroids should not exceed 2 weeks.
Third line	Ophthalmic ketorolac	
Vernal/Atopic Conjunctivitis		
First line	Ophthalmic antihistamine or oral antihistamine *or* Mast cell stabilizer	
Second line	For acute exacerbations: Addition of a brief course of low-potency topical corticosteroid to the first-line agent	
Viral Conjunctivitis		
First line	Topical antihistamines *or* Artificial tears *or* Cold compresses	There is no effective treatment for viral conjunctivitis; treatment is for symptom mitigation.
Second line	In severe cases: A low-potency topical corticosteroid	Use of the topical corticosteroids should not exceed 2 weeks.
Giant Papillary Conjunctivitis		
Mild disease	One or more of the following: Replace contact lenses more frequently, decrease contact lens wearing time, increase the frequency of enzyme treatment, use preservative-free lens care systems, switch to disposable lenses, administer mast cell stabilizer, change the contact lens polymer	
Moderate or severe disease	Same as mild disease *and* Discontinuation of contact lens wear for several days to weeks or a brief course of topical corticosteroid treatment	

PATIENT EDUCATION

It is important to instruct patients with bacterial or viral conjunctivitis to wash their hands carefully to prevent spreading infection. Organisms in bacterial conjunctivitis remain active (and contagious) for 24 to 48 hours after therapy begins, while patients with viral conjunctivitis can remain contagious for up to 14 days. Patients should be taught how to apply the medication in the inner aspect of the lower eyelid. The tip of the container should not touch the eyelashes, as it may contaminate the medication and result in therapy failure or reinfection. Patients should not share eye medications because this can spread the infection. To improve the effectiveness of an ophthalmic antibiotic, crusted eyelids should be gently cleansed before instilling medication. Regardless of the etiology, contact lens wearers should refrain from wearing contact lenses during an acute case of conjunctivitis.

DRY EYE SYNDROME: KERATOCONJUNCTIVITIS SICCA

Keratoconjunctivitis sicca, commonly referred to as dry eye syndrome (DES), is a common ophthalmologic abnormality involving bilateral disruption of tear film on the ocular surface. While estimates vary about the prevalence of dry eye in the United States, the figure of 10 to 14 million Americans with DES is generally accepted (Ekong & Foster, 2004). The prevalence of DES increases with age: 14.4% of Americans over the age of 48 have symptoms of DES, with the prevalence of DES doubling for patients aged 60 and above (Moss et al., 2000). DES can occur intermittently or as a chronic condition that becomes a self-perpetuating syndrome. Patients with DES are at direct risk for potentially blinding infections, including bacterial keratitis (Sheppard, 2003).

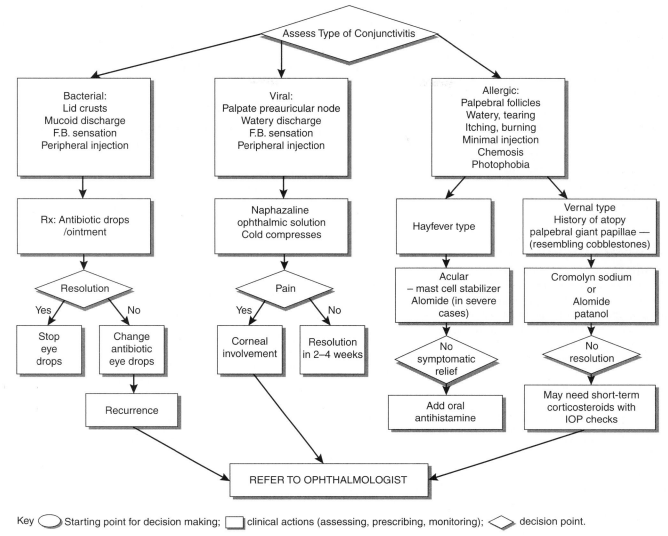

Figure 16–1 Treatment algorithm for conjunctivitis.

CAUSES

DES is a multifactorial disease. It can be the result of decreased tear production, excessive tear evaporation, or abnormality in the production of mucus or lipids found in the tear layer. In addition, decreased tear secretion and clearance initiate an inflammatory response on the ocular surface, and research suggests that this inflammation plays a role in the pathogenesis of DES (Pflugfelder et al., 2000).

Risk factors for DES include advanced age, female gender, and smoking history (Moss et al., 2000). Individuals with concomitant inflammatory conditions (allergies, asthma, or collagen vascular disease), autoimmune disease (rheumatoid arthritis, lupus, colitis), or conditions such as Sjögren's syndrome or Bell's palsy are also at increased risk for DES (AAO, 2003c).

Symptoms caused by dry eye may be exacerbated by environmental factors such as wind, reduced humidity, cigarette smoke, and air conditioning. Systemic medications such as antihistamines, diuretics, anticholinergics, antidepressants, statins, systemic retinoids, and isotretinoin can also exacerbate dry eye symptoms (AAO, 2003c).

PATHOPHYSIOLOGY

Tears are composed of three layers: a mucus layer that coats the cornea, allowing the tear to adhere to the eye; a middle aqueous layer, which provides moisture and supplies oxygen and nutrients to the cornea; and an outer lipid film layer that seals the tear film on the eye and prevents evaporation. Normally, the integrity of the lacrimal system is maintained by a precise interplay of secretions from primary and secondary lacrimal glands located under the eyelids and from sebaceous glands on the flat rims of the eyelid (Wilson, 2003).

Disruptions to the integrity of the lacrimal system can lead to DES. Tear deficiency can be due to poor production of watery tears (resulting from age, hormonal changes, or autoimmune diseases) or excessive evaporation of the watery tear layer (resulting from an insufficient overlying lipid layer). Excessive tear evaporation can result from episodes of decreased blinking (experienced during reading, watching TV, or performing tasks that require intense visual attention) or conditions in which the eyelids cannot be closed (eg, Parkinson's disease and Bell's palsy) (AAO, 2003c). Abnormalities in the production of mucin (resulting from chemical burns to the eye or autoimmune disease) or lipids (due to meibomian gland dysfunction) in the tear layer result in uneven distribution of the tear film across the corneal surface.

Recently, a neurologic/inflammatory component has been promoted as contributing to the pathophysiology of DES. In this theory, the lacrimal glands suffer from neurogenic inflammation, resulting in T-cell activation and cytokine secretion into lacrimal glands, tear film, and conjunctiva (Baudouin, 2001; Wilson, 2003). The resulting inflammation of the ocular surface disrupts sensory signals from the surface of the eye, and the normal stimulus for tear secretion is minimized. The lacrimal glands may also be damaged or destroyed, shutting down the lacrimal system and inciting a self-perpetuating inflammation that the eye's normal defense mechanism cannot repair.

DIAGNOSTIC CRITERIA

Family physicians should always refer patients reporting dry eye to an ophthalmologist (Sheppard, 2003). Making the diagnosis of DES, particularly the mild form, can be difficult because of the inconsistent correlation between reported symptoms and clinical signs, and the relatively poor sensitivity/specificity of existing diagnostic tests (AAO, 2003c). Because most dry eye conditions are chronic, repeat observation will allow a more accurate clinical diagnosis of DES.

Signs and symptoms of DES include a dry eye sensation, ocular irritation, redness, burning, and stinging, a foreign body or gritty sensation, blurred vision, contact lens intolerance, an increased frequency of blinking, and, paradoxically, increased tearing (Pflugfelder et al., 2000). The inability to cry under emotional distress has also been reported among DES patients. DES symptoms tend to worsen in dry climates, in the wind, during air travel, with prolonged visual efforts, and toward the end of the day (AAO, 2003c).

No single diagnostic test or set of tests can confirm or rule out DES (Bron, 2001). However, after a slit-lamp biomicroscopy to rule out other causes of ocular irritation (AAO, 2003c), several tests can be used to lend some objectivity to the diagnosis (Ekong & Foster, 2004). Tear break-up time testing or ocular surface dye staining (rose bengal, fluorescein, sulforhodamine B, or lissamine green) can be useful for patients with mild symptoms. Tear break-up time testing may detect an unstable tear film, while ocular surface dye testing may detect epitheliopathy. For patients with moderate to severe aqueous tear deficiency, the diagnosis can be made with one or more of the following tests (in order of recommendation): tear break-up time, ocular surface dye staining, or the Schirmer wetting test (AAO, 2003c).

INITIATING DRUG THERAPY

Before starting drug therapy, the patient should try nonpharmacologic interventions such as environmental control (increasing air humidity, avoiding drafts) and scheduling regular breaks during computer use and reading. Unfortunately, these interventions result in limited effectiveness and produce few lasting improvements in DES symptoms. Exogenous medical factors that can cause DES (eg, blepharitis) should be addressed, and prescription medications that can exacerbate DES symptoms should be discontinued when possible (AAO, 2003c).

If the nonpharmacologic interventions fail to eliminate DES symptoms, drug therapy is appropriate. Table 16-5 gives information about the drugs used to treat DES.

Goals of Drug Therapy

The goals of drug therapy in DES are to relieve discomfort and prevent complications (vision loss, infection, and structural damage) (AAO, 2003c). Therapy should attempt to normalize tear volume and composition so that the eye tissues are properly lubricated, nourished, and protected, resulting in improved patient satisfaction and clinical outcomes (Wilson, 2003).

Artificial Tears and Lubricants

Artificial tears and lubricants can be used as palliative therapies to relieve DES symptoms. The goal of using tear substitutes is to increase humidity at the ocular surface and to improve lubrication (Calonge, 2001). Designed to mimic the composition of natural tears, artificial tears contain lipids, water with dissolved salts and proteins, and mucin. Artificial tears and lubricants are over-the-counter products, available in a variety of formulations (solutions, gels, ointments). Ointments and gels may make the eyelids sticky and blur vision, and are often used only at bedtime.

For patients with mild DES, use of artificial tears four times daily plus a lubricating ointment at bedtime may be useful. As the severity of dry eye increases, administration of artifical tears can increase to hourly. Preservative-free preparations should be used if the patient applies tears more than four to six times a day (AAO, 2003c; Calonge, 2001).

Pilocarpine

The cholinergic agonist pilocarpine is indicated for the treatment of dry mouth in patients with Sjögren's syndrome. Pilocarpine binds to muscarinic receptors, stimulating secretion of the salivary and sweat glands and improving tear function. Given at 5 mg four times a day, pilocarpine improves tear production and flow and improves the symptoms of dry eye and dry mouth in patients with Sjögren's syndrome (Vivino et al., 1999). The main adverse event is excessive sweating, reported in 40% of patients. Its use is contraindicated in patients with uncontrolled asthma and when miosis is undesirable (acute iritis, narrow-angle glaucoma).

Topical Cyclosporine

Cyclosporine ophthalmic emulsion has been reported to increase aqueous tear production and decrease ocular irritation symptoms in patients with DES. It prevents T cells from activating and releasing cytokines that incite the inflammatory component of dry eye. Side effects include ocular burning, conjunctival hyperemia, discharge, itching, and blurred vision. It is contraindicated in patients with active ocular infections.

Table 16.5

Overview of Dry Eye Syndrome Agents

Generic (Trade) Name and Dosage	Selected Adverse Events	Contraindications	Special Considerations
Artificial Tear Substitutes solutions containing preservatives: Comfort Tears, Dry Eyes, GenTeal, Isopto Tears, Liquifilm Tears, Murine, Murocel, Nu-Tears, Refresh Tears, Teargen, Tears Naturale, Ultra Tears	Stinging, blurred vision		Should not be used more than 4–6 times per day; if use in excess of 4–6 times a day is necessary, use a preservative-free preparation
preservative-free solutions: AquaSite, Bion Tears, Celluvisc, Hypotears PF, Refresh, Refresh Plus, OcuCoat PF, Tears Naturale Free, Viva-Drops	Stinging, blurred vision		
Ocular Lubricants ointments containing preservatives: LubriTears, Stye, Paralube, Lacri-Lube S.O.P.	Blurred vision		
preservative-free ointments: Dry Eyes, Duratears Naturale, HypoTears, Tears Renewed, Lacri-Lube NP, Moisture Eyes PM, Refresh PM	Blurred vision		
Cholinergic pilocarpine 5-mg tablets (Salagen) Dosing: 1 tablet 4 times a day	Excessive sweating, headache, urinary frequency, nausea, flushing, dyspepsia	Uncontrolled asthma Acute iritis Narrow-angle glaucoma	Dehydration may develop from excessive sweating. Visual disturbances may impair the ability to drive, especially at night.
Anti-inflammatory cyclosporine 0.05% emulsion (Restasis) Dosing: 1 drop in each eye twice a day, approximately 12 hours apart	Ocular burning, blurred vision, conjunctival hyperemia, discharge, eye pain, foreign body sensation, pruritus, stinging	Active ocular infection	Use the emulsion from a single-use vial immediately after opening; discard the remaining contents.

Topical Corticosteroids

Topical corticosteroids have been shown to reduce inflammation in DES by reducing cytokine levels in the conjunctival epithelium. Low-dose corticosteroid therapy can be used at infrequent intervals for short-term (2 weeks) suppression of irritation secondary to inflammation (AAO, 2003c). Long-term use of topical corticosteroids is associated with severe side effects, including ocular hypertension, cataract formation, glaucoma, and infection (Calonge, 2001).

Selecting the Most Appropriate Agent

Agent selection is determined by the severity of DES and the underlying pathophysiology (Table 16-6).

First-Line Therapy

For patients with mild DES, the use of a tear substitute four times a day is appropriate. For moderate or severe DES, artificial tears can be used as often as hourly. Preservative-free preparations should be used if the patient uses tears more than four to six times a day. A lubricating ointment applied at bedtime may also be useful.

A patient with DES and underlying Sjögren's syndrome may benefit from therapy with oral pilocarpine 5 mg four times daily.

Second-Line Therapy

Patients who fail to experience any improvement in DES symptoms with artificial tears may benefit from therapy with cyclosporine ophthalmic emulsion 1 drop in each eye twice a day. Due to the side effect profile, corticosteroid therapy is limited to second-line therapy for short-term (2 weeks) suppression of irritation secondary to inflammation.

Table 16.6

Recommended Order of Treatment for Dry Eye

Order	Agent	Comments
First line	Mild DES: artificial tear substitute 4 times a day *or* Moderate to severe DES: preservative-free artificial tear substitute, administered up to hourly	If the patient has underlying Sjögren's syndrome, administer pilocarpine tablets 5 mg 4 times a day.
Second line	Cyclosporine 0.05% ophthalmic emulsion twice a day	Ophthalmic corticosteroid therapy may be useful for the short-term (2-week) suppression of irritation secondary to inflammation.

Third-Line Therapy

Patients with severe DES that fails to respond to drug therapy are candidates for punctate occlusion or tarsorrhaphy.

MONITORING PATIENT RESPONSE

The frequency and extent of follow-up will depend upon the severity of DES and the therapeutic approach selected. Patients with mild DES can be seen once or twice per year for follow-up if symptoms are controlled by therapy. Patients with sterile corneal ulceration associated with DES require careful, sometime daily, monitoring (AAO, 2003c).

PATIENT EDUCATION

Patients with DES should be educated about the chronic nature of the disease and given specific instructions about their therapeutic regimens.

GLAUCOMA (PRIMARY OPEN-ANGLE GLAUCOMA)

Glaucoma is a group of eye diseases involving optic neuropathy characterized by irreversible damage to the optic nerve and retinal ganglion cells. Over time, this deterioration results in the loss of visual sensitivity and field, which frequently goes unnoticed until a significant amount of damage has occurred. An estimated 3 to 4 million Americans have glaucoma, half of whom who are not aware they have the disease. Glaucoma is the second leading cause of irreversible blindness in the United States and the leading cause of blindness among blacks (Quigley & Vitale, 1997; Tielsch et al., 1991a).

There are numerous types of glaucoma, including primary open-angle glaucoma (POAG), acute closed-angle glaucoma, normal-tension glaucoma, and narrow-angle glaucoma. Approximately 70% of glaucoma cases in the United States are POAG; as such, this section will specifically review POAG.

CAUSES

Several studies have shown that the prevalence of POAG increases with increasing IOP (Mitchell et al., 1996; Sommer et al., 1991). The median IOP in large populations is 15.5 ± 2.5 mm Hg. Previously, it was thought that increased IOP was the sole cause of POAG, but it is now recognized that IOP is one of several factors associated with the development of POAG, and an increased IOP is not required for the diagnosis of POAG.

Additional risk factors for the development of POAG include increasing age, black race (four times greater than whites), a family history of glaucoma, a thin central cornea, extreme nearsightedness, and diabetes mellitus (AAO, 2003d; National Eye Institute, 2002; Tielsch et al., 1991a; Tielsch et al., 1994).

PATHOPHYSIOLOGY

Aqueous humor is produced by the ciliary body and secreted into the posterior chamber of the eye. A pressure gradient in the posterior chamber forces the aqueous humor between the iris and lens and through the pupil into the anterior chamber. Aqueous humor in the anterior chamber leaves the eye through two methods: filtration through the trabecular meshwork to Schlemm's canal (80% to 85%), or traversal of the anterior face of the iris and absorption into iris blood vessels (uveoscleral outflow) (Lesar, 2002). In POAG, the increase in IOP is a result of a decrease in the outflow of the aqueous humor through the trabecular meshwork.

DIAGNOSTIC CRITERIA

Symptoms of POAG do not manifest until substantial damage has already occurred. The diagnosis of any glaucoma should be made by an eye care professional. Any patients reporting visual field loss should be referred to an eye care professional for prompt evaluation.

During the physical examination, IOP is measured in each eye, preferably with a Goldmann-type applanation tonometer, before gonioscopy or dilation of the pupil (AAO, 2003d). Unfortunately, the measurement of IOP is not an effective method for screening populations for glaucoma. At an IOP cutoff of 21 mm Hg, the sensitivity for the diagnosis of POAG by tonometry was 47.1% (Tielsch et al., 1991b). As such, the AAO recommends, in addition to the measurement of IOP, that a physical examination include the following elements: patient history, test of pupil reactivity, slit-lamp biomicroscopy of the anterior segment, determination of central corneal thickness, gonioscopy, evaluation of the optic nerve head and retinal nerve fiber layer, documentation of the optic nerve head appearance, evaluation of the fundus, and evaluation of the visual field (AAO, 2003d).

INITIATING DRUG THERAPY

The goal of therapy for POAG is to enhance the patient's health and quality of life by preserving visual function without causing untoward effects of therapy (AAO, 2003d). Most cases of glaucoma can be controlled and vision loss prevented with early detection and treatment. Treatment of POAG entails decreasing aqueous humor production, increasing aqueous outflow, or a combination of both.

Over the past 10 years, glaucoma management has changed significantly, primarily due to the introduction of pharmaceutical agents that have shown clinical effectiveness (Table 16-7). These agents have been associated with a significant reduction in surgery rates among glaucoma patients (Bateman et al., 2002).

Once a target IOP has been determined, treatment may include drug therapy, laser surgery, or incisional surgery. Topical medication is, in most cases, indicated as first-line therapy. Several trials have clearly shown that reducing IOP by treatment with ocular hypotensive medication can prevent or reduce the risk of progression of glaucoma. Further, the greater the reduction in IOP, the greater the reduction in risk for glaucomatous eye damage.

Table 16.7

Overview of Glaucoma Agents

Generic (Trade) Name and Dosage	Selected Adverse Events	Contraindications	Special Considerations
Beta Blockers			
betaxolol 0.25% suspension or 0.5% solution (Betopic, Betopic S) Dosing: 1–2 drops in the affected eye(s) twice daily	Discomfort on instillation, tearing, allergic reactions, decreased corneal sensitivity, edema, bradycardia, hypotension, dizziness	Cardiogenic shock Second- or third-degree AV block Sinus bradycardia Overt cardiac failure	A cardioselective (beta-1) blocker, it has fewer effects on pulmonary and cardiovascular parameters.
carteolol 1% solution (Ocupress) Dosing: 1 drop in the affected eye(s) twice daily	Transient eye irritation, burning, tearing, conjunctival hyperemia, edema, bradycardia, hypotension, arrhythmia, palpitations	Bronchial asthma or severe COPD Sinus bradycardia Second- or third-degree AV block Overt cardiac failure Cardiogenic shock	May be absorbed systemically; the same adverse reactions seen with oral beta blockers may occur May mask the symptoms of acute hypoglycemia or hyperthyroidism
levobunolol 0.25% or 0.5% solution (AKBeta, Betagan Liquidfilm) Dosing: 1–2 drops in the affected eye(s) once daily (0.5%) or twice daily (0.25%).	Burning and stinging, blepharoconjunctivitis, urticartia, ataxia, bradycardia, arrhythmia, hypotension, syncope, heart block	Bronchial asthma or severe COPD Sinus bradycardia Second- or third-degree AV block Overt cardiac failure Cardiogenic shock	May be absorbed systemically; the same adverse reactions seen with oral beta blockers may occur May mask the symptoms of acute hypoglycemia or hyperthyroidism
metipranolol 0.3% solution (OptiPranolol) Dosing: 1 drop in the affected eye(s) twice a day	Transient local discomfort, conjunctivitis, eyelid dermatitis, blepharitis, blurred vision, headache, asthenia, angina, palpitation, bradycardia	Bronchial asthma or severe COPD Symptomatic sinus bradycardia Second- or third-degree AV block Overt cardiac failure Cardiogenic shock	May be absorbed systemically; the same adverse reactions seen with oral beta blockers may occur May mask the symptoms of acute hypoglycemia or hyperthyroidism
timolol 0.25% or 0.5% solution (Timpotic, Betimol) or gel-forming solution (Timoptic-XE) Dosing Solution: 1 drop in the affected eye(s) twice daily Gel-forming solution: 1 drop in the affected eye(s) once daily	Ocular irritation, decreased corneal sensitivity, visual disturbances, conjunctivitis, tearing, headache, dizziness, bradycardia, arrhythmia	Bronchial asthma or severe COPD Sinus bradycardia Second- or third-degree AV block Overt cardiac failure Cardiogenic shock	May be absorbed systemically; the same adverse reactions seen with oral beta blockers may occur May mask the symptoms of acute hypoglycemia or hyperthyroidism Other ophthalmic medications should be administered 10 minutes before the gel-forming solution.
Carbonic Anhydrase Inhibitors			
dorzolamide 1% solution (Trusopt) Dosing: 1 drop in the affected eye(s) 3 times a day	Ocular burning and stinging, bitter taste, keratitis, ocular allergy, blurred vision, tearing, photophobia	Sulfa allergy	
brinzolamide 1% suspension (Azopt) Dosing: 1 drop in the affected eye(s) 3 times a day	Blurred vision, bitter taste, blepharitis, dermatitis, dry eye, headache, hyperemia ocular pain, pruritus	Sulfa allergy	
Prostaglandins			
latanoprost 0.005% solution (Xalatan) Dosing: 1 drop in the affected eye(s) once daily in the evening	Iris discoloration, blurred vision, burning and stinging, conjunctival hyperemia, itching, eyelash changes, eyelid skin darkening		Iris discoloration is irreversible. Requires refrigeration until dispensed.
travoprost 0.004% solution (Travatan) Dosing: 1 drop in the affected eye(s) once daily in the evening	Ocular hyperemia, decreased visual acuity, eye discomfort, foreign body sensation, eye pain, pruritus		Iris discoloration is irreversible. May interfere in pregnancy; should not be used during pregnancy or by those attempting to become pregnant
bimatoprost 0.03% solution (Lumigan) Dosing: 1 drop in the affected eye(s) once daily in the evening	Conjunctival hyperemia, growth of eyelashes, ocular pruritus, dry eye, iris discoloration, visual disturbance, eye pain, pigmentation of the periocular skin, foreign body sensation		Iris discoloration is irreversible; incidence less than with latanoprost.

(continued)

Table 16.7

Overview of Glaucoma Agents (*Continued*)

Generic (Trade) Name and Dosage	Selected Adverse Events	Contraindications	Special Considerations
unoprostone 0.15% solution (Rescula) Dosing: 1 drop into the affected eye(s) twice daily	Burning and stinging, dry eye, itching, increased length of eyelashes, injection, abnormal vision, corneal edema, hyperpigmentation of eyelid or iris		Iris discoloration is irreversible.
Adrenergic Agonists brimonidine 0.15% or 0.2% solution (Alphagan, Alphagan P) Dosing: 1 drop in the affected eye(s) 3 times a day, approximately 8 hours apart	Ocular hyperemia, ocular pruritus, visual disturbance, somnolence, headache, fatigue, drowsiness, dry mouth	Patients receiving MAO inhibitors	Not recommended in children <2 years old
apraclonidine 0.5% solution (Iopidine) Dosing: 1–2 drops in the affected eye(s) 3 times a day	Hyperemia, tearing, pruritus, lid edema, dry mouth, foreign body sensation, eyelid retraction	Hypersensitivity to clonidine Patients receiving MAO inhibitors	For short-term use only A 1% solution is available for prevention of postsurgical elevations in IOP.
epinephrine 0.1%, 0.5%, 1%, or 2% solution (Epifrin, Glaucon) Dosing: 1 drop in the affected eye(s) once or twice daily	Stinging and burning, brow ache, eye pain, headache, conjunctival hyperemia, conjunctival or corneal pigmentation, palpitations, tachycardia	Narrow- or shallow-angle glaucoma Aphakia Patients for whom the nature of the glaucoma is not clearly established	Do not administer while wearing soft contact lenses. Use with caution in patients with hypertension, hyperthyroidism, diabetes, heart disease, cerebral arteriosclerosis, and asthma.
dipivefrin 0.1% solution and liquid (Propine, AKPro) Dosing: 1 drop into the eye(s) every 12 hours	Stinging and burning, conjunctival injection, follicular conjunctivitis, mydriasis, tachycardia, arrhythmias	Narrow-angle glaucoma	A prodrug of epinephrine Caution should be used in aphakic patients.
Cholinergic Blocking Agents carbachol 0.75%, 1.5%, 2.25%, or 3% solution (Isopto Carbachol, Carboptic) Dosing: 2 drops into eye(s) 3 times a day	Blurred vision or change in near or distance vision, eye pain, stinging and burning, headache, stomach cramps, salivation	Acute iritis or other conditions where papillary constriction is undesirable	Patients should use caution while night driving or performing hazardous tasks in poor light.
demecarium 0.125% or 0.25% solution (Humorsol) Dosing: 1–2 drops in affected eye(s) from twice daily to twice weekly	Iris cysts, burning, lacrimation, lid muscle twitching, brow ache, nausea, diarrhea, retinal detatchment	Pregnancy Acute uveal inflammation Glaucoma associated with iridocyclitis	Very long-acting agent If the patient does not respond within 24 hours of initial therapy, other measures should be considered.
pilocarpine 0.25%, 0.5%, 1%, 2%, 3%, 4%, 5%, 6%, 8%, or 10% solution (Pilocar, Piloptic, Pilostat, Isopto Carpine) or 4% gel (Pilopine HS) Dosing: Solution: 1–2 drops 3 or 4 times a day Gel: ½-inch ribbon in the lower conjunctival sac of affected eye(s) once daily at bedtime	Stinging and burning, tearing, ciliary spasm, blurred vision, brow ache, hypertension, tachycardia, bronchospasm, salivation	Acute iritis or other conditions where papillary constriction is undesirable	A weekly pilocarpine ocular insert (Ocusert) is available.
Combination Products pilocarpine and epinephrine 1%-1%, 2%-1%, 4%-1%, or 6%-1% solutions (P$_1$E$_\#$, E-Pilo-#) Dosing: 1–2 drops into the eye(s) 1–4 times daily	See individual components.	See individual components.	Opposing actions on the pupil may prevent marked miosis and mydriasis.
dorzolamide and timolol 2%-0.5% solution (Cosopt) Dosing: 1 drop into the affected eye(s) 2 times a day	See individual components.	See individual components.	Combined effect results in greater IOP lowering than either agent alone, but not as great as dorzolamide 3 times a day and timolol 2 times a day administered concomitantly.

AV, atrioventricular mode; COPD, chronic obstructive pulmonary disease; MAO, monoamine oxidase.

Goals of Drug Therapy

The goals of drug therapy for POAG are to reduce IOP to a target level and to prevent or slow the progression of vision loss. In patients with POAG, the initial IOP target should be 20% to 30% lower than baseline. Additional IOP lowering to 40% or more below baseline is justified by the severity of existing optic nerve damage, the height of the measured IOP and the rapidity at which the damage occurred, and the presence of other risk factors such as family history and race (AAO, 2003d). Visual fields and optic nerve photographs should be monitored for signs of change; if progression is detected, the IOP target should be lowered an additional 15% (AAO, 2003d).

Beta Blockers

Beta-blockers are the benchmark against which other IOP-lowering medications are measured. Beta blockers reduce adenylyl cyclase activity, which in turn reduces the production of aqueous humor in the ciliary body. Beta blockers lower IOP an average of 20% to 30%. There are five ophthalmic beta blockers available in the United States: timolol, levobunolol, carteolol, and metipranolol are nonselective beta blockers, while betaxolol is a beta$_1$-selective agent. Although nonselective beta blockers may be more efficacious in lowering IOP, selective beta blockers appear to be better tolerated systemically, particularly in patients with chronic obstructive pulmonary disease.

The ophthalmic beta blockers are typically applied twice daily. Timolol is available in a solution that forms a gel upon application, allowing once-daily dosing. Side effects include stinging, burning, dry eye, and blurred vision. Topical beta blockers can be absorbed systemically and may cause bradycardia, reduced blood pressure, aggravation of congestive heart failure, heart block, bronchospasm in asthma patients, and central nervous system side effects such as hallucinations and depression. Betaxolol is less likely to cause these systemic side effects, but a risk still exists. All of the ophthalmic beta blockers are contraindicated in patients with sinus bradycardia, second- or third-degree atrioventricular node block, overt cardiac failure, and cardiogenic shock, and all except betaxolol are contraindicated in patients with bronchial asthma or severe chronic obstructive pulmonary disease.

Prostaglandins

The prostaglandin F$_{2\alpha}$ analogs bimatoprost, latanoprost, and travoprost and the docosonoid unoprostone reduce IOP by improving the uveoscleral outflow of aqueous humor. Given once a day, the prostaglandin F$_{2\alpha}$ analogs reduce IOP by 25% to 35%; unoprostone is given twice daily and is substantially less effective than either timolol or latanoprost in reducing IOP. A study of bimatoprost, latanoprost, and travoprost found no statistical difference in IOP lowering between agents (Parrish et al., 2003).

These agents are more effective when given at bedtime rather than in the morning. Further, dosing in excess of once a day may decrease the IOP-lowering effect. Latanoprost requires refrigeration until dispensed; latanoprost and travoprost should be discarded within 6 weeks of the time the package is opened. Side effects of the prostaglandins and unoprostone include ocular hyperemia, blurred vision, pruritus, dry eye, lengthening and thickening of the eyelashes, and conjunctival hyperemia. These agents are also associated with irreversible iris discoloration, most often affecting patients with mixed-color irises. Iris discoloration is reported by 7% to 12% of latanoprost users, with discoloration starting between 18 and 26 weeks after commencement of therapy. Compared to latanoprost, the incidence of iris discoloration is lower for bimatoprost, travoprost, and unoprostone. In addition, darkening of the eyelid skin can occur with these agents.

Carbonic Anhydrase Inhibitors

The topical carbonic anhydrase inhibitors (CAIs) brinzolamide and dorzolamide work through the reversible and competitive binding of carbonic anhydrase. Carbonic anhydrase acts as a catalyst for the reversible hydration of carbonic acid, which plays a role in fluid transport in various cell systems. By decreasing bicarbonate formation, movement of sodium and fluid into the posterior chamber declines and less aqueous fluid is generated, reducing IOP (Fischella, 2002). While the topical CAIs reduce IOP to a lesser extent (15% to 26%) than beta blockers, prostaglandins, or systemic CAIs, they are rarely associated with systemic side effects.

The topical CAIs are given three times a day. Side effects include ocular burning and stinging, bitter taste, blurred vision, itching, tearing, and keratitis. The topical CAIs are contraindicated in patients with hypersensitivity to sulfonamides, and are not recommended for use in patients with severe renal impairment, respiratory acidosis, and electrolyte disorders.

The systemic CAIs (acetazolamide, methazolamide, and dichlorphenamide) are the most potent agents for reducing IOP, producing a 25% to 40% decrease in IOP. However, these agents produce severe side effects such as paresthesias, gastrointestinal disturbances (anorexia, nausea, and weight loss), metallic taste, central nervous system effects (lethargy, malaise, and depression), electrolyte disturbances, and renal calculi, which limit their use. Elderly patients do not tolerate systemic CAIs as well as younger patients (Lesar, 2002).

Adrenergic Agonists

The adrenergic agonists (apraclonidine, epinephrine, dipivefrin, and brimonidine) vary in their level of alpha and beta selectivity. Agents with alpha-2 activity (apraclonidine, brimonidine) activate the presynaptic alpha-2 receptors, inhibiting the release of norepinephrine. As less norepinephrine is available for activation of postsynaptic beta receptors on the ciliary epithelium, the formation of aqueous humor is reduced. The nonselective adrenergic agonists epinephrine and dipivefrin (epinephrine prodrug) have both alpha- and beta-adrenergic activity; the alpha activity results in decreased aqueous production, while the beta activity increases aqueous production and may also stimulate conventional and uveoscleral outflow.

Apraclonidine and brimonidine reduce IOP by 18% to 27%. Brimonidine is a highly selective alpha-2 agonist, causing little or no alpha-1 activity. In addition to decreasing aqueous humor, it increases uveoscleral outflow. Side effects include dry mouth, fatigue, ocular hyperemia, somnolence, and headache. Apraclonidine is a relatively selective alpha-2 agonist; it is associated with some alpha-1 activity, which can lead to mydriasis, conjunctival bleeding, and eyelid retraction. Apraclonidine is primarily indicated for short-term adjunctive therapy, as the efficacy of apraclonidine diminishes over time; the benefit for most patients lasts less than 1 to 2 months. Both agents are contraindicated in patients taking monoamine oxidase inhibitors. In addition, brimonidine has been associated with respiratory and cardiac depression in infants, and should be used with caution in children under age 2.

Epinephrine and dipivefrin provide poor IOP control. Side effects include stinging and tearing, brow ache, and the formation of black conjunctival spots and conjunctival deposits. Epinephrine is contraindicated in aphakic patients and patients for whom the nature of the glaucoma is not clearly established. Use should be avoided in patients with hyperthyroidism or cardiac disease and in those taking monoamine oxidase inhibitors or tricyclic antidepressants (Bendel & Juzych, 2001). Because of the side effects and limited efficacy, these agents are rarely used today.

Cholinergic Blocking Agents

There are two types of cholinergic blocking agents: direct acting (pilocarpine) and indirect acting (eg, demecarium). Direct-acting cholinergics stimulate the parasympathetic muscarinic receptor site to increase aqueous outflow through the trabecular meshwork. While effective in lowering IOP by 20% to 30%, pilocarpine usually needs to be given four times a day. Side effects include eye pain, brow ache, blurred vision, and accommodative spasms. It can also provoke miotic responses such as papillary constriction, which can decrease night vision. The intense dosing regimen and the side effect profile make adherence difficult. A once-daily pilocarpine gel may be helpful when therapy adherence is an issue.

The indirect-acting cholinergics promote the accumulation of acetylcholine at the muscarinic receptors, stimulating increased aqueous outflow. In addition to the side effects of the direct-acting cholinergics, the indirect-acting agents may produce cataracts, iris cysts, occlusion of the nasolacrimal ducts, and corneal toxicity. Demecarium is a very long-acting agent and should only be used when shorter-acting agents have proven inadequate. Further, if the patient fails to respond within 24 hours of initial therapy, other measures should be considered. Demecarium is contraindicated during pregnancy, in patients with acute uveal infiltration, and for glaucoma associated with iridocyclitis.

Carbachol possesses the properties of both direct-acting and indirect-acting cholinergic blocking agents. It is most similar to pilocarpine but is more potent and can produce more pronounced side effects, including brow pain.

Combination Products

Combination products simplify administration and can promote adherence to therapy. Solutions of pilocarpine are available in a variety of strengths (1%, 2%, 4%, or 6%) with epinephrine 1%. When administered together, the opposing actions on the pupil may prevent marked miosis and mydriasis. A solution of dorzolamide 2% and timolol 0.5% is also available; the combined effect results in additional IOP reduction compared to either agent alone, but the result is less than dorzolamide three times a day and timolol two times a day administered separately.

Selecting the Most Appropriate Agent

The AAO does not recommend a specific agent as first-line therapy. When the first-line agent drug fails to reduce IOP, the AAO recommends that it be discontinued in favor of another therapy before the original agent is supplanted by other medications. When selecting the first-line therapy for glaucoma, factors such as efficacy, side effects, cost, and dosing frequency should all be considered. About 70% of patients need new or extra medications within 2 years after the start of drug treatment. Table 16-8 lists the recommended order of treatment for these agents.

First-Line Therapy

The prostaglandins have been recommended as first-line therapy for POAG, as they possess the best balance between efficacy, safety, and ease of dosing regimen (Schwartz & Budenz, 2004).

Second-Line Therapy

If the prostaglandin fails to decrease IOP to a significant extent, the patient should be switched to a different class of medicine. Beta blockers are recommended because of their efficacy, tolerability, and ease of dosing (Schwartz & Budenz, 2004). If the IOP decreases with a prostaglandin but fails to reach the target IOP, a beta blocker should be added.

Table 16.8

Recommended Order of Treatment for Glaucoma

Order	Agent	Comments
First line	Prostaglandin ophthalmic solution (bimatorpost, latanoprost, or travoprost)	An ophthalmic beta blocker may be substituted if the patient cannot afford the prostaglandins.
Second line	Substitution of an ophthalmic beta blocker (if failure to decrease IOP to a significant extent) *or* Addition of an ophthalmic beta blocker (if IOP is significantly decreased but not to goal)	
Third line	Addition of an ophthalmic carbonic anhydrase inhibitor *or* Addition of brimonidine	Dorzolamide is available in a combination product with timolol.

Third-Line Therapy

If a patient fails to reach the target IOP with the first-line and second-line therapies, a topical CAI (usually the fixed combination of timolol and dorzolamide to keep the dosing regimen simple) can be added. If this fails, dorzolamide should be discontinued in favor of brimonidine (Schwartz & Budenz, 2004).

MONITORING PATIENT RESPONSE

Patients with POAG should receive follow-up evaluations and care from their eye care professional to determine the effectiveness of therapy. In addition to a recent history, a physical examination including a slit-lamp biomicroscopy and tests of visual acuity and IOP in each eye should be performed (AAO, 2003d). The practitioner must distinguish between the impact of a prescribed agent on IOP and ordinary background fluctuations of IOP.

PATIENT EDUCATION

Patients should wash their hands before administering glaucoma medications. Patients should be taught how to apply the medication in the inner aspect of the lower eyelid. The tip of the container should not touch the eyelashes or any part of the eye, as this may contaminate the medication. Contact lenses should be removed prior to administration, and patients should separate administration of different glaucoma medications by at least 10 minutes.

■ Case Study

J.S., age 7, presents with a feeling that there is sand in his eye. He had a cold a week ago and woke up this morning with his left eye crusted with yellowish drainage. On physical examination, he has injected conjunctiva on the left side, no adenopathy, and no vision changes. His vision is 20/20. Fluorescein staining reveals no abrasion. He is allergic to sulfa.

Diagnosis: Conjunctivitis

1. List specific goals of treatment for J.S.
2. What drug therapy would you prescribe? Why?
3. What are the parameters for monitoring the success of the therapy?
4. List one or two adverse reactions for the selected agent that would cause you to change therapy.
5. What would be the choice for second-line therapy?
6. Describe one or two drug/drug or drug/food interactions for the selected agent.
7. Discuss the education you would give to the parents regarding drug therapy.
8. What over-the-counter or alternative medications would be appropriate for J.S.?
9. What dietary and lifestyle changes should be recommended for J.S.?

Bibliography

Starred references are cited in the text.

*American Academy of Ophthalmology Cornea/External Disease Panel, Preferred Practice Guidelines Committee. (2003a). *Blepharitis*. San Francisco: AAO.

*American Academy of Ophthalmology Cornea/External Disease Panel, Preferred Practice Guidelines Committee. (2003b). *Conjunctivitis*. San Francisco: AAO.

*American Academy of Ophthalmology Cornea/External Disease Panel, Preferred Practice Guidelines Committee. (2003c). *Dry eye syndrome*. San Francisco: AAO.

*American Academy of Ophthalmology Cornea/External Disease Panel, Preferred Practice Guidelines Committee. (2003d). *Primary open-angle glaucoma*. San Francisco: AAO.

*American Academy of Pediatrics. (2000). Chlamydial infections. In: L. K. Pickering (Ed.), *Red Book: report of the Committee on Infectious Diseases* (25th ed., pp. 208–211). Elk Grove Village, IL: American Academy of Pediatrics.

*Bateman, D. N., Clark, R., Azuara-Blanco, A., et al. (2002). The effects of new topical treatments of management of glaucoma in Scotland: an examination of ophthalmological health care. *British Journal of Ophthalmology*, 86, 551–554.

*Baudouin, C. (2001). The pathology of dry eye. *Survey of Ophthalmology*, 45(Suppl. 2), S211–S220.

*Bendel, R. E., & Juzych, M. S. (2001). Principles and complications of medical therapy of glaucoma. In: T. J. Zimmerman & K. S. Kooner (Eds.), *Clinical pathways in glaucoma*. New York: Thieme.

Brewitt, H., & Sistani, F. Dry eye disease: the scale of the problem. *Survey of Ophthalmology*, 45(Suppl. 2), S199–S202.

*Bron, A. J. (2001). Diagnosis of dry eye. *Survey of Ophthalmology*, *45*(Suppl. 2), S221–S226.

*Calonge, M. (2001). The treatment of dry eye. *Survey of Ophthalmology*, *45*(Suppl. 2), S227–S239.

*Chen, J. Y. (1992). Prophylaxis of ophthalmia neonatorium: comparison of silver nitrate, tetracycline, erythromycin, and no prophylaxis. *Pediatric Infectious Disease*, *11*, 1026–1030.

Dalzell, M. D. (2002). Glaucoma: prevalence, utilization, and economic implications. *Pharmacy and Therapeutics*, *27*(Suppl. 11), 10–15.

Dalzell, M. D. (2003). Dry eye: prevalence, utilization, and economic implications. *Managed Care*, *12*(Suppl. 12), 9–13.

*Ekong, A. S., & Foster, C. S. (2004). Dry eye syndrome. E-medicine: http://www.emedicine.com/oph/topic597.htm Accessed July 30, 2004.

*Fischella, R. G. (2002). Glaucoma medications: a drug-therapy review. *P&T*, *27*(Suppl. 11), 25–31.

Goldberg, L. D. (2002). Clinical guidelines for the treatment of glaucoma. *P&T*, *27*(Suppl. 11), 16–24.

*Horton, J. C. (1998). Disorders of the eye. In: A. S. Fauci (Ed.), *Harrison's principles of internal medicine* (14th ed., pp 158–172). New York: McGraw-Hill.

Lemp, M. A. (2003). Contact lenses and associated anterior segment disorders: dry eye, blepharitis, and allergy. *Ophthalmology Clinics of North America*, *16*(3), 463–469.

*Lesar, T. S. (2002). Glaucoma. In: J. T. Dipiro (Ed.), *Pharmacotherapy: a pathophysiologic approach* (5th ed., pp. 1665–1678). New York: McGraw-Hill.

*McCulley, J. P., Dougherty, J. M., & Deneau, D. G. (1982). Classification of chronic blepharitis. *Ophthalmology*, *89*, 1173–1180.

McCulley, J. P., & Shine, W. E. (2000). Changing concepts in the diagnosis and management of blepharitis. *Cornea*, *19*(5), 650–658.

McCulley, J. P., & Shine, W. E. (2003). Eyelid disorders: the meibomian gland, blepharitis, and contact lenses. *Eye & Contact Lens*, *29*(1S), S93–S95.

*Mitchell, P., Smith, W., Attebo, K., & Healey, P. R. (1996). Prevalence of open-angle glaucoma in Australia. *Ophthalmology*, *103*, 1661–1669.

*Morrow, G. L., & Abbott, R. L. (1998). Conjunctivitis. *American Family Physician*, *57*(4), 735–746.

*Moss, S. E., Klein, R., & Klein, B. E. (2000). Prevalence and risk factors for dry eye syndrome. *Archives of Ophthalmology*, *118*, 1264–1268.

*National Eye Institute. (2002). *Vision problems in the U.S.* Bethesda, MD: Prevent Blindness America.

*Parrish, R. K., Palmberg, P., Sheu, W. P., et al. (2003). A comparison of latanoprost, bimatoprost, and travoprost in patients with open-angle glaucoma or ocular hypertension: a 12-week, randomized, masked-evaluator multicenter study. *American Journal of Ophthalmology*, *135*, 688–703.

*Pflugfelder, S. C., Solomon, A., & Stern, M. E. (2000). The diagnosis and management of dry eye: a twenty-five year review. *Cornea*, *19*, 644–649.

*Quigley, H. A., & Vitale, S. (1997). Models of glaucoma prevalence and incidence in the United States. *Investigative Ophthalmology & Visual Science*, *38*, 83–91.

*Schwartz, K., & Budenz, D. (2004). Current management of glaucoma. *Current Opinion in Ophthalmology*, *15*, 119–126.

*Sheppard, J. D. (2003). Dry eye moves beyond palliative care. *Managed Care*, *12*(Suppl. 12), 6–8.

*Shields, S. R. (2000). Managing eye disease in primary care. *Postgraduate Medicine*, *108*(5), 83–96.

*Shovlin, J. P., & DePaolis, M. D. (Sept. 15, 2002). Managing lid disease in lens wearers. *Review of Optometry*, *139*(9).

*Silverman, M. A., & Bessman, E. (2003). Conjunctivitis. E-medicine: http://www.emedicine.com/emerg/topic110.htm Accessed July 30, 2004.

*Sommer, A., Tielsch, J. M., Katz, J., et al. (1991). Racial differences in cause-specific prevalence of blindness in East Baltimore. *New England Journal of Medicine*, *325*, 1412–1417.

*Song, P. I., Abraham, T. A., Park, Y., et al. (2001). The expression of functional LPS receptor proteins CD14 and toll-like receptor 4 in human corneal cells. *Investigative Ophthalmology & Visual Science*, *42*, 2867–2877.

*Teoh, D. L., & Reynolds, S. (2003). Diagnosis and management of pediatric conjunctivitis. *Pediatric Emergency Care*, *19*(1), 48–55.

*Tielsch, J. M., Katz, J., Sommer, M., et al. (1994). Family history and risk of primary open-angle glaucoma. *Archives of Ophthalmology*, *112*, 69–73.

*Tielsch, J. M., Sommer, A., Katz, J., et al. (1991a). Racial variations in the prevalence of primary open-angle glaucoma. *JAMA*, *266*, 369–374.

*Tielsch, J. M., Katz, J., Singh, K., et al. (1991b). A population-based evaluation of glaucoma screening: the Baltimore Eye Survey. *American Journal of Epidemiology*, *134*, 1102–1110.

*Vivino, F. B., Al-Hashima, I., Khan, Z., et al. (1999). Pilocarpine tablets for the treatment of dry mouth and dry eye symptoms in patients with Sjögren syndrome. *Archives of Internal Medicine*, *159*, 174–181.

*Wilson, S. E. (2003). Inflammation: a unifying theory for the origin of dry eye syndrome. *Managed Care*, *12*(Suppl. 12), 14–19.

Visit the Connection web site for the most up-to-date drug information.

17

OTITIS MEDIA AND OTITIS EXTERNA

■ LINDA ZIMMERMAN AND ANDREW M. PETERSON

Infections of the ear are a common problem in children, but they can also affect adults. Otitis media, chronic otitis, and serous otitis media are common middle ear infections. Otitis externa, also known as *swimmer's ear*, is usually associated with recent water exposure or trauma.

Diagnosis and treatment of both otitis media and otitis externa are essential to prevent hearing loss and other serious complications, including mastoiditis, bacteremia, and meningitis. Factors differentiating acute otitis media (AOM), serous otitis media, and otitis externa are summarized in Table 17-1.

OTITIS MEDIA

In 1990, more than 25 million physician visits were attributed to otitis media, resulting in 809 antibacterial prescriptions per 1,000 visits. By the year 2000, the number of office visits decreased to 16 million, yet the number of prescriptions remained relatively the same, at 802 per 1,000 visits (AAP/AAFP Guidelines, 2004). AOM is most common in infants and children between the ages of 6 months and 2 years, but the infection may occur at any age. Otitis media occurs in 60% to 70% of all children by the end of the first year of life and in more than 90% by age 7 (Hoberman et al., 2002). Some children who are "susceptible" to ear infections may experience three or four episodes of otitis yearly. Recurrent otitis media is more common in children who experience their first ear infection by 6 months of age.

The disorder is more common in the fall, winter, and spring and also more common in boys than girls. It is very common and often serious in the Eskimo and Native American populations. Most AOM infections in children resolve with appropriate treatment, but chronic effusions develop in 10% to 20% of these children as a result of reinfection because of incomplete eradication of the organism (Karver, 1998).

CAUSES

AOM frequently follows an upper respiratory infection in which the eustachian tube closes secondary to swollen mucous membranes. The swelling obstructs the eustachian tube, which normally drains secretions into the nasopharynx. This causes eustachian tube dysfunction and negative pressure in the middle ear, which then permits fluid and bacteria to be pulled into the middle ear from the mucosal lining. The result is the inflammation known as AOM.

The bacteria most frequently associated with AOM are *Streptococcus pneumoniae* (35% of infections), *Haemophilus influenzae* (25% of infections), and *Moraxella catarrhalis* (15% of infections). These bacteria are most common in neonates and children. *S. pneumoniae* and *H. influenzae* are the most common organisms affecting the adult population. Most ear infections are viral, but it is difficult to distinguish between the etiologies.

Risk factors for AOM include male sex, upper respiratory infections, smoking, allergies, and congenital defects, such as cleft palate. Children who have not been breast-fed or who have been breast-fed for only a short time are at greater risk. Infant feeding methods are also factors in otitis media. For infants, breast-feeding has a protective effect against respiratory viruses, thereby limiting the exposure of the eustachian tube to microbial pathogens. Reflux of milk into the eustachian tube is also less likely in breast-fed infants because of the feeding position. Adults with tonsils and adenoids are at risk for otitis media when they have upper respiratory infections, allergies, and barotrauma (eg, from airplane travel).

Serous otitis media, also known as otitis media with effusion, results from prolonged blockage of the eustachian tube, which causes negative pressure that allows fluid to accumulate in the middle ear. Fluid that was once thought to be bacteria-free and nonpurulent has now been identified as harboring *Pseudomonas aeruginosa*, *Proteus* species, *Staphylococcus aureus*, and mixed anaerobic organisms, but the effusion may persist for several months without signs of infection.

The etiology of noninfectious otitis media is unknown. The inflammation does, however, frequently result from eustachian tubes blocked by edema related to allergic rhinitis, viral illness, previous acute episodes of otitis media, or hypertrophic adenoids.

PATHOPHYSIOLOGY

The eustachian tube protects the middle ear from nasopharyngeal secretions, provides drainage of secretions produced in the middle ear into the nasopharynx, and permits equilibration of air pressure to atmospheric pressure in the middle ear. The structure of a child's eustachian tube differs from

Table 17.1

Comparing Kinds of Otitis

Acute Otitis Media	Serous Otitis Media	Otitis Externa
Etiology		
Streptococcus pneumoniae	Eustachian tube obstruction causing sterile effusion in the middle ear	Infectious: *Pseudomonas aeruginosa, Staphylococcus aureus, Streptococcus* sp.
Haemophilus influenzae		Malignant: *P. aeruginosa*
Moraxella catarrhalis		
Mycoplasma pneumoniae is associated with bullous myringitis.		
Symptoms*		
Otalgia	Hearing loss that may be manifested by delayed language development in young children or decreased school performance in older children	Infectious: Erythema and swelling of the external canal with otalgia and itching; muffled hearing; watery or thick discharge from the ear
Ear pulling		
Upper respiratory infection symptoms	Feeling of ear fullness	Malignant: Persistent foul-smelling discharge, and deep ear pain
Fever	Popping sensation with swallowing, yawning, or blowing the nose	
Vertigo		
Otorrhea		
Decreased hearing		
Clinical Findings		
Diffuse redness and bulging of the tympanic membrane	Clear, yellowish, or bluish-gray fluid behind the tympanic membrane, with or without air bubbles	Infectious: Pain with movement of tragus; raised area of induration on the tragus; swollen external auditory canal; red pustular lesions
Decreased movement of the tympanic membrane	The tympanic membrane may be retracted with decreased movement.	Malignant: Progressive cranial nerve palsies; granulations in the external ear canal
Possibly, perforation of the tympanic membrane		
Reddish-purple blister on the tympanic membrane or at the junction of the membrane and the canal (bullous myringitis)		

* Note: Some patients with acute otitis media or serous otitis media do not have symptoms.

that of an adult's. The adult eustachian tube lies at 45 degrees to the horizontal plane. The bony portion of the tube is always open, with the exception of the medial cartilaginous portion, which is usually closed. At least four muscles are involved in opening the tube.

The middle ear is covered with respiratory epithelial mucosa that secretes mucus. An adult ear clears this mucus as it is produced. The child's eustachian tube, however, is short and horizontal and does not function as well as the adult's. In addition, a child has a cartilaginous tube that is not as stiff as an adult's, and the muscles that open the tube are poorly developed. When a child has mild inflammation or edema of the eustachian tube, the ear has difficulty clearing the mucus that is normally produced by the epithelial mucosa.

Often the precursor to AOM is a viral upper respiratory tract infection (Hoberman et al., 2002). The viral infection causes an inflammation of the mucosa, causing eustachian tube dysfunction and leading to a retention of bacteria, ending up as an AOM. If the inflammation subsides and the eustachian tube function returns, an AOM may not develop.

DIAGNOSTIC CRITERIA

AOM, which is commonly bilateral in children and unilateral in adults, causes otalgia that may be aggravated by sucking and chewing. Fever, postauricular and cervical lymphadenopathy, dizziness, and nausea can accompany the ear pain. Infants may become irritable and hold or pull their ears. On inspection, the tympanic membrane appears bulging, with unidentifiable landmarks, erythema, and limited mobility of the membrane (Table 17-2).

Increased pressure from the accumulated exudate may rupture the tympanic membrane. When this occurs, pain relief is almost immediate, fever dissipates, and purulent drainage appears in the external auditory canal.

Children with serous otitis media do not appear ill. They may complain of a full sensation in the ear or they may report cracking or popping sounds. Parents may notice that the child's hearing seems reduced. The tympanic membrane may appear retracted, with identifiable fluid levels or bubbles. Decreased tympanic membrane mobility can be detected during pneumatic otoscopy.

INITIATING DRUG THERAPY

AOM resolves spontaneously in approximately 80% of children. Studies show no difference in results between antibiotic treatment, myringotomy, or combinations of both. Observation without the use of antibiotics is an option for children over the age of 2 if the diagnosis is uncertain (not meeting all

Table 17.2

Diagnostic Criteria for Acute Otitis Media

1. History of acute onset of signs/symptoms
2. Presence of middle ear effusion (indicated by one of the following)
   a. Bulging of tympanic membrane
   b. Limited or absent tympanic membrane mobility
   c. Otorrhea
   d. Air–fluid level behind tympanic membrane
3. Signs and symptoms of middle ear inflammation
   a. Erythema of tympanic membrane
   b. Otalgia

three criteria in Table 17-2). Observation can also be an option if the child is displaying mild otalgia or fever less than 39°C in the past 24 hours. If the observation option is chosen, then the practitioner must make sure of appropriate follow-up and treatment if necessary. Typically, observation is coupled with symptomatic treatment. Supportive therapy with analgesics, antipyretics, and local heat applications is helpful. Analgesic ear drops (eg, Auralgan Otic or Americaine Otic Drops) may be indicated for pain relief if the tympanic membrane is intact. Symptoms that persist after 3 or 4 days, however, justify antibiotic use. Because of increasing antibiotic resistance, strict adherence to the diagnostic guidelines and a justified trial of observation should be considered.

Prevention

AOM is associated with a number of risk factors, some modifiable and others not. Bottle-feeding within the first 6 months, feeding in the supine position ("bottle propping"), persistent use of a pacifier after the first 6 months, and exposure to second-hand smoke have all been implicated as risk factors for AOM. The non-modifiable risk factors include premature birth, male gender, Native American heritage, presence of siblings, and a history of recurrent AOM.

The pneumococcal vaccine is recommended for all children younger than 2 years of age, as well as other patients at high risk for developing AOM. Children 6 weeks to 6 months of age should receive four doses (at 2, 4, 6, and 12 to 15 months), children 7 to 11 months of age three doses, children 12 to 23 months of age two doses, and children 2 years through 9 years of age one dose.

Goals of Drug Therapy

The goals of treating acute and serous otitis media are to relieve symptoms, prevent chronic otitis media with effusion, and avoid complications. Antibiotic treatment can help achieve rapid symptom resolution, decrease the likelihood of relapsing infections, and decrease complications such as mastoiditis, hearing loss, and delayed language development. However, increased bacterial resistance to antibiotics has prompted practitioners in the United States to research and consider the antibiotic therapy changes adopted by practitioners in other countries, although controversy exists concerning changes in treatment protocols. Shorter treatment courses of 5 days are being suggested for children older than 6 years of age who have a mild episode of AOM and whose response to therapy is rapid. Symptomatic care with observation and initiation of antibiotic therapy if symptoms persist or become more severe is becoming an acceptable management method.

Antibiotic treatment includes typically 10 days of treatment, but mild to moderate disease in older children (more than 6 years old) may be appropriately treated with 5- to 7-day courses. Typical antibiotics include amoxicillin, amoxicillin–clavulanate potassium, cefuroxime, azithromycin, or parenteral ceftriaxone (Table 17-3). When hearing loss is detected or

Table 17.3

Overview of Antibiotics for Acute Otitis Media

Generic (Trade) Name and Dosage	Selected Adverse Events	Contraindications	Special Considerations
amoxicillin (various) 80–90 mg/kg/day PO divided into two doses per day	Abnormal taste, anemia, diarrhea, headache	Type I hypersensitivity to penicillins, cephalosporins, imipenem, or β-lactamase inhibitors (piperacillin/tazobactam).	Used as first line in patients with temperatures <39°C
amoxicillin/clavulanate (Augmentin) 80–90 mg/kg/day plus 6.4 mg/kg/day clavulanate PO divided into two doses per day	Abnormal taste, anemia, cholestatic jaundice/hepatic dysfunction, diarrhea, headache, thrombocytosis	As above plus amoxicillin/clavulanate-associated cholestatic jaundice/hepatic dysfunction	Used as first line in patients with temperatures ≥39°C or if severe otalgia present. Also used as primary alternative if amoxicillin alone failed in first 48–72 hours.
azithromycin (Zithromax) 10 mg/kg load on day 1 followed by 5 mg/kg/day for 4 more days or 10 mg/kg per day for 3 days or 30 mg/kg once (max 500 mg)	Diarrhea, nausea, rash, vomiting	Hypersensitivity to macrolide antibiotics	Often used as an alternative in penicillin-sensitive patients (type I hypersensitivity)
ceftriaxone (Rocephin) 50 mg/kg/day IV or IM for 3 days	Serum sickness, seizures, coagulation disturbances, superinfection, rash	Type I hypersensitivity to penicillins or cephalosporins	Used third line after treatment failure with amox/clav
Cefdinir (Omnicef) 14 mg/kg/day PO once a day or 7 mg/kg dose twice a day	Serum sickness, seizures, superinfection, rash	As above	Often used as an alternative in penicillin-sensitive patients (non-type I hypersensitivity reaction)
cefpodoxime (Vantin) 10 mg/kg/day once daily	As above	As above	As above
cefuroxime (Ceftin) 30 mg/kg/day PO divided into two doses per day	As above	As above	As above
clindamycin (various)			

effusion persists beyond 4 months, the patient should be referred to an otolaryngologist.

Practitioners need to evaluate each episode of otitis media individually when considering observation or a shorter treatment protocol. In cases involving children younger than 6 years, severe episodes, or otitis media that occurs in the winter, changes from the routine 10- to 14-day treatment regimen should be approached thoughtfully and cautiously. See Table 17-3 for an overview of medications used for AOM.

If an episode of AOM in a child completely resolves but then recurs after 1 month, it may be treated the same as the initial infection. When treating a patient whose symptoms do not resolve in 2 to 3 days, whose signs of infection remain after a 10-day treatment period, or whose otitis recurs, the diagnosis of AOM should be confirmed and a different class of antibiotics should be prescribed if appropriate.

Drugs of choice for patients with chronic otitis media with a perforated tympanic membrane or a tympanotomy tube are amoxicillin–clavulanate (Augmentin), cefuroxime axetil (Ceftin), or cefixime (Suprax). Most perforations heal within a few weeks after AOM. Perforations that do not heal within 3 to 6 months may require surgical correction.

In children, the tympanic membrane is usually repaired between 7 and 9 years of age and when auditory function improves. Repair may be indicated for younger children if the remaining tympanic membrane does not become infected or effusion does not occur for 1 year.

Serous otitis media that follows AOM may resolve spontaneously within a few weeks to 3 months with control of environmental risk factors. The patient should be observed for resolution of the problem. The Agency for Health Care Policy and Research (AHCPR, 1994) suggests either observation or antibiotic treatment for an effusion that persists for fewer than 12 to 18 weeks without hearing loss.

Cephalosporins

Cefdinir, cefuroxime, and cefpodoxime are all oral agents useful in the treatment of AOM. Further intramuscular ceftriaxone for 1 to 3 days may also be used when oral therapy is not acceptable or when amoxicillin–clavulanate fails. Drugs of choice for patients with chronic otitis media involving a perforated tympanic membrane or a tympanotomy tube are cefuroxime axetil, cefaclor, and cefixime.

Macrolides

Otitis media has also been treated with erythromycin–sulfisoxazole, but the increasing level of resistance makes this agent less useful. Azithromycin (Zithromax) or clarithromycin (Biaxin) is useful when *M. catarrhalis* or certain strains of *H. influenzae* are the suspected infecting organisms. Azithromycin may be given as a 5-day regimen (10 mg/kg on day 1, followed by 4 days of 5 mg/kg), a 3-day regimen (10 mg/kg daily for 3 days), or a 1-day regimen (30 mg/kg once). The obvious benefits of increased compliance with shorter and shorter regimens may be counterbalanced by a potentially decreased efficacy or an increase in side effects. For example, 4.3% of patients receiving the single-day regimen reported diarrhea, versus 1.8% of those receiving the 5-day regimen. Similarly, vomiting occurred in 4.9% of patients on the single-day regimen and only 1.1% of those on the 5-day regimen.

Penicillins

Amoxicillin remains the drug of choice for treating AOM when the infecting organism is unknown. Most guidelines recommend using high-dose amoxicillin (80 to 90 mg/kg/day), particularly if drug-resistant *S. pneumoniae* (DRSP) is suspected or if the patient received antibiotics within the past month (AAP/AAFP, 2004; Hoberman et al., 2002). Amoxicillin has potent activity against *S. pneumoniae* and *H. influenzae*. Amoxicillin at half the usual dosage may be used for prophylactic treatment of otitis media. Amoxicillin–clavulanate is used when *M. catarrhalis* or certain strains of *H. influenzae* are suspected; it also may be used for treating chronic otitis media with tympanic perforation. When otitis media with effusion persists for less than 12 to 18 weeks, amoxicillin–clavulanate therapy may be considered.

Topical Anesthetics

Local topical anesthetics such as Americaine (benzocaine 20%) otic drops or Auralgan (antipyrine and benzocaine) otic solution can be used to control otalgia. Four or five drops should be instilled into the ear canal. These analgesic drops may be used every 1 to 2 hours if needed.

Selecting the Most Appropriate Agent

The most appropriate agent is selected based on the suspected causative organism. As appropriate, selection is also affected by the patient's allergies and dosing convenience (Fig. 17-1).

First-Line Therapy

The first-line agent for the treatment of AOM is high-dose amoxicillin. If the patient presents with severe otalgia or a fever of 39°C or higher, then the combination of amoxicillin and clavulanate is indicated. Patients who have chronic otitis media with a perforated tympanic membrane or a tympanotomy tube are treated with amoxicillin–clavulanate, cefuroxime axetil, cefaclor, and cefixime as drugs of choice (Table 17-4). Alternatives for patients with penicillin allergy include cephalosporin if the reaction is not a type I hypersensitivity reaction or azithromycin if a type I reaction exists.

Table 17.4

Recommended Order of Treatment for Acute Otitis Media

Order	Agents	Comments
First line	High-dose amoxicillin or High-dose amoxicillin/clavulanate	For patients with severe otalgia or a fever ≥39°, use amoxicillin–clavulanate. If allergic to penicillin, consider a cephalosporin or a macrolide.
Second line	High-dose amoxicillin/clavulanate	If allergic to penicillin, consider a cephalosporin or a macrolide.
Third line	IM ceftriaxone or tympanocentesis	Clindamycin may be an alternative if type I hypersensitivity to penicillin exists.

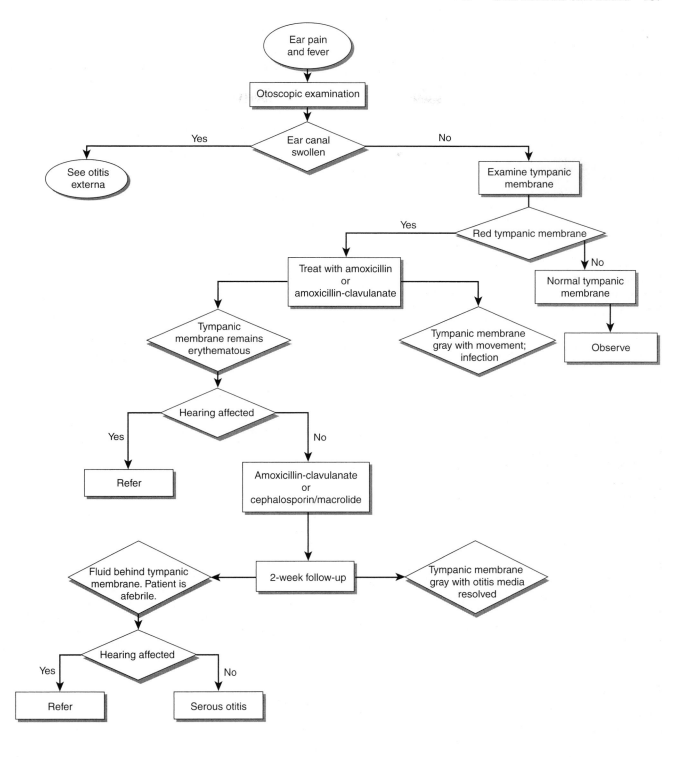

Figure 17–1 Treatment algorithm for acute otitis media.

Second-Line Therapy

Amoxicillin–clavulanate is indicated if treatment failure with amoxicillin is seen within 48 to 72 hours. If the patient was started on amoxicillin–clavulanate, then the next treatment would be cefuroxime axetil (Dohar, 2003) or parenteral ceftriaxone (AAP/AAFP, 2004).

Third-Line Therapy

Third-line therapy consists of parenteral ceftriaxone (AAP/AAFP, 2004) or tympanocentesis. Alternatively, oral clindamycin may be instituted. In addition, antibiotic–corticosteroid drops containing neomycin, polymyxin B or ofloxacin, and hydrocortisone (PediOtic, Floxin, Cortisporin) may be instilled directly into the external auditory canal as second-line treatment when the tympanic membrane is perforated in patients with chronic otitis media. Some practitioners, however, do not recommend this because of the potential for ototoxicity.

Special Population Considerations

Pediatric

Antibiotics are prescribed and administered with caution for children. Cefaclor is not recommended for infants younger than 1 month of age, and cefixime is not recommended for infants younger than 6 months. Ciprofloxacin (Cipro HC) is not recommended for children younger than age 18 years. Fluoroquinolones have been considered effective for the treatment of *S. pneumoniae* infections in adults. However, animal evidence suggests that fluoroquinolones may induce arthropathy in children and growing adults, essentially contraindicating their use.

Acetic acid, 2% solution, is not recommended for children younger than 3 years of age. Acetic acid and Auralgan Otic drops should not be used in children who have a perforated tympanic membrane.

Pregnant Women

Ampicillin, amoxicillin, amoxicillin–clavulanate, cephalosporins, and macrolide antibiotics are pregnancy category B drugs. Auralgan, ciprofloxacin, antibiotic–corticosteroid drops, and dexamethasone (Decadron) are all category C drugs. They are recommended for cautious use or not for use by breast-feeding mothers.

MONITORING PATIENT RESPONSE

Treatment of AOM should be followed by a re-evaluation of tympanic membrane status in 2 to 3 weeks. If fluid remains behind the tympanic membrane but erythema and signs and symptoms of acute otitis are absent, the patient should be re-evaluated in another 2 weeks. If erythema of the tympanic membrane remains, a 10-day course of a different antibiotic should be prescribed. Serous otitis media that does not resolve with time (3 to 4 months) or with antibiotic therapy, or patients with hearing loss, should be referred to a specialist (Jackson, Todd, & Turner, 1997). A specialist also should be suggested for patients who fail to respond to prophylactic treatment for AOM.

Children with persistent middle ear effusions who demonstrate delayed language skills and hearing loss should also be referred for special intervention, such as tympanotomy tube insertion.

PATIENT EDUCATION

Patient teaching is an important aspect of care for patients taking antibiotics. The following information and recommendations should be stressed when initiating treatment:

- Take antibiotics as prescribed; do not double the dose.
- Complete the entire course of prescribed medication to ensure eradication of the infecting organism.

- To maintain consistently accurate levels of drug in the blood, take antibiotics at equal intervals around the clock.
- Wear or carry medical identification, such as a MedicAlert bracelet, to identify penicillin allergies.

Patients who are taking a penicillin should report sore throat, fever, fatigue, and diarrhea, which may indicate a superimposed infection or agranulocytopenia. Patients taking cephalosporins should report sore throat, bruising, bleeding, or joint pain, which may indicate blood dyscrasias.

Drug Information

The Centers for Disease Control and Prevention (CDC) and the American Academy of Pediatrics publish recommendations on the treatment of AOM. For specific drug information, the practitioner should consult references such as "Facts and Comparisons" or the FDA website (http://www.fda.gov).

Patient-Oriented Information Sources

The patient may be directed to the FDA website for information. The American Academy of Pediatrics has an excellent patient information site on ear infections (http://www.aap.org/healthtopics/earinfections.cfm).

Complementary and Alternative Medications

There are no complementary or alternative medications useful in the treatment of AOM (AAP/AAFP, 2004).

OTITIS EXTERNA

Acute otitis externa usually occurs during the summer and may be a result of decreased auditory canal acidity, promoting bacterial overgrowth. Otitis externa rarely causes hearing deficits but is responsible for pruritus and otalgia; however, it can be life-threatening if it becomes invasive.

Factors predisposing to otitis externa include allergy, humidity, trauma, and excessive fluid in the ear canal, such as from swimming. Early diagnosis and treatment are needed to reduce morbidity.

CAUSES

Otitis externa is usually caused by *P. aeruginosa, Staphylococcus* species, and, to a less extent, fungi that grow in a neutral or basic environment. The acidic environment of the external ear can be changed by persistent moisture in the canal, by mechanical trauma such as scratching, or by foreign bodies.

Malignant otitis externa, associated with infections in diabetic or immunocompromised patients, is caused by *P. aeruginosa*. Persistent otitis externa can deteriorate into osteomyelitis of the underlying bone of the external auditory canal.

PATHOPHYSIOLOGY

Viscid secretions of the sebaceous glands protect the outer portion of the auditory canal. The secretions of the apocrine gland combine with exfoliated surface cells of the skin and form a protective, waxy coating. This protection of the external canal can be disturbed by moisture in the canal or mechanical trauma such as a break in the skin (Arnold, 1996; Beers & Abramo, 2004; Jackler & Kaplan, 1999).

DIAGNOSTIC CRITERIA

Otitis externa commonly presents with pain on movement of the pinna or tragus and a painful, erythematous auditory canal with occasional otorrhea. Hearing is usually unaffected unless pressure and fullness in the ear exist, producing an occasional conductive or sensorineural hearing loss. Severely swollen and tender auditory canals may prevent otoscopic examination. The tympanic membrane is unaffected and moves normally during pneumatic otoscopy. The patient with malignant otitis externa typically has fever, excruciating pain, foul discharge, granulation tissue in the ear canal, and cranial nerve palsies.

INITIATING DRUG THERAPY

Otitis externa resulting from prolonged exposure to water or humidity is treated with otic drops applied to the external canal. If edema prevents application of the drops, cotton gauze saturated with antibiotic drops can be placed into the ear. The medication should be applied to the cotton wick as often as possible. After 24 to 48 hours, the cotton can be removed and the medication applied directly into the canal. Malignant otitis externa is usually treated with prolonged antipseudomonal antibiotic therapy (Table 17-5).

Goals of Drug Therapy

Whereas the goal of treating acute and serous otitis media is to relieve symptoms, prevent chronic otitis media with effusion, and avoid complications, otitis externa treatment aims to eradicate the organisms responsible for the infection and decrease the accompanying pain. This can be accomplished by re-establishing an acidic environment in the external auditory canal or through direct antimicrobial activity.

Antibiotic Agents

Fluoroquinolones

The fluoroquinolone antibiotics, ciprofloxacin and ofloxacin, are often used to treat infections associated with otitis externa. The antipseudomonal activity of these agents, coupled with the gram-positive coverage of *Staphylococcus* species, makes these agents useful. These agents are comparable in efficacy to the gold standard, neomycin/polymyxin B, with a clinical cure rate ranging from 84% to 96% (Dohar, 2003). In addition,

Table 17.5

Overview of Treatment for Otitis Externa

Generic (Trade) Name and Dosage	Selected Adverse Events	Contraindications	Special Considerations
polymyxin B sulfate, neomycin, and hydrocortisone (PediOtic) Children: 3 drops into ear canal 3–4 times daily for maximum of 10 days Adults: 4 drops into ear canal 3–4 times daily for maximum of 10 days	Superinfection, contact dermatitis, and ototoxicity with prolonged use	Herpes simplex, fungal, tubercular, or viral otic infections Perforated eardrum Prescribe with caution in pregnancy (category C drug) and in breast-feeding patients.	Use otic drops for a maximum of 10 days.
ofloxacin (Floxin) Children 1–12 y: 5 drops into ear canal bid for 10 days Children >12 y and adults: 10 drops bid for 10 d	Pruritus, site reaction, dizziness, earache, vertigo, taste perversion, paresthesia, and rash	Not recommended for patients <1 y of age Prescribe with caution in pregnancy (category C drug) and in breast-feeding patients.	Use otic drops for a maximum of 10 days.
polymyxin B sulfate, neomycin, and hydrocortisone (Cortisporin) Children: 3 drops into ear canal 3–4 times daily for maximum of 10 days Adults: 4 drops into ear canal 3–4 times daily for maximum of 10 days	Viral infection in ear	Perforated eardrum Prescribe with caution in pregnancy (category C drug) and in breast-feeding patients.	Use otic drops for a maximum of 10 days.
acetic acid, propylene glycol diacetate (Vosol) Children >3 y: 3–5 drops into ear canal 3–4 times daily Adults: 5 drops into ear canal 3–4 times daily	Contact dermatitis, transient stinging	Perforated eardrum, viral otic infections	
acetic acid in aluminum sulfate (Otic Domeboro) Adults and children: 4–6 drops into ear canal every 2–3 h	Ear discomfort	Perforated eardrum	Discontinue in presence of excessive irritation.

Table 17.6

Recommended Order of Treatment for Otitis Externa

Order	Agents	Comments
First line	Fluoroquinolone drops	Floxin is not recommended for patients <1 y. Use all otic drops for a maximum of 10 days. All drops are contraindicated in cases of perforated eardrum.
Second line	Combination neomycin/polymyxin B drops	Vosol is not recommended for patients <3 y. All drops are contraindicated in cases of perforated eardrum.

these agents offer a potential decrease in adverse effects compared to neomycin/polymyxin B.

The dosage of Ciprodex (ciprofloxacin/dexamethasone) is four drops (0.42 mg ciprofloxacin, 0.14 mg dexamethasone) into the affected ear twice daily for 7 days. This regimen should show a response within 3 to 4 days of initiation. Typical adverse events include ear discomfort or pain, ear pruritus, and irritability. Floxin Otic (ofloxacin) is administered as 5 drops once daily (children 6 months to 13 years) or 10 drops once daily (children older than 13 years and adults).

The addition of a corticosteroid to the antibiotic formulation is controversial. The anti-inflammatory effects potentially include reduced pain, swelling, and itching. Dohar (2003) reported on a controlled study suggesting that the addition of hydrocortisone decreases duration of pain by about 1 day. However, additional studies should be conducted to confirm this point. The risk of local immunosuppression and potential hypersensitivity reactions should be studied in light of the potential benefit. The Floxin Otic preparation does not contain a corticosteroid.

Aminoglycoside Antibiotics

The combination product Cortisporin (neomycin sulfate/polymyxin B/hydrocortisone acetate) has been used for more than 20 years. The combination of the gram-positive coverage of the aminoglycoside neomycin and the antipseudomonal activity of polymyxin has made this combination the gold standard of treatment. The same controversy regarding the addition of a corticosteroid exists with this combination. Treatment consists of instilling three drops in the affected ear three or four times a day for a maximum of 10 days. The clinical cure rate of this regimen is 83% to 96% (Beers & Abramo, 2004; Dohar, 2003). However, the side effect profile, particularly the hypersensitivity reactions related to neomycin (and possibly the thimerosal preservative), is high (Dohar, 2003). Further, ototoxicity with neomycin has been reported, though the number of reports is low and the data are speculative, particularly when the patient's tympanic membrane is intact.

Topical Otic Agents

A 2% solution of acetic acid may be used as an alternative to antibiotic solution for otitis externa, primarily because acetic acid is not associated with allergic or toxic affects, has no cross-reactivity with other medications, and is affordable. Acetic acid can be used for both fungal and pseudomonal infections.

Selecting the Most Appropriate Agent

First-Line Therapy

Otitis externa is treated initially with a fluoroquinolone antibiotic. The selection of ciprofloxacin versus ofloxacin depends on the formulary status of the agents as well as the clinician's experience with added corticosteroids. See Table 17-6 and Figure 17-2 for more information.

Second-Line Therapy

Neomycin/polymyxin B combinations are considered second-line agents, primarily due to their side effect profile. The lower cost of these agents, though, warrants consideration, particularly in patients without insurance or other means of paying for the more expensive fluoroquinolones.

Third-Line Therapy

Otitis externa is treated with antibacterial–antifungal and astringent and solvent agents (Domeboro and Vosol) when a third-line medication is needed.

Special Population Considerations

Acetic acid 2% solution is not recommended for children younger than 3 years of age. The concern related to the use of systemic fluoroquinolones in children is not relevant due to the minimal systemic absorption.

MONITORING PATIENT RESPONSE

A gallium scan should be performed to ensure reduction in the inflammatory process of malignant otitis externa. Cleansing of the local affected area is needed, but extensive débridement can be reserved until the initial antibiotic therapy is completed.

PATIENT EDUCATION

Drug Information

The otic solution should be warmed before instilling it in the ear, as a cold solution may induce dizziness. To warm the otic solution, the patient should hold the bottle in the hand for 1 to 2 minutes. To instill the drops, the patient should lie with the affected ear upward and remain in this position for about 5 minutes to help the solution penetrate into the ear canal.

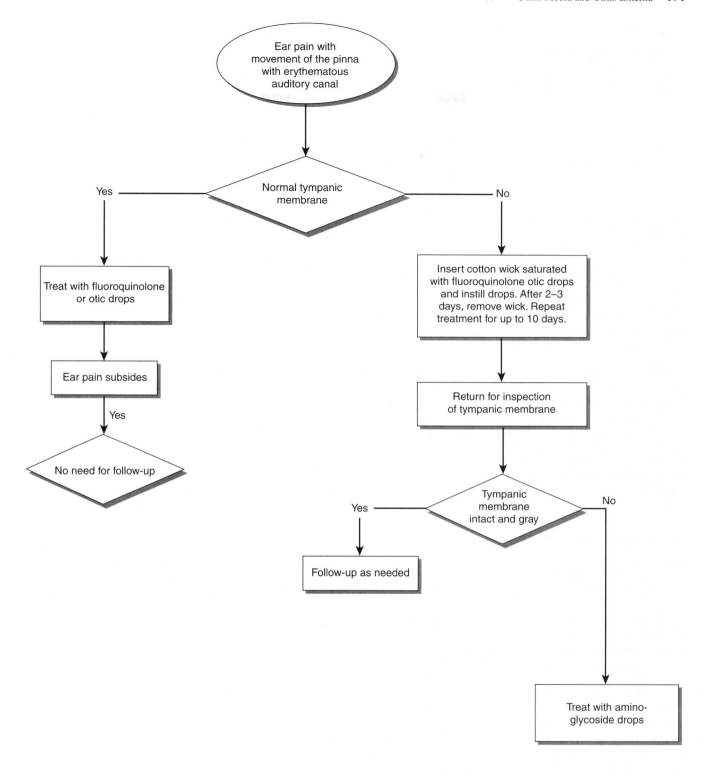

Figure 17–2 Treatment algorithm for otitis externa.

Patient-Oriented Information Sources

The Centers for Disease Control & Prevention (CDC) website (http://www.cdc.gov/healthyswimming/swimmers_ear.htm) and the KidsHealth website (http://kidshealth.org/parent/infections/bacterial_viral/swimmer_ear.html) have sections on swimmer's ear.

Nutrition/Lifestyle Changes

Otitis externa can be prevented by wearing ear plugs when swimming or showering. Drying the ears with a hair dryer if they get water in them is also beneficial. The patient should avoid trying to remove ear wax mechanically with cotton-tipped swabs, hairpins, or the like. If the ear is very swollen, the patient can insert a wick of cotton into the ear and apply the medication to the wick. It is important for the patient to keep water away from the ear until the infection clears (usually 5 to 7 days) and for 4 to 6 weeks afterward. To accomplish this, hair can be washed in a sink instead of a shower or tub, and the patient can use a shower cap or ear plugs when bathing.

Complementary and Alternative Medications

If the patient is susceptible to recurrent otitis externa, instillation of a few drops of a 1:1 solution of white vinegar and rubbing alcohol before and after contact with water is good prophylaxis. Prolonged use of ear plugs may also prevent otitis externa.

■ Case Study

C. J., age 17, is on his high school swim team. He presents with sudden onset of right ear pain that worsens at night. He says that the pain intensifies when he touches his ear and that he has a feeling of fullness in the ear. On examination, the auditory canal is edematous and erythematous, with yellow crusting. His temperature is 97.8°F and his tympanic membranes are pearly gray with landmarks intact.

Diagnosis: Otitis externa

→ 1. List two specific treatment goals for C. J.

→ 2. What drug therapy would you prescribe? Why?

→ 3. Would you recommend a complementary or alternative medication? If so, what?

→ 4. What would indicate that treatment is successful?

→ 5. What would you tell C. J. about the medication?

→ 6. What adverse reactions should you be concerned about?

→ 7. What lifestyle changes would you recommend to prevent this from happening again?

→ 8. If C. J. returns in 2 weeks with the same symptoms, what would you prescribe?

Bibliography

Starred references are cited in the text.

*Agency for Health Care Policy and Research [AHCPR]. (1994). Managing otitis media with effusion in young children (AHCPR Publication No. 94-0623). Rockville, MD: U.S. Department of Health and Human Services.

*American Academy of Pediatrics (AAP) and American Academy of Family Physicians (AAFP) (2004). Clinical practice guidelines: diagnosis and management of acute otitis media. *Pediatrics, 113,* 1451–1465.

*Arnold, J. (1996). Otitis media and its complications. In R. Behrman, R. Kliegman, & A. Arvin (Eds.), *Textbook of pediatrics* (pp. 1816–1818). Philadelphia: W. B. Saunders.

*Beers, S. L., & Abramo, T. J. (2004). Otitis externa review. *Pediatric Emergency Care, 20*(4), 250–256.

Behrman, R., Kliegman, R., & Arvin, A. (Eds.). (2000). *Textbook of pediatrics* (pp. 1813–1819). Philadelphia: W. B. Saunders.

Berman, S. (1995). Otitis media in children. *New England Journal of Medicine, 332,* 1560–1564.

Berman, S., & Chan, K. (1999). Ear, nose, and throat. In W. Hay, A. Hayward, M. Levin, & J. Sondheimer (Eds.), *Pediatric diagnosis and treatment* (pp. 394–402). Stamford, CT: Appleton & Lange.

Bredfeldt, R. (1996). Chronic serous otitis media. In R. Rackel (Ed.), *Manual of medical practice* (pp. 80–81). Philadelphia: W. B. Saunders.

Culpepper, L., & Froom, J. (1997). Routine antimicrobial treatment of AOM: is it necessary? *New England Journal of Medicine, 278,* 1643–1645.

Daiichi Pharmaceutical Corporation. (1997). *Floxin Otic: the safe and sound solution.* Fort Lee, NJ: Author.

*Dohar, J. E. (2003). Evolution of management approaches for otitis externa. *Pediatric Infectious Disease Journal, 22*(4), 299–308.

Dowell, S. F., Marcy, S. M., Phillips, W. R., Gerber, M. A., & Schwartz, B. (1998). Otitis media: principles of judicious use of antimicrobial agents. *Pediatrics, 101,* 165–171.

Durand, M., Joseph, M., & Baker, A. (1998). Infections of the upper respiratory tract. In A. Fauci, E. Braunwald, K. Isselbacker, J. Wilson, J. Martin, D. Kasper, S. Hauser, & D. Longo (Eds.), *Principles of internal medicine* (pp. 179–182). New York: McGraw-Hill.

*Hoberman, A., Marchant, C., Kaplan, S. L., & Feldman, S. (2002). Treatment of acute otitis media consensus recommendations. *Clinical Pediatrics, 41*(6), 373–390.

*Jackler, R., & Kaplan, M. (1999). Ears, nose, and throat. In L. Tierney, S. McPhee, & M. Papadakis (Eds.), *Current medical diagnosis and treatment* (pp. 215–219). Stamford, CT: Appleton & Lange.

*Jackson, R., Todd, N., & Turner, J. (1997). Ears, nose and throat diseases. In T. Speight & N. Holford (Eds.), *Drug treatment* (pp. 563–567). Philadelphia: Adis International.

*Karver, S. B. (1998). Otitis media: primary care. *Clinics in Office Practice, 25,* 619–632.

Kristiansen, P. (1999). Diagnosis of malignant otitis externa. *Journal of American Academy of Nurse Practitioners, 11,* 297–300.

Kuhn, M. (1998). Medications used in ear disorders. In M. Kuhn (Ed.), *Pharmacotherapeutics: a nursing process approach* (pp. 978–981). Philadelphia: F. A. Davis.

La Rosa, S. (1998). Primary care management of otitis externa. *Nurse Practitioner, 23,* 125–133.

Maxson, S., & Yamaguchi, T. (1996). Acute otitis media. *Pediatrics in Review, 17,* 191–195.

McEvoy, G., Litvak, K., & Welsh, O. (1998). *Drug information.* Bethesda, MD: American Society of Health-System Pharmacists.

Melnyk, B. M., & Herendeen, P. (1998). Inside and out: the latest on otitis media and otitis externa. *Advance for Nurse Practitioners, 6,* 36–38, 43–45.

Murphy, J. L. (Ed.). (1998, Feb.). *Monthly prescribing reference.* New York: Prescribing Reference, Inc.

Neu, H. (1995). Selection of an antibacterial agent. In T. Brody, J. Larner, K. Minneman, & H. Neu (Eds.). *Human pharmacology: molecular to clinical* (pp. 697–699). Philadelphia: C. V. Mosby.

Niederman, M., Skerrett, S., Yamauchi, T., & Pinkowish, M. (1998). Antibiotics or not? Managing patients with respiratory infections. *Patient Care,* 60–70.

O'Handley, J. (1996). Acute otitis media. In R. Rackel (Ed.), *Manual of medical practice* (pp. 78–79). Philadelphia: W. B. Saunders.

Paradisise, J. (1997). Short-course antimicrobial treatment for acute otitis media: not best for infants and young children. *New England Journal of Medicine, 278,* 1640–1642.

Patterson, M., & Paparella, M. M. (1999). Otitis media with effusion and early sequelae. *Otolaryngologic Clinics of North America, 32,* 391–400.

Pichichero, M., & Cohen, R. (1997). Shortened course of antibiotic therapy for acute otitis media, sinusitis and tonsillopharyngitis. *Pediatric Infectious Disease Journal, 16,* 680–692.

Redwood, D. (1996). Chiropractic. In M. Micozzi (Ed.), *Fundamentals of complementary and alternative medicine* (p. 107). New York: Churchill Livingstone.

Richer, M., & Deschenes, M. (1999). Upper respiratory tract infections. In J. Dipiro, R. Talbert, G. Yee, G. Matzke, B. Wells, & L. Posey (Eds.), *Pharmacotherapy: a pathophysiologic approach* (3rd ed., pp. 1671–1675). Stamford, CT: Appleton & Lange.

Richer, M., & LeBel, M. (1997). Upper respiratory tract infections. In J. Dipiro, R. Talbert, G. Yee, G. Matzke, B. Wells, & L. Posey (Eds.), *Pharmacotherapy: a pathophysiologic approach* (4th ed., pp. 1763–1783). Stamford, CT: Appleton & Lange.

Silko, G. (1996). Otitis externa. In R. Rackel (Ed.), *Manual of medical practice* (pp. 82–83). Philadelphia: W. B. Saunders.

Skid-More, L., & McKenry, L. (1997). *Drug guide for nurses.* Philadelphia: C. V. Mosby.

Stool, S., Mount, M., & Medellin, G. (1996). Diagnosing otitis media: a workshop. *Comprehensive Therapy, 22,* 776–777.

Tracy, J., Demain, J., Hoffman, K., & Goetz, D. (1998). Intranasal beclomethasone as an adjunct to treatment of chronic middle ear effusion. *Annals of Allergy, Asthma, and Immunology, 80,* 198–205.

Turner, J. (1996). Otitis media. In J. Hurst (Ed.), *Medicine for the practicing physician* (pp. 1861–1864). Stamford, CT: Appleton & Lange.

Wetmore, R. (1997). Otitis media. In M. Swartz, T. Curry, A. Sargent, N. Blum, & J. Fein (Eds.), *Pediatric primary care: a problem-oriented approach* (pp. 670-673). Philadelphia: C. V. Mosby.

Visit the Connection web site for the most up-to-date drug information.

IV

Pharmacotherapy for Cardiovascular Disorders

HYPERTENSION

■ KELLY BARRINGER, EVA VIVIAN, AND ANDREW M. PETERSON

Hypertension is a chronic disease that affects approximately 50 million Americans. Many people are unaware that they have hypertension because the disease rarely causes symptoms; hence, the disease is appropriately nicknamed "the silent killer." Hypertension is a serious health concern for all Americans because it is associated with renal and cardiovascular disease as well as with type 2 diabetes mellitus.

Hypertension affects all ethnic groups, but African-Americans suffer disproportionately from hypertension and its effects, leading to high rates of cardiovascular morbidity and mortality. Hypertension in African-Americans occurs at an earlier age, is more severe, and results in organ damage such as coronary heart disease, stroke, and end-stage renal disease more often than it does in whites.

CAUSES

Hypertension is classified as primary, essential, or idiopathic when there is no identifiable cause for elevation in blood pressure (BP). Over 90% of hypertensive cases fall into this category. The lifestyle of a patient with documented hypertension should be evaluated to reveal identifiable causes of hypertension. Several factors may contribute to primary hypertension: environmental factors (eg, obesity, dietary sodium, stress), hyperinsulinemia, defective natriuresis, abnormal neural and peripheral autoregulation, and defects in the renin-angiotensin-aldosterone system.

When a cause for elevated BP is identified, hypertension is classified as secondary hypertension. Identifiable causes include chronic renal disease, pheochromocytoma, primary aldosteronism, sleep apnea, coarctation of the aorta, and renovascular disease, to name a few (Box 18-1).

Medications that may increase BP include oral contraceptives, steroids, appetite suppressants, tricyclic antidepressants, the antidepressant venlafaxine (Effexor), cyclosporine (Sandimmune), nonsteroidal anti-inflammatory drugs (NSAIDs), and some nasal decongestants. Herbal products that affect BP include capsicum, goldenseal, licorice root, ma huang (ephedra), scotch broom, witch hazel, and yohimbine.

PATHOPHYSIOLOGY

Role of Nervous System

The central and autonomic nervous systems play a key role in regulating BP. Centrally located beta receptors stimulate the release of norepinephrine, whereas alpha-2 receptors inhibit norepinephrine release, which produces vasodilation and therefore reduces BP.

Receptors located in the periphery also regulate BP. These receptors are located on effector cells that are innervated by sympathetic neurons. Alpha-1 receptors located on arterioles and venules cause vasoconstriction, while the beta-2 receptors on these vessels produce vasodilation. Beta-1 receptors, which are located on the heart and kidneys, regulate heart rate and contractility, which ultimately has an effect on cardiac output. Because BP is the product of cardiac output and peripheral resistance, any reduction in cardiac output results in a decrease in BP. Blockade of beta-1 receptors decreases cardiac output, peripheral resistance, and BP. When stimulated, beta-2 receptors located in the venules and arterioles cause vasodilation.

Baroreceptors, which are nerve endings located in large arteries such as the aortic arch and carotids, play a significant role in regulating BP. These receptors are sensitive to changes in BP. When BP drops drastically, the baroreceptors send an impulse to the brain stem that results in vasoconstriction and increased heart rate and contractility. In contrast, elevation in BP increases baroreceptor firing, which results in vasodilation and decreased heart rate and contractility. Any disturbance in this system can result in elevated BP.

Peripheral autoregulatory components also play a role in controlling BP. Normally, rises in BP result in sodium and water being eliminated by the kidney. In turn, plasma volume, cardiac output, and BP decrease. Any defect in this mechanism, however, could raise plasma volume and BP.

Role of Renal System

The renin-angiotensin-aldosterone system regulates sodium, potassium, and fluid balance in the body. Renin, an enzyme secreted by the juxtaglomerular cells of the afferent arterioles

BOX 18–1. IDENTIFIABLE CAUSES OF HYPERTENSION

Adrenal steroids
Chronic kidney disease
Chronic steroid therapy and Cushing syndrome
Coarctation of the aorta
Cocaine, amphetamines, other illicit drugs
Cyclosporine and tacrolimus
Drug-induced or drug-related
Erythropoietin
Inadequate doses
Inappropriate combinations
Licorice (including some chewing tobacco)
Nonadherence
Nonsteroidal anti-inflammatory drugs; cyclo-oxygenase-2 inhibitors
Oral contraceptives
Pheochromocytoma
Primary aldosteronism
Renovascular disease
Selected over-the-counter dietary supplements and medicines (eg, ephedra, ma huang, bitter orange)
Sleep apnea
Sympathomimetics (decongestants, anorectics)
Thyroid or parathyroid disease

of the kidney, is released in response to changes in BP resulting from reduced renal perfusion, decreased intravascular volume, or increased circulation of catecholamines. Renin catalyzes the conversion of angiotensinogen to angiotensin I. Angiotensin I is converted to the potent vasoconstrictor angiotensin II by angiotensin-converting enzyme (ACE).

Angiotensin II causes direct vasoconstriction and stimulation of the sympathetic nervous system. Angiotensin II also stimulates release of aldosterone from the adrenal gland, which results in the retention of sodium and water. In normotensive patients, angiotensin II directly inhibits further release of renin through a negative feedback system. If the negative feedback system fails, BP rises.

Hyperinsulinemia may contribute to hypertension by causing sodium retention and stimulating the sympathetic nervous system.

DIAGNOSTIC CRITERIA

Hypertension is generally defined as an elevation in systolic and/or diastolic BP. A new category of hypertension (prehypertension) has been identified by the Joint National Committee on Prevention, Detection, Evaluation and Treatment of High Blood Pressure in its Seventh Report (JNC VII) guidelines. Prehypertension is a systolic BP of 120 to 139 mm Hg and a diastolic BP of 80 to 89 mm Hg. Stage 1 hypertension is a systolic BP of at least 140 mm Hg and a diastolic BP of at least 90 mm Hg. Stage 2 hypertension is a systolic BP of at least 160 mm Hg or a diastolic BP of at least 100 (Table 18-1).

Hypertension is not diagnosed on an initial reading; rather, it is confirmed after two or more properly measured, seated BP readings on each of two or more office visits. BP measurements should be obtained after the patient has had time to relax for at least 5 minutes. Patients should be seated in a chair rather than on an examination table, with feet on the floor and arm supported at heart level. Patients should avoid smoking cigarettes or drinking coffee for at least 30 minutes before the BP measurement. For an accurate reading, the appropriate-size sphygmomanometer cuff should be used. The cuff should encompass 80% of the arm, and the width of the cuff should be at least 60% of the length of the upper arm (JNC VII, 2003).

Table 18.1

Classification and Management of Blood Pressure for Adults*

BP Classification	SBP* (mm Hg)	DBP* (mm Hg)	Lifestyle Modification	Initial Drug Therapy Without Compelling Indication	Initial Drug Therapy With Compelling Indications
Normal	<120	and <80	Encourage		
Prehypertension	120–139	or 80–89	Yes	No antihypertensive drug indicated	Drug(s) for compelling indications‡
Stage 1 Hypertension	140–159	or 90–99	Yes	Thiazide-type diuretics for most. May consider ACEI, ARB, BB, CCB, or combination.	Drug(s) for the compelling indications.‡ Other antihypertensive drugs (diuretics, ACEI, ARB, BB, CCB) as needed.
Stage 2 Hypertension	≥160	or ≥100	Yes	Two-drug combination for most† (usually thiazide-type diuretic and ACEI or ARB or BB or CCB)	

DBP, diastolic blood pressure; SBP, systolic blood pressure.
ACEI, angiotensin-converting enzyme inhibitor; ARB, angiotensin receptor blocker; BB, beta blocker; CCB, calcium channel blocker.
*Treatment determined by highest BP category.
†Initial combined therapy should be used cautiously in those at risk for orthostatic hypotension.
‡Treat patients with chronic kidney disease or diabetes to BP goal of <130/80 mm Hg.

Ambulatory BP monitoring (ABPM) is recommended not only for patients with suspected "white coat hypertension" but also for those in whom drug resistance is a possibility. Patients with "white coat hypertension" have a persistently elevated BP in the doctor's office but a persistently normal BP at other times. ABPM readings correlate better with target-organ damage than clinical measurements. ABPM also identifies patients in whom BP does not drop significantly during sleep. More aggressive treatment may be necessary for these patients, who are known to be at higher cardiovascular risk. An elevated systolic BP is a more potent cardiovascular risk factor than an elevated diastolic BP.

Physical Examination

A thorough examination should be performed, including a history of personal and family risk factors (Box 18-2) and a history of prescription medications, over-the-counter medications, and herbal products. For patients with documented hypertension, lifestyle should be evaluated, other cardiovascular risk factors or concomitant disorders should be identified, and the presence of target-organ damage and cardiovascular disease should be assessed.

Physical examination includes two or more measured seated BP readings with verification in the contralateral arm, body mass index (calculated as weight in kilograms divided by the square of height in meters; measurement of waist circumference may also be useful); auscultation for carotid, abdominal, and femoral bruits; palpation of the thyroid gland; thorough examination of the heart and lungs; examination of the abdomen for enlarged kidneys, masses, and abnormal aortic pulsation; palpation of the lower extremities for edema and pulses; and neurologic assessment.

Diagnostic Tests

The following laboratory tests are recommended before initiating therapy: electrocardiogram, blood glucose, hemoglobin, hematocrit, complete urinalysis, serum potassium and creatinine, liver function tests, calcium and magnesium, glycosylated hemoglobin (hemoglobin A1c), and fasting lipid panel (9- to 12-hour fast), which includes low-density lipoprotein cholesterol, high-density lipoprotein cholesterol, and triglycerides. Optional tests include urinary albumin excretion or albumin/creatinine ratio. More extensive testing for identifiable causes is not indicated unless BP control is not achieved.

INITIATING THERAPY

Initial therapy is determined by categorizing the patient's BP as prehypertension or stage 1 or stage 2 hypertension, and assessing for the presence of target-organ damage and cardiovascular disease. Table 18-1 and Figure 18-1 show the current recommendations for initiating therapy.

All patients diagnosed with hypertension should be counseled about the benefits of lifestyle modifications (Box 18-3). Patients are encouraged to maintain appropriate body weight (body mass index 18.5 to 24.9) and adopt the Dietary Approaches to Stop Hypertension (DASH) diet. The DASH diet is rich in fruits, vegetables, and low-fat dairy products, with a reduced content of saturated and total fat; dietary sodium is restricted to less than 100 mmol/d (2.4 g sodium or 6 g sodium chloride daily); and physical activity is encouraged, while reducing alcohol consumption. Since patients with prehypertension are at increased risk for progression to hypertension, preventive measures such as the dietary considerations mentioned above should be taken. However, if the prehypertensive patient has a concomitant disease that should also be treated, then an appropriate antihypertensive agent should be selected. If the patient progresses to stage 1 hypertension, then drug therapy is initiated.

Antihypertensive medication is initiated for patients with stage 1 hypertension. The JNC VII recommends one of the thiazide-type diuretics as initial therapy. If the goal BP is not achieved, a second drug should be added to the regimen. The diuretic should be continued and a second drug can be selected from among the ACE inhibitors, angiotensin receptor II blockers (ARBs), beta blockers, or calcium channel blockers (CCBs).

For stage 2 hypertension, the JNC VII guidelines strongly suggest starting drug therapy with two medications, usually a thiazide-type diuretic plus an ACE inhibitor, ARB, beta blocker, or CCB. Care should be taken to avoid orthostatic hypotension. Combination drug products, such as ACE inhibitors and diuretics and ARBs and diuretics, often make adhering to therapy easier for the patient.

Patients with a compelling indication (Table 18-3) should be started on the indicated medication, regardless of the stage of hypertension.

BOX 18–2. CARDIOVASCULAR RISK FACTORS

Major Risk Factors
 Hypertension*
 Cigarette smoking
 Obesity (BMI ≥ 30)*
 Physical inactivity
 Dyslipidemia*
 Diabetes mellitus*
 Microalbuminuria or estimated GFR < 60 mL/min
 Age (>55 years for men, >65 years for women)
 Family history of premature cardiovascular disease
  (men <55 years or women <65 years)

Target-Organ Damage
 Heart
  Left ventricular hypertrophy
  Angina or prior myocardial infarction
  Prior coronary revascularization
  Heart failure
 Brain
  Stroke or transient ischemic attack
 Chronic kidney disease
 Peripheral arterial disease
 Retinopathy

BMI, body mass index; GFR, glomerular filtration rate.
*Components of the metabolic syndrome.

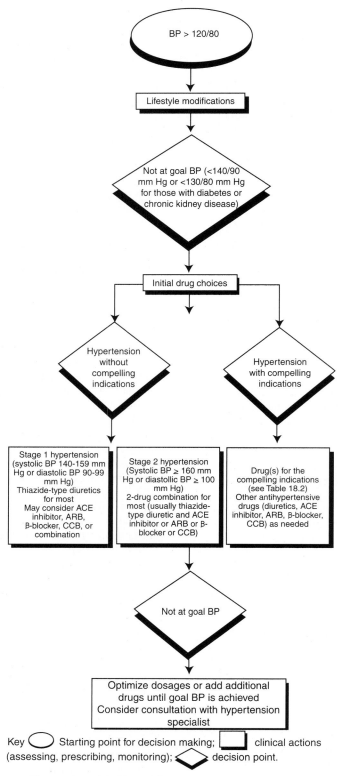

Figure 18–1 Modified JNC VII treatment for hypertension.

Goals of Drug Therapy

The goal of antihypertensive therapy is to reduce cardio-vascular and renal morbidity and mortality. Reducing BP to less than 140/90 mm Hg is associated with a decrease in the risk of cardiovascular disease (CVD). Beginning at 115/75 mm Hg, the risk of CVD doubles with each 20-mm Hg increment above systolic BP or 10-mm Hg increment above diastolic BP. Individuals who are normotensive at age 55 years have a 90% lifetime risk of developing hypertension.

In patients with hypertension and comorbidities (diabetes or renal disease), the BP goal is less than 130/80 mm Hg. This goal is endorsed by the JNC VII as well as the American Diabetes Association, the National Kidney Foundation, and the Canadian Hypertensive Society. The American College

BOX 18–3. LIFESTYLE MODIFICATIONS TO MANAGE HYPERTENSION*

Modification	Recommendation	Approximate Systolic BP Reduction, Range
Weight reduction	Maintain normal body weight (BMI, 18.5–24.9).	5–20 mm Hg/10-kg weight loss
Adopt DASH eating plan	Consume a diet rich in fruits, vegetables, and low-fat dairy products with a reduced content of saturated and total fat.	8–14 mm
Dietary sodium reduction	Reduce dietary sodium intake to no more than 100 mEq/L (2.4 g sodium or 6 g sodium chloride).	2–8 mm Hg
Physical activity	Engage in regular aerobic physical activity such as brisk walking (at least 30 minutes per day, most days of the week).	4–9 mm Hg
Moderation of alcohol consumption	Limit consumption to no more than 2 drinks per day (1 oz or 30 mL ethanol [eg, 24 oz beer, 10 oz wine, or 3 oz 80-proof whiskey]) in most men and no more than 1 drink per day in women and lighter-weight persons.	2–4 mm Hg

*For overall cardiovascular risk reduction, stop smoking. The effects of implementing these modifications are dose and time dependent and could be higher for some individuals.

of Physicians' goal for systolic BP is slightly higher, at 135 mm Hg.

Diuretics

There are five classes of diuretics: carbonic anhydrase inhibitors (which are not used for hypertension because of their weak antihypertensive effects), thiazides, thiazide-like diuretics, loop diuretics, and potassium-sparing diuretics. Diuretics decrease BP by causing diuresis, which results in decreased plasma volume, stroke volume, and cardiac output (Table 18-2). During chronic therapy their major hemodynamic effect is reduction of peripheral vascular resistance. As a result of drug-induced diuresis, hypokalemia and hypomagnesemia may lead to cardiac arrhythmias. Patients at greatest risk are those receiving digitalis therapy, those with left ventricular hypertrophy, and those with ischemic heart disease.

Thiazide Diuretics

Mechanism of Action

Thiazide diuretics work by increasing the urinary excretion of sodium and chloride in equal amounts (see Table 18-2). They inhibit the reabsorption of sodium and chloride in the thick ascending limb of the loop of Henle and the early distal tubules. Thiazide diuretics also increase potassium and bicarbonate excretion and decrease calcium excretion and uric acid retention. The thiazide diuretics are the preferred agents to reduce BP unless there are compelling or specific indications for another drug. The antihypertensive action requires several days to produce effects. The duration of action of the thiazides requires a single daily dose to control BP. Caution should be used in patients with a history of gout or hyponatremia. Diuretic-induced hyperuricemia may produce gouty arthritis or uric acid stones.

Contraindications

Diuretics are contraindicated in patients who are anuric (creatinine clearance less than 30 mL/min), who have renal decompensation, or who are hypersensitive to thiazides or sulfonamides.

Adverse Events

Side effects include hypokalemia, hypomagnesemia, hypercalcemia, hyperuricemia, hyperglycemia, and hyperlipidemia. As a result of drug-induced diuresis, hypokalemia occurs in 15% to 20% of patients taking low-dose thiazide diuretics; therefore, potassium (K^+) supplements are needed by some patients. Combination therapy with thiazide and potassium-sparing diuretics (eg, hydrochlorothiazide [HydroDIURIL] and triamterene [Dyrenium]) may be prudent when potassium levels are less than 4.0 mEq/L and the patient is taking a thiazide diuretic or when a low potassium level may potentiate drug toxicity, as in patients concurrently taking digoxin (Lanoxin). Other side effects include tinnitus, paresthesias, abdominal cramps, nausea, vomiting, diarrhea, muscle cramps, weakness, and sexual dysfunction.

Loop Diuretics

Loop diuretics are indicated in the presence of edema associated with congestive heart failure, hepatic cirrhosis, and renal disease (see Table 18-2). This class of drug is useful when greater diuretic potential is desired. In general, loop diuretics should be reserved for hypertensive patients with chronic renal insufficiency.

Furosemide and ethacrynic acid inhibit the reabsorption of sodium and chloride, not only in proximal and distal tubules but also in the loop of Henle. In contrast, bumetanide is more chloruretic than natriuretic and may have an additional action in the proximal tubule.

Contraindications

Loop diuretics are contraindicated in patients who are anuric, in patients hypersensitive to these compounds or to sulfonylureas, and in patients with hepatic coma or in states of severe electrolyte depletion. Ethacrynic acid is contraindicated in infants.

Adverse Events

Loop diuretics may cause the same side effects as thiazides, although the effects on serum lipids and glucose are not as

Table 18.2

Overview of Selected Antihypertensive Agents

Generic (Trade) Name and Dosage	Selected Adverse Events	Contraindications	Special Considerations
Selected Diuretics			
THIAZIDE AND THIAZIDE-LIKE			
chlorthalidone (Hygroton) 12.5–100 mg qd	Hyperuricemia, hypokalemia, hypomagnesemia, hyperglycemia, hyponatremia, hypercalcemia, hypercholesterolemia, hypertriglyceridemia, pancreatitis, rashes and other allergic reactions	High doses are relatively contraindicated in patients with hyperlipidemia, gout, and diabetes.	Preferred in patients with creatinine clearance >30 mL/min
hydrochlorothiazide (HydroDIURIL, Microzide) 12.5–25 mg qd	Same as chlorthalidone	Same as chlorthalidone	Same as chlorthalidone
indapamide (Lozol) 1.25–5 mg qd	Same as chlorthalidone	Same as chlorthalidone	Same as chlorthalidone
metolazone (Zaroxolyn) 2.5–5 mg qd	Less or no hypercholesterolemia	Same as chlorthalidone	Same as chlorthalidone
LOOP DIURETICS			
bumetanide (Bumex) 0.5–5 mg bid–tid	Dehydration, circulatory collapse, hypokalemia, hyponatremia, hypomagnesemia, hyperglycemia, metabolic alkalosis, hyperuricemia (short duration of action, no hypercalcemia)	High doses are relatively contraindicated in patients with hyperlipidemia, gout, and diabetes.	Effective in patients with creatinine clearance <30 mL/min
ethacrynic acid (Edecrin) 25–100 mg bid–tid	Same as bumetanide (only nonsulfonamide diuretic, ototoxicity)	Same as bumetanide	Same as bumetanide
furosemide (Lasix) 20–320 mg qd	Same as bumetanide	Same as bumetanide	Same as bumetanide
torsemide (Demadex) 5–20 mg qd	Short duration of action, no hypercalcemia	Same as bumetanide	Same as bumetanide
POTASSIUM-SPARING DIURETICS			
amiloride (Midamor) 5–10 mg qd–bid	Hyperkalemia, GI disturbances, rash	High doses are relatively contraindicated in patients with hyperlipidemia, gout, and diabetes.	Same as bumetanide
spironolactone (Aldactone) 12.5–100 mg qd–bid	Hyperkalemia, GI disturbances, rash, gynecomastia	Same as amiloride	Ideal in patients with heart failure
triamterene (Dyrenium) 50–150 mg qd–bid	Hyperkalemia, GI disturbances, nephrolithiasis	Same as amiloride	Same as bumetanide
Beta-Adrenergic Blocking Agents			
SELECTED BETA BLOCKERS			
atenolol (Tenormin) 25–100 mg qd	Fatigue, depression, bradycardia, decreased exercise tolerance, congestive heart failure, aggravates peripheral arterial insufficiency, bronchospasm; masks symptoms of and delays recovery from hypoglycemia, Raynaud's phenomenon, insomnia, vivid dreams or hallucinations, acute mental disorder, impotence; increased serum triglycerides, decreased high-density lipoprotein cholesterol; sudden withdrawal can lead to exacerbation of angina and myocardial infarction	Contraindicated in first trimester of pregnancy; heart failure (except carvedilol and metoprolol); relatively contraindicated in patients with asthma, diabetes; hyperlipidemia	Abrupt cessation should be avoided; taper the dose of beta blocker over a 2-wk period. Advantageous in patients with angina, tachycardia, acute myocardial infarction; hypertensive patients with left ventricular hypertrophy
betaxolol (Kerlone) 5–20 mg qd	Same as atenolol	Same as atenolol	Same as atenolol
bisoprolol (Zebeta) 2.5–10 mg qd	Same as atenolol	Same as atenolol	Same as atenolol
timolol (Blocadren) 10–60 mg bid	Same as atenolol	Same as atenolol	Same as atenolol
metoprolol tartrate (Lopressor) 50–100 qd–bid	Same as atenolol	Same as atenolol	Same as atenolol
nadolol (Corgard) 40–120 mg qd	Same as atenolol	Same as atenolol	Same as atenolol

Table 18.2

Overview of Selected Antihypertensive Agents (*Continued*)

Generic (Trade) Name and Dosage	Selected Adverse Events	Contraindications	Special Considerations
propranolol (Inderal, Inderal LA) 40–160 mg bid 60–180 mg bid	Same as atenolol	Same as atenolol	Same as atenolol
metoprolol succinate (Lopressor, Topral-XL) 50–100 mg qd–bid	Same as atenolol	Same as atenolol	Same as atenolol
pindolol (Visken) 10–40 mg bid	Same as atenolol, but with less resting bradycardia and lipid changes	Same as atenolol	Same as atenolol
penbutolol sulfate (Levatol) 10–40 mg qd	Same as atenolol, but with less resting bradycardia and lipid changes	Same as atenolol	Same as atenolol
acebutolol (Sectral) 200–600 mg bid	Same as atenolol, but with less resting bradycardia and lipid changes; positive antinuclear antibody test and occasional drug-induced lupus	Same as atenolol	Same as atenolol
carteolol (Cartrol) 2.5–10 mg qd	Same as atenolol, but with less resting bradycardia and lipid changes	Same as atenolol	Same as atenolol
COMBINED BLOCKERS			
carvedilol (Coreg) 12.5–50 mg bid	Similar to atenolol but more postural hypotension, bronchospasm	Same as atenolol	Same as atenolol
labetalol (Normodyne, Trandate) 200–800 mg bid	Hepatotoxicity	Same as atenolol	Same as atenolol; does not affect serum lipids

Selected Angiotensin-Converting Enzyme Inhibitors

benazepril (Lotensin) 10–40 mg qd–bid	Common: cough; hypotension, particularly with a diuretic or volume depletion; hyperkalemia, rash, loss of taste, leukopenia, angioedema, neutropenia, and agranulocytosis in <1% of patients	Contraindicated in pregnancy; avoid in patients with bilateral renal artery stenosis or unilateral stenosis	First line in hypertensive diabetic patients with proteinuria; congestive heart failure patients with systolic dysfunction. Check potassium levels within 1 mo of initiating therapy. May decrease excretion of lithium
captopril (Capoten) 25–100 mg bid–tid	Same as benazepril; rash in 10% of patients; loss of taste	Same as benazepril	Same as benazepril
enalapril maleate (Vasotec) 2.5–40 mg qd–bid	Same as benazepril	Same as benazepril	Same as benazepril
fosinopril (Monopril) 10–40 mg qd	Same as benazepril	Same as benazepril	Same as benazepril
lisinopril (Prinivil, Zestril) 10–40 mg qd	Same as benazepril	Same as benazepril	Same as benazepril
moexipril (Univasc) 7.5–30 mg qd	Same as benazepril	Same as benazepril	Same as benazepril
quinapril (Accupril) 10–80 mg qd	Same as benazepril	Same as benazepril	Same as benazepril
ramipril (Altace) 2.5–20 mg qd	Same as benazepril	Same as benazepril	Same as benazepril
trandolapril (Mavik) 1–4 mg qd	Same as benazepril	Same as benazepril	Same as benazepril

Angiotensin II Receptor Blockers

losartan (Cozaar) 25–100 mg qd–bid	Similar to ACE inhibitors but does not cause cough; angioedema (very rare), hyperkalemia		
valsartan (Diovan) 80–320 mg qd			
candesartan cilexetil (Atacand) 8–32 mg qd			
irbesartan (Avapro) 150–300 mg qd			
telmisartan (Micardis) 20–80 mg qd			
eprosartan (Teveten) 400–800 mg qd–bid			
olmesartan (Benicar) 20–40 mg qd			

(*continued*)

Table 18.2

Overview of Selected Antihypertensive Agents (*Continued*)

Generic (Trade) Name and Dosage	Selected Adverse Events	Contraindications	Special Considerations
Calcium Channel Blocking Agents			
NONDIHYDROPYRIDINES			
diltiazem HC1 (Cardizem SR, Cardizem CD) (Dilacor XR) (Tiazac) 180–420 mg qd (Diltia XT) 120–480 mg qd Cardizemla 120–540 mg qd	Dizziness, headache, edema, constipation (especially verapamil); lupus-like rash with diltiazem; conduction defects, worsening of systolic dysfunction, gingival hyperplasia (nausea, headache)	Avoid in patients with atrio-ventricular node dysfunction (second- or third-degree heart block), or left ventricular (systolic) dysfunction	Swallow whole; do not chew, divide, or crush. Hypertensive diabetic patients with proteinuria Increased levels of cyclosporine may occur with concomitant use.
verapamil HC1 (Isoptin SR, Calan SR, Verelan) 120–480 mg qd (Covera HS) 180–480 mg qd	Constipation	Same as diltiazem	Swallow whole; do not chew, divide, or crush. Hypertensive diabetic patients with proteinuria
DIHYDROPYRIDINES			
amlodipine (Norvasc) 2.5–10 mg qd	Dizziness, headache, rash, peripheral edema, flushing, headache, gingival hypertrophy		Swallow whole; do not chew, divide, or crush. Elderly patients with isolated systolic hypertension
felodipine (Plendil) 2.5–20 mg qd	Same as amlodipine		Swallow whole; do not chew, divide, or crush.
isradipine (DynaCirc) 2.5–10 mg bid (DynaCirc CR) 5–10 mg bid	Same as amlodipine		Swallow whole; do not chew, divide, or crush.
nicardipine (Cardene SR) 60–120 mg bid	Same as amlodipine		Swallow whole; do not chew, divide, or crush.
nifedipine (Procardia XL, Adalat CC) 30–60 mg qd	Same as amlodipine		Swallow whole; do not chew, divide, or crush. Do not use sublingually.
nisoldipine (Sular) 10–40 mg qd	Same as amlodipine		Swallow whole; do not chew, divide, or crush.
Other			
ALPHA BLOCKERS			
doxazosin (Cardura) 1–16 mg qd	First-dose phenomenon, postural hypotension, lassitude, vivid dreams, depression, headache, palpitations, fluid retention, weakness, priapism, drowsiness		Administer initially at bedtime; start with low dose and titrate slowly. Ideal for hypertensive patients with benign prostatic hypertrophy
prazosin (Minipress) 2–20 mg bid–tid	Same as doxazosin		Same as doxazosin
terazosin (Hytrin) 1–20 mg qd–bid	Same as doxazosin		Same as doxazosin
CENTRAL AGONISTS			
clonidine (Catapres) 0.1–0.8 mg bid–tid Transdermal (Catapres TTS) one patch weekly (0.1–0.3 mg/d)	Sedation, dry mouth, bradycardia, withdrawal hypertension, bradycardia, heart block	Avoid prescribing for noncompliant patients	Do not stop therapy abruptly without consulting health care provider first.
guanabenz (Wytensin) 4–64 mg bid	Similar to clonidine	Similar to clonidine	Tolerance of alcohol may decrease.
guanfacine (Tenex) 0.5–2.0 mg qd	Similar to clonidine	Similar to clonidine	Take at bedtime. Tolerance of alcohol may decrease.
methyldopa (Aldomet) 250–1000 mg bid	Drowsiness, sedation, fatigue, depression, dry mouth, orthostatic hypotension, bradycardia, heart block, autoimmune disorders, including colitis; hepatitis, hemolytic anemia <1% of patients		Urine may darken after voiding when exposed to air.
DIRECT VASODILATORS			
hydralazine (Apresoline) 25–100 mg bid	Tachycardia, aggravation of angina, headache, dizziness, fluid retention, nasal congestion, lupus-like syndrome, dermatitis, drug fever, hepatitis, peripheral neuropathy		May precipitate angina in patients with coronary artery disease

Table 18.2

Overview of Selected Antihypertensive Agents (*Continued*)

Generic (Trade) Name and Dosage	Selected Adverse Events	Contraindications	Special Considerations
minoxidil (Loniten) 2.5–80 mg qd–bid	Tachycardia, aggravation of angina, dizziness, fluid retention, hypertrichosis	Avoid in patients taking nitrates	Restrict to patients with refractory hypertension.
ADRENERGIC ANTAGONISTS guanadrel (Hylorel) 10–75 mg bid	Postural hypotension, exercise hypotension, diarrhea, weight gain, syncope, retrograde ejaculation		Restrict to patients with refractory hypertension.
guanethidine (Ismelin) 10–50 mg qd	Similar to guanadrel, but greater incidence of diarrhea	Relatively contraindicated in depression	Maximal effect not seen for 2–4 wk Avoid doses above 0.25 mg daily in patients with depression.
reserpine (Serpasil) 0.5–0.25–0.1 mg qd	Nasal stuffiness, drowsiness, GI disturbances, bradycardia, nightmares with high doses, fluid retention, depression, activation of peptic ulcer		

significant, and hypocalcemia may occur instead. The metabolic abnormalities, such as hyperlipidemia and hyperglycemia, usually occur with high doses of diuretics and can be avoided by using low doses of the drug. Loop diuretics may lead to electrolyte and volume depletion more readily than thiazides; they have a short duration of action, but the thiazide diuretics are more effective than loop diuretics in reducing BP in patients with normal renal function. Therefore, loop diuretics should be reserved for hypertensive patients with renal dysfunction (serum creatinine of more than 2.5).

Potassium-Sparing Diuretics

In the kidney, potassium is filtered at the glomerulus and then absorbed parallel to sodium throughout the proximal tubule and thick ascending limb of the loop of Henle, so that only minor amounts reach the distal convoluted tubule. As a result, potassium appearing in urine is secreted at the distal tubule and collecting duct. The potassium-sparing diuretics interfere with sodium reabsorption at the distal tubule, thus decreasing potassium secretion (see Table 18-2).

The Randomized Spironolactone Evaluation Study (RALES) showed the benefits of low-dose spironolactone (Aldactone) to improve morbidity and mortality rates in patients with severe heart failure. Potassium-sparing diuretics have the potential for causing hyperkalemia and hyponatremia, especially in patients with renal insufficiency or diabetes and in patients receiving concurrent treatment with an ACE inhibitor, NSAIDs, or potassium supplements.

Contraindications

Contraindications are the same as for the diuretic class. Additionally, aldosterone antagonists and potassium-sparing diuretics can cause hyperkalemia and hyponatremia and should be avoided in patents with serum potassium levels of more than 5 mEq/L.

Adverse Events

Side effects of spironolactone include gynecomastia, hirsutism, and menstrual irregularities.

Beta-Adrenergic Blockers

Mechanism of Action

Beta-1 receptors, located predominantly in the heart and kidney, regulate heart rate, renin release, and cardiac contractility (see Table 18-2). Beta-2 receptors, located in the lungs, liver, pancreas, and arteriolar smooth muscle, regulate bronchodilation and vasodilation. Beta blockers reduce BP by blocking central and peripheral beta receptors, which results in decreased cardiac output and sympathetic outflow. Blockade of beta-1 receptors on the surface of juxtaglomerular cells located on the afferent arteriole of the kidney results in reduced renin release and decreased stimulation of the renin-angiotensin-aldosterone system.

Despite several pharmacologic differences in the available beta blockers, they are all effective in treating hypertension. Beta blockers that bind specifically to beta-1 receptors are referred to as *cardioselective* because they do not block beta-2 receptors and therefore do not stimulate bronchoconstriction. These agents, which include metoprolol (Lopressor), betaxolol (Kerlone), atenolol (Tenormin), acebutolol (Sectral), and bisoprolol (Zebeta), may be safer than nonselective beta blockers for patients with asthma, chronic obstructive pulmonary disease, and peripheral vascular disease. At higher doses, selective beta blockers lose cardioselectivity and may aggravate a pre-existing condition.

Some beta blockers possess intrinsic sympathomimetic activity (ISA); these agents are partial beta-receptor agonists that reduce heart rate and contractility during excessive sympathetic outflow. In resting states, heart rate and contractility are maintained. Typical medications include pindolol (Visken), penbutolol (Levatol), carteolol (Cartrol), and acebutolol.

Studies suggest that beta blockers may decrease sympathetic activity involved with the progression of heart failure. For example, carvedilol (Coreg) decreased mortality rates in patients with heart failure. Moreover, carvedilol and metoprolol decreased ventricular remodeling (which results in left ventricular hypertrophy). Beta blockers should be used only in patients with stable congestive heart failure. Practitioners should refer any patient with heart failure to a cardiologist for evaluation of therapy.

Patients should be cautioned not to discontinue therapy abruptly. The dose of beta blockers should be tapered gradually over 14 days to prevent withdrawal symptoms, which include unstable angina, myocardial infarction, or even death in patients with underlying cardiovascular disease. Patients without coronary artery disease may experience sinus tachycardia, palpations, increased sweating, and fatigue.

Contraindications

Beta blockers should be avoided in patients who have sinus bradycardia, asthma, chronic obstructive pulmonary disease, second- or third-degree heart block, or overt cardiac failure. Non-ISA beta blockers are the preferred agents for treating hypertension in patients with coexisting coronary artery disease, and especially in patients after myocardial infarction. Beta blockers should be used cautiously in patients with resting ischemia or severe claudication secondary to peripheral vascular disease, reactive airway disease, systolic congestive heart failure, diabetes mellitus, or depression.

Adverse Events

The most common side effects of beta blockers are fatigue, drowsiness, dizziness, bronchospasm, nausea, and vomiting. Serious side effects include bradycardia, atrioventricular conduction abnormalities, and the development of congestive heart failure.

ACE Inhibitors

Mechanism of Action

ACE inhibitors such as captopril, enalapril, and lisinopril exert an antihypertensive effect by inhibiting ACE, which is responsible for converting angiotensin I to angiotensin II, a potent vasoconstrictor (see Table 18-2). ACE inhibitors also inhibit the degradation of bradykinin and increase the synthesis of vasodilating prostaglandins. This class of antihypertensive agents is indicated as first-line therapy in hypertensive diabetic patients who have proteinuria. ACE inhibitors decrease morbidity and mortality rates in patients with congestive heart failure and systolic dysfunction. The Second Australian National BP trial reported slightly better outcomes in white men with a regimen that began with an ACE inhibitor compared with one starting with a diuretic.

Contraindications

ACE inhibitors should be avoided in patients with bilateral renal artery stenosis or unilateral stenosis because of the risk of acute renal failure. They are also contraindicated in patients who have experienced angioedema and during pregnancy because of their teratogenic effects.

Adverse Events

The most common side effects associated with ACE inhibitors include chronic dry cough, rashes (most common with captopril [Capoten]), and dizziness. Hyperkalemia can occur in patients with renal disease or diabetes. Angioedema is a rare but dangerous side effect that occurs most frequently in African-Americans; it is reversible on discontinuation of the agent (Brown, Ray, Snowden, & Griffin, 1996;

Burkhart, Brown, Griffin, et al., 1996; He, Klag, Appek, et al., 1999). Laryngeal edema, another rare adverse effect, is life-threatening and requires immediate medical attention.

Angiotensin II Receptor Blockers

ARBs block the vasoconstriction and aldosterone-secreting effects of angiotensin II by selectively blocking the binding of angiotensin II to the angiotensin II receptor found in many tissues (see Table 18-2). They are indicated for patients with hypertension, nephropathy in type 2 diabetes, and heart failure and those who cannot tolerate the side effects associated with ACE inhibitors.

The results of the Losartan Intervention for Endpoint reduction in hypertension study (LIFE) suggest that losartan is more effective than atenolol in reducing cardiovascular morbidity and mortality in diabetic patients with hypertension and left ventricular hypertrophy. Available ARBs are losartan (Cozaar), valsartan (Diovan), candesartan (Atacand), telmisartan (Micardis), eprosartan (Teveten), olmesartan (Benicar), and irbesartan (Avapro). The incidence of cough and hyperkalemia associated with this class of drugs is lower than with ACE inhibitors.

Contraindications

Caution should be used in patients with renal and hepatic function impairment. Angioedema can also be seen with ARB therapy, but with much less frequency than with ACE inhibitors. There should be some justification (heart failure or proteinuric nephropathic) for the use of ARBs in patients having experienced ACE inhibitor-related angioedema.

Adverse Events

Adverse reactions include dizziness, upper respiratory tract infections, cough, viral infection, fatigue, diarrhea, pain, sinusitis, pharyngitis, and rhinitis. Like ACE inhibitors, ARBs are contraindicated in pregnancy.

Calcium Channel Blockers

CCBs share the ability to inhibit the movement of calcium ions across the cell membrane (see Table 18-2). The effects on the cardiovascular system include depression of mechanical contraction of myocardial and smooth muscle and depression of both impulse formation and conduction velocity. The result is muscle relaxation and vasodilation. Common CCBs, such as verapamil (Calan) and diltiazem (Cardizem), decrease heart rate and slow cardiac conduction at the atrioventricular node. The dihydropyridines (amlodipine [Norvasc], felodipine [Plendil], nifedipine [Procardia XL], nicardipine [Cardene SR], nisoldipine [Sular], and isradipine [DynaCirc]) are potent vasodilators. CCBs are effective as monotherapy and are especially effective in African-American patients. CCBs are indicated for treating hypertension associated with ischemic heart disease. The long-acting dihydropyridines are second-line therapy for elderly patients with isolated systolic hypertension. The CCBs are similar in antihypertensive effectiveness but differ in other pharmacodynamic effects.

Contraindications

First-generation CCBs such as verapamil and diltiazem may accelerate the progression of congestive heart failure in a patient with cardiac dysfunction. Therefore, these agents should be avoided unless they are being used to treat angina, hypertension, or arrhythmia. Two trials with amlodipine in patients with severe heart failure showed that this agent is safe (Tierney et al., 2004).

Diltiazem and verapamil should also be avoided in patients with atrioventricular node dysfunction (second- or third-degree heart block) or left ventricular (systolic) dysfunction when the ejection fraction measures less than 45%. Short-acting nifedipine should not be used for treating essential hypertension or hypertensive emergencies because of its association with erratic fluctuations in BP and reflex tachycardia.

Adverse Events

The most common side effects of CCBs are headache, peripheral edema, and bradycardia. The dihydropyridine agents (nifedipine, nicardipine, isradipine, felodipine, nisoldipine, and amlodipine) produce symptoms of vasodilation, such as headache, flushing, palpations, and peripheral edema. Other side effects of nifedipine include dizziness, gingival hyperplasia, mood changes, and various gastrointestinal complaints. Nifedipine may cause reflex tachycardia as a result of stimulating the baroreceptors in response to an acute drop in BP.

Diltiazem and verapamil can cause gastrointestinal upset, peripheral edema, and hypotension. Rare side effects include bradycardia, atrioventricular block, and congestive heart failure. Verapamil can cause constipation in the elderly.

Peripheral Alpha-1 Receptor Blockers

Doxazosin (Cardura), prazosin (Minipress), and terazosin (Hytrin) are selective alpha-1 receptor blockers that are effective in patients with benign prostatic hypertrophy (see Table 18-2). Peripheral alpha-1 receptor blockers act peripherally by dilating both arterioles and veins, causing relaxation of smooth muscle. In clinical studies, this class of antihypertensive agents is associated with a small decrease in LDL and cholesterol.

Contraindications

In the presence of cardiovascular disease, alpha-1 receptor blockers should be avoided, as the ALLHAT study showed that these patients had an increase in mortality. The use of tadalafil (Cialis) and vardenafil (Levitra) is contraindicated with the use of alpha-1 receptor blockers. Sildenafil (Viagra) should be avoided within 4 hours of administration of alpha-1 receptor blockers due to an increased risk of symptomatic hypotension.

Adverse Events

The most common side effect associated with this class of antihypertensive medications is the first-dose phenomenon, which consists of dizziness or faintness, palpitations, or syncope. These agents should be administered initially at bedtime and the dosage should be adjusted slowly. With chronic administration, even at low doses, fluid and sodium accumulate, requiring concurrent diuretic therapy. Other side effects include vivid dreams and depression.

Central Alpha-2 Receptor Agonists

Central alpha-2 agonists stimulate alpha-2-adrenergic receptors in the brain, resulting in decreased sympathetic outflow, cardiac output, and peripheral resistance (see Table 18-2). These agents may cause fluid retention and in most cases should be used in combination with a diuretic. Clonidine (Catapres), methyldopa (Aldomet), guanabenz (Wytensin), and guanfacine (Tenex) should not be used as initial monotherapy. Abrupt cessation of alpha-2 agonist therapy may result in a compensatory increase in the norepinephrine level, which in turn raises BP. This effect is commonly referred to as *rebound hypertension* (JNC VI, 1997).

Adverse Events

These agents may cause fluid retention, sedation, and dry mouth. Also, the first-dose effect of dizziness and syncope are possible.

Direct Vasodilators

The direct vasodilators hydralazine (Apresoline) and minoxidil (Loniten) cause arteriolar smooth muscle relaxation, resulting in reduced BP (see Table 18-2). Direct vasodilators should be reserved for patients with essential or severe hypertension.

Both hydralazine and minoxidil may cause fluid retention and reflex tachycardia. Their use should be combined with a diuretic and a beta blocker or other agent (clonidine, diltiazem, or verapamil) that slows the heart rate.

Contraindications

Hydralazine is contraindicated in patients with coronary artery disease and mitral valvular rheumatic heart disease. Minoxidil is contraindicated in patients with pheochromocytoma, acute myocardial infarction, and dissecting aortic aneurysm.

Adverse Events

Hydralazine is associated with a lupus-like syndrome that is dose-related at dosages greater than 300 mg/day. Other adverse reactions include dermatitis, drug fever, and peripheral neuropathy. Minoxidil may cause a drug-induced hirsutism, which is unacceptable to most female patients.

Adrenergic Antagonists

Reserpine (Serpasil), guanethidine (Ismelin), and guanadrel (Hylorel) inhibit the sympathetic system by depleting norepinephrine stores in the central nervous system (see Table 18-2). This results in a decrease in peripheral vascular resistance and a reduction in BP. In patients who use these agents, depression may result from decreased catecholamine and serotonin levels in the central nervous system. Reserpine's use is limited because of its side effect profile, which includes depression, impotence, diarrhea, bradycardia, drowsiness, and nasal stuffiness.

Guanadrel and guanethidine also produce numerous adverse effects, such as diarrhea, impotence, orthostatic hypotension, and syncope. They should be used with caution.

SELECTING THE MOST APPROPRIATE AGENT

First-Line Therapy

First-line therapy with diuretics is preferred in most cases of stage 1 hypertension (see Fig. 18-1). The NHLBI and the JNC VII endorsed the result of ALLHAT using diuretics as monotherapy in preference of other antihypertensive agents. BP was brought under control in 60% of the participants in the ALLHAT trail. ACE inhibitors, ARBs, beta blockers, CCBs, or combinations may be considered if the BP goal is not reached. However, patients with concomitant diseases may be treated with other agents as the first line, depending on the compelling indication (Table 18-3). The following discussion addresses some of the more common compelling indications.

Ischemic Heart Disease

Ischemic heart disease is the most common form of target-organ damage associated with hypertension. For patients who also have stable angina, the first choice agent is a beta blocker followed by a long-acting CCB. In patients with acute coronary syndrome, a beta blocker and an ACE inhibitor are the initial therapy. Patients recovering from a myocardial infarction are candidates for treatment with ACE inhibitors, beta blockers, and/or aldosterone antagonists. Aggressive therapy with lipid management and aspirin is also indicated in these patients.

Heart Failure

Heart failure (systolic or diastolic ventricular dysfunction) results from systolic hypertension and ischemic heart disease. Preventive measures for those at high risk include BP and cholesterol control. ACE inhibitors and beta blockers are recommended in asymptomatic individuals. For patients with symptomatic ventricular dysfunction of end-stage heart disease, ACE inhibitors, beta blockers, ARBs, and aldosterone blockers are recommended, along with loop diuretics (JNC VII, 2003).

The Metoprolol CR/XL Randomized Intervention Trial in Heart Failure (MERIT-HF) and the Carvedilol Prospective Randomized Cumulative Survival (COPERNICUS) trial showed favorable results using beta blockers to treat heart failure. Chapter 21 gives more detail.

Diabetes Mellitus

In patients with diabetic hypertension, the targeted BP goal is 130/80; achieving this goal usually requires a combination of two or more drugs. Thiazide diuretics, beta blockers, ACE inhibitors, ARBs, and CCBs are beneficial in reducing the incidence of cardiovascular disease and stroke. Studies have shown favorable effects of ACE inhibitors and ARBs on the progression of diabetic nephropathy and cardiovascular disease and in the reduction of albuminuria. Chapter 49 gives more detail.

Chronic Kidney Disease

Chronic kidney disease is defined by either reduced excretory function with an estimated glomerular filtration rate of 60 mL/min per 1.73 m^2 (creatinine of above 1.5 mg/dL in men or above 1.3 mg/dL in women) or the presence of albuminuria (above 300 mg/d or 200 mg albumin per gram of creatinine). Aggressive BP management with three or more drugs is required to reach a target BP goal of less than 130/80 mm Hg and to slow the deterioration of renal function. ACE inhibitors and ARBs offer the best renal protection, as recommended by JNC VII, the National Kidney Foundation, and the American Diabetes Association.

Cerebrovascular Disease

The rate of recurrent stroke is lowered by the combination of an ACE inhibitor and a thiazide-type diuretic. The HOPE Study and the Perindopril Protection Against Recurrent Stroke Study (PROGRESS) provided compelling evidence that treatment with an ACE inhibitor or an ACE inhibitor and a diuretic can further reduce the risk of stroke.

Obesity and the Metabolic Syndrome

Obesity is a risk factor for the development of hypertension and cardiovascular disease. The Adult Treatment Panel III

Table 18.3

Compelling Indications

High-Risk Conditions with Compelling Indication	Recommended Drugs					
	Diuretic	Beta Blocker	ACE Inhibitor	ARB	CCB	Aldosterone Antagonist
Heart failure	•	•	•	•		•
Post–myocardial infarction		•	•			•
High coronary disease risk	•	•	•		•	
Diabetes	•	•	•	•	•	
Chronic kidney disease			•	•		
Recurrent stroke prevention	•		•			
Atrial fibrillation		•			•	

guidelines for cholesterol management define metabolic syndrome as abdominal obesity (more than 40 inches in men, more than 35 inches in women), glucose intolerance (fasting glucose of above 110), BP of at least 130/85 mm Hg, triglyceride level of more than 150, and a low level of high-density lipoprotein cholesterol (less than 40 mg/dL in men or less than 50 mg/dL in women). Aggressive lifestyle modification should be pursued in all patients with the metabolic syndrome, and appropriate drug therapy should be instituted for each of its components.

Left Ventricular Hypertrophy (LVH)

LVH increases the risk of subsequent cardiovascular disease. Aggressive BP management as well as weight loss and sodium restriction can slow the regression of LVH. Treatment with all classes of antihypertensive agents is acceptable except for direct vasodilators such as hydralazine or minoxidil.

Peripheral Arterial Disease

Peripheral arterial disease is equivalent in risk to ischemic heart disease. Treatment can include any class of antihypertensive drugs. Aspirin should be used and other risk factors should be treated aggressively.

Benign Prostatic Hypertrophy (BPH)

BPH can be treated with an alpha antagonist (doxazosin, prazosin, terazosin). The preferred drug for BPH is tamsulosin (Flomax). The ALLHAT study found alpha blockers increased the mortality rate in cardiovascular disease.

Second-Line Therapy

When the patient's systolic BP exceeds 160 (stage 2 hypertension), antihypertensive treatment begins with combination therapy. Combination therapy can include a diuretic with an ACE inhibitor, ARB, CCB, or beta blocker, or any other combination. The second agent should be a drug from another class; typically, a diuretic is one of the two agents, unless other reasons prohibit its use or a compelling indication exists. Low-dose combination therapy has gained wide support due to its efficacy, ease of administration, compliance rate, and decreased risk of side effects. If the patient's BP remains elevated, dosages should be adjusted and additional drugs included until the goal BP is achieved.

Special Population Considerations

Pediatric

Treatment of hypertension in children can be approached in the same manner as for adults, with the appropriate agent selected for specific indications. Dosages of antihypertensive medication should be adjusted for children.

Geriatric

The Trial of Nonpharmacological Interventions in the Elderly (TONE) showed that in older patients with hypertension, BP can be reduced by low-sodium diets and weight loss. In some instances, patients could discontinue

their antihypertensive medications or reduce the number of medications required to remain normotensive (Sander, 2002).

Elderly patients are very sensitive to medications that cause sympathetic inhibition and are at greater risk of becoming volume depleted than their younger counterparts. Decreased renal and hepatic function increases the risk of adverse events in this population. Antihypertensive medications should be started at half the recommended starting dose to decrease the risk of adverse effects.

Diuretics and beta blockers are effective in elderly patients because they have been shown to reduce morbidity and mortality rates. Patients with isolated systolic hypertension should start hypertensive therapy with a diuretic unless there is a compelling reason to avoid its use. The long-acting dihydropyridine CCBs are also effective and are an alternative in these patients.

Women

There are no significant differences in BP response between the sexes. Women taking oral contraceptives may have an increase in BP, and the risk of hypertension may increase with the duration of oral contraceptive use. If hypertension develops as a result of oral contraceptive use, an alternate contraception method should be used. Because of the risk of stroke associated with oral contraceptive use and cigarette smoking, women taking oral contraceptives should be encouraged not to smoke cigarettes, and women older than 35 years of age should not take oral contraceptives if they continue to smoke.

Women diagnosed with hypertension before pregnancy can continue taking antihypertensive agents throughout pregnancy. Most but not all antihypertensive agents are safe for use during pregnancy. ACE inhibitors and ARBs should be avoided during pregnancy because they are teratogenic. Beta blockers should also be avoided during early pregnancy because of the risk of fetal growth retardation, but beta blockers may be used during the second or third trimester. Methyldopa is recommended for women who are diagnosed with hypertension during pregnancy.

African-Americans

The incidence of hypertension and hypertension-related complications is believed to be higher in African-Americans than in any ethnic group. Some African-Americans experience hypertension before age 10. This is attributed to two major risk factors, obesity and inactivity. Other risk factors include a diet high in sodium and low in potassium. This has resulted in the greatest incidence of stroke, end-stage renal disease, cardiovascular disease, and death in this population. African-Americans who are diagnosed and treated have a lower incidence of complications.

African-Americans have physiologic characteristics that contribute to this risk, including low circulating renin levels with excessive levels of angiotensin II; endothelial dysfunction as a result of reduced bradykinin and nitric oxide; abnormal sympathetic nervous system activation; and higher levels of intracellular calcium stores. African-Americans are more responsive to monotherapy with diuretics. Results from the ALLHAT found that chlorthalidone and amlodipine were superior to ACE inhibitors in treating African-Americans (Papademetriou et al., 2003). Alpha blockers should not be used as initial monotherapy. ACE inhibitors may induce angioedema, which occurs two to four times more frequently in African-Americans.

Diabetic Patients

Diuretics are underprescribed in patients with diabetes mellitus and hyperlipidemia because of the risk of increasing insulin resistance. However, the SHEP trial showed that morbidity and mortality rates were reduced in diabetic patients treated with low-dose diuretics (Moser, 1998; SHEP Cooperative Research Group, 1991). The goal BP in diabetic patients with hypertension is 130/85 mm Hg.

HYPERTENSIVE EMERGENCY

Hypertensive emergency or malignant hypertension is defined as a severe elevation in diastolic BP, usually higher than 120 mm Hg, in the presence of target-organ damage. Immediate treatment with an intravenous antihypertensive agent is needed to salvage viable tissue. The marked elevation in BP results in arteriolar fibrinoid necrosis, endothelial damage, platelet and fibrin deposition in the media of smooth muscle, and loss of autoregulatory function. This results in end-organ ischemia such as encephalopathy, myocardial infarction, unstable angina, pulmonary edema, eclampsia, stroke, intracranial hemorrhage, life-threatening arterial bleeding, or aortic dissection. These patients require hospitalization and parenteral drug therapy. How rapidly BP should be lowered, and to what level, remains controversial.

The drug of choice to treat hypertensive emergencies depends on the clinical situation. Commonly used medications include nitroprusside, intravenous nitroglycerine, diazoxide, trimethaphan, labetalol, and hydralazine.

In cases of hypertensive urgency without evidence of target-organ damage, the BP can be reduced over 24 hours. Fast-acting oral agents such as captopril and clonidine (Table 18-4) are commonly used. Most patients with hypertensive urgency are those who are newly diagnosed or who do not adhere to the therapeutic regimen. After BP is lowered, the patient's drug regimen is assessed to determine possible causes of nonadherence, such as adverse effects that interfere with the patient's lifestyle or a complex regimen that could be simplified.

MONITORING PATIENT RESPONSE

Follow-Up and Monitoring

Patients should be followed at 1-month intervals after the initiation of treatment until the goal BP is attained. Patients with a higher BP may need more frequent visits until the target BP is achieved. Patient with complicated conditions should be seen more often. Once the desired BP is attained, patients should return for visits at 3- to 6-month intervals. The patient's efforts and lifestyle modifications should be discussed at each visit. Serum creatinine and potassium levels should be monitored once or twice a year in patients taking antihypertensive medications.

Patients with stage 1 or stage 2 hypertension should be scheduled for a follow-up visit 2 to 4 weeks after initiation of drug therapy or a change in the drug regimen. Patients with stage 3 hypertension and hypertensive urgency should be seen within 2 weeks. Once BP returns to a normal range, the patient should be monitored every 3 to 6 months.

The importance of adhering to the drug regimen cannot be overemphasized. The practitioner needs to be alert for signs of nonadherence and should ask patients about their experiences or problems with adhering to the drug regimen. Side effects should be discussed, and changes in medications may or may not be considered at each visit.

PATIENT EDUCATION

Patient education is a vital part of hypertension treatment. Because most patients are free of symptoms, they must be educated about the disease, the importance of adhering therapy, and the consequences of uncontrolled hypertension. Patient education booklets available from most pharmaceutical companies may be used to reinforce the information provided by the practitioner.

Because each antihypertensive medication has some side effects, the patient needs to be informed about what they are, what actions to take to relieve minor side effects, and what to do about intolerable or dangerous side effects. Because the objective of drug therapy is to lower BP without intolerable effects, the patient needs to know which adverse reactions should be reported to the practitioner and which ones may be relieved by switching to an alternative drug in a different class. The patient also needs to know that several different agents may be tried before finding the one that best controls his or her BP with minimal or no side effects. Other important teaching involves information

Table 18.4

Oral Drugs Commonly Used to Treat Hypertensive Urgencies

Drug	Dose/Route	Onset of Action	Duration of Action	Major Side Effects	Mechanism of Action
captopril	25–50 mg PO	15 min	4–6 h	Rash, pruritus, proteinuria, loss of taste, hypotension	ACE inhibitor
clonidine	0.2 mg PO initially, then 0.1 mg/h up to 0.8 mg total	0.5–2 h	6–8 h	Sedation, dry mouth, dizziness, constipation	Alpha-2 antagonist
labetalol	200–400 mg PO 2–3 h	0.5–2 h	4 h	Orthostatic hypertension, nausea and vomiting	Alpha- and beta-adrenergic blocker
minoxidil	5–20 mg PO	0.5–1 h (max: 2–4 h)	12–16 h	Tachycardia, fluid retention	Vasodilator

about lifestyle changes and the consequences of uncontrolled hypertension.

Nutrition/Lifestyle Changes

Hypertensive adults should lose weight and increase their physical activity levels as needed. Patients should maintain an appropriate body weight, follow the DASH eating plan, and restrict sodium and alcohol consumption.

Complementary and Alternative Medications

To date, there is no evidence that alternative medications reduce BP.

■ Case Study

M.R., a 55-year-old African-American man, was referred to the hypertension clinic for evaluation of high BP noted on an initial screening. He reports having headaches and occasional nosebleeds. He states that he has gained 15 pounds over the last year.

Past medical history
  Appendectomy 30 years ago
  Peptic ulcer disease 10 years ago
  Type 2 diabetes mellitus for 5 years

Family history
  Father had hypertension; died of myocardial infarction at age 55 years
  Mother had diabetes mellitus and hypertension; died of cerebrovascular accident at age 60 years

Physical examination
  Height 69 in, weight 108 kg
  BP: 164/98 mm Hg (left arm), 168/96 mm Hg (right arm)
  Pulse: 84 beats/min, regular
  Funduscopic examination: mild arterial narrowing, sharp discs, no exudates or hemorrhages

Laboratory findings
  Blood urea nitrogen: 24 mg/dL
  Serum creatinine: 2.0 mg/dL
  Glucose: 95 mg/dL
  K^+: 4.0 mEq/L
  Total cholesterol: 224 mg/dL
  High-density lipoprotein cholesterol: 30 mg/dL
  Triglycerides: 125 mg/dL
  Urinalysis: 1+ proteinuria
  Electrocardiogram and chest radiograph: mild left ventricular hypertrophy

Social history
  Tobacco: 35 pack/years
  Alcohol: pint of vodka/week
  Coffee: 2 cups/day

Diagnosis: Stage 2 hypertension

→ 1. List specific goals for treating M.R.'s hypertension.

→ 2. What would you consider as first-line therapy for M.R., and why?

→ 3. What dietary and lifestyle changes would you consider recommending for M.R.?

→ 4. What over-the-counter and/or alternative medications would be appropriate for M.R.?

→ 5. Beside BP, what else will you monitor to determine whether your therapy is successful? When you monitor these?

→ 6. Describe one or two drug/drug or drug/food interactions that you would be wary of when prescribing your selected first-line agent.

(Continued)

■ Case Study (*Continued*)

→ 7. List one or two adverse reactions for the selected agent that would cause you to change therapy.

→ 8. If your first-line agent was unsuccessful or a significant adverse drug event occurred, what would be your second-line agent for M.R., and why?

→ 9. Discuss specific patient education based on both your first- and second-line choices.

Bibliography

Starred references are cited in the text.

Basile, J. (2003). High-risk hypertensive patients: how to optimize therapy using ACE inhibitors and ARBs. *Consultant*, 139–140.

Bloch, M. J. (2003). The diagnosis and management of renovascular disease: a primary care perspective. *Journal of Clinical Hypertension, 5*, 210–218.

*Brown, N. J., Ray, W. A., Snowden, M., & Griffin, M. R. (1996). Black Americans have an increased rate of angiotensin-converting enzyme inhibition associated angioedema. *Clinical Pharmacology and Therapeutics, 60*, 8–13.

*Burkhart, G. A., Brown, N. J., Griffin, M. R., Ray, W. A., Hammerstrom, T., et al. (1996). Angiotensin-converting enzyme inhibitor-associated angioedema: higher risk in blacks than whites. *Pharmacoepidemiology and Drug Safety, 5*, 149–154.

CAPRICORN Investigators. (2001). Effects of carvedilol on outcome after myocardial infarction in patients with left-ventricular dysfunction: the CAPRICORN randomised trial. *Lancet, 357*, 1385–1390.

Drug facts and comparisons 2004 (8th ed.). Missouri: Wolters Kluwer Health.

Ferdinand, K. (2003). Treatment guidelines for hypertension in African Americans. *The Clinical Advisor*, 2–14.

Flack, J. M. (2003). Hypertension in the African-American population. *Therapeutic Spolight*, 4–10.

Hawkins, D. W., Bussey, H. I., & Prisant, L. M. (1999). Hypertension. In J. T. Dipiro, R. L. Talbert, G. C. Yee, G. R. Matzke, B. G. Wells, & L. M. Posey (Eds.), *Pharmacotherapy: a pathophysiologic approach* (4th ed., pp. 131–152). Stamford, CT: Appleton & Lange.

*He, J., Klag, M. J., Appek, L. J., Charleston, J., & Whelton, P. K. (1999). The renin-angiotensin system and BP: differences between blacks and whites. *American Journal of Hypertension, 12*(6), 555–562.

Kang-Sha, L. (2002). Angioedema associated with candesartan. *Pharmacotherapy, 22*(9), 1176–1179.

*Joint National Committee on Prevention, Detection, Evaluation, and Treatment of High BP. (1997). Sixth report of the Joint National Committee on Prevention, Detection, Evaluation, and Treatment of High BP (JNC VI). *Archives of Internal Medicine, 157*, 2413–2446.

*Joint National Committee on Prevention, Detection, Evaluation, and Treatment of High BP. (2003). Seventh report of the Joint National Committee on Prevention, Detection, Evaluation, and Treatment of High BP (JNC VI). *Journal of the American Medical Association, 289*, 2560–2572.

*Moser, M. (1998). Why are physicians not prescribing diuretics more frequently in the management of hypertension? *Journal of the American Medical Association, 279*, 1813–1816.

National High Blood Pressure Education Program [NHBPEP] Working Group. (1994). National High Blood Pressure Education Program Working Group report on hypertension in diabetes. *Hypertension, 23*, 145–158.

Oparil, S. (2003). Hypertension in African Americans: reducing the risks. *Clinical Advisor*, 11–14.

*Papademetriou, V., Piller, L., Ford, C., et al. (2003). Characteristics and lipid distribution of a large, high-risk, hypertension population: the lipid-lowering component of the antihypertensive and lipid-lowering treatment to prevent heart attack trail (ALLHAT). *Journal of Clinical Hypertension, 5*, 377–385.

Poole-Wilson, P., Swedberg, K., Cleland, J., et al. (2003). Comparison of carvedilol and metoprolol on clinical outcomes in patients with chronic heart failure in the Carvedilol Or Metoprolol European Trial (COMET): randomised controlled trial. *Lancet, 362*, 7–13.

*Sander, G. (2002). High blood pressure in the geriatric population: treatment considerations. *American Journal of Geriatric Cardiology, 11*, 223–232.

*SHEP Cooperative Research Group. (1991). Prevention of stroke by antihypertensive drug treatment in older persons with isolated systolic hypertension. *Journal of the American Medical Association, 265*, 3255–3264.

Sica, D. (2002). ACE inhibitors and stroke: new considerations. *Journal of Clinical Hypertension, 4*, 126–129.

Sica, D., & Black, H. (2002). ACE inhibitor-related angioedema: can angiotensin-receptor blockers be safely used? *Journal of Clinical Hypertension, 4*(5), 375–380.

*Tierney, L., McPhee, S., & Papadakis, M. (2004). *Current medical diagnosis and treatment*. New York: McGraw-Hill.

Tucker, C. A. (2003) Hidden dangers: self-medication by hypertension patients. *Advance*, 61–63.

Yancy, C., Fowler M., Colucci, W., et al. (2001). Race and the response to adrenergic blockade with carvedilol in patients with chronic heart failure. *New England Journal of Medicine, 344*, 1358–1365.

Whelton, P. K., Appel, L. J., Espeland, M. A., et al. (1998). Sodium reduction and weight loss in the treatment of hypertension in older persons. *Journal of the American Medical Association, 279*, 839–846.

Williams, G. (2001). Hypertensive vascular disease. In *Harrison's principles of internal medicine* (pp. 1414–1430). New York: McGraw-Hill.

Visit the Connection web site for the most up-to-date drug information.

HYPERLIPIDEMIA

■ JOHN BARRON

Hyperlipidemia is a blood disorder characterized by elevations in blood cholesterol levels. The term is often used synonymously with *dyslipidemia* and *hypercholesterolemia*. Hyperlipidemia is one of the major contributing risk factors in the development of coronary heart disease (CHD). It is estimated that approximately 12.6 million people in the United States have CHD, with approximately 530,000 deaths each year (National Heart, Lung and Blood Institute, 2002). In addition, approximately $112 billion is spent each year on healthcare expenditures and lost productivity secondary to CHD.

Informed estimates indicate that approximately 105 million adults aged 20 and older have total cholesterol levels above 200 mg/dL (50.7%), and 37 million (18.3%) have levels above 240 mg/dL (American Heart Association, 2003). Less than half of the patients eligible for lipid-lowering therapy receive it, and only about one third are at their low-density lipoprotein (LDL) cholesterol goal (Expert Panel, National Cholesterol Education Program, 2001). In addition, approximately 50% of patients discontinue therapy within 6 months of initiating treatment, with only 30% to 40% remaining on therapy after 12 months.

Multiple large studies have shown that reducing elevated cholesterol levels reduces morbidity and mortality rates in patients with and without existing CHD (Downs et al., 1998; Frick, Elo, Kaapa, et al., 1987; Heart Protection Study Collaborative Group, 2002; Lewis, Moye, Sacks, et al., 1998; Long-Term Intervention With Pravastatin in Ischaemic Disease [LIPID] Study Group, 1998; Scandinavian Simvastatin Survival Study Group, 1994; Shepherd et al., 1995). Advances in CHD therapies, including treatment of high cholesterol levels and preventive measures such as aspirin and beta-blocker therapy in patients with previous myocardial infarction (MI), have reduced mortality associated with acute MI and have improved long-term survival in patients after MI (Pearson & Swan, 1996). As a result of these advances, deaths from cardiovascular disease have decreased by approximately 50% since the early 1980s, although cardiovascular disease still remains the leading cause of death in the United States.

CAUSES

In hyperlipidemia, serum cholesterol levels may be elevated as a result of an increased level of any of the lipoproteins (see section on Pathophysiology: Lipoproteins and Lipid Metabolism). The mechanisms for hyperlipidemia appear to be genetic (primary) and environmental (secondary). In fact, the most common cause of hyperlipidemia (95% of all those with hyperlipidemia) is a combination of genetic and environmental factors.

Some individuals are genetically predisposed to elevated cholesterol levels. They may inherit defective genes that lead to abnormalities in the synthesis or breakdown of cholesterol. These may include abnormalities in LDL receptors and mutations in apolipoproteins that lead to increased production of cholesterol or decreased clearance of cholesterol from the bloodstream (see section on Pathophysiology: Lipoproteins and Lipid Metabolism).

Secondary factors may include medications (eg, beta blockers and oral contraceptives), concomitant disease states or other conditions (eg, diabetes mellitus and pregnancy), diets high in fat and cholesterol, lack of exercise, obesity, and smoking (Box 19-1).

PATHOPHYSIOLOGY

The major plasma lipids are cholesterol, triglycerides, and phospholipids. Cholesterol is a naturally occurring substance that is required by the body to synthesize bile acids and steroid hormones and to maintain the integrity of cell membranes. Although cholesterol is found predominantly in the cells, approximately 7% circulates in the serum. It is this serum cholesterol that is implicated in atherosclerosis. Triglycerides are made up of free fatty acids and glycerol and serve as an important source of stored energy. Phospholipids are essential for cell function and lipid transport. Because these lipids are insoluble in plasma, they are surrounded by special fat-carrying proteins, called *lipoproteins*, for transport in the blood.

Lipoproteins are produced in the liver and intestines, but endogenous production of lipoproteins occurs primarily in the liver. Lipoproteins consist of a hydrophobic (water-insoluble) inner core made of cholesterol and triglycerides and a hydrophilic (water-soluble) outer surface composed of apolipoproteins and phospholipids. Apolipoproteins are specialized proteins that identify specific receptors to which the lipoprotein will bind. They are thought to play a role in the development or prevention of hyperlipidemia because they control the interaction and metabolism of the lipoproteins.

BOX 19–1. SECONDARY CAUSES OF HYPERLIPIDEMIA

Disease States	Drugs
Acute hepatitis	Alcohol
Diabetes mellitus	Beta blockers
Hypothyroidism	Glucocorticoids
Nephrotic syndrome	Oral contraceptives
Primary biliary cirrhosis	Progestins
Systemic lupus erythematosus	Thiazide diuretics
Uremia	

Lipoproteins and Lipid Metabolism

The major lipoproteins are named according to their density. They include chylomicrons, very–low-density lipoproteins (VLDL), intermediate-density lipoproteins (IDL), LDL, high-density lipoproteins (HDL), and lipoprotein (a).

Chylomicrons

Chylomicrons, the largest lipoproteins, are composed primarily of triglycerides. Chylomicrons are produced in the gut from dietary fat and cholesterol that has been solubilized by bile acids (exogenous pathway). Chylomicrons normally are not present in the blood after a 12- to 14-hour fast.

Very–Low-Density Lipoproteins

Very–low-density lipoproteins are primarily composed of cholesterol and triglycerides. VLDLs are the major carrier of endogenous triglycerides. On secretion into the bloodstream, lipoprotein lipase and hepatic lipase hydrolyze the triglyceride core by a mechanism similar to that which occurs with chylomicrons. As the triglyceride content decreases, the lipoprotein becomes progressively smaller with a higher percentage of cholesterol; it is now referred to as an IDL. IDL is a short-lived lipoprotein that is converted to LDL or is taken up by LDL receptors on the liver. LDL, the final product of the metabolism of VLDL, contains the most cholesterol by weight of all the lipoproteins. It is estimated that 60% to 75% of the total cholesterol is contained in LDLs (Talbert, 1997).

Approximately 50% of LDL is taken up by the liver, and the remaining 50% is taken up by peripheral cells. Increased levels of LDL cholesterol are directly related to the probability that atherosclerosis will develop. Thus, LDL cholesterol is usually referred to as "bad" cholesterol.

High-Density Lipoproteins

High-density lipoprotein particles are produced in the liver and intestine. The primary function of HDL cholesterol is to remove LDL cholesterol from the peripheral cells and to remove triglycerides that result from the degradation of chylomicrons and VLDL particles. The HDL then transports these particles to the liver for metabolism. This process is termed reverse cholesterol transport. For this reason, HDL is often referred to as "good" cholesterol.

Lipoprotein (a)

Lipoprotein (a) is an LDL-like lipoprotein that contains an additional apolipoprotein, apo (a). Although the exact mechanism by which lipoprotein (a) contributes to CHD is unknown, many experts believe that lipoprotein (a) is an independent risk factor for the development of CHD.

Pathogenesis of Atherosclerosis

Atherosclerosis is characterized by the development of lesions resulting from accumulations of cholesterol in the blood vessel wall. Atherosclerosis primarily affects the larger arteries, including the coronary arteries.

The atherogenic process begins with the accumulation of LDL cholesterol under the endothelial lining of the innermost arterial layer, the intima. As LDLs accumulate, circulating monocytes attach to the endothelial lining and penetrate between the endothelial cells into the subendothelial space. On entry into the subendothelial space, the monocytes form into macrophages, which then ingest the LDLs. Macrophages, in particular, have a high affinity for modified (oxidized) LDL, which is believed to be more atherogenic than nonoxidized LDL. Thus, by preventing the oxidation of LDL, antioxidants such as vitamin E may be beneficial in preventing CHD, although the efficacy of antioxidants in this capacity remains unproven.

As the macrophages ingest the modified LDL, they are converted into foam cells and form the fatty streak, which is the initial lesion in the atherogenic process. These lesions commonly affect the coronary arteries. Formation begins in the mid-teens, and the lesions grow as the person ages.

Once the fatty streak forms, the oxidized LDL and macrophages act in other ways that promote the progression of the atherogenic lesion. Oxidized LDL appears to act as a chemotactic agent, recruiting other circulating monocytes and preventing macrophages from leaving the subendothelial space. Macrophages also produce chemotactic factors as well as growth factors. The growth factors cause proliferation of smooth muscle cells from the media into the fatty streak, leading to the formation of a fibrous plaque (Ross & Glomset, 1976). Fibrous plaques are usually raised and protrude into the lumen of the artery, thereby compromising blood flow.

As the foam cells grow, the endothelium stretches and may become damaged. This leads to platelet aggregation and clot formation. In many instances, these fissures heal and incorporate the thrombi inside the plaque. This process may occur dozens of times and eventually may produce a complicated lesion. The formation of complicated lesions is the major cause of acute cardiovascular events. However, in some instances, rupture of a small, unstable plaque may also cause the formation of a single large clot that totally occludes the vessel. The fibrous plaques that are most likely to rupture are those that have large lipid cores and a thin fibrous cap, a layer of smooth muscle cells directly over the lipid core. Large plaques with a strong fibrous cap may be more stable and less likely to rupture (Cooke & Bhatnagar, 1997; McKenney & Hawkins, 1995).

The primary symptom associated with atherosclerosis is the chest pain known as angina. Symptoms occur when the lesion compromises blood flow in the vessel lumen. A lesion that occludes approximately 50% of the lumen usually causes symptoms when more blood flow is required (ie, exercise-induced angina). As the lesions grow and occlude more than 70% of the vessel, anginal symptoms may occur even when the person is resting (Cooke & Bhatnagar, 1997).

RISK ASSESSMENT

The National Cholesterol Education Program's Third Report on the Detection, Evaluation and Treatment of High Cholesterol in Adults (NCEP ATP III) recommends that all adults 20 years of age or older should have a fasting lipoprotein panel (total cholesterol, LDL cholesterol, HDL cholesterol, and triglycerides) measured at least once every 5 years (Table 19-1). If the patient was not fasting, only total and HDL cholesterol are usable. In this instance, if the total cholesterol is 200 mg/dL or more or HDL cholesterol is less than 40 mg/dL, the patient should have a fasting lipoprotein profile performed. Patients should also be evaluated for CHD risk factors (Box 19-2) and for clinical evidence of CHD or CHD risk equivalents (Box 19-3).

Evaluation of patients with suspected hyperlipidemia should include a complete history and physical examination, fasting lipoprotein analysis to determine LDL and triglyceride levels, and determination of secondary causes of hyperlipidemia. For accurate results, the patient undergoing lipoprotein analysis must fast for at least 12 hours. The reason for this is that triglyceride levels can be falsely elevated in a patient who has not fasted because of circulating chylomicrons. Normal triglyceride levels are lower than 150 mg/dL. Levels of 150 to 199 mg/dL are considered borderline high. Levels of 200 to 499 mg/dL are considered high, those above 500 mg/dL are considered very high, and those above 1,000 mg/dL could lead to complications such as pancreatitis.

Total and HDL cholesterol values are minimally affected if a patient does not fast. However, because most laboratories calculate LDL cholesterol, the patient must be fasting because elevations in the triglyceride level may lead to falsely low LDL cholesterol levels.

The formula for calculating LDL is LDL = total cholesterol - HDL - VLDL (VLDL is equivalent to triglycerides/5). However, as triglyceride levels approach or exceed 400 mg/dL, this formula is not accurate. In this case, the patient may require a direct LDL cholesterol level analysis. A second analysis should be performed within 1 to 8 weeks to confirm the results of the first test before a definitive diagnosis is made.

The treatment of patients who require a fasting lipoprotein analysis is based on LDL cholesterol values. The LDL cholesterol goal is determined by presence of CHD risk factors (see Box 19-2) or by presence of CHD or CHD risk equivalents (see Box 19-3). Patients at highest risk are those with CHD or CHD risk equivalents. These patients have a greater than 20% risk of having a coronary event within 10 years. CHD risk equivalents include patients with diabetes mellitus and patients with a 10-year risk of CHD that exceeds 20%. This includes patients with two or more risk factors and increased risk based upon Framingham risk score. To calculate the 10-year risk for a patient, see Table 19-2.

BOX 19–2. CORONARY HEART DISEASE RISK FACTORS*

Positive CHD Risk Factors
1. **Age:** Men ≥45 years old
          Women ≥55 years old
2. **Family History of Premature CHD:**
   Male first-degree relative—MI or sudden death before **55** years old
   Female first-degree relative—MI or sudden death before **65** years old
3. **Current cigarette smoking**
4. **Hypertension:**
   Blood pressure >140/90 mm Hg on several occasions or taking antihypertensive medications
5. **Low HDL cholesterol** (<40 mg/dL)

Negative CHD Risk Factors
1. **High HDL cholesterol** (≥60 mg/dL or 1.6 mmol/L)

Total Risk Factors = Positive risk factors minus Negative risk factors

* Diabetes mellitus is considered a CHD risk equivalent.

BOX 19–3. ATHEROSCLEROTIC VASCULAR DISEASE AND CHD RISK EQUIVALENTS

Coronary Heart Disease (CHD)
Myocardial infarction
Significant myocardial ischemia (angina pectoris)
History of coronary artery bypass graft (CABG)
History of coronary angioplasty
Angiographic evidence of lesions

Peripheral Vascular Disease
Claudication

Carotid Artery Disease
Thrombotic stroke
Transient ischemic attack

CHD Risk Equivalent
Diabetes mellitus

Table 19.1

Classification of LDL, Total, and HDL Cholesterol

	Cholesterol Level (mg/dL)	Initial Classification
LDL cholesterol	<100	Optimal
	100–129	Near or above optimal
	130–159	Borderline high
	160–189	High
	≥190	Very high
Total cholesterol	<200	Desirable
	200–239	Borderline high
	≥240	High
HDL cholesterol	<40	Low
	≥60	High

Table 19.2

Calculation of Estimate of 10-Year Risk

Estimate of 10-Year Risk for Men
(Framingham Point Scores)

Age	Points
20–34	−9
35–39	−4
40–44	0
45–49	3
50–54	6
55–59	8
60–64	10
65–69	11
70–74	12
75–79	13

Total Cholesterol	Points Age 20–39	Age 40–49	Age 50–59	Age 60–69	Age 70–79
<160	0	0	0	0	0
160–199	4	3	2	1	0
200–239	7	5	3	1	0
240–279	9	6	4	2	1
≥280	11	8	5	3	1

	Points Age 20–39	Age 40–49	Age 50–59	Age 60–69	Age 70–79
Nonsmoker	0	0	0	0	0
Smoker	8	5	3	1	1

HDL (mg/dL)	Points
≥60	−1
50–59	0
40–49	1
<40	2

Systolic BP (mm Hg)	If Untreated	If Treated
<120	0	0
120–129	0	1
130–139	1	2
140–159	1	2
≥160	2	3

Point Total	10-Year Risk %
<0	<1
0	1
1	1
2	1
3	1
4	1
5	2
6	2
7	3
8	4
9	5
10	6
11	8
12	10
13	12
14	16
15	20
16	25
≥17	≥30

10-Year risk_____%

Estimate of 10-Year Risk for Women
(Framingham Point Scores)

Age	Points
20–34	−7
35–39	−3
40–44	0
45–49	3
50–54	6
55–59	8
60–64	10
65–69	12
70–74	14
75–79	16

Total Cholesterol	Points Age 20–39	Age 40–49	Age 50–59	Age 60–69	Age 70–79
<160	0	0	0	0	0
160–199	4	3	2	1	1
200–239	8	6	4	2	1
240–279	11	8	5	3	2
≥280	13	10	7	4	2

	Points Age 20–39	Age 40–49	Age 50–59	Age 60–69	Age 70–79
Nonsmoker	0	0	0	0	0
Smoker	9	7	4	2	1

HDL (mg/dL)	Points
≥60	−1
50–59	0
40–49	1
<40	2

Systolic BP (mm Hg)	If Untreated	If Treated
<120	0	0
120–129	1	3
130–139	2	4
140–159	3	5
≥160	4	6

Point Total	10-Year Risk %
<9	<1
9	1
10	1
11	1
12	1
13	2
14	2
15	3
16	4
17	5
18	6
19	8
20	11
21	14
22	17
23	22
24	27
≥25	≥30

10-Year risk_____%

U.S. DEPARTMENT OF HEALTH AND HUMAN SERVICES   NIH Publication No. 02-3305
Public Health Service   May 2001
National Institutes of Health
National Heart, Lung, and Blood Institute

Table 19.3

LDL Cholesterol Goals Based Upon CHD Risk Factors

Risk Factors	LDL Goal
CHD and CHD risk equivalents	<100 mg/dL with desirable <70 mg/dL
Multiple (2+) risk factors	<130 mg/dL
0 or 1 risk factor	<160 mg/dL

INITIATING DRUG THERAPY

Management of patients with no evidence of CHD or CHD risk equivalents is termed *primary prevention*. Management of patients with CHD or CHD risk equivalents is termed *secondary prevention*. Management of patients with hyperlipidemia consists of nonpharmacologic and pharmacologic therapy. The decision to treat hyperlipidemia with drug therapy is based on LDL levels (Table 19-3), as is follow-up treatment (Table 19-4).

Lifestyle Modification

Most patients with newly diagnosed hyperlipidemia should attempt to make lifestyle modifications before beginning pharmacologic therapy. The primary lifestyle modifications include dietary therapy, exercise, weight loss, moderation of alcohol intake, and smoking cessation. Before initiating any lifestyle modifications, the patient's current lifestyle needs to be evaluated to determine what modifications would be beneficial. This evaluation should also include the patient's understanding of the disease and the importance of treating it and his or her ability to learn and follow these lifestyle modifications. Evaluation of social, cultural, and economic factors also is necessary, especially if drug therapy may be warranted.

Diet

The primary goal of dietary therapy is to reduce the intake of fat, especially saturated fat, and cholesterol and to achieve a desirable body weight. The Third National Health and Nutrition Examination Survey (NHANES III) stated that 36% or 37% of calories in the typical American diet comes from fat. All adults with hyperlipidemia should follow a "therapeutic lifestyle changes" (TLC) diet. The primary targets of the

Table 19.5

Therapeutic Lifestyle Changes (TLC) diet

Nutrient	Recommended Intake
Total fat	25–35% total calories
Saturated fat	<7% total calories
Polyunsaturated fat	Up to 10% of total calories
Monounsaturated fat	Up to 20% of total calories
Carbohydrates	50–60% total calories
Protein	15% total calories
Fiber	20–30 g/day
Cholesterol	<200 mg/day
Total calories	Amount to maintain desired weight/prevent weight gain

TLC diet are to reduce intake of saturated fats to less than 7% of total calories and cholesterol intake to less than 200 mg per day (Table 19-5). Total daily fat intake should represent 25% to 35% of total calories. The patient should follow this diet for at least 6 weeks. If the LDL cholesterol goal is not met, increased intake of plant stanol/sterols and viscous fiber is recommended.

In addition to decreasing dietary fat and cholesterol, overweight patients should attempt to lose weight. The ability to lose weight depends on the amount of calories consumed and the amount of calories burned. To lose weight, most people need to reduce their caloric intake by approximately 500 calories daily and increase physical activity. The goal for overweight patients should be a realistic, gradual, and steady loss of weight. Once an ideal weight is achieved, caloric intake is adjusted to maintain that weight.

Exercise

Regular physical exercise may provide several benefits in patients with hyperlipidemia. As mentioned, it should be used along with dietary therapy to promote weight loss. Exercise may benefit the lipid profile by reducing triglycerides and raising HDL levels. Exercise may also improve control of diabetes and coronary blood flow. The most effective exercise is aerobic activity, such as walking, swimming, jogging, and tennis. The optimal schedule for aerobic exercise is 30 to 45 minutes a day, 5 to 7 days a week, but any exercise is beneficial.

Table 19.4

Treatment Decisions Based on LDL Cholesterol Levels

	LDL Goal	Initiate Dietary Therapy	Initiate Pharmacologic Therapy
0 or 1 risk factor	<160 mg/dL	≥160 mg/dL	≥190 mg/dL (160–189: drug therapy optional
2+ risk factors			
10-year risk <10%	<130 mg/dL	≥130 mg/dL	≥160 mg/dL
10-year risk 10–20%	<130 mg/dL	≥130 mg/dL	≥130 mg/dL
Patients with CHD or CHD risk equivalents (10-year risk >20%)	<100 mg/dL or <70 mg/dL*	≥100 mg/dL	≥130 mg/dL (100–129: drug therapy optional)

* For patients with established CVD plus multiple risk factors (eg, diabetes and continued smoking).

Moderation of Alcohol Intake and Smoking Cessation

Excessive alcohol intake may elevate serum lipid levels, specifically triglyceride levels, but in moderation (no more than two drinks per day), alcohol may improve HDL levels and has been associated with lower CHD rates (Jackson & Beaglehole, 1993). Despite these benefits, alcohol should not be recommended for CHD prevention because the consequences associated with excessive alcohol use outweigh any benefits.

Cigarette smoking is an independent risk factor in the development of CHD (Hjermann, Byre, Holme, & Leren, 1981). Although smoking minimally affects cholesterol levels, it contributes to the development of CHD by damaging the vascular endothelium and promoting platelet aggregation, which results in increased risk of clot formation. Smoking cessation can reduce this risk and should be encouraged by all health care professionals. The risk for development of CHD decreases by approximately 50% within 1 to 2 years of smoking cessation.

Goals of Drug Therapy

Drug therapy should be used in patients who do not attain their LDL cholesterol goal with lifestyle modifications alone. As mentioned, most patients without CHD should try lifestyle changes for approximately 6 months before initiating drug therapy. Patients with very high LDL cholesterol levels who are unlikely to attain their LDL cholesterol goal with lifestyle changes alone may require drug therapy before this 6-month period. Because patients with CHD are at higher risk for future cardiovascular events, these patients should be managed more aggressively. Often, drug therapy should be considered after a trial of lifestyle modifications of 3 months or less.

The medication classes used to treat abnormal cholesterol levels are the HMG-CoA reductase inhibitors (statins), bile acid resins, nicotinic acid (niacin), cholesterol absorption inhibitors, and fibric acid derivatives. All of the major drugs with the exception of gemfibrozil (fibric acid derivative) promote a decrease in LDL cholesterol and a slight increase in HDL levels, but they differ in their potency and effects on triglyceride levels.

The primary goal of drug therapy in treating hyperlipidemia is to reduce cardiovascular-related morbidity and mortality without affecting quality of life. The primary surrogate marker for predicting morbidity and mortality is cholesterol levels. As mentioned previously, patients with fewer than two risk factors and no evidence of CHD or CHD risk equivalents have an LDL cholesterol goal of less than 160 mg/dL. Patients with two or more risk factors and without evidence of CHD or CHD risk equivalents and 10-year risk of less than 20% have an LDL cholesterol goal of less than 130 mg/dL, with the ideal being less than 100 mg/dL. The intensity of LDL-lowering drug therapy for high-risk and moderately high-risk patients should be sufficient to achieve at least a 30% to 40% reduction in LDL levels, either with statins alone or a combination of lower doses of statins and other drugs, or with food products containing plant stanol/sterols. Patients with any evidence of CHD, CHD risk equivalents, or a 10-year risk of CHD that exceeds 20% are treated most aggressively and have an LDL cholesterol goal of 100 mg/dL or less, with a desired rate of below 70 mg/dL.

HMG-CoA Reductase Inhibitors (Statins)

The statins are the newest class of lipid-lowering drugs. Lovastatin (Mevacor), the first drug in this class, became available in the United States in 1987. Since then, five additional medications have been approved for use. The statins are the most heavily used class of lipid-lowering drugs because of their ability to lower LDL cholesterol and, more important, associated morbidity and mortality rates. These drugs are well tolerated by most patients.

Mechanism of Action

The selection of a statin is based in general on its ability to lower cholesterol levels. The current guidelines from NCEP ATP III suggest that patients be treated to reach a certain LDL cholesterol goal. Trying to lower the LDL cholesterol level beyond this does not necessarily reduce morbidity and mortality. For this reason, the most potent agent may not always be necessary. Several agents in this class also lower triglyceride levels, primarily at the higher doses. (For patients who require significant lowering of triglyceride levels, niacin or fibric acid derivatives should be used.)

Primarily, the statins block the conversion of HMG-CoA to mevalonate, which is the rate-limiting step in the production of cholesterol in the liver. Blocking the production of cholesterol in the liver leads to an increase in the number of LDL cholesterol receptors on the liver. As a result, a larger amount of LDL cholesterol is taken up by the liver, thereby decreasing the amount of LDL cholesterol in the bloodstream (Fig. 19-1).

Low-density lipoprotein receptors are also involved with the uptake of VLDL and IDL, thus leading to a decrease in triglyceride levels. In addition, modest increases in HDL tend to occur. Despite having the same mechanism of action, there are differences between the agents, including their ability to lower cholesterol (Table 19-6). For example, fluvastatin (Lescol) can lower LDL cholesterol levels up to approximately 36% with the maximum dose, whereas atorvastatin (Lipitor) and rosuvastatin (Crestor) can lower LDL cholesterol levels up to 60% at maximum doses.

Maximum effects usually are seen after 4 to 6 weeks of therapy. For this reason, dosage adjustments should not be made more frequently than every 4 weeks.

Contraindications

There are several instances when statins are contraindicated or should be used with caution. Although no studies have been conducted in pregnant women, lovastatin causes skeletal malformations in rats, so statins are contraindicated during pregnancy. These agents should be used with extreme caution in women who are breast-feeding because they may be excreted in breast milk.

Statins are also contraindicated in patients with active liver disease or with unexplained elevated aminotransferase levels. They should be used with caution in patients who consume large amounts of alcohol or have a history of liver disease.

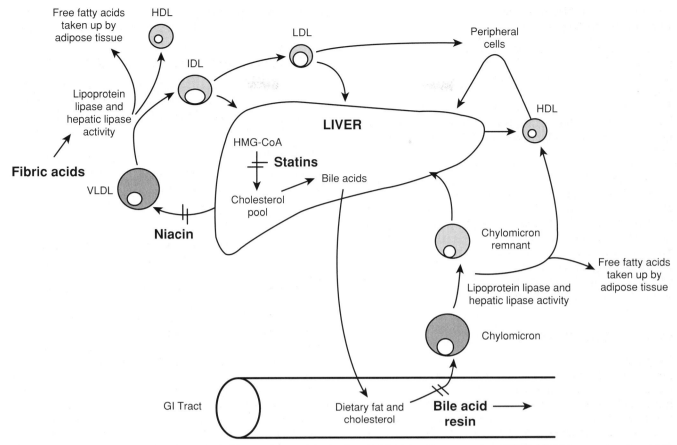

Figure 19–1 How lipid-lowering drugs work. The statins work in the liver by blocking the conversion of HMG–Co A to mevalonate, which is involved in producing cholesterol. The bile acid resins bind bile acid in the intestines for excretion in the feces so that lipids are not absorbed by the intestinal tract and returned to the liver. Niacin works to decrease circulating triglyceride and LDL cholesterol and fibric acid derivatives appear to lower triglyceride levels and stimulate lipoprotein lipase, which enhances the breakdown of VLDL to LDL cholesterol.

Adverse Events

The statins are well tolerated by most patients and long-term therapy does not appear to have any serious risks. Gastrointestinal (GI) complaints and headache are the two most commonly reported adverse events, but they are usually mild and transient. The most common adverse event that occurs with the statins is asymptomatic elevations in liver function test (LFT) values. LFTs should be checked at baseline (before starting therapy), at 6 and 12 weeks after starting or titrating therapy, and periodically thereafter. Several agents, including atorvastatin (Lipitor), pravastatin (Pravachol), and simvastatin (Zocor), do not require LFTs to be performed at 6 weeks after initiation or titration of therapy. Therapy should be discontinued if two consecutive tests disclose values that are two to three times above upper normal limits.

Other adverse effects include muscle pain and weakness, which may be a sign of myopathy. If myopathy is suspected, the patient's creatinine phosphokinase level should be

---

Table 19.6

Doses and Lipid-Lowering Ability of Currently Available Statins

Generic Name (Trade Name)	Usual Daily Dose	LDL*	HDL*	Triglycerides*
Lovastatin (Mevacor)	10–80 mg	↓24–48%	↑7%	↓10–14%
Pravastatin (Pravachol)	10–40 mg	↓22–34%	↑2–12%	↓11–24%
Simvastatin (Zocor)	20–80 mg	↓24–40%	↑7–16%	↓12–21%
Fluvastatin (Lescol)	20–80 mg	↓22–36%	↑3–6%	↓12–18%
Cerivastatin (Baycol)	0.2–0.4 mg	↓25–34%	↑7–8%	↓11–16%
Atorvastatin (Lipitor)	10–80 mg	↓39–60%	↑5–9%	↓19–37%
Rosuvastatin[†] (Crestor)	5–40 mg	↓47–65%	↑2–9%	↓20%

* Effects on lipid levels are dose dependent.
† Based on results from the STELLAR Study (McKenney, Jones, Adamczyk, et al., 2003).

checked and drug therapy discontinued if levels exceed 10 times the upper normal limits. Additionally, proteinuria and renal failure have been noted in a few patients, specifically those taking rosuvastatin. Renal function tests should be monitored with doses of 40 mg or higher.

Interactions

The risk of myopathy increases when the statins are used with erythromycin (E-mycin), niacin, gemfibrozil (Lopid), and cyclosporine (Sandimmune). Moreover, myopathy may occur at any time during therapy. Patients should be instructed to report any unusual muscle pain or weakness during therapy.

The practitioner should encourage the patient to take the statins in the evening or at bedtime because a significant amount of cholesterol production seems to occur during sleep. By taking the medication before bedtime, peak concentrations of medication occur during sleep. Two exceptions are lovastatin, which has an increased bioavailability when taken with food and is usually taken with the evening meal, and atorvastatin, which can be taken at any time during the day because of its long half-life.

Bile Acid Resins

Bile acid resins decrease cholesterol absorption through the exogenous pathway. These agents are not absorbed from the GI tract. They act to bind bile acids in the intestines, forming an insoluble complex that is excreted in the feces. This decreases the return of cholesterol to the liver. The body responds to this by increasing LDL receptors on the liver, which in turn increases the amount of LDL cholesterol taken up by the liver and thus decreases LDL cholesterol levels in the bloodstream (see Fig. 19-1). Unfortunately, this process also leads to increased production of VLDL particles. As a result, triglyceride levels rise, especially in patients with elevated baseline triglyceride levels. Bile acid resins can decrease LDL cholesterol levels by 15% to 30%, increase HDL levels by approximately 3%, and increase triglyceride levels by up to 15% (Table 19-7). As with the statins, these effects are dose related.

Maximum effects of cholesterol lowering are seen in approximately 3 weeks. Bile acid resins are indicated as adjunct therapy for patients who do not respond to dietary therapy alone. Because of their safety with long-term use, they are extremely useful in young adult men and premenopausal women who are at relatively low cardiovascular risk. These agents are contraindicated in patients with biliary obstruction or chronic constipation.

Adverse Events

Bile acid resins are not absorbed, and therefore systemic adverse events are minimal. Monitoring for abnormal LFT values is not required. The most common adverse events are GI related and include flatulence, bloating, abdominal pain, heartburn, and constipation. For these reasons, some patients, such as elderly patients, may not be good candidates for bile acid resins.

Interactions

Because bile acid resins block the absorption of cholesterol from the GI tract, they should be taken with meals to maximize effectiveness. These agents are usually administered once or twice daily but can be taken up to four times a day. If taken once a day, a bile acid resin should be taken with the largest meal. The two major agents in this class are cholestyramine (Questran, Questran Light, Prevalite) and colestipol (Colestid).

Cholestyramine is available as a powder and colestipol is available as granules or tablets. The powder and granules should be mixed with water, noncarbonated beverages, soups, or pulpy fruits such as applesauce. The tablets should be swallowed whole with water or other fluids. These agents should not be taken dry because they can cause esophageal distress. Patients should avoid taking these agents with carbonated beverages because it may result in increased GI discomfort. Medications taken concomitantly, such as thyroid hormones, antibiotics, and fat-soluble vitamins, should be taken at least 1 hour before or 4 hours after the bile acid resin because of the bile acid resin's potential to bind to other medications and decrease their bioavailability.

Niacin

Niacin (nicotinic acid) is a naturally occurring B vitamin that can improve cholesterol levels when used at doses 100 to 300 times the recommended daily allowance as a vitamin. Niacin's mechanism of action is uncertain, but the substance appears to decrease VLDL synthesis in the liver, inhibit lipolysis in adipose tissue, and increase lipoprotein lipase activity. This results in decreased triglyceride and LDL cholesterol levels in the bloodstream (see Fig. 19-1). LDL cholesterol levels can be decreased by 15% to 25% and triglycerides by up to 50%, whereas HDL cholesterol levels may be increased by up to 35% (see Table 19-6). Although niacin is one of the most effective agents in improving cholesterol levels, most patients cannot tolerate the adverse events associated with its use (see Adverse Events).

Table 19.7

Doses and Lipid-Lowering Ability of Currently Available Bile Acid Resins

Generic Name (Trade Name)	Usual Daily Dose	LDL*	HDL*	Triglycerides*
Cholestyramine (Questran, Questran Light, Prevalite)	4–16 g	↓13–32%	↑3–5%	↑0–15%
Colestipol (Colestid)	Tablets: 2–16 g Granules: 5–30 g	↓12–25%	↑0–1%	↑0–24%

*Effects on lipid levels are dose dependent.

Dosage

Doses of at least 1.5 g niacin daily are usually required to achieve beneficial effects on lipid levels. However, to minimize adverse events, dosages need to be titrated gradually. The usual starting dose is 50 to 100 mg two or three times a day. The dose can be increased every 1 to 2 weeks until a dosage of 1.0 to 1.5 g daily is reached; this should take approximately 4 to 5 weeks. This dosage range provides significant increases (15% to 30%) in HDL cholesterol levels and decreases (20% to 30%) in triglyceride levels. However, for maximal LDL cholesterol lowering, dosages of 3 g/day or more may be necessary. Niacin is available in both immediate-release and sustained-release formulations. Maximum effects usually are seen after 4 to 6 weeks of therapy on the aforementioned dosages.

Contraindications

Niacin is contraindicated in patients with hepatic dysfunction, severe hypotension, or active peptic ulcers. In addition, niacin can elevate uric acid levels and worsen glucose control. Therefore, niacin is not a first-line treatment agent in patients with gout or diabetes mellitus, and it should be used cautiously in this population.

Adverse Events

Niacin use has been limited primarily because of its extensive adverse events. Although it is one of the most effective agents for improving lipid profiles, most patients cannot tolerate the adverse events. The most common adverse events are attributed to an increase in prostaglandin activity and include pruritus and flushing of the face and neck. A dose of aspirin, 325 mg, taken 30 minutes before the niacin dose may decrease the severity. As mentioned earlier, niacin can also increase uric acid levels and worsen glucose control and should be used cautiously, if at all, in patients with a history of gout or diabetes mellitus. Baseline glucose and uric acid levels should be checked in all patients starting niacin therapy.

Other adverse events include GI side effects (it is contraindicated in patients with an active peptic ulcer), rash, hepatotoxicity, and, rarely, acanthosis nigricans (hyperpigmentation of the skin, usually in the axilla, neck, or groin). As with the statins, LFTs should be monitored at 6 and 12 weeks after initiating or titrating therapy and periodically thereafter.

Cholesterol Absorption Inhibitors

Currently, there is only one cholesterol absorption inhibitor on the market, ezetimibe (Zetia). Ezetimibe appears to act at the brush border of the small intestine and inhibits the absorption of cholesterol, leading to a decrease in the delivery of intestinal cholesterol to the liver. This causes a reduction of hepatic cholesterol stores and an increase in clearance of cholesterol from the blood; this distinct mechanism is complementary to that of HMG-CoA reductase inhibitors.

Zetia, introduced in April 2003, is indicated for use as monotherapy or as combination therapy with a statin. LDL cholesterol levels are reduced by up to 18% with monotherapy and up to an additional 25% when added to ongoing statin therapy. Together with a statin, LDL cholesterol reductions of more than 50% have been noted. The recommended dosage of ezetimibe is 10 mg daily. If taken with a bile acid sequestrant, ezetimibe should be taken 2 hours before or 4 hours after the bile acid (Table 19-8).

Contraindications

Ezetimibe is contraindicated in patients who have a hypersensitivity to any component of the medication. The combination of ezetimibe with an HMG-CoA reductase inhibitor is contraindicated in patients with active liver disease or unexplained persistent elevations in serum transaminases. There are no adequate, controlled studies of ezetimibe in pregnant women, so use during pregnancy is indicated only if the potential benefit outweighs any potential risk to the fetus.

Adverse Events

Adverse events with ezetimibe are minimal. Adverse events noted in clinical trials include headache, diarrhea, and abdominal pain. In addition, myopathy and rhabdomyolysis have been noted when given in combination with statins. The incidence of elevated liver enzymes was similar to placebo.

Fibric Acid Derivatives

Fibric acid derivatives are not considered a major class of lipid-lowering drugs because they have minimal effects on LDL cholesterol levels. The exact mechanism of action of fibric acid derivatives is unclear, but the principal effect of triglyceride lowering appears to result from the stimulation

Table 19.8

Doses and Lipid Lowering Ability of Other Available Agents

Class	Generic Name (Trade Name)	Usual Daily Dose	LDL[*]	HDL[*]	Triglycerides[*]
Cholesterol absorption inhibitors	Ezetimibe (Zetia)[‡]	10 mg	↓16–19%	↑3–4%	↓5%
			↓33–60%	↑8–11%	↓19–40%
Niacin[†]	Niacin (various)	1.5–3.0 g	↓12–21%	↑18–30%	↓15–44%
Fibric acid derivatives	Gemfibrozil (Lopid)	600 mg BID	0	↑6%	↓31%
	Fenofibrate (TriCor)	67–201 mg QD	↓20%	↑11%	↓38%

[*]Effects on lipid levels are dose dependent.
[†]Dose must be titrated slowly (usually weekly) to avoid side effects.
[‡]Results in first line are those seen when used as monotherapy (Bays, 2001). Second results are those seen when used with statin therapy (Kerzner, 2003 [lovastatin]; Davidson, 2002 [simvastatin]; Ballantyne; 2003 [atorvastatin]).

of lipoprotein lipase, which enhances the breakdown of VLDL to LDL cholesterol (see Fig. 19-1).

These agents may also inhibit hepatic VLDL production, and they lower triglyceride levels up to 60% and increase HDL cholesterol by up to 30%. Although gemfibrozil and clofibrate (Atromid-S) have minimal effects on LDL cholesterol lowering, fenofibrate (TriCor) has been shown to decrease LDL cholesterol by up to 20%. Fibric acid derivatives are primarily indicated in patients who have severely elevated triglyceride levels and who have not responded to dietary therapy (see Table 19-8).

Gemfibrozil, clofibrate, and fenofibrate are the currently available fibric acid derivatives.

Dosage

Gemfibrozil is given in 600-mg doses twice daily with breakfast and dinner. A total of 2 g of clofibrate is taken in divided doses two or four times a day without regard to meals. No titration of dose is necessary for either agent, although some patients may respond at lower doses. Fenofibrate therapy is initiated at 67 mg/day. The dosage can be increased to a maximum of 201 mg/day. Because its absorption is increased when taken with food, fenofibrate should be taken with meals. Clofibrate is not commonly used because of a lack of studies showing its benefit in reducing the risk for atherosclerosis. Maximum effects usually are seen after 4 to 6 weeks of therapy.

Contraindications

Fibric acid derivatives are contraindicated in patients with a history of gallstones and in those with severe hepatic or renal dysfunction. No studies have been conducted in pregnant women, so therefore these agents should be used only if the benefits clearly outweigh any risks to the fetus.

Adverse Events

The fibric acid derivatives usually are well tolerated. The most common adverse events are GI related and include epigastric pain, nausea and vomiting, dyspepsia, flatulence, and constipation. Myopathy can occur and is diagnosed by a creatinine phosphokinase level 10 times above the upper normal limits. The incidence of myopathy is increased when fibric acid derivatives are used with lovastatin and, to a lesser degree, other statins and niacin. As with the other systemic lipid-lowering agents, hepatotoxicity can occur, and LFTs should be monitored at 6 and 12 weeks and periodically thereafter. If LFT values increase to more than two or three times the upper normal limits, the fibric acid derivative should be discontinued. Other adverse events include rhabdomyolysis, cholestatic jaundice, gallstones, and, rarely, leukopenia, anemia, and thrombocytopenia.

Interactions

As mentioned previously, the incidence of myopathy is increased when fibric acids are used in combination with lovastatin and, to a lesser degree, other statins and niacin. Fenofibrate should be used with caution in patients taking anticoagulant therapy because it can increase the effects of the anticoagulant. Doses of the anticoagulant should be lowered and levels monitored closely if fenofibrate therapy is initiated (see Table 19-8).

Combination Therapy

Some patients may require combination lipid-lowering therapy to achieve desired cholesterol goals, particularly those with severe hypertriglyceridemia or severely elevated LDL cholesterol levels. Combination therapy may also allow the patient to take lower doses of each of the individual drugs. Bile acid resins can be used safely and effectively with statins, niacin, and fibric acid derivatives to enhance LDL cholesterol lowering. The only concern with using bile acid resins in combination is ensuring that the concomitant medications are taken at least 1 hour before or 4 hours after the resin to ensure adequate GI absorption. Combining statins with a cholesterol absorption inhibitor has shown added benefits in reducing LDL cholesterol.

Other combination therapies are associated with a higher risk of adverse actions, but most can still be used with close monitoring. Statins and niacin have been used together for patients with severely elevated LDL cholesterol and hypertriglyceridemia, but patients may be at higher risk for myopathy and hepatotoxicity. In general, combining lovastatin with gemfibrozil should be avoided because of the high incidence of myopathy with this combination. However, other agents, such as fluvastatin, have been used successfully with gemfibrozil with close monitoring. Patients with severe hypertriglyceridemia may require the combination of a fibric acid derivative with niacin, with close monitoring for hepatotoxicity. In any case, combination therapy should be used only if the risk–benefit ratio is favorable.

Alternative Therapy

Antioxidant therapy has been a major focus of studies on preventing CHD, but its preventive benefits have yet to be determined. In theory, antioxidants block the conversion of LDL cholesterol to a modified (oxidized) LDL in the vascular endothelium. As mentioned previously, modified LDL cholesterol appears to be more atherogenic than nonoxidized LDL cholesterol. Thus, blocking the production of oxidized LDL cholesterol may slow the atherogenic process. The major antioxidants that have been studied include vitamin E, vitamin C, and beta carotene, a precursor of vitamin A. Most of the beneficial evidence has been seen with the use of vitamin E, but there is no strong evidence to support vitamin E use.

Other alternatives include garlic, vinegar, and fish oils. Although some evidence suggests that these are beneficial, no conclusive evidence exists to support their use.

Selecting the Most Appropriate Agent

Choosing which drugs to use in which order is individualized and based on the patient's clinical status, the amount of cholesterol lowering that is required, and an assessment of potential patient compliance. Factors that affect compliance include side effects, cost of therapy, health beliefs supporting the need to lower high cholesterol levels, and the understanding that this is lifelong treatment. It is estimated that

Table 19.9

Selecting the Most Appropriate Agent

	Agents	Comments
First line	Statins	Most experts agree that the benefits of treatment with statins are a class-wide effect. Choice of an agent depends upon the amount of LDL lowering required to reach goal.
Second line	Bile acid resins, cholesterol absorption inhibitors	Bile acids are not systemically absorbed and can be used in patients who cannot tolerate the effects of statins or in combination with statins for patients who are unable to reach LDL goal on a statin alone. Cholesterol absorption inhibitors can be used alone or in combination with statins. When used in combination, LDL cholesterol lowering of approximately 60% has been shown.
Third line	Niacin, fibric acid derivatives	Niacin has beneficial effects on each of the lipoproteins, but most patients cannot tolerate the side effects of the drug. Fibric acid derivatives are reserved for patients with very high triglyceride levels (>1,000 mg/dL) who do not respond to dietary interventions or in combination with other agents for patients with elevated triglyceride levels that cannot be controlled with other agents.

15% to 46% of patients who start lipid-lowering therapy discontinue their medication within 1 year (Andrade, Walker, Gottlieb, et al., 1995).

Table 19-9 and Figure 19-2 give more information. Because of its favorable effects on all lipoproteins, niacin is especially useful in patients with mixed hyperlipidemia, although severe adverse effects may lead to discontinuation of therapy. The kind of hyperlipidemia the patient has is another factor in selecting the most effective drug therapy:

- Patients who have polygenic hyperlipidemia and desired triglyceride and HDL levels are usually treated with bile acid resins, niacin, statins, or cholesterol absorption inhibitors.
- Patients with polygenic hyperlipidemia and isolated low HDL levels may benefit from niacin, a statin, or a combination of a statin and niacin.
- Patients who have familial hyperlipidemia and desired triglyceride and HDL levels may receive a statin, bile acid resin, cholesterol absorption inhibitor, or niacin.
- Nondiabetic patients with mixed hyperlipidemia may benefit from niacin, a statin, or a fibric acid derivative, such as gemfibrozil, or a combination of niacin–statin, statin–gemfibrozil, niacin–bile acid resin, or niacin–gemfibrozil.
- Diabetic patients with mixed hyperlipidemia may need a statin or fibric acid derivative, such as gemfibrozil, or combination therapy with statin–gemfibrozil, statin–cholesterol absorption inhibitor, statin–bile acid resin, or gemfibrozil–bile acid resin.

Special Population Considerations

Pediatric

Pharmacologic therapy may be considered in children older than 10 years of age if lifestyle modifications cannot adequately lower cholesterol levels. Use in children younger than 10 years usually is not recommended because atherosclerotic lesions are not thought to develop before this age. A consultation with a lipid specialist is recommended for any child with elevated cholesterol levels.

Geriatric

The age limit at which lipid-lowering therapy should or should not be initiated is a highly debatable issue. A sub-analysis from the Cholesterol and Recurrent Events (CARE) trial showed that patients between 65 and 75 years of age with a previous cardiovascular event benefit from lipid-lowering drugs, specifically the statins (Lewis et al., 1998). There is no strong evidence to support initiating these agents in patients older than 75 years of age.

Women

Lipid-lowering therapy should usually be avoided in women who are pregnant unless the benefits outweigh the risks of use. Statins are classified as category X by the FDA and should not be used by pregnant women because of the potential for fetal abnormalities. Most other agents are classified as category C, meaning that tests have not been performed in humans.

MONITORING PATIENT RESPONSE

Monitoring for the beneficial effects of lipid-lowering therapy is done by a fasting lipid panel analysis. A fasting lipid panel identifies total cholesterol, HDL cholesterol, triglycerides, and a calculated LDL cholesterol level. Because the LDL cholesterol is a calculated value, inaccurate results can occur in patients with triglyceride levels approaching or exceeding 400 mg/dL. These patients may require a separate test to measure LDL cholesterol directly.

Because maximal effects are seen by 4 to 6 weeks after starting drug therapy, fasting lipid panel results should be reviewed approximately 6 weeks after starting or titrating drug therapy. If no changes are made in therapy, a fasting lipid panel test should be repeated at 3 and 6 months and yearly thereafter if the patient has achieved the LDL cholesterol goal.

PATIENT EDUCATION

Patient education consists of a thorough explanation of the value of modifying habits and making lifestyle changes (diet, exercise) to avoid or enhance drug therapy in reducing lipid levels. Equally important is thorough teaching about the need for regular laboratory tests to evaluate the effect of drug therapy on body systems and organs, such as the liver. Such education will encourage the patient to cooperate with the therapeutic plan.

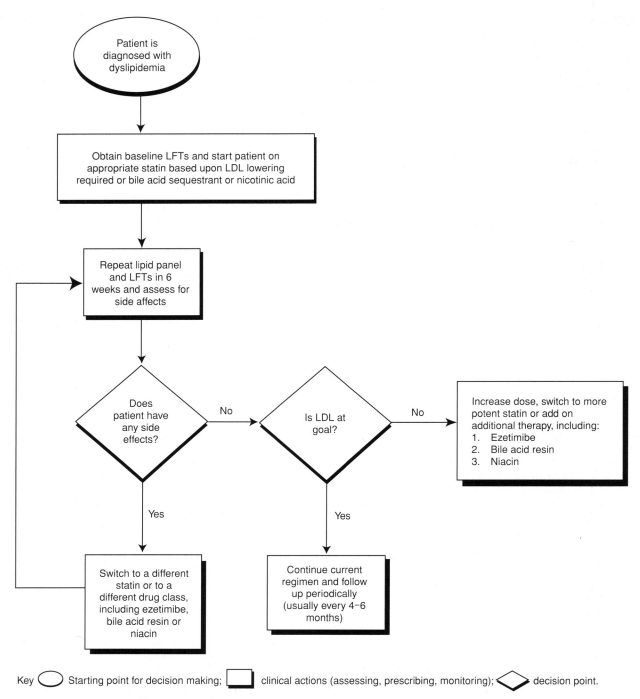

Figure 19–2 Treatment algorithm for initiating cholesterol-lowering therapy.

Two websites that provide useful information for patients are www.americanheart.org (American Heart Association) and www.nhlbi.nih.gov (Department of Health and Human Services, National Institute of Health, National Heart, Lung and Blood Institute). On the latter site, the patient can calculate his or her 10-year risk of having a heart attack.

Cholesterol screening should begin at age 20 and should be done every 5 years if it is normal unless there has been a significant lifestyle change, such as significant weight gain. Children should be screened if their parents have a choles-terol level greater than 240 or they have grandparents age 55 or younger with overt coronary heart disease.

Drug Information

Grapefruit juice may increase the potency of all statins except pravastatin. It may be taken occasionally with other statins, but not on a daily basis. Patients taking statins should report any new muscle pain, since these drugs can cause myopathy and, rarely, rhabdomyolysis.

Nutrition

The patient should eat a diet low in saturated fats and cholesterol. The diet can include up to 35% daily fats, but no more than 7% saturated fats. Cholesterol intake should be less than 200 mg/day.

Complementary and Alternative Medications

Dietary supplements thought to lower cholesterol include flax seed, garlic, oil of evening primrose, and wine (in moderation), but there are no good clinical studies that provide supportive evidence.

■ Case Study

J.J., age 55, has come in for his annual physical. He is healthy except for hypertension, which is controlled with enalapril 10 mg daily. His father died at age 55 of a myocardial infarction, and his brother, age 57, just underwent angioplasty. J.J. eats fast food at least 5 times a week because of his work schedule. He weighs 245 lb and stands 5-foot-11. His blood pressure is 134/80. His total cholesterol is 272 (LDL, 162; HDL, 32; triglycerides, 154).

1. List the specific goals of therapy for J.J. What are his ideal values for total cholesterol, LDL, HDL, and triglycerides?

2. What drug therapy would you prescribe, and why?

3. What are the parameters for monitoring the success of the therapy for lowering J.J.'s cholesterol level?

4. Discuss the specific patient education that you would provide to J.J.

5. List one or two adverse reactions for the drug therapy that you prescribed for J.J. that would cause you to change therapy.

6. When rechecked, J.J.'s total cholesterol is 234 (LDL, 135; HDL, 35). What would be your second line of therapy?

7. What over-the-counter or dietary supplements would you recommend to J.J.?

8. What dietary and lifestyle changes would you recommend for J.J.?

9. Describe one or two drug/drug or drug/food interactions for the selected agent.

Bibliography

*Starred references are cited in the text.

American Heart Association. (2004). *Heart disease and stroke statistics*. www.Americanheart.org.

*Andrade, S. E., Walker, A. M., Gottlieb, L. K., et al. (1995). Discontinuation of antihyperlipidemic drugs: do rates reported in clinical trials reflect rates in primary care settings? *New England Journal of Medicine, 332*, 1125–1131.

Ballantyne, C. M., Houri, J., Notarbartolo, A., et al. (2003). Effect of ezetimibe coadministered with atorvastatin in 628 patients with primary hypercholesterolemia: a prospective, randomized, double-blind trial. *Circulation, 107*(19), 2409–2415.

Bays, H. E., Moore, P. B., Drehobl, M. A., et al. (2001). Effectiveness and tolerability of ezetimibe in patients with primary hypercholesterolemia: pooled analysis of two phase II studies. *Clinical Therapy, 23*(8), 1209–1230.

*Cooke, J. P., & Bhatnagar, R. (1997). Pathophysiology of atherosclerotic vascular disease. *Disease Management and Health Outcomes, 2*(Suppl. 1), 1–8.

Davidson, M. H., McGarry, T., Bettis, R., et al. (2002). Ezetimibe coadministered with simvastatin in patients with primary hypercholesterolemia. *Journal of the American College of Cardiology, 40*(12), 2125–2134.

*Downs, J. R., et al. (1998). Primary prevention of acute coronary events with lovastatin in men and women with average cholesterol levels: results of AFCAPS/TexCAPS. *Journal of the American Medical Association, 279*, 1615–1622.

*Expert Panel, National Cholesterol Education Program. (2001). Executive summary of the third report of the National Cholesterol Education Program (NCEP) Expert Panel on Detection, Evaluation and Treatment of High Blood Cholesterol in Adults (Adult Treatment Panel III). *Journal of the American Medical Association, 285*, 2486–2497.

*Frick, H., Elo, O., Kaapa, K., et al. (1987). Helsinki Heart Study: primary prevention trial with gemfibrozil in middle-aged men with dyslipidemia. *New England Journal of Medicine, 257*, 3233–3240.

Grundy, S. M., Cleeman, J. I., Merz, N. B., et al. (2004). NCEP report. *Circulation, 110*, 227–239.

*Heart Protection Study Collaborative Group. (2002) MRC/BHF Heart Protection Study of cholesterol lowering with simvastatin in 20536 high-risk individuals: a randomised placebo-controlled trial. *Lancet, 360*, 7–22.

*Hjermann, I., Byre, K. V., Holme, I., & Leren, P. (1981). Effect of diet and smoking intervention on the incidence of coronary heart disease: report from the Oslo Study Group of a randomized trial in healthy men. *Lancet, 2,* 1303–1310.

*Jackson, R., & Beaglehole, R. (1993). The relationship between alcohol and coronary heart disease: is there a protective effect? *Current Opinion in Lipidology, 4,* 21–26.

Kerzner, B., Corbelli, J., Sharp, S., et al. (2003). Efficacy and safety of ezetimibe coadministered with lovastatin in primary hypercholesterolemia. *American Journal of Cardiology, 91*(4), 418–424.

*Lewis, S. J., Moye, L. A., Sacks, F. M., et al. (1998). Effect of pravastatin on cardiovascular events in older patients with myocardial infarction and cholesterol levels in the average range: results of the Cholesterol and Recurrent Events (CARE) Trial. *Annals of Internal Medicine, 129,* 681–689.

*Long-Term Intervention With Pravastatin in Ischaemic Disease (LIPID) Study Group. (1998). Prevention of cardiovascular events and death with pravastatin in patients with coronary heart disease and a broad range of initial cholesterol levels. *New England Journal of Medicine, 339,* 1349–1357.

*McKenney, J. M., & Hawkins, D. W. (1995). *Handbook on the management of lipid disorders.* National Pharmacy Cholesterol Council. Springfield, NJ: Scientific Therapeutics Information, Inc.

McKenney, J. M., Jones, P. H., Adamczyk, M. A., et al. (2003). Comparison of efficacy of rosuvastatin vs atorvastatin, simvastatin and pravastatin in achieving lipid goals. Results from STELLAR trial. *Current Medical Research, 19*(8), 689–698.

*National Heart, Lung and Blood Institute. (2002). *Morbidity and mortality: 2002 chartbook on cardiovascular, lung and blood disease.* Bethesda, MD: U.S. Department of Health and Human Services, Public Health Service.

*Pearson, T. A., & Swan, H. J. C. (1996). Lipid lowering: the case for identifying and treating high-risk patients. *Cardiology Clinics, 14,* 117–130.

*Ross, R., & Glomset, J. A. (1976). The pathogenesis of atherosclerosis (first of two parts). *New England Journal of Medicine, 295,* 369–377.

Rubins, H. B., Robins, S. J., Collins, D., et al. (1999). Gemfibrozil for the secondary prevention of coronary heart disease in men with low levels of high-density lipoprotein cholesterol. *New England Journal of Medicine, 341,* 410–418.

Sacks, F. M., Pfeffer, M. A., Moye, L. A., et al. (1996). The effect of pravastatin on coronary events after myocardial infarction in patients with average cholesterol levels: the Cholesterol and Recurrent Events Trial. *New England Journal of Medicine, 335,* 1001–1009.

*Scandinavian Simvastatin Survival Study Group. (1994). Randomized trial of cholesterol lowering in 4444 patients with coronary heart disease: the Scandinavian Simvastatin Survival Study (4S). *Lancet, 344,* 1383–1389.

*Shepherd, J., et al. (1995). Prevention of coronary heart disease with pravastatin in men with hypercholesterolemia: the West of Scotland Coronary Prevention Study. *New England Journal of Medicine, 333,* 1301–1307.

*Talbert, R. L. (1997). Hyperlipidemia. In J. T. Dipiro, R. L. Talbert, G. C. Yee, G. R. Matzke, B. G. Wells, & L. M. Posey (Eds.), *Pharmacotherapy: a pathophysiologic approach* (3rd ed., pp. 459–489). Stamford, CT: Appleton & Lange.

Visit the Connection web site for the most up-to-date drug information.

20

ANGINA

■ ALICIA REESE, NANCY YOUNGBLOOD, AND ANDREW M. PETERSON

Cardiovascular disease was responsible for nearly 40% of deaths recorded in 2001, making it the leading cause of death in the United States (American Heart Association, 2004). Angina is a clinical syndrome caused by coronary artery disease (CAD) that can result in substantial morbidity. In 2004, the cost of cardiovascular disease is estimated to be nearly $240 billion, with CAD accounting for over $133 billion (American Heart Association, 2004).

Fortunately, the overall mortality rate from CAD has been declining. The reason for this decline is the improved treatments for cardiovascular disease, including angina. Despite this hopeful note, angina remains a significant challenge for primary care management. Successful management depends on an in-depth understanding of the pathologic process, diagnosis, and treatment of this symptom complex.

Angina is a syndrome, a constellation of symptoms, that results from myocardial oxygen demand being greater than the oxygen supply (myocardial ischemia). By definition, angina is associated with reversible ischemia, so it does not result in permanent myocardial damage. Myocardial infarction is the result of irreversible ischemia when myocardial tissue is permanently damaged.

Patients with angina may report chest pain, discomfort, heaviness, or pressure, and the sensation may radiate to the back, neck, jaw, and throat or arms. Usually these sensations last 1 to 15 minutes. Patients may also experience shortness of breath or fatigue. It is important to note, however, that not all patients present with "angina" in a typical fashion. For example, dyspnea on exertion may be the only presenting symptom. If a patient presents with unique symptoms, his or her group of symptoms associated with identified ischemia is called that patient's "anginal equivalent." Box 20-1 lists common and unique terms used to describe angina. Typical stable angina is often precipitated by physical exertion or emotional stress and relieved by rest or nitroglycerin. Unstable angina is experienced when the patient is at rest or is prolonged or progressive. Other types of angina include variant angina, nocturnal angina, angina decubitus, and postinfarction angina (Box 20-2). Stable angina is most commonly managed in the primary care setting and is the focus of this chapter.

CAUSES

The development of angina is directly related to the risk factors that have been identified for CAD. Nonmodifiable risk factors for CAD cannot be altered or improved by the patient; they include age, family history, and gender. Modifiable risk factors may be controlled or treated by lifestyle modifications or pharmacologic therapy to reduce the risk of morbidity or mortality from CAD. Modifiable risk factors include cigarette smoking, hypertension, dyslipidemia, diabetes, obesity, and physical inactivity. Box 20-3 lists the risk factors for CAD.

Nonmodifiable Risk Factors

Age

It is uncommon for men younger than 40 years of age and premenopausal women to have symptomatic CAD, but the incidence increases with age and is increased in women after menopause. This increasing incidence of CAD with age is likely linked to age-related changes in the vasculature and the higher prevalence of other CAD risk factors among older persons.

Family History

A family history of premature CAD in a first-degree relative (i.e., mother, father, sister, or brother) is a strong predictor for CAD in an individual. Premature CAD is defined as occurring in a man under 55 years or in a woman under 65 years. The strong association between family history and the development of CAD has been consistently demonstrated in a large number of studies. Therefore, individuals with a family history of CAD should be carefully screened for other CAD risk factors and managed appropriately.

Gender

In general, the risk of CAD is higher for men than women. Male gender is considered a nonmodifiable risk factor for CAD.

BOX 20–1. WORDS PATIENTS USE TO DESCRIBE ANGINA

Ache, toothache-like, dull
Burning, heartburn, soreness, bursting, searing indigestion
Choking, strangling, compressing, constricting, tightness, viselike
Discomfort, fullness, swelling, heaviness, pressure, weight, uncomfortable

---

Differences for CAD susceptibility diminish, however, when comparing postmenopausal women and older men. In fact, after 65 years of age, the incidence of CAD increases in women to be much closer to that of similarly aged men.

Modifiable Risk Factors

Cigarette Smoking

Cigarette smoking increases the risk of CAD by at least two- to threefold (Maron, Grundy, Ridler, & Pearson, 1998). Smoking increases the incidence of atherosclerosis by a mechanism that is not clearly understood. It is thought to increase the release of catecholamines, which leads to elevated blood pressure due to an increased workload of the heart caused by an increase in the heart rate and peripheral vascular constriction. Catecholamines also increase the release of free fatty acids, which increases the amount of lipids in the blood. Smoking lowers high-density lipoprotein (HDL) levels and increases low-density lipoprotein (LDL) levels, and is thought to enhance platelet adhesiveness, which increases the risk of clot formation in the arteries. All patients with CAD risk factors or established disease should be instructed to stop smoking. See Chapter 58 for a more detailed discussion of smoking cessation.

Hypertension

It is estimated that over 50 million Americans have elevated blood pressure (American Heart Association, 2004). Hypertension is a major risk factor for CAD and can lead to vascular complications that increase morbidity and mortality. Additionally, the higher the blood pressure, the higher the risk of MI and other cardiovascular events.

Atherosclerotic changes in the vasculature are exacerbated by increased pressure. Increased blood pressure alone also causes injury to the inner lining of the arteries, resulting in atherosclerotic changes and thrombus formation. As the arteries become more stiff and narrow, the blood flow that normally increases during physical activity is restricted to a greater degree, resulting in ischemic symptoms. Chapter 18 provides further discussion of drug therapy for hypertension.

Dyslipidemia

Nearly half of the American population has high cholesterol (American Heart Association, 2004). Cholesterol plays a

---

BOX 20–2. CLASSIFICATION OF CLASSIC ANGINA

Stable Angina
Angina is called *stable* when the paroxysmal chest pain or discomfort is provoked by physical exertion or emotional stress and is relieved by rest and/or nitroglycerin. Stable angina exists when the stimulating factors or activities and the degree and duration of discomfort have not changed for the past 60 days (Schant & Alexander, 1998).

Unstable Angina
Unstable angina is also called *preinfarction angina, crescendo angina,* or *intermittent coronary syndrome.* It is differentiated from stable angina by the fact that the symptoms may be triggered by minimal physical exertion or symptoms may be present at rest. Anginal episodes that are increasing in frequency, duration or severity are also referred to as "unstable." Patients who experience unstable angina are at high risk of developing an MI.

Nocturnal Angina
Nocturnal angina occurs during sleep. It is associated with rapid eye movement (REM) sleep and the dreaming that occurs during that state.

Angina Decubitus
Angina decubitus (also called *lying-down angina*) occurs when the patient reclines and is relieved when the patient assumes an upright position.

Postinfarction Angina
Postinfarction angina occurs after a myocardial infarction when residual ischemia may cause anginal episodes.

Variant Angina (Prinzmetal's Angina)
Variant angina is caused by coronary artery spasm.

BOX 20–3. RISK FACTORS FOR ANGINA

Nonmodifiable Risk Factors
Age
Family history
Gender

Modifiable Risk Factors
Cigarette smoking
Hypertension
Dyslipidemia
Diabetes
Obesity
Physical inactivity

substantial role in the pathophysiology of atherosclerosis and CAD. High levels of LDL cholesterol and low levels of HDL cholesterol are associated with an increased risk of cardiovascular disease and occurrence of MI or other poor cardiovascular outcomes. Treatment of dyslipidemia in patients with CAD using pharmacologic and non-pharmacologic means has been shown in multiple large-scale studies to reduce the risk of cardiovascular death. See Chapter 19 for more detailed information on the treatment of dyslipidemia.

Diabetes

Cardiovascular disease is the most common cause of death in patients with diabetes. In fact, patients with diabetes have the same risk of having an MI as a patient who already has a history of an MI. Although data have not shown a clear or conclusive link between glucose control and cardiovascular risk reduction, an effort should be made to prevent or treat diabetes in these patients. For a complete discussion of diabetes treatment, see Chapter 49.

Obesity

In the United States, nearly two-thirds of the population is considered overweight or obese. The increasing incidence of obesity has been attributed to poorer nutrition and a more sedentary lifestyle.

Obesity is a risk factor for CAD in both men and women. Hypertension, dyslipidemia, and diabetes are more common in patients who are obese, but obesity also increases cardiovascular risk independent of these other risk factors by a mechanism that is not well understood. Even modest weight loss can improve blood pressure, hypertension, and insulin resistance and reduce cardiovascular risk. Weight loss is discussed in Chapter 61.

Physical Inactivity

A sedentary lifestyle predisposes patients to CAD. Regular physical exercise reduces blood pressure, maintains a healthy weight, and improves dyslipidemia, but it also reduces the risk of CAD independent of these changes. Patients should be carefully screened and counseled before beginning an exercise program. Exercise may include walking, running, cycling, or formalized aerobic exercise routines. The risk of CAD is reduced by as little as 30 minutes of aerobic activity 3 or 4 days a week. Ideally, a patient should participate in daily aerobic exercise.

PATHOPHYSIOLOGY

Angina is a symptomatic manifestation of reversible myocardial ischemia, which occurs when demand for oxygen in the myocardium exceeds available supply. This imbalance between oxygen supply and demand is caused by limited blood supply due to narrowing of the blood vessels that supply the heart muscle. The most common cause of this narrowing of the coronary arteries is atherosclerotic disease. Rarely, vasospasm of the coronary arteries narrows the arteries, thereby limiting the blood supply to the heart muscle. Other even more uncommon sources of anginal symptoms

are thrombosis, aortic stenosis, primary pulmonary hypertension, and severe hypertension.

Atherosclerotic Disease

The pathophysiology of angina involves atherosclerosis, a disorder of lipid metabolism resulting in the deposit of cholesterol in the blood vessel. Over time, this causes a reactive endothelial injury that eventually results in a narrowing of the vessels by episodes of acute thrombosis. The narrow arteries impair the ability of oxygen and nutrients to reach the myocardium. This reduction in blood supply, or ischemia, impairs myocardial metabolism. The myocardial cells remain alive but cannot function normally. Once the blood supply is restored, cardiac function returns to normal. If the ischemia is caused by complete occlusion of the coronary artery, a myocardial infarction (cell death) occurs.

Regardless of the risk factors that cause the development of atherosclerosis and resulting restriction of coronary blood supply, the pathophysiologic process is essentially the same. The three layers of the arterial wall—intima, media, and adventitia—are affected by structural changes that lead to CAD. The intima is a single layer of endothelial cells, comprising the innermost surface of the artery. It is impermeable to the substances in the blood. The media is the middle layer of the artery and is made up almost entirely of smooth muscle. The outer layer, or adventitia, consists mainly of smooth muscle cells, fibroblasts (which are normally only in this layer), and loose connective tissue. Atherosclerotic changes in the artery occur in stages. Normally, the intima is thin and contains only an occasional muscle cell. As a person ages, the intima slowly increases in thickness and muscle cells proliferate.

Atherosclerosis primarily affects the intima of the arterial wall. It normally takes years to develop and clinical manifestations do not occur until the disorder is well advanced. CAD progresses through three developments—the fatty streak, the fibrous plaque, and the complicated lesion.

The Fatty Streak

Thought to begin in childhood, the fatty streak is caused by the development of fatty, lipid-rich lesions that result from macrophages adhering to the intact endothelial surface. The macrophages take in lipids, which leads to a thickening of the intimal layer. Smooth muscle cells migrate to the intima and become lipid laden. The lesions at this stage do not obstruct the artery. However, on examination, fatty streaks appear in the coronary arteries as early as 15 years of age. They continue to enlarge through the third decade of life and appear to be a precursor to plaque formation, although the process is not clearly understood.

The Fibrous Plaque

The raised fibrous plaque is a white, elevated area on the surface of the artery. It signals the beginning of progressive changes in the arterial wall, including protrusion of the lesion into the lumen of the artery. These more advanced lesions begin to develop at approximately 30 years of age in most patients. The major change in the arterial intima during this phase is the migration and proliferation of smooth muscle cells and the formation of a fibrous cap over a deeper deposit of extracellular lipid and cell debris. The lipid accumulation directly or indirectly reduces the blood supply. The decrease in blood supply is permanent and results in cell necrosis and cell debris.

The Complicated Lesion

A complicated lesion contains a fibrous plaque, calcium deposits, and a thrombus formed by hemorrhage into the plaque. The complicated lesion results from continuing cell degeneration. As the complicated lesion, with its lipid, necrotic center, becomes larger, it calcifies. The intimal surface may develop open or ruptured areas that degenerate into an ulcer. The damage is most likely to occur in areas where blood flow creates the greatest amount of stress in the vessel, such as at branches and bifurcations. The damaged surface allows blood from the artery lumen to enter the lipid core. Then platelets adhere and thrombus formation begins. The thrombus expands and distorts the plaque, which becomes larger and begins to block the lumen of the artery. The blockage impedes the blood flow needed to supply extra oxygen and nutrients to meet the increased workload of the heart. The result is cardiac ischemia and anginal symptoms. These symptoms are relieved when either the workload of the heart is decreased or administration of vasodilating drugs increases blood flow to the myocardium. Complete blockage can cause permanent myocardial death because the cells are entirely deprived of oxygen and blood flow cannot be restored in time to revive the cardiac cells, resulting in a myocardial infarction (MI).

Coronary Artery Vasospasm

A less common cause of restricted coronary blood supply may be coronary vasospasm, a narrowing of the coronary artery lumen. This narrowing is produced by an arterial muscle spasm and limits the blood supply to the myocardium. The exact cause is unknown, but it is thought to occur when the smooth muscles of the coronary arteries contract in response to neurogenic stimulation. Cigarette smoking and hyperlipidemia appear to play a role in this type of angina because they interfere with normal neurogenic control of the arterial intima.

Spasm is suspected of playing a role in acute MI, as well as in triggering anginal episodes. Coronary artery spasm also can occur with abrupt nitrate withdrawal, cocaine use, and direct mechanical irritation from cardiac catheterization. However, the exact mechanisms leading to spasm are still unclear.

Activation of Ischemic Episodes

Regardless of the existing pathophysiologic process, ischemic episodes that result in anginal pain are usually activated by two situations occurring simultaneously or independently: (1) ambient factors that increase myocardial oxygen demand, and (2) circumstances that decrease oxygen supply. For example, the person with atherosclerosis (noncompliant arteries) climbs a flight of stairs. The activity increases the workload of the heart and the myocardium needs more oxygen. The damaged

arteries are unable to meet this demand. In some situations, the arteries may be so constricted that they are unable to deliver an adequate amount of oxygen even if the person is in a resting state. Therapy is directed at resolution or control of these situations so that the heart can receive the oxygen it needs to meet the physical demands of the body. Control of the blood flow to the heart by increasing it when necessary prevents the pathophysiologic process responsible for the myocardial ischemia.

DIAGNOSTIC CRITERIA
Health History

The health history is an important part of the diagnosis and management of angina. The chief complaint for most patients is usually chest pain or discomfort, but other symptoms may predominate, such as neck or jaw pain or shortness of breath. The patient should be asked to describe the duration, quality, location, severity, and radiation of the pain. Additionally, the practitioner should inquire about potential triggers of the pain and any accompanying symptoms, such as dyspnea, diaphoresis, nausea, or palpitations. The practitioner also should explore what interventions relieved the patient's pain or symptoms, such as rest or nitroglycerin (NTG).

For all patients with angina, an assessment of CAD risk factors should be performed to determine an individual patient's risk for CAD and to better target pharmacologic and nonpharmacologic management. Practitioners should ask patients about both nonmodifiable and modifiable risk factors, including family history, cigarette smoking, hypertension, dyslipidemia, diabetes, and physical inactivity. A past history of cerebrovascular disease or the presence of peripheral vascular disease also increases a patient's risk of CAD.

Physical Findings

Most commonly, practitioners will not have the opportunity to examine a patient during an acute anginal episode. In that case, the physical examination should focus on the assessment of risk factors and the cardiovascular system as a whole. For example, the practitioner should assess a patient for obesity during the physical examination. Additionally, the vasculature may be evaluated by looking for fundoscopic changes or decreased peripheral pulses. Hypertension may be evident from taking the patient's blood pressure, and clinical signs and symptoms of heart failure may include murmurs, changes in the heart sounds, edema, rales, or organomegaly. Patients with dyslipidemia may exhibit xanthomas or cholesterol nodules.

If a physical exam is performed during an episode of anginal pain, a variety of findings may be present. These may include extra heart sounds, mild hypertension, tachycardia, or tachypnea. A paradoxical split of S_2 may indicate altered left ventricular heart function associated with the ischemic discomfort.

Diagnostic Tests

Before therapy for angina can be properly prescribed, diagnostic testing is necessary to identify a cardiac cause of the patient's chest pain. Diagnostic testing includes electrocardiography (ECG), echocardiography, exercise tolerance testing, radioisotope imaging, and coronary artery angiography.

Patients with new, current, or recent chest pain should have an ECG to detect signs of cardiac ischemia. During an acute anginal episode, ST segment depressions with symmetric T-wave inversions may be noted in the leads that correspond to the myocardium affected. During pain-free intervals, however, the ECG reverts to baseline. ECG changes that may be present in the patient with chronic CAD include evidence of a prior MI, LV hypertrophy, and repolarization abnormalities.

Echocardiography is recommended if valvular disease or heart failure is suspected, if the patient has a history of myocardial infarction, or if the patient experiences ventricular arrhythmias. All patients with intermittent episodes of chest pain should undergo an exercise tolerance test with ECG monitoring (also called a "stress test") to evaluate the risk of future cardiac events. Those suspected of having coronary ischemia based on the presence of anginal symptoms should undergo testing within 72 hours of symptoms. Further testing with radioisotope perfusion testing or coronary artery angiography may be indicated for subgroups of patients. If diagnostic testing confirms cardiac ischemia as the cause of anginal symptoms, drug therapy is warranted.

INITIATING DRUG THERAPY

The treatment goals for the management of angina include relieving the acute anginal episode, preventing additional anginal episodes, preventing progression of CAD, reducing the risk of MI, improving functional capacity, and prolonging survival. These goals should be accomplished while maintaining the patient's quality of life and avoiding adverse events associated with therapy.

Nonpharmacologic therapy is the cornerstone of treatment for patients with angina. The clinician must assess the patient's modifiable risk factors and work with him or her to reduce the risk for CAD. Practitioners should counsel patients on smoking cessation at each clinic visit and provide support and access to pharmacologic treatment if necessary. Patients should be instructed to maintain a normal weight by consuming a low-fat, low-cholesterol diet, and practitioners should provide dietary counseling and refer interested patients to dieticians for further support. Finally, practitioners should encourage patients to engage in regular aerobic exercise. Further details on these lifestyle modifications are provided in Chapters 18, 19, and 58.

The practitioner should emphasize to the patient that nonpharmacologic therapy and lifestyle modifications supplement drug therapy and should continue indefinitely.

Goals of Drug Therapy

After the patient has been properly instructed on nonpharmacologic therapy for angina, appropriate drug therapy may be initiated. A summary of selected agents is provided in Table 20-1 and Table 20-2. Several classes of medications are used to treat angina, including nitrates, beta blockers, calcium channel blockers, and antiplatelet agents.

Table 20.1

Drugs That Ameliorate Pathophysiologic Processes Associated With Angina

Pathophysiologic Changes	Drugs Used
Narrowing of the blood vessels	*Beta-adrenergic blockers* reduce oxygen demand. *Calcium channel blockers* inhibit the entrance of calcium into cardiac and smooth muscle cells of arteries, causing vasodilation. *Nitrates* cause marked relaxation of vessels, thereby decreasing preload and end diastolic volume.
Fibrous plaques	*Antiplatelet therapy* prevents platelet aggregation and thrombus generation at the site of ruptured fibrous plaques.
Coronary artery vasospasm	*Calcium channel blockers* inhibit the entrance of calcium into cardiac and smooth muscle cells of the arteries, causing vasodilation. *Nitrates* moderate the effect of vasospasm.

Nitrates

The nitrates are one of the original medications used for controlling angina, and they are still commonly used to halt an acute anginal attack, to prevent predictable episodes, and for chronic treatment to prevent anginal episodes.

Mechanism of Action

Nitrates and their analogs are potent agents and have profound effects on vascular smooth muscle. The nitrates cause dilation throughout the vasculature—in the peripheral arteries and veins as well as the coronary arteries. When dilated, the veins return less blood to the heart, thereby reducing left ventricular filling volume and pressure (preload). This decreases the workload of the heart. Another primary effect of the nitrates is coronary arterial dilation, which results in increased blood flow and oxygen supply to the myocardium. Nitrates do not directly influence the chronotropic or inotropic actions of the heart, so their administration does not affect or alter cardiac function, but rather decreases the work of the heart and increases myocardial oxygenation. Nitrates are moderately effective in lessening coronary vasospasm.

Rapid-Acting Nitrates

The sublingual forms of NTG are rapid acting (see Table 20-2). These medications are used for acute attacks of angina. Short-acting nitrates are also used for prophylaxis of angina in situations when an anginal episode can be reasonably predicted by the patient, such as during walking, climbing stairs, or sexual activity. To be effective, NTG must be administered sublingually to avoid hepatic first pass metabolism, which would inactivate the medication.

Sublingual NTG (Nitrol, Isordil, others) remains the first-line therapy for managing acute angina episodes. NTG may

Table 20.2

Overview of Agents Used to Treat Angina

Generic (Trade) Name and Dosage	Selected Adverse Events	Contraindications	Special Considerations
Short-Acting Nitrates			
Nitroglycerin (Nitrostat, Nitroquick) 0.4 mg SL prn	Headache, dizziness, tachycardia, hypotension, edema	Combination with phosphodiesterase-5 inhibitors (e.g., sildenafil, vardenafil, and tadalafil)	For acute treatment of anginal episodes
Isosorbide dinitrate (ISDN; Isordil, Sorbitrate) 5 mg SL prn	Above notes also apply	Above notes also apply	Above notes also apply
Long-Acting Nitrates			
Nitroglycerin Topical ointment (Nitro-bid) ½–1 in bid–tid Transdermal patch (Minitran, Nitro-Dur, Nitrol, Transderm-Nitro) 0.2–0.8 mg/hr	Above notes also apply Local irritation and erythema with topical application	Above notes also apply	For chronic prevention of anginal episodes Use nitrate-free interval to reduce risk of nitrate tolerance Potential hypotensive effect with vasodilators Tapering is recommended after long-term use Onset of action with transdermal application is approximately 60 minutes
Isosorbide mononitrate (ISMN) Immediate release (Ismo, Monoket) 5–20 mg bid Extended release (Imdur) 30–120 mg bid	Above notes also apply	Above notes also apply	Above notes also apply Extended-release formulations should be swallowed whole
Beta-blockers			
Propranolol Immediate release (Inderal) 40–160 mg bid Extended release (Inderal LA) 80–240 mg qd	Fatigue, dizziness, decreased exercise tolerance, bradycardia, hypotension, dyspnea	Use with caution in patients with reactive airway disease Bradycardia (heart rate <45 beats per minute) Acutely decompensated heart failure	Abrupt cessation of beta-blocker therapy should be avoided Extended-release formulations should be swallowed whole
Atenolol 25–100 mg qd	Above notes also apply	Above notes also apply	Above notes also apply
Metoprolol Immediate release (metoprolol tartrate, Lopressor) 25–200 mg tid Extended release (metoprolol succinate, Toprol XL) 50–100 mg qd	Above notes also apply	Above notes also apply	Toprol XL tablets may be split, but should not be chewed or crushed
Calcium Channel Blockers			
Amlodipine 2.5–10 mg qd	Headache, dizziness, flushing, edema, gingival hyperplasia	Severe conduction abnormalities Use with caution in patients with pre-existing bradycardia or CHF	Useful for patients with isolated systolic hypertension
Nifedipine (extended release, Adalat CC, Procardia XL) 30–60 mg qd	Above notes also apply	Above notes also apply	Should be swallowed whole
Diltiazem (extended release, Cardizem CD, Dilacor XR, Tiazac) 180–420 mg qd	Headache, nausea, conduction abnormalities, gingival hyperplasia	Above notes also apply	Should be swallowed whole
Verapamil Immediate release (Calan, Isoptin) 80–320 mg bid Extended release (Calan SR, Isoptin SR) 120–480 mg qd	Above notes also apply Constipation	Above notes also apply	Extended-release formulations should be swallowed whole
Antiplatelet Agents			
Aspirin 81–325 mg qd	Nausea, dyspepsia	Allergy to aspirin Bleeding disorders	For primary and secondary prevention of cardiovascular events
Clopidogrel (Plavix) 75 mg qd	Nausea	Allergy to clopidogrel Bleeding disorders	Alternative antiplatelet agent for aspirin-intolerant patients

be adequate treatment for patients who experience angina no more frequently than once a week. NTG usually relieves anginal symptoms within 1 to 5 minutes and provides short-term (up to 30 minutes) relief. NTG tablets or spray (0.3 to 0.6 mg) is used sublingually for immediate symptomatic treatment of anginal episodes. The practitioner instructs the patient to rest at the time of pain, take a single dose, repeat the dose if the pain does not resolve within 5 minutes, and to call emergency medical services if the pain is not relieved with 3 doses.

Patients should be instructed to mark the date they open a bottle of NTG tablets or first use a NTG spray canister. Tablets in an opened glass bottle of NTG retain efficacy for only 1 year and should be discarded after that time period. NTG canisters retain their efficacy for up to 3 years.

The main advantage of rapid-acting nitrates is their ability to halt an episode of angina once it has begun. Generally, the adverse effects of short-acting nitrates are related to their vasodilatory effects; however, patients may also experience burning under the tongue with sublingual preparations.

Long-Acting Nitrates

Due to their short duration of action, short-acting nitrates such as sublingual NTG are not suitable for mantainance therapy; long-acting nitrates must be used for chronic prophylaxis of anginal episodes. Long-acting nitrates act to maintain vasodilation, thereby continuously decreasing the workload of the heart and maintaining blood flow to the heart. The most prescribed long-acting nitrates are ISDN (oral [Cedocard SR, Isordil, others]), isosorbide mononitrate (ISMN; oral [Imdur, Ismo, Monoket, others]), and long-acting NTG preparations (transdermal [Minitran, Nitro-Dur, Transderm-Nitro, others], topical [Nitro-Bid, others]).

Isosorbide Dinitrate (Oral)

Single oral doses of 20 to 40 mg significantly improve hemodynamic parameters and exercise tolerance, and the effect continues for several hours. The starting dose should be low (e.g., ISDN 5 mg three times a day) and the dosage should be advanced slowly in small increments every 1 to 2 weeks to minimize side effects. The dose is increased until control is obtained, side effects become intolerable, systolic blood pressure falls to $\leq$100 mm Hg, resting heart rate increases more than 10 beats per minute, or postural hypotension occurs.

Intestinal absorption with ISDN is unpredictable, especially when taken with food, so oral nitrates should be taken on an empty stomach, 1 hour before or 2 hours after food intake. A drawback to ISDN products is the short half-life (approximately 2 to 4 hours) and duration of action, which necessitates multiple doses during the day.

Isosorbide Mononitrate (Oral)

ISMN is a long-acting metabolite derivative of ISDN. Formulated in extended-release tablets, ISMN can be administered in fewer doses (Imdur, once daily; other products, twice daily). A common twice-daily starting regimen is 20 mg (immediate-release) orally at 7 AM and 3 PM, allowing for a nitrate-free period to reduce the risk of nitrate tolerance. A starting dose using extended-release ISMN (Imdur) is 30 to 60 mg orally in the morning. Like ISDN, ISMN should also be taken on an empty stomach. Extended-release formulations of ISMN must be taken whole, without crushing or chewing the tablet.

Nitroglycerin (Transdermal)

Transdermal NTG is long-acting and effective for treating and preventing anginal pain. Two percent (2%) NTG ointment may be applied to the skin as an adjunct to isosorbide therapy for nocturnal pain or, with repeated daily dosing, used alone for anginal treatment. One half to one inch of the ointment is applied to a clean, hairless area of the torso before bed. Alternatively, the ointment may be applied every 4 to 6 hours while awake, allowing for an 8- to 12-hour nitrate-free interval. Measurement guides are provided with the product to assist in dosing. The dose is increased by a half inch at a time until pain relief is achieved.

Transdermal NTG patches may also be used as a long-acting nitrate. Therapy is typically initiated with a 5-mg (0.2 mg/ hr) or 10-mg (0.4 mg/hr) patch, which should be left in place for 12 to 14 hours and then removed to prevent nitrate tolerance. Nitrate patches should be applied to the torso intact, since cutting a patch destroys the drug delivery system. Care should be taken to assure a previously applied patch is removed before applying a new patch.

Nitrate Tolerance

A drawback to the use of nitrates to treat angina is the potential for the development of nitrate tolerance. Nitrate tolerance refers to the loss of ability of the smooth muscles to respond to the action of the nitrates. Tolerance develops to both the peripheral and coronary vasodilator effects of nitrates. This phenomenon occurs with continuous nitrate use over prolonged periods. Tolerance is both dose- and time-dependent. Nitrate tolerance can be seen after as few as 7 to 10 days of continuous administration. Nitrate tolerance may also develop with frequent sublingual administration of nitrates, if the oral tablets are given four times daily in evenly spaced intervals, or if the transdermal patches are left on the skin for 24-hour periods.

Prevention of nitrate tolerance is based on a treatment plan that provides for rapid changes in blood nitrate levels over a given time, usually 24 hours. To prevent nitrate tolerance, one 10- to 12-hour nitrate-free interval per day is necessary. In this manner, the intervals between doses need not be equal. For example, the patch can be applied in the morning and removed in the evening. The same schedule can be developed for patients taking oral medications. The medication is given three times during the day when the patient is awake. The patient does not receive any medication during the night to minimize the risk of nitrate tolerance. Combination anti-anginal therapy (e.g., beta-blocker plus a long-acting nitrate) should be used for patients whose anginal symptoms are not controlled during the nitrate-free interval.

Adverse Events

The common side effects of the nitrates are related to their vasodilatory effects: headache, flushing, dizziness, weakness, and orthostatic hypotension. Additionally, since all segments of the vascular system relax in response to nitrates, reflex tachycardia often results as the heart compensates for the blood pressure drop to maintain cardiac output. Transdermal nitrate products may also cause irritation of the skin at the site of application.

Most of the side effects associated with nitrates abate or disappear with continuation of therapy. By starting therapy at a low dose and slowing titrating the dose upward, side effects are minimized and may not present at all. However, starting with a high dose can produce severe side effects (especially headache), and if side effects are intolerable, the patient may self-discontinue the medication.

If a patient has been receiving nitrate therapy long-term, it should not be abruptly discontinued because of the risk of rebound hypertension and angina. If discontinuation of nitrate therapy is required, it should be done by tapering the dose over a period of time.

Caution should be exercised when using nitrates in combination with vasodilators due to additive hypotensive effects. Concurrent use of nitrates and phosphodiesterase-5 inhibitors such as sildenafil (Viagra), vardenafil (Levitra), or tadalafil (Cialis) is contraindicated due to the potential for severe hypotension.

Beta-blockers

Beta-blockers are very effective in managing angina. They reduce the workload of the heart and decrease overall myocardial oxygen demand and consumption through antagonism of adrenergic receptors. This is accomplished by a reduction in the heart rate and myocardial contractility, both at rest and during periods of normal exercise. As such, they are particularly beneficial for treating exertional angina.

Nitrates and beta-blockers have complementary effects on myocardial oxygen supply and demand and therefore are often used together. Because beta-blockers reduce the heart rate, they can be used to control the reflex tachycardia that sometimes occurs with the administration of nitrates. This reduction in heart rate also allows more time for myocardial perfusion during diastole.

Mechanism of Action

Beta-blockers can be categorized according to their cardioselectivity, that is, the degree of preferential affinity for beta$_1$ receptors, which predominate in the heart and are the principal target of these medications. Beta antagonists that block only beta$_1$ receptors are considered *cardioselective* beta-blockers. Those that block both beta$_1$ and beta$_2$ receptors are *nonselective*. There are many beta-blockers available, all of which block beta$_1$ receptors. However, many agents also block beta$_2$ receptors, which predominate in the lungs.

Beta$_1$-receptor blockade is desirable in a patient with angina because it causes a slowing of the heart rate and a reduction in myocardial contractility. These effects reduce myocardial oxygen demand and therefore improve and prevent anginal symptoms.

Blockage of beta$_2$ receptors can lead to bronchoconstriction; therefore, nonselective beta-blockers should be used with caution in patients with uncontrolled or unstable reactive airway disease. At low to intermediate doses, cardioselectivity is demonstrated by atenolol (Tenormin) and metoprolol (Lopressor). Propranolol (Inderal) is an example of a nonselective beta-blocker. However, even cardioselective beta-blockers show nonselective action at high doses.

Propranolol is a nonselective beta-blocker with a short half-life (4 to 6 hours). Immediate-release formulations of propranolol must be dosed multiple times per day, but sustained-release preparations for once-daily dosing are also available. Other nonselective beta-blockers include nadolol and timolol.

Atenolol and metoprolol are selective beta$_1$ antagonists. These drugs, which preferentially block beta$_1$ receptors, were developed to eliminate the unwanted bronchoconstriction effect of the agents that also block beta$_2$ receptors. These agents may be a better choice for patients with severe or uncontrolled asthma or chronic obstructive pulmonary disease (COPD). However, when these agents are prescribed at high dosage levels, they lose their cardioselective properties. Atenolol has a long duration of action, and therefore may be dosed once daily. Immediate-release metoprolol tartrate (Lopressor) must be given two to three times daily, but extended-release metoprolol succinate (Toprol XL) is given only once daily. Both atenolol and metoprolol tartrate are available in generic forms and are relatively inexpensive.

Pindolol and acebutolol are beta-blockers that also possess some agonist activity. They are not completely blockers in that they have the ability also to stimulate weakly both beta$_1$ and beta$_2$ receptors, possessing so-called *intrinsic sympathomimetic activity* (ISA). Drugs possessing ISA can stimulate the beta receptor to which they are bound, yet as antagonists they block the activation of the receptor by the more potent endogenous catecholamines, epinephrine and norepinephrine. Because of the agonist action, there is a diminished effect on cardiac rate and cardiac output. Patients who cannot tolerate the other beta-blockers because of pre-existing bradycardia or heart block may tolerate these agents.

Contraindications

Beta-blockers are contraindicated and therefore should not be used in patients with pre-existing bradycardia because beta-blockade may lower the heart rate further. Additionally, beta-blockers should not be used if a patient is experiencing an acute episode of decompensated heart failure. Addition of a beta-blocker in this situation has the potential to negatively impact the patient by further reducing heart rate and contractility. Finally, as discussed above, beta-blockers should be used with caution in patients with reactive airway disease. In patients with stable or controlled asthma or COPD, a selective beta-blocker may be a better choice to minimize the risk of bronchospasm.

Adverse Events

Beta-blockers have the potential to adversely affect cardiac function. These effects include slowing the sinoatrial node and atrioventricular (AV) conduction, leading to symptomatic bradycardia and heart block. Sinus arrest is possible. If the patient has pre-existing cardiac conduction system disease, a preparation with some intrinsic beta-agonist activity may be chosen to minimize these adverse events. These patients require close and frequent monitoring to ensure that early conduction system disease is managed promptly. Beta-blockers should not be given to patients with a slow heart rate at baseline due to the potential for severe bradycardia.

Since beta-blockers attenuate the "fight or flight" response, the clinical manifestations of hypoglycemia may be masked. Therefore, patients with diabetes should be instructed to more closely monitor their serum glucose to avoid severe hypoglycemic reactions. Typical symptoms of hypoglycemia, including tachycardia, tremor, or sweating, may be decreased or absent when these patients are taking a beta-blocker.

Abrupt withdrawal of beta-blockers can precipitate tachycardia, hypertensive crises, angina exacerbation, acute coronary insufficiency, or even MI (Goroll et al., 1998). For this reason, beta-blocker therapy should always be tapered. Withdrawal is of particular concern in the anginal patient on large doses of beta-blockers who is faced with an emergency situation that makes it impossible to continue taking the prescribed beta-blocker for more than 48 hours.

Beta-blockers may also cause adverse CNS effects, including drowsiness and depression. These effects may occur more frequently in the elderly or in patients with pre-existing depression or psychiatric disorders. In these patients, careful monitoring of mood, sleep pattern, and sexual and cognitive functioning is necessary.

Calcium Channel Blockers

Calcium channel blockers are effective in managing angina because they exert vasodilatory effects on the coronary and peripheral vessels. Depending on the specific agent, they have the potential to depress cardiac contractility, heart rate, and conduction, which may mediate their antianginal effects. These drugs are effective in relieving coronary constriction associated with vasospastic angina.

Mechanism of Action

Calcium plays a major role in the electrical excitation and contraction of cardiac and vascular smooth muscle cells. The calcium channel blockers inhibit the entrance of calcium into smooth muscle cells of the coronary and systemic arterial vessels, which inhibits muscular contraction and therefore causes vasodilation. These vasodilatory effects are more pronounced on arteries than veins because of the relatively large amount of smooth muscle found in the arteries. Because calcium channel blockers do not cause substantial venous dilation, they do not reduce preload. Calcium channel blockers reduce heart rate by slowing conduction through the sinoatrial and atrioventricular nodes, and they depress cardiac contractility.

Two major groups of calcium channel blockers are available, the dihydropyridines and the nondihydropyridines.

Dihydropyridines

The dihydropyridine calcium channel blockers are potent dilators of the coronary and peripheral arteries. Due to the vasodilatory effect of these agents, they may cause reflex tachycardia due to a reduction in systemic blood pressure. Since dihydropyridines do not alter conduction, they do not slow the sinus rate.

There are many dihydropyridine calcium channel blockers available. Nifedipine is an example of a first-generation dihydropyridine; nicardipine, felodipine, isradipine, and amlodipine are second-generation dihydropyridines. In general, the second-generation agents are better tolerated than the first-generation agents.

All of these agents are administered orally, and they have relatively short half-lives. Doses should be titrated upward slowly to minimize orthostasis or other adverse events. Several dihydropyridines (e.g., nifedipine, nicardipine) must be administered as multiple daily doses unless the sustained formulations are used. Amlodipine is administered once daily.

Nondihydropyridines

Although diltiazem and verapamil are both nondihydropyridine calcium channel blockers, they display different effects on the cardiovascular system. Verapamil has a pronounced effect on cardiac conduction, reducing the rate of electrical conduction through the AV node. Verapamil also exerts negative inotropic and chronotropic effects, suppressing contractility, reducing heart rate, and therefore causing a reduction in oxygen demand. However, due to this effect, verapamil should be used with caution in those patients with depressed cardiac function or AV conduction abnormalities. Immediate-release formulations of verapamil must be administered as divided doses, but sustained-release products are administered once daily.

Like verapamil, diltiazem reduces the heart rate, but to a lesser extent. Diltiazem also has a less potent effect than verapamil on conduction and contractility, but it is a more potent vasodilator. Diltiazem has immediate- and sustained-release formulations. The immediate-release formulation usually is taken four times a day before meals; the sustained-release formulation is taken daily on an empty stomach.

Contraindications

Before a calcium channel blocker can be selected for treating angina, a careful assessment must be done to determine a patient's left ventricular and conduction system function. Calcium channel blockers with negative inotropic properties may worsen pre-existing LV dysfunction. Patients with conduction system disease are poor candidates for calcium channel blocker therapy because of the risk of bradyarrhythmias.

The nondihydropyridine calcium channel blockers are contraindicated in patients with heart block because of the significant depression of AV node conduction. Additionally, calcium channel blockers should be used with caution in patients with sick sinus syndrome and hypotension.

Adverse Events

In general, adverse events accompanying the dihydropyridine calcium channel blockers are more common with the first-generation than the second-generation agents. Leg edema, a common problem, results from vasodilation, which causes fluid to pool in the legs. In some cases, the edema may be so severe that new-onset heart failure may be suspected. In this situation, dosage reduction or drug discontinuation may be considered. Other common side effects of the calcium channel blockers include fatigue, dizziness, headache, flushing, and gingival hyperplasia. Verapamil is associated with constipation much more often than the other calcium channel blockers.

Antiplatelet Therapy

Antiplatelet drugs inhibit platelet aggregation through a variety of mechanisms. Aspirin inhibits platelet activation through irreversible enzyme antagonism to block prostaglandin synthesis, and clopidogrel reduces ADP-induced platelet activation. Aggregation is a normal process that causes disease when the platelets adhere to vessel walls, causing thrombus formation. Antiplatelet therapy limits the formation of the thrombus, thereby decreasing the risk of progressive CAD. When antiplatelet medications are used to treat patients with angina, the chances of having an MI are reduced by 50% (Black & Matassarin-Jacobs, 1997).

In patients with stable angina, the risk of myocardial infarction can be lowered with daily aspirin therapy. Aspirin acts by blocking prostaglandin synthesis, which prevents formation of the platelet-aggregating substance thromboxane A_2. Current angina recommendations suggest that all patients with acute or chronic ischemic heart disease receive aspirin as primary or secondary prevention of cardiovascular disease (Gibbons et al., 2002).

The usual dosage of aspirin for antiplatelet therapy is 81 to 325 mg taken once daily. Adverse events associated with aspirin use include dyspepsia, bruising, and bleeding. Enteric-coated aspirin may be prescribed to minimize gastrointestinal symptoms. Aspirin is contraindicated in patients with a known aspirin hypersensitivity.

Clopidogrel is another antiplatelet agent that may be used in patients with angina. It reduces ADP-induced platelet activation by antagonizing the platelet ADP receptors. Clopidogrel is recommended for prevention of myocardial infarction in angina patients who have contraindications to aspirin. Like aspirin, clopidogrel has been shown to reduce the incidence of morbidity and mortality in patients with established cardiovascular disease.

The dose of clopidogrel is 75 mg daily. Since it is only commercially available as a branded product, clopidogrel is more expensive than aspirin for most patients. Bleeding events associated with clopidogrel are similar to aspirin, although it typically exhibits better gastrointestinal tolerance.

For further discussion of antiplatelet agents, refer to Chapter 54.

Selecting the Most Appropriate Anti-anginal Therapy

Choosing the appropriate medications for treating a patient with angina can be challenging. The primary goal is to design a regimen that will reduce the frequency and severity of anginal episodes. Subsequent adjustments are made empirically based on the patient's response to treatment, disease progression, risk factor modification, and patient satisfaction and adherence (Fig. 20-1).

Acute Treatment of Anginal Episodes

All patients with angina should be provided a short-acting nitrate for acute treatment of anginal episodes. Additionally, patients with infrequent episodes of angina can be managed effectively with short-acting nitrates alone. They are a good choice for the patient who has infrequent attacks or predictable pain on exertion.

Chronic Prevention of Anginal Episodes

Patients with repeated episodes of angina should receive long-acting therapy for chronic prophyaxis. There are three classes of agents that may be used for chronic anti-anginal therapy: the beta-blockers, calcium channel blockers, and long-acting nitrates. The initial choice of an anti-anginal agent should be based on the patient's specific characteristics, such as physical exam findings and coexisting medical conditions. Treatment with a single agent is generally used for initial anti-anginal therapy, whereas combination therapy is instituted for patients who fail monotherapy.

First-Line Therapy

In the absence of contraindications, beta-blockers are the agents of choice for prevention of acute anginal episodes in patients with or without a history of MI. Beta-blockers reduce the frequency and likelihood of anginal episodes and reduce CAD-related morbidity and mortality. Additionally, beta-blockers are useful as antihypertensive and antiarrhythmic agents. Beta-blockers are particularly useful in patients whose anginal symptoms are related to physical exertion.

For patients whose anginal symptoms have been linked to coronary vasospasm, a calcium channel blocker may be considered for initial treatment. See Table 20-3 for more information.

Second-Line Therapy

For patients who do not respond sufficiently to therapy with a single anti-anginal agent, combination therapy should be attempted. When initial treatment with a beta-blocker is not successful, either a calcium channel blocker or a long-acting nitrate may be added to beta-blocker therapy.

A long-acting nitrate/beta-blocker program is safe, effective, and low in cost. Nitrates and beta-blockers are well tolerated, and their effects are complementary. Reflex tachycardia caused by nitrates is blunted by a beta-blocker. The control of reflex tachycardia is beneficial because a decrease in heart rate lowers myocardial oxygen demand. The combination of nitrates and beta-blockers is an accepted treatment of angina, and they are often used together.

A beta-blocker plus a calcium channel blocker is another typical combination. Patients who have anginal symptoms that cannot be controlled by beta-blocker or calcium channel blocker monotherapy often respond to a combination of the two. However, a beta-blocker plus calcium channel blocker combination should be used with caution. When drugs from these two classes are given together, the additive effect is the potent suppression of AV conduction, which may be problematic in patients with pre-existing cardiac conduction abnormalities. It is best to start with low doses of each drug and monitor each dosage increase so that side effects can be identified early.

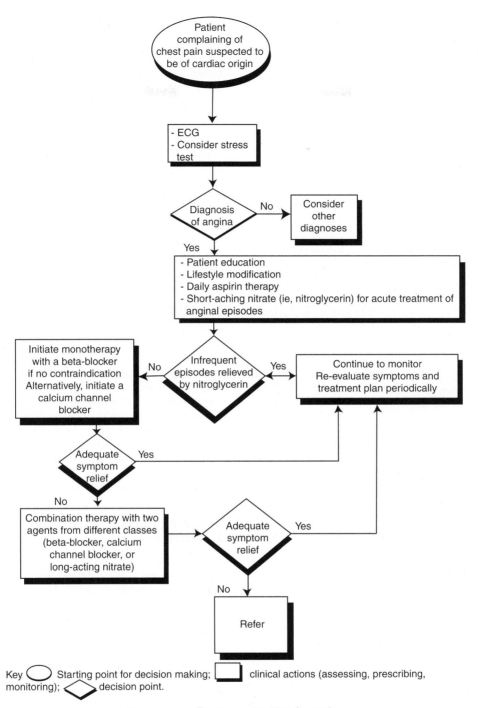

Figure 20–1 Treatment algorithm for angina.

Nitrates are often combined with a nondihydropyridine calcium channel blocker, such as diltiazem or verapamil, or a second-generation dihydropyridine calcium channel blocker, such as amlodipine. Since nitrates and first-generation dihydropyridine calcium channel blockers are potent vasodilators, they should be used together with extreme caution and only if no other treatment option is available.

Third-Line Therapy

In patients who are refractory to a two-drug regimen, a three-drug regimen of a calcium channel blocker, beta-blocker, and a long-acting nitrate may be used. In general, patients whose anginal symptoms do not respond to two anti-anginal agents should be referred to a specialist's care.

MONITORING PATIENT RESPONSE

In patients with angina, monitoring is important to evaluate for progression or stability of the disease, response to therapy, and presence or absence of adverse events.

Patient monitoring begins when a stress test is performed to confirm the diagnosis of angina. Once the diagnosis is made, stress tests may be repeated if there is a change in the

Table 20.3

Recommended Order of Treatment for Angina

Order	Agents	Comments
For all patients	Short-acting nitrate	For acute treatment of anginal episodes May be used to prevent predictable episodes May be used alone in patients with infrequent episodes
Chronic prevention of anginal episodes		
First line	Beta-blocker	Reduces workload of heart by decreasing overall myocardial oxygen consumption
	Calcium channel blocker	Useful for patients who cannot tolerate a beta-blocker
Second line	Combination therapy	If monotherapy fails, add another agent from a different class: beta-blocker, calcium channel blocker, long-acting nitrate (e.g., beta-blocker and long-acting nitrate)

pattern of anginal symptoms. Additionally, patients with stable angina should have an ECG if the history or physical examination changes or if the practitioner suspects new myocardial ischemia or development of a conduction abnormality (Gibbons et al., 2002).

Routine follow-up depends on the frequency and severity of the patient's complaints. Stable patients should be seen every 2 to 6 months, but visits should be more frequent if the patient's symptoms change or become more severe or more frequent. Medication initiation and adjustment also requires more office visits. At each office visit, vital signs should be taken and a complete physical examination performed. The patient should be questioned about anginal pain and associated symptoms and side effects of the drug regimen. Additional monitoring parameters should be determined by the specific drug regimen. Ideally, a patient's anti-anginal regimen should make him or her symptom-free.

PATIENT EDUCATION

For optimal control of anginal symptoms, the patient should be educated on his or her disease and medications. Patients should be informed of the seriousness of coronary artery disease and the potential consequences of leaving their angina untreated. Education about lifestyle modification strategies should be provided to all patients as often as possible. Additionally, patients need to know how to rec-

ognize worsening or escalating symptoms so they know when to seek emergency care.

Drug Information

There are many sources of information relating to the treatment of angina. Several therapeutic guidelines are available to the practitioner, including those from the American College of Cardiology and American Heart Association, the American College of Chest Physicians, the European Society of Cardiology, and many other organizations. Specific questions relating to pharmacologic agents used in the treatment of angina may be addressed using the *Physician's Desk Reference, Drug Facts and Comparisons, Micromedex,* or another drug reference. Finally, information regarding ongoing clinical trials for angina and other conditions may be obtained from a website provided by the National Institutes of Health (www.clinicaltrials.gov).

Patient-Oriented Information Sources

Practitioners may provide disease- and treatment-related information to patients with information from a variety of sources. The website for the American Heart Association (www.americanheart.org) has many resources available to explain cardiovascular disease and angina in a fashion patients will understand. Also, the American Academy of Family Physicians (www.aafp.org) provides on its website a variety of resources under the heading of "Patient Ed." Finally, the National Heart, Lung, and Blood Institute describes for patients the disease of angina, its causes, and appropriate treatments under the "Diseases and Conditions Index" (http://www.nhlbi.nih.gov/health/dci/Diseases/Angina/ Angina_WhatIs.html).

Complementary and Alternative Medications

Although there are a variety of complementary medications that allege to provide symptom relief for patients with angina, no herbal medication has been shown to have efficacy similar to that of the traditional agents described above. If at all possible, practitioners should counsel patients to adhere to treatment regimens that have shown efficacy in the treatment of angina.

Patients should be educated on each of the medications they are provided. They should know the importance of taking their medications as prescribed. They should be informed of each medication's indication and possible side effects, and what to do if they miss one or more doses of a scheduled medication, such as a long-acting nitrate. Additionally, practitioners should educate patients about the proper storage of all medications.

■ Case Study

E.H. is a 45-year-old African-American man who recently moved to the community from another state. He requests renewal of a prescription for a calcium channel blocker, prescribed by a physician in the former state. He is unemployed and lives with a woman, their son, and the woman's two children. His past medical history is remarkable for asthma and six "heart attacks" that he claims occurred because of a 25-year history of drug use (primarily cocaine). He states that he used drugs as recently as 2 weeks ago. He does not have any prior medical records with him. He claims that he has been having occasional periods of chest pain. He is unable to report the duration or pattern of the pain.

Before proceeding, explore the following questions: What further information would you need to diagnose angina (substantiate your answer)? What is the connection between cocaine use and angina? Identify at least three tests that you would order to diagnose angina.

Diagnosis: Angina

1. List specific goals of treatment for E.H.

2. What dietary and lifestyle changes should be recommended for this patient?

3. What drug therapy would you prescribe for E.H. and why?

4. How would you monitor for success in E.H.?

5. Describe one or two drug–drug or drug–food interactions for the selected agent.

6. List one or two adverse reactions for the selected agent that would cause you to change therapy.

7. What would be the choice for the second-line therapy?

8. Discuss specific patient education based on the prescribed first-line therapy.

9. What over-the-counter and/or alternative medications would be appropriate for E.H.?

Bibliography

*Starred references are cited in the text.

*American Heart Association. (2004). *Heart and stroke facts: 2004 update.* Dallas, Texas: American Heart Association.

*Black, J., & Matassarin-Jacobs, E. (1997). *Medical-surgical nursing: Clinical management for community care* (5th ed.). Philadelphia: W. B. Saunders.

Bullock, B., & Henge, R. (2000). *Focus on pathophysiology.* Philadelphia: Lippincott Williams & Wilkins.

Ellsworth, A., Witt, D., Dugdale, D., & Oliver, L. (1997). *Mosby's medical drug reference.* Philadelphia: Mosby–Year Book.

*Gibbons, R. J., Abrams, J., Chatterjee, K., et al. (2003). ACC/AHA 2002 guideline update for the management of patients with chronic stable angina: a report of the American College of Cardiology/American Heart Assocation Task Force on Practice Guidelines (Committee to Update the 1999 Guidelines for the Management of Patients with Chronic Stable Angina). *Journal of the American College of Cardiology, 41,* 159–168.

*Goroll, A., May, L., & Mulley, A. (1998). Management of chronic stable angina. In *Primary care medicine.* Philadelphia: Lippincott Williams & Wilkins (update on CD, Vol. 2, no. 1).

Katzung, B., & Chatterjee, M. (1998). Vasodilators and the treatment of angina pectoris. In B. Katzung (Ed.), *Basic and clinical pharmacology* (7th ed.). Stamford, CT: Appleton & Lange.

*Maron, D. J., Grundy, S. M., Ridler, P. M., & Pearson, T. A. (2004). Dyslipidemia, other risk factors, and the prevention of coronary heart disease. In V. Fuster, R. W. Alexander, & R. A. O'Rourke (Eds.), *Hurst's the heart* (11th ed., pp. 1093-1122). New York: McGraw-Hill.

Mycek, M., Harvey, R., & Champe, P. (1997). *Lippincott's illustrated reviews: Pharmacology.* Philadelphia: Lippincott–Raven.

O'Rourke, R. A., O'Gara, P., & Dougles, J. S. (2004). Diagnosis and management of patients with chronic ischemic heart disease. In V. Fuster, R. W. Alexander, & R. A. O'Rourke (Eds.), *Hurst's the heart* (11th ed., pp. 1465–1494). New York: McGraw-Hill.

Patrano, C., Coller, B., FitzGerald, G. A., Hirsh, J., & Roth, G. (2004). Platelet-active drugs: The relationships among dose, effectiveness, and side effects: The seventh ACCP conference on antithrombotic and thrombolytic therapy. *Chest, 126*(3, Suppl.), 234S–264S.

Ross, R. (1998). Factors influencing atherogenesis. In R. Alexander, R. Schant, & V. Fuster (Eds.), *Hurst's the heart* (9th ed., pp. 1139–1160). New York: McGraw-Hill.

Uphold, C., & Graham, M. (1998). *Clinical guidelines in family practice* (3rd ed.). Gainesville, FL: Barmarrae Books.

Walker, B. F. (2004). Nonatherosclerotic coronary heart disease. In V. Fuster, R. W. Alexander, & R. A. O'Rourke (Eds.), *Hurst's the heart* (11th ed., pp. 1173–1214). New York: McGraw-Hill.

HEART FAILURE

■ SANDRA CHASE AND ANDREW M. PETERSON

Heart failure (HF), one of the most serious consequences of cardiovascular disease, has rapidly become one of the most important health problems in cardiovascular medicine. It affects 4.8 million people in the United States alone (1.5% to 2% of the U.S. adult population), and between 400,000 and 700,000 new cases are diagnosed each year (American Heart Association [AHA], 1998; Massie & Shah, 1997). The incidence more than doubles each decade in people between 45 and 75 years of age, and the disease represents the most common medical discharge diagnosis for patients older than 65 years of age (Massie & Shaw, 1997; O'Connell & Bristow, 1994). HF is more common in men than in women, probably because of the higher incidence of ischemic heart disease in men. Approximately 75% of all ambulatory patients with HF are 60 years of age or older (AHA, 1998). The disorder is associated with significant mortality from sudden death and progressive HF, with approximately 250,000 patients dying each year (O'Connell & Bristow, 1994).

The economic impact of HF also is significant. The large number and often high complexity of hospitalizations for HF make this diagnosis very costly. The total cost of HF hospitalizations in the U.S. has been estimated at $8 billion. After hypertension, HF is the second most common indication for physician office visits. Thus, the overall cost of managing HF can be conservatively estimated at $10 to $15 billion, but estimates run as much as two to three times higher (Massie & Shaw, 1997). Consequently, improved quality of life is considered a worthy health care goal, and the therapeutic approach to HF is directed toward increasing the patient's ability to maintain a positive quality of life with symptom-free activity and to enhance survival. Vasodilator therapy, especially with the angiotensin-converting enzyme (ACE) inhibitors, has made significant contributions toward achieving this goal.

CAUSES

The development of HF may be related to many etiologic variables. Coronary artery disease, hypertension, and idiopathic cardiomyopathy are the most frequently cited risk factors for HF (Braunwald, 1988; Franciosa et al., 1983; Packer & Cohn, 1999). Acute conditions that may result in HF include acute myocardial infarction (MI), arrhythmias, pulmonary embolism, sepsis, and acute myocardial ischemia (Braunwald, 1988). Gradual development of HF may be caused by liver or renal disease, primary cardiomyopathy, cardiac valve disease, anemia, bacterial endocarditis, viral myocarditis, thyrotoxicosis, chemotherapy, excessive dietary sodium intake, and ethanol abuse.

Drugs also can worsen HF. Drugs that may cause fluid retention, such as nonsteroidal anti-inflammatory drugs (NSAIDs), steroids, hormones, antihypertensives (eg, hydralazine [Apresoline], nifedipine [Procardia XL]), sodium-containing drugs (eg, carbenicillin disodium [Geopen]), and lithium (Eskalith, others) may cause congestion. Beta blockers, antiarrhythmics (eg, disopyramide [Norpace], flecainide [Tambocor], amiodarone [Cordarone], sotalol [Betapace]), tricyclic antidepressants, and certain calcium channel blockers (eg, diltiazem [Cardizem], nifedipine, verapamil [Calan]) have negative inotropic effects and further decrease contractility in an already depressed heart. Direct cardiac toxins (eg, amphetamines, cocaine, daunorubicin [DaunoXome], doxorubicin [Adriamycin], ethanol) also can worsen or induce HF (Covinsky & Willett, 1999).

PATHOPHYSIOLOGY

HF is a pathophysiologic state in which abnormal myocardial function inhibits the ventricles from delivering adequate quantities of blood to metabolizing tissues at rest or during activity. It results not only from a decrease in intrinsic systolic contractility of the myocardium, but also from alterations in the pulmonary and peripheral circulations (Braunwald, 1988).

When the heart fails as a pump and cardiac output (the volume of blood pumped out of the ventricle per unit of time) decreases, a complex scheme of compensatory mechanisms to raise and maintain cardiac output occurs. These compensatory mechanisms include increased preload (volume and pressure or myocardial fiber length of the ventricle prior to contraction [end of diastole]); increased afterload (vascular resistance); ventricular hypertrophy (increased muscle mass); and dilatation, activation of the sympathetic nervous system (SNS), and activation of the renin–angiotensin–aldosterone system (RAAS) (Covinsky & Willett, 1999).

Although initially beneficial for increasing cardiac output, these compensatory mechanisms are ultimately associated with further pump dysfunction. In effect, the consequence of

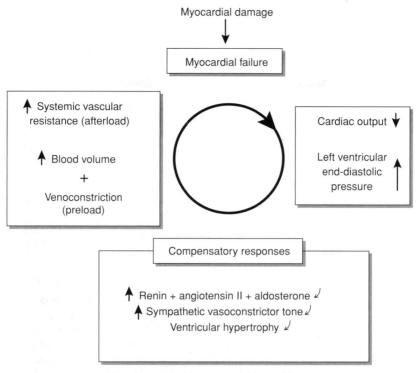

Figure 21–1 Vicious circle of heart failure.

activating the compensatory systems is a worsening of the HF. This is often referred to as the *vicious cycle of HF* (Fig. 21-1). Without therapeutic intervention, some of the compensatory mechanisms continue to be activated, ultimately resulting in a reduced cardiac output and a worsening of the patient's symptoms. An understanding of the compensatory mechanisms makes it clear why one goal in treating HF is to interrupt this vicious cycle and why various drugs are used in managing patients with HF.

DIAGNOSTIC CRITERIA

The signs and symptoms of HF are useful in diagnosing and assessing a patient's clinical response to therapy. The clinical manifestations of HF are in part due to pulmonary or systemic venous congestion and edema. When the left ventricle malfunctions, congestion initially occurs proximally in the lungs. When the right ventricle functions inadequately, congestion in the supplying systemic venous circulation results in peripheral edema, liver congestion, and other indicators of right HF (Box 21-1). Both pulmonary and systemic congestion eventually develop in most patients with left HF. In fact, the chief cause of right HF is left HF (Covinsky & Willett, 1999).

Depressed ventricular function may be confirmed by echocardiography, radionuclide ventriculography, or cardiac catheterization. Abnormalities in the electrocardiogram (ECG) are common and include dysrhythmias, conduction delays, left ventricular (LV) hypertrophy and nonspecific ST-T changes, which typically reflect the underlying etiology. Laboratory findings from liver function or other tests disclose such abnormalities as elevated blood urea nitrogen (BUN) and creatinine levels, hyponatremia, and elevated

serum enzymes of hepatic origin. The circumstances in which the symptoms of HF occur are also particularly important in determining the severity of disease in a particular patient.

BOX 21–1. CLINICAL MANIFESTATIONS OF HEART FAILURE

Left Ventricular Failure–Pulmonary Congestion
Symptoms: Cough, dyspnea, dyspnea on exertion, orthopnea, paroxysmal nocturnal dyspnea, nocturia
Signs: Cardiomegaly, S_3 heart sound, bibasilar rales, signs of pulmonary edema, tachycardia, increased respiratory rate
Right Ventricular Failure–Systemic Congestion
Symptoms: Peripheral pitting edema, abdominal pain, anorexia, bloating, constipation, nausea, vomiting
Signs: Hepatomegaly, distention of the jugular veins, hepatojugular reflex, signs of portal hypertension, ascites, splenomegaly

Decreased Cardiac Output
Peripheral cyanosis, fatigue, decreased tissue perfusion, decrease in metabolism and renal elimination of drugs, decreased appetite, angina, increased risk for thromboembolism

Table 21.1

New York Heart Association Functional Classification for Heart Failure

Class	Definition
I	No limitation of physical activity. Ordinary physical activity does not cause undue fatigue or dyspnea.
II	Slight limitation of physical activity. Comfortable at rest, but ordinary physical activity results in fatigue or dyspnea.
III	Marked limitation of physical activity. Comfortable at rest, but less than ordinary activity causes fatigue or dyspnea.
IV	Unable to carry on any physical activity without symptoms. Symptoms are present even at rest. If any physical activity is undertaken, symptoms are increased.

The New York Heart Association (NYHA) classifies the functional incapacity of patients with cardiac disease into four levels depending on the degree of effort needed to elicit symptoms (Table 21-1):

- *Class I*: Patients may have symptoms of HF only at levels that would produce symptoms in normal people.
- *Class II*: Patients may have symptoms of HF on ordinary exertion.
- *Class III*: Patients may have symptoms of HF on less than ordinary exertion.
- *Class IV*: Patients may have symptoms of HF at rest.

INITIATING DRUG THERAPY

In the past, digitalis, glycosides, and diuretics were the mainstays of therapy for HF. However, the concept of HF has changed dramatically from a narrow focus on the weakened heart to a broadened view of the systemic pathophysiologic state, with peripheral as well as myocardial factors playing important roles. The goals of therapy are to improve the quality of life, decrease mortality, and reduce the compensatory mechanisms causing the symptoms. Three general approaches are used:

1. An underlying cause of HF is treated if possible (eg, surgical correction of structural abnormalities or medical treatment of conditions such as infective endocarditis or hypertension).
2. Precipitating factors that produce or worsen HF are identified and minimized (eg, fever, anemia, arrhythmias, medication noncompliance, or drugs).
3. After these two steps, drug therapy to control the HF and improve survival becomes important.

Nonpharmacologic management techniques should be used along with pharmacologic therapy in patients with HF. In the past, reduced activities and bed rest were considered a standard part of the care of patients with HF. However, it has been determined that even short periods of bed rest result in reduced exercise tolerance and aerobic capacity. There is insufficient evidence to recommend a specific type of training program or the routine use of supervised rehabilitation programs. Although most patients should not participate in heavy labor or exhausting sports, aerobic activity

should be encouraged (except during periods of acute decompensation). For example, according to the Agency for Health Care Policy and Research (AHCPR), regular exercise (eg, walking or cycling) is recommended for patients with stable class I to III disease.

Goals of Drug Therapy

Pharmacologic management of patients with HF is critical in reducing symptoms and decreasing mortality. In most cases, drug therapy is long term and consists of ACE inhibitors, diuretics, digoxin (Lanoxin), beta blockers, and others. Table 21-2 gives an overview of drugs used to treat HF.

Angiotensin-Converting Enzyme Inhibitors

Patients who have HF resulting from LV systolic dysfunction and who have an LV ejection fraction less than 35% to 40% should be given a trial of ACE inhibitors, unless they cannot tolerate treatment with these drugs. The ACE inhibitors may be considered sole therapy in the subset of patients who present with fatigue or mild dyspnea on exertion and who do not have any other signs or symptoms of volume overload. In patients with evidence for, or a prior history of, fluid retention, ACE inhibitors are usually used together with diuretics (see section on Selecting the Most Appropriate Agent). ACE inhibitors are also recommended for use in patients with LV systolic dysfunction who have no symptoms of HF (Packer & Cohn, 1999). The clinical and mortality benefits of the ACE inhibitors have been shown in numerous uncontrolled and controlled, randomized clinical trials.

ACE inhibitors have a positive effect on cardiac function (ie, reduced preload and afterload, increased cardiac index, and ejection fraction) and the signs and symptoms of HF (eg, dyspnea, fatigue, orthopnea, and peripheral edema). As a result, exercise capacity is increased, NYHA functional classification is significantly improved, and morbidity and mortality rates in patients with HF, including those who have suffered an MI, is reduced because these drugs can attenuate ventricular dilation and remodeling.

Captopril (Capoten), enalapril (Vasotec), fosinopril (Monopril), lisinopril (Zestril), quinapril (Accupril), and Ramipril (Altace) are the ACE inhibitors currently indicated for treating HF (see Table 21-2). The ACE inhibitors that are approved for use in patients with LV dysfunction, and have been shown to prolong survival, are enalapril, captopril, and lisinopril. Quinapril and fosinopril are labeled for symptom reduction in HF, but data are lacking as to their effect on mortality rates.

Mechanism of Action

"Balanced" vasodilators, including the ACE inhibitors and angiotensin II receptor blockers, cause vasodilation on both the venous and arterial sides of the heart and therefore provide the hemodynamic and clinical benefits of both preload and afterload reduction.

Activation of the RAAS is an important compensatory mechanism in HF (Fig. 21-2). ACE catalyzes the conversion of angiotensin I to angiotensin II, a potent vasoconstrictor

Table 21.2

Overview of Selected Agents Used to Treat Heart Failure

Generic (Trade) Name and Dosage	Selected Adverse Events	Contraindications	Special Considerations
Selected Angiotensin-Converting Enzyme Inhibitors			
captopril (Capoten) Start: 6.25 mg or 12.5 mg tid Therapeutic range: 25–100 mg tid	Common: cough; hypotension, particularly with a diuretic or volume depletion; hyperkalemia, loss of taste, leukopenia; angioedema, neutropenia, and agranulocytosis in <1% of patients; rash in >10% of patients	Contraindicated in pregnancy Avoid in patients with bilateral renal artery stenosis or unilateral stenosis.	Renal impairment related to ACE inhibitors is seen as an increase in serum creatinine and azotemia, usually in the beginning of therapy. Monitor BUN, creatinine, and K levels when starting.
enalapril (Vasotec) Start: 2.5 mg qd or bid Range: 5–20 mg qd or bid daily	Same as above	Same as above	Same as above Use only 2.5 mg/d in patient with impaired renal function or hyponatremia.
fosinopril (Monopril) Start: 10 mg qd Range: 10–40 mg qd	Same as above	Same as above	Same as above Use only 5 mg/d in patient with impaired renal function or hyponatremia.
lisinopril (Zestril, Prinivil) Start: 5 mg qd Range: 5–20 mg qd	Same as above	Same as above	Same as above Use only 2.5 mg/d in patient with impaired renal function or hyponatremia.
quinapril (Accupril) Start: 5 mg bid Range: 20–40 bid	Same as above	Same as above	Same as above Use only 2.5 mg/d in patient with impaired renal function or hyponatremia.
ramipril (Altace) Start: 1.25 mg twice daily Range: 1.25–5 mg twice daily	Same as above	Same as above	Same as above
Selected Thiazide and Thiazide-like Diuretics			
chlorthalidone (Hygroton) 12.5–50 mg qd	Hyperuricemia, hypokalemia, hypomagnesemia, hyperglycemia, hyponatremia, hypercalcemia, hypercholesterolemia, hypertriglyceridemia, pancreatitis, rashes and other allergic reactions	High doses are relatively contraindicated in patients with hyperlipidemia, gout, and diabetes.	Thiazide diuretics preferred in patients with CrCl >30 mL/min
hydrochlorothiazide (HydroDIURIL, Microzide) 12.5–50 mg qd	Same as chlorthalidone	Same as chlorthalidone	Same as chlorthalidone
metolazone (Zaroxolyn) 2.5–10 mg qd	Less or no hypercholesterolemia	Same as chlorthalidone	Same as chlorthalidone
Loop Diuretics			
bumetanide (Bumex) 0.5–5 mg qd–bid	Dehydration, circulatory collapse, hypokalemia, hyponatremia, hypomagnesemia, hyperglycemia, metabolic alkalosis, hyperuricemia (short duration of action, no hypercalcemia)	High doses are relatively contraindicated in patients with hyperlipidemia, gout, and diabetes.	Effective in patients with CrCl <30 mL/min Monitor BUN, creatinine, and K levels when starting and with dosage changes.
ethacrynic acid (Edecrin) 25–100 mg bid–tid	Same as bumetanide (only nonsulfonamide diuretic, ototoxicity)	Same as bumetanide	Same as bumetanide
furosemide (Lasix) 20–320 mg bid–tid	Same as bumetanide	Same as bumetanide	Same as bumetanide
torsemide (Demadex) 5–20 mg qd–bid	Short duration of action, no hypercalcemia	Same as bumetanide	Same as bumetanide
Potassium-Sparing Diuretics			
amiloride (Midamor) 5–20 mg qd–bid	Hyperkalemia, GI disturbances, rash	High doses are relatively contraindicated in patients with hyperlipidemia, gout, and diabetes.	Same as bumetanide
spironolactone (Aldactone) 12.5–100 mg qd–bid	Hyperkalemia, GI disturbances, rash, gynecomastia	Same as amiloride	Spironolactone ideal in patients with heart failure
triamterene (Dyrenium) 50–150 mg qd–bid	Hyperkalemia, GI disturbances, nephrolithiasis	Same as amiloride	Same as bumetanide
Other Agents			
digitalis/digoxin (Lanoxin) 0.25 mg qd	Ventricular tachycardia, paroxysmal atrial tachycardia, fatigue, anorexia, nausea	Allergy, ventricular tachycardia, ventriular fibrillation, heart block, sick sinus syndrome, idiopathic hypertrophic subaortic stenosis, acute MI, renal insufficiency, electrolyte abnormalities	Check potassium levels before starting. Check serum levels once a year.

(continued)

Table 21.2

Overview of Selected Agents Used to Treat Heart Failure (*Continued*)

Generic (Trade) Name and Dosage	Selected Adverse Events	Contraindications	Special Considerations
isosorbide dinitrate (ISDN) (Isordil) 10–40 mg tid	Headache, dizziness, tachycardia, retrosternal discomfort, blurred vision, rash, flushing	Use with caution in pregnancy and lactation. Hypersensitivity to nitrates, closed-angle glaucoma, early MI, head trauma, pregnancy (category C)	Advise patient to avoid rapid changes in position.
hydralazine (Apresoline) 25–75 mg tid	Postural hypotension, tachycardia	Coronary artery disease, aortic stenosis	Advise patient to avoid rapid changes in position. Patient can be started on 10 mg tid if elderly, with severe heart failure, or hypotensive.
Beta-blockers carvedilol (Coreg) 3.125–50 mg bid	Bradycardia, congestive heart failure, atrioventricular block, postural hypotension, vertigo, fatigue, depression, bronchospasm, impotence, insomnia, decreased exercise tolerance, impaired peripheral circulation, generalized edema, sinusitis	Sinus bradycardia, second- or third-degree heart block, asthma, liver abnormalities	Advise patient to avoid abrupt cessation of therapy. Observe for signs of dizziness for 1 h when dose is increased.
metoprolol Start: 6.25 mg 2–3 times daily Range: 50–100 mg 2–3 times daily	Same as above	Same as above	Same as above
bisoprolol (ZeBeta) Start: 5 mg daily Range: 5–20 mg daily	Same as above	Same as above	Same as above
Selected Angiotensin Receptor Blockers (ARBs) losartan (Cozaar) Start: 12.5 mg/day Range: 50–100 mg/day	Dyspnea, hypotension, hyperkalemia	Angioedema secondary to ACE inhibition	May be used in patients experiencing cough due to ACE inhibitor
valsartan (Diovan) Start: 80 mg/day Range: 80–160 mg twice daily	Same as above	Same as above	Same as above
Other Agents dobutamine (Dobutrex) 2–5 mcg/kg/min intravenously	Elevated blood pressure, increased heart rate, angina, hypotension	Idiopathic hypertrophic subaortic stenosis	May increase insulin requirements

and stimulant of aldosterone secretion. ACE inhibitors are uniquely effective in managing HF by interrupting stimulation of the RAAS, inhibiting the contributions of this system to the downward spiral of HF. The pharmacodynamic properties of ACE inhibitors involve specific competitive binding to the active site of ACE.

Angiotensin II interacts with at least two known membrane receptors, type 1 and type 2 (AT$_1$ and AT$_2$). By blocking formation of angiotensin II, ACE inhibitors indirectly produce vasodilation and a decrease in systemic vascular resistance (LV afterload). In addition, because angiotensin II stimulates aldosterone secretion by the adrenal cortex and provides negative feedback for plasma renin, inhibition of angiotensin II may lead to decreased aldosterone and increased renin activity. This prevents aldosterone-mediated sodium and water retention and may produce a small increase in serum potassium levels. The reduction in volume expansion due to ACE inhibition decreases ventricular end-diastolic volume (ie, preload). Because ACE (kininase II) is involved in the breakdown of bradykinin, a vasodilator, a decrease in kininase II activity by an ACE inhibitor could increase bradykinin as well as prostaglandin production, either of which can lead to vasodilation (Borek et al., 1989).

ACE inhibitors produce vasodilation, inhibit fluid accumulation, and increase blood flow to vital organs, such as the brain, kidney, and heart, without precipitating reflex tachycardia. The hemodynamic effects of ACE inhibitors in

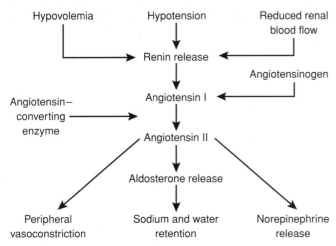

Figure 21–2 The renin–angiotensin–aldosterone (RAA) syndrome.

HF include decreased preload, afterload, and mean arterial pressure, as well as increased cardiac output. Ejection fraction is also improved. Clinical benefits to patients with HF include improvement in exercise duration, NYHA functional class, dyspnea/fatigue focal index, and signs and symptoms of HF, as well as increased survival.

Dosage

ACE inhibitors should be initiated at low doses followed by gradual dosage increases if the lower doses have been well tolerated. Renal function and serum potassium should be assessed within 1 to 2 weeks of starting therapy and periodically thereafter, especially in patients with pre-existing hypotension, hyponatremia, diabetes, or azotemia, or if they are receiving potassium supplementation. Doses should be titrated to the target doses shown in clinical trials to decrease morbidity and mortality (eg, at least 150 mg/day of captopril or at least 20 mg/day of enalapril or lisinopril). The doses of ACE inhibitors can be increased to these effective doses unless the patient cannot tolerate high doses. The practitioner should provide the following information to patients taking ACE inhibitors:

- Adverse effects may occur early in therapy but do not usually prevent long-term use of the drug.
- Symptomatic improvement may not be seen for several weeks or months.
- ACE inhibitors may reduce the risk of disease progression even if the patient's symptoms have not responded favorably to treatment (Packer & Cohn, 1999).

Captopril, lisinopril, ramipril (Altace), and trandolapril (Mavik) have been shown to reduce mortality rates in patients who have had an MI and who have HF symptoms. The indications for these ACE inhibitors in this population vary slightly and the dosing in patients after MI differs from the dosing for patients with chronic HF. Captopril is indicated to improve survival after MI in clinically stable patients with LV dysfunction manifested as an ejection fraction of 40% or less and to reduce the incidence of overt HF and subsequent hospitalizations for HF. Captopril may be initiated as early as 3 days after an MI with a single dose of 6.25 mg. If the patient tolerates this dose, he or she should receive 12.5 mg three times a day, increasing to 25 mg three times a day over the next several days. Over the next several weeks, the dose should be increased to a target of 50 mg three times a day. Other post-MI therapies (eg, thrombolytics, aspirin, and beta blockers) may be used concurrently.

Lisinopril has been shown to decrease mortality rates in both acute and post-MI patients. Lisinopril also is indicated for treating hemodynamically stable patients within 24 hours of an acute MI to improve survival. Patients should receive, as appropriate, the standard recommended treatments, such as thrombolytics, aspirin, and beta blockers. The first 5-mg dose of lisinopril may be given to hemodynamically stable patients within 24 hours of the onset of symptoms of acute MI, followed by 5 mg after 24 hours, 10 mg after 48 hours, and then 10 mg once daily. Dosing should be continued for 6 weeks. At that time, the patient should be assessed for signs and symptoms of HF and therapy should be continued if necessary. The dose should be decreased to 2.5 mg in patients with a low systolic blood pressure (below 120 mm Hg) when treatment is started, or during the first 3 days after the MI. If hypotension occurs (systolic blood pressure below 100 mm Hg), a daily maintenance dose of 5 mg may be given with temporary reductions to 2.5 mg if needed. If prolonged hypotension occurs (systolic blood pressure below 90 mm Hg for at least 1 hour), lisinopril therapy should be discontinued. Patients who develop symptoms of HF should receive the usual effective dose of lisinopril for HF, with a goal of 20 mg/day.

Ramipril has also been approved for stable patients who have shown clinical signs of HF within the first few days after an acute MI. It is used to decrease the risk of death (principally cardiovascular death) and to decrease the risks of failure-related hospitalization and progression to severe or resistant HF. The starting dose is 2.5 mg twice daily. A patient who becomes hypotensive at this dose may be switched to 1.25 mg twice daily, but all dosages should then be titrated, as tolerated, toward a target dose of 5 mg twice daily. In patients with a creatinine clearance less than 40 mL/minute/1.73 m^2 (serum creatinine level of less than 2.5 mg/dL), the dose should be decreased to 1.25 mg once daily. The dosage may be increased to 1.25 mg twice daily up to a maximum dose of 2.5 mg twice daily, depending on clinical response and tolerability.

Trandolapril also is approved for use in stable patients who have evidence of LV systolic dysfunction (identified by wall motion abnormalities) or who have symptoms of HF within the first few days after an acute MI. However, this drug is not used for chronic HF. In white patients, trandolapril decreases the risk of death (principally cardiovascular death) and of HF-related hospitalization (Kober et al., 1995), but data regarding outcomes in other patients are insufficient. The recommended starting dose is 1 mg once daily. Dosages should be titrated, as tolerated, toward a target dose of 4 mg/day. If the 4-mg dose is not tolerated, patients can continue therapy with the highest tolerated dose.

Contraindications

Patients should not receive an ACE inhibitor if they have experienced life-threatening adverse effects (eg, angioedema or anuric renal failure) during previous exposure, or if they are pregnant. Angioedema is a potentially fatal allergic reaction that may cause sudden difficulty in breathing, speaking, and swallowing accompanied by obvious swelling of the lips, face, and neck. Patients should receive an ACE inhibitor with caution if they have any of the following:

- Very low systemic blood pressure (systolic blood pressure less than 80 mm Hg)
- Markedly increased serum creatinine levels (above 3 mg/dL)
- Bilateral renal artery stenosis (previously considered a contraindication)
- Elevated serum potassium levels (above 5.5 mmol/L)

In addition, ACE inhibitors should not be given to hypotensive patients who are at immediate risk of cardiogenic shock and who require intravenous pressor support (eg, dobutamine [Dobutrex] or epinephrine [Adrenalin, others]). These patients should receive treatment for their pump failure first; then, once they are stabilized, the HF should be re-evaluated (Packer & Cohn, 1999).

When taken by pregnant women during the second and third trimesters, ACE inhibitors can cause injury and even death to the fetus. When pregnancy is detected, the ACE inhibitor should be discontinued immediately.

Adverse Events

The most common adverse reactions of ACE inhibitors are dizziness, headache, fatigue, diarrhea, cough, and hypotension. Angioedema of the face, extremities, lips, tongue, glottis, or larynx also has been reported in patients treated with ACE inhibitors. Angioedema associated with throat or laryngeal edema may be fatal because of airway blockage, which causes suffocation. Patients should be advised about this possible adverse effect and told to go to an emergency department immediately if they experience any of the symptoms suggesting angioedema.

Hypotension may occur with any of the ACE inhibitors and is usually observed after the first dose. It is more common in patients who are sodium or volume depleted, such as those treated vigorously with diuretics or those on dialysis, and in patients with severe HF. Hypotension can be minimized by starting with a very low dose, then increasing it slowly (usually every 3 to 7 days based on response) to the highest clinically effective level that does not produce hypotension. The diuretic dose may also need to be decreased or discontinued before starting the ACE inhibitor. Blood pressure should be followed closely after the first dose (until the blood pressure is stabilized), for the first 2 weeks of therapy, and whenever the dose of the ACE inhibitor or diuretic is increased. Hypotension, an anticipated problem among older patients with HF because of blunted baroreceptor reflexes, is no more common in the elderly than in other age groups.

Changes in renal function may occur in susceptible patients (ie, patients with hyponatremia; those taking high doses of diuretics; those with low cardiac output, diabetes mellitus, severe HF, or pre-existing renal impairment) because of inhibition of the RAAS. Patients with bilateral or unilateral renal artery stenosis should receive ACE inhibitors with extreme caution and should be monitored closely because renal failure may occur. The increases in serum creatinine and BUN that may occur are usually reversible by adjusting the dose of the ACE inhibitor, diuretic, or both. Furthermore, an increase in serum creatinine not exceeding 30% of the basal value is now being viewed as an indicator that the drug is working (ie, there is adequate ACE inhibition) and not that it has caused renal failure. However, the initial dose of an ACE inhibitor should be reduced with increasing severity of HF and the titration period should be monitored carefully. Age-related declines in renal function may slow the elimination of ACE inhibitors and thus increase the level and duration of their effects. Therefore, it may be necessary to reduce the initial dose of ACE inhibitors in the elderly or in patients with a serum creatinine level of 2.5 mg/dL or more. These patients may not tolerate as high a dose as other patients with HF, but should be titrated to the highest possible dose.

Diuretic-induced potassium loss (hypokalemia) may be reduced when an ACE inhibitor is used in combination with a diuretic. However, hyperkalemia may occur in patients with renal impairment or in those receiving a potassium-sparing diuretic, a potassium supplement, or potassium-containing salt substitutes. ACE inhibitors should be administered cautiously if hypokalemia exits. Frequent monitoring of serum potassium levels should be performed.

A cough is a common adverse event associated with ACE inhibitor therapy, occurring in 5% to 15% of patients. It is thought to be due to increased production of bradykinins or substance P, both of which lower the cough reflex. The cough is described as an annoying, ticklish, dry cough that is reversible on discontinuation of the ACE inhibitor. In patients with HF, cough is rarely severe enough to require discontinuation of therapy. Patients who experience cough should be questioned to determine whether this symptom is due to the ACE inhibitor or to pulmonary edema. The ACE inhibitor should be implicated only after other causes have been excluded. The cough severity may be lessened with the use of inhaled cromolyn (Intal), although this does add another medication to an already complicated regimen. In most cases, the patient and family can be advised that if the cough is bothersome but not intolerable, the benefits of ACE inhibitor therapy outweigh this adverse effect. However, if the cough is persistent and troublesome, the clinician can suggest withdrawing the ACE inhibitor and trying alternative medications (eg, an AT_1 receptor antagonist or a combination of hydralazine and isosorbide dinitrate [HYD/ISDN]).

Because HF is common among the elderly and increases in prevalence with age, safety and efficacy in this population is important. When ACE inhibitors first became available, many experts believed that because elderly patients tend to have low plasma renin activity, these agents would be relatively ineffective. Furthermore, the physiologic consequences of aging may alter the absorption, distribution, and elimination of drugs, as well as the sensitivity of the patient to drugs. Thus, it was recognized that safety and efficacy studies should be conducted in this important patient population. A number of studies have been completed, and they document that ACE inhibitors are well tolerated and effective for elderly patients with HF. Studies have not yet identified differences in response between the elderly and younger patients. However, greater sensitivity of some older patients cannot be ruled out. Older patients receiving ACE inhibitors do not experience more adverse effects than younger patients (Giles, 1990; SOLVD Investigators, 1991, 1992).

Interactions

The ACE inhibitors have been associated with very few significant drug–drug interactions. One or all of the ACE inhibitors have been used in combination with digoxin, methyldopa (Aldomet), prazosin (Minipress), hydralazine, beta blockers, nitrates, and calcium channel blockers. The drug interactions that should be kept in mind are listed in Table 21-3.

Diuretics

During initial evaluation, the clinician should determine whether the patient manifests symptoms (eg, orthopnea, paroxysmal nocturnal dyspnea, or dyspnea on exertion) or signs (eg, pulmonary rales, a third heart sound, or jugular venous distention) of volume overload. Patients with HF and significant volume overload should be started immediately on a diuretic in conjunction with an ACE inhibitor and a beta blocker (see Table 21-2).

Table 21.3

Drug Interactions Associated With the Angiotensin-Converting Enzyme Inhibitors

Interacting Agent	Potential Effect
antacids	Decrease the bioavailability of captopril; therefore, separate administration times by 2 h
aspirin	Decreases hemodynamic response of ACE inhibitor
capsaicin	Triggers or exacerbates the coughing that is associated with ACE inhibitor treatment
lithium	In combination with ACE inhibitor, causes increased serum lithium levels and symptoms of lithium toxicity
nonsteroidal anti-inflammatory drugs	In combination with ACE inhibitor, promotes sodium and water retention and diminishes control of hypertension and heart failure
potassium supplements/ potassium-sparing diuretics/salt substitutes	In combination with ACE inhibitor, increases risk of hyperkalemia
rifampin	Reduces the pharmacologic effects of enalapril
tetracycline	In combination with quinapril, tetracycline undergoes decreased absorption (28% to 37%), possibly from the high magnesium content in quinapril.

Mechanism of Action

Diuretics cause an increase in sodium and water excretion by the kidney. Thiazide diuretics work at the distal tubule of the kidney. Loop diuretics exert their effect at the loop of Henle as well as the proximal and distal tubules. Thus, loop diuretics are more potent in inhibiting sodium, chloride, and water excretion. Diuretics decrease preload by reducing the volume overload. An immediate effect (extrarenal) is an increase in venous capacity, with resultant redistribution of venous blood away from the lungs toward the periphery, which results in a decrease in pulmonary capillary pressure.

Dosage

Therapy is commonly initiated with low doses of a diuretic (eg, furosemide [Lasix] 20 to 40 mg/day), and the dose is increased until urine output increases and weight decreases, usually by 0.5 to 1.0 kg daily. Increases in the dose of the diuretic may be required to sustain the loss of weight. The goal is to reduce symptoms as well as eliminate physical signs of fluid retention by restoring jugular venous pressures toward normal, by eliminating edema, or both (Packer & Cohn, 1999). Patients with persistent volume overload despite initial medical management may require one of the following:

- More aggressive administration of the current diuretic (eg, intravenous administration)
- A combination of diuretics (eg, loop diuretic and metolazone [Zaroxolyn])
- Short-term use of drugs that increase renal blood flow (eg, dopamine [Intropin])

Although patients are commonly prescribed a fixed dose of diuretic, the dose of these drugs should be adjusted ideally on a daily basis. This can be accomplished in most cases by having the patient record his or her weight daily and allowing the patient or an appropriately trained health professional to adjust the dosage if the weight increases or decreases beyond a specified range for that patient (Packer & Cohn, 1999). Thus, the most useful approach for practitioners to select the dose of, and monitor the response to, diuretic therapy is by measuring body weight, preferably on a daily basis. Practitioners should educate patients on the importance of weighing themselves and contacting a health care professional when weight increases or symptoms return. This may help to avoid hospitalization of the patient with HF.

Patients with pulmonary edema or with marked volume overload should be given an intravenous loop diuretic initially. Diuretics should then be titrated to achieve resolution or improvement of signs and symptoms of volume overload. There is no standard target dose. Excessive diuresis should be avoided before starting an ACE inhibitor. Volume depletion may lead to hypotension or renal insufficiency when ACE inhibitors are started (Konstam et al., 1994).

The ACTION HF recommendations addressed the use of spironolactone (Aldactone) to block the effects of aldosterone as another approach to inhibit one of the actions of the RAAS. In the Randomized Aldactone Evaluation Study (RALES) clinical trial, spironolactone was associated with a 27% reduction in mortality, a 36% decrease in the hospitalization rate for HF, and a 22% reduction in the combined risk of death or hospitalization for any reason. Therefore, low doses (25 to 50 mg/day) of spironolactone merit consideration in patients with recent or current NYHA class IV symptoms (Packer & Cohn, 1999; Pitt et al., 1999). The efficacy and safety of aldosterone antagonists in patients with mild or moderate HF remain unknown.

Adverse Events

Potassium depletion commonly occurs when patients are treated chronically with diuretics. However, ACE inhibitors decrease renal potassium losses and raise serum potassium levels, so many patients with HF who are treated with both agents may not have potassium depletion. Concomitant administration of ACE inhibitors alone or in combination with potassium-sparing agents (eg, spironolactone) can prevent electrolyte depletion in most patients with HF. Diuretics may also cause magnesium depletion, which often accompanies potassium depletion. If high doses of diuretics are used, magnesium levels should be followed and oral supplementation given when needed (Mg 1.5 mEq/L) (Konstam et al., 1994).

Interactions

The NSAIDs (including aspirin) may blunt the natriuretic effect of diuretics. Therefore, patients receiving daily therapy with NSAIDs may need an increase in the dose of the diuretic to compensate for fluid retention. Diuretics may decrease lithium clearance, which may raise lithium levels into the toxic range. Lithium levels should be monitored in patients receiving both drugs. Patients may be at an increased risk of ototoxicity when high doses of loop diuretics and other ototoxic drugs (eg, aminoglycosides) are used concomitantly.

Angiotensin II Type 1 Receptor Blockers (ARBs)

These antagonists were developed to offer the advantages of increased selectivity and specificity and to maintain blockade of the circulating and tissue RAAS at the AT_1 receptor level, without the adverse reactions associated with ACE inhibitors. AT_1 receptor antagonists do not block the degradation of vasoactive substances (eg, bradykinin, enkephalins, and substance P) and may not cause the adverse effects, such as cough, related to ACE inhibitor–induced bradykinin accumulation.

Of the five currently approved AT_1 receptor antagonists, losartan (Cozaar) has been the most extensively studied in patients with HF. Losartan lowers blood pressure, systemic vascular resistance, pulmonary capillary wedge pressure, and heart rate and raises the cardiac index. Dyspnea on exertion and HF exacerbation decrease with losartan. Compared with the ACE inhibitor enalapril, losartan shows no significant difference in terms of altered exercise capacity (6-minute walk test), clinical status (dyspnea–fatigue index), neurohumoral activation (norepinephrine, N-terminal atrial natriuretic factor), laboratory evaluation, or incidence of adverse effects. Comparisons with another ACE inhibitor, captopril, show that losartan has the same incidence of persistent renal dysfunction and no difference in the incidence of death or HF hospital admissions. However, losartan was associated with fewer hospital admissions for any reason and less all-cause mortality than captopril in one small clinical trial in elderly patients with HF (Pitt et al., 1997).

Further studies with other ACE inhibitors in various patient populations are needed to determine whether losartan reduces morbidity and mortality to a greater degree than the ACE inhibitors. The initial studies of losartan for treating HF seem promising. In addition, studies with other AT_1 receptor antagonists for HF are ongoing, and studies of the combination of AT_1 receptor antagonists and ACE inhibitors are also being conducted. However, the effect of AT_1 receptor antagonists on mortality rates is unknown. Because there is no persuasive evidence that AT_1 receptor antagonists are equivalent or superior to ACE inhibitors in treating HF, they should not be used for treating HF in patients who have no prior use of ACE inhibitors. In addition, they should not be substituted for ACE inhibitors in patients who tolerate ACE inhibitors without difficulty. It is reasonable to prescribe AT_1 receptor antagonists instead of ACE inhibitors only in patients who cannot tolerate ACE inhibitors because of angioedema or intractable cough.

Mechanism of Action

Angiotensin II receptor blockers (ARBs) block the physiologic effects of angiotensin II by inhibiting receptor stimulation. The currently marketed ARBs—candesartan (Atacand), eprosartan (Teveten), losartan (Cozaar), olmesartan (Benicar), telmisartan (Micardis), valsartan (Diovan), irbesartan (Avapro)—are FDA approved for the management of hypertension. These antagonists were developed to offer the advantages of increased selectivity and specificity and to maintain blockade of the circulating and tissue RAAS at the AT_1 receptor level, without the adverse reactions associated with ACE inhibitors. ARBs do not block the degradation of vasoactive substances (eg, bradykinin, enkephalins, and substance P) and may not cause the adverse effects, such as cough, related to ACE inhibitor–induced bradykinin accumulation.

When ARBs were introduced into practice, there was a theoretical consideration that reducing the production of angiotensin II with an ACE inhibitor and blocking the remaining angiotensin II with an ARB would be better than either therapy alone. However, the VAL-HeFT study showed that adding an ARB to ACE inhibitor therapy is not beneficial.

Dosage

The doses of these agents vary. Table 21-2 lists selected ARBs and their doses, but a more complete review of these agents can be found in Chapter 18. Regardless of which agent is selected, the practitioner should monitor the patient's renal function and blood pressure.

Adverse Events

ARB therapy may be associated with hypotension. This usually occurs with the first dose but may also occur during upward titration or when clinical status worsens. This situation is most common among patients with hyponatremia, hypovolemia, low baseline blood pressure, renal impairment, and high baseline levels of renin or aldosterone (SOLVD Investigators, 1991, 1992). Potentiation of the vasodilator effects of bradykinin and prostaglandins appears to contribute to this hypotension. Theoretically, AT_1 receptor antagonists, which do not interfere with the degradation of these peptides, should result in fewer episodes of first-dose hypotension (Lang et al., 1997). However, this beneficial effect remains to be proven in clinical trials. In addition, specific AT_1 receptor antagonists could block the deleterious effects of angiotensin II produced by non–ACE-dependent pathways that are not blocked by ACE inhibitors (Lang et al., 1997).

The most common adverse events with losartan include dyspnea, worsening of HF, hypotension, dizziness, cough, and upper respiratory tract infection (Dickstein et al., 1995; Lang et al., 1997). The AT_1 receptor antagonists appear as likely as the ACE inhibitors to produce hypotension, worsening renal function, and hyperkalemia. Also, like ACE inhibitors, these agents are contraindicated in pregnancy, especially during the second and third trimesters.

Beta Blockers

Historically, beta blockers have been contraindicated for treating HF. The negative inotropic effect, bradycardic effect, and peripheral constriction of the beta blockers can all exacerbate HF. However, observations from experimental studies and controlled clinical trials indicate that prolonged activation of the SNS can accelerate the progression of HF. The studies also determined that the risks of such progression can be substantially decreased through the use of pharmacologic agents that interfere with the actions of the SNS on the heart and peripheral blood vessels. Thus, the use of beta blockers is gaining acceptance as a treatment for HF.

The AHCPR clinical practice guideline states that beta blockers may improve functional status and natural history in patients with HF but should be considered experimental therapy at this time. For patients with HF and angina or hypertension, the practice guideline states that beta blockers should be given only under the care of practitioners experienced in prescribing these agents. However, the AHCPR clinical practice guideline was written before carvedilol (Coreg) was approved for treating HF. The new recommendations strongly advocate using beta blockers for treating patients with HF.

As stated previously, the recommendations state that all patients with stable NYHA class II to class IV HF due to LV systolic dysfunction should receive a beta blocker unless they have a contraindication to its use or have shown to be unable to tolerate treatment with the drug. Beta blockers should not be used in unstable patients or in acutely ill patients ("rescue" therapy), including those who are in the intensive care unit with refractory HF requiring intravenous support. There are clinical trials underway that will help define the role of beta blockers in such patients. Beta blockers are recommended to improve symptoms and clinical status and to decrease the risk of death and hospitalization in patients with mild to moderate (NYHA class II) or moderate to severe (NYHA class III) HF who have an LV ejection fraction of less than 35% to 40%. Beta blockers should be added to pre-existing treatment with diuretics and an ACE inhibitor, and may be used together with digitalis or vasodilators (Packer & Cohn, 1999).

Carvedilol, a nonselective beta-adrenergic receptor blocker with vasodilating action (through alpha-adrenergic blocking action) previously approved for the management of essential hypertension, has become the first beta blocker approved in the United States for treating HF. It is intended to reduce the progression of disease as evidenced by cardiovascular death, cardiovascular hospitalization, or the need to adjust other HF medications. Similarly, the extended-release formulation of metoprolol, metoprolol succinate, was shown to be superior to placebo in decreasing mortality in HF patients. There are no trials comparing this extended-release agent to the immediate-release version (metoprolol tartrate). However, most clinicians use either of these formulations interchangeably, depending on the cost and the patient's insurance coverage. Bisoprolol (Zebeta) is also a beta blocker used in the treatment of HF that decreases mortality.

Mechanism of Action

Catecholamines can cause peripheral vasoconstriction that can exacerbate loading conditions in the failing heart and may precipitate myocardial ischemia and ventricular arrhythmias. In addition, activation of the SNS can increase heart rate, which may adversely affect the relation between myocardial supply and demand and more importantly may exacerbate the abnormal force–frequency relation that exists in HF. In addition, catecholamines activate cellular pathways that can lead to the loss of myocardial cells by a process of programmed cell death (apoptosis), which has been implicated in the progression of HF.

In experimental models of HF, pharmacologic interference with the SNS can favorably alter the natural history of the disease, similar to the manner in which antagonism of the RAAS by ACE inhibitors can modify the course of HF. Extensive research implicating the target mechanism, increased adrenergic drive, as being unfavorable to the natural history of systolic dysfunction and the HF clinical syndrome has been done. This has led to the conclusion that the primary mechanism of action of beta blockers in chronic HF is to prevent and reverse adrenergically mediated intrinsic myocardial dysfunction and remodeling. This occurs through a time-dependent, biologic effect involving inhibition of beta-adrenergic mechanisms directly or indirectly responsible for the development of cellular contractile dysfunction and remodeling (Bristow, 1997). In addition, one of the beta blockers used in patients with HF, carvedilol, has direct antioxidant effects that may decrease the role played by apoptosis in the progression of HF (Bristow, 1993).

Studies have shown that carvedilol and metoprolol improve LV function, hemodynamic parameters, and various symptoms of HF. Carvedilol also improves submaximal exercise tolerance and NYHA classification (Krum et al., 1995; Metra et al., 1994). In multicenter clinical trials, carvedilol was associated with a highly significant 65% reduction in the risk of death versus placebo (all patients received conventional therapy in addition to carvedilol or placebo). This was due to a decrease in both death due to pump failure and sudden death (Packer & Cohn, 1999). In addition, carvedilol decreases the risk of hospitalization for cardiovascular causes and the combined risk of all-cause mortality and cardiovascular hospitalization.

Dosage

Adverse effects with carvedilol usually occur early in therapy and are more frequent and severe with higher doses. Because of this, the starting dose of carvedilol is 3.125 mg twice daily, and each dose titration should be done slowly over a 2-week period, doubling the dose each time. At initiation of each new dosage, the patient should be observed for 1 hour for signs of dizziness or lightheadedness. In addition, blood pressure should be monitored. The maximum recommended dosage is 25 mg twice daily in patients weighing less than 85 kg, and 50 mg twice daily in patients weighing 85 kg or greater. In addition, patients should be seen in the office during titration and evaluated for symptoms of worsening HF, vasodilation (ie, dizziness, lightheadedness, and symptomatic hypotension), or bradycardia to determine their tolerance for carvedilol. Treatment with metoprolol starts at 6.25 mg two or three times daily and the dose is titrated slowly up to a target of 100 mg two or three times daily.

Initiation of therapy with a beta blocker may produce fluid retention, which may be severe enough to cause pulmonary or peripheral congestion and worsening symptoms of HF. Increases in body weight may occur after 3 to 5 days of starting treatment and if untreated may lead to worsening symptoms within 1 to 2 weeks. For this reason, practitioners should ask patients to weigh themselves daily. The amount of weight gain then guides the practitioner in prescribing an increase in the diuretic dosage until the patient's weight is restored to pretreatment levels. The dose of carvedilol may also have to be decreased; occasionally, the drug must be temporarily discontinued.

Excessive vasodilation may occur with initiation of therapy. It is usually asymptomatic but may be accompanied by dizziness, lightheadedness, or blurred vision. Vasodilatory adverse effects are usually seen within 24 to 48 hours of the first dose or increments in dose but usually subside with repeated dosing without any change in the dose of carvedilol or other medications. The risk of hypotension may be minimized by taking the beta blocker, ACE inhibitor, or vasodilator (if used) at different times during the day. Practitioners can work with patients to develop a regimen that is convenient and minimizes adverse effects. The practitioner may need to reduce the dose of the ACE inhibitor or vasodilator if hypotension is excessive. If the patient's heart rate decreases to less than 50 beats per minute or second- or third-degree heart block occurs, the patient should contact the practitioner, who may then decrease the dose of the beta blocker. Practitioners should evaluate the patient's concomitant medications for drug interactions that also may decrease heart rate or cause heart block (eg, diltiazem or flecainide).

Contraindications

Beta blockers should not be used in patients with bronchospastic disease, symptomatic bradycardia, or advanced heart block (unless treated with a pacemaker). Patients should receive a beta blocker with caution if they have asymptomatic bradycardia (heart rate below 60 beats per minute). Despite concerns that beta blockade may mask some of the signs of hypoglycemia, patients with diabetes mellitus may be particularly likely to experience a reduction in morbidity and mortality with beta-blocker therapy.

Adverse Events

The adverse effect profile of beta blockers in patients with HF is consistent with the pharmacology of the drug and the health status of the patient. The most common adverse effects are dizziness, fatigue, and worsening of HF. Other adverse reactions that occur less frequently include bradycardia, hypotension, generalized edema, dependent edema, sinusitis, and bronchitis (Packer et al., 1996c). Rare cases of liver function abnormalities have been reported in patients receiving carvedilol, but no deaths due to these abnormalities have been reported. Mild hepatic injury related to carvedilol has been reversible and has occurred after short- and long-term therapy. Carvedilol should be discontinued if a patient has laboratory evidence of liver function abnormalities or jaundice.

Practitioners should advise patients receiving therapy with carvedilol or other beta blockers of the following:

- Adverse effects may occur early in therapy but usually do not prevent long-term use of the drug.
- Symptomatic improvement may not be seen for 2 to 3 months.
- Beta blockade may reduce the risk of disease progression even if the patient's symptoms have not responded favorably to treatment.

Digoxin

Digoxin can prevent clinical deterioration in patients with HF due to LV systolic dysfunction and can improve these patients' symptoms. However, it does not decrease the mortality rate. The latest large trial, the Digitalis Investigation Group (DIG) study, showed that survival was not changed by use of digoxin (0.125 to 0.5 mg) in NYHA class II and III patients with HF who were taking diuretics and ACE

inhibitors. However, digoxin significantly decreased the number of hospitalizations compared with placebo. This effect seemed to be more pronounced in patients with the lowest ejection fractions and the most enlarged hearts. However, digoxin increased the risk of non-HF causes of cardiac death from presumed arrhythmia or MI (Digitalis Investigation Group, 1997).

The AHCPR guidelines state that digoxin should be used in patients with severe HF and should be added to the medical regimen of patients with mild or moderate failure who remain symptomatic after optimal management with ACE inhibitors and diuretics. The ACTION HF organization recommends digoxin to improve the clinical status of patients with HF due to LV systolic dysfunction, and recommends that it should be used in conjunction with diuretics, an ACE inhibitor, and a beta blocker. In addition, digoxin is recommended in patients with HF who have rapid atrial fibrillation, even though beta blockers may be more effective in controlling the ventricular response during exercise (Packer & Cohn, 1999). If a patient is receiving digoxin but not an ACE inhibitor or a beta blocker, treatment with digoxin should not be withdrawn, but appropriate therapy with the neurohormonal antagonists should be instituted. Patients should not receive digoxin if they have significant sinus or atrioventricular (AV) block, unless the block has been treated with a permanent pacemaker. Digoxin should be used cautiously in patients receiving other drugs that can depress sinus or AV nodal function (eg, amiodarone or a beta blocker), although these patients usually tolerate digoxin without difficulty. In addition, digoxin is not indicated for the stabilization of patients with acutely decompensated HF (unless they have rapid atrial fibrillation). There are no data to recommend using digoxin in patients with asymptomatic LV dysfunction (NYHA class I).

Mechanism of Action

Digoxin produces a mild inotropic effect by inhibiting cell membrane sodium–potassium adenosine triphosphatase activity and thereby enhancing calcium entry into the cell. Calcium enhances contractile protein activity, allowing for a greater force and velocity of contraction.

Dosage

Loading doses of digoxin usually are not needed in patients with HF. The typical dosage of 0.25 mg daily may be initiated if there is no evidence of renal dysfunction. Patients who have reduced renal function, who have baseline conduction abnormality, or who are small or elderly should be started on 0.125 mg daily or lower and titrated to an adequate serum digoxin level. Levels of 0.9 to 1.2 mg/mL are considered therapeutic, but levels as high as 2.5 mg/mL may be tolerated. It is not clear whether the beneficial effects of digoxin are greater at higher serum levels. Although it has been suggested that serum levels may be used to guide the selection of an appropriate dose of digoxin, there is no evidence to support this approach (Packer & Cohn, 1999).

Steady state is reached in approximately 1 week in patients with normal renal function, although 2 to 3 weeks may be required in patients with renal impairment. When steady state is achieved, the patient should be evaluated for symptoms of toxicity. In addition, an ECG, serum digoxin level, serum electrolytes, BUN, and creatinine should be obtained. It is not clear whether regular serum digoxin monitoring is necessary, but levels should be checked once a year after a steady state is achieved. In addition, levels should be checked if HF status worsens, renal function deteriorates, signs of toxicity develop (eg, confusion, nausea, anorexia, visual disturbances, arrhythmias), or additional medications are added that could affect the digoxin level (Konstam et al., 1994).

Adverse Events

Signs of digoxin toxicity develop in approximately 20% of patients, and up to 18% of digoxin-toxic patients die from the arrhythmias that occur. Noncardiac symptoms are related to the central nervous system and gastrointestinal tract. Anorexia is often an early manifestation, with nausea and vomiting following. The central nervous system adverse effects include headache, fatigue, malaise, disorientation, confusion, delirium, seizures, and visual disturbances. The noncardiac symptoms do not always precede the cardiac symptoms. Cardiac toxicity manifested by arrhythmias can take the form of almost every known rhythm disturbance (eg, ectopic and re-entrant cardiac rhythms and heart block).

Digoxin should be discontinued (often with consideration of reinstitution at a lower dose after 2 to 3 days if the patient is benefiting from therapy) if any of the following is noted:

- Elevated digoxin level
- Substantial reduction in renal function
- Symptoms of toxicity
- Significant conduction abnormality (eg, symptomatic bradycardia due to second- or third-degree AV block or high-degree AV block in atrial fibrillation)
- An increase in ventricular arrhythmias (Konstam et al., 1994)

Practitioners should counsel patients about the potential adverse effects of digoxin. They also should stress the importance of taking digoxin exactly as it is prescribed to avoid toxicity or a subtherapeutic effect.

Interactions

The medications that most often cause an increase in digoxin levels are quinidine (Cardioquin, others), amiodarone, flecainide, propafenone (Rythmol), spironolactone, and verapamil. It may be necessary to decrease the dose of digoxin when treatment with these drugs is initiated (Packer & Cohn, 1999). Antibiotics may decrease gut flora and prevent bacterial inactivation of digoxin, and anticholinergic agents may decrease intestinal motility. Both of these drug classes also may increase digoxin levels. Antacids, cholestyramine (Questran), neomycin (Mycifradin Sulfate), and kaolin--pectin (Kaopectate) may inhibit the absorption of digoxin and decrease digoxin levels. Patients should be advised to take digoxin at least 2 hours before these medications. Diuretics can enhance digoxin toxicity by decreasing renal clearance of digoxin and by causing electrolyte changes, including hypokalemia, hypomagnesemia, and hypercal-cemia (thiazides). Before any new medications are added to a patient's regimen, the prescriber should determine whether the medication interacts with digoxin.

Hydralazine/Isosorbide Dinitrate

The HYD/ISDN combination of vasodilators is an appropriate alternative in patients with contraindications to or intolerance of ACE inhibitors (Konstam et al., 1994). The combination should not be used for treating HF in patients who have not tried ACE inhibitors, and should not be substituted for ACE inhibitors in patients who are tolerating ACE inhibitors without difficulty (Packer & Cohn, 1999). No studies have specifically addressed the use of HYD/ISDN for patients who cannot take or tolerate ACE inhibitors, and the FDA has not approved HYD/ISDN for use in patients with HF. Isosorbide mononitrate also is not approved for HF and has not been studied for treating HF. HYD/ISDN is not as beneficial as the ACE inhibitor enalapril in reducing mortality rates during the first 2 years of treatment. However, this combination has been shown to achieve an absolute reduction in mortality rates compared with placebo during the first 3 years of treatment. The combination increases exercise capacity as much as enalapril, but adverse effects are a significant problem.

Mechanism of Action

Vasodilators may be classified by their mechanism of action or their site of action (venodilators, arteriolar dilators, or "balanced" vasodilators). ISDN is a venodilator that redistributes blood volume to the venous side of the heart to the systemic circulation, away from the lungs, which decreases the ventricular blood volume (preload). Hydralazine, along with prazosin and minoxidil (Loniten), which are not used for treating HF, is an arteriolar dilator. Hydralazine decreases the resistance the heart encounters during contraction (afterload), which allows for increased stroke volume (volume of blood leaving the heart) and increased cardiac output. Balanced vasodilators, including the ACE inhibitors and angiotensin II receptor blockers, cause vasodilation on both the venous and arterial sides of the heart and therefore provide the hemodynamic and clinical benefits of both preload and afterload reduction (as discussed in other sections).

Dosage

Isosorbide dinitrate usually should be initiated at 10 mg three times a day and increased weekly to 40 mg three times a day as tolerated (up to 160 mg/day). Hydralazine should be initiated at 25 mg three times a day and increased weekly to 75 mg three or four times a day (up to 300 mg/day) (Konstam et al., 1994; Packer & Cohn, 1999). Patients with low blood pressure, severe HF, or advanced age can be started on 10 mg three times a day for both agents.

Adverse Events

Adverse events include reflex tachycardia, headache, flushing, nausea, dizziness, syncope, nitrate tolerance, and sodium and water retention. Nitrate tolerance can be avoided by providing a nitrate-free period of 10 to 14 hours.

Interactions

Other drugs that lower blood pressure, including diuretics, may cause additive hypotension, and blood pressure should be monitored.

Other Agents

Amiodarone

Amiodarone is approved in the United States for treating refractory life-threatening ventricular arrhythmias. Amiodarone has been studied in patients with HF with ventricular arrhythmias to assess whether it reduces mortality rates. Some studies demonstrated that low-dose amiodarone (300 mg/day) reduced mortality rates, whereas others found no improvement (Doval et al., 1994; Singh et al., 1995). A meta-analysis of 13 randomized, controlled trials of prophylactic amiodarone in patients with recent MI (8 trials) or HF (5 trials) found that amiodarone reduced the rate of arrhythmic/sudden death in high-risk patients with recent MI or HF (Amiodarone Trials Meta-Analysis Investigators, 1997).

The FDA has not approved amiodarone for treating HF. Further studies are needed to determine whether it is useful for routine prophylactic treatment of patients with ventricular arrhythmias and nonischemic HF. It may be beneficial in patients at high risk for arrhythmic/sudden death, patients with primary cardiomyopathy, or patients with both (Amiodarone Trials Meta-Analysis Investigators, 1997; Gheorghiade et al., 1998). The recommendations suggest that some class III antiarrhythmic agents (eg, amiodarone) do not appear to increase the risk of death in patients with chronic HF. Such drugs are preferred over class I agents when used for treating atrial fibrillation in patients with LV systolic dysfunction. Because of its known toxicity and equivocal evidence for efficacy, amiodarone is not recommended for general use to prevent death (or sudden death) in patients with HF already treated with drugs that reduce mortality rates (eg, ACE inhibitors or beta blockers).

Mechanism of Action

Amiodarone is classified as a Vaughn-Williams class III (potassium channel blocking) antiarrhythmic drug, but it also possesses class I (sodium blocking), class II (beta blocking), and class IV (calcium channel blocking) antiarrhythmic effects. It also has vasodilatory properties (Doval et al., 1994). The therapeutic benefit of amiodarone may be due to its beta-blocking effects and not to an antiarrhythmic effect.

Dosage

Before treatment with amiodarone starts, the practitioner should make sure the patient does not have hyperthyroidism or advanced liver disease. In addition, pulmonary function tests, chest radiography, ophthalmologic examination, and neurologic assessment are recommended before initiating therapy. The maintenance dosage should be 200 to 300 mg/day. High doses of amiodarone may cause initial cardiac decompensation with abnormal hemodynamics; therefore, use of high loading doses in patients with very severe forms of HF should be avoided (Gheorghiade et al., 1998).

Interactions

Amiodarone interacts with warfarin (Coumadin; increases the international normalized ratio) and digoxin (increases digoxin levels).

Calcium Channel Blockers

Because vasodilator therapy with ACE inhibitors or the HYD/ISDN combination reduces symptoms and improves survival in patients with HF, it was thought that the vasodilatory effects of calcium channel blockers would be beneficial also. However, early short-term and long-term studies with calcium channel blockers have shown that these agents may actually worsen HF and increase the risk of death in patients with advanced LV dysfunction. This effect, which was found with most of the calcium channel blockers, may be due to a baroreceptor-mediated catecholamine release that is seen with short-acting dihydropyridine agents or to the negative inotropic effects of some calcium channel blockers. Thus, health care practitioners were advised to avoid calcium channel blockers in patients with HF, even if the drugs would treat coexisting angina or hypertension (Gheorghiade et al., 1998; Konstam et al., 1994).

It was not clear whether longer-acting dihydropyridines or more vascular-selective calcium channel blockers would have the same effect when trials with amlodipine (Norvasc) and felodipine (Plendil) extended release (ER) were conducted. A trial using amlodipine found that patients with ischemic HF had no decrease in mortality or morbidity rates with the drug. Amlodipine was safe in patients with ischemic HF, did not increase the mortality rate, and decreased anginal symptoms. In contrast, among patients with nonischemic cardiomyopathy, amlodipine significantly reduced the combined risk of fatal and nonfatal events by 31% and decreased the risk of death by 46%. The possibility that amlodipine prolongs survival in patients with nonischemic dilated cardiomyopathy requires further study. The investigators concluded that amlodipine can be used with relative safety in patients with severe HF with concomitant hypertension or angina. This is an important finding because these diseases can be difficult to treat in patients with LV dysfunction.

Felodipine ER was also studied to evaluate whether a long-acting, vascular-selective calcium channel blocker would benefit patients with HF. Felodipine significantly reduced blood pressure and, at 3 months, increased the ejection fraction. Exercise tolerance, quality of life, and the need for hospitalization did not improve. During long-term follow-up, the favorable effects on ejection fraction did not persist, but felodipine prevented worsening of exercise tolerance and quality of life. Mortality and hospitalization rates were similar between the two groups. The researchers concluded that felodipine ER therapy was not associated with clear-cut short- or long-term clinical benefit or reduction in mortality rates, but that it can be used safely in patients with HF if used for another indication. In addition, it confirmed the results of the trial with amlodipine that long-acting dihydropyridine therapy did not cause an excess of cardiovascular events (Cohn et al., 1997b).

In addition, despite more recent study findings and FDA approval, the ACTION HF recommendations remain consistent with the AHCPR guidelines. They do not recommend using calcium channel blockers to treat HF because of the lack of evidence supporting efficacy and because large-scale trials of newer agents have not provided evidence that long-term treatment with these drugs can improve the symptoms of HF or prolong survival. Because of concerns about safety, most calcium channel blockers should be avoided in patients with HF, even when used to treat angina or hypertension. The possibility that amlodipine might have a favorable effect on survival in patients with a nonischemic cardiomyopathy requires further study before such a finding is applied to the care of patients with HF (Packer & Cohn, 1999).

Dosage

Amlodipine and felodipine ER should be prescribed for treating hypertension or angina at a dosage of 5 to 10 mg/day.

Adverse Events

The most common adverse effects with these drugs include hypotension, dizziness, flushing, headache, and edema. Patients should be monitored for hypotension and worsening of HF.

Selecting the Most Appropriate Agent

The revised AHCPR clinical practice guidelines changed the approach to the management of patients with HF. Instead of digoxin, an ACE inhibitor is now the drug of first choice. Table 21-4 and Figure 21-3 summarize therapeutic regimens.

First-Line Therapy

The ACE inhibitors are now considered the first-line choice for routine use in patients with HF. According to the clinical practice guidelines, patients with systolic dysfunction should receive a trial of an ACE inhibitor unless contraindications are present (see discussion of ACE inhibitors). The ACE inhibitors may be considered sole therapy in HF patients who have fatigue or mild dyspnea on exertion and who do not have any other signs or symptoms of volume overload. However, if these symptoms persist after the target dose of the ACE inhibitor is reached, a diuretic should be added (see Second-Line Therapy). Thus, ACE inhibitor therapy is appropriate for patients in NYHA class I as a means of preventing HF and in patients in NYHA class II to IV

with symptoms to decrease mortality rates (see discussion of ACE inhibitors). They may be used alone or in conjunction with other drugs, such as beta blockers, which some practitioners consider first-line therapy.

The AHCPR guidelines state that beta blockers should be used with caution, however, because these drugs have a negative inotropic effect. However, since the publication of the AHCPR clinical practice guidelines, a beta blocker with vasodilating action has been approved for treating HF (see discussion of beta blockers). Until the recent ACTION HF organization recommendations, there were no published guidelines to address the role of beta blockers in managing patients with HF (Packer & Cohn, 1999). These latest recommendations have elevated the use of beta blockers to initial therapy.

The recommendations state that all patients with stable NYHA class II or III HF due to LV systolic dysfunction should receive a beta blocker unless the drug is contraindicated or cannot be tolerated. Beta blockers should be used with diuretics and ACE inhibitors. Blockers should not be used in unstable patients or in acutely ill patients (rescue therapy), including those who are in the intensive care unit with refractory HF requiring intravenous support (Packer & Cohn, 1999). Studies of beta-blocker therapy in various types of patients with HF are continuing to define their role.

Second-Line Therapy

Diuretics are used to increase sodium and water excretion, correct volume overload (which manifests as dyspnea on exertion), and maintain sodium and water balance. Patients with HF and signs of significant volume overload should be started immediately on a diuretic in addition to an ACE inhibitor. Patients with mild HF or concomitant hypertension may be managed adequately on thiazide diuretics. However, a loop diuretic is preferred in most patients, particularly those with renal impairment or marked fluid retention. A potassium-sparing diuretic or potassium supplement should be used for patients with serum potassium concentrations less than 4.0 mEq/L. Patients with persistent volume overload despite initial medical management may require more aggressive administration of the current diuretic (eg, intravenous administration), more potent diuretics, or a combination of diuretics (eg, furosemide and metolazone, or furosemide and spironolactone) (Konstam et al., 1994; Packer & Cohn, 1999).

Table 21.4

Recommended Order of Treatment for Heart Failure

Order	Agents	Comments
First line	ACE inhibitor, beta blocker with or without a diuretic (depends on patient)	Monitor patient's response carefully.
Second line	ACE inhibitor, with a diuretic and digoxin	In patient with mild heart failure, use a potassium-sparing diuretic when serum potassium level is <4.0 mEq/L.
Third line	ACE inhibitor, beta blocker, diuretic, and digoxin	An angiotensin II receptor antagonist can be substituted if ACE inhibitor cannot be tolerated.

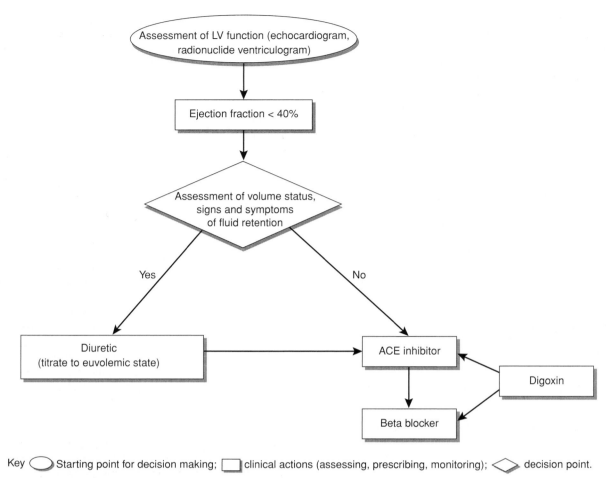

Key ⬭ Starting point for decision making; ▢ clinical actions (assessing, prescribing, monitoring); ◇ decision point.

Figure 21–3   Treatment algorithm for chronic heart failure. (Modified from Packer, M., & Cohn, J. N. [1999] on behalf of the steering Committee and Membership of the Advisory Council to Improve Outcomes Nationwide in Heart Failure. Consensus recommendations for the management of chronic heart failure. *American Journal of Cardiology, 83*[2A], 1A–38A.)

Third-Line Therapy

Although digitalis preparations have been used for more than 200 years in managing chronic HF, only recently has the FDA approved digoxin for use in patients with HF who are in sinus rhythm or atrial fibrillation (AHA, 1999).

The AHCPR clinical practice guidelines state that digoxin should be used in patients with severe HF and should be added to the medical regimen of patients with mild or moderate failure who remain symptomatic after optimal management with ACE inhibitors and diuretics. The ACTION HF recommendations state that digoxin is recommended to improve the clinical status of patients with HF due to LV systolic dysfunction and should be used with diuretics, an ACE inhibitor, and a beta blocker (Packer & Cohn, 1999). Both groups suggest that digoxin may be beneficial in patients with HF when there is a second indication for digoxin therapy (eg, a supraventricular arrhythmia for which digoxin is specifically indicated) (Konstam et al., 1994). However, there remains a question of whether the benefits of digoxin therapy outweigh its risks.

Fourth-Line Therapy

Fourth-line therapy consists of angiotensin II receptor antagonists (ARA), such as losartan, the HYD/ISDN com-

bination of vasodilators, or an aldosterone antagonist, such as spironolactone.

According to the AHCPR guidelines and the ACTION HF recommendations, the HYD/ISDN combination is an appropriate alternative in patients with contraindications to or intolerance of ACE inhibitors (Konstam et al., 1994; Packer & Cohn, 1999). There is little evidence to support using nitrates alone or hydralazine alone in treating HF (Packer & Cohn, 1999). The AHCPR guidelines note that nitrates and aspirin may be used to treat patients with both angina and HF (Konstam et al., 1994).

According to the Guideline Committee for the Heart Failure Society of America (2000), spironolactone at a low dosage of 12.5 to 25 mg once daily should be considered for patients who are receiving standard therapy and who have severe HF (with recent or current NYHA class IV standing) caused by LV systolic dysfunction. Patients should have a normal serum potassium level (5.0 mmol/L) and adequate renal function (serum creatinine 2.5 mg/dL).

Special Populations

Pediatric

Children with HF usually have maturational differences in contractile function or congenital structural or genetic heart dysfunction. Drug data for children with HF are not well established. In general, treatment for class I acute HF includes intravenous inotropes (excluding digoxin) and intravenous diuretics. For class II failure, digoxin may be added, and for class III oxygen may be administered. Drug therapy in children is highly individualized according to the child's condition and setting and is usually managed by a specialist in pediatric cardiology.

Geriatric

Because of age-related reductions in renal function, elderly patients may be particularly susceptible to drug-induced decreases in blood pressure, making careful monitoring essential not only at baseline but also when dosage or drug adjustments are instituted. Blood pressure, renal function, and potassium levels should be monitored regularly. Changes in renal function may also affect the elimination of digoxin, and patients should be monitored for digoxin toxicity and educated to recognize its signs and symptoms.

An important issue in drug therapy for elderly patients with HF is therapeutic compliance. In one study, investigators identified the primary reason for hospitalization of elderly patients with HF as noncompliance with diet and medication therapy; moreover, the investigators concluded that up to 40% of readmissions could be prevented by therapeutic compliance and appropriate discharge planning, follow-up, and adequate patient and caregiver education (SOLVD Investigators, 1991).

Women

In pregnant women, ACE inhibitor therapy may pose the risk of congenital birth defects. The same is true for angiotensin II receptor antagonist therapy.

MONITORING PATIENT RESPONSE

A careful history and a physical examination guide outcomes and direct therapy. The patient's symptoms and activities should be explored; any worsening suggests the need to adjust therapy. Although ECG exercise testing is not recommended, repeated testing may be ordered if the patient has a new heart murmur or a new MI, or suddenly deteriorates despite compliance with the medication regimen. Serum electrolyte levels, renal function, blood pressure, and diuretic use should be monitored regularly, particularly in patients taking ACE inhibitors. Within 2 weeks of initial ACE inhibitor therapy, serum potassium, creatinine, and BUN measurements should be repeated. If values are stable, monitoring can occur at 3-month intervals or within 1 week of a change in dosage of the ACE inhibitor or diuretic drug.

Response to initial ACE inhibitor therapy should be monitored by blood pressure measurements at 1 to 2 hours (captopril) and 4 to 6 hours for long-acting drugs (enalapril or lisinopril). Blood pressure and heart rate should be monitored for 1 hour after initiating carvedilol to assess tolerance to the drug; clinical re-evaluation should occur at each increase in dose and with any worsening of symptoms (increasing fatigue, decreased exercise tolerance, weight gain).

Patients taking spironolactone should have their serum potassium level measured after the first week of therapy, at regular intervals thereafter, and after any change in dose or concomitant medications that may affect potassium balance.

PATIENT EDUCATION

Practitioners must take an active role in patient education to enhance compliance and help prevent medication errors and adverse effects. Patients taking ACE inhibitors should take captopril and moexipril (Univasc) 1 hour before meals. They should also be advised of potential adverse effects, particularly the effects that signal a dangerous reaction: sore throat, fever, swelling of hands or feet, irregular heartbeat, chest pains, and signs of angioedema (swelling of the face, eyes, lips, or tongue; difficulty swallowing or breathing; hoarseness). If these occur, the patient should notify the health care professional at once.

Patients taking diuretics need to know that they can take the medication with food or milk to prevent gastrointestinal upset and they can schedule administration so that the need to urinate does not interrupt sleep. Because some diuretics cause photosensitivity, patients should use sunblock or avoid extensive exposure to sunlight. The practitioner can show the patient how to rise slowly from a lying or sitting position to avoid orthostatic hypotension.

Patients taking digoxin should understand that discontinuing the medication can be dangerous and that they should consult their health care provider before doing so. They should avoid taking over-the-counter medications, such as antacids, cold and allergy products, and diet drugs. Reportable signs and symptoms are loss of appetite, low stomach pain, nausea, vomiting, diarrhea, unusual fatigue or weakness, headache, blurred or yellow vision, rash or hives, or mental depression.

Women of childbearing age need to know that angiotensin II receptor antagonists should be avoided if pregnancy is a possibility. Patients taking spironolactone should know the signs and symptoms to report (muscle weakness or cramps and fatigue).

Nutrition/Lifestyle Changes

Dietary sodium intake should be limited to 2 or 3 g daily. Although a 2-g daily sodium intake is preferred, patient compliance may be poor because most patients find such a diet unpalatable. Patients with mild or moderate (NYHA class II or III) HF may tolerate 3 g daily. Alcohol decreases myocardial contractility, and therefore consumption of alcoholic beverages should be discouraged or limited to one drink (ie, a glass of beer or wine or a cocktail containing 1 ounce or less of alcohol) per day. Patients with HF should avoid excessive fluid intake, but fluid restriction is not advisable unless hyponatremia develops.

Patients should stop smoking because cigarettes cause cardiac injury. Some patients with HF experience severe limitation or repeated hospitalizations despite aggressive drug therapy. If revascularization (eg, bypass surgery or angioplasty) is unlikely to be beneficial, consideration should be given to cardiac transplantation (Konstam et al., 1994).

■ Case Study

I.W., age 62, is a white man who is new to your practice. He is reporting shortness of breath on exertion, especially after climbing steps or walking three to four blocks. His symptoms clear with rest. He also has difficulty sleeping at night (he tells you he needs two pillows to be comfortable).

He tells you that 2 years ago, he suddenly became short of breath after hurrying for an airplane. He was admitted to a hospital and treated for acute pulmonary edema. Three days before the episode of pulmonary edema, he had an upper respiratory tract infection with fever and mild cough. After the episode of pulmonary edema, his blood pressure has been consistently elevated. His previous physician started him on a sustained-release preparation of diltiazem 180 mg/day. His medical history includes moderate prostatic hypertrophy for 5 years, adult-onset diabetes mellitus for 10 years, hypertension for 10 years, and degenerative joint disease for 5 years. His medication history includes hydrochlorothiazide (HydroDIURIL) 50 mg/day, atenolol (Tenormin) 100 mg/day, controlled-delivery diltiazem 180 mg/day, glyburide (DiaBeta) 5 mg/day, and indomethacin (Indocin) 25 to 50 mg three times a day as needed for pain. While reviewing his medical records, you see that his last physical examination revealed a blood pressure of 160/95 mm Hg; a pulse of 95 bpm; a respiratory rate of 18; normal peripheral pulses; mild edema bilaterally in his feet; a prominent S3 and S4; neck vein distention; and an enlarged liver.

Diagnosis: Heart failure

1. List specific goals of treatment for I.W.

2. What drug(s) would you prescribe? Why?

3. What are the parameters for monitoring the success of your selected therapy?

4. Discuss specific patient education based on the prescribed therapy.

5. Describe one or two drug/drug or drug/food interactions for the selected agent(s).

6. List one or two adverse reactions for the selected agent(s) that would cause you to change therapy.

7. What would be the choice for the second-line therapy?

8. What over-the-counter or alternative medications would be appropriate for this patient?

9. What dietary and lifestyle changes should be recommended for I.W.?

Bibliography

Starred references are cited in the text.

Acute Infarction Ramipril Efficacy (AIRE) study investigators. (1993). Effect of ramipril on mortality and morbidity of survivors of acute myocardial infarction with clinical evidence of heart failure. *Lancet, 342,* 821–828.

Ahmed, A., & Dell'Italia, L. J. (2004). Use of beta-blockers in older adults with chronic heart failure. *American Journal of the Medical Sciences, 328*(2), 100–111.

*American Heart Association. (1999). *2000 Heart and stroke statistical update* (pp. 1–30). Dallas: American Heart Association.

American Society of Health-System Pharmacists. (1997). ASHP therapeutic guidelines on angiotensin-converting-enzyme inhibitors in patients with left ventricular dysfunction. *American Journal of Health-System Pharmacists, 54,* 299–313.

*Amiodarone Trials Meta-Analysis Investigators. (1997). Effect of prophylactic amiodarone on mortality after acute myocardial infarction and in congestive heart failure: meta-analysis of individual data from 6500 patients in randomized trials. *Lancet, 350,* 1417–1424.

Australia–New Zealand Heart Failure Research Collaborative Group. (1997). Randomised, placebo-controlled trial of carvedilol in patients with congestive heart failure due to ischaemic heart disease. *Lancet, 349,* 375–380.

*Borek, M., Charlap, S., & Frishman, W. H. (1989). Angiotensin-converting enzyme inhibitors in congestive heart failure. *Medical Clinics of North America, 73,* 315–338.

*Braunwald, E. (1988). Clinical manifestations of heart failure. In E. Braunwald (Ed.), *Heart disease* (pp. 471–484). Philadelphia: W. B. Saunders.

*Bristow, M. R. (1993). Pathophysiologic and pharmacologic rationales for clinical management of chronic heart failure with beta-blocking agents. *American Journal of Cardiology, 71,* 12C–22C.

*Bristow, M. R. (1997). Mechanisms of action of beta-blocking agents in heart failure. *American Journal of Cardiology, 80,* 26L–40L.

Bristow, M. R., Gilbert, E. M., Abraham, W. T., et al., for the MOCHA investigators. (1996). Carvedilol produces dose-related improvements in left ventricular function and survival in subjects with chronic heart failure. *Circulation, 94*, 2807–2816.

Brown, E. J., Chew, P. H., MacLean, A., et al. (1995). Effects of fosinopril on exercise tolerance and clinical deterioration in patients with chronic congestive heart failure not taking digitalis. *American Journal of Cardiology, 75*, 596–600.

Cohn, J. N., Fowler, M. B., Bristow, M. R., et al. (1997a). Safety and efficacy of carvedilol in severe heart failure. *Journal of Cardiac Failure, 3*, 173–199.

Cohn, J. N., Johnson, G., Ziesche, S., et al. (1986). Effect of vasodilator therapy on mortality in chronic congestive heart failure: result of a Veterans Administration Cooperative Study. *New England Journal of Medicine, 314*, 1547–1552.

Cohn, J. N., Johnson, G., Ziesche, S., et al. (1991). A comparison of enalapril with hydralazine-isosorbide dinitrate in the treatment of chronic HF. *New England Journal of Medicine, 325*, 303–310.

*Cohn, J. N., Ziesche, S., Smith, R., et al., for the Vasodilator-Heart Failure Trial (V-HeFT) Study Group. (1997b). Effect of the calcium antagonist felodipine as supplementary vasodilator therapy in patients with chronic heart failure treated with enalapril (V-HeFT III). *Circulation, 96*, 856–863.

Colucci, W. S., Packer, M., Bristow, M. R., et al. (1996). Carvedilol inhibits progression in patients with mild symptoms of heart failure. *Circulation, 94*, 2800–2806.

CONSENSUS Trial Study Group. (1987). Effects of enalapril on mortality in severe HF: results of the Cooperative North Scandinavian Enalapril Survival Study (CONSENSUS). *New England Journal of Medicine, 316*, 1429–1435.

*Covinsky, J. O., & Willett, M. S. (1999). Congestive heart failure. In J. T. DiPiro, R. L. Talbert, G. C. Yee, G. R. Matzke, B. G. Wells, & L. M. Posey (Eds.), *Pharmacotherapy: a pathophysiologic approach* (pp. 153–181). Stamford, CT: Appleton & Lange.

Crozier, I., Ikram, H., Awan, N., et al. (1995). Losartan in heart failure: hemodynamic effects and tolerability. *Circulation, 91*, 691–697.

*Dickstein, K., Chang, P., Willenheimer, R., et al. (1995). Comparison of the effects of losartan and enalapril on clinical status and exercise performance in patients with moderate or severe chronic heart failure. *Journal of the American College of Cardiology, 26*, 438–445.

*Digitalis Investigation Group. (1997). The effect of digoxin on mortality and morbidity in patients with heart failure. *New England Journal of Medicine, 336*, 525–533.

*Doval, H. C., Nul, D. R., Grancelli, H. O., et al. (1994). Randomized trial of low-dose amiodarone in severe congestive heart failure. *Lancet, 344*, 493–498.

*Franciosa, J. A., Wilen, M., Ziesche, S., et al. (1983). Survival in men with severe chronic left ventricular failure due to either coronary heart disease or idiopathic dilated cardiomyopathy. *American Journal of Cardiology, 51*, 831–836.

*Gheorghiade, M., Cody, R. J., Francis, G. S., McKenna, W. J., Young, J. B., & Bonow, R. O. (1998). Current medical therapy for advanced heart failure. *American Heart Journal, 135*, S2231–S248.

*Giles, T. D. (1990). Clinical experience with lisinopril in congestive heart failure. Focus on the older patient. *Drugs, 39*(Suppl. 2), 17–22.

Gottlieb, S. S., Dickstein, K., Fleck, E., et al. (1993). Hemodynamic and neurohormonal effects of the angiotensin II antagonist losartan in patients with congestive heart failure. *Circulation, 88*, 1602–1609.

Gruppo Italiano per lo Studio della Sopravvivenza nell'Infarto Miocardico (GISSI-3). (1994). GISSI-3: effects of lisinopril and transdermal glyceryl trinitrate singly and together on 6-week mortality and ventricular function after acute myocardial infarction. *Lancet, 343*, 1115–1122.

*Guideline Committee for the Heart Failure Society of America. (2000). HFSA guidelines for the management of patients with heart failure caused by left ventricular systolic dysfunction—pharmacologic approaches. *Journal of Cardiac Failure, 5*, 357–382.

Hargreaves, M. R., & Benson, M. K. (1995). Inhaled sodium cromoglycate in angiotensin-converting enzyme inhibitor cough. *Lancet, 345*, 13–16.

Hood, W. B., Jr., Dans, A. L., Guyatt, G. H., Jaeschke, R., & McMurray, J. J. (2004). Digitalis for treatment of congestive heart failure in patients in sinus rhythm. *Cochrane Database of Systematic Reviews*, (2), 002901.

Hunt, S. A., Baker, D. W., Chin, M. H., Cinquegrani, M. P., Feldman, A. M., & Francis, G. S., et al. (2002). ACC/AHA guidelines for the evaluation and management of chronic heart failure in the adult: executive summary. *Journal of Heart & Lung Transplantation, 21*(2), 189–203.

ISIS-4 (Fourth International Study of Infarct Survival) Collaborative Group. (1995). ISIS-4: a randomized factorial trial assessing early oral captopril, oral mononitrate, and intravenous magnesium sulphate in 58050 patients with suspected acute myocardial infarction. *Lancet, 345*, 669–685.

Johnston, C. I. (1995). Angiotensin receptor antagonists: focus on losartan. *Lancet, 346*, 1403–1407.

*Kober, L., Torp-Pedersen, C., Carlsen, J. E., Bagger, H., Eliasen, P., Lyngborg, K., et al. (1995). A clinical trial of the angiotensin-converting-enzyme inhibitor trandolapril in patients with left ventricular dysfunction after myocardial infarction. *New England Journal of Medicine, 333*, 1670–1676.

*Konstam, M., Dracup, K., Baker, D., et al. (1994). *Heart failure: evaluation and care of patients with left-ventricular systolic dysfunction.* Clinical practice guideline no. 11 (AHCPR Publication No. 94-0612). Rockville, MD: Agency for Health Care Policy and Research, Public Health Service, U. S. Department of Health and Human Services.

*Krum, H., Sackner-Bernstein, J. D., Goldsmith, R. L., et al. (1995). Double-blind, placebo-controlled study of the long-term efficacy of carvedilol in patients with severe heart failure. *Circulation, 92*, 1499–1506.

LacourciPre, Y., Brunner, H., Irwin, R., et al., for the Losartan Cough Study Group. (1994). Effects of modulators of the renin-angiotensin-aldosterone system on cough. *Journal of Hypertension, 12*, 1387–1393

*Lang, R. M., Elkayam, U., Yellen, L. G., et al., for the Losartan Pilot Exercise Study Investigators. (1997). Comparative effects of losartan and enalapril on exercise capacity and clinical status in patients with heart failure. *Journal of the American College of Cardiology, 30*, 983–991.

*Massie, B. M., & Shah, N. B. (1997). Evolving trends in the epidemiologic factors of heart failure: rationale for preventive strategies and comprehensive disease management. *American Heart Journal, 133*, 703–712.

*Metra, M., Nardi, M., Giubbini, R., et al. (1994). Effects of short- and long-term carvedilol administration on rest and exercise hemodynamic variables, exercise capacity, and clinical conditions in patients with idiopathic dilated cardiomyopathy. *Journal of the American College of Cardiology, 24*, 1678–1687.

*O'Connell, J. B., & Bristow, M. R. (1994). Economic impact of heart failure in the United States: time for a different approach. *Journal of Heart and Lung Transplantation, 13*, S107–S112.

Olsen, S. L., Gilbert, E. M., Renlund, D. G., et al. (1995). Carvedilol improves left ventricular function and symptoms in chronic heart failure: a double-blind randomized study. *Journal of the American College of Cardiology, 25*, 1225–1231.

Packer, M., Bristow, M.R., Cohn, J.N., et al., for the U.S. Carvedilol Heart Failure Study Group. (1996a). The effect of carvedilol on morbidity and mortality in patients with chronic heart failure. *New England Journal of Medicine, 334,* 1349–1355.

*Packer, M., Cohn, J.N., on behalf of the Steering Committee and Membership of the Advisory Council to Improve Outcomes Nationwide in Heart Failure. (1999). Consensus recommendations for the management of chronic heart failure. *American Journal of Cardiology, 83,* 1A–38A.

Packer, M., Colucci, W. S., Sackner-Bernstein, J.D., et al., for the PRECISE Study Group. (1996b). Double-blind, placebo-controlled study of the effects of carvedilol in patients with moderate to severe heart failure: the PRECISE Trial. *Circulation, 94,* 2793–2799.

*Packer, M., O'Connor, C. M., Ghali, J.K., et al., for the Prospective Randomized Amlodipine Survival Evaluation Study Group. (1996c). Effect of amlodipine on morbidity and mortality in severe chronic heart failure. *New England Journal of Medicine, 335,* 1107–1114.

Pfeffer, M. A., Braunwald, E., Moye, L. A., et al. (1992). Effect of captopril on mortality and morbidity in patients with left ventricular dysfunction after myocardial infarction: results of the Survival and Ventricular Enlargement Trial. *New England Journal of Medicine, 327,* 669–677.

*Pitt, B., Segal, R., Martinez, F. A., et al. (1997). Randomised trial of losartan versus captopril in patients over 65 with heart failure (Evaluation of Losartan in the Elderly Study, ELITE). *Lancet, 349,* 747–752.

*Pitt, B., Zannad, F., Remme, W. J., et al. (1999). The effect of spironolactone on morbidity and mortality in patients with severe heart failure. *New England Journal of Medicine, 341*(10), 709–717.

*Singh, S. N., Fletcher, R. D., Fischer, S. G., et al. (1995). Amiodarone in patients with congestive heart failure and symptomatic ventricular arrhythmias. *New England Journal of Medicine, 333,* 77–82.

Smith, T. W., Braunwald, E., & Kelly, R. A. (1988). The management of heart failure. In: E. Braunwald (Ed.), *Heart disease* (pp. 485–543). Philadelphia: W. B. Saunders.

*SOLVD Investigators. (1991). Effect of enalapril on survival in patients with reduced left ventricular ejection fractions and HF. *New England Journal of Medicine, 325,* 303–310.

*SOLVD Investigators. (1992). Effect of enalapril on mortality and the development of congestive heart failure in asymptomatic patients with reduced left ventricular ejection fractions. *New England Journal of Medicine, 327,* 685–691.

Williams, J. F., Bristow, M. R., Fowler, M. B., et al. (1995). Guidelines for the evaluation and management of heart failure: report of the American College of Cardiology/American Heart Association Task Force on Practice Guidelines (Committee on Evaluation and Management of Heart Failure). *Journal of the American College of Cardiology, 26,* 1376–1398.

Visit the Connection web site for the most up-to-date drug information.

22

DYSRHYTHMIAS

■ CYNTHIA SANOSKI, MARY BOWEN, AND ANDREW M. PETERSON

Dysrhythmia is any abnormal cardiac rhythm, including tachyarrhythmia (an increase in heart rate) and bradyarrhythmia (a decrease in heart rate). Dysrhythmias may be asymptomatic or symptomatic, causing palpitations, weakness, loss of consciousness, heart failure, and sudden death. Searching for a reversible cause of the dysrhythmia is the first step in patient care. However, in many cases, antiarrhythmic drugs are necessary to permit stabilization until the underlying condition is normalized. Many patients require chronic drug therapy for a dysrhythmia due to an underlying disease condition that makes them chronically susceptible to cardiac dysrhythmias that are associated with high morbidity and mortality rates.

CAUSES

Dysrhythmias may result from structural or electrical/conduction system changes in the heart, which may compromise cardiac function and output. Conditions that give rise to dysrhythmia include myocardial ischemia, chronic heart failure, hypertension, valvular heart disease, hypoxemia, hypercapnia, thyroid abnormalities, electrolyte disturbances, drug toxicity, excessive caffeine or ethanol ingestion, anxiety, and exercise. Some of these conditions are reversible, and some cause structural changes that are not reversible.

PATHOPHYSIOLOGY

Basic Electrophysiology

Electrically active myocardial cells (non–pacemaker-type cells) at rest maintain a potential difference between their intracellular fluid and the extracellular fluid. When excited, these cells manifest a characteristic sequence of transmembrane potential changes called the *action potential*. The resting membrane potential is 280 mV with respect to the extracellular fluid. The activity of the Na^+-K^+ pump and the permeability of the membrane to Na^+, K^+, and Ca^{2+} ions determine the membrane potential of a cardiac cell at any given time. Permeability is defined by the diffusion of ions across the membrane through various ion-selective channels. The phases of the action potential correspond to the excitation state of a myocardial cell (Box 22-1).

Dysrhythmias are considered to result from disorders of impulse formation, impulse conduction, or both. Several factors are believed to be involved in precipitating dysrhythmias. There may be a defect in the normal mechanism of spontaneous phase 4 depolarization, or an increased automaticity of pacemaker cells. In addition, ectopic pacemakers in normally quiescent tissue are responsible for dysrhythmias originating from disorders of impulse formation. Impulse conduction defects occur when the impulse is slowed or blocked because of functional unidirectional block, a change in conduction velocity, or a change in the refractory period. Furthermore, simultaneous abnormalities of impulse formation and conduction may occur.

Antiarrhythmic drugs are used to treat abnormal electrical activity of the heart. The drugs outlined in this chapter are used to treat, suppress, or prevent two major mechanisms of dysrhythmias—an abnormality in impulse formation (ie, increased automaticity) or an abnormality in impulse conduction (ie, reentry).

Automaticity

Automaticity refers to the ability of the cardiac cells to depolarize spontaneously. Three factors determine automaticity: maximum diastolic depolarization, the rate of depolarization, and the level of the threshold potential. Dysrhythmias resulting from abnormal automaticity include sinus bradycardia or tachycardia and irregular sinus rhythm. The sinoatrial (SA) node has the most rapid rate of depolarization during diastole and reaches threshold first. Cells of the atrioventricular (AV) node and His-Purkinje system have automaticity but a slower rate of phase 4 depolarization. The primary role of the SA node is as the pacemaker of the heart. The SA node is sensitive to alterations in autonomic nervous system output and in its biochemical surroundings. Catecholamine stimulation leads to shorter action potential duration and increases the spontaneous rate of depolarization. Vagal stimulus and endogenous purines such as adenosine (Adenocard) increase outward K^+ currents, thus inhibiting depolarization. Increased adrenergic innervation produces major changes in ionic current activity in the SA node.

Another mechanism for dysrhythmias due to abnormal impulse formation is intracellular calcium overload, called *after-depolarization*. If after-depolarizations reach threshold, a

BOX 22–1. PHASES OF THE ACTION POTENTIAL

- **Phase 0** is when rapid depolarization occurs due to the rapid influx of Na^+.
- **Phase 1** is a brief initial repolarization period. Inactivation of the inward Na^+ current and activation of the outward K^+ current cause this brief but rapid phase of repolarization.
- **Phase 2** is a plateau period during which there is little change in membrane potential. The outward K^+ current and the influx of Ca^{2+} through calcium channels typify the plateau period. The offsetting effect of these currents creates only a small net change in potential, thus creating a plateau.
- **Phase 3** is a period of repolarization that is characterized primarily by K^+ efflux.
- **Phase 4** is a gradual depolarization of the cell, with Na^+ gradually leaking into the intracellular space, balanced by decreasing efflux of K^+. As the cell is slowly depolarized during this phase, an increase in Na^+ permeability occurs, which again leads to phase zero.

BOX 22–2. CATEGORIES OF SUPRAVENTRICULAR, JUNCTIONAL, AND VENTRICULAR DYSRHYTHMIAS

Supraventricular Dysrhythmias
Sinus tachycardia
Paroxysmal supraventricular tachycardia (a site originating above or within the AV node and conducting to the His-Purkinje system) (eg, AV nodal reentrant tachycardia, AV reentrant tachycardia)
Sinus bradycardia
Atrial fibrillation
Atrial flutter
Atrial tachycardia
Premature atrial contractions
Wolff-Parkinson-White syndrome

Junctional Dysrhythmias
Nonparoxysmal AV junctional tachycardia (heart rate > 60 beats/min)
Junctional escape rhythm (heart rate 40–60 beats/min)
Premature AV junctional complexes
AV dissociation
First-degree heart block
Second-degree heart block (Mobitz type I [Wenckebach], Mobitz type II)
Third-degree (complete) heart block

Ventricular Dysrhythmias
Premature ventricular contractions
Ventricular tachycardia
Ventricular fibrillation
Torsades de pointes (a rapid form of polymorphic ventricular tachycardia associated with a long QT interval)

new action potential is generated and propagated in adjacent cells. After-depolarizations may occur in response to hypothermia, electrolyte imbalance, catecholamine excess, or stretch. Late after-depolarizations may also be of particular importance in some of the dysrhythmias due to digitalis intoxication.

Reentry

Reentry involves indefinite propagation of the impulse and continued activation of previously refractory tissue (Wit, Rosen, & Hoffman, 1974). Reentrant foci occur if there are two pathways for impulse conduction, an area of unidirectional block (prolonged refractoriness) in one of these pathways, and slow conduction in the other pathway. A refractory period occurs when the cell cannot be activated after having already fired. Excitability determines the strength of a stimulus required to initiate a new action potential at any given point during the action potential cycle.

Types of Dysrhythmias

Dysrhythmias evolve either above or below the ventricles and can be regular or irregular. *Supraventricular dysrhythmias* evolve above the ventricles in the atria, SA node, or AV node. These dysrhythmias may present with either tachycardia or bradycardia or with regularity or irregularity.

Atrioventricular nodal dysrhythmias originate at or within the AV node and are caused by delayed or absent SA node conduction to the AV node. Supraventricular and AV nodal dysrhythmias are not usually life-threatening; however, they may become troublesome and lead to reduced cardiac output related to decreased ventricular filling.

Ventricular dysrhythmias originate in the ventricles or the bundle of His. These types of dysrhythmias may be sympto-

matic, causing loss of consciousness or death. Therefore, dysrhythmias in this category require immediate intervention. Underlying clinical conditions that usually give rise to these dysrhythmias are myocardial ischemia/infarction, dilated and hypertrophic cardiomyopathies, electrolyte disorders, hypoxia, hyperthyroidism, valvular diseases, and drug toxicity. Box 22-2 lists dysrhythmias by category.

DIAGNOSTIC CRITERIA

The practitioner must first assess the patient through a thorough and sometimes urgent history and physical examination. There may be no symptoms, or the patient may report symptoms such as chest pain, shortness of breath, decreased level of consciousness, syncope, confusion, diaphoresis, weakness, and palpitations. The practitioner should ask when the symptoms started, how long they lasted, their frequency, and how the patient tolerated the symptoms.

It also is important to assess the patient's risk factors for development of dysrhythmias, such as previous coronary artery disease, myocardial infarction (MI), dilated or hypertrophic cardiomyopathy, hypertension, valvular heart disease, alcohol or drug abuse, or prescription drug use (eg, digoxin [Lanoxin], antiarrhythmics). The practitioner should focus the physical examination on heart rate, rhythm, and pattern; presence of extra beats or skipped beats; rate, rhythm, amplitude, and symmetry of peripheral pulses; response to exercise; and orthostatic hypotension.

Laboratory and diagnostic studies also are vital in diagnosing dysrhythmias. The practitioner should examine the electrocardiogram (ECG) for evidence of myocardial ischemia, calculation of the PR interval, QRS interval, and QT interval, presence of premature contractions, characteristics of Wolff-Parkinson-White (WPW) syndrome, presence or absence of atrial activity, and relationship between P waves and QRS complexes. In addition, long rhythm strips in leads II or V_1 help identify P waves, which aid in diagnosing the type of dysrhythmia. Continuous cardiac monitoring is needed for patients who have episodes of life-threatening dysrhythmias so that antiarrhythmic drugs can be administered as an immediate intervention.

A complete blood count, chemical profile (to assess electrolyte concentrations), thyroid profile, and digoxin laboratory tests should be performed as necessary to determine any underlying causes of the dysrhythmia. In addition, an echocardiogram should be performed to assess left ventricular function. If myocardial ischemia is suspected as a cause of the dysrhythmia, the patient should undergo further evaluation with cardiac stress testing and possibly even cardiac catheterization.

INITIATING DRUG THERAPY

The past two decades have seen the introduction of numerous agents to treat dysrhythmias, but there have been no "miracle cures" in terms of drug therapy. In fact, more recent studies disclose that many of these drugs are themselves pro-arrhythmic. Therefore, the decision to administer antiarrhythmic drugs must be based on whether the morbidity and mortality associated with the dysrhythmia outweigh the potential adverse events associated with the drugs.

Treatable conditions may cause the dysrhythmia. Identification of treatable causes before administering an antiarrhythmic agent is a priority. Conditions that may cause dysrhythmias are electrolyte imbalance, drug overdose, drug interactions with other medications or herbs, renal failure, thyroid disorders, metabolic acidosis, hypovolemia, MI, pulmonary embolism, cardiac tamponade, tension pneumothorax, dissecting aneurysm, hypoxemia, fever, and valvular or congenital defects in the heart.

Most antiarrhythmic drugs are used to treat tachyarrhythmias; atropine is the drug used to treat bradyarrhythmia. Antiarrhythmic management of these dysrhythmias is focused on relieving the acute episode of cardiac irregularity, establishing normal sinus rhythm, and preventing further attacks. Certain antiarrhythmic drugs are known to be more effective for one type of arrhythmia than another.

Nonpharmacologic therapies, such as radiofrequency (RF) catheter ablation and implantable cardioverter–defibrillators (ICDs), are also available to treat various dysrhythmias. ICDs are used to treat ventricular dysrhythmias, and their benefits have been demonstrated in several clinical trials (eg, Antiarrhythmics Versus Implantable Defibrillators [AVID] Investigators, 1997; Connolly et al, 2000; Kuck et al, 2000). RF catheter ablation permanently terminates the dysrhythmia by ablating the focal area where the dysrhythmia occurs. This procedure can be used for atrial fibrillation, atrial flutter, and symptomatic drug-refractory ventricular tachycardia (VT).

Goals of Drug Therapy

The overall goals of antiarrhythmic drug therapy are to relieve the acute episode of irregular rhythm, establish sinus rhythm, and prevent further attacks. This is usually achieved through modification of the ion fluxes described previously by blocking Na^+, K^+, or Ca^{2+} channels and beta-adrenergic receptors. Typical agents used to treat dysrhythmias include antiarrhythmics (classes I through IV), digoxin, adenosine, and atropine (Table 22-1).

Drug Classification

Antiarrhythmic drugs are organized into four classes, I (IA, IB, IC), II, III, and IV (Vaughan Williams, 1984). Although the Vaughan Williams classification system is the most widely used classification system for grouping antiarrhythmic agents based on their electrophysiologic actions, using this classification system requires some points of exception to be made. This system is somewhat incomplete, and it excludes such drugs as digoxin, adenosine, and atropine. In addition, the classification is not pure, and there is some overlapping of drugs into more than one category. For instance, amiodarone has electrophysiologic properties of all four Vaughan Williams classes. Furthermore, this system does not take into account that the active metabolites of antiarrhythmics may have different electrophysiologic effects than their parent drugs. For example, N-acetyl-procainamide (NAPA), the major active metabolite of procainamide, blocks outward K^+ channels and therefore can be considered a class III drug. Although procainamide blocks outward K^+ channels, it also primarily blocks inward Na^+ currents, thereby making it a class IA antiarrhythmic. Therefore, the overall electrophysiologic effect produced by procainamide depends upon the relative concentrations of procainamide and NAPA that are present in the body, which can vary based on several clinical factors. The Vaughan Williams classification scheme (Box 22-3) identifies drugs that block fast Na^+ channels (class IA, IB, and IC), those that are beta blockers (class II), those that block K^+ channels (class III), and those that are calcium channel blockers (class IV).

Class I Antiarrhythmic Drugs

This class of drugs, known as the sodium channel blockers, may be subdivided into classes IA, IB, and IC according to the rate of sodium channel dissociation. These agents vary in the rate at which they bind and then dissociate from the Na^+ channel receptor. Class IB antiarrhythmics bind to and dissociate from the Na^+ channel receptor quickly ("fast on-off"), while class IC antiarrhythmics slowly bind to and dissociate from this receptor ("slow on-off"). The binding kinetics of the class IA antiarrhythmics are intermediate between those of the class IB and IC agents. In addition, class I antiarrhythmics possess rate dependence, whereby Na^+ channel blockade is greatest at fast heart rates (ie, tachycardia) and least during slower heart rates (ie, bradycardia) (see Table 22–1).

Table 22.1

Overview of Selected Antiarrhythmic Agents

Generic (Trade) Name and Dosage	Selected Adverse Events	Contraindications	Special Considerations
acebutolol (Sectral) Adult: 200–600 mg PO bid	Hypotension, bradycardia, heart block, heart failure exacerbation, fatigue, bronchospasm, depression, decreased exercise tolerance, aggravated peripheral arterial insufficiency, masking of symptoms of and delayed recovery from hypoglycemia, Raynaud's phenomenon, insomnia, vivid dreams or hallucinations, impotence, increased serum triglyceride levels, decreased high-density lipoprotein levels	2nd or 3rd degree heart block or sick sinus syndrome in the absence of a pacemaker, LV systolic dysfunction Relatively contraindicated in asthma	Because sudden withdrawal can lead to exacerbation of angina and myocardial infarction, instruct patient not to discontinue drug abruptly. Teach patient how to take pulse and blood pressure, weigh self daily and report weight gain, and report any dyspnea on exertion or when lying down.
adenosine (Adenocard) Adult: 6 mg IV push over 1–2 sec; repeat with 12 mg IV push if sinus rhythm not obtained within 1–2 min after first dose; may repeat 12 mg dose a second time if no response in 1–2 min	Headache, chest pain, lightheadedness, dizziness, nausea, flushing, dyspnea, blurred vision	2nd or 3rd degree heart block or sick sinus syndrome in the absence of a pacemaker	Monitor ECG during administration. Use cautiously in patients with asthma as bronchoconstriction may occur. Instruct patient to report adverse reactions immediately or any discomfort at IV site. Each dose should be immediately followed with a 10-mL saline flush.
amiodarone (Cordarone) *Atrial Fibrillation* Adult IV: 5–7 mg/kg over 30–60 min, then 1,200–1,800 mg/d given via continuous infusion; convert to PO therapy when hemodynamically stable and able to take PO medications Adult PO: 800–1,200 mg/d in 2 or 3 divided doses for 1 week, until patient receives ~ 10 g total, then 200 mg PO daily *Pulseless VT/VF* Adult IV: 300 mg IV push, followed by 10–20 mL saline flush; may repeat with 150 mg IV push every 3–5 min, if necessary (followed by 10–20 mL saline flush); if stable rhythm achieved, can initiate continuous infusion at 1 mg/min for 6 h, then 0.5 mg/min (maximum dose = 2.2 g/24 h); convert to PO therapy when hemodynamically stable and able to take PO medications (see PO dose under Stable VT) *Stable VT* Adult IV: 150 mg (diluted in 100 mL of D5W or saline) over 10 min; may repeat dose every 10 min, if necessary for breakthrough VT; if stable rhythm achieved, can	IV: hypotension, phlebitis, bradycardia, heart block PO: corneal microdeposits, optic neuritis, nausea, vomiting, anorexia, pulmonary fibrosis, bradycardia, tremor, ataxia, paresthesias, insomnia, constipation, abnormal liver function tests, hypothyroidism, hyperthyroidism, blue-gray discoloration of skin, photosensitivity		Instruct patient to report adverse reactions immediately. Advise patient to apply sunscreen and to minimize areas of exposure to sun. Patients should have a chest x-ray and ophthalmologic exam performed on an annual basis. In addition, liver function and thyroid function tests shoud be performed every 6 months. Pulmonary function tests should be performed if the patient becomes symptomatic or if the chest x-ray is abnormal. All of these tests should also be performed at baseline when amiodarone is initiated.

Table 22.1

Overview of Selected Antiarrhythmic Agents (*Continued*)

Generic (Trade) Name and Dosage	Selected Adverse Events	Contraindications	Special Considerations
initiate continuous infusion at 1 mg/min for 6 hr, then 0.5 mg/min (maximum dose = 2.2 g/24 h); convert to PO therapy when hemodynamically stable and able to take PO medications Adult PO: 1,200–1,600 mg/d in 2 or 3 divided doses for 1 week, until patient receives ∼ 15 g total, then 300–400 mg PO daily			
atropine Adult: 0.5–1 mg IV every 3–5 min; not to exceed 2 mg total dose	Palpitations, tachycardia, dry mouth, dizziness	Acute angle-closure glaucoma, obstructive uropathy, tachycardia, obstructive disease of GI tract	Administer IV over 1 min. Monitor ECG during administration.
digoxin (Lanoxin) Adult LD (IV or PO): 0.25–0.5 mg over 2 min; may give 0.125–0.25 mg q6h for 2 more doses for a total dose of 1 mg or 10–15 μg/kg Adult MD: 0.125–0.25 mg IV or 0.125–0.5 mg PO daily in normal renal function	Anorexia, nausea, vomiting, diarrhea, headache, fatigue, dizziness, vertigo, visual disturbances (yellow-green halos), confusion, hallucinations, dysrhythmias, AV conduction disturbances (heart block, AV junctional rhythm, bradycardia)	2nd or 3rd degree heart block or sick sinus syndrome in the absence of a pacemaker	Instruct patient to report adverse reactions immediately. Teach patient how to take pulse. Dose adjustment required in renal insufficiency
diltiazem (Cardizem) Adult IV: 0.25 mg/kg over 2 min; if ventricular rate remains uncontrolled after 15 min, can repeat with 0.35 mg/kg over 2 min; initiate continuous infusion of 5–15 mg/h Adult PO: Start with 30 mg qid and increase to 180–480 mg/d in divided doses (SR form can be given once daily)	Dizziness, headache, edema, heart block, bradycardia, heart failure exacerbation, hypotension	2nd or 3rd degree heart block or sick sinus syndrome in the absence of a pacemaker, LV systolic dysfunction	Teach patient how to take pulse and blood pressure. Increased levels of cyclosporine may occur with concomitant use.
disopyramide (Norpace) Adult (<50 kg): 100 mg PO q6h or SR form, 200 mg PO q12h Adult (>50 kg): 150 mg PO q6h or SR form, 300 mg PO q12h; may increase up to 800 mg/d	Hypotension, heart failure, exacerbation, nausea, anorexia, dry mouth, urinary retention, blurred vision, constipation, torsades de pointes	2nd or 3rd degree heart block or sick sinus syndrome in the absence of a pacemaker, heart failure	Dose adjustment required in patients with renal insufficiency (CrCl ≤40 mL/min)
dofetilide (Tikosyn) Adult: 125–500 μg PO bid	Chest pain, headache, dizziness, insomnia, nausea, diarrhea, dyspnea, torsades de pointes	CrCl < 20 mL/min, QT > 440 msec	Specialized training and facilities are required for initiation of therapy. Dose adjustment required in patients with renal insufficiency (CrCl ≤ 60 mL/min) Dose must also be adjusted based on QT interval.
esmolol (Brevibloc) Adult: 500 μg/kg/min IV for 1 min followed by a maintenance infusion of 50 μg/kg/min; if inadequate response, rebolus with 500 μg/kg/min for 1 min and increase infusion rate by	Hypotension, wheezing, bronchospasm, heart block, bradycardia, heart failure exacerbation	2nd or 3rd degree heart block in the absence of a pacemaker, decompensated heart failure, sinus bradycardia	Instruct patient to report adverse reactions immediately or any discomfort at IV site.

(continued)

Table 22.1

Overview of Selected Antiarrhythmic Agents *(Continued)*

Generic (Trade) Name and Dosage	Selected Adverse Events	Contraindications	Special Considerations
50 μg/kg/min; repeat this process until desired response achieved or maximum infusion rate of 300 μg/kg/min is reached			
flecainide (Tambocor) Adult: 50 mg PO q12h up to a maximum of 300 mg/d	Dizziness, headache, lightheadedness, syncope, blurred vision or other visual disturbances, dyspnea, heart failure exacerbation, dysrhythmias	2nd or 3rd degree heart block in the absence of a pacemaker, recent myocardial infarction, ischemic heart disease, cardiogenic shock, heart failure	Instruct patient to report adverse reactions immediately.
ibutilide (Corvert) Adult (≥60 kg): 0.01 mg/kg IV over 10 min; can repeat with another dose if atrial fibrillation/flutter does not terminate within 10 min after end of initial dose Adult (<60 kg): 1 mg IV over 10 min; can repeat with another dose if atrial fibrillation/flutter does not terminate within 10 min after end of initial dose	Torsades de pointes, hypotension, heart block, headache, nausea	Pre-existing hypokalemia or hypomagnesemia, QT > 440 msec	Stop infusion if the QT interval increases or ventricular arrhythmias occur. Monitor ECG during administration. Monitor electrolytes before administering.
lidocaine (Xylocaine) *Pulseless VT/VF* Adult: 1–1.5 mg/kg IV push; may give additional 0.5–0.75 mg/kg IV push in 3–5 min, if necessary (maximum total dose = 3 mg/kg); if stable rhythm achieved, can initiate continuous infusion of 1–4 mg/min *Stable VT* Adult: Dose depends upon patient's left ventricular systolic function. If LVEF >40%, can use dose for Pulseless VT/VF. If LVEF <40%, administer 0.5–0.75 mg/kg IV push; may repeat every 5–10 min, if necessary (maximum total dose = 3 mg/kg). If stable rhythm achieved, can initiate continuous infusion of 1–4 mg/min	Seizures, confusion, stupor, dizziness, bradycardia, respiratory depression, slurred speech, blurred vision, muscle twitching, tinnitus	Hypersensitivity to amide local anesthetics, 2nd or 3rd degree heart block in the absence of a pacemaker	A lower infusion rate should be used in elderly patients or patients with heart failure or hepatic disease.
metoprolol (Lopressor) Adult IV: 2.5–5 mg over 2 min; can repeat every 2 min up to a total of 3 doses Adult PO: 25 mg bid or 50 mg daily (SR form); may increase up to 400 mg/d	Bradycardia, heart failure exacerbation, heart block, bronchospasm, fatigue, dizziness, hypotension	2nd or 3rd degree heart block in the absence of a pacemaker, decompensated heart failure, heart rate <45 beats/min	Use with caution in patients with severe LV systolic dysfunction, diabetes, or respiratory disease. Teach patient how to take pulse and blood pressure. Because sudden withdrawal can lead to exacerbation of angina and myocardial infarction, instruct patient not to discontinue drug abruptly. Instruct patient to report adverse reactions immediately.

Table 22.1

Overview of Selected Antiarrhythmic Agents (*Continued*)

Generic (Trade) Name and Dosage	Selected Adverse Events	Contraindications	Special Considerations
mexiletine (Mexitil) Adult: 200 mg PO q8h; may increase up to 400 mg PO q8h	Dizziness, drowsiness, paresthesias, blurred vision, tremor, seizures, confusion, dysrhythmias, nausea, vomiting	2nd or 3rd degree heart block in the absence of a pacemaker, cardiogenic shock	Instruct patient to report adverse reactions immediately.
moricizine (Ethmozine) Adult: 200–300 mg PO q8h	Blurred vision, dizziness, headache, fatigue, heart block, dysrhythmias, heart failure exacerbation, nausea, diarrhea	2nd or 3rd degree heart block in the absence of a pacemaker, cardiogenic shock	Use with caution in patients with renal or hepatic impairment or sick sinus syndrome. Advise patient to avoid hazardous activities if blurred vision or CNS reactions occur.
phenytoin (Dilantin) Adult: 50–100 mg IV over 1–2 min every 10–15 min until the dysrhythmia subsides (not to exceed a total of 15 mg/kg)	Ataxia, slurred speech, dizziness, confusion		Tell patient that this drug is given to correct acute ventricular dysrhythmias caused by digoxin toxicity. Monitor heart rate and blood pressure closely during administration because hypotension may occur. Inform patient of CNS effects that may occur and advise reporting these effects immediately.
procainamide (Pronestyl, Procanbid) *Supraventricular Arrhythmias* Adult IV: 15–17 mg/kg over 25–60 min, then continuous infusion of 1–4 mg/min (or can convert to PO after initial loading dose) Adult PO: Immediate release, 250–500 mg q3–6h; SR form (Procanbid), 500–2,000 mg q12h; usual dose = 50 mg/kg/day *Refractory VT/VF* Adult IV: 15–17 mg/kg infused at 30 mg/min (maximum total dose = 17 mg/kg); if stable rhythm achieved, can initiate continuous infusion at 1–4 mg/min; convert to oral therapy when hemodynamically stable and able to take oral medications (see PO dose under Stable VT) *Stable VT* Adult IV: 20 mg/min infusion given until arrhythmia suppressed, hypotension occurs, QRS widens by >50%, or total dose of 17 mg/kg administered; if stable rhythm achieved, can initiate continuous infusion at 1–4 mg/min; convert to oral therapy when hemodynamically stable and able to take oral medications	Dizziness, diarrhea, nausea, vomiting, lupus-like syndrome, torsades de pointes, agranulocytosis	Hypersensitivity to procaine, 2nd or 3rd degree heart block in the absence of a pacemaker	Use with caution, if at all, in patients with renal insufficiency. Instruct patient to report adverse reactions immediately.

(continued)

Table 22.1

Overview of Selected Antiarrhythmic Agents *(Continued)*

Generic (Trade) Name and Dosage	Selected Adverse Events	Contraindications	Special Considerations
Adult PO: Immediate release, 250–500 mg q3–6h; SR form (Procanbid), 500–2,000 mg q12h; usual dose = 50 mg/kg/day			
propafenone (Rythmol) Adult: 150 mg PO q8h; up to a maximum of 300 mg PO q8h	Dizziness, drowsiness, heart failure exacerbation, dysrhythmias, heart block, bradycardia, blurred vision, taste disturbances, bronchospasm	2nd or 3rd degree heart block in the absence of a pacemaker, bradycardia, cardiogenic shock, heart failure, bronchospastic disorders	Instruct patient to report adverse reactions immediately.
propranolol (Inderal) Adult IV: 1 mg over 1 min; may repeat every 5 min up to a total dose of 5 mg Adult PO: 10–20 mg q6–8h; can increase to 80–240 mg/d in 2–4 divided doses	Same as acebutolol	Same as acebutolol	Same as acebutolol
quinidine (Quinidex, Quinaglute) Adult: Quinidine sulfate, 200–400 mg PO q6h, up to a maximum of 600 mg PO q6h; quinidine gluconate, 324 mg PO q8–12h, up to a maximum of 972 mg PO q8–12h	Torsades de pointes, heart block, hypotension, tinnitus, diarrhea, nausea, vomiting, fever, heart failure exacerbation, thrombocytopenia	Allergy or sensitivity to quinidine or cinchona derivatives, long QT syndrome (may predispose to torsades de pointes)	Instruct patient to take drug with food if GI distress occurs. Instruct patient to report adverse reactions immediately.
sotalol (Betapace) **Atrial Fibrillation** Adult: 80 mg PO bid, up to a maximum of 160 mg PO bid **Ventricular Arrhythmias** Adult: 80 mg PO bid, up to a maximum of 320 mg PO bid	Bradycardia, heart block, heart failure exacerbation, torsades de pointes, bronchospasm	2nd or 3rd degree heart block in the absence of a pacemaker, bradycardia, heart failure, asthma, long QT syndrome (may predispose to torsades de pointes)	Dosing interval must be adjusted in patients with renal insufficiency. Instruct patient to take drug on an empty stomach. Instruct patient not to discontinue drug abruptly.
tocainide (Tonocard) Adult: 1,200–1,800 mg PO divided into three doses daily	Dizziness, vertigo, confusion, heart failure exacerbation, dysrhythmias, bradycardia, pulmonary edema, agranulocytosis	Hypersensitivity to lidocaine or other amide drugs, 2nd or 3rd degree heart block in the absence of a pacemaker	Instruct patient to report adverse reactions and pulmonary symptoms immediately.
verapamil (Calan) Adult IV: 2.5–5 mg over 2 min; if ventricular rate remains uncontrolled after 15–30 min, can double initial dose and administer over 2 min; initiate continuous infusion of 5–10 mg/hr Adult PO: 240–360 mg/d in three divided dosesa	Constipation, bradycardia, heart block, heart failure exacerbation, hypotension, dizziness, peripheral edema	2nd or 3rd degree heart block or sick sinus syndrome in the absence of a pacemaker, LV systolic dysfunction	Encourage patient to increase fluid and fiber intake to combat constipation. Teach patient how to take pulse and blood pressure.

AV, atrioventricular; BID, twice daily; CNS, central nervous system; CrCl; creatinine clearance; D5W, 5% dextrose in water; ECG, electrocardiogram; GI, gastrointestinal; IV, intravenous; LD, loading dose; LV, left ventricular; LVEF, left ventricular ejection fraction; MD, maintenance dose; PO, oral; QID, four times daily; SR, sustained release; VF, ventricular fibrillation; VT, ventricular tachycardia.

Class IA Drugs

Quinidine

Quinidine is a broad-spectrum antiarrhythmic drug that may be used to treat supraventricular and ventricular dysrhythmias. This drug decreases automaticity (phase 4), slows conduction velocity (phase 0), and prolongs refractoriness (phase 3). Quinidine widens the QRS complex, prolongs the QT interval, and slightly prolongs the PR interval. Quinidine has been used in the management of atrial flutter or fibrillation, AV nodal reentrant tachycardia, and VT.

Quinidine has potent anticholinergic properties that affect the SA and AV nodes. Therefore, quinidine can increase the SA nodal discharge rate and AV nodal conduction. Consequently,

BOX 22–3. CLASSIFICATION OF ANTIARRHYTHMIC DRUGS

Class I—Na+ Channel Blockers
IA (intermediate onset/offset)
   disopyramide (Norpace)
   procainamide (Pronestyl, Procanbid [sustained release]) quinidine (Quinidex [sulfate], Quinaglute [gluconate])
IB (fast onset/offset)
   lidocaine (Xylocaine)
   mexiletine (Mexitil)
   phenytoin (Dilantin)
   tocainide (Tonocard)
IC (slow onset/offset)
   flecainide (Tambocor)
   moricizine (Ethmozine)
   propafenone (Rythmol)*

Class II—Beta Blockers
acebutolol (Sectral)
atenolol (Tenormin)
esmolol (Brevibloc)
metoprolol (Lopressor)
pindolol (Visken)
propranolol (Inderal)

Class III—K+ Channel Blockers
amiodarone (Cordarone)†
bretylium (Bretylol)
dofetilide (Tikosyn)
ibutilide (Corvert)
sotalol (Betapace)*

Class IV—Ca2+ Channel Blockers
diltiazem (Cardizem)
verapamil (Calan)

* Also has beta-blocking properties (class II)
† Also has Na+-channel blocking (class I), beta-blocking (class II), and Ca2+-channel blocking (class IV) properties

in patients with atrial flutter or fibrillation, these anticholinergic effects may lead to a more rapid ventricular rate. Therefore, the AV node should be adequately inhibited with the use of an AV nodal blocking drug, such as a beta blocker, non-dihydropyridine calcium channel blocker (eg, diltiazem or verapamil), or digoxin prior to administering quinidine in these patients. Quinidine also blocks α_1 receptors, which can lead to vasodilation and subsequent dose-related hypotension, especially when administered intravenously (IV).

The most common adverse events associated with quinidine are gastrointestinal (nausea, vomiting, and diarrhea). As with other class IA drugs, quinidine can cause proarrhythmia, specifically torsades de pointes. Other adverse events reported with quinidine use include hypersensitivity, thrombocytopenia, hepatitis, cinchonism (tinnitus, blurred vision, headache), worsening of underlying heart failure, and hemolytic anemia.

Quinidine is a substrate of the cytochrome P-450 (CYP) 3A4 enzyme as well as an inhibitor of the CYP 2D6 enzyme. Therefore, quinidine can interact with any other drug that inhibits or induces CYP 3A4 (eg, inhibitors: ketoconazole, erythromycin, amiodarone, verapamil, diltiazem; inducers: rifampin, phenobarbital, phenytoin) or is a substrate of CYP 2D6 (eg, beta blockers). Quinidine can also significantly increase serum digoxin concentrations.

Procainamide

Procainamide (Pronestyl) has basically the same electrophysiologic effects as those of quinidine, except that procainamide does not have the anticholinergic activity of quinidine. Procainamide decreases automaticity (phase 4), slows conduction velocity (phase 0), and prolongs refractoriness (phase 3). Procainamide widens the QRS complex, lengthens the QT interval, and slightly prolongs the PR interval. NAPA, the major metabolite of procainamide, blocks outward K+ currents and thereby has class III electrophysiologic properties. NAPA causes lengthening of the QT interval (Coyle, Carnes, & Schaal, 1992). Procainamide is a broad-spectrum antiarrhythmic and has been used to treat supraventricular and ventricular dysrhythmias.

Cardiac adverse events associated with procainamide include bradycardia, AV block, worsening of underlying heart failure, and torsades de pointes. The most common adverse event associated with procainamide is the development of a clinical syndrome that resembles systemic lupus erythematosus (SLE) (Coyle et al., 1992). During chronic therapy, positive antinuclear antibodies develop in 50% to 80% of patients. Common signs and symptoms of SLE include rash, arthralgias, fever, pericarditis, and pleuritis. The syndrome is usually reversible if the drug is discontinued; however, symptoms may be persistent and require treatment with salicylates or corticosteroids. Hematologic effects such as agranulocytosis and pancytopenia are reported occasionally. Other adverse events associated with procainamide use include nausea, vomiting, diarrhea, and drug fever.

Both procainamide and NAPA can accumulate in patients with renal insufficiency. Therefore, serum concentrations of both procainamide and NAPA must be monitored regularly to assess for efficacy and toxicity. The therapeutic ranges of procainamide and NAPA are 4 to 10 mcg/mL and 15 to 25 mcg/mL, respectively.

Disopyramide

Disopyramide (Norpace) decreases conduction velocity (phase 0) and automaticity (phase 4) and prolongs refractoriness (phase 3). These effects are manifested as a prolonged QT interval and a slightly prolonged QRS complex on the ECG. Disopyramide has direct and indirect effects on heart rate similar to those of quinidine. Disopyramide is a broad-spectrum antiarrhythmic and has been used to treat supraventricular and ventricular dysrhythmias. However, the clinical use of this agent is limited because of its potent anticholinergic and negative inotropic effects. If it is used to treat atrial flutter or fibrillation, the practitioner should give an AV nodal blocking agent (eg, beta blocker, diltiazem, verapamil, or digoxin) to minimize its vagolytic effect. The primary adverse events associated with disopyramide are precipitation of heart failure and anticholinergic effects (eg, dry mouth, urinary retention, constipation, blurred vision). Disopyramide is contraindicated in patients with a left ventricular ejection fraction of less than 40% because of significant myocardial depression. Disopyramide can also cause torsades de pointes.

Class IB Drugs

Class IB antiarrhythmic agents are lidocaine (Xylocaine), mexiletine (Mexitil), tocainide (Tonocard), and phenytoin (Dilantin). These agents decrease automaticity and conduction velocity and shorten refractoriness. These agents primarily exert their electrophysiologic effects on the ventricular myocardium since they have little or no effect on atrial tissue.

Lidocaine

Lidocaine is categorized as a class IB antiarrhythmic; however, its electrophysiologic effects are different in that it is selective to ischemic tissue, and especially to active fast sodium channels in the bundle of His, Purkinje fibers, and ventricular myocardium. Thus, lidocaine has little effect on conduction in non-ischemic tissue and the atrial myocardium. Lidocaine also has very little effect on the automaticity of the SA node. However, lidocaine does suppress the automaticity of ectopic ventricular pacemakers and Purkinje fibers. In normal tissues, the action potential duration is shortened and conduction velocity shows little change with lidocaine. However, in depolarized fibers or in fibers damaged by ischemia, lidocaine prolongs the action potential and slows conduction.

Lidocaine is primarily effective in treating ventricular dysrhythmias, especially those associated with acute MI. Prophylactic administration in patients with acute MI demonstrated a decreased incidence of ventricular fibrillation (VF) but no difference in prehospital treatment outcomes of acute MI and no improvement or even higher mortality rates in hospitalized patients. Selective administration of lidocaine to patients with VF associated with MI or cardiac arrest similarly demonstrated no improvement in survival rates (Teo, Yusuf, & Furberg, 1993; Wyse, Kellen, & Rademaker, 1988). The use of lidocaine as prophylaxis against VT or VF in patients with MI is not warranted. Its use should be reserved for the treatment of ventricular dysrhythmias.

Lidocaine is not effective in the treatment of supraventricular dysrhythmias such as atrial flutter or fibrillation. However, lidocaine can be used for treatment of digitalis-induced dysrhythmias (atrial and ventricular) because of its selectivity for depolarized myocardium.

Lidocaine is eliminated chiefly by hepatic metabolism, with the metabolic rate proportional to hepatic blood flow. In congestive heart failure, the volume of distribution in the central compartment is decreased and hepatic blood flow may be decreased if cardiac output is depressed. Hepatic failure slows the clearance rate but does not affect the volume of distribution.

The principal adverse events associated with lidocaine are central nervous system effects of dizziness, paresthesia, disorientation, tremor, and agitation. At higher concentrations, seizures and respiratory arrest may occur. Adverse events are more frequent in the elderly, patients with congestive heart failure or hepatic disease, and during prolonged administration (more than 24 hours). Therefore, these patients should be closely monitored for signs and symptoms of lidocaine toxicity. Lidocaine concentrations should also be closely monitored in these patients. The therapeutic range of lidocaine is 1.5 to 6 mg/L. Lidocaine toxicity is most commonly observed at concentrations greater than 5 mg/L.

Mexiletine

Mexiletine is a structurally related oral analog of lidocaine and has similar electrophysiologic effects, antiarrhythmic benefits, and adverse events. Mexiletine decreases conduction velocity (phase 0) preferentially in ischemic tissue. Mexiletine can be used in combination with class IA and III agents for the treatment of refractory ventricular dysrhythmias.

Mexiletine was developed as an anticonvulsant in Europe and was used initially in the United States in the mid-1980s. Mexiletine is effective in the treatment of VT. However, its use as a single agent in refractory ventricular dysrhythmias has not proved effective (Duff, Roden, & Primm, 1983). Combining mexiletine with a second antiarrhythmic agent (class IA or III) has proven more effective with sustained VT. However, its clinical use is limited by a high incidence of gastrointestinal reactions such as nausea and vomiting. Neurologic side effects of dizziness, confusion, ataxia, and speech disturbances may lead the practitioner to discontinue antiarrhythmic treatment with this drug. Mexiletine can also cause proarrhythmia, although the incidence is lower when compared to other antiarrhythmic agents.

Tocainide

Tocainide is the chemically related oral analog of lidocaine and has similar antiarrhythmic and electrophysiologic effects. However, one main difference between lidocaine and tocainide is that the latter may shorten the tachycardic cycle in VT and cause degeneration to VF (Engler & LeWinter, 1981; Roden & Woosley, 1986). Tocainide is of little value in treating sustained VT and has little benefit during acute MI (Campbell, Hutton, & Elton, 1983). Unlike mexiletine and lidocaine, tocainide can produce blood dyscrasias such as agranulocytosis. In addition, pulmonary fibrosis and interstitial pneumonitis have been associated with the use of tocainide. The central nervous system and gastrointestinal side effects of tocainide are similar to those of lidocaine and mexiletine. Like mexiletine, tocainide can also be pro-arrhythmic. Because of the potential to cause serious toxicities, the use of tocainide should be limited to the treatment of life-threatening ventricular dysrhythmias that are refractory to other antiarrhythmics.

Phenytoin

Phenytoin can be used to correct acute arrhythmias caused by digitalis toxicity. Phenytoin is useful as an antiarrhythmic agent in refractory VT, in tricyclic antidepressant and digoxin toxicity, and in torsades de pointes because of its unique effect in increasing AV nodal conduction (Vukmir & Stein, 1991). It has an action similar to that of lidocaine, with decreased automaticity (phase 4) and conduction velocity (phase 0) in ischemic tissue. However, refractoriness is essentially unchanged. Adverse reactions include hypotension caused by the phenol vehicle and occasional central nervous system toxicity after excessive dosing (Vukmir & Stein, 1991).

Class IC Drugs

Flecainide

Flecainide (Tambocor) is a potent blocker of fast Na^+ channels during phase 0 of the action potential, slowing conduction velocity in the Purkinje fibers and AV node and diminishing automaticity in the Purkinje fibers. Because of the slowed cardiac conduction, increases in the PR interval and QRS duration may be seen.

Flecainide is most commonly used in clinical practice for the treatment of supraventricular arrhythmias, such as atrial fibrillation/flutter. Although flecainide is FDA approved for the treatment of life-threatening ventricular arrhythmias, its efficacy is rather poor and the potential for serious adverse events is rather high (Anderson, Lutz, & Allison, 1983). In fact, flecainide has been known to cause a rapid, sustained VT that is resistant to resuscitation. The results of the CAST I (CAST Investigators, 1989) study suggest that patients who have ischemic heart disease and poor left ventricular function are predisposed to this type of sustained VT.

The CAST I study was a prospective, double-blinded, randomized study of survivors of MI who were asymptomatic or had mildly symptomatic ventricular dysrhythmias. This trial was conducted to determine if the suppression of asymptomatic or mildly symptomatic premature ventricular contractions (PVCs) with the class IC antiarrhythmics flecainide, encainide, or moricizine would decrease the incidence of death from arrhythmia in survivors of MI. In the study, 730 patients were randomized to flecainide and 725 patients were randomized to placebo. Despite adequate suppression of ventricular dysrhythmias, flecainide significantly increased mortality from dysrhythmia or cardiac arrest and significantly increased total mortality rates. Older age increased the likelihood of adverse events, including death, in patients receiving flecainide (Akiyama et al., 1992). Overall, the results of this trial demonstrated that the use of antiarrhythmic therapy to suppress asymptomatic PVCs in patients after an MI does not improve survival and is most likely detrimental. The use of flecainide should be avoided in patients with any form of structural heart disease, which includes evidence of coronary artery disease, left ventricular dysfunction, valvular heart disease, or left ventricular hypertrophy.

Adverse events associated with flecainide use include blurred vision, dizziness, headache, tremor, nausea, vomiting, conduction disturbances, and ventricular dysrhythmias (sustained VT) that prove resistant to cardioversion. Flecainide also has potent negative inotropic effects that may lead to worsening heart failure.

Propafenone

Propafenone (Rythmol) has the same ability to block Na^+ channels, slow conduction velocity, and diminish automaticity in the AV node and Purkinje fibers as flecainide. However, propafenone also has a mild, nonselective beta-adrenergic blocking effect. Although propafenone is FDA approved for the treatment of life-threatening ventricular arrhythmias, its use in clinical practice has been limited to the management of supraventricular arrhythmias such as atrial fibrillation. Oral propafenone has been shown to be effective for restoring and maintaining sinus rhythm in patients with atrial fibrillation (Miller et al., 2000; Roy et al., 2000). The use of single, oral loading doses of propafenone (450 to 600 mg) in patients with recent-onset atrial fibrillation has been associated with conversion rates of 72% to 76% at 8 hours (Slavik et al., 2001). Although propafenone was not evaluated in the CAST study and has not been associated with increased mortality in other trials, there still tends to be an overall negative perception of this drug's safety in patients with structural heart disease. Until the safety of propafenone can be demonstrated conclusively in a large, randomized, prospective trial in patients with structural heart disease, its use should be avoided in this population.

Adverse events associated with propafenone use include blurred vision, dizziness, headache, nausea, vomiting, fatigue, bronchospasm, taste disturbances (metallic taste), conduction disturbances (bradycardia, heart block, QRS prolongation), and ventricular dysrhythmias (sustained VT) that prove resistant to cardioversion. Propafenone also has potent negative inotropic effects that may lead to worsening heart failure.

Moricizine

Moricizine hydrochloride is used to treat life-threatening ventricular dysrhythmias such as sustained VT. Class IC drugs are local anesthetic agents that have as their predominant effect a depression of Na^+ conductance during phase 0 of the action potential. Conduction velocity is slowed, and this class of antiarrhythmic agents decreases excitability.

The use of moricizine in treating ventricular dysrhythmias was studied in the second Cardiac Arrhythmia Suppression Trial (CAST II) (CAST II Investigators, 1992), a prospective, double-blinded, randomized study. The study comprised 1,155 survivors of MI with poor left ventricular function who were asymptomatic or had mildly symptomatic ventricular dysrhythmias. In the study, 581 patients were randomized to moricizine and 574 patients were randomized to placebo. The prevalence of nonsustained VT was 30%. Thirty-eight percent of the patients were between 66 and 79 years of age. Adequate suppression of ventricular dysrhythmias was required before randomization. The investigators concluded that the use of moricizine was not only ineffective but also harmful. In fact, mortality (likely due to proarrhythmia) was significantly higher in the moricizine group compared to the placebo group, even within the first 2 weeks of the trial. Older age increased the likelihood of adverse events, including death, in patients receiving moricizine (Akiyama et al., 1992). On the basis of these data, the practitioner should not use moricizine for the treatment of ventricular dysrhythmia in patients younger than 65 or those with heart disease.

Class II Antiarrhythmic Drugs

The beta blockers are useful in suppressing ventricular dysrhythmias. They also are used for treating many supraventricular dysrhythmias because of their ability to block receptor sites in the conduction system by slowing AV nodal conduction and the SA nodal rate, which in turn slows the ventricular rate. Furthermore, beta blockers are helpful when used in combination with other antiarrhythmic agents or in treating the underlying cause of some dysrhythmias (ischemia, catecholamine excess) (see Table 22-1).

Beta blockers decrease automaticity (decreasing the slope of phase 4 depolarization in the sinus node and in the Purkinje fibers) and conduction velocity (phase 0) and prolong refractoriness (phase 3). This occurs because of their effect on exogenous autonomic stimuli and internal membrane stabilization (Ebihara & Fujimura, 1991). Changes in the ECG caused by beta blockers are a sinus bradycardia, consisting of a normal or slightly prolonged PR interval and occasional shortening of the QT interval. In addition to being negative chronotropic drugs (decrease AV nodal conduction), beta blockers are negative inotropic agents (decrease cardiac contractility) as well. Both of these properties enable beta blockers to decrease myocardial oxygen consumption, which is useful especially in patients with underlying ischemic heart disease. Exercise-related or stress-related sinus tachycardia is usually modulated by beta blockers. Patients with sinus node dysfunction or AV conduction system defects may have significant sinus bradycardia.

In general, beta blockers lower the heart rate and blood pressure, decrease myocardial contractility, decrease oxygen consumption in the myocardium, and lower cardiac output. Beta blockers have a diverse range of uses, including supraventricular tachycardia, atrial fibrillation or flutter, arrhythmias caused by catecholamine excess, ischemia, mitral valve prolapse, hypertrophic cardiomyopathy, and MI. Beta blockers also reduce complex ventricular dysrhythmias, including VT (Lichstein, Morganroth, Harrist, & Hubble, 1983). The VF threshold is increased with the use of beta blockers in animal models, and beta blockers have been found to decrease VF in patients with acute MI. Beta blockers reduce myocardial ischemia, which may reduce the likelihood of VF. In the CAST study, patients receiving beta blockers had a 66% decrease in the incidence of death or cardiac arrest at 30 days, a 53% decrease at 1 year, and a 36% decrease at 2 years (Kennedy, Brooks, & Barker, 1994). Multivariate analysis has shown beta blockers to be an independent factor for a 40% decreased incidence of arrhythmic death or cardiac arrest, and a reduction in all-cause mortality by 33%. The practitioner should strongly consider the use of beta blockers in the treatment of MI and ischemia. All beta blockers (without intrinsic sympathomimetic activity) are relatively similar in efficacy for the treatment of supraventricular and ventricular arrhythmias. Selection of a particular beta blocker is usually based on the safety profile of the individual agent.

The adverse events associated with beta blockers depend on their selectivity for beta$_1$ receptors or beta$_2$ receptors. Bronchospasm may be seen in patients with asthma and chronic obstructive pulmonary disease, and this is not eliminated by the use of selective beta$_1$ antagonists. Heart failure, hypotension, bradycardia, and depression also are common side effects. In addition, patients receiving beta blockers often report fatigue and impotence.

Class III Antiarrhythmic Drugs

Class III antiarrhythmic drugs include bretylium tosylate (Bretylol), amiodarone hydrochloride (Cordarone), sotalol, ibutilide (Corvert), and dofetilide (Tikosyn). Ibutilide and dofetilide are used to treat atrial fibrillation or atrial flutter. Amiodarone and sotalol can be used to treat both supraventricular and ventricular arrhythmias. While bretylium is indicated for the treatment of life-threatening ventricular arrhythmias, due to lack of availability this drug is no longer used in clinical practice and therefore will not be discussed in detail.

Patients receiving class III antiarrhythmics should be monitored closely for ECG changes such as increased ventricular ectopy and changes in PR interval, QRS duration, and QT interval. Practitioners should avoid using class III antiarrhythmics concomitantly with other drugs that can prolong the QT interval to minimize the risk of torsades de pointes (see Table 22-1).

Amiodarone

Amiodarone is a unique drug in that it possesses electrophysiologic characteristics of all four classes of antiarrhythmic agents. While amiodarone is primarily a K$^+$ channel blocker (blocks the rapid and slow component of the delayed rectifier potassium current), it also blocks Na$^+$ channels, has nonselective beta-blocking activity, and has weak calcium-channel blocking properties. As a result, amiodarone reduces automaticity (phase 4) and conduction velocity (phase 0) and prolongs refractoriness (phase 3). Its binding characteristics to the Na$^+$ channels are similar to those of the class IB antiarrhythmics ("fast on/fast off"). When administered IV, amiodarone's beta-blocking and calcium-channel blocking activity is more predominant. Amiodarone has minimal to no negative inotropic effects, which makes it one of the few antiarrhythmic drugs that can be safely used in patients with left ventricular dysfunction. The PR and QT intervals are prolonged and there is a widening of the QRS complex. Amiodarone is used to treat both supraventricular and ventricular arrhythmias.

Since the proportion of patients with atrial fibrillation who have concomitant structural heart disease appears to be increasing, amiodarone use for this particular arrhythmia has dramatically increased, because this is one of the few antiarrhythmics that has been proven to be safe in this population. Amiodarone is often given IV for acute treatment of life-threatening ventricular arrhythmias, such as VT or VF. IV amiodarone can also be used to terminate atrial fibrillation acutely. Even though ICDs now play a primary role in the chronic management of ventricular arrhythmias, amiodarone is still used in patients who refuse or are not candidates for these devices. Also, amiodarone can also be used as adjunctive therapy in these patients if frequent ICD discharges occur.

Because of amiodarone's poor oral bioavailability, large volume of distribution, and long half-life, its onset of action may not be apparent for several months. To achieve efficacy more quickly, loading doses of oral amiodarone must be initially used to saturate the myocardial stores. Once the patient is appropriately loaded with oral amiodarone, the dose should be reduced to the recommended maintenance dose to minimize the incidence of adverse events.

Because of its extremely large volume of distribution and high lipophilicity, amiodarone has the potential to accumulate and cause adverse effects in numerous organs, with the lungs, thyroid, eyes, heart, liver, skin, gastrointestinal tract, and central nervous system being most notably affected. Unlike other amiodarone-induced adverse effects, pulmonary toxicity can be life-threatening. Definitive diagnosis of amiodarone-induced pulmonary toxicity is difficult, since many of the subjective and objective findings are nonspecific. Patients may present with cough, dyspnea, or fever. The chest radiograph may reveal diffuse infiltrates; pulmonary function tests may demonstrate a reduction in the diffusion capacity. If pulmonary toxicity is detected, amiodarone should be immediately discontinued. Corticosteroids may be needed to treat the pulmonary inflammation. To screen for pulmonary toxicity in patients receiving amiodarone, pulmonary function tests and a chest radiograph should be obtained at baseline. Subsequently, a chest radiograph should be obtained on an annual basis, while pulmonary function tests can be repeated if symptoms develop (Goldschlager et al., 2000).

Because it contains approximately 38% iodine by weight, amiodarone may also cause thyroid abnormalities that can manifest as either hypothyroidism or hyperthyroidism. Hypothyroidism is the more common form of amiodarone-induced thyroid dysfunction. Although patients often report increased lethargy, the diagnosis of amiodarone-induced hypothyroidism is made upon detection of elevated levels of thyroid-stimulating hormone (TSH). Patients developing hypothyroidism can generally be treated with thyroid hormone supplementation. The diagnosis of amiodarone-induced hyperthyroidism should be suspected if patients present with new or recurrent arrhythmias. Patients developing hyperthyroidism have abnormally low TSH levels and can usually be treated with antithyroid medications. To screen for thyroid dysfunction in patients receiving amiodarone, thyroid function tests should be performed at baseline and then at 6-month intervals throughout therapy (Goldschlager et al., 2000).

Ocular complications induced by amiodarone often manifest as corneal and lens opacities. Although these opacities rarely produce visual disturbances, photophobia, halos, and blurred vision have been reported. Because of their relatively benign nature, these opacities do not require discontinuation of amiodarone. Chronic amiodarone therapy has also been associated with optic neuritis and optic neuropathy. Since these ocular disturbances are vision-threatening, amiodarone must be discontinued once the diagnosis is confirmed. To screen for this complication, ophthalmologic examinations should be performed at baseline and then on an annual basis (Goldschlager et al., 2000).

Gastrointestinal adverse effects are relatively common and occur most frequently when amiodarone loading doses are administered. Typically, patients report nausea, vomiting, loss of appetite, and abdominal pain. Constipation can also occur during long-term therapy. These gastrointestinal disturbances can be minimized by dividing the total daily dose and by taking the drug with food. Liver function test abnormalities can also develop. Although elevations in aspartate aminotransferase and alanine aminotransferase levels are relatively common, only rarely do patients develop clinical hepatitis. The liver enzyme levels usually return to baseline following reduction of the dose or discontinuation of the drug. To screen for these hepatic abnormalities, liver function tests should be performed at baseline and then every 6 months throughout therapy with amiodarone (Goldschlager et al., 2000).

Although laboratory tests cannot detect amiodarone-induced cardiovascular, neurologic, and dermatologic toxicities, patients should still be clinically evaluated on a routine basis. Compared with other antiarrhythmics, amiodarone produces fewer cardiovascular adverse effects. The bradycardia and heart block that can develop merely represent an accentuation of amiodarone's pharmacologic and electrophysiologic properties. Additionally, even though amiodarone markedly prolongs the QT interval, torsades de pointes is rare. Neurologic toxicities associated with amiodarone occur frequently and may include tremors, ataxia, peripheral neuropathy, fatigue, and insomnia. The most common dermatologic reactions observed during amiodarone therapy are photosensitivity and a blue/gray skin discoloration. Photosensitivity reactions can range from extremely tanned areas to sunburned areas with erythema and edema. Blue/gray skin discoloration, which often appears on the patient's face and hands, may be related to the cumulative dose and duration of therapy. To prevent these dermatologic toxicities, patients should use opaque sunscreens such as zinc oxide while outdoors.

Patients receiving amiodarone also need to be monitored for drug interactions. Amiodarone is a potent inhibitor of the CYP 3A4, 2C9, 2D6, and 1A2 isoenzymes. Amiodarone also significantly interacts with digoxin and warfarin, which are commonly used in patients with atrial fibrillation. Amiodarone potentiates the anticoagulant effects of warfarin, which results in an increased INR and an increased risk of bleeding (Sanoski & Bauman, 2002). Amiodarone can also double serum digoxin concentrations. Close monitoring of patients receiving digoxin and/or warfarin is essential, as dosage adjustments may be needed.

Sotalol

Sotalol (Betapace, Betapace AF) is a class III antiarrhythmic agent that also has nonselective beta-adrenergic blocking properties. Sotalol blocks the rapid component of the delayed rectifier potassium current, which prolongs atrial and ventricular refractoriness. Sotalol increases the QT interval by prolonging ventricular repolarization and may give rise to torsades de pointes (Anderson & Prystowsky, 1999; Soyka, Wirtz, & Spangenberg, 1990). The QT interval prolongation with sotalol is a dose-dependent effect. The practitioner should monitor the QT interval closely during treatment. Sotalol should be discontinued if the QT interval exceeds 550 msec. The practitioner should avoid combining sotalol with other drugs that increase the QT interval. Because sotalol is eliminated primarily by the kidneys, the initial dose must be based on the patient's creatinine clearance. The practitioner should routinely monitor the patient's renal function throughout therapy to determine if any dosing adjustments are necessary. The practitioner should also routinely monitor electrolytes, especially if the patient is concomitantly receiving diuretics, since hypokalemia and hypomagnesemia can increase the risk for torsades de pointes. Most of the adverse effects associated with sotalol can be attributed to its beta-blocking activity (eg, bradycardia, fatigue, dyspnea). The beta-blocking effect of sotalol may decrease cardiac contractility, so this drug should be avoided in patients with left ventricular dysfunction.

Sotalol is effective for the treatment of supraventricular (ie, atrial fibrillation, atrial flutter) and ventricular arrhythmias. Although sotalol is not effective for conversion of atrial fibrillation, it is an effective agent for maintaining sinus rhythm (Roy et al., 2000). In patients with an ICD, sotalol has also been shown to significantly reduce arrhythmia recurrence and discharge from the device (Pacifico et al., 1999).

Dofetilide

Dofetilide acts as a selective K^+ channel blocker, affecting the rapid component of the delayed rectifier potassium current. This results in a prolonged action potential and an increased QT interval. It affects the atrium more than the ventricle. Dofetilide exhibits reverse-use dependence, whereby its action potential-prolonging effects are lessened at higher heart rates and increased at lower heart rates.

Dofetilide appears to be a pure class III agent, with few to no hemodynamic effects. The agent has no negative inotropic activity. Like amiodarone, dofetilide is also safe to use in patients with left ventricular dysfunction (Køber et al., 2000).

Dofetilide is approved for the conversion of atrial fibrillation or atrial flutter to sinus rhythm and for the maintenance of sinus rhythm in patients with atrial fibrillation or atrial flutter of greater than 1 week's duration who have been converted to sinus rhythm. In the Symptomatic Atrial Fibrillation Investigative Research on Dofetilide (SAFIRE-D) trial, approximately 6%, 10%, and 30% of patients receiving 125 mcg, 250 mcg, and 500 mcg of dofetilide, respectively, converted to sinus rhythm. At 1 year, slightly more than 50% of patients in the group taking 500 mcg remained in normal sinus rhythm (Singh et al., 2000).

As with other antiarrhythmics, the main concern with dofetilide is the dose-dependent onset of torsades de pointes and other ventricular dysrhythmias. Other adverse events include headache, dizziness, insomnia, chest pain, nausea, diarrhea, and dyspnea.

Dofetilide has a number of important drug interactions. The concomitant use of cimetidine, ketoconazole, megestrol, prochlorperazine, trimethoprim–sulfamethoxazole, or verapamil with dofetilide is contraindicated since these drugs can significantly increase plasma concentrations of dofetilide. Since dofetilide is metabolized to a small extent by the CYP 3A4 isoenzyme, drugs that are inhibitors of this isoenzyme should be used cautiously with dofetilide because they can increase dofetilide concentrations. Examples of such inhibitors include macrolide antibiotics, azole antifungals, protease inhibitors, selective serotonin reuptake inhibitors, diltiazem, grapefruit juice, nefazodone, and zafirlukast. Similarly, drugs that prolong the QT interval should not be used concomitantly with dofetilide.

The recommended dosage is 500 mg twice daily. The dosage should be lowered in patients with impaired renal function or an already extended QT interval. The drug should not be given to patients with a creatinine clearance of less than 20 mL/min or a QT interval greater than 440 msec. Because of concerns over torsades de pointes, the manufacturer recommends that patients be started on dofetilide in a setting where creatinine clearance testing, ECG monitoring, and cardiac resuscitation are available consistently for 3 days. Therefore, this agent is available only to facilities and prescribers who have undergone appropriate dosing and initiation training (Pfizer Laboratories, 2000).

Ibutilide

Ibutilide is structurally related to L-sotalol, but it has no beta-adrenergic blocking action. It prolongs the action potential by increasing the slow inward Na^+ current and blocking the rapid component of the delayed rectifier potassium current.

Electrophysiologic studies have demonstrated increases in atrial and ventricular effective refractory periods and suppression of induction of dysrhythmias (Buchanan, Turcotte, Kabell, & Gibson, 1993). Ibutilide is available only in IV form. It is indicated only for the acute termination of atrial fibrillation or atrial flutter.

Ibutilide restores sinus rhythm in approximately 50% of patients with these arrhythmias. However, it is more effective for restoring sinus rhythm in patients with atrial flutter than in those with atrial fibrillation (Stambler et al., 1996; Volgman et al., 1998). Ibutilide also appears to be effective for facilitating direct-current cardioversion of atrial fibrillation (Oral et al., 1999). The major adverse effect associated with ibutilide is torsades de pointes. Patients with left ventricular dysfunction and electrolyte abnormalities (eg, hypokalemia or hypomagnesemia) are especially at risk for developing proarrhythmia with ibutilide.

Class IV Antiarrhythmic Drugs

The class IV antiarrhythmic agents, verapamil and diltiazem (Cardizem), are non-dihydropyridine calcium channel blockers used to treat supraventricular dysrhythmias, usually of reentry origin. These dysrhythmias include paroxysmal supraventricular tachycardia (PSVT), atrial fibrillation, and atrial flutter. These agents have the ability to slow conduction, prolong refractoriness, and decrease automaticity in the SA and AV nodes. In atrial fibrillation or atrial flutter, these drugs slow conduction through the AV node and thereby slow the ventricular rate. The cardiac effects are vascular relaxation, a negative inotropic effect, and a negative chronotropic effect. Verapamil has more potent negative inotropic effects than diltiazem.

The primary action of these drugs is to inhibit the inward movement of Ca^{2+} through Ca^{2+} channels located in cell membranes. The AV node depends on the influx of Ca^{2+} through voltage-dependent Ca^{2+} channels or "slow" channels; therefore, supraventricular tachycardias are sensitive to treatment with calcium channel blockers. Although these agents rarely affect normal sinus node function, they may produce sinus arrest or sinus block in patients with SA nodal disease. Use of verapamil or diltiazem in these patients may lead to severe hypotension, bradycardia, or asystole. These drugs also should not be used in patients with an accessory pathway or WPW syndrome since they can shorten the refractory period of the accessory pathway and subsequently increase the ventricular rate, which may lead to VF (see Table 22-1).

Because of their potent negative inotropic effects, both verapamil and diltiazem should be avoided in patients with left ventricular dysfunction, since they are likely to precipitate worsening heart failure symptoms. The practitioner should use caution when using IV verapamil, since significant hypotension can occur (Phillips et al., 1997). It is recommended that IV verapamil be slowly administered over at least 2 minutes to minimize the risk of hypotension; use in the elderly may require an even slower rate of administration. Bradycardia, heart block, headache, flushing, dizziness, and peripheral edema are the most common adverse effects of diltiazem and verapamil. Verapamil can also cause constipation. The practitioner should be cautious when administering these agents concomitantly with beta blockers because of the increased risk for bradycardia and heart block. Since diltiazem and verapamil are substrates and inhibitors of the CYP 3A4 isoenzyme, the practitioner should use caution when concomitantly administering either of these drugs with other agents that are also metabolized by this isoenzyme.

Other Antiarrhythmic Agents

Several other classifications of antiarrhythmic agents are commonly used to treat abnormal cardiac impulse formation or conduction. Digoxin, adenosine, and atropine are used in the treatment of cardiac dysrhythmias (see Table 22-1).

Digoxin

Digoxin is a digitalis glycoside whose predominant antiarrhythmic effect is on the AV node of the conduction system. It can be used for ventricular rate control in atrial fibrillation and as a weak inotrope in chronic heart failure. Digoxin affects the automatic nervous system by stimulating the parasympathetic division, which increases vagal tone. This vagal effect slows conduction through the AV node and prolongs the AV nodal refractory period. ECG changes are seen in an increased PR interval, a downward-sloping ST depression, and a shortened QT interval.

Digoxin is commonly used to slow electrical impulse conduction through the AV node, thus slowing the ventricular rate in supraventricular dysrhythmias such as atrial fibrillation/flutter. Digoxin is not effective for converting atrial fibrillation/flutter to sinus rhythm. Although digoxin is frequently used to control ventricular rate in patients with left ventricular dysfunction and concomitant atrial fibrillation/flutter, its use does tend to be limited by its relatively slow onset of action and its inability to control heart rate during exercise and even during normal daily activities. Even after an appropriate loading dose is administered, digoxin's peak onset of effect is delayed for up to 6 to 8 hours. Achievement of steady-state concentrations may take up to a week in patients with normal renal function, even longer in patients with renal insufficiency. The increased sympathetic tone that is generated during exercise tends to offset the vagal effects of digoxin, which limits its efficacy under these conditions. In patients with left ventricular dysfunction and concomitant atrial fibrillation/flutter, digoxin can provide effective heart rate control without increasing the risk for worsening heart failure symptoms because of its additional positive inotropic effects.

Digoxin toxicity can be precipitated by declining renal function, electrolyte disturbances, and drug interactions. Because digoxin is primarily excreted unchanged by the kidneys, a decline in the creatinine clearance can predispose a patient to digoxin toxicity. Hypokalemia, hypomagnesemia, and hypercalcemia can also predispose the myocardium to the toxic effects of digoxin. Concomitant drug therapy with agents such as amiodarone and verapamil can also increase serum digoxin concentrations. Potential signs and symptoms of digoxin toxicity include heart block, AV junctional tachycardia, ventricular arrhythmias, visual disturbances (eg, blurred vision, yellow/green halos), dizziness, weakness, nausea, vomiting, diarrhea, and anorexia. Digoxin toxicity can essentially precipitate the development of virtually any type of supraventricular or ventricular arrhythmia. Cardiac glycosides have a narrow therapeutic index. Therefore, to prevent digitalis toxicity, the dosage should be individualized based on the patient's serum digitalis concentration. The therapeutic range is 0.5 to 2 ng/mL.

Adenosine

Adenosine is an antiarrhythmic agent used for converting PSVT to sinus rhythm. It activates K^+ channels and by increasing the outward K^+ current hyperpolarizes the membrane potential, decreasing spontaneous SA nodal depolarization. The nucleoside may also decrease the inward Ca^{2+} current by blocking adenylate cyclase, which normally increases the inward Ca^{2+} current. Automaticity (phase 4) and conduction (phase 0) are inhibited in the SA and AV nodes. The most common adverse effects of adenosine include chest discomfort, dyspnea, flushing, and headache. Sinus arrest can also occur. However, because of adenosine's short half-life of 10 seconds, these adverse effects are short-lived. Adenosine is administered IV because of its short half-life.

Atropine

Atropine sulfate is a parasympatholytic drug that enhances both sinus nodal automaticity and AV nodal conduction through direct vagolytic action. Atropine blocks acetylcholine at parasympathetic neuroeffector sites. Atropine is used almost exclusively in the monitored clinical setting for slow dysrhythmias causing symptomatic bradycardia.

Patients who do not experience symptoms or signs of hemodynamic compromise, ischemia, or frequent ventricular ectopy do not require atropine in bradycardic events. Atropine has been reported to be harmful in some patients with AV block at the His-Purkinje level (type II AV block and third-degree AV block with a new wide QRS complex). Atropine can be used in these situations, but the practitioner must monitor the patient closely for paradoxical slowing of the heart rate.

Atropine may induce tachycardia, which may result in poor outcomes in patients with myocardial ischemia or infarction. Therefore, atropine should be used cautiously in patients with myocardial ischemia.

Selecting the Most Appropriate Agent

Determining the cause and type of the dysrhythmia is essential to selecting the most appropriate agent. Figures 22-1 to 22-5, as well as Table 22-1, guide the practitioner in the initial assessment of which drug to use for each patient. The practitioner should know how to manage dysrhythmias in cardiovascular and cardiopulmonary conditions in which the patient is not in cardiovascular compromise or collapse. These dysrhythmias could lead to life-threatening dysrhythmias and cardiac arrest. This discussion presents the initial approach to dysrhythmias that, unless identified and treated, may deteriorate to cardiac arrest. These dysrhythmias can be categorized as serious, nonlethal dysrhythmias that are either "too fast" or "too slow."

The first main question to ask when selecting drug therapy is whether the slow or fast rate of the dysrhythmia

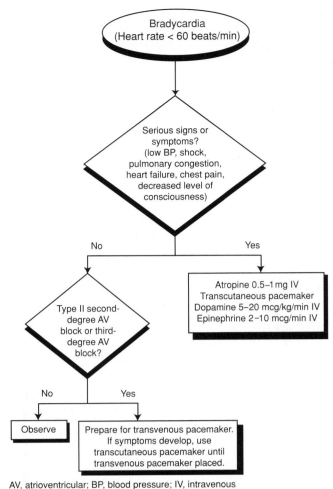

AV, atrioventricular; BP, blood pressure; IV, intravenous

Key ⬭ Starting point for decision making; ☐ clinical actions (assessing, prescribing, monitoring); ◇ decision point.

Figure 22–1 Treatment algorithm for bradycardia. (Adapted from The American Heart Association in Collaboration with the International Liaison Committee on Resuscitation [ILCOR]. [2000]. *Circulation, 102* [Suppl. I], I-156.)

makes the patient ill or symptomatic. A symptomatic patient is one with a dysrhythmia characterized by low blood pressure, shock, chest pain, shortness of breath, decreased level of consciousness, pulmonary congestion, heart failure, or acute MI. The practitioner should not make clinical decisions or take clinical actions based only on the monitor display. For instance, atrial fibrillation may be a stable rhythm from a hemodynamic perspective and may not need immediate treatment. However, treatment of a new onset of atrial fibrillation, even though the patient's heart rate is not too slow or too fast, is important. Treatment is discussed in the first-line and second-line therapy sections. Table 22-2 consolidates the various treatment regimens.

Second, the practitioner must think of treatable conditions that might be causing the dysrhythmia. This is where serum laboratory values and history are important. Some possible causes of dysrhythmias are electrolyte imbalance, drug overdose, drug interactions with other medications, renal failure, endocrine disorders such as hypothyroidism or hyperthyroidism, metabolic acidosis, hypovolemia, MI, pulmonary embolism, cardiac tamponade, tension pneumothorax, dissecting aneurysm, hypoxemia related to pulmonary disorders,

fever, or structural defects in the heart itself. The practitioner should consider the whole picture presented by the patient, not just the cardiac monitor.

The practitioner may have to correct the cause of the dysrhythmia before initiating the drug therapy, especially if the patient is asymptomatic and not ill. However, time may be a critical factor when treating symptomatic dysrhythmias.

Initial vagal maneuvers may serve both a diagnostic and therapeutic purpose. For example, carotid sinus massage may make the flutter waves in atrial flutter more apparent. Appearance of flutter waves allows the practitioner to differentiate atrial flutter from atrial fibrillation, PSVT, or other tachycardias. Vagal maneuvers may include some of the following: unilateral carotid sinus massage, breath holding, facial immersion in ice water, coughing, nasogastric tube placement, gag reflex stimulation by tongue blade or fingers, eyeball pressure, squatting, digital sweep of the anus, and bearing down during a bowel movement. Many patients who have recurrent PSVT with disorders such as mitral valve prolapse learn how to do these maneuvers and terminate the dysrhythmia themselves.

Note: Eyeball massage should never be taught, encouraged, or performed, because it may cause a retinal detachment. Carotid massage (firm massage of the carotid sinus that never lasts for more than 5 to 10 seconds) should be performed only with continuous ECG monitoring and an IV line in place. The procedure should be avoided in elderly patients and should not be performed on patients with carotid bruits because it may occlude already impaired circulation to the brain. Likewise, the practitioner should avoid ice water facial immersion in patients with ischemic heart disease.

Atrial Fibrillation/Flutter

Atrial fibrillation and atrial flutter may be stable or unstable. If the patient has hemodynamic instability (severe hypotension, syncope, heart failure, or angina), the practitioner should prepare for immediate electrical (direct current [DC]) cardioversion. When the patient is hemodynamically stable, the practitioner should consider acute conditions that might cause the atrial fibrillation/flutter that may be reversible. Such conditions include acute MI, hypoxia, pulmonary embolism, electrolyte imbalance, medication toxicity (especially digoxin or sympathomimetic agents), thyrotoxicosis, and alcohol intoxication. Since new-onset atrial fibrillation can be due to acute MI, the practitioner should look for ischemic changes on the 12-lead ECG. If acute ischemic changes appear, admission of the patient to the hospital in a monitored bed may be needed. Obviously, correction and treatment of acute causes of atrial fibrillation/flutter should be a priority.

If not treated, atrial fibrillation/flutter can lead to serious hemodynamic and thromboembolic consequences. A rapid ventricular rate can induce angina in patients with ischemic heart disease or worsening signs and symptoms of heart failure in patients with systolic or diastolic dysfunction. A persistently rapid ventricular rate may lead to the development of a tachycardia-induced cardiomyopathy. Loss of synchronized atrial contraction can lead to a significant reduction in cardiac output, which can especially affect patients with underlying heart failure. In addition, loss of coordinated atrial contraction can lead to the pooling of blood and subsequent thrombus formation. Therefore, these arrhythmias can lead to serious thromboembolic complications, particularly ischemic stroke. Overall, the treatment goals for atrial fibrillation/flutter are

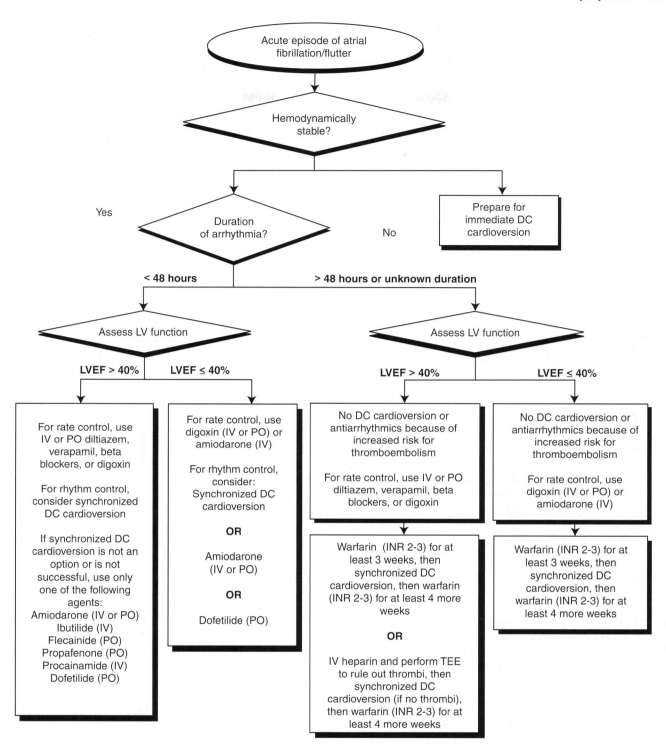

DC, direct current; INR, International Normalized Ratio; IV, intravenous; LV, left ventricular; LVEF, left ventricular ejection fraction; PO, oral; TEE, transesophageal echocardiogram

Key ⬭ Starting point for decision making; ▭ clinical actions (assessing, prescribing, monitoring); ◇ decision point.

Figure 22–2 Treatment algorithm for acute atrial fibrillation/flutter. (Adapted from The American Heart Association in Collaboration with the International Liaison Committee on Resuscitation [ILCOR]. [2000]. *Circulation, 102* [Suppl. I], I-158–I-165 and Fuster, V., et al. [2001]. *Journal of the American College of Cardiology, 38*, 1231.)

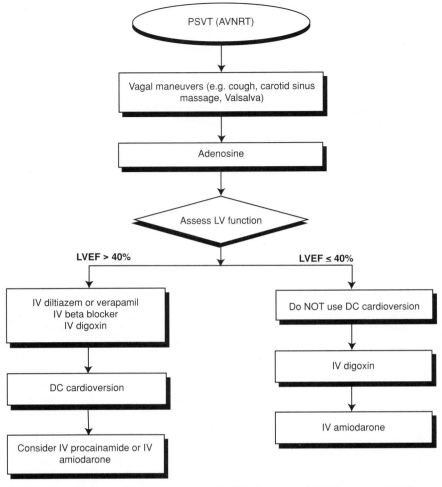

AVNRT, atrioventricular nodal reentrant tachycardia; DC, direct current; IV, intravenous; LV, left ventricular; LVEF, left ventricular ejection fraction; PSVT, paroxysmal supraventricular tachycardia

Key ⬭ Starting point for decision making; ▭ clinical actions (assessing, prescribing, monitoring); ◇ decision point.

Figure 22–3 Treatment algorithm for paroxysmal supraventricular tachycardia (due to atrioventricular nodal reentrant tachycardia). (Adapted from The American Heart Association in Collaboration with the International Liaison Committee on Resuscitation [ILCOR]. [2000]. *Circulation, 102* [Suppl. I], I–162.)

controlling the ventricular rate, restoring and maintaining sinus rhythm, and preventing thromboembolic events.

First-Line Therapy

If the patient is hemodynamically unstable (ie, severe hypotension, syncope, heart failure, or angina), immediate DC cardioversion is first-line therapy. If the patient is hemodynamically stable and has a rapid ventricular rate, the first priority is to control the ventricular rate. In the acute treatment of atrial fibrillation, the selection of a drug to control the ventricular rate depends on the patient's left ventricular function (American Heart Association, 2000). In patients with preserved left ventricular function (left ventricular ejection fraction more than 40%), IV diltiazem, verapamil, beta blockers, or digoxin can be used. Of these options, IV diltiazem, verapamil, or a beta blocker is usually preferred because of digoxin's relatively slow onset of action. Beta blockers are especially useful in high adrenergic states (ie, postoperative patients, hyperthyroidism). The use of digoxin

is limited by its relatively slow onset of action and its inability to control heart rate in high adrenergic states (ie, exercise). In patients with left ventricular dysfunction (left ventricular ejection fraction 40% or less), IV digoxin or amiodarone can be used to control the ventricular rate acutely (American Heart Association, 2000). Digoxin is often used as first-line therapy in this setting because of its added positive inotropic effects. IV amiodarone can be used as an alternative in patients with left ventricular systolic dysfunction. Since amiodarone is a class III antiarrhythmic agent, the practitioner should be aware that the patient may convert to sinus rhythm when using this agent. Patients with atrial fibrillation that has persisted for longer than 48 hours are at risk for thromboembolic events if conversion to sinus rhythm occurs in the absence of therapeutic anticoagulation. Therefore, in these patients who have not been therapeutically anticoagulated, IV amiodarone should be used with caution or avoided. The use of non-dihydropyridine calcium channel blockers and beta blockers for acute ventricular rate control should be avoided in patients with left ventricular systolic

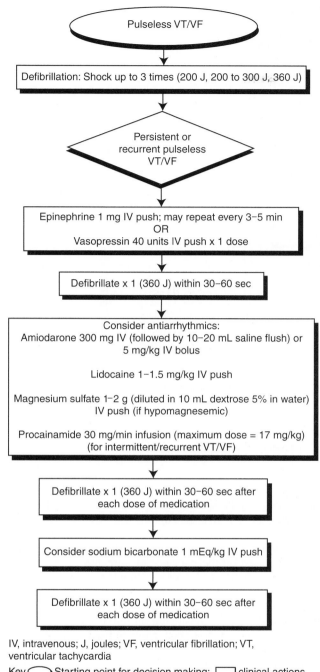

IV, intravenous; J, joules; VF, ventricular fibrillation; VT, ventricular tachycardia

Key ⬭ Starting point for decision making; ▭ clinical actions (assessing, prescribing, monitoring); ◇ decision point.

Figure 22–4 Treatment algorithm for pulseless ventricular tachycardia/ventricular fibrillation. (Adapted from The American Heart Association in Collaboration with the International Liaison Committee on Resuscitation [ILCOR]. [2000]. *Circulation, 102* [Suppl. I], I-147.)

dysfunction because their inotropic effects may precipitate worsening heart failure symptoms.

Second-Line Therapy

Once the ventricular rate is acutely controlled, in patients with a first episode of atrial fibrillation or in those who experience severe symptoms during episodes of recurrent atrial fibrillation, it is reasonable to consider cardioversion as an initial manage-

ment strategy. Because patients with underlying left ventricular dysfunction tend to develop worsening heart failure symptoms when atrial fibrillation develops, these patients should also be considered for cardioversion as an initial management strategy. Restoration of sinus rhythm in patients with atrial fibrillation can be achieved by either DC or pharmacologic cardioversion. Direct current cardioversion appears to be associated with higher success rates than pharmacologic cardioversion. The decision of whether to proceed acutely with cardioversion usually depends on the duration of the arrhythmia.

If the atrial fibrillation has been present for more than 48 hours or for an unknown duration, cardioversion should not be performed acutely because of the risk of thromboembolism (American Heart Association, 2000). Restoration to sinus rhythm may dislodge thrombi in the atria. These patients should be therapeutically anticoagulated with warfarin for at least 3 weeks. After that time, the patient can then undergo DC or pharmacologic cardioversion, which should be followed by at least another 4 weeks of therapeutic anticoagulation with warfarin. Specifically, in patients with preserved left ventricular function (left ventricular ejection fraction more than 40%) and atrial fibrillation that has been present for more than 48 hours or an unknown duration, a transesophageal echocardiogram could alternatively be performed initially (while the patient is being anticoagulated with IV heparin) to rule out the presence of thrombi. By performing this procedure, the practitioner could avoid the initial 3 weeks of anticoagulation, thus accelerating the time to cardioversion. If no thrombi are present in these patients, DC or pharmacologic cardioversion can be performed within 24 hours, followed by the use of therapeutic anticoagulation with warfarin for at least 4 additional weeks. If a thrombus is detected, then the patient should receive at least 3 weeks of therapeutic anticoagulation with warfarin prior to DC or pharmacologic cardioversion. (See Chapter 54 for a discussion of anticoagulation in atrial fibrillation.)

If the atrial fibrillation has been present for less than 48 hours, the practitioner may proceed with cardioversion without anticoagulation, since the risk of thromboembolism is low (American Heart Association, 2000). The practitioner can consider DC cardioversion as initial therapy in patients with either preserved or depressed left ventricular function. However, if the practitioner decides to use pharmacologic cardioversion as the initial therapy, the selection of drug should be based on the patient's left ventricular function. In patients with preserved left ventricular function (left ventricular ejection fraction above 40%), IV amiodarone, ibutilide, or procainamide can be used. Additionally, oral flecainide or propafenone can be used in these patients. In patients with left ventricular dysfunction (left ventricular ejection fraction 40% or less), amiodarone (given IV or orally) or dofetilide can be used.

If the practitioner does not wish to proceed with cardioversion, an initial management strategy of ventricular rate control and anticoagulation is also reasonable. This strategy, whereby the patient is left in atrial fibrillation, has been shown to be an acceptable alternative to rhythm control for the chronic management of atrial fibrillation, especially in patients with recurrent atrial fibrillation and risk factors for stroke (Wyse et al., 2002). The selection of an oral drug for chronic ventricular rate control is primarily based on the patient's left ventricular function. In patients with preserved left ventricular function (left ventricular ejection fraction

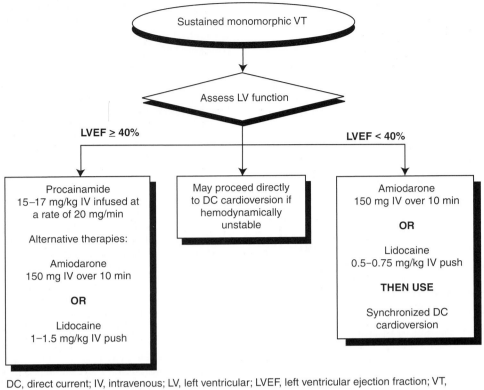

Figure 22–5   Treatment algorithm for sustained monomorphic ventricular tachycardia. (Adapted from The American Heart Association in Collaboration with the International Liaison Committee on Resuscitation [ILCOR]. [2000]. *Circulation, 102* [Suppl. I], I-163.)

above 40%), an oral beta blocker, diltiazem, or verapamil is preferred over digoxin. In patients with left ventricular dysfunction (left ventricular ejection fraction 40% or less), an oral beta blocker or digoxin is preferred because these agents can also concomitantly be used to treat chronic heart failure. The non-dihydropyridine calcium channel blockers should be avoided in patients with left ventricular systolic dysfunction because of their potent negative inotropic effects. In patients with atrial fibrillation and stable heart failure symptoms, the beta blockers, carvedilol, metoprolol, or bisoprolol should be used as first-line therapy because of their documented survival benefits in patients with heart failure (CIBIS II Investigators and Committees, 1999; MERIT-HF Study Group, 1999; Packer et al., 1996). Other beta blockers should be avoided in these patients, since their effects on survival in heart failure are unknown. Digoxin should be used as first-line therapy in patients with atrial fibrillation and worsening heart failure symptoms, since beta-blocker therapy may exacerbate the heart failure symptoms. Because chronic tachycardia can increase a patient's chance of developing a cardiomyopathy, the goal heart rate should be less than 80 beats/min at rest and less than 100 beats/min during exercise.

Third-Line Therapy

For patients who develop severe symptoms during atrial fibrillation episodes, it is reasonable to consider antiarrhythmic drug therapy to maintain sinus rhythm once they have been converted to sinus rhythm. Once again, because patients

with underlying left ventricular dysfunction tend to feel better when they are in sinus rhythm, chronic antiarrhythmic therapy should be considered in this population. The selection of an antiarrhythmic drug to maintain sinus rhythm is primarily based on the presence of structural heart disease (Fuster et al., 2001). In patients without structural heart disease, any oral class IA, IC, or III antiarrhythmic can be used to maintain sinus rhythm. However, flecainide, propafenone, or sotalol should be considered as initial therapy in these patients because of their better adverse effect profiles. In patients with any type of structural heart disease, the class IC antiarrhythmics, flecainide and propafenone, should be avoided. In these patients, the selection of antiarrhythmic drug therapy is based upon the type of structural heart disease present. In patients with left ventricular dysfunction (left ventricular ejection fraction 40% or less), either oral amiodarone or dofetilide can be used. In patients with coronary artery disease, sotalol can be used as initial therapy as long as the left ventricular function is normal. Amiodarone or dofetilide can be considered as an alternative therapy in these patients if sotalol is not tolerated. In patients with left ventricular hypertrophy, amiodarone is the drug of choice.

For patients with permanent atrial fibrillation, a treatment strategy of ventricular rate control and anticoagulation should be used, since the efficacy of antiarrhythmics is extremely poor in this population. The oral drugs used for ventricular rate control are discussed in the "Second-Line Therapy" section. Drug-refractory patients may also be considered for AV nodal ablation.

Table 22.2

Recommended Order of Treatment for Dysrhythmias

Order	Agents	Comments
Atrial Fibrillation/Flutter		
First line	Hemodynamically unstable patient: synchronized DC cardioversion. Start with 100 J and proceed to 200, 300, and 360 J if not successful in the preceding cardioversions. Hemodynamically stable patient with rapid ventricular rate: • Normal LV systolic function (EF > 40%): IV diltiazem, IV verapamil, IV beta blocker, or IV digoxin • LV systolic dysfunction (EF ≤ 40%): IV digoxin or IV amiodarone	Start with 50 J in patients with atrial flutter. Premedicate whenever possible when performing DC cardioversion. Avoid the use of IV amiodarone for rate control in patients with LV dysfunction if the atrial fibrillation/flutter has been present >48 h as these patients may be at risk for thromboembolic events induced by conversion to sinus rhythm.
Second line	Patients with 1st episode of arrhythmia or with severe symptoms associated with arrhythmia: Electrical or pharmacologic cardioversion can be considered once ventricular rate acutely controlled. Decision of whether to proceed acutely with cardioversion depends on the duration of the arrhythmia: • <48 hrs: May proceed with cardioversion without anticoagulation. For pharmacologic cardioversion, the antiarrhythmic used depends on patient's LV function. • >48 hrs or unknown duration: Anticoagulate with warfarin (INR 2–3) for at least 3 weeks before proceeding with cardioversion. Anticoagulate with warfarin (INR 2–3) for at least 4 weeks following cardioversion.	A TEE can be performed in patients with atrial fibrillation (>48 hrs or unknown duration) and preserved LV function to exclude the presence of thrombi and to facilitate cardioversion. IV heparin should be started in these patients. If a thrombus is detected, the patient should be anticoagulated with warfarin (INR 2–3) for at least 3 weeks prior to cardioversion. If no thrombus is detected, cardioversion can be performed within 24 h without the need for the initial 3-week period of anticoagulation. These patients will still require anticoagulation after cardioversion for at least 4 weeks. For antiarrhythmics to be used for acute pharmacologic cardioversion, see Figure 22-2.
	For patients with recurrent atrial fibrillation and risk factors for stroke, a strategy of ventricular rate control and anticoagulation is a reasonable alternative to rhythm control. Selection of PO drug for ventricular rate control (diltiazem, verapamil, beta blocker, or digoxin) depends on patient's LV function. Warfarin therapy should be maintained at INR of 2–3.	Goal heart rate is <80 beats/min at rest and <100 beats/min during exercise. PO agents for ventricular rate control: • Normal LV systolic function (EF > 40%): diltiazem, verapamil, or beta blockers • LV systolic dysfunction (EF ≤ 40%): beta blockers or digoxin PO antiarrhythmic agents for chronic rhythm control:
Third line	Chronic antiarrhythmic therapy can be considered for patients who develop severe symptoms during episodes of atrial fibrillation. The antiarrhythmic used depends on patient's LV function and the type of structural heart disease that may be present. For patients with permanent atrial fibrillation, a strategy of ventricular rate control and anticoagulation should be considered. Selection of PO drug for ventricular rate control (diltiazem, verapamil, beta blocker, or digoxin) depends on patient's LV function. Warfarin therapy should be maintained at INR of 2–3. If the patient's heart rate remains uncontrolled, an AV nodal ablation can be performed.	• No structural heart disease: flecainide, propafenone, sotalol, amiodarone, dofetilide, procainamide, quinidine, or disopyramide • LV systolic dysfunction (EF ≤ 40%): amiodarone or dofetilide • Coronary artery disease: sotalol, amiodarone, or dofetilide • LV hypertrophy: amiodarone Avoid flecainide and propafenone in patients with *any* form of structural heart disease.
Paroxysmal Supraventricular Tachycardia (due to AVNRT)		
First line	Hemodynamically unstable patient: synchronized DC cardioversion. Start with 100 J and proceed to 200, 300, and 360 J if not successful in the preceding cardioversions. Hemodynamically stable patient: vagal maneuvers	Premedicate whenever possible when performing DC cardioversion. Examples of vagal maneuvers include unilateral carotid sinus massage, Valsalva maneuver, facial immersion in ice water, and coughing. Carotid sinus massage should be avoided in patients with carotid bruits or history of cerebrovascular disease.
Second line	IV adenosine Subsequent antiarrhythmic therapy depends on patient's LV function • Normal LV systolic function (EF > 40%): IV diltiazem, IV verapamil, or IV beta blockers; if PSVT is persistent, can attempt synchronized DC cardioversion; if PSVT remains persistent, can use IV procainamide or IV amiodarone • LV systolic dysfunction (EF ≤ 40%): IV digoxin or IV amiodarone	

(continued)

Table 22.2

Recommended Order of Treatment for Dysrhythmias (Continued)

Order	Agents	Comments
Third line	If patient continues to have frequent episodes of PSVT or infrequent episodes accompanied by severe symptoms, refer for possible radiofrequency catheter ablation. If patient is not a candidate for or refuses radiofreqency catheter ablation, PO diltiazem, verapamil, beta blocker, or digoxin can be used for chronic therapy.	If PSVT is infrequent and/or accompanied by only mild symptoms, no chronic therapy is needed.
Premature Ventricular Contractions		
First line	No structural heart disease: • Asymptomatic or minimal symptoms: No drug therapy • Symptomatic: PO beta blocker Structural heart disease: • Asymptomatic or minimal symptoms: PO beta blocker (especially patients who are post-MI or those with LV systolic dysfunction (EF ≤ 40%) • Symptomatic: PO beta blocker	Patients who are post-MI or with LV systolic dysfunction (EF ≤ 40%), should receive a beta blocker even if they have no or minimal symptoms associated with the PVCs to reduce mortality associated with these disease states.
Second line	Same as first line	
Third line	Same as first line	
Nonsustained Ventricular Tachycardia		
First line	No structural heart disease: • Asymptomatic or minimal symptoms: No drug therapy • Symptomatic: PO beta blocker Post-MI patients: • Normal LV systolic function (EF > 40%): PO beta blocker regardless of the presence of symptoms • LV systolic dysfunction (EF ≤ 40%): EP testing; if sustanied VT/VF, ICD should be placed; if sustained VT/VF noninducible, PO beta blocker or amiodarone may be used.	Correct reversible causes. Post-MI patients with normal LV systolic function should receive a beta blocker even if they have no or minimal symptoms associated with the NSVT to reduce mortality associated with the MI. If frequent shocks occur in patients with an ICD, PO amiodarone (preferred for patients with LV systolic dysfunction) or sotalol can be started.
Second line	Same as first line	
Third line	Same as first line	
Sustained Ventricular Tachycardia		
First line	Hemodynamically unstable patient: synchronized DC cardioversion. Start with 100 J and proceed to 200, 300, and 360 J if not successful in the preceding cardioversions. Hemodynamically stable patient: • Normal LV systolic function (EF > 40%): IV procainamide • LV systolic dysfunction (EF ≤ 40%): IV amiodarone or lidocaine, then synchronized DC cardioversion	Premedicate whenever possible when performing DC cardioversion. Correct reversible causes.
Second line	Normal LV systolic function (EF > 40%): IV amiodarone or lidocaine Once arrhythmia acutely terminated, patient should be considered for ICD placement. If patient refuses or is not a candidate for an ICD, oral amiodarone or a beta blocker (as an alternative to amiodarone) can be considered.	If frequent shocks occur in patients with an ICD, PO amiodarone (preferred for patients with LV systolic dysfunction) or sotalol can be started.
Pulseless Ventricular Tachycardia/Ventricular Fibrillation		
First line	Establish an airway, start CPR, and defibrillate with up to three shocks, if needed (200 J, 200–300 J, and 300 J).	Correct reversible causes.
Second line	If patient remains in pulseless VT/VF, continue CPR and give epinephrine 1 mg IV push or vasopressin 40 units IV push, then shock with 360 J within 30–60 sec.	
Third line	The epinephrine 1 mg IV push can be continued every 3–5 min for as long as the arrhythmia persists. Only one dose of vasopressin should be given.	

(continued)

Table 22.2

Recommended Order of Treatment for Dysrhythmias *(Continued)*

Order	Agents	Comments
	If patient remains in pulseless VT/VF, consider antiarrhythmic therapy (IV amiodarone, lidocaine, IV magnesium sulfate, IV procainamide, IV sodium bicarbonate).	
Bradycardia		
First line	If patient is successfully resuscitated, ICD placement should be considered. Patient with unstable bradycardia (heart rate <60 beats/min accompanied by symptoms): atropine 0.5–1 mg IV push	Correct reversible causes.
Second line	Patient with stable bradycardia: • 2nd or 3rd degree heart block: Transcutaneous pacing should be used until transvenous pacer can be inserted. • No 2nd or 3rd degree heart block: Observe the patient.	
Third line	If unstable bradycardia persists, consider transcutaneous pacing. If unstable bradycardia persists, dopamine or epinephrine continuous infusion may be started.	

AV, atrioventricular; CPR, cardiopulmonary resuscitation; DC, direct current; EF, ejection fraction; ICD, implantable cardioverter-defibrillator; INR, International Normalized Ratio; IV, intravenous; J, joules; LV, left ventricular; MI, myocardial infarction; NSVT, nonsustained ventricular tachycardia; PO, oral; PSVT, paroxysmal supraventricular tachycardia; PVC, premature ventricular contraction; TEE, transesophageal echocardiogram; VF, ventricular fibrillation; VT, ventricular tachycardia.

Paroxysmal Supraventricular Tachycardia (Due to Atrioventricular Nodal Reentrant Tachycardia)

First-Line Therapy

Hemodynamically unstable PSVT requires first-line therapy of DC cardioversion to restore sinus rhythm and correct hemodynamic compromise. Unless contraindicated, patients with mild to moderate symptoms can be initially managed with vagal maneuvers (eg, unilateral carotid sinus massage, Valsalva maneuver, facial immersion in ice water, and coughing).

Second-Line Therapy

If vagal maneuvers are unsuccessful or if the PSVT recurs after successful vagal maneuvers, second-line therapy is antiarrhythmic therapy. The first-choice drug for PSVT is adenosine. Clinical studies have shown that adenosine is as effective as IV verapamil in initial conversion of PSVT. Adenosine does not produce hypotension to the degree that verapamil does, and it has a short half-life. If a total of 30 mg of adenosine does not successfully terminate PSVT, further doses of this agent are unlikely to be effective. Therefore, in patients with persistent PSVT, other antiarrhythmic agents will need to be used. The selection of a subsequent treatment regimen depends on the patient's left ventricular function (American Heart Association, 2000). In patients with preserved left ventricular function (left ventricular ejection fraction above 40%), IV diltiazem, verapamil, or a beta blocker is preferred. IV digoxin can be considered if these agents are ineffective or contraindicated. If these drugs fail to terminate the PSVT, DC cardioversion can be considered. If the PSVT continues despite these treatment measures, the use of IV procainamide or amiodarone can also be considered. In patients with left ventricular dysfunction (left ventricular ejection fraction 40% or less), IV digoxin is the preferred agent. IV amiodarone can be considered an alternative in these patients if digoxin is ineffective or contraindicated.

Third-Line Therapy

Third-line therapy focuses on the management of chronic PSVT. Chronic preventive therapy is usually necessary if the patient has either frequent episodes of PSVT that require therapeutic intervention or infrequent episodes of PSVT that are accompanied by severe symptoms. RF catheter ablation is considered first-line therapy for most of these patients because of its effectiveness in preventing recurrence of PSVT and its relatively low complication rate. Drug therapy with oral diltiazem, verapamil, beta blockers, or digoxin can also be considered if the patient is not a candidate for or refuses to undergo RF catheter ablation.

Premature Ventricular Contractions

Occasional PVCs occur in most people and rarely compromise cardiac output or function. Correcting reversible causes such as an electrolyte imbalance sometimes eliminates these benign PVCs. Asymptomatic or minimally symptomatic PVCs in patients without associated heart disease carry little or no risk. PVCs in patients with heart disease were traditionally treated in the past: decreasing the number and frequency of PVCs was thought to diminish the risk of sudden cardiac death. However, the results of the CAST study showed that the use of antiarrhythmic drug therapy to suppress asymptomatic PVCs in patients after MI may increase mortality rates (CAST Investigators, 1989). Therefore, if patients with structural heart disease have symptomatic PVCs, drug therapy should be limited to beta blockers. These agents have been associated with a reduction in mortality and sudden cardiac death in post-MI patients. These agents are also effective for suppressing symptomatic PVCs in patients without structural heart disease. Asymptomatic PVCs do not require treatment.

Nonsustained Ventricular Tachycardia

Ventricular tachycardia that spontaneously terminates within 30 seconds is known as nonsustained VT. Given the poor survival of patients who experience cardiac arrest, it is essential to identify the most effective treatment strategies to prevent the initial episode of sustained VT or sudden cardiac death from occurring.

The presence of nonsustained VT in patients without structural heart disease is not associated with an increased risk of sudden cardiac death. Therefore, drug therapy is not necessary in these patients if they are asymptomatic. However, if these patients do become symptomatic, beta-blocker therapy can be initiated. Post-MI patients (especially those with left ventricular dysfunction) who develop nonsustained VT are at increased risk for sudden cardiac death. For these patients, the selection of therapy is based on the patient's left ventricular function. In post-MI patients with preserved left ventricular function (left ventricular ejection fraction above 40%), drug therapy is not necessary to treat the arrhythmia if they are asymptomatic. However, these patients should still chronically receive a beta blocker specifically to reduce mortality associated with the MI. Beta blockers are also effective if these patients develop significant symptoms associated with the nonsustained VT. In post-MI patients with left ventricular dysfunction (left ventricular ejection fraction 40% or less), electrophysiologic testing is often performed when asymptomatic nonsustained VT occurs (Moss et al., 1996; Buxton et al., 1999). If sustained ventricular tachyarrhythmia is induced, an ICD is then recommended. If sustained ventricular tachyarrhythmia is not induced, a beta blocker or amiodarone can be initiated.

Sustained Ventricular Tachycardia

VT that persists for at least 30 seconds or that requires electrical or pharmacologic termination because of hemodynamic instability is known as sustained VT. Since sustained VT can degenerate into VF, the treatment goals are to terminate the VT acutely and then prevent recurrence of the arrhythmia.

First-Line Therapy

If the patient is hemodynamically unstable (ie, severe hypotension, syncope, heart failure, or angina), immediate DC cardioversion is first-line therapy. If the patient is hemodynamically stable, the selection of antiarrhythmic drug therapy to terminate the VT acutely is based on the patient's left ventricular function (American Heart Association, 2000). For patients with preserved left ventricular function (left ventricular ejection fraction above 40%), IV procainamide is the antiarrhythmic of first choice. In patients

with left ventricular dysfunction (left ventricular ejection fraction 40% or less), the first-line antiarrhythmic therapy to terminate the VT acutely is either IV amiodarone or lidocaine. After administering either of these agents, synchronized cardioversion should be used.

Second-Line Therapy

For the acute termination of sustained VT, second-line therapy is recommended only for patients with preserved left ventricular function (left ventricular ejection fraction above 40%) (American Heart Association, 2000). In these patients, either IV amiodarone or lidocaine is acceptable. Because IV amiodarone and lidocaine possess relatively minimal negative inotropic effects in comparison to the other IV antiarrhythmic agents, these are the only antiarrhythmics recommended for the acute termination of sustained VT in patients with left ventricular dysfunction.

Once the acute episode is terminated, measures should be taken to prevent recurrent episodes of VT. Based on the results of several trials, ICDs are clearly indicated as first-line therapy in patients with a history of sustained VT or VF (AVID Investigators, 1997; Connolly et al., 2000; Kuck et al., 2000). If patients with an ICD experience frequent discharges because of recurrent ventricular arrhythmias or new-onset supraventricular arrhythmias, oral amiodarone or sotalol therapy can be initiated. For patients who refuse or are not candidates for an ICD, oral amiodarone should be used as an alternative therapy. If a patient refuses or is not a candidate for either an ICD or amiodarone, beta-blocker therapy can then be used.

Pulseless Ventricular Tachycardia/Ventricular Fibrillation

The majority of cases of sudden cardiac death can be attributed to VF. Sustained VT usually precedes VF and most commonly occurs in patients with ischemic heart disease. VF is usually not preceded by any symptoms and always results in a loss of consciousness and eventually death if not treated. Immediate treatment is necessary in patients who develop VF or pulseless VT, since survival is reduced by 10% for every minute that the patient remains in the arrhythmia.

First-Line Therapy

First-line therapy for pulseless VT/VF is defibrillation up to three times at 200, 200 to 300, and 360 J successively. Obviously, the practitioner must correct any reversible causes for the arrhythmia, if possible.

Second-Line Therapy

If the pulseless VT/VF is persistent or recurrent, second-line therapy is vasopressor therapy, which includes either epinephrine or vasopressin (American Heart Association, 2000). In this situation, vasopressin can be considered as an alternative to epinephrine. Vasopressin's half-life of approximately 10 to 20 minutes is considerably longer than the 3- to 5-minute half-life of epinephrine, which suggests that its vasopressor effects may be more sustained than those of epinephrine during cardiac arrest. Unlike epinephrine, vasopressin also maintains its vasoconstrictive effects under acidotic and hypoxic conditions, which suggests that this agent may continue to work during prolonged cardiac arrest situations. The recommended dosage of epinephrine for pulseless VT/VF is 1 mg IV push every 3 to 5 minutes. The recommended dosage of vasopressin for pulseless VT/VF is 40 units IV push for one dose only. If there is no response 5 to 10 minutes after the dose of vasopressin is administered, the routine use of epinephrine 1 mg IV push every 3 to 5 minutes should be continued for as long as the arrhythmia persists. Each dose of either vasopressin or epinephrine should be followed by a single defibrillation of 360 J.

Third-Line Therapy

If the patient remains in pulseless VT/VF, third-line therapy is to consider antiarrhythmic therapy. IV amiodarone is recommended as first-line antiarrhythmic therapy for the treatment of pulseless VT/VF (American Heart Association, 2000). This agent has been proven to be safe and effective in the management of both in-hospital and out-of-hospital pulseless VT/VF (Dorian et al, 2002; Kudenchuck et al., 1999). Compared to lidocaine, IV amiodarone has been associated with a significantly higher rate of survival to hospital admission in patients with out-of-hospital cardiac arrest due to VF (Dorian et al., 2002). Therefore, lidocaine is now considered as second-line antiarrhythmic therapy for the treatment of pulseless VT/VF (American Heart Association, 2000). IV magnesium sulfate can be considered for patients who have or are thought to have hypomagnesemia. For patients with intermittent or recurrent pulseless VT/VF despite the above therapies, IV procainamide can be used as last-line therapy. In addition, the administration of IV sodium bicarbonate can be considered as the cardiac arrest persists, since the patient is likely to become acidotic. Each dose of all of these medications should be followed by a single defibrillation of 360 J.

If the patient is resuscitated from the pulseless VT/VF episode, measures should be taken to prevent recurrent episodes of cardiac arrest. Based on the results of several trials, ICDs are clearly indicated as first-line therapy in patients with a history of sustained VT or VF (AVID Investigators, 1997; Connolly et al., 2000; Kuck et al., 2000). If patients with an ICD experience frequent discharges because of recurrent ventricular arrhythmias or new-onset supraventricular arrhythmias, oral amiodarone or sotalol therapy can be initiated. For patients who refuse or are not candidates for an ICD, oral amiodarone should be used as an alternative therapy. If a patient refuses or is not a candidate for amiodarone, beta-blocker therapy can then be used.

Bradycardia

Patients with unstable bradycardia can experience hypotension, dizziness, and syncope. First-line therapy for unstable bradycardia is atropine 0.5 to 1 mg IV. If the bradycardia persists, transcutaneous pacing may be considered. If the symptomatic bradycardia continues despite atropine and transcutaneous pacing, a dopamine continuous infusion (5 to 20 mcg/kg/min) can be initiated, followed by an epinephrine continuous infusion (2 to 10 mcg/min), if needed (American Heart Association, 2000). Patients with second- or

third-degree AV block (even in the absence of serious signs and symptoms) should be initially managed with a transcutaneous pacemaker until a transvenous pacer can be inserted.

Special Population Considerations

Pediatric

The epidemiology of dysrhythmias is different between adults and children. Adults have dysrhythmias primarily of a cardiac origin, whereas children have dysrhythmias primarily of a respiratory origin.

Tachyarrhythmias occasionally compromise infants and young children. PSVT is the most common dysrhythmia in young children. It typically occurs during infancy or in children with congenital heart disease. PSVT with ventricular rates exceeding 180 to 220/min can produce signs of shock. If signs of shock appear, synchronized cardioversion or administration of adenosine can be done in an emergency situation. Common causes of PSVT in young children and infants are congenital heart disease (preoperative) such as Ebstein's anomaly, transposition of the great arteries, or a single ventricle. Postoperative PSVT also can occur after atrial surgery for correction of congenital defects of the heart. Other common causes of PSVT in children are drugs such as sympathomimetics (cold medications, theophylline, beta agonists). WPW syndrome and hyperthyroidism also can cause PSVT. Common causes of atrial fibrillation/flutter in children are intra-atrial surgery, Ebstein's anomaly, heart disease with dilated atria (AV valve regurgitation), cardiomyopathy, WPW syndrome, sick sinus syndrome, and myocarditis.

Bradycardia is a common dysrhythmia in seriously ill infants or children. It is usually associated with a fall in cardiac output and is an ominous sign, suggesting that cardiac arrest is imminent. The first-line therapy for this dysrhythmia in infants and young children is administration of oxygen, support respiration, and epinephrine.

Pulseless VT and VF are treated much the same way as in adults. The recommended dose of epinephrine for a pulseless child is 0.01 mg/kg, administered as 0.1 mL/kg of a 1:10,000 dilution.

Geriatric

With aging, body fat increases, lean body tissue decreases, and hepatic and renal system changes set the stage for potential overdosage and toxicity, particularly in the case of antiarrhythmic drugs. Similarly, declining function affects the amount and dosage of the drug prescribed as well as the occurrence of adverse effects. Cardiac disease and chronic conditions such as heart failure exacerbate the decline in organ function. Together, these factors can increase the risk of an adverse effect from the antiarrhythmic medications the practitioner prescribes.

For example, digoxin toxicity is relatively common in elderly patients who are not receiving a reduced dosage to accommodate for the reduced renal function. The practitioner must always have a baseline renal panel to identify abnormalities in the blood urea nitrogen and serum creatinine, and a hepatic panel to identify impairment in liver function. These two tests are important in prescribing the proper dosage of many of the antiarrhythmic medications discussed in this chapter.

Signs and symptoms of adverse effects of many drugs are confusion, weakness, and lethargy. These signs and symptoms are often attributed to senility or disease. Therefore, it is important for the practitioner to take a thorough drug history and to document accurately the dosages and frequencies prescribed in the patient record. If the practitioner merely attributes confusion to old age, the patient may continue to receive the drug while actually experiencing drug toxicity. Furthermore, the practitioner may add another drug to treat the complications caused by the original antiarrhythmic, compounding the issue of polypharmacy and excessive medication.

In elderly patients taking antiarrhythmic medications, the practitioner must be particularly alert to adverse effects from diuretics, digoxin, sleeping aids, and nonprescription drugs.

Antiarrhythmic drugs sometimes require accurate and timely dosing. If an elderly patient forgets to take a dose or cannot remember when he or she took the last dose, undermedication or overmedication may occur. This can be dangerous when antiarrhythmic drugs are prescribed. Many of the elderly have multiple prescriptions, even for the same medication, and therefore take an overdose of the drug. Consequently, it is essential to review medications with elderly patients and make sure they understand and can follow a safe drug therapy regimen.

MONITORING PATIENT RESPONSE

The goals of antiarrhythmic therapy are to restore sinus rhythm and prevent recurrences of the original dysrhythmia or development of new dysrhythmias. Evaluating the outcomes of antiarrhythmic therapy requires the practitioner to schedule regular follow-up visits after initial treatment of the dysrhythmia. The outcomes to be closely monitored include impulse generation and conduction from the SA node to the AV node, time interval for conduction, heart rate within a normal range that is age-specific, and patterns of AV and ventricular conduction.

Data to be monitored to evaluate therapeutic outcomes vary from the simple to complex. The patient may monitor some of them and needs to be taught the signs and symptoms to look for and the expectations from the therapeutic regimen. Patients with dysrhythmias may be monitored on a regular or periodic basis with 12-lead ECG, 24-hour Holter monitors, electrophysiologic testing, monitoring of vital signs (blood pressure, pulse rate), echocardiograms for cardiac function, and electrolytes and serum drug levels.

In addition, the patient needs to self-monitor for symptoms such as lightheadedness, dizziness, syncopal episodes, palpitations, chest pain, shortness of breath, or weight gain. Other clinical outcomes to be monitored are those that affect quality of life, such as activity tolerance, tissue perfusion, cognitive function, fear, anxiety, and depression.

PATIENT EDUCATION

Drug Information

Included in the therapeutic plan for dysrhythmia is patient education. Learning outcomes can be evaluated by monitoring compliance with the medication regimen, recurrences of dysrhythmia, adverse effects, weight gain, blood pressure, heart rate, and emergency department visits or hospitalizations.

Cardiac drugs have prolonged half-lives and narrow therapeutic windows. Toxicity is common at normal dosages. Consequently, patient education is essential for providing maximal benefits and avoiding adverse effects and accidental overdosing or underdosing.

The patient, family, and significant others should be taught the basics, such as the name of the drug (both the generic and trade name), the dose, the frequency and timing of the dose, and the reason the drug is needed. This may avoid duplicate prescribing and administration of antiarrhythmics. The patient should communicate, either verbally or in writing, the names and dosages of these drugs to all other health care providers and should wear a medical identification device listing all medications. In addition, the patient should inform his or her health care provider when any new prescription, over-the-counter, or complementary or alternative medications are started so that potential drug interactions can be minimized or avoided.

The practitioner should provide written instructions for the medication regimen. Providing instructions in large print and simple language may be helpful to patients who have difficulty with memory, hearing, or vision. Instructions should include what to do when the patient misses a dose of medication, has an adverse response to the medication, or wants to stop taking the drug. If beta blockers are prescribed, the patient should be warned that abrupt discontinuance may result in rebound angina, an increased heart rate, and hypertension. The symptoms associated with these adverse effects also should be identified.

The practitioner can also teach the patient or caregiver how to take blood pressure and pulse readings, how to interpret the readings, and how to recognize and respond to signs and symptoms of hypotension, dizziness, chest pain, shortness of breath, peripheral edema, or palpitations. The patient should take his or her weight each day and call the practitioner if a weight gain greater than 2 pounds occurs. If the patient has difficulty learning these monitoring techniques or cannot perform them, he or she may need to schedule regular follow-up appointments for monitoring. Patients with atrial fibrillation or flutter should know the signs and symptoms of a stroke.

In today's health care environment, the insurance plan's pharmacy provider sometimes makes substitutions with generics or less expensive brands of medications. To prevent harmful drug effects, the patient needs to be aware of this practice and should be cautioned not to change brands of the prescribed antiarrhythmic without the approval of the practitioner.

An important teaching point from an ethical and legal perspective is to warn the patient to avoid hazardous activities such as driving, using electrical tools, climbing ladders, or any activity that would put the patient or others in harm's way until the effects of the drug are demonstrated. Patients with an ICD should refrain from driving for at least 6 months after either implantation of the device or an appropriate discharge from the device for a ventricular arrhythmia. Documentation of patient teaching on risks, benefits, lifestyle modification, and safety issues with antiarrhythmic treatment should always be entered in the patient's record. Documenting a review of this information on a follow-up visit aids health care providers who follow up on the patient's progress in the future.

Nutrition

Clear instructions should be given to avoid alcohol, excessive salt intake, and caffeine during treatment for dysrhythmias. Many antiarrhythmics may cause periods of hypotension resulting in dizziness, or the dose of the drug may need to be regulated, especially in the initial weeks.

Complementary and Alternative Medications

The practitioner must emphasize to the patient the importance of reporting the use of any of these agents so that interactions with antiarrhythmic therapy can be minimized or avoided. While the information regarding potential interactions between antiarrhythmic drugs and specific complementary and alternative medications is relatively sparse, there are a few notable interactions of which practitioners should be aware. Patients taking antiarrhythmics should avoid licorice root. Licorice has mineralocorticoid effects, which can promote hypokalemia. In patients taking digoxin, the presence of hypokalemia may predispose the patient to digoxin toxicity. In patients taking other antiarrhythmic agents, the presence of hypokalemia may promote the development of atrial or ventricular arrhythmias. In addition, certain licorice preparations have been shown to cause QT interval prolongation, which may be additive in patients receiving class IA or III antiarrhythmics. This interaction could lead to torsades de pointes. The use of Siberian ginseng or oleander should also be avoided in patients receiving digoxin, as digoxin toxicity may result. The use of St. John's wort may decrease digoxin concentrations; therefore, digoxin concentrations should be closely monitored when concomitant therapy is used. St. John's wort may also decrease plasma concentrations of amiodarone, which may predispose the patient to arrhythmia recurrence. Consequently, the use of St. John's wort in patients receiving amiodarone should be discouraged. Patients with a history of atrial or ventricular arrhythmias should also be instructed to avoid the use of any medication containing ephedra (eg, Ma Huang), since it can promote the development of arrhythmias.

Bibliography

Starred references are cited in the text.

*Akiyama, T., Pawtin, Y., & Campbell, W. B. (1992). Effects of the advancing age on the efficacy and side effects of antiarrhythmic drugs in post myocardial infarction patients with ventricular arrhythmias. *Journal of the Geriatric Society, 40*, 666–672.

*American Heart Association in Collaboration with the International Liaison Committee on Resuscitation (ILCOR) (2000). Guidelines 2000 for cardiopulmonary resuscitation and emergency cardiovascular care: an international consensus on science. *Circulation, 102*(Suppl I), I-142–I-165.

*Anderson, J. L., Lutz, J. R., & Allison, S. B. (1983). Electrophysiologic and antiarrhythmic effects of oral flecainide in patients with inducible ventricular tachycardia. *Journal of the American College of Cardiology, 2*, 105–114.

*Anderson, J. L., & Prystowsky, E. N. (1999). Sotalol: an important new antiarrhythmic. *American Heart Journal, 137*, 3.

*Antiarrhythmics Versus Implantable Defibrillators (AVID) Investigators (1997). A comparison of antiarrhythmic-drug therapy with implantable defibrillators in patients resuscitated from near-fatal ventricular arrhythmias. *New England Journal of Medicine, 337*, 1576–1583.

*Buchanan, L. V., Turcotte, U. M., Kabell, G. G., & Gibson, J. K. (1993). Antiarrhythmic and electrophysiologic effects of ibutilide in a chronic canine model of atrial flutter. *Journal of Cardiovascular Pharmacology, 33*, 10–14.

*Buxton, A. E., Lee, K. L., Fisher, J. D., et al. (1999). A randomized study of the prevention of sudden death in patients with coronary artery disease. *New England Journal of Medicine, 341*, 1882–1890.

Cairns, J. A., Connolly, S. J., & Roberts, R. (1997). Randomized trial of outcome after myocardial infarction in patients with frequent or repetitive ventricular premature depolarizations: CAMIAT. *Lancet, 349*, 675–682.

*Campbell, R. W., Hutton, I., & Elton, R. A. (1983). Prophylaxis of primary ventricular fibrillation with tocainide in acute myocardial infarction. *British Heart Journal, 49*, 557–563.

*Cardiac Suppression Trial Investigators (1989). Preliminary report: effect of encainide and flecainide on mortality in a randomized trial of arrhythmia suppression after myocardial infarction. *New England Journal of Medicine, 321*, 406–412.

*Cardiac Suppression Trial II Investigators (1992). Effect of the antiarrhythmic agent moricizine on survival after myocardial infarction. *New England Journal of Medicine, 327*, 227–233.

*CIBIS II Investigators and Committees (1999). The Cardiac Insufficiency Bisoprolol Study II (CIBIS-II): a randomised trial. *Lancet, 353*, 9–13.

*Connolly, S., Gent, M., Roberts, R. S., et al. (2000). Canadian Implantable Defibrillator Study (CIDS): a randomized trial of the implantable cardioverter defibrillator versus amiodarone. *Circulation, 101*, 1297–1302.

*Coyle, J. D., Carnes, C. A., & Schaal, S. F. (1992). Electrophysiologic interactions of procainamide and N-acetyl-procainamide in isolate canine cardiac Purkinje fibers. *Journal of Cardiovascular Pharmacology, 20*, 197–205.

*Dorian, P., Cass, D., Schwartz, B., et al. (2002). Amiodarone as compared with lidocaine for shock-resistant ventricular fibrillation. *New England Journal of Medicine, 346*, 884–890.

*Duff, H. J., Roden, D., & Primm, R. K. (1983). Mexiletine in the treatment of resistant ventricular arrhythmias: enhancement of efficacy and reduction of dose-related side effects by combination with quinidine. *Circulation, 67*, 1124–1128.

*Ebihara, A., & Fujimura, A. (1991). Metabolites of antihypertensive drugs: an updated review of their clinical pharmacokinetic and therapeutic implications. *Clinical Pharmacokinetics, 21*, 331–343.

*Engler, R. L., & LeWinter, M. (1981). Tocainide-induced ventricular fibrillation. *American Heart Journal, 101*, 494–496.

*Fuster, V., Ryden, L. E., Asinger, R. W., et al. (2001). ACC/AHA/ESC guidelines for the management of patients with atrial fibrillation: a report of the American College of Cardiology/American Heart Association Task Force on Practice Guidelines and the European Society of Cardiology Committee for Practice Guidelines and Policy Conferences. *Journal of the American College of Cardiology, 38*, 1231–1266.

*Goldschlager, N., Epstein, A. E., Naccarelli, G., et al. (2000). Practical guidelines for clinicians who treat patients with amiodarone. *Archives of Internal Medicine, 160*, 1741–1748.

Gray, R. J., Bateman, T. M., & Ozer, L. S. (1985). Esmolol: a new ultrashort-acting beta-adrenergic blocking agent for rapid control of heart rate in postoperative supraventricular tachyarrhythmias. *Journal of the American College of Cardiology, 5*, 141–156.

Gunnar, R. M., Passamani, E. R., Bourdillon, P. D., Pitt, B., Dixon, D. W., Rappaport, E., Fuster, V., Reeves, T. J., Russell, R. O., & Karp, R. B. (1998). Guidelines for the early management of patients with acute myocardial infarction: a report of the American College of Cardiology and American Heart Association Task Force on Assessing Diagnostic and Therapeutic Cardiovascular Procedures (subcommittee to develop guidelines for the early management of patients with acute myocardial infarction). *Journal of the American College of Cardiology, 16,* 249–292.

Julian, D. G., Camm, A. J., & Fragnin, G. (1997). Randomized trial of effect of amiodarone on mortality inpatients with left ventricular dysfunction after recent myocardial infarction: EMIAT. *Lancet, 349,* 667–674.

*Kennedy, H. L., Brooks, M. M., & Barker, A. H. (1994). Beta blocker therapy in the Cardiac Arrhythmia Suppression Trial. *American Journal of Cardiology, 74,* 674–680.

*Køber, L., Bloch-Thomsen, P. E., Møller, M., et al (2000). Danish Investigations of Arrhythmia and Mortality on Dofetilide (DIAMOND) Study Group. Effect of dofetilide in patients with recent myocardial infarction and left-ventricular dysfunction: a randomised trial. *Lancet, 356,* 2052–2058.

*Kuck, K. H., Cappato, R., Siebels, J., et al. (2000). Randomized comparison of antiarrhythmic drug therapy with implantable defibrillators in patients resuscitated from cardiac arrest: the Cardiac Arrest Study Hamburg (CASH). *Circulation, 102,* 748–754.

*Kudenchuck, P. J., Cobb, L. A., Copass, M. K., et al. (1999). Amiodarone for resuscitation after out-of-hospital cardiac arrest due to ventricular fibrillation. *New England Journal of Medicine, 341,* 871–879.

*Lichstein, E., Morganroth, J., Harrist, R., & Hubble, M. S. (1983). Effect of propranolol on ventricular arrhythmia: the beta blocker heart attack trial experience. *Circulation, 67* (Suppl. I), 5–10.

*MERIT-HF Study Group (1999). Effect of metoprolol CR/XL in chronic heart failure: Metoprolol CR/XL Randomized Intervention Trial in Congestive Heart Failure (MERIT-HF). *Lancet, 353,* 2001–2007.

*Miller, M. R., McNamara, R. L., Segal, J. B., et al. (2000). Efficacy of agents for pharmacological conversion of atrial fibrillation and subsequent maintenance of sinus rhythm: a meta-analysis of clinical trials. *Journal of Family Practice, 49,* 1033–1046.

Morganroth, J., & Goin, J. E. (1991). Quinidine related mortality in the short- to medium-term treatment of ventricular arrhythmias: a meta-analysis. *Circulation, 84,* 1977–1983.

*Moss, A. J., Hall, W. J., Cannom, D. S., et al. (1996). Improved survival with an implanted defibrillator in patients with coronary disease at high risk for ventricular arrhythmia. *New England Journal of Medicine, 335,* 1933–1940.

*Oral, H., Souza, J. J., Michaud, G. F., et al. (1999). Facilitating transthoracic cardioversion of atrial fibrillation with ibutilide pretreatment. *New England Journal of Medicine, 340,* 1849–1854.

*Pacifico, A., Hohnloser, S. H., Williams, J. H., et al. (1999). Prevention of implantable-defibrillator shocks by treatment with sotalol: Sotalol Implantable Cardioverter-Defibrillator Study Group. *New England Journal of Medicine, 340,* 1855–1862.

*Packer, M., Bristow, M. R., Cohn, J. N., et al. (1996). The effect of carvedilol on morbidity and mortality in patients with chronic heart failure. *New England Journal of Medicine, 334,* 1349–1355.

*Pfizer Laboratories. (2000). *Tikosyn (dofetilide) package insert.* New York: Author.

*Phillips, B. G., Gandhi, A. J., Sanoski, C. A., et al. (1997). Comparison of intravenous diltiazem and verapamil for the acute treatment of atrial fibrillation and flutter. *Pharmacotherapy, 17,* 1238–1245.

Pinkowish, M. D. (1999). Ventricular arrhythmias: a new era in management. *Patient Care, 33*(14), 152–170.

Pritchett, E. L., McCarthy, E. A., & Wilkinson, W. E. (1991). Propafenone treatment of symptomatic paroxysmal supraventricular arrhythmias: a randomized, placebo-controlled crossover trial in patients tolerating oral therapy. *Annals of Internal Medicine, 114,* 539–544.

*Roden, D. M., & Woosley, R. L. (1986). Drug therapy: tocainide. *New England Journal of Medicine, 315,* 41–45.

*Roy, D., Talajic, M., Dorian, P., et al. (2000). Amiodarone to prevent recurrence of atrial fibrillation. *New England Journal of Medicine, 342,* 913–920.

*Sanoski, C. A., & Bauman, J. L. (2002). Clinical observations with the amiodarone/warfarin interaction: dosing relationships with long-term therapy. *Chest, 121,* 19–23.

*Singh, S., Zoble, R. G., Yellen, L., et al. (2000). Efficacy and safety of oral dofetilide in converting to and maintaining sinus rhythm in patients with chronic atrial fibrillation or atrial flutter: the Symptomatic Atrial Fibrillation Investigative Research on Dofetilide (SAFIRE-D) Study. *Circulation, 102,* 2385–2390.

*Slavik, R. S., Tisdale, J. E., & Borzak, S. (2001). Pharmacological conversion of atrial fibrillation: a systematic review of available evidence. *Progress in Cardiovascular Diseases, 44,* 121–152.

*Soyka, L. F., Wirtz, C., & Spangenberg, R. B. (1990). Clinical safety profile of sotalol in patients with arrhythmias. *American Journal of Cardiology, 65*(Suppl.), 74A–81A.

*Stambler, B. S., et al. (1996). Efficacy and safety of repeated intravenous doses of ibutilide for rapid conversion of atrial flutter or fibrillation. *Circulation, 94,* 1613–1621.

Stroke Prevention in Atrial Fibrillation Investigators. (1991). Stroke prevention in atrial fibrillation study: final report. *Circulation, 84,* 527–539.

*Teo, K. K., Yusuf, S., & Furberg, C. D. (1993). Effects of prophylactic antiarrhythmic drug therapy in acute myocardial infarction: an overview of results from randomized controlled trials. *Journal of the American Medical Association, 270,* 1589–1595.

*Vaughan Williams, E. M. (1984). A classification of antiarrhythmic actions reassessed after a decade of new drugs. *Journal of Clinical Pharmacology, 24,* 129–147.

*Volgman, A. S., et al. (1998). Conversion efficacy and safety of intravenous ibutilide compared with intravenous procainamide in patients with atrial flutter or fibrillation. *Journal of the American College of Cardiology, 31,* 1414–1419.

*Vukmir, R. B., & Stein, K. L. (1991). Torsades de pointes therapy with phenytoin. *Annals of Emergency Medicine, 20,* 198–200.

*Wit, A. L., Rosen, M. R., & Hoffman, B. F. (1974). Electrophysiology and pharmacology of cardiac arrhythmias: relationship of normal and abnormal electrical activity of cardiac fibers to the genesis of arrhythmias. *American Heart Journal, 88,* 664–670, 798–806.

Witterchein, G. (1998). Ready or not, here comes multicultural care. *Physicians Management, 38*(7), 34–39.

*Wyse, D. G., Kellen, J., & Rademaker, A. W. (1988). Prophylactic versus selective lidocaine for early ventricular arrhythmias of myocardial infarction. *Journal of the American College of Cardiology, 12,* 507–513.

*Wyse, D. G., Waldo, A. L., DiMarco, J. P., et al. (2002). A comparison of rate control and rhythm control in patients with atrial fibrillation. *New England Journal of Medicine, 347,* 1825–1833.

Visit the Connection web site for the most up-to-date drug information.

V

Pharmacotherapy for Respiratory Disorders

23

UPPER RESPIRATORY INFECTIONS

■ VIRGINIA P. ARCANGELO AND SILVANA POLETAJEV

Upper respiratory tract infections (URIs), including the common cold and sinusitis, are some of the most common problems seen in primary care. URIs are usually self-limiting, minor illnesses that account for half or more of all acute illnesses. It is difficult to differentiate the common cold from sinusitis or allergic rhinitis (see Chapter 51). URIs share common symptoms, such as nasal discharge, nasal congestion, tenderness over the sinuses, fever, headache, malaise, sore throat and myalgias, sneezing, a full feeling around the eyes and ears, and coughing. Symptoms may present individually or in combination, and it is difficult to determine whether the cause is viral or bacterial.

URIs can progress to acute or chronic complications. In children especially, URIs may progress to otitis media. In 5% to 10% of cases, the viral or bacterial cause may travel, causing sinusitis and bronchitis. There is an enormous economic burden associated with URIs.

COMMON COLD

Acute infectious rhinitis (coryza), or the common cold, is a viral URI. One of the most common infections, it is self-limiting. Coryza is an acute inflammation of the mucous membranes of the respiratory passages, particularly of the nose, sinuses, and throat, and is characterized by sneezing, rhinorrhea (watery nasal discharge), and coughing.

Approximately 100 million colds occur annually in the United States, resulting in approximately 26 million days off from school, 23 million absent days from work, 27 million visits to a primary care provider, and 250 million days of restricted activities. Nearly $1 billion is spent on cold remedies and $1.5 billion on analgesics. Adults average three colds per year. Children average six episodes per year, and the common cold is more common in children who attend day care or preschool (where they are in contact with other children and groups that may spread disease) than in those who spend more time at home and have less contact with crowds. Exposure to smoke is also a predisposing factor.

CAUSES

The pathogens most frequently associated with common colds are rhinovirus (30% to 40% of cases), especially during the fall and spring, and coronavirus (10% to 15%), which is most prevalent during the winter. The respiratory syncytial virus, influenza virus, parainfluenza virus, and adenovirus are also responsible, but the rhinovirus is the single most pervasive cause of colds. The rhinovirus is a single-stranded RNA virus that replicates well at 95°F or below but poorly at 99°F to 100°F, which is probably why it causes URIs and not pneumonia.

Predisposition to viral infections can be attributed to many factors, including frequent exposure to viral infectious agents; in children, the age of the child; and the inability to resist invading organisms because of allergies, malnutrition, immune deficiencies, physical abnormalities, or other comorbid conditions. Some experts propose a relationship between host response to the virus and the production of cold symptoms. Studies show that common colds are more frequent or more severe in those under increased stress, probably as a result of stress weakening the immune system (Lorber, 1996).

PATHOPHYSIOLOGY

If the protective barriers of the upper respiratory tract (ie, cough, gag, and sneeze reflexes, lymph nodes, immunoglobulin A antibodies, and rich vasculature) fail, viral pathogens trigger an acute inflammatory reaction with release of vasoactive mediators and increased parasympathetic stimuli. This produces congestion and rhinorrhea. Rhinoviruses grow in the upper airway and attach and gain entry to host cells by binding to an intracellular adhesion molecule (ICAM-1). Infection begins in the adenoidal area and spreads to the ciliated epithelium in the nose. Rhinoviruses are hardy and remain infectious for at least 3 hours after drying on hard surfaces such as telephones or countertops, but they do not last as long on porous surfaces such as tissues.

Transmission of the virus has been attributed to three methods: airborne transmission by small particles (droplets), airborne transmission by large particles, and direct contact. Large particle transmission is not efficient and requires prolonged exposure. The major means of transmission is by direct contact from a donor's nose to a donor's hand, and from there to the recipient's hand and subsequently to the nose or eye. Although conjunctival cells are not thought to harbor rhinovirus, it probably can be passed through the tear duct into the nose. Incubation of the rhinovirus is 1 to 10 days. Onset of signs and symptoms occurs 1 to 2 days after viral infection, and they peak in approximately 2 to 4 days. The virus may remain present for a week or longer after the onset of symptoms.

DIAGNOSTIC CRITERIA

Diagnostic tests have no cost/benefit effect in diagnosing the common cold. Symptoms consist primarily of clear nasal discharge, sneezing, nasal congestion, cough, low-grade fever (below 102°F), scratchy or sore throat, mild aches, chills, headache, watery eyes, tenderness around the eyes, full feeling in the ears, and fatigue. In children, the presentation could also include nasal blockage, fever with seizures, anorexia, vomiting, diarrhea, and abdominal pain. Symptoms usually resolve in approximately 1 week, but they may linger for 2 weeks.

INITIATING DRUG THERAPY

Mistreatment of the common cold by clinicians is common for two reasons:

- It is difficult to determine whether the cause is viral or bacterial.
- Patients often have preconceived notions and demand antibiotics for their URI even though it is simply the common cold, which is caused by a virus.

There is no cure for the common cold. Treatment is geared toward minimizing symptoms (Table 23-1).

Nonpharmacologic alternatives to treating the common cold are the first line. For example, rest allows the body to gain strength and be more effective in defending itself against the pathogen. The body can then dictate the increase in activities. An alternative to decongestants and expectorants is increasing water or juice intake. This assists in liquefying tenacious secretions, making expectoration easier, soothing scratchy, sore throats, and relieving dry skin and lips. Saline gargles also are effective for soothing sore throats.

Coughing caused by chest congestion can cause a muscular chest pain. Menthol rubs can soothe this ache and open airways for some congestion relief. Menthol lozenges also have been effective in soothing scratchy throats and clearing nasal passages. Saline nasal flushes are also effective for clearing nasal passages without the rebound side effect. Petrolatum-based ointments for raw and macerated skin around the nose and upper lip ease the drying effects of dehydration and the use of multiple tissues (see Table 23-1).

Other measures, such as drinking chicken soup, taking a hot shower, or using a room humidifier, may prove helpful. Inhaling warm, moist heat helps raise the temperature of the nasal mucosa to at least 37°C, a temperature at which the virus does not replicate so readily.

Goals of Drug Therapy

The main goals of treatment for the common cold are relief of symptoms, reduction of the risk for complications, and prevention of spread to others (Box 23-1). Polypharmacy is often used to treat intolerable symptoms.

Table 23.1

Alternative Therapies for Cold Symptoms

Symptoms	Nonpharmacologic	Pharmacologic	Alternative Therapy
Any cold symptoms	Eat proper diet, rest, drink fluids.		Echinacea (prevention) Zinc lozenges (decreased duration of symptoms)
Rhinorrhea Nasal obstruction	Use disposable paper tissues. Decrease ingestion of milk products. Inhale warm, moist heat, such as showers. Increase fluid intake.	Anticholinergic nasal spray Children: saline nose drops by bulb syringe Apply topical decongestants. If nasal obstruction is still a problem after 3 days, take oral decongestants unless contraindicated by hypertension or coronary artery disease.	Bayberry tea
Serous otitis media or sensation of fullness in ears		Decongestants (oral)	
Headache, sore throat, malaise, myalgia, fever	Gargle with salt water, drink plenty of fluids, suck on menthol lozenges.	Nonsteroidal anti-inflammatory drugs	Chaparral, aromatherapy rubs, boneset
Chest congestion	Drink fluids, have menthol rubs, and humidify room air.	Expectorants	
Sneezing and watery eyes	Humidify room air.	Two schools of thought: antihistamine of choice, but critics say antihistamines not needed in treating colds, especially in children	
Cough	Humidify room air.	Antitussives, naproxen	

Decongestants

Mechanism of Action

Decongestants are sympathomimetic agents that stimulate alpha- and beta-adrenergic receptors, causing vasoconstriction in the respiratory tract mucosa and thereby improving ventilation (Table 23-2). Decongestants come in topical or oral preparations. Topical decongestants in the form of nasal sprays slow ciliary motility and mucociliary clearance. Topical agents have little systemic absorption. However, topical decongestants should not be used for more than 3 days because prolonged use can cause rhinitis medicamentosa (rebound congestion), which is characterized by severe nasal edema, rebound congestion, and increased discharge due to decreased receptor sensitivity.

Oral decongestants are frequently used and are sold over the counter (OTC) alone or in combination with other drugs. A common example of a combination preparation is an antihistamine and a decongestant. The most common oral decongestant is pseudoephedrine (Sudafed, others). Oral decongestants have the same mode of action as topical agents but can cause more systemic responses. Decongestants assist in clearing nasal obstruction. Their use may be encouraged to prevent sinusitis and eustachian tube blockage.

Contraindications

Decongestants are contraindicated in patients with narrow-angle glaucoma, hypertension, and severe coronary artery disease. Caution is recommended in patients with hyperthyroidism, diabetes, and prostatic hypertrophy (causes difficulty with urination).

Adverse Events

Adverse events include increased blood pressure, increased heart rate, palpitations, headache, dizziness, gastrointestinal distress, and tremor. These reactions are especially seen at doses above 210 mg.

Interactions

Decongestants interact with appetite suppressants, monoamine oxidase (MAO) inhibitors (hypertensive crisis), and beta-adrenergic agents (bradycardia and hypertension). Decongestants are less effective when taken with drugs that acidify the urine and more effective when taken with drugs that alkalize the urine.

Expectorants

One of the most important nondrug considerations in treating coughs is discovering its cause, because the prolonged use of OTC expectorants or other cough products may mask symptoms of a serious underlying disorder. The drug should not be used for more than a week. If the cough persists, additional measures may be investigated.

Mechanism of Action

Expectorants, including water, increase the output of respiratory tract fluid by decreasing the adhesiveness and surface tension of the respiratory tract and by facilitating removal of viscous mucous (see Table 23-2). The effect is noted within 1 to 2 hours.

Adverse Events

Adverse events include drowsiness, headache, and gastrointestinal symptoms.

Antitussives

Cough is a frequent complaint of a person with an URI. Cough can be stimulated from congestion or can occur as a result of postnasal drip.

Mechanism of Action

Antitussives diminish the cough reflex by direct inhibition of the cough center in the medulla (see Table 23-2). There are narcotic antitussives and non-narcotic antitussives. Onset of action is noted within 15 to 30 minutes. Many practitioners believe that cough suppressants are ineffective in children.

Contraindications

Antitussives are contraindicated in a patient with a productive cough, a history of substance abuse, or chronic obstructive pulmonary disease.

Table 23.2

Overview of Agents for Upper Respiratory Infections

Generic (Trade) Name and Dosage	Selected Adverse Events	Contraindications	Special Considerations
Decongestants			
oxymetazoline hydrochloride (Afrin) ≥6 y: 2–3 sprays bid 2–6 y (use children's spray): 2–3 sprays bid	Palpitations, headaches		These drugs may cause rebound congestion. Use only 2 to 3 days, then switch to oral decongestants.
phenylephrine hydrochloride (Neo-Synephrine) Adults: 1 spray q3–4h as needed	Palpitations, headaches	Not recommended for children	These drugs may cause rebound congestion. Use only 2 to 3 days, then switch to oral decongestants.
pseudophedrine (Sudafed, Benalyn decongestant) Adults: short acting: 60 mg q4–6h; long acting: 120 mg q12h Children 7–12 y: short acting: 30 mg q4–6h Children 3–6 y: 15 mg q4–6h	Palpitations, headaches, increased blood pressure, dizziness, GI upset, tremor	Hypertension, coronary artery disease	Give at least 2 h before bedtime. Do not crush, break, or chew tablets.
Expectorants			
guaifenesin (Anti-Tus, Humabid sprinkles, Robitussin, Unitussin) Adults: short acting: 200–400 mg q4h long acting: 600–1,200 mg q12h Children 7–12 y: short acting: 100–200 mg q4h long acting: 600 mg q12h Children 2–6 y: 50–100 mg q4h	GI upset, drowsiness, headache, rash, dizziness	Breast-feeding mothers, pregnancy category C	Not given for prolonged time if cough persists or accompanied by high fever Humabid sprinkles may be swallowed whole or opened and sprinkled on soft food.
Antitussives			
dextromethorphan (Benylin—15 mg/5 mL) 10 mL q6–8h (Delsym—30 mg/5 mL) Adults: 10 mL q12h Children 2–5 y: 2.5 mL q12h 6–12 y: 5 mL q12h	Drowsiness, palpitations, excitability in children	Hypertension, diabetes, asthma	None
Narcotic Antitussives			
codeine phosphate 10 mg, guaifenesin 300 mg tablets and liquid (Brontex) Adults: 20 mL q4h Children 6–12 y: 10 mL q4h	Lightheadedness, dizziness, sedation, sweating, nausea, vomiting	Known addiction, cautious use in asthmatics, COPD, cardiac disease, seizure disorders, renal/hepatic impairment, BPH, head injuries, hypothyroidism, and pregnancy	Increased CNS depression if used with alcohol or other narcotics Usually used with antihistamines, expectorants, decongestants, or analgesics Controlled substance (Drug Enforcement Agency number required for prescription)
phenergan with codeine (codeine 10 mg and promethazine 6.25 mg/5 mL) Adults: 5 mL Children: 2–5 y: 1.25–2.5 mL q4h 6–12 y: 2.5–5 mL q4h	Same as above	Same as above	Same as above
codeine 10 mg, guaifenesin 100 mg/5 mL (Robitussin AC) or codeine 10 mg, pseudoephedrine 30 mg, and guaifenesin 100 mg/5 mL (Tussar SF) Adults: 10 mL q4h to maximum of 40 mL/d	Same as above	Children: not recommended	Same as above
hydrocodone (in combination with other agents) 5 mg up to 4 qid	Same as above	Known addiction; cautious use in asthmatics, COPD, cardiac disease, seizure disorders, renal/hepatic impairment, BPH, head injuries, hypothyroidism, and pregnancy	Same as above

Table 23.2

Overview of Agents for Upper Respiratory Infections (*Continued*)

Generic (Trade) Name and Dosage	Selected Adverse Events	Contraindications	Special Considerations
hydrocodone 2.5 mg, guaifenesin 100 mg, pseudoephedrine 30 mg/5 mL (Duratuss HD) Adults: 10 mL q4–6h Children 6–12 y: 5 mL q2–6h Maximum of 4 doses/d	Same as above	Same as above	Same as above
hydrocodone 5 mg and homatropine 1.5 mg (Hycodan tablets and syrup) Adults: 1 tablet or 5 mL q4–6h Children: 6–12 y: ½ tablet or 2.5 mL q4–6h	Same as above	Same as above	Same as above
hydrocodone 5 mg and guaifenesin 100 mg/5 mL (Hycotuss) Adults: 5 mL after meals and hs Children: 6–12 y: 2.5–5 mL after meals and hs	Same as above	Same as above	Same as above
hydrocodone 10 mg and chlorpheniramine maleate 8 mg/5 mL (Tussionex) Adults: 5 mL q12h Children: 6–12 y: 2.5 mL q12h	Same as above	Same as above	Same as above
hydrocodone 5 mg guaifenesin 100 mg per 5 mL (Vicodin Tuss) Adults: 5 mL at meals and hs Children 6–12 y: 2.5 mL at meals and hs	Same as above	Same as above	Same as above
Combination Products—Non-narcotic			
dextromethorphan hydrobromide 10 mg, brompheniramine maleate 2 mg, pseudoephedrine 30 mg/5 mL (Bromfed-D, Dimetane-DX) Adults: 10 mL q4h Children: 2–5 y: 2.5 mL q4h 6–12 y: 5 mL q4h	Drowsiness, sedation, nausea, dizziness, palpitations, increased blood pressure, excitation in children, constipation	Asthma, lower respiratory disorders, neonates, severe hypertension, severe cardiovascular disease, within 14 days of monoamine oxidase inhibitors, nursing mothers; use cautiously in patients with history of urinary obstruction, mild hypertension, and hyperthyroidism	These drugs are combination antitussives, antihistamines, and sympathomimetics. Used for cough and congestion Pregnancy category C Not recommended for children <2 y These drugs are sold over the counter.
dextromethorphan Hbr 10 mg, pseudoephedrine HCl 30 mg, guaifenesin 100 mg/5 mL (Novahistamine DMX, Robitussin-DM) Adults: 10 mL q4h to maximum of 4 doses/d Children: 2–5 y: 2.5 mL q4h 6–12 y: 5 mL q4h to maximum of 4 doses/d Robitussin-DM indicated for infants in the following doses: 6–11 mo (14–17 lbs): 1.25 mL 12–23 mo (18–23 lbs): 2.5 mL q6–8h	Same as above	Same as above	Same as above

(continued)

Table 23.2

Overview of Agents for Upper Respiratory Infections (*Continued*)

Generic (Trade) Name and Dosage	Selected Adverse Events	Contraindications	Special Considerations
carbinoxamine maleate 4 mg, pseudoephedrine HCl 60 mg per tab or per 5 mL (Rondec syrup) Over 6 y: 5 mL or 1 tab qid 18 mo–6 y: 2.5 mL qid Comes in drops for infants and the drops should be used for children ≤18 mo Drops are dextromethorphan Hbr 4 mg, carbinoxamine maleate 4 mg, pseudoephedrine HCl 60 mg per 5 mL Children 1–3 mo: 0.25 mL 3–6 mo: 0.5 mL 6–9 mo: 0.75 mL 9–18 mo: 1 mL qid	Same as above	Same as above	Same as above
carbetapentane tannate 60 mg, chlorpheniramine tannate 5 mg, ephedrine tannate 10 mg, phenylephrine tannate 10 mg (Rynatuss) Tablets Adults: 1–2 tablets q12h carbetapentane tannate 30 mg, chlorpheniramine tannate 5 mg, ephedrine tannate 5 mg, phenylephrine tannate 5 mg (Rynatuss Pediatric Syrup) 2–5 y: 2.5–5 mL q12h 6–12 y: 5–10 mL q12h	Same as above	Same as above	Same as above Is a prescription medication
Anti-inflammatories and Antipyretics			
naproxen sodium (Naprosyn, Alleve) Adults: 500 mg q12h or 250 mg q6–8h; maximum 1 g/d Children >2 y may take suspension form 10 mg/kg in two divided doses	Nausea, vomiting, dyspepsia	Not for children <2 y	Take on full stomach to reduce side effects of possible GI discomfort.
Anticholinergics			
ipratropium bromide (Atrovent) Adults: two 36-μg inhalations qid or two sprays of 0.06% per nostril tid–qid Spray: two 0.03% sprays per nostril bid–tid	Headache, epistaxis, pharyngitis, nasal dryness	Hypersensitivity to atropine Use caution in patients with narrow-angle glaucoma, BPH, bladder neck obstruction, pregnancy, and lactation.	Protect inhalable solution from light
Antibiotics			
amoxicillin (Amoxil) Adults: 500 mg tid for 10 d Children: 20–40 mg/kg/d in divided doses	Nausea, vomiting, diarrhea, rash, allergic reactions, fungal infections, pseudomembranous colitis, Stevens-Johnson syndrome, seizures (high doses)	Hypersensitivity or allergy to penicillin or cephalosporins Use cautiously in renal impairment.	Therapy should continue for at least 10 d or 1 wk after symptoms subside.
amoxicillin with clavulanic acid (Augmentin) Adults: 500 mg tid or 875 mg bid for 10 d Children: same as amoxicillin for adults	Same as above	Same as above	Same as above Combination drug Clavulanic acid protects amoxicillin from breakdown by bacterial beta-lactamase enzymes.
cefpodoxime (Vantin) Adults: 200 mg q12h Children (>2 mo.): 5 mg/kg q12h	GI upset, rash, abdominal pain, headache	Caution with penicillin allergy	Interacts with antacids, H2 antagonists. Avoid diuretics.
cefuroxime (Ceftin) Adults: 250 mg q12h Children (>6 mo.): 7.5–15 mg/kg q12h	As above	As above	As above

Table 23.2

Overview of Agents for Upper Respiratory Infections (*Continued*)

Generic (Trade) Name and Dosage	Selected Adverse Events	Contraindications	Special Considerations
trimethoprim–sulfamethoxazole (TMP-SMZ, Bactrim, Septra) Adults: 160 mg trimethoprim and 800 mg sulfamethoxazole orally q12h for up to 14 d Children: 8 mg/kg/d; trimethoprim in 2 doses × 10 d	Nausea, vomiting, anorexia, megaloblastic anemia, hallucinations, depression, seizures	Megaloblastic anemia, pregnancy category C, breast-feeding, sulfa allergy	Hemolysis may develop in patients with glucose-6-phosphate dehydrogenase deficiency. May cause falsely elevated creatinine level Advise patient to increase fluid intake.
clarithromycin (Biaxin) Adults: 500 mg bid for 10 d Biaxin XL 1000 mg qd for 7 d	Nausea, vomiting, diarrhea, dyspepsia, abnormal taste, allergic reactions, fungal infection Serious: pseudomembranous colitis	Allergy to macrolides Pregnancy and lactation Use with caution in severe hepatic or renal disease.	Take with or without food. Monitor for drug interactions with other agents that are metabolized by the cytochrome P450 3A4 isoenzyme. Interactants: warfarin, digoxin, carbamazepine, theophylline, cisapride
telithromycin (Ketex) 800 mg daily for 5 days	Diarrhea, nausea, headache, dizziness, elevated LFTs	Hypersensitivity to macrolides, visapride use, caution if hypokalemia, QT prolongation	Pregnancy category C May decrease efficacy of oral contraceptives

BPH, benign prostatic hypertrophy; COPD, chronic obstructive pulmonary disease; GI, gastrointestinal.

Adverse Events

Adverse events include dizziness, nausea, drowsiness, and sedation.

Interactions

Drug–drug interactions occur with concomitant use of amiodarone (Cordarone), MAO inhibitors, quinidine (Cardioquin, others), selective serotonin reuptake inhibitors, and other antidepressants.

Anti-inflammatories and Antipyretics

Nonsteroidal anti-inflammatory drugs (NSAIDs) inhibit prostaglandin secretions, which serves to decrease mucus secretion. Effects are noted within 1 to 2 hours.

NSAIDs alleviate constitutional symptoms such as headache, sore throat, malaise, myalgia, and fever. The NSAID naproxen (Naprosyn) is given 500 mg every 12 hours or 250 mg every 6 to 8 hours, not to exceed 1 g/day. Naproxen alleviates symptoms without increasing viral shedding. NSAIDs are contraindicated in patients with asthma, renal disease, severe hepatic disease, and ulcers. Adverse events include nausea, gastrointestinal ulceration, bleeding, nephrotoxicity, and blood dyscrasias. NSAIDs may increase the action of heparin.

Aspirin (Bayer, others), a common NSAID, should not be used in children because of the secondary risk of Reye's syndrome. The patient should also refrain from taking acetaminophen (Tylenol) and nonprescription doses of ibuprofen (Motrin) because these drugs are believed to shed the virus. NSAIDs are discussed in greater detail in Chapter 38.

Anticholinergic Agents

Ipratropium bromide (Atrovent) nasal spray (0.03% and 0.06%) has been recommended for rhinorrhea associated with the common cold. It can be prescribed in both strengths for adults and in the 0.03% strength for children 6 years of age and older. It inhibits vagally mediated reflexes by antagonizing the action of acetylcholine at the cholinergic receptor, thereby inhibiting secretions from the serous and seromucous glands lining the nasal mucosa. The result is a decrease in nasal discharge. The dosage is two sprays per nostril three or four times a day.

Ipratropium bromide is not used in patients with a history of sensitivity to atropine or in pregnant or lactating women. It is used with caution in patients with narrow-angle glaucoma, prostatic hypertrophy, or bladder neck obstruction. Adverse events include epistaxis, dry mouth, nasal congestion, and nasal dryness.

Antihistamines

For sneezing and rhinorrhea, a combination of pseudoephedrine and a first-generation antihistamine seems to be effective. Some critics say the use of antihistamines is irrational and has no place in treatment of the common cold (Berman & Chan, 1999). They state that their drying effect might exacerbate symptoms of congestion and cause upper airway obstruction by impairing the flow of mucous. In contrast, antihistamines have been effective in controlling the symptoms of watery eyes, runny nose, and a feeling of fullness in the ears. Antihistamines are discussed further in Chapter 51.

Selecting the Most Appropriate Agent

Because symptoms of a cold are manifest individually or in combination, depending on the patient, not everyone has the same signs and symptoms. Therefore, the therapeutic approach is to treat symptoms as specifically as possible. In addition, if the cold is caused by a bacterial infection, as evidenced by throat culture results and the like, antibiotic treatment is prescribed (Fig. 23-1).

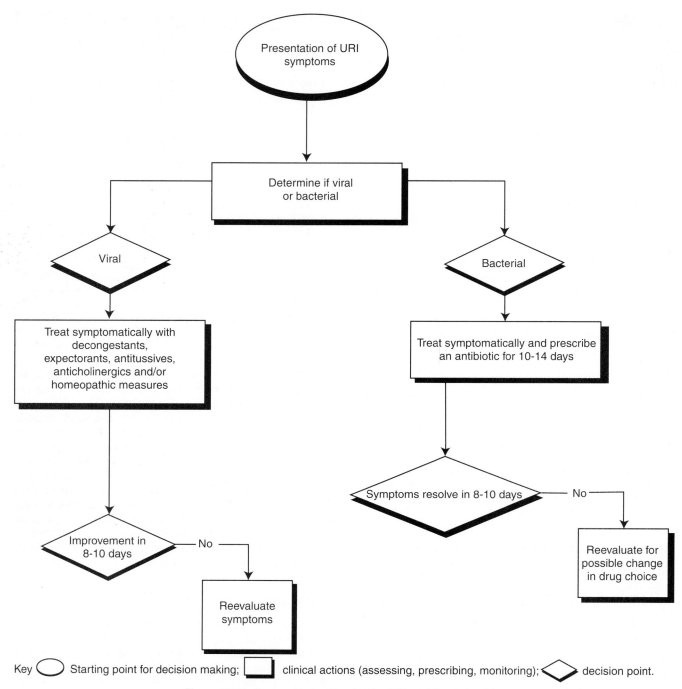

Figure 23–1   Treatment algorithm for the URIs: cold and sinusitis.

First-Line Therapy

Initial therapy consists of symptom relief. For nasal obstruction and rhinorrhea, which are caused by secretions and increased vascular permeability with leakage of serum into the nasal mucosa, topical decongestants, such as oxymetazoline hydrochloride (Afrin) or phenylephrine hydrochloride (Neo-Synephrine), are often used for the first 3 days, when the patient feels the worst (Table 23-3). Topical vasoconstrictors are recommended for only 3 days because they predispose many patients to rebound congestion. Rebound congestion interferes with ciliary action and dries the nasal mucosa. If other symptoms are diminished but nasal obstruction remains a problem, the use of an oral decongestant, such as pseudoephedrine, or a combination decongestant and antihistamine, or an antihistamine alone may relieve symptoms and help prevent complications such as sinusitis and eustachian tube blockage. Antipyretics, such as acetaminophen, or anti-inflammatories, such as ibuprofen, may be recommended to relieve fever and accompanying aches and discomfort.

Second-Line Therapy

Second-line therapy may be instituted if first-line therapy fails to relieve symptoms or if complications, such as secondary infection (ear infections, sinusitis, bronchitis, or pneumonia), develop. The therapy should be specific to the disorder.

Table 23.3

Recommended Order of Treatment for the Common Cold

Order	Agent	Comments
First line	Symptom relief with oral and topical decongestants, topical vasoconstrictors, antihistamines, expectorants or antitussives, anti-inflammatories, and antipyretics as indicated	Cold treatment is symptom specific. There is no cure. The disorder is self-limiting.
Second line	Specific drug therapy aimed at treating complications if symptoms progress to sinusitis, bronchitis, or other disorders	Patient should be advised to contact practitioner if cold symptoms do not subside in approximately 7 days.

Special Population Considerations

Pediatric

In infants, using saline nose drops with a bulb syringe before feedings may be helpful. Saline nose drops may be prepared by adding one quarter of a teaspoon of salt to 8 ounces of water. Children younger than 7 years of age should not be encouraged to blow their nose because the pressure of blowing increases the risk of ear congestion great enough to promote infection. Aspirin is not given to children because of the risk of Reye's syndrome. There is controversy over whether antitussives are effective in children.

MONITORING PATIENT RESPONSE

Patient response is monitored by the decrease of symptoms. If symptoms decrease without onset of complications, then therapy was successful. If the common cold does not improve in 8 to 10 days, a bacterial cause is suspected and antibiotic therapy is considered.

PATIENT EDUCATION

The most important aspect of patient education is to prevent contracting the virus by practicing good hygiene, such as frequent hand washing, getting adequate sleep and exercise, avoiding contact with infected people, eating a nutritious diet, and so on. Another important aspect of patient education is teaching patients to prevent spreading the virus through correct tissue disposal, hand washing, covering the mouth when coughing, and so on (see Box 23-1).

Alternative Therapies

There is a growing interest in alternative or complementary therapies for treating colds. The root of the bayberry bush in large doses has been used to increase the secretion of nasal mucus during head colds. Echinacea's medicinal properties inhibit microbial infections by stimulating the body's immune system. It is used for prevention. However, prolonged use can lead to immune system overstimulation and eventual suppression.

The use of zinc lozenges in treating the common cold is becoming more popular. A study by Mossad, Macknin, Medendorp, and Mason (1996) showed that zinc, taken at least every 2 hours in lozenge form, can reduce the duration of cold symptoms. The mechanism of action remains unknown (see Table 23-1).

SINUSITIS

Sinusitis, also called rhinosinusitis, is a bacterial URI characterized by inflammation of the mucous membranes that line the paranasal sinuses. Air trapped within a blocked sinus, along with pus or other secretions, can cause pressure on the sinus wall. The result is the sometimes-intense sinus pain. Similarly, when air is prevented from entering a paranasal sinus by a swollen membrane at the opening, a vacuum can be created that also causes pain.

It can be acute or chronic. Acute sinusitis often results from progression of the common cold (5% to 10% of cases) and lasts for 3 weeks or less. Chronic sinusitis is defined as episodes of prolonged inflammation or repeatedly treated acute sinus infections. Symptoms last for 3 to 8 weeks but may be present for longer than 3 months. Bacterial infections can occur from impaired drainage resulting from polyps, enlarged turbinates, a deviated septum, the common cold, anatomic abnormalities, tooth infections, exacerbation of allergic rhinitis, and so on. Health care experts estimate that 37 million Americans are affected by sinusitis every year.

CAUSES

Rhinosinusitis is a more appropriate term than either rhinitis or sinusitis to describe inflammatory disease involving the upper respiratory tract. The nasal and sinus mucosa are contiguous; sinusitis rarely occurs in the absence of rhinitis.

Most cases of acute sinusitis start with a common cold of viral etiology that inflames the sinuses. Both the cold and the sinus inflammation usually resolve without treatment in 2 weeks. The nose reacts to an invasion by viruses that cause infections such as the common cold or flu by producing mucus and sending white blood cells to the lining of the nose, which congest and swell the nasal passages.

When this swelling involves the adjacent mucous membranes of the sinuses, air and mucus are trapped behind the narrowed openings of the sinuses. When sinus openings become too narrow, mucus cannot drain properly. This increase in mucus sets up prime conditions for bacteria to multiply.

The most common causes are the bacterial pathogens *Streptococcus pneumoniae* and *Haemophilus influenzae*, which account for 75% of cases of rhinosinusitis. *Moraxella catarrhalis* is most common in children. Other organisms that may cause sinusitis, but less frequently, are group A

Streptococcus, *Chlamydia pneumoniae*, and *Streptococcus pyogenes*.

Most healthy persons harbor bacteria such as *S. pneumoniae* and *H. influenzae* in their upper respiratory tracts with no problems until the body's defenses are weakened or drainage from the sinuses is blocked by a cold or other viral infection. Then, bacteria that may have been living harmlessly in the nose or throat can multiply and invade the sinuses, causing an acute sinus infection.

Chronic inflammation of the nasal passages also can lead to sinusitis. Persons with allergic rhinitis or hay fever can also experience episodes of acute sinusitis. Vasomotor rhinitis, caused by humidity, cold air, alcohol, perfumes, and other environmental conditions, can also be complicated by sinus infections.

Persons with asthma may have frequent episodes of chronic sinusitis. Persons who are allergic to airborne allergens, such as dust, mold, and pollen, that trigger allergic rhinitis, may develop chronic sinusitis. Persons vulnerable to chronic sinusitis can also be affected by damp weather (especially in northern temperate climates) or pollutants in the air and in buildings. In addition, persons with nasal polyps or a severe asthmatic response to aspirin and aspirin-like medicines such as ibuprofen may develop chronic sinusitis often.

Other risks for developing sinusitis include the following: overuse of nasal decongestants, presence of deviated nasal septum, presence of a nasal foreign body, frequent swimming or diving, dental work, pregnancy, changes in altitude, exposure to air pollution and cigarette smoke, gastroesophageal reflux disease (GERD), and hospitalization.

PATHOPHYSIOLOGY

There are four paired, air-filled cavities that make up the sinuses. Small tubular openings, the sinus ostia, connect the sinus cavities and facilitate drainage of the sinuses into the nasal cavity using ciliated cells. Proper sinus functioning requires motile cilia, patent ostia, and mucus of a low viscosity that allows transport. Inflammation causes dysfunctional cilia, obstruction of the ostia, or both. Negative pressure develops in the clogged sinuses, facilitating the transport of intranasal bacteria into the sinuses. This can promote bacterial growth and inflammation and bacterial sinusitis.

DIAGNOSTIC CRITERIA

Bacterial infections (ie, sinusitis) share the same symptoms of a viral cold with respect to nasal congestion, cough, fever, sore throat, aches, chills, headaches, tenderness around the eyes, a full feeling in the ears, and fatigue. The distinction lies with the severity and duration of symptoms with a bacterial URI. In sinusitis, there is persistent rhinitis without resolution and a cough that lasts more than 8 to 10 days after a cold. The nasal discharge increases in quantity, viscosity, and purulence. In addition, there is often malodorous breath without poor dental hygiene, and by morning periorbital swelling may be present. The patient reports facial pain on movement. Fever and malaise also may occur.

Differentiation between infectious and noninfectious disease usually can be made by history. The typical patient reports a URI that has been unusually severe and failed to resolve or improve after 7 to 10 days. The general course of the disease may be biphasic. Major symptoms include facial pain, pressure, congestion, fullness, obstruction, blockage, or discharge with a temperature greater than 38°C. Purulent drainage in the middle meatus may be a strong indicator of acute sinus disease; however, nasal purulence does not differentiate viral from bacterial infection. There may be a lack of response to decongestants. Symptoms may include headache, fatigue, dental pain, halitosis, otalgia, or cough.

Williams and Simel (1993) identified a classic method of diagnosing sinusitis. Characteristic symptoms include toothache and poor response to decongestants. Characteristic signs are purulent, green or yellow nasal discharge and abnormal sinus illumination. Acute bacterial sinusitis is a consideration in patients who report cold symptoms lasting more than 8 days or with prolonged nasal obstruction, or a cold that seems to have gotten better but returns with more severe symptoms.

Chronic sinusitis is a persistent, low-grade infection involving the paranasal sinuses with mucosal thickening. It is diagnosed with sinus x-ray or computed tomography scan. Characteristics of chronic sinusitis include nasal discharge, nasal congestion, cough lasting more than 30 days, or a combination of all three.

INITIATING DRUG THERAPY

In sinusitis, antibiotic treatment is used in addition to symptomatic treatment. Antibiotic therapy should be considered when the patient has a combination of the following: temperature above 102°F; pain or tenderness in the ears, sinuses, or face; purulent, colorful sputum; sore throat; dyspnea and pleuritic chest pain; and symptoms that persist with no improvement for over 10 days.

Nonpharmacologic therapies are the same as those for the common cold, particularly when the symptoms are the same. Surgical intervention is avoided in acute cases, but irrigation and surgical drainage may be necessary in recurrent chronic cases of sinusitis in which complications are present and the patient fails to respond to medical therapy.

Goals of Drug Therapy

The primary treatment goal is eradication of bacterial infection with antibiotics to prevent life-threatening complications. Other goals include reducing mucosal swelling and relieving pain. Decongestants are often prescribed to treat intolerable symptoms of acute sinusitis, and topical corticosteroids may be used to treat mucosal swelling associated with acute or chronic sinusitis.

Antibiotics

Antibiotics are indicated if the diagnosis of sinusitis is made. The appropriate antibiotic is selected based on causative organisms. Most cases of sinusitis are responsive to amoxicillin (Amoxil) for 10 to 14 days, or 1 week after resolution of symptoms, with notable improvement in 2 to 3 days. This drug is safe for use during pregnancy and lactation (see Table 23-2).

Patients with penicillin allergies can be given trimethoprim–sulfamethoxazole (TMP-SMZ). Some strains of bacteria are beta-lactamase–producing (100% of *M. catarrhalis*, 10% to 50% of *S. pneumoniae*, and 25% of *H. influenzae*) and must be treated with amoxicillin combined with clavulanic acid (Augmentin). Cefprozil (Cefzil) is a cephalosporin antibiotic that can be used in general for treating sinusitis. For chronic sinusitis, an antibiotic with anaerobic coverage is needed. Treatment lasts for 3 to 4 weeks.

Symptomatic Therapy

Therapy is also initiated to relieve the symptoms of sinusitis. For the most part, drug choices are the same as for the common cold: aspirin or acetaminophen for fever and aches and decongestants for stuffy nose and the like, unless contraindicated. Topical corticosteroids usually are not used because they may impede the immune system's response to infection.

Selecting the Most Appropriate Agent

Due to the increasing levels of antimicrobial resistance worldwide, clinicians must re-evaluate their approaches to URIs by using evidence-based methods of diagnosis and treatment. Although clinical diagnosis is necessary for most URIs, bacterial and nonbacterial diseases are difficult to distinguish on clinical grounds. When a bacterial pathogen is suspected or diagnosed, antibiotics are not always indicated as a first-line therapy. Patients need to be educated regarding the appropriate initial treatment regimens. When prescribing antibiotics, the regimen should be tailored to the patient. If a patient is not at risk for resistant bacteria, an agent with proven efficacy, narrow spectrum, and low cost is indicated.

First-Line Therapy

Amoxicillin is the first-line antibiotic for treating sinusitis (Table 23-4). Amoxicillin–clavulanate (Augmentin) is also appropriate because it provides coverage for *H. influenza* and *M. catarrhalis*. For penicillin-allergic patients, TMP-SMZ, telithromycin (Ketex), erythromycin, doxycycline, and clarithromycin (Biaxin) are used. Antibiotic treatment lasts 10 to 14 days or 1 week after resolution of symptoms.

Nasal steroid sprays are indicated in sinusitis if there is mucosal swelling. Topical and systemic decongestants may be used to help relieve congestion.

Second-Line Therapy

If there is no relief of symptoms in 8 days, the antibiotic may need to be changed. A different antibiotic should also be used if the patient was treated with antibiotics in the past 4 to 6 weeks. If the organism is thought to be beta-lactamase–producing, amoxicillin–clavulanate may be prescribed. Clarithromycin (Biaxin), cefpodoxime (Vantin), and cefuroxime (Ceftin) are other choices.

Decongestants may be administered topically (oxymetazoline or phenylephrine) or orally (pseudoephedrine), and mucolytics (guaifenesin) may facilitate drainage of involved sinuses. In patients with atopy, reactive airways disease, or nasal polyposis, oral steroid therapy may help decrease mucosal inflammation and work synergistically with antibiotics in re-establishing drainage through the frontal recess and ostiomeatal complex.

MONITORING PATIENT RESPONSE

The patient who has sinusitis and who is taking an antibiotic should notice relief from symptoms in 48 to 72 hours. If there is no response, the patient should be advised to return as soon as feasible for adjustment in medication and a general assessment of the condition. If symptoms resolve, the patient can be seen for a general checkup in 10 to 14 days.

Special Population Considerations

The challenges in diagnosis and management of rhinosinusitis in children are greater than those in adults. Although the typical adult has two or three acute viral rhinosinusitis episodes annually, the typical child has six to eight episodes that must be distinguished from acute bacterial rhinosinusitis. More than half of patients are given an antibiotic prescription, even though antibiotic therapy does not hasten resolution or prevent bacterial complications of viral rhinosinusitis. Education and counseling are important components in the response to demands by parents to resolve purulent rhinorrhea, which is part of the natural course of viral rhinosinusitis. Bacterial infection is suggested when symptoms persist without improvement for more than 10 days or when they are unusually severe. Facial tenderness, transient periorbital swelling, daytime cough, or fever of 39°C or higher in combination with purulent rhinorrhea is suggestive of bacterial infection.

The high frequency of acute infection in children also may lead to overdiagnosis of chronic rhinosinusitis. Although structural problems play a central role in the etiology of adults with chronic rhinosinusitis, they do not in children, so surgery plays a minor role in management. Immaturity of the immune system, evidenced by higher frequency of viral infection and

Table 23.4

Recommended Order of Treatment for Sinusitis

Order	Agents	Comments
First line	Antibiotic therapy (depends on suspected or confirmed bacterial organisms) Common selections include amoxicillin, trimethoprim–sulfamethoxazole, and symptom relief with decongestants, such as pseudoephedrine; nasal sprays, such as Neo-synephrine (no more than 3 days); and antihistamines, only if allergic process exists	Treatment lasts for 10–14 d. If the patient is severely penicillin allergic, clarithromycin may be substituted.
Second line	Change antibiotic therapy, for example, to amoxicillin with clavulanic acid. Continue symptom relief.	

atopic disease, is a significant etiologic factor in this population. Gastroesophageal reflux is also an important etiologic factor for pediatric chronic rhinosinusitis. The prevalence of reflux disease is higher in children with chronic rhinosinusitis, and treatment of reflux improves sinus symptoms.

As in purulent otitis media, most cases of acute rhinosinusitis are caused by *S. pneumoniae*, *H. influenzae*, and *M. catarrhalis*. In addition, they can be caused by anaerobic organisms and *S. aureus*. Resistance patterns are important in predicting response to antimicrobial therapy: *H. influenzae* and *M. catarrhalis* can be resistant to beta-lactam antibiotics such as ampicillin due to beta-lactamase production. In contrast, *S. pneumonia* and *S. aureus* can be resistant to the penicillins and most other antibiotics by a genetic alteration in penicillin-binding proteins. This form of resistance is much more significant because it is not treated successfully by the typical "second-line" agents such as cephalosporins, macrolides, and amoxicillin–clavulanate. Oral antibiotic options include high-dose amoxicillin and clindamycin.

More than 80% of children with sinusitis have a family history of allergy, as opposed to a general population frequency of 15% to 20%. More than half of the cases of sinusitis are closely associated with asthma. Allergy can contribute to sinusitis by either nasal congestion and subsequent ostia obstruction, or direct allergic effects on sinus-lining cells. Although not IgE mediated, cow's milk protein allergy may be present in very young children with a history of rashes or colic and can be a contributing factor to rhinosinusitis in these children.

For young children with mild to moderate sinusitis, amoxicillin is recommended at the normal dose (45 mg/kg) or high dose (90 mg/kg). Patients with amoxicillin allergy should be treated with a cephalosporin such as cefdinir, cefuroxime, or cefpodoxime, whereas severely allergic patients should be treated with a macrolide such as clarithromycin or azithromycin. Children who do not respond to first-line therapy, children with more severe initial disease, and children who are considered at high risk for resistant *S. pneumoniae* (those who recently have used antibiotics or attend day care) should be treated with high-dose amoxicillin–clavulanate (90 mg/kg of amoxicillin component).

Adjuvant therapies are not necessary in the treatment of uncomplicated acute rhinosinusitis, although saline spray may make children feel better by clearing out secretions, and the newer nonsedating antihistamines may be beneficial in children where allergy is suspected as the causative factor.

PATIENT EDUCATION

The role of the practitioner is to make the patient aware not only of the importance of the therapeutic regimen but also of prevention (see Box 23-1). Education needs to begin before cold and flu season so that patients can take steps to prevent disease and to make educated decisions on whether a health care visit is needed or whether the symptoms are likely to be self-limiting.

Patients also need to know that symptoms of viral and bacterial URIs are similar, but that viral URIs and allergies are more prevalent than bacterial sinusitis. Decongestants may be used in almost all situations, unless the patient has hypertension or coronary artery disease, and they may even be helpful in preventing sinusitis in patients with recurrent symptoms.

Drug Information

Possibly the most important thing for patients to learn is to complete the full course of antibiotic therapy and not to stop taking the medication because symptoms subside in 48 to 72 hours. The patient also needs to know how to recognize and respond to adverse effects of antibiotic therapy, especially because allergic reactions are more prevalent with these drugs than other drugs. The patient should be encouraged to schedule a follow-up visit to assess the potential for chronic sinusitis or other complications, especially if he or she does not feel completely better.

Lifestyle Changes

Although sinusitis cannot be completely prevented, certain measures can reduce the number and severity of the attacks and may prevent acute sinusitis from becoming chronic. These measures include the following: use of a humidifier, particularly if the environment is heated by a dry forced-air system; use of air conditioners to help provide an even temperature; and use of electrostatic filters attached to heating and air conditioning equipment to help remove allergens from the air.

Persons prone to developing sinus disorders, especially persons with allergies, should avoid cigarette smoke and other air pollutants. If allergies inflame the nasal passages, the likelihood for a strong reaction to all irritants is increased.

Drinking alcohol also causes nasal and sinus membranes to swell. For persons prone to sinusitis, it may be uncomfortable to swim in pools treated with chlorine because it irritates the lining of the nose and sinuses. Divers often get sinus congestion and infection when water is forced into the sinuses from the nasal passages.

Air travel may pose a problem for persons with acute or chronic sinusitis. As the air pressure in a plane is reduced, pressure can build up in the head, blocking sinuses or eustachian tubes. The patient may feel discomfort in the sinus or middle ear during the plane's ascent or descent.

■ Case Study

M. R., a 28-year-old Asian-American, presents with complaints of a cold. He states he has been sick for 6 days and is feeling worse. He complains of a thick, green nasal discharge, congestion, and inability to breathe through his nose. He also says he has had a thick, yellow-green expectoration for 4 days, and has chills off and on. He complains of a pounding headache all over his head with sudden movement. He has pain in his neck over the submaxillary and submental nodes when touched, but he is able to swallow. He has tried "flu medicine," but it is not effective. Nothing makes it better or worse.

Objective data include:

Vital signs: temperature, 100.4°F; pulse rate 88; respiratory rate 18; blood pressure 120/70
Ears: tympanic membrane intact bilaterally, landmarks visible
Eyes: conjunctivae pale and moist
Nose: anterior nasal turbinates erythematous and boggy
Throat: pharynx injected without exudate
Neck: (+) tenderness and lymphadenopathy submaxillary and submental cervical nodes, (2) thyroid
Sinuses: frontal and maxillary sinuses tender on palpation; minimal transillumination
Lungs: anterior upper lobes bilaterally with scattered rhonchi—clears with coughing
Other lobes clear to auscultation; (+) thoracic expansion and thorax symmetric; resonance on percussion; no shortness of breath
Neurologic: cranial nerves 2 to 12 intact

Diagnosis: Acute sinusitis

1. List specific goals for treatment for M.R.

2. What drug therapy would you prescribe? Why?

3. What are the parameters for monitoring the success of the therapy?

4. Discuss specific patient education based on the prescribed therapy.

5. List one or two adverse reactions for the selected agent that would cause you to change therapy.

6. What would be the choice for the second-line therapy?

7. What OTC or alternative medications would be appropriate for this patient?

8. What dietary and lifestyle changes should be recommended for this patient?

9. Describe one or two drug/drug or drug/food interactions for the selected agent.

Bibliography

Starred references are cited in the text.

Agency for Health Care Policy and Research. (1999). *Diagnosis and treatment of acute bacterial rhinosinusitis. Evidence report/technology assessment no. 9* (ACHPR publication no. 9). Rockville, MD: Author.

*Berman, S. & Chan, K. (1999). Infections: Viral and rickettsial. In W. Hay, A. Hayward, M. Levine, & J. Sondheimer (Eds.), *Pediatric diagnosis and treatment* (pp. 406, 960–967). Stanford, CT: Appleton & Lange.

Dykewicz, M. S. (2003). Rhinitis and sinusitis. *Journal of Allergy and Clinical Immunology, 111*(2), S520–529.

Gilbert, D. M., Moellering, R. C., Eliopoulos, G. M., & Sande, M. A. (2004). *The Sanford guide to antimicrobial therapy* (34th ed.). Hyde Park, VT: Antimicrobial Therapy.

Goldsmith, A. J., & Rosenfeld, R. M. (2003). Treatment of pediatric sinusitis. *Pediatric Clinics of North America, 50*(2), 413–426.

Hemila, H. (1996). Vitamin C supplementation and common cold symptoms: problems with inaccurate reviews. *Nutrition, 12,* 804–809.

*Lorber, B. (1996). The common cold. *Journal of General Internal Medicine, 11,* 229–236.

Maccabee, M., & Hwang, P. (2001). Medical therapeutics of acute and chronic frontal rhinosinusitis. *Otolaryngologic Clinics of North America, 34*(1), 41–47.

Maltinski, G. (1998). Nasal disorders and sinusitis. *Primary Care: Clinics in Office Practice, 25,* 663–683.

*Mossad, S. B., Macknin, M. L., Medendorp, S. V., & Mason, P. (1996). Zinc gluconate lozenges for treating the common cold: a randomized, double-blind, placebo-controlled study. *Annals of Internal Medicine, 125*(2), 81–88.

Whitman, J. H. (2004). Upper respiratory tract infections. *Clinics in Family Practice, 6*(1), 35–40.

*Williams, J. W., & Simel, D. L. (1993). Does this patient have sinusitis? Diagnosing acute sinusitis by history and physical examination. *Journal of the American Medical Association, 270,* 1242–1246.

Winstead, W. (2003). Rhinosinusitis. *Primary Care Clinics in Office Practice, 30*(1), 137–154.

Visit the Connection web site for the most up-to-date drug information.

24

ASTHMA

■ VIRGINIA P. ARCANGELO

Asthma is a chronic inflammatory disease of the airways that affects 6 per 100 people in the United States. Approximately 4.8 million of these people are children. It is one of the leading causes for both outpatient and hospital care, with approximately 500,000 hospitalizations and more than 5,000 deaths annually. At greatest risk for hospitalization with asthma are African-Americans and children. Death rates from asthma are highest among African-Americans between the ages of 15 and 24 years. The cost for asthma-related treatment is estimated to be $14.5 billion. Approximately half of all cases of asthma develop during childhood and another third before 40 years of age. However, asthma can begin at any age, and it can affect both sexes and all cultures.

CAUSES

Childhood-onset asthma is strongly related to atopy. Approximately 80% of all people with asthma have allergies. Adult-onset asthma can be caused by factors such as coexisting sinusitis, nasal polyps, sensitivity to aspirin or nonsteroidal anti-inflammatory drugs (NSAIDs), and occupational exposure to workplace materials. Those with the greatest risk for development of asthma are children with atopy and a family history of asthma.

Several factors increase the severity of asthma. These include untreated rhinitis or sinusitis, gastroesophageal reflux disorder (GERD), aspirin sensitivity, exposure to sulfites or beta blockers, and influenza.

PATHOPHYSIOLOGY

Asthma is a chronic inflammatory disorder of the airways characterized by airway obstruction, inflammation, and hyperresponsiveness. There is increased resistance to airflow and a decreased flow rate from airway obstruction. Hyperinflation distal to the obstruction, altered pulmonary mechanics, and increased difficulty breathing are a result of the airway obstruction.

There are complex interactions among inflammatory cells, mediators, and the cells and tissues in the airways. Atopic asthma causes bronchospasm, resulting from increased responsiveness of the smooth muscle in the bronchioles to external stimuli. This, in turn, promotes a release of endoge-

nous allergic mediators from the mast cells. These mediators include histamine, leukotrienes, and eosinophil chemotactic factor. There are two phases of symptoms, the acute-phase response and the late-phase response. The acute phase occurs within a few minutes and lasts for several hours, during which there is an interaction of allergens and macrophages. Upregulation of T cells causes the production of interleukins. The response in this phase is bronchospasm. The late-phase response occurs in 2 to 6 hours and lasts approximately 12 to 24 hours.

Long-lived cytokines, such as interleukins, activate eosinophils and T lymphocytes in the airways and release mediators that reproduce the acute asthma attack. Nonatopic asthma does not have an allergic cause but can be a result of exposure to drugs, such as aspirin, NSAIDs, or beta-adrenergic antagonists; chemical irritants; chronic obstructive pulmonary disease; dry air; excessive stress; and exercise. These cause stimulation of the parasympathetic reflex pathway with release of acetylcholine, which constricts bronchial smooth muscle.

Increased permeability and sensitivity to inhaled allergens, irritants, and inflammatory mediators is a consequence of epithelial injury. The chronic inflammation of the airways that is characteristic of asthma can cause thickening of the basement membrane and the deposition of collagen in the bronchial wall. These changes cause the chronic small airway obstruction seen in asthma. The release of inflammatory mediators causes bronchospasm, vascular congestion, vascular permeability, edema, production of thick mucus, and impaired mucociliary function.

Diagnostic Criteria

Key indicators for diagnosing asthma include:

- Wheezing on exhalation
- History of cough that is worse at night, recurrent chest tightness, and recurrent shortness of breath
- Reversible airflow restriction with variability during the day
- Increased symptoms with exercise, viral infections, exposure to allergens, and change in weather
- Awakening at night with symptoms

When the practitioner suspects asthma, further evaluation is called for by measuring pulmonary function. Obstruction of small airways is indicated if there is a reduction in forced expiratory volume in 1 second (FEV$_1$), in peak expiratory flow (PEF), in the ratio of FEV$_1$ to fluid volume capacity (FEV$_1$:FVC), or in the mid-expiratory flow rate. If asthma is suspected, a beta-adrenergic agonist is administered and pulmonary function tests are repeated in 15 to 30 minutes to see if there is an improvement in test values. An increase of PEF or FEV$_1$ exceeding 12% from baseline values strongly supports the diagnosis of asthma.

Asthma is classified according to four steps, which are based on the frequency and intensity of presenting symptoms: mild intermittent, mild persistent, moderate persistent, and severe persistent (Table 24-1). There can be movement up and down the steps, depending on symptoms.

INITIATING DRUG THERAPY

Because asthma is a chronic disease, medication is needed for treatment. However, nonpharmacologic management of asthma also is an essential part of therapy. Patients must be aware of what triggers their asthma symptoms and should remove or avoid all precipitating factors. Smoke, seasonal allergies, animal dander, and cockroach droppings are strong triggers for asthma exacerbations. Outdoor exercise and exertion also should be avoided when pollution levels are high or temperatures are extreme.

Because GERD plays a role in asthma symptoms, the clinician should evaluate the patient for GERD and treat for the problem (see Chapter 29 for a discussion of GERD).

Tight medication control of asthma is desired. Two categories of drugs are used in asthma: long-term medications to control symptoms and quick-relief medications (or rescue medications) to treat acute exacerbations. Long-term control medications include inhaled steroids, cromolyn sodium (Intal, others) and nedocromil (Tilade), leukotriene modifiers, and methylxanthines. Quick-relief medications are bronchodilators (beta$_2$-adrenergic agonists) and systemic (oral) corticosteroids. Medications are available in oral forms, nebulizer solutions, and metered-dose inhalers (MDIs), which deliver a predetermined amount of medication with each inhalation.

Goals of Asthma Therapy

The goals of asthma therapy, as determined by the National Asthma Education and Prevention Program (NAEPP) (2002), include the following:

- Minimal or no symptoms
- Normal PEF rate with variations of less than 20%
- Minimal episodes of exacerbation
- No emergency visits
- Minimal need for prn beta$_2$-adrenergic agonists
- No limitation of activities
- Minimal adverse effects from medications
- Decrease in or amelioration of the long-term airway remodeling leading to irreversible lung changes
- Reduced morbidity and mortality

Inhaled Steroids

Inhaled steroids are the most effective therapy in the treatment of asthma and are indicated for long-term prevention of symptoms and the suppression, control, and reversal of inflammation (Table 24-2).

Mechanism of Action

Inhaled steroids are very lipophilic and quickly enter target cells of the airway and bind to cytosolic glucocorticoid

---

Table 24.1

Classification of Asthma

	Clinical Features Before Treatment*		
	Symptoms†	Nighttime Symptoms	Lung Function
Step 4: Severe persistent	Continual symptoms Limited physical activity Frequent exacerbations	Frequent	FEV$_1$ or PEF ≤60% predicted PEF variability >30%
Step 3: Moderate persistent	Daily symptoms Daily use of inhaled short-acting beta$_2$ agonist Exacerbations affect activity Exacerbations ≥2 times a week; may last days	>1 time a week	FEV$_1$ or PEF >60%–<80% predicted PEF variability >30%
Step 2: Mild persistent	Symptoms >2 times a week but <1 time a day Exacerbations may affect activity	>2 times a month	FEV$_1$ or PEF ≥80% predicted PEF variability 20–30%
Step 1: Mild intermittent	Symptoms ≤2 times a week Asymptomatic and normal PEF between exacerbations Exacerbations brief (from a few hours to a few days); intensity may vary	≤2 times a month	FEV$_1$ or PEF ≥80% predicted PEF variability <20%

FEV$_1$, forced expiratory volume in 1 second; PEF, peak expiratory flow.

* The presence of one of the features of severity is sufficient to place a patient in that category. An individual should be assigned to the most severe grade in which any feature occurs. The characteristics noted in this table are general and may overlap because asthma is highly variable. Furthermore, an individual's classification may change over time.

† Patients at any level of severity can have mild, moderate, or severe exacerbations. Some patients with intermittent asthma experience severe and life-threatening exacerbations separated by long periods of normal lung function and no symptoms.

(From National Asthma Education and Prevention Program, National Health, Lung and Blood Institute, National Institutes of Health. [1997]. *Expert Panel Report II: Guidelines for the diagnosis and management of asthma.* Bethesda, MD; U.S. Department of Health and Human Services.)

Table 24.2

Overview of Selected Drugs Used to Treat Asthma

Generic (Trade) Name and Dosage	Selected Adverse Events	Contraindications	Special Considerations
Inhaled Corticosteroids			
beclomethasone 40 µg/inh 80 µg/inh (GVAR) >6 y: 1 inh bid Children: not for use <5 y Max. 160 mcg/d for Children 320 mcg/d for adults	Hoarseness, dry mouth, oral candidiasis, dysphonia, throat irritation, coughing, headache. GI upset, dizziness	Not for primary treatment of acute attack	Early intervention with inhaled corticosteroids can improve asthma control, normalize lung function, and may prevent irreversible airway injury. They must be used on a regular basis to be effective. It is most effective when administered with a spacer. Patients should rinse their mouths after use. Monitor growth with children. High doses of inhaled corticosteroids have some potential for suppression of growth. Consider calcium supplements or hormone replacement for postmenopausal women on doses >1,000 µg/d.
flunisolide (Aerobid) 250 µg/inh Adult: 2–4 inh bid Children: not for use <6 y 6–15 y: as adult dosage	Same as above	Same as above	Same as above
fluticasone propionate (Flovent) 44, 110, 220 µg/inh 88–440 µg bid Rotadisk—50, 100, 250 µg/inh Rotadisk—100–500 µg bid Children 4–11 y: 50–100 µg bid	Same as above	Same as above	Same as above Not used for children <4 y Caution with ketoconazole
triamcinolone acetonide 100 µg/inh (Azmacort) Adults: 2 inh, tid–qid Children: 1–2 inh, tid–qid or 2–4 inh bid	Same as above	Same as above	Same as above
budesonide (Pulmicort Turbuhaler) 200 µg/inh Adults: 1–2 inh, qd–bid Max. 4 inh bid Children ≤6 y: 1–2 inh bid	Same as above	Same as above	Inhalation powder Use once a day in intermittent or mild persistent asthma.
Mast Cell Stabilizers			
cromolyn sodium (Intal) MDI: 1 mg/inh Nebulizer solution: 20 mg/ampule Adults: MDI: 2–4 inh tid–qid Nebulizer: 1 ampule tid–qid Children: same as adult	Transient bronchospasm, coughing, dry throat, laryngeal edema, joint swelling and pain, dizziness, dysuria, nausea, headache, rash, unpleasant taste, nasal irritation	Not for treatment of acute attacks	Used for long-term control Very effective for exercise-induced asthma One dose before exposure to irritant or before exercise provides protection for 1–2 h.
nedocromil (Tilade) MDI: 1.75 mg/inh nebulizer solution Adults: 2–4 inh bid–qid Children: 1–2 inh bid–qid	Distinctive taste, dizziness, headache, nausea and vomiting	Same as above	Same as above
Leukotriene Modifers			
zafirlukast (Accolate) 10/20 mg tablets Adults: 20 mg bid Children: >75 yrs old 10 mg bid	Headache, respiratory tract infection, GI upset, pain, fever, elevated liver enzymes (rare), dizziness	Potentiates warfarin Increases prothrombin time Potentiated by aspirin May be antagonized by erythromycin and theophylline Not for acute asthma attack	Administration with meals decreases bioavailability; take at least 1 h before meals or 2 h after meals. Not for treatment of acute attacks
montelukast sodium (Singular) 4 mg, 5 mg chewable, drug granules 10 mg tablets Children 12–23 mo 4 mg 2–5 yr 4 mg, 14 y: 5 mg in PM Adults: 10 mg in PM	Headache, asthenia/fatigue, fever, GI disturbances, laryngitis, pharyngitis		Use chewable or granules in children. Pregnancy category B Monitor closely with phenobarbital and rifampin.

Table 24.2

Overview of Selected Drugs Used to Treat Asthma (*Continued*)

Generic (Trade) Name and Dosage	Selected Adverse Events	Contraindications	Special Considerations
Beta$_2$-Adrenergic Agonists albuterol (2 and 4 mg tablets, 2 mg/5 mL syrup, 90 μg/inh, 0.5% and 0.83% solution for nebulizers) (Proventil) 4 mg sustained release (Proventil Repetabs) (Ventolin) same doses as above except: (Rotacaps) 200 μg Adults: Tablets: 2–4 mg tid–qid with a max of 32 mg/d Syrup: 5–10 mL tid–qid Inhaler: 1–2 inh q4–6h Nebulizer solu: 1.25–5 mg in 2–3 mL saline q4–6h Elderly: Tablets: 2 mg tid–qid Syrup: 5 mL tid–qid Children: Tablets: Not recommended <6 y 6–12 y: 2 mg tid–qid with gradual increase to max of 24 mg/d Syrup: not recommended <2 y 2–6 y: 0.1 mg/kg tid to max. of 5 mL tid; may increase gradually to 0.2 mg/kg tid to max. of 10 mL tid 6–14 y: 5 mL tid–qid with gradual increase to 60 mL/d in divided doses (Rotacap) Adults: 1–2 capsules q4–6h Children: <4 y not recommended >4 y: 1 capsule q4–6h	Tachycardia, skeletal muscle tremor, hypokalemia, hyperglycemia, increased lactic acid, dizziness	Patients with preexisting cardiovascular disease may have adverse cardiovascular reactions with inhaled therapy. Antagonized by beta blockers Use with caution in patients taking other sympathomimetics, monoamine oxidase inhibitors, tricyclics.	Very few systemic effects with inhaled therapy Drug of choice for acute bronchospasm Regularly scheduled daily use is not recommended because it does not affect asthma control. Increased use indicates poor asthma control (use of >1 canister per month). At least 1 min should lapse between inhalations. Must use Rotahaler with Rotacaps
pirbuterol (Maxair Autoinhaler) (200 μg/inh) Adults: 1–2 inh q4–6h with a max of 12 inh/d Children: not recommended terbutaline (Brethine) (0.2 mg/inh) (2.5 and 5 mg tablets and mg/mL) Adults: 2 inh q4–6h Adults: 2.5–5 mg tid 0.25 mg into deltoid; may repeat after 15–30 min with max. 0.5 mg/4 h Children 12–15 y: 2.5 mg tid, otherwise not recommended	Paradoxical bronchospasms, nervousness, tremors, headache, dizziness, cough, nausea	Not to be used with other inhaled beta agonists Same as above	
levalbuterol (Xopenex) 0.31 mg/3 mc, 0.63 mg/3 mc, 1.25 mg 6–11 yrs old 0.31 mg tid >11 yrs old 61.3–1.25 mg	Same as above	Same as above	May increase serum digoxin levels
Combination long-acting beta$_2$-agonist and inhaled steroid (Advair Diskus) Fluticasone propionate and salmeterol 100/50, 250/50 and 500/50 4–11 years: 100/50 one inhalation bid	URI, hoarseness, dry mouth, headache, cough, palpitations, pharyngitis, dizziness	Acute asthma attack, caution with cardiac disease	Rinse mouth after use.

(continued)

Table 24.2

Overview of Selected Drugs Used to Treat Asthma (*Continued*)

Generic (Trade) Name and Dosage	Selected Adverse Events	Contraindications	Special Considerations
Adults: start at 100/50 bid and increase if symptoms persist			
Systemic Corticosteroids methylprednisolone (Medrol) (2, 4, 8, 16, 32-mg tablets) prednisolone (5-mg tablets or 5-mg/mL, 15-mg/mL solutions) prednisone (Deltasone) (1, 2.5, 5, 10, 20, 25-mg tablets or 5-mg/mL solution) Adults: 7.5–60 mg/d Short course: 30–60 mg/d as single dose or 2 divided doses for 5–14 d Children: 0.25–2.0 mg/kg/d in single dose or qid as needed for control Short course: 1–2 mg/kg/d to a maximum of 60 mg/d for 3–10 d	*Skin:* acne, decreased wound healing, ecchymosis, petechiae, hirsutism *Central nervous system:* depression, euphoria, headache, personality changes *Cardiovascular:* hypertension *GI:* anorexia, nausea, peptic ulcer *Endocrine:* hyperglycemia, adrenal suppression, weight gain, moon face *Hematologic:* thromboembolism *Musculoskeletal:* muscle wasting, osteoporosis, muscle pain *Fluid and electrolyte:* fluid retention, hypokalemia	Herpes, varicella, tuberculosis, hypertension, peptic ulcer, untreated infections, lactation (with chronic use)	Lowest effective dose should be used. Alternate-day or AM dosing reduces toxicity. Increased efficacy if administered at 3 PM May increase requirements of hypoglycemics Oral contraceptives may block metabolism. Increased risk of tendon rupture with fluoroquinolones Decreased effectiveness of phenytoin, phenobarbital, and rifampin

receptors. Glucocorticoid receptors may directly bind certain transcription factors that are activated by cytokines. Inhaled steroids reduce the number of circulating eosinophils and the number of mast cells in the airways. In addition, they reduce airway hyperresponsiveness by reducing airway inflammation. Chronic treatment with inhaled steroids reduces responsiveness to histamine, cholinergic agonists, exercise, allergens, and irritants. They also reduce symptoms and improve pulmonary function. These drugs provide long-term prevention of symptoms and suppression, control, and reversal of inflammation when taken regularly.

However, inhaled steroids are *not* effective for relieving acute episodes.

Dosage

The lowest dose required to control symptoms is recommended. The recommended dose is two to four inhalations two to four times a day. Inhaled corticosteroids now come in powder form, which is thought to deliver more of the drug to the lungs (budesonide [Pulmicort Turbuhaler]). Table 24-3 lists comparative doses for inhaled corticosteroids.

Table 24.3

Estimated Comparative Daily Dosages for Inhaled Corticosteroids

Drug	Low Daily Dose Adult	Low Daily Dose Child*	Medium Daily Dose Adult	Medium Daily Dose Child*	High Daily Dose Adult	High Daily Dose Child*
beclomethasone CFC 42 or 84 mcg/puff	168–504 mcg	84–336 mcg	504–840 mcg	336–672 mcg	>840 mcg	>672 mcg
beclomethasone HFA 40 or 80 mcg/puff	80–240 mcg	80–160 mcg	240–480 mcg	160–320 mcg	>480 mcg	>320 mcg
budesonide DPI 200 mcg/inhalation	200–600 mcg	200–400 mcg	600–1,200 mcg	400–800 mcg	>1,200 mcg	>800 mcg
Inhalation suspension for nebulization (child dose)		0.5 mg		1.0 mg		2.0 mg
flunisolide 250 mcg/puff	500–1,000 mcg	500–750 mcg	1,000–2,000 mcg	1,000–1,250 mcg	>2,000 mcg	>1,250 mcg
fluticasone MDI: 44, 110, or 220 mcg/puff	88–264 mcg	88–176 mcg	264–660 mcg	176–440 mcg	>660 mcg	>440 mcg
DPI: 50, 100, or 250 mcg/inhalation	100–300 mcg	100–200 mcg	300–600 mcg	200–400 mcg	>600 mcg	>400 mcg
triamcinolone acetonide 100 mcg/puff	400–1,000 mcg	400–800 mcg	1,000–2,000 mcg	800–1,200 mcg	>2,000 mcg	>1,200 mcg

*Children ≤12 years of age
National Asthma Education and Prevention Program. (2002). National Heart, Lung and Blood Institute.

Onset of Action

It takes approximately 2 weeks of continuous therapy for inhaled steroids to achieve maximum effectiveness.

Contraindications

These drugs are contraindicated for use in acute attacks and should be used cautiously in children because of the potential impact on linear growth. However, low-dose inhaled steroids can be used in children younger than 5 years of age with a spacer and a mask if mast call stabilizers are not effective.

Adverse Events

Inhaled steroids usually are well tolerated. Side effects are minimal; the most common adverse events are oropharyngeal candidiasis, dysphonia, hoarseness, cough, and headache. Most of these effects are dose-dependent and can be minimized by using a spacer for delivery and rinsing the mouth after use. Spacers also increase the amount of the drug delivered to the airways.

Mast Cell Stabilizers

Mechanism of Action

Cromolyn sodium and nedocromil inhibit the release of mediators from mast cells, probably by preventing calcium influx across the mast cell membrane (see Table 24-2). They suppress the influx of inflammatory cells and antigen-induced bronchial hyperactivity. These drugs are especially useful in reducing bronchospasm induced by stimuli such as exercise and dry air.

These are used as first-line therapy in children because they do not have the potential for negatively affecting linear growth. These agents are not used for the immediate relief of bronchospasm but for long-term control and for exercise-induced asthma. Cromolyn is effective only as an inhaled agent.

Dosage

The recommended dosage is two to four inhalations three or four times a day.

Time Frame for Response

Plasma concentrations are seen approximately 15 minutes after inhalation; the half-life is 45 to 100 minutes. Any of the medication that is absorbed is excreted unchanged in the bile and urine. It takes 1 to 2 weeks for the medication to become effective, but it may take longer to achieve maximum benefit.

Contraindications

These agents are contraindicated in acute asthma exacerbations for immediate relief.

Adverse Events

Adverse events include headache, nasal irritation, transient bronchospasm, cough, an unpleasant taste, rash, and dry throat.

Leukotriene Modifiers

Levels of the leukotrienes, potent inflammatory mediators, are increased in asthma.

Mechanism of Action

Zafirlukast (Accolate), a receptor antagonist, and montelukast sodium (Singular) block binding of leukotrienes to the receptor. These medications reduce symptoms, improve pulmonary function, and inhibit acute asthma attacks. They are also thought to have anti-inflammatory properties because they reduce the eosinophil count.

Contraindications

The leukotriene modifiers, which dilate the bronchial pathways from the beginning of use, are contraindicated for the reversal of acute bronchospasm. Their effect on breast milk is not determined, so caution should be used in lactating women. Patients with liver impairment may require lower doses.

Adverse Events

Adverse events include headache, dizziness, weakness, gastrointestinal symptoms, elevated liver enzyme levels, back pain, myalgias, fever, and infection.

Interactions

Blood levels of zafirlukast are increased by aspirin and decreased by erythromycin (Eramycin, others) and theophylline (Theo-Dur, others). There is an increased effect of warfarin (Coumadin) when taken with zafirlukast. Food decreases the absorption of zafirlukast. Increased blood levels of theophylline, propranolol (Inderal), and warfarin are found when administered with leukotrienes (see Table 24-2).

Methylxanthines

Methylxanthines inhibit the enzyme phosphodiesterase, preventing the breakdown of cyclic adenosine monophosphate (cAMP). This relaxes bronchial smooth muscle and may prevent the release of endogenous allergens, such as histamine and leukotrienes, from mast cells. The methylxanthines are thought to antagonize prostaglandin-mediated bronchoconstriction and block receptors for adenosine. The main effects are smooth muscle relaxation, central nervous system excitation, and cardiac stimulation. They also increase cardiac output and lower venous pressure. The most common methylxanthine is theophylline. In elderly patients, use of theophylline is considered unsafe because of concomitant disease that may alter theophylline pharmacokinetics, multiple drug interactions, and the frequent inability to tolerate the medication. These are discussed in Chapter 25.

Beta₂-Adrenergic Agonists

In asthma, short-acting beta₂-adrenergic agonists are considered rescue medications that relieve bronchospasm. Long-acting beta₂-adrenergic agonists last for 12 hours but do not act rapidly (see Table 24-2).

For the most part, beta₂-adrenergic agonists are inhaled through a nebulizer or MDI, although they come in oral form. It is important that the patient learn the proper inhalation technique to ensure optimal benefit of the medication. The patient who uses more than one canister of these drugs every month is poorly controlled.

Mechanism of Action

Beta₂-adrenergic agonists provide smooth muscle relaxation after adenylate cyclase activation and an increase in cAMP. This relieves bronchoconstriction.

Dosage

The usual dosage is two or three inhalations every 3 to 4 hours from an MDI (see Table 24-2 for doses of oral and nebulizer solutions). Beta₂-adrenergic agonists work rapidly to increase airflow.

Contraindications

Caution is recommended in patients with ischemic heart disease, hypertension, cardiac arrhythmia, seizure disorder, and hyperthyroidism.

Adverse Events

Adverse events include tachycardia, skeletal muscle tremor, hypokalemia, hyperglycemia, increased lactic acid, headache, hyperglycemia, and dizziness. These drugs can interact with other sympathomimetics, tricyclic antidepressants, and monoamine oxidase inhibitors; they are antagonized by beta blockers.

Systemic Corticosteroids

Systemic corticosteroids are effective in treating an acute asthma exacerbation (see Table 24-2).

Mechanism of Action

These drugs inhibit cytokine and mediator release, attenuation of mucus secretion, and upregulation of beta-adrenergic receptor numbers. They also inhibit immunoglobulin E synthesis, decrease microvascular permeability, and suppress inflammatory cell influx and the inflammatory process. Airway reactivity is reduced by the suppression of airway inflammation, which in turn inhibits mucus secretion, reduces edema of the airway mucosa, and decreases denudation of airway epithelia.

Time Frame for Response

Although these medications are readily absorbed when taken orally, peak plasma concentrations are not achieved for 1 to 2 hours. Short-term (5 days to 2 weeks) therapy with systemic corticosteroids is recommended for acute exacerbations that cannot be controlled with bronchodilators. Symptoms usually improve quickly with oral corticosteroids, within 24 hours.

Dosage

Treatment is usually initiated with an oral dose of 30 to 60 mg of prednisone daily. The daily dose can be tapered or a short course of therapy (5 to 14 days) can be given without tapering. The corticosteroid therapy usually can be discontinued in 5 to 14 days. When symptoms are controlled, the patient is then maintained on inhaled corticosteroids and bronchodilators. If corticosteroids are used in the short term for treating an asthma exacerbation, there is improved efficacy when they are administered at 3 PM because the drug mimics the body's natural cortisone level. Short-term treatment should be continued until the patient achieves 80% PEF or the symptoms resolve.

If corticosteroids are prescribed for long-term therapy to maintain pulmonary function, the lowest possible dose should be used. Corticosteroids can be administered in the morning, either daily or every other day. Dosing late in the day may cause insomnia. Dosing every other day may produce less adrenal suppression.

Contraindications

Oral corticosteroids are contraindicated in untreated infections, lactation (chronic use), and known alcohol intolerance.

Adverse Events

Serious adverse events include psychosis and peptic ulcer. Less serious adverse events include nausea, vomiting, dyspepsia, edema, headache, mood swings, hypokalemia, elevated blood pressure, hyperglycemia, ecchymosis, and acne. Adverse events affecting all body systems are much more common in long-term corticosteroid therapy than in short-term therapy (see Table 24-2).

Interactions

Systemic corticosteroid therapy may increase the dosage requirements of insulin or oral hypoglycemic agents. Metabolism of corticosteroids may be blocked with oral contraceptives. Corticosteroids combined with quinolones may increase the risk of tendon rupture. The effectiveness of phenytoin (Dilantin), phenobarbital (Luminal), and rifampin (Rifadin) may be decreased when using corticosteroids.

Selecting the Most Appropriate Agent

Asthma treatment consists of a stepwise approach that corresponds to the patient's asthma classification (ie, the features or severity of asthma; Fig. 24-1 and Table 24-4). Control of asthma symptoms should be achieved as quickly as possible. To gain control, treatment may be started at the step most appropriate to the severity of symptoms, or a higher level. When control of symptoms is achieved, therapy should be prescribed that includes the least amount of medication needed.

A rescue course of systemic corticosteroids may be needed at any time and for patients diagnosed in any step for quick symptomatic relief. Acute exacerbations of asthma

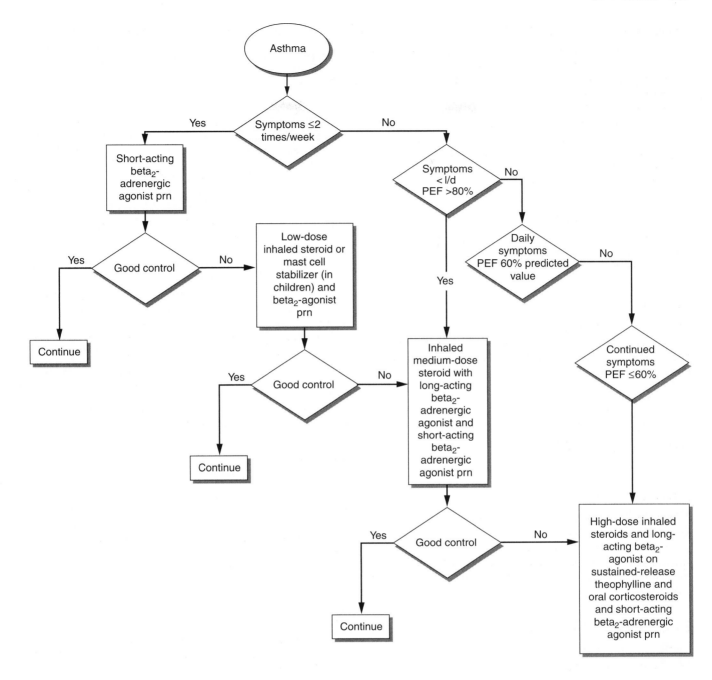

Key ⬭ Starting point for decision making; ▢ clinical actions (assessing, prescribing, monitoring); ◇ decision point.

Figure 24–1 Treatment algorithm for asthma.

can be treated with inhaled, short-acting beta₂-adrenergic agonists. If the patient has a good response to systemic corticosteroid therapy (PEF 70% normal), it may be used to manage the condition with close follow-up. The dose of systemic corticosteroids is 1 to 2 mg/kg/day in a single dose for children and 30 to 60 mg/day for adults.

First-Line Therapy (Step 1)

In the patient with mild intermittent asthma (symptoms no more than twice a week), the recommended treatment is an

inhaled short-acting bronchodilator as needed. No daily medication is needed. If beta₂-adrenergic agonists are used more than twice a week, or a canister is used in a month, the patient should move up to second-line therapy.

Second-Line Therapy (Step 2)

The next step is for mild persistent asthma (symptoms more than twice a week but less than once a day). The treatment recommendation is a low-dose inhaled corticosteroid with a short-acting bronchodilator once a day as needed for symptom

Table 24.4

Stepwise Approach for Managing Asthma in Adults and Children Older Than 5 Years of Age: Treatment

Classify Severity: Clinical Features Before Treatment or Adequate Control			Medications Required To Maintain Long-Term Control
	Symptoms/Day Symptoms/Night	PEF or FEV₁ PEF Variability	Daily Medications
Step 4 **Severe Persistent**	Continual Frequent	≤60% >30%	• **Preferred treatment:** –**High-dose inhaled corticosteroids** AND –**Long acting inhaled beta₂-agonists** AND, if needed, –Corticosteroid tablets or syrup long term (2 mg/kg/day, generally do not exceed 60 mg per day). (Make repeat attempts to reduce systemic corticosteroids and maintain control with high-dose inhaled corticosteroids.)
Step 3 **Moderate Persistent**	Daily >1 night/week	>60% – <80% >30%	• **Preferred treatment:** –**Low to medium-dose inhaled corticosteroids and long-acting inhaled beta₂-agonists** • Alternative treatment –Increase inhaled corticosteroids within medium-dose range OR –Low- to medium-dose inhaled corticosteroids and either leukotriene modifier or theophylline If needed (particularly in patients with recurring severe exacerbations): • **Preferred treatment:** –**Increase inhaled corticosteroids within medium-dose range and add long-acting inhaled beta₂ agonists.** • Alternative treatment –Increase inhaled corticosteroids within medium-dose range and add either leukotriene modifier or theophylline.
Step 2 **Mild Persistent**	>2/week but <1x/day >2 nights/month	≥80% 20–30%	• **Preferred treatment:** –**Low-dose inhaled corticosteroids** • Alternative treatment: cromolyn, leukotriene modifier, nedocromil, OR sustained-release theophylline to serum concentration of 5–15 mcg/mL
Step 1 **Mild Intermittent**	≤2 days/week ≤2 nights/month	≥80% <20%	• **No daily medication needed** • Severe exacerbations may occur, separated by long periods of normal lung function and no symptoms. A course of systemic corticosteroids is recommended.

Quick Relief **All Patients**	• Short-acting bronchodilator: 2–4 puffs **short-acting inhaled beta₂-agonists** as needed for symptoms • Intensity of treatment will depend on severity of exacerbation; up to 3 treatments at 20-minute intervals or a single nebulizer treatment as needed. Course of systemic corticosteroids may be needed. • Use of short-acting beta₂-agonists >2 times a week in intermittent asthma (daily, or increasing use in persistent asthma) may indicate the need to initiate (increase) long-term-control therapy.

Step down
Review treatment every 1 to 6 months; a gradual stepwise reduction in treatment may be possible.

Step up
If control is not maintained, consider step up. First, review patient medication technique, adherence, and environmental control.

Note

• The stepwise approach is meant to assist, not replace, the clinical decision making required to meet individual patient needs.

• Classify severity: assign patient to most severe step in which any feature occurs (PEF is % of personal best: FEV₁ is % predicted).

• Gain control as quickly as possible (consider a short course of systemic corticosteroids); then step down to the least medication necessary to maintain control.

• Minimize use of short-acting inhaled beta₂-agonists. Overreliance on short-acting inhaled beta₂-agonists (e.g., use of approximately one canister a month even if not using if every day) indicates inadequate control of asthma and the need to initiate or intensify long-term-control therapy.

• Provide education on self-management and controlling environmental factors that make asthma worse (e.g., allergens and irritants).

• Refer to an asthma specialist if there are difficulties controlling asthma or if step 4 care is required. Referral may be considered if step 3 care is required.

Goals of Therapy: Asthma Control
• Minimal or no chronic symptoms day or night
• Minimal or no exacerbations
• No limitations on activities; no school/work missed
• Maintain (near) normal pulmonary function
• Minimal use of short-acting inhaled beta₂-agonist
• Minimal or no adverse effects from medications

National Asthma Education and Prevention Program. (2002). National Heart, Lung and Blood Institute.

relief. An alternative to inhaled anti-inflammatory therapy (but not a preferred therapy) is sustained-release theophylline or leukotriene modifiers. If symptoms are not controlled with this regimen, there is a need to move to third-line therapy.

Third-Line Therapy (Step 3)

The third step is for moderate persistent (daily symptoms) asthma. Evidence shows that the use of a long-acting beta$_2$-agonist added to a low or medium dose of inhaled corticosteroid improves lung function. Use of the short-acting beta$_2$-adrenergic agonist more than once a day indicates failure of this regimen and necessitates movement to fourth-line therapy. Adding a leukotriene modifier or theophylline to inhaled corticosteroids or doubling the dose of the inhaled corticosteroid improves outcomes also, but the evidence is not as strong.

In children younger than 5, either a long-acting beta$_2$-agonist should be added to a low-dose inhaled corticosteroid or a medium-dose inhaled corticosteroid should be used as monotherapy.

Fourth-Line Therapy (Step 4)

The fourth step is for severe persistent asthma (continual symptoms). The treatment recommendation is the use of a high-dose inhaled corticosteroid and a long-acting beta$_2$-agonist. Oral corticosteroids are added as needed. A short-acting bronchodilator is used as needed for symptom control. At this step, the patient should be under the care of a specialist.

Special Population Considerations

Pediatric

There is strong evidence from clinical trials that inhaled corticosteroids improve the control of asthma for children with mild to moderate persistent asthma. The lowest effective dose is used and growth is monitored carefully. It is the opinion of the National Asthma Education and Prevention Program Expert Panel that the initiation of long-term control therapies should be considered in infants and young children who have had more than three episodes of wheezing in the past year that lasted more than 1 day and affected sleep and who have risk factors for the development of asthma. Risk factors include parental history of asthma or diagnosed atopic dermatitis, allergic rhinitis, wheezing apart from colds, and peripheral blood eosinophils. This applies also to infants and young children who require symptomatic treatment more than twice per week or who have severe exacerbations less than 6 weeks apart.

Data in children followed for 6 years suggest that low to medium doses of inhaled corticosteroids may decrease growth by about 1 cm in the first year of treatment, but this effect is not sustained in subsequent years of treatment and the final predicted height is reached. The height of any child taking corticosteroids, either oral or inhaled, should be monitored; if growth retardation is seen, the benefits of asthma control should be weighed against the possibility of growth delay.

Oral corticosteroids can cause growth retardation in young children and are used only if the exacerbation of asthma is moderate to severe. Instead of using inhalers, children 5 years of age and younger should use nebulizers or MDIs with a face mask to promote maximum delivery of inhaled medications. Table 24-5 summarizes asthma treatment for infants and children younger than 5 years of age.

Women

There may be a decrease in bone mineral content with inhaled corticosteroids, increasing the risk for osteoporosis. Postmenopausal women are already at risk for osteoporosis, so the practitioner should prescribe supplemental calcium, 1,000 to 1,500 mg/day, and vitamin D, 400 U/day.

Asthma management during pregnancy is similar to management in nonpregnant women, with medications that are safe and well tolerated by the mother and fetus. If oral corticosteroids are prescribed, blood glucose levels should be monitored regularly because of the drug's association with an increased risk for gestational diabetes.

Geriatric

Because older patients with cardiovascular disease may experience tremors and tachycardia with beta$_2$-adrenergic agonists, it is helpful to use combination beta$_2$-adrenergic agonists and anticholinergics to prevent this. Because theophylline clearance is decreased in elderly patients, the build-up of theophylline may exacerbate a pre-existing heart condition, so the drug should be used cautiously in the elderly.

In elderly patients, prolonged use of systemic corticosteroids can have an adverse effect on bone metabolism by decreasing calcium deposition and enhancing calcium resorption, predisposing some patients to osteoporosis.

MONITORING PATIENT RESPONSE

After beginning therapy, the patient should be evaluated in 1 to 2 weeks. Subsequent evaluations every 1 to 6 months are necessary to determine if the asthma is well controlled. If there is good control, the patient should be moved down a treatment step; if control is poor, the patient should be moved up a treatment step. Before moving the patient up to the next step, a careful history of medication use and technique and exposure to triggers is taken. For instance, if the patient has been diagnosed with moderate persistent asthma and has been well controlled on a low-dose inhaled steroid and a long-acting beta$_2$-adrenergic agonist with a short-acting beta$_2$-adrenergic agonist as needed, he or she can be tried on a low-dose inhaled steroid with the short-acting beta$_2$-adrenergic agonist used as needed. The patient monitors his or her PEF and uses the short-acting beta$_2$-adrenergic agonist if the PEF drops below 80% of predicted value or if there is increased wheezing. If asthma is not controlled with the intervention initiated, the prescriber must assume that the patient is at the next step and initiate treatment accordingly.

PATIENT EDUCATION

Medication

The various types of delivery systems for inhaled medications include inhalers, nebulizers, disks, and rotosystems. Each product includes information on how many inhalations are contained in the device. It is important that the patient does not run out of medications. The patient must learn the correct way to use each system and should have an extra system on hand as a backup for use at all times. These systems are described and a detailed description of their use is provided in Box 24-1.

Internet sites for information on asthma include www.AAAAI.org (American Academy of Allergy, Asthma

Table 24.5

Stepwise Approach for Managing Infants and Young Children (5 Years of Age and Younger) With Acute or Chronic Asthma

Classify Severity: Clinical Features Before Treatment or Adequate Control		Medications Required To Maintain Long-Term Control
	Symptoms/Day Symptoms/Night	Daily Medications

Step 4
Severe Persistent
	Continual
	Frequent
		• **Preferred treatment:**
		  –**High-dose inhaled corticosteroids**
		    AND
		  –**Long-acting inhaled beta₂-agonists**
		    AND, if needed,
		  –Corticosteroid tablets or syrup long term (2 mg/kg/day, generally do not exceed 60 mg per day). (Make repeat attempts to reduce systemic corticosteroids and maintain control with high-dose inhaled corticosteroids.)

Step 3
Moderate Persistent
	Daily
	>1 night/week
		• **Preferred treatments:**
		  –**Low-dose inhaled corticosteroids and long-acting inhaled beta₂-agonists.**
		    OR
		  –**Medium-dose inhaled corticosteroids**
		• Alternative treatment:
		  –Low-dose inhaled corticosteroids and either leukotriene receptor antagonist or theophylline
		
		If needed (particularly in patients with recurring severe exacerbations):
		• **Preferred treatment:**
		  –**Medium-dose inhaled corticosteroids and long-acting beta₂-agonists**
		• Alternative treatment:
		  –Medium-dose inhaled corticosteroids and either leukotriene receptor antagonist or theophylline

Step 2
Mild Persistent
	>2 week but <1x/day
	>2 nights/month
		• **Preferred treatment:**
		  –**Low-dose inhaled corticosteroid (with nebulizer or MDI with holding chamber with or without face mask or DPI)**
		• Alternative treatment
		  –Cromolyn (nebulizer is preferred or MDI with holding chamber)
		    OR leukotriene receptor antagonist

Step 1 **Mild Intermittent**	≤2 days/week ≤2 nights/month	• **No daily medication needed**

Quick Relief
All Patients
	• Bronchodilator as needed for symptoms. Intensity of treatment will depend upon severity of exacerbation.
	  –Preferred treatment: **Short-acting inhaled beta₂-agonists** by nebulizer or face mask and space/holding chamber
	  –Alternative treatment: Oral beta₂-agonist
	• With viral respiratory infection
	  –Bronchodilator q 4–6 hours up to 24 hours (longer with physician consult); in general, repeat no more than once every 6 weeks
	  –Consider systemic corticosteroid if exacerbation is severe or patient has history of previous severe exacerbations
	• Use of short-acting beta₂-agonists >2 times a week in intermittent asthma (daily, or increasing use in persistent asthma) may indicate the need to initiate (increase) long-term-control therapy.

 Step down
Review treatment every 1 to 6 months; a gradual stepwise reduction in treatment may be possible.

 Step up
If control is not maintained, consider step up. First, review patient medication technique, adherence, and environmental control.

Note
• The stepwise approach is intended to assist, not replace, the clinical decision making required to meet individual patient needs.
• Classify severity: assign patient to most severe step in which any feature occurs.
• There are very few studies on asthma therapy for infants.
• Gain control as quickly as possible (a course of short systemic corticosteroids may be required): then step down to the least medication necessary to maintain control.
• Minimize use of short-acting inhaled beta₂-agonists. Overreliance on short-acting inhaled beta₂-agonists (e.g., use of approximately one canister a month even if not using if every day) indicates inadequate control of asthma and the need to initiate or intensify long-term-control therapy.
• Provide parent education on asthma management and controlling environmental factors that make asthma worse (e.g., allergies and irritants).
• Consultation with an asthma specialist is recommended for patients with moderate or severe persistent asthma. Consider consultation for patients with mild persistent asthma.

Goals of Therapy: Asthma Control
• Minimal or no chronic symptoms day or night
• Minimal or no exacerbations
• No limitations on activities; no school/parent's work missed
• Minimal use of short-acting inhaled beta₂-agonist
• Minimal or no adverse effects from medications

National Asthma Education and Prevention Program. (2002). National Heart, Lung and Blood Institute.

BOX 24–1. DIRECTIONS FOR USE OF DELIVERY DEVICES FOR ASTHMA MEDICATIONS

Metered-Dose Inhaler
1. Remove the cap and hold the inhaler upright.
2. Shake the inhaler.
3. Tilt your head back slightly and breathe out.
4. Use the inhaler in any of these ways:
   a. Open mouth with inhaler 1 to 2 inches away
   b. Use spacer
   c. In the mouth
5. Press down on the inhaler to release the drug as you start to breathe in slowly.
6. Breathe in slowly for 3 to 5 seconds.
7. Hold your breath for 10 seconds to allow the drug to reach deeply into your lungs.
8. Repeat puffs as directed, waiting 1 minute between puffs.
9. Rinse your mouth after use if using an inhaled corticosteroid.

Turbuhaler
1. Unscrew the cover and lift it off.
2. Hold inhaler upright with the mouthpiece up.
3. Turn the colored base as far as it will go, then back, until it clicks to release a measured dose of the drug.
4. Breathe out to empty your lungs.
5. Place the mouthpiece between your teeth with lips snug around it and your tongue out of the way.
6. Breathe in deeply.
7. Hold your breath for 10 seconds to allow the drug to reach deeply into your lungs.
8. Repeat as directed.
9. Rinse your mouth after use.
10. A red dot in the little window indicates that there are 20 doses left.

Diskhaler
1. Lift the back of the lid until it points straight up and down to pierce the blister of drug.
2. Breathe out to empty your lungs.
3. With the diskhaler level, place the mouthpiece between your teeth with lips snug around it and tongue out of the way. Keeping the device horizontal prevents the powder from spilling.
4. Breathe deeply and quickly.
5. Hold your breath for 10 seconds to allow the drug to reach deeply into your lungs.
6. Repeat as directed.
7. Clean the device regularly with the brush provided.
8. Don't cover the air inlet holes at the base.
9. Rinse your mouth after use.

Diskus
1. Open the diskus by holding the outer case in one hand and putting the thumb of the other hand on the thumb grip and push as far as it will go. Keep the diskus horizontal.
2. Slide the lever away until you hear a click.
3. Breathe out to empty your lungs.
4. Place the mouthpiece between your teeth with your lips snug around it.
5. Breathe in as deeply and as quickly as possible.
6. Hold your breath for 10 seconds to allow the drug to reach deeply into your lungs.
7. Close the diskus by sliding the thumb grip backwards as far as it will go. This automatically resets the lever to its initial position.
8. If a second dose is needed, close the diskus and repeat.
9. Rinse your mouth after use.

Spacer with Mask for Children Under 3
1. Remove the cap from the canister.
2. Shake the canister.
3. Place the canister upside down with the mouthpiece in the rubber opening of the spacer device.
4. Place the mask of the spacer over the child's mouth and nose, making a good seal.
5. Press down on the canister, releasing a puff of medication into the spacer.
6. Hold the mask in place until the child has taken at least 6 breaths, as seen from movement of a window on the mask.
7. Rinse the mask with warm water weekly and let it dry in room air.

BOX 24–1. DIRECTIONS FOR USE OF DELIVERY DEVICES FOR ASTHMA MEDICATIONS (*continued*)

Spacer with Mouthpiece for Children Over 3
1. Remove the cap from the canister.
2. Shake the canister.
3. Place the canister upside down with the mouthpiece in the rubber opening of the spacer device.
4. Have the child take a deep breath out to empty the lungs.
5. Place the mouthpiece in the child's mouth.
6. Press down on the canister, releasing a puff of medication into the spacer.
7. Have the child breathe in deeply and slowly.
8. Have the child hold his or her breath for 10 seconds.
9. Repeat to be sure that all of the drug is used.

Nebulizer with Mask or Mouthpiece
1. Measure the drug into the cup below the mask or mouthpiece.
2. Put the mask over the mouth and nose or the mouthpiece between the teeth with the tongue out of the way.
3. Switch on the machine.
4. Use the nebulizer for 10 to 15 minutes until all of the drug in the cup has been used.
5. Rinse the nebulizer with warm water after each use.

and Immunology), www.lungusa.org/asthma (American Lung Association), and www.nhlbl.gov/guidelines/asthma (guidelines from the National Asthma Education and Prevention Program).

The patient with asthma is prescribed a peak flow meter, which measures PEF, and is instructed to monitor and record PEF. PEF rates measure control and exacerbations of asthma. This monitoring allows the patient to determine when additional intervention is warranted. The practitioner should bring the record of PEF readings for review at each office visit. Predicted PEF values are shown in Table 24-6, although these may vary by individual. The

TABLE 24.6

Normal Predicted Average Peak Expiratory Flow (PEF) (liters per minute)

Age (y)	Men[1*] Height (in) 60	65	70	75	80	Age (y)	Women[1*] Height (in) 55	60	65	70	75	Adolescents[2†] Height (in)	Boys	Girls
15	511	531	548	564	578	15	423	438	451	463	473	50	249	248
20	554	575	594	611	626	20	444	460	474	486	497	51	262	261
25	580	603	622	640	656	25	455	471	485	497	509	52	276	275
30	594	617	637	655	672	30	458	475	489	502	513	53	289	288
35	599	622	643	661	677	35	458	474	488	501	512	54	303	302
40	597	620	641	659	675	40	453	469	483	496	507	55	316	315
45	591	613	633	651	668	45	446	462	476	488	499	56	329	328
50	580	602	622	640	656	50	437	453	466	478	489	57	343	342
55	566	588	608	625	640	55	427	442	455	467	477	58	356	355
60	551	572	591	607	622	60	415	430	443	454	464	59	370	369
65	533	554	572	588	603	65	403	417	430	441	451	60	383	382
70	515	535	552	568	582	70	390	404	416	427	436	61	397	395
75	496	515	532	547	560	75	377	391	402	413	422	62	410	409
												63	423	422
												64	437	436
												65	450	449
												66	464	462
												67	477	476
												68	491	489
												69	504	503
												70	517	516

* Computed from the equations of Nunn and Gregg.[1]
† Computed from the equations of Godfrey et al.[2]
Courtesy of 1. Nunn, A.J. & Gregg, I. (1989). New regression equations for predicting peak expiratory flow in adults. *British Medical Journal, 298,* 1068–1070;2. Godfrey, S., Kamburoff, P.L., Naim, J.R. et al. (1970). Spirometry, lung volumes and airway resistance in normal children aged 5 to 18 years. *British Journal of Diseases of the Chest, 64,* 15–24.
NOTE: All tables are averages and are based on tests with a large number of people. The peak flow of an individual can vary widely. Individuals at altitudes above sea level should be aware that peak flow readings may be lower than those provided in the tables. (Reproduced with permission of Glaxo Wellcome Inc., Research Triangle Park, NC.)

BOX 24–2. HOW TO USE YOUR PEAK FLOW METER

A peak flow meter is a device that measures how well air moves out of your lungs. During an asthma episode, the airways of the lungs usually begin to narrow slowly. The peak flow meter may tell you if there is narrowing in the airways hours—sometimes even days—before you have any asthma symptoms.

By taking your medicine(s) early (before symptoms), you may be able to stop the episode quickly and avoid a severe asthma episode. Peak flow meters are used to check your asthma the way that blood pressure cuffs are used to check high blood pressure.

The peak flow meter also can be used to help you and your doctor:

- Learn what makes your asthma worse
- Decide if your treatment plan is working well
- Decide when to add or stop medicine
- Decide when to seek emergency care

A peak flow meter is most helpful for patients who must take asthma medicine daily. Patients age 5 and older are usually able to use a peak flow meter. Ask your doctor or nurse to show you how to use a peak flow meter.

How To Use Your Peak Flow Meter
- Do the following five steps with your peak flow meter:
  1. Move the indicator to the bottom of the numbered scale.
  2. Stand up.
  3. Take a deep breath, filling your lungs completely.
  4. Place the mouthpiece in your mouth and close your lips around it. Do not put your tongue inside the hole.
  5. Blow out as hard and fast as you can in a single blow.
- Write down the number you get. If you cough or make a mistake, don't write down the number, do it over again.
- Repeat steps 1 through 5 two more times and write down the best of the three blows in your asthma diary.

Find Your Personal Best Peak Flow Number
Your personal best peak flow number is the highest peak flow number you can achieve over a 2- to 3-week period when your asthma is under good control. Good control is when you feel good and do not have any asthma symptoms.

Each patient's asthma is different, and your best peak flow may be higher or lower than the peak flow of someone of your same height, weight, and sex. This means that it is important for you to find your own personal best peak flow number. Your treatment plan needs to be based on your own personal best peak flow number.

To find out your personal best peak flow number, take peak flow readings:

- At least twice a day for 2 to 3 weeks
- When you wake up and between noon and 2:00 pm
- Before and after you take your short-acting inhaled beta$_2$-agonist for quick relief, if you take this medicine
- As instructed

From National Asthma Education and Prevention Program, National Health, Lung and Blood Institute, National Institutes of Health. (1997) *Expert Panel Report II: Guidelines for the diagnosis and management of asthma.* Bethesda, MD: U.S. Department of Health and Human Services.

BOX 24–3. PEAK FLOW ZONE SYSTEM

Green Zone
- Peak flow is greater than 80% of personal best.
- No symptoms of asthma are present.
- Medications are taken normally.

Yellow Zone
- Peak flow is 50% to 80% of personal best.
- Control is not good, which may indicate one of the following:
  - An exacerbation with need for intervention
  - Poor control with need for change of regimen

Red Zone
- Peak flow is below 50% of personal best.
- This is a medical alert.
- Take inhaled beta$_2$-agonist immediately.
- Contact the primary care provider if intervention does not return peak flow to the yellow or green zone.

best personal value is determined by having the patient measure PEF rates twice a day for 2 weeks during a symptom-free period, or after maximum therapy. The patient is instructed to do three measurements and take the best of the three. Instructions on using a peak flow meter are found in Box 24-2.

The patient is then taught the concept of zones as they pertain to PEF monitoring. The zones are green, yellow, and red (Box 24-3). If the patient is in the green zone, treatment remains as usual. If he or she is in the yellow zone, an inhaled beta$_2$-adrenergic agonist should be taken right away. The red zone signals a medical emergency, and the patient should take an inhaled beta$_2$-adrenergic agonist at once and seek medical treatment.

Lifestyle Changes

Since asthma is associated with allergies and is exacerbated when the patient is exposed to allergens, the patient should be aware of triggers and avoid them. Many asthmatics are sensitive to scents and should avoid them when possible.

■ Case Study

M.L. is a 15-year-old boy who plays soccer for his school team. He has noticed that when running, he sometimes has trouble catching his breath. He also reports an increased runny nose and itchy eyes. He has a frequent dry cough and is awakened with coughing spells at least four times a week. His mother and father have seasonal allergies and his mother has asthma. This morning he woke up and heard "funny sounds" when he took a breath. His coughing increased when he took a deep breath. In his nose, the mucosa is pale and swollen bilaterally. His lungs have bilateral expiratory wheezing; respirations are 22 and PEF is 400. His heart shows a normal sinus rhythm, with no murmurs or gallops; pulse is 72; and there is no cyanosis.

Diagnosis: Mild persistent asthma

1. List specific goals of therapy for M.L.
2. What drug therapy would you prescribe?
3. What are the parameters for monitoring the success of the therapy?
4. Discuss specific patient education based on the prescribed therapy.
5. List one or two adverse reactions for the selected agent(s) that would cause you to change therapy.
6. If the patient is still having symptoms with the prescribed therapy, what would be your next course of action?
7. What lifestyle changes would you recommend for M.L.?
8. When would you instruct him to return for evaluation?
9. If upon return his symptoms have resolved, what would be your course of action?

Bibliography

Starred references are cited in the text.

Apter, A. (2003). Clinical advances in adult and pediatric asthma. *Journal of Allergy and Clinical Immunology, 111*(3 Suppl), 780–784.

Apter, A., & Szefler, S. (2004). Advances in adult and pediatric asthma. *Journal of Allergy and Clinical Immunology, 113*(3), 407–411.

Centers for Disease Control and Prevention (1998). Surveillance for asthma—United States, 1960–1995. *MMWR, 47*(SS1), 1–28.

National Asthma Education and Prevention Program, National Heart, Lung and Blood Institute, National Institutes of Health (1999). *Expert Panel Report II: guidelines for the diagnosis and management of asthma.* Bethesda, MD: U.S. Department of Health and Human Services.

*National Asthma Education and Prevention Program, National Heart, Lung and Blood Institute, National Institutes of Health (2002). *Expert Panel Report II: guidelines for the diagnosis and management of asthma. Update on selected topics.* Bethesda, MD: U.S. Department of Health and Human Services.

National Institutes of Health (1997). *Teach your patients about asthma: a clinician's guide.* Bethesda, MD: U.S. Department of Health and Human Services.

Stafford, R. S., et al. (2003). National trends in asthma visits and asthma pharmacotherapy. *Journal of Allergy and Clinical Immunology, 111*(4), 729–735.

Williams, S. G., Schmidt, D. K., Reed, S. C., & Storm, W. (2002). Key clinical activities for quality asthma care. Recommendations of National Asthma Education and Prevention Program. *MMWR, 52*(RR-6), 1–8.

Visit the Connection web site for the most up-to-date drug information.

CHRONIC OBSTRUCTIVE PULMONARY DISEASE

■ VIRGINIA P. ARCANGELO

Chronic obstructive pulmonary disease (COPD), also called chronic obstructive lung disease (COLD), is a pulmonary disorder characterized by small airway obstruction and reduction in expiratory flow rate. Approximately 12.1 million Americans were diagnosed with COPD in 2001, and almost as many have early asymptomatic disease. It is the fourth leading cause of death in the United States, rating second as a cause of disability. By 2020, it is expected to be the third leading cause of death. The estimated cost of COPD in 2002 was $32.1 billion (U.S. Department of Health and Human Services, 2003). COPD begins early in life, but significant symptoms do not usually appear until the middle years. The prevalence of COPD increases with age. Prevalence is also higher in men than in women and in whites compared with other racial groups. One of the biggest problems with COPD is that there are no clinical findings during the early stages of the disease process, and by the time the patient is symptomatic, the disease has progressed significantly.

The most common forms of COPD are chronic bronchitis and emphysema. Chronic bronchitis is diagnosed in patients who have a history of excessive secretion of bronchial mucus with a productive cough for 3 months or longer in at least 2 consecutive years. The lungs of patients with emphysema are characterized by an abnormal, permanent enlargement of the air spaces distal to the terminal bronchiole, with destruction of the acinar wall. The patient usually demonstrates some features of both types of COPD, but one dominates.

CAUSES

The most common cause is smoking: smokers have a 30 times greater risk of death from COPD. Other risk factors are air pollution, occupational exposure to respiratory irritants, chronic respiratory infections, and hyperresponsive airways due to asthma.

Emphysema, unlike chronic bronchitis, may also result from a genetic deficiency of the protein alpha$_1$-antitrypsin. This protein deficiency can trigger early-onset emphysema, even in nonsmokers. Both parents must carry the gene for the disease to be acquired by offspring. The genetic factor accounts for only approximately 3% of cases.

PATHOPHYSIOLOGY

Chronic bronchitis is marked by thickened bronchial walls, hyperplastic and hypertrophied mucus glands, and mucosal inflammation in the bronchial walls and airways. Emphysema is characterized by permanent destruction of the alveoli as a result of irreversible destruction of elastin, a protein in the lung that maintains the strength of the alveolar walls. The destruction of elastin causes enlargement of air spaces as the walls of the small airways and alveoli lose elasticity. In addition, there is a narrowing of the bronchioles, limiting airflow to the lungs. The walls of the airways thicken, closing off some of the smaller air passages and narrowing larger ones. Air enters the alveoli during expansion of the lung in inhalation but cannot escape during exhalation because the air passages collapse. Air is trapped in the lungs, causing uneven blood flow and airflow to the walls of the alveoli. In some alveoli, there is adequate blood flow but little air; in others, there is adequate air but inadequate blood flow. This results in a decreased oxygen exchange. It becomes more difficult for air to flow through narrow airways, and the patient's respiratory muscles tire. Inadequate air reaches the alveoli, causing inadequate removal of carbon dioxide from the lungs. This results in a buildup of carbon dioxide and a decreased level of oxygen in the blood.

Diagnostic Criteria

The symptoms of COPD depend on whether the disease results from chronic bronchitis or pulmonary emphysema. Chronic bronchitis presents with wheezing; copious, purulent sputum production; and shortness of breath. For a diagnosis of chronic bronchitis to be made, there must be cough and sputum production on most days for more than 3 months during 2 consecutive years. Emphysema presents with dyspnea with light exertion; scant, thick sputum production; and possibly a slight cough with little sputum production. A patient presenting with symptoms of COPD usually has lost between 50% and 70% of lung tissue.

Pulmonary function studies are essential in diagnosing COPD. Forced vital capacity is the maximum volume of air that can be exhaled with force. This indicates lung size. Forced expiratory volume measures the maximum volume of air expired in 1 second (FEV$_1$). Lung function as measured

Table 25.1

Stages of COPD

Stage 0	At risk	Chronic cough and sputum production Lung function normal
Stage I	Mild	Mild airflow limitation $FEV_1/FVC < 70\%$ but $FEV_1 \geq 80\%$ predicted value Usually chronic cough and sputum production
Stage II	Moderate	Airflow limitation $FEV_1/FVC > 70\%$ $50\% \leq FEV_1 < 80\%$ predicted value Progression of symptoms with shortness of breath, especially on exertion
Stage III	Severe	Further worsening of airflow limitation $FEV_1/FVC < 70\%$ $30\% \leq FEV_1 < 50\%$ predicted value Increased shortness of breath, repeated exacerbations
Stage IV	Very severe	Severe airflow limitation $FEV_1/FVC < 70\%$ $FEV_1 < 30\%$ predicted value plus chronic respiratory failure

by FEV_1 diminishes with age at a rate of approximately 25 mL/year from 35 years of age on. Smoking increases the rate of decline. FEV_1 and symptoms are used to stage COPD (Table 25-1).

INITIATING DRUG THERAPY

COPD is a progressive disease, but early intervention is beneficial in relieving symptoms and slowing disease progression. Avoidance of irritants such as allergens and smoke is essential in managing asthma and COPD. Outdoor exercise and exertion should be avoided when pollution levels are high or temperatures are extreme. The patient with COPD is taught how to conserve energy to maintain quality of life. For example, the most strenuous activity should be done in the early morning, when the patient has the most energy.

Drug therapy is initiated when the patient becomes symptomatic. Patients with COPD usually are older and are more susceptible to the side effects of medications, so a stepwise approach is useful in treatment.

Goals of Drug Therapy

Although COPD is not reversible, the major goals of therapy are to slow the progression of the disease, prevent acute exacerbations, maintain quality of life (ie, minimize limitation of activities and loss of productivity), improve the symptoms associated with obstruction, and reduce mortality. Drug therapy relieves cough and bronchospasm and enhances airflow. Drugs used to treat COPD include beta$_2$ agonists, anticholinergics, theophylline, corticosteroids, and antibiotics for infectious process (Table 25-2).

Inhaled Beta$_2$ Agonists

Beta$_2$ agonists relax smooth muscle, dilate airways, and improve pulmonary function. These drugs are used for symptom relief in patients with COPD. The dosage should not exceed 12 inhalations a day for short-acting preparations.

The short-acting beta$_2$ agonist albuterol (Proventil) can be used in combination with the inhaled anticholinergic agent ipratropium. If this combination therapy is used, ipratropium should be taken 2 hours before albuterol. Inhaled beta$_2$ agonists are discussed in more detail in Chapter 24.

Anticholinergics

Mechanism of Action

Inhaled anticholinergics relax the bronchial muscles and act as a bronchodilator. They also block the contraction of bronchial smooth muscle and decrease the mucus secretion from parasympathetic activity. Anticholinergics prevent the acetylcholine-induced release of allergenic mediators from mast cells. The most common anticholinergic is ipratropium (Atrovent). There is also a long-acting anticholinergic tiotropium (Spiriva HandiHaler).

Dosage and Time Frame for Response

The dosage of ipratropium is two to four puffs four to six times a day. Onset of action after inhalation is 15 minutes, with a peak response of 1 to 2 hours and a duration of action of 3 to 4 hours.

The dosage of tiotropium is 1 capsule daily. Onset of action is within 5 minutes; it is effective for 24 hours.

Contraindications

Anticholinergics are not used in a patient with hypersensitivity to atropine. They also are not used for acute episodes of bronchospasm. Caution is used in a patient with narrow-angle glaucoma or benign prostatic hypertrophy, and in pregnancy and lactation. It should not be used in people with soy or peanut allergies.

Adverse Events

Common adverse events associated with anticholinergic use include restlessness, dizziness, headache, gastrointestinal distress, blurred vision, hoarseness, cough, palpitations, and urinary obstruction.

Methylxanthines (Theophyllines)

Theophylline is a third-line therapy for treating the reversible component of airway obstruction in chronic bronchitis and COPD. Other therapies are preferred because of the adverse event profile of the theophyllines, particularly the potential for toxicity.

Mechanism of Action

Methylxanthines inhibit the enzyme phosphodiesterase, preventing the breakdown of cyclic adenosine monophosphate. This relaxes bronchial smooth muscle and may prevent the release of endogenous allergens such as histamine and leukotrienes from mast cells. The methylxanthines are thought to antagonize prostaglandin-mediated bronchoconstriction and block receptors for adenosine. The main effects are smooth muscle relaxation, central nervous system excitation, and

Table 25.2

Overview of Selected Agents Used to Treat COPD

Generic (Trade) Name and Dosage	Selected Adverse Events	Contraindications	Special Considerations
Beta$_2$ Agonists			
albuterol (Proventil) 2–4-mg tablets, 2 mg/5 mL syrup, 90-µg/inhalation, 0.5% and 0.83% solution for nebulizers; (Proventil Repetabs) 4-mg sustained release; (Ventolin Rotocaps) 200 µg *Adults* Tablets: 2–4 mg tid or qid with a maximum of 32 mg/d Syrup: 5–10 mL tid or qid Inhaler: 1–2 inhalations q4–q6 Inhalable solution: 2.5 mg (0.5 mL of 0.5% solution diluted to 3 mL with normal saline solution or 3 mL of 0.083% solution *Elderly* Tablets: 2 mg tid or qid Syrup: 5 mL tid or qid *Children* Tablets not recommended <6 y 6–12 y: 2 mg tid or qid with gradual increase to maximum of 24 mg/d Syrup not recommended <2 y; ages 2–6 y: 0.1 mg/kg tid to maximum of 5 mL tid, may increase gradually to 0.2 mg/kg tid; ages 6–14 y: 5 mL tid or qid with gradual increase to 60 mL/d in divided doses	Tachycardia, skeletal muscle tremor, increased lactic acid levels, hypokalemia, hyperglycemia, dizziness	Antagonized by beta blockers in patients taking other sympathomimetic drugs, monoamine oxidase inhibitors, tricyclic antidepressants Patients with pre-existing cardiovascular disease may have adverse cardiovascular reactions with inhaled therapy.	Very few systemic effects with inhaled therapy Drug of choice for acute bronchospasm At least 1 min should elapse between inhalations.
pirbuterol (Maxair Autoinhaler) 200 µg/inhalation 1–2 inhalations q4–6h with a maximum of 12 inhalations/day	Paradoxical bronchospasms, nervousness, tremors, headache, dizziness, cough, nausea		Same as above Also, avoid use with other inhaled beta agonists.
terbutaline (Brethaire) 0.2 mg/inhalation *Adults* 2 inhalations q4–6h (Brethine) 2.5- and 5-mg tablets; also injectable preparation *Adults* 2.5–5 mg tid or 0.25 mg into deltoid; may repeat after 15 to 30 min with maximum 0.50 mg/4 h *Children* 12–15 y: 2.5 mg tid; otherwise not recommended	Same as above Also, prolongation of QT interval	Same as above	Long acting; not to be used to treat acute symptoms Not to be used in place of anti-inflammatory therapy
Combination Long-Acting Beta$_2$-Agonist and Inhaled Steroid Advair Diskus Fluticasone propionate and salmeterol 100/50, 250/50, and 500/50 4–11 years: 100/50 one inhalation bid Adults: start at 100/50 bid and increase if symptoms persist	URI, hoarseness, dry mouth, headache, cough, palpitations, pharyngitis, dizziness	Acute asthma attack, caution with cardiac disease	Rinse mouth after use.

(continued)

Table 25.2

Overview of Selected Agents Used to Treat COPD (*Continued*)

Generic (Trade) Name and Dosage	Selected Adverse Events	Contraindications	Special Considerations
Anticholinergics			
ipratropium bromide (Atrovent) 18 µg/inhalation 2 inhalations qid	Exacerbation of symptoms, cough, nervousness, dizziness, GI upset, headache, palpitations, rash, urinary retention	Allergy to atropine Allergy to peanuts Caution with BPH & narrow-angle glaucoma	Patients using this drug for the first time need to learn how to use inhaler device properly for best effect.
ipratropium bromide (18 µg) and albuterol (90 µg) (Combivent) 2 inhalations qid	Same as above Also, upper respiratory infection and rhinitis	Same as above	Antagonized by beta blockers
tiotropium bromide (Spiriva) 18 mcg/capsule 1 capsule inhaled daily	Same as above	Same as above	Use with HandiHaler device only.
Methylxanthines			
theophylline (SloPhyllin) 200–400 mg bid or 400–800 mg at night for nocturnal symptoms	Exacerbation of symptoms, cough, nervousness, dizziness, GI upset, headache, palpitations, rash	Allergy to atropine Allergy to peanuts	Monitor theophylline levels regularly to detect potential toxicity early.

cardiac stimulation. They also increase cardiac output and lower venous pressure. The most commonly used methylxanthine is theophylline.

Dosage and Time Frame for Response

The dosage of the sustained-release preparation is 200 to 400 mg twice a day or 400 to 800 mg at night for nocturnal symptoms. The drug is usually taken at 8 PM for relief of nocturnal symptoms. Smokers may require a dose 50% higher than the recommended dose. The dosage prescribed for patients with hypoxia, congestive heart failure, or liver disease is 25% to 50% lower than the normal dose.

The half-life of theophylline is 3 to 15 hours (4 to 5 hours in smokers), with extended-release formulas having the longer half-life.

Contraindications

Theophylline is contraindicated in peptic ulcer disease, seizure disorders, arrhythmias, and severe respiratory obstruction. Theophylline is metabolized in the liver and excreted in the urine, so it is used cautiously in patients with heart failure, liver disease, and thyroid dysfunction, and theophylline levels are carefully monitored.

Adverse Events

Adverse effects include headache, irritability, and insomnia. The patient also may experience palpitations, loss of appetite, gastrointestinal distress, tachypnea, urinary retention, and flushing. Toxicity can produce cardiac arrhythmias and seizures.

Interactions

Excessive caffeine intake (greater than the equivalent of six cups of coffee a day) can cause increased concentration of the drug. Theophylline interacts with many drugs, including cimetidine (Tagamet), erythromycin, quinolones, oral contracep-

tives, and barbiturates. Food may alter bioavailability of the sustained-release theophylline preparation; therefore, the prescriber may recommend taking the medication 1 hour before or 2 hours after a meal.

Corticosteroids

Systemic corticosteroids suppress inflammation of the airways and inhibit prostaglandin-induced narrowing of the airways. Systemic corticosteroids are used only for severe flare-ups and are most useful in patients with chronic bronchitis. They enhance the effects of the bronchodilators. If the corticosteroids are used for long-term therapy, the lowest possible dose should be used. They can be administered either daily or every other day, in the morning or early afternoon because they may cause insomnia. Dosing every other day may produce less adrenal suppression.

Inhaled steroids diminish airway inflammation. Their use in COPD is questionable, but they might allow for withdrawal of systemic steroids. They do appear to lower the exacerbation rate, although this response is seen primarily in patients with severe disease who have frequent exacerbations. It is unclear whether they have an effect on symptoms or exercise capacity. The use of the combination salmeterol (50 mcg) and fluticasone (250 mcg) (Advair) has been shown to increase lung function but does not reduce exacerbations or decrease symptoms.

Antibiotics

Patients with chronic bronchitis are predisposed to repeated respiratory infections resulting from mucus stagnation due to impaired ciliary movement and plugging. Aggressive management of respiratory infections is paramount to the management of COPD. The most common bacterial causes of respiratory infection in patients with COPD are *Haemophilus influenzae, Streptococcus pneumoniae, Chlamydia pneumoniae,* and *Legionella pneumophila.* Treatment of these infections is discussed in Chapter 26.

Table 25.3

Recommended Order of Treatment for COPD

Order	Agent	Comments
First line	Inhaled short-acting bronchodilator	
Second line	Inhaled beta₂ agonists and anticholinergics	The combination drug ipratropium and albuterol (Combivent) can be used.
Third line	Theophylline with beta₂ agonist rescue	Serum theophylline levels must be monitored (recommended range: 8–12 µg/mL).
	Inhaled corticosteroids	
Fourth line	Managed by a specialist with corticosteroids at a tapering dose for 2 wk	Use for acute exacerbations and as long-term therapy in patients not responsive to other therapeutic regimens. Once symptoms improve, the patient may be switched to inhaled steroids.

Selecting the Most Appropriate Agent

Medications cannot alter the course of COPD, but they can control symptoms and improve quality of life. A stepwise approach to therapy is recommended, adding medications as symptoms increase (Table 25-3 and Fig. 25-1).

First-Line Therapy

A short-acting bronchodilator is recommended when needed for mild COPD. This can be either an anticholinergic or a beta₂ agonist. It can be used on a regular basis for patients with persistent symptoms.

Second-Line Therapy

Many patients with COPD do not get relief from just one medication. If the patient does not respond adequately to an anticholinergic medication, an inhaled beta₂ agonist can be added, or vice versa. If the patient has coexisting heart disease, inhaled beta₂ agonists should be administered carefully. The combination ipratropium and albuterol preparation (Combivent) is also used as second-line therapy.

Third-Line Therapy

When anticholinergics and beta₂ agonists do not control symptoms, theophylline can be added to the regimen. Theophylline is a third-line drug choice because it has a limited bronchodilatory effect and a narrow therapeutic range. However, theophylline has been shown to decrease dyspnea and improve quality of life (Celli, 1998). Beta₂ agonists are used only for acute symptoms. Sustained-release theophylline is used in doses of 200 to 400 mg two times a day or 400 to 800 mg at bedtime for control of nocturnal symptoms. A smoker usually needs a dose 50% higher than that for a nonsmoker.

Inhaled corticosteroids may be helpful if the patient's FEV_1 is less than 50% predicted or if the patient has repeated exacerbations.

Fourth-Line Therapy

Corticosteroids are used for patients with acute exacerbations of COPD and as long-term therapy in patients who do not respond to bronchodilators and anticholinergics. Systemic corticosteroids are prescribed at a tapering dose for 14 days, starting with 40 mg. If there is no improvement, these drugs are discontinued. If improvement occurs, inhaled steroids can be added to the regimen when the oral steroids are discontinued, or the patient can be maintained on the minimum effective dose of oral systemic corticosteroids. Approximately 20% to 30% of patients with COPD improve if given long-term oral corticosteroids (Celli, 1998). These patients should be managed along with a specialist.

Special Population Considerations

Geriatric

In older patients with cardiovascular disease, tremors and tachycardia may develop with beta₂ agonist therapy. The combination of ipratropium and albuterol may be prescribed to help prevent tremors and tachycardia. Theophylline clearance is decreased in elderly patients, and the subsequent buildup of theophylline may exacerbate a preexisting heart condition. Therefore, this drug should be prescribed cautiously for elderly patients.

Women

Inhaled corticosteroids may promote a decrease in bone mineral content, thereby increasing the risk for osteoporosis. Postmenopausal women are already at risk for osteoporosis, so they may be advised to take 1,000 to 1,500 mg of supplemental calcium and 400 units of vitamin D daily. Hormone replacement therapy may be considered when appropriate.

MONITORING PATIENT RESPONSE

Patients taking theophylline on a regular basis need to have their blood theophylline levels monitored routinely. Safe theophylline levels in patients with COPD are 8 to 12 mg/dL. Theophylline levels are analyzed 2 weeks after initiation of therapy, then every 6 to 12 months. If theophylline levels are too low, the dose is increased by 25% and levels are rechecked after 2 weeks. If the levels are too high, the next dose is withheld if it is 20 to 25 mg/L and the dosage decreased by 10%. At 25 to 30 mg/L, the next dose is withheld and subsequent doses are decreased by 25%. Levels are rechecked in several days. If the level is greater than 30 mg/L, the next two doses are withheld and the dosage is decreased by 50% and levels are rechecked in several days. Theophylline levels should be checked 1 to 2 hours after administration of a

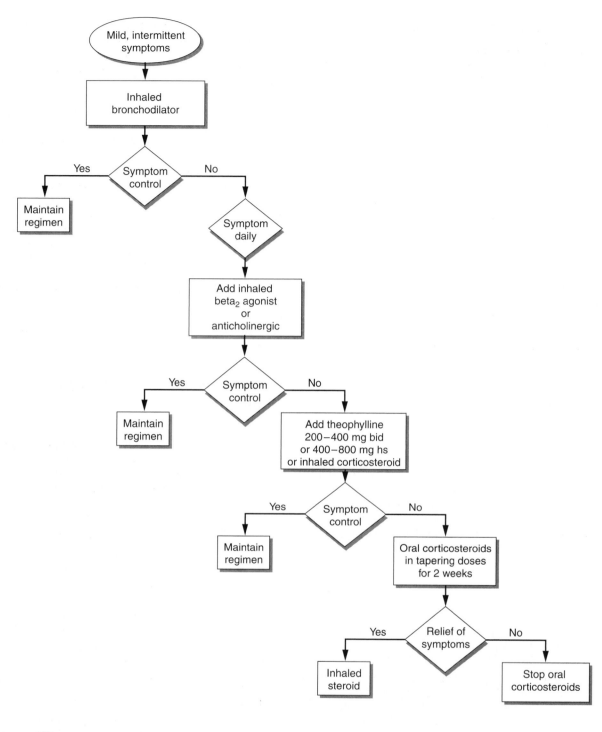

Figure 25–1   Treatment algorithm for COPD.

short-acting preparation or 4 hours after administration of a long-acting preparation.

Follow-up examinations should be scheduled at 2 to 3 months. Meanwhile, the patient needs to be aware of the warning signs of respiratory infection and symptoms that suggest worsening of the condition. Pulmonary function tests are recommended every 1 to 2 years to determine the efficacy of therapy.

PATIENT EDUCATION

Drug Information

Patients with COPD are cautioned to avoid antihistamines, cough suppressants, sedatives, tranquilizers, beta blockers, and narcotics because these may further compromise the patient's already depressed respiratory state. All patients with COPD should be immunized against pneumonia and influenza.

Patient-Oriented Information Sources

The best source for patients about COPD is the National Heart, Lung and Blood Institute's website, www.nhlbi.nih.gov. Other sources are the American College of Chest Physicians (www.chest.net.org/education/patient/guide/copd) and the American Lung Association (www.lungusa.org/lungprofilers/copdlungprofiler.html).

Nutrition/Lifestyle Changes

The practitioner should explain to the patient that preventing respiratory infection is very important in COPD management. This is because serious consequences—and most deaths—result from respiratory failure caused by infection. The patient should be advised to stay away from anyone with a respiratory infection, and the practitioner should ensure that the patient can recognize the warning sings of infection, including a change in the color, consistency, and amount of sputum. If symptoms develop, treatment should be sought immediately.

The practitioner should also discuss the advantages of conserving energy to maintain activities of daily living. Activities should be attempted early in the day, when the patient has the most energy. The patient can do aerobic exercises using the arms and legs to increase endurance.

Another important aspect of management of COPD is rehabilitation: the patient should partake in at least 2 months of pulmonary rehabilitation.

Additional teaching involves showing the patient how to use inhalers, nebulizers, or spacer devices (see Chapter 24 for more information).

Weight loss frequently occurs in patients with COPD and is a determining factor of functional capacity, health status, and mortality. As many as one third to one half of patients with COPD are undernourished. Low body weight in patients with COPD is associated with an impaired pulmonary status, reduced diaphragmatic mass, lower exercise capacity, and a higher mortality rate than in adequately nourished individuals with COPD. Weight loss occurs because of increased energy requirements unbalanced by dietary intake. Both metabolic and mechanical inefficiency contribute to the elevated energy expenditure. An imbalance between protein synthesis and protein breakdown may cause a disproportionate depletion of fat-free mass in some patients. Patients need to eat a high-calorie diet and should be encouraged to use supplemental feedings to maintain a desirable weight.

■ Case Study

R.W. is a 64-year-old postal clerk who has smoked a pack of cigarettes a day for the past 35 years. He presents with progressive difficulty getting his breath while doing simple tasks. He is having difficulty doing any manual work, but he has no symptoms when working behind his desk. He also reports a cough, fatigue, and weight loss. He has been treated for three respiratory infections a year for the past 3 years and feels like another one is developing now.

On physical examination, you notice clubbing of his fingers, use of accessory muscles for respiration, wheezing in the lungs, and hyperresonance on percussion of the lungs. Pulmonary function studies show an FEV_1 of 58%.

Diagnosis: Chronic obstructive pulmonary disease

1. List specific treatment goals for R.W.
2. What drug therapy would you prescribe? Why?
3. What are the parameters for monitoring the success of the therapy?
4. Describe specific patient education based on the prescribed therapy.
5. List one or two adverse reactions for the selected agent that would cause you to change therapy.
6. What would be the choice for second-line therapy?
7. What dietary and lifestyle changes should be recommended for this patient?
8. Describe one or two drug/drug or drug/food interactions for the selected agent.

Bibliography

Starred references are cited in the text.
Barnes, P. J. (2003). Therapy of chronic obstructive pulmonary disease. *Pharmacological Therapy, 97*(1), 87–94.

*Celli, B. R. (1998). Standards for optimal management of COPD: A summary. *Chest, 113,* 283S–287S.
Global Initiative for Chronic Obstructive Lung Disease (GOLD). Accessed at www.goldcopd.com on July 30, 2004.

McEvoy, C. E., & Niewoebner, D. E. (2000). Corticosteroids in chronic obstructive pulmonary disease: clinical benefits and risks. *Clinical Chest Medicine, 21*(4), 739–752.

Schols, A. M., & Wouters, E. F. (2000). Nutritional abnormalities and supplements in chronic obstructive pulmonary disease. *Clinical Chest Medicine, 21*(4), 753–762.

Sin, D. D., McAlister, F. A., Man, S. F. P், & Anthonisen, N. R. (2003). Contemporary management of chronic obstructive pulmonary disease. *Journal of the American Medical Association, 290,* 2301–2312.

Thomas, D. R. (2002). Dietary prescription for chronic obstructive pulmonary disease. *Clinical Geriatric Medicine, 18*(4), 835–839.

*U.S. Department of Health and Human Services. National Institute of Health, National Heart, Lung and Blood Institute (2003). *Chronic obstructive pulmonary disease. Data fact sheet.* NIH Publication 03-5229.

Visit the Connection web site for the most up-to-date drug information.

BRONCHITIS AND PNEUMONIA

■ ERIC WITTBRODT AND TEEN EAPPEN-ABRAHAM

One of the most commonly occurring upper respiratory tract infections is bronchitis, which may present as an acute or a chronic infection.

ACUTE BRONCHITIS

Acute bronchitis is a frequently diagnosed condition and is the ninth most common outpatient illness in the United States. The disease is a reversible inflammatory condition of the tracheobronchial tree that occurs in all age groups and is usually self-limiting. Typically, acute bronchitis occurs during the winter months. Predisposing factors for acute bronchitis include cold air, damp climates, fatigue, malnutrition, and inhalation of irritating substances, such as polluted air and cigarette smoke.

CAUSES

Viral infections cause 95% of acute bronchitis episodes; the most common respiratory viruses associated with acute bronchitis are rhinovirus, coronavirus, influenza virus A, parainfluenza virus, adenovirus, and respiratory syncytial virus (RSV) (Bartlett, 1997; Hueston & Mainous, 1998).

Bacterial infections cause 5% to 20% of acute bronchitis. The only bacterial microorganisms implicated in the pathogenesis of uncomplicated acute bronchitis are *Bordetella pertussis*, *Chlamydia pneumoniae*, and *Mycoplasma pneumoniae*. Limited evidence indicates that other common respiratory tract pathogens such as *Streptococcus pneumoniae* can contribute to acute bronchitis.

PATHOPHYSIOLOGY

Acute bronchitis is characterized by infection of the tracheobronchial tree. This infection results in hyperemic and edematous mucous membranes, yielding an increase in bronchial secretions. Destruction of the respiratory epithelial lining and reduced mucociliary function result from these changes. This process is usually transient and resolves after the infection clears.

DIAGNOSTIC CRITERIA

Signs and symptoms of acute bronchitis are preceded by manifestations of an upper respiratory tract infection such as coryza, malaise, chills, back and muscle pain, headache, and sore throat. If fever is present, it rarely exceeds 39°C and lasts for 3 to 5 days. Fever is more commonly seen with adenovirus, influenza virus, and *M. pneumoniae* infection. The hallmark of acute bronchitis is a cough that is initially dry and nonproductive; however, as the production of bronchial secretions increases, the cough becomes more abundant and mucoid. The cough usually lasts for 7 to 10 days, although in some patients it can persist for weeks to months.

Pulmonary examination may reveal signs of coarse, moist bilateral crackles, rhonchi, and wheezing. The chest x-ray typically reveals no active disease. The usefulness of cultures to identify the causative microorganisms is limited because most cases of acute bronchitis are viral in origin, and cultures usually are negative or grow normal nasopharyngeal flora. Laboratory tests may reveal a normal or slightly elevated white blood cell (WBC) count.

The high reported incidence of acute bronchitis can be correlated with the absence of definitive diagnostic signs or laboratory tests. Thus, the diagnosis is based purely on the patient's risk factors and signs and symptoms. In many patients an upper respiratory tract infection (sinusitis or allergic rhinitis) may be misdiagnosed as acute bronchitis.

INITIATING DRUG THERAPY

The general treatment for acute bronchitis is symptomatic and supportive (Fig. 26-1). Patients should be encouraged to drink plenty of fluids to prevent dehydration and decrease the viscosity of bronchial secretions. Bed rest is indicated until fever subsides. Mild analgesic/antipyretic therapy is effective for relief of fever and musculoskeletal pains. Aspirin or acetaminophen (Tylenol; 650 mg in adults or 10-15 mg/kg per dose in children) or ibuprofen (Advil, others; 200-400 mg in adults or 10 mg/kg per dose in children) administered every 4 to 6 hours can be used as analgesic/antipyretic therapy. Acetaminophen is the agent of choice because aspirin should be avoided owing to the correlation of aspirin and the development of Reye

325

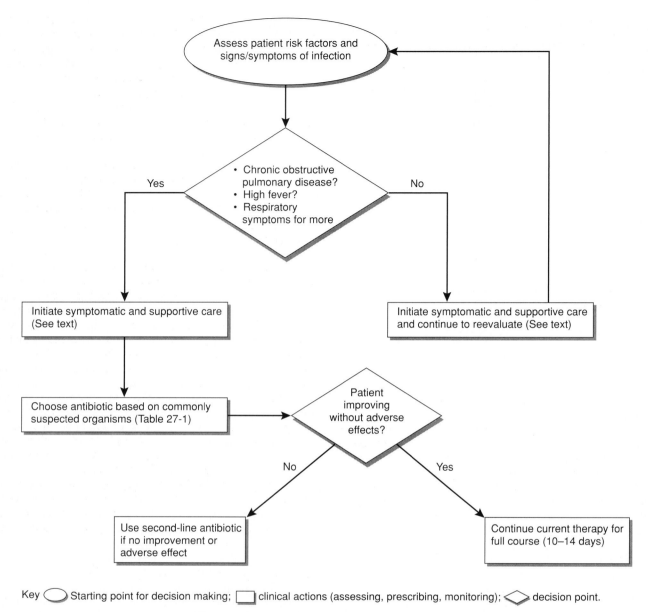

Figure 26–1   Treatment algorithm for acute bronchitis.

syndrome in children. Aspirin and ibuprofen should also be used cautiously in elderly patients, patients with a history of peptic ulcer disease, and patients with renal insufficiency.

Nonprescription cough and cold medications (see Chap. 23) often are used by patients to help reduce the signs and symptoms of acute bronchitis. The use of nonprescription medications that contain various combinations of antihistamines, sympathomimetic agents, and antitussives can result in dehydration of bronchial secretions. This could lead to further aggravation of symptoms, which prolongs the recovery process. Cough that is associated with acute bronchitis can become bothersome for the patient. Dextromethorphan, an antitussive agent, is recommended to help treat mild, persistent cough. Severe cough may require more potent cough medications that contain codeine or similar agents.

Goals of Drug Therapy

The goals of pharmacotherapy include providing the patient with comfort and, in severe cases, treating associated dehydration and respiratory compromise. If antibiotics are administered, minimizing side effects is also a goal.

Antibiotics

Antibiotics often are prescribed for patients with acute bronchitis; however, they offer little relief from the respiratory symptoms of the disease and do not shorten the course of the illness.

The routine use of antibiotics for acute bronchitis is discouraged. Antibiotics are indicated if the patient has concomitant chronic obstructive pulmonary disease (COPD), high fevers, purulent sputum, or respiratory symptoms for

Table 26.1

Acute Bronchitis: Drug Therapy for Selected Microorganisms

Microorganism	Treatment
Haemophilus influenzae	aminopenicillin (ampicillin or amoxicillin)
Maraxella catarrhalis, *H. influenzae* (beta-lactamase producing)	aminopenicillin + clavulanic acid (Augmentin)
Mycoplasma pneumoniae, *Chlamydia* spp.	macrolide (erythromycin, clarithromycin, or azithromycin) or doxycycline
Bordetella pertussis	erythromycin
Influenza A	amantadine or rimantadine or oseltamivir or zanamivir
Influenza B	amantadine or rimantadine or oseltamivir or zanamivir

more than 4 to 6 days. Empiric antibiotic therapy should be directed against the microorganisms commonly suspected to cause acute bronchitis.

Selecting the Most Appropriate Agent

Table 26-1 lists the antibiotics that are commonly used to treat acute bronchitis caused mostly by bacteria. Aminopenicillins such as ampicillin (Omnipen) and amoxicillin (Amoxil) are effective against infections caused by pneumococci, streptococci, and *Haemophilus influenzae.*

For microorganisms that produce β-lactamase, such as *Moraxella catarrhalis,* and *H. influenzae,* aminopenicillins given in combination with a β-lactamase inhibitor such as clavulanate (Augmentin) should be administered.

For acute bronchitis due to atypical bacteria such as *M. pneumoniae* and *Chlamydia* species, macrolides (eg, erythromycin [Eryc], clarithromycin [Biaxin], or azithromycin [Zithromax]) or doxycycline (Vibramycin) are usually efficacious. Doxycycline should not be used in children younger than 8 years of age. In this population, the agent of choice is erythromycin. If *B. pertussis* is the likely microorganism, erythromycin is the drug of choice. Fluoroquinolone antibiotics (eg, gatifloxacin [Tequin], levofloxacin [Levaquin], moxifloxacin [Avelox]) are effective against typical and atypical organisms, but are usually reserved for acute bronchitis refractory to macrolides or doxycycline. Their use is not recommended for patients younger than 18 years.

During epidemics caused by influenza A virus, amantadine (Symmetrel) or rimantadine (Flumadine) may be administered early in the course of the illness to minimize symptoms. Oseltamivir (Tamiflu) and zanamivir (Relenza) are two new antiviral agents that can be used for the symptomatic treatment of complicated acute bronchitis caused by influenza A or B in adults who have been symptomatic for no longer than 2 days (see Fig. 26-1; for more information about antibiotic/antimicrobial therapy, refer to Chapter 8).

CHRONIC BRONCHITIS

Chronic bronchitis is a component of COPD, which is the fourth leading cause of death in the United States. (See Chapter 25 for a discussion of COPD.) The standard description/definition of chronic bronchitis is productive cough and sputum production for 3 months per year for at least 2 years, and an acute exacerbation of chronic bronchitis is defined as worsening of respiratory symptoms such as increased cough, sputum, and dyspnea. Chronic bronchitis primarily affects adults and occurs more commonly in men than in women. Between 10% and 25% of the adult population in the United States 40 years of age or older is afflicted with chronic bronchitis, which accounts for a large amount of health care expenditures and lost wages.

Because many infections are untreated, the exact morbidity of acute exacerbations of chronic bronchitis is unknown. Patients with chronic bronchitis are more likely to have frequent and severe episodes of acute bacterial bronchitis.

CAUSES

Several factors are implicated in the pathogenesis of chronic bronchitis; however, the precise cause of this disease is unknown. The predominant factor in chronic bronchitis is cigarette smoke, a well-known respiratory irritant, and most patients with chronic bronchitis have a history of cigarette smoking. Occupational dust, fumes, and environmental pollution also contribute to the etiology of the disease. The phrase industrial bronchitis refers to chronic bronchitis acquired from occupational and environmental exposure to pollutants. Cold, damp climates can provoke acute exacerbations of chronic bronchitis; hypersecretion of mucus in patients with asthma has also been shown to yield symptoms of chronic bronchitis. Evidence suggests that recurrent respiratory infections may predispose a person to development of chronic bronchitis, although the exact reason for this is unclear.

Colonization of the lower airways with bacteria such as *H. influenzae, M. catarrhalis,* and *S. pneumoniae* has been frequently detected in patients with chronic lung disease. Viral infections may account for nearly one third of acute exacerbations of chronic bronchitis.

PATHOPHYSIOLOGY

Several physiologic abnormalities of the bronchial mucosa may lead to chronic bronchitis. It has been suggested that patients with chronic bronchitis are predisposed to respiratory infections because of impaired mucociliary clearance due to chronic inhalation of irritating substances. Factors that can lead to impaired mucociliary clearance are the proliferation of mucous-secreting goblet cells and the replacement of ciliated epithelium with nonciliated metaplastic cells. The latter event results in the inability of the bronchi to clear the profuse, thick, sticky secretions present in patients with chronic bronchitis.

Other changes in the bronchial mucosa of patients with chronic bronchitis that predispose them to infection are hypertrophy and dilation of the glands that produce mucus. In addition, inhalation of toxic irritants results in bronchial obstruction because of stimulation of cholinergic activity and increased bronchomotor tone.

Bacteria residing in the tracheobronchial tree also predispose patients to acute exacerbations of chronic bronchitis. *H. influenzae* and other microorganisms harbored in the bronchial epithelium act as reservoirs for infection when the patient's host defenses are compromised. Compromised host defenses include decreased phagocytosis of bacteria by polymorphonuclear neutrophils, deficient bactericidal activity, reduced numbers of macrophages, and decreased amounts of immunoglobulin A.

Diagnostic Criteria

As with acute bronchitis, cough is the hallmark of chronic bronchitis. Cough can be mild or severe (with purulent sputum) and may be stimulated by factors such as simple conversation. Many patients with chronic bronchitis expectorate a large quantity of white to yellow, tenacious sputum in the morning. Because of the characteristics of sputum, many patients complain of a foul taste in the mouth.

The earliest symptom in patients with acute exacerbations of chronic bronchitis is an increase in frequency and severity of cough. Other symptoms include greater sputum production, purulent sputum, hemoptysis, chest congestion and discomfort, increased dyspnea, and wheezing. Malaise, loss of appetite, chills, and fever may also be present. True chills (rigors) and fever suggest pneumonia rather than acute exacerbations of chronic bronchitis; these findings require further diagnostic investigation (chest x-ray study, sputum culture).

Clinical assessment and the patient's medical history contribute to the diagnosis of chronic bronchitis. Other diseases such as bronchiectasis, cardiac failure, cystic fibrosis, tuberculosis, and lung carcinoma must be excluded before diagnosing a patient with chronic bronchitis. Patients with chronic bronchitis must have had a sputum-producing cough for at least 3 consecutive months each year for 2 consecutive years. An additional criterion for diagnosis is loss of wages for 3 or more weeks in a year due to cough and sputum production.

Physical examination of patients with chronic bronchitis is usually unremarkable except that chest auscultation reveals inspiratory and expiratory rales, rhonchi, and mild wheezing; normal breath sounds are diminished. As the severity of the disease progresses, an increase in the anteroposterior diameter of the thoracic cage (barrel chest appearance), hyperresonance on percussion, and limited mobility of the diaphragm are observed. Pulmonary function tests demonstrate a decrease in vital capacity and prolongation of expiratory flow. Other features of disease progression include clubbing of the fingers, cor pulmonale, hepatomegaly, and edema of the lower extremities.

To determine the need for antibiotic treatment or hospitalization during an acute exacerbation of chronic bronchitis, the severity of the patient's symptoms needs to be evaluated. A sputum culture is necessary to identify the causative microorganism. To determine the presence of infection, the following two criteria must be present: the Gram stain must exhibit a significant concentration of bacterial growth that is not present when the patient is stable, and the increased bacterial concentration seen on the Gram stain must be accompanied by a doubling of the neutrophil count in the sputum.

Culture and sensitivity findings are not needed, although these results may guide the clinician in choosing appropriate antibiotic therapy. Culture and sensitivity are recommended if any of the following is present:

- The Gram stain reveals a significant amount of *Staphylococcus* species.
- Antibiotic resistance is suspected.
- A decrease in bacteria is detected by Gram stain after 3 to 5 days of antibiotic therapy, and the infection is hospital-acquired.
- Laboratory test results reveal a normal or slightly elevated WBC count during an acute exacerbation of chronic bronchitis.

Finally, a chest x-ray should be performed in patients who have fever or crackles on auscultation to rule out pneumonia.

A proposed classification system for patients with chronic bronchitis has been developed to help clinicians identify high-risk patients and select the appropriate antimicrobial therapy according to the suspected microorganism. Table 26-2 outlines the classification system, taking into consideration the baseline clinical status, risk factors, and most likely common pathogens.

Patients with uncomplicated chronic bronchitis have little or no lung impairment. The forced expiratory volume in 1 second (FEV_1) of these patients is greater than 50%, and they have increased purulent sputum production. The most common pathogens include *H. influenzae, M. catarrhalis*, and β-lactam–resistant *S. pneumoniae*. Viral infections should be considered before bacterial infections in this category of patients.

Patients with moderate to severe chronic bronchitis include those with moderate (FEV_1 between 50% and 80% of predicted) to severe (FEV_1 <50% of predicted) lung impairment, those who are elderly (>65 years of age), those who have frequent exacerbations (more than four episodes per year), and those who have comorbid illnesses such as congestive heart failure, diabetes mellitus, chronic renal failure, or chronic liver disease. The most common pathogens isolated in severe chronic bronchitis are *H. influenzae, S. pneumoniae*, and *M. catarrhalis*.

Patients with chronic bronchial infections have characteristics similar to those in the previous group, but they have increased sputum production, cough, and worsening dyspnea. The same microorganisms that were found in the other groups should be considered in these patients; however, gram-negative microorganisms should also be suspected.

Table 26.2

Classification of Chronic Bronchitis

Clinical Status	Risk Factors	Microorganisms
Simple chronic bronchitis	FEV_1 >50%, increased sputum production and purulence	*Haemophilus influenzae, Moraxella catarrhalis, Streptococcus pneumoniae* (possible beta-lactam resistance)
Complicated chronic bronchitis	FEV_1 <50%, advanced age, ≥4 exacerbations/year	*H. influenzae, M. catarrhalis, S. pneumoniae* (resistance to beta-lactam common)
Chronic bronchial infection	Complicated chronic bronchitis and continuous sputum production throughout year	The above microorganisms and enterobacteria + *Pseudomonas aeruginosa*

Adapted from Grossman, R. F. (1997). Guidelines for the treatment of acute exacerbations of chronic bronchitis. *Chest, 112*, 310S–313S.

INITIATING DRUG THERAPY

A complete assessment of the patient's occupational and environmental history should be performed to treat chronic bronchitis properly. Patients should reduce or eliminate cigarette smoking and their exposure to second-hand smoke. This can be accomplished by counseling sessions and the use of nicotine replacement therapy. Also, exposure to inhaled irritants at work or home should be reduced or eliminated.

The approach to treatment of acute exacerbations of chronic bronchitis is multifactorial (Fig. 26-2). The therapies listed in Box 26-1 should be initiated in combination with antibiotic therapy by the clinician. Prompt initiation of therapy with antimicrobial agents is important for the

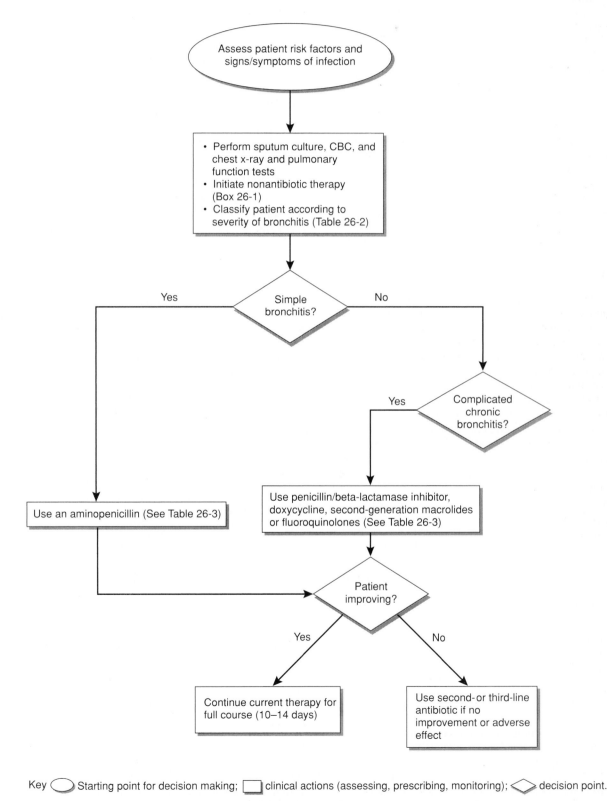

Figure 26–2 Treatment algorithm for chronic bronchitis.

BOX 26–1. NONANTIBIOTIC THERAPY FOR ACUTE EXACERBATIONS OF CHRONIC BRONCHITIS

- Stop smoking
- Avoid inhalation of polluted air
- Increase ingestion of fluids (nonalcoholic)
- Humidify atmosphere
- Use expectorants (guaifenesin)
- Use bronchodilators
- Treat any associated asthma

effective treatment of most acute exacerbations of chronic bronchitis.

Goals of Drug Therapy

There are two goals for the treatment of chronic bronchitis: to reduce the severity of the chronic symptoms and to ameliorate acute exacerbations with prolonged infection-free intervals.

Antimicrobial Therapy

The concentration of the antimicrobial agent in the sputum does not reflect the success of treating the invading microorganism; the penetration of the antimicrobial agent into bronchial tissues is a better indicator of clinical success. Among the antimicrobial agents used to treat chronic bronchitis are the aminopenicillins (ampicillin), cephalosporins, and fluoroquinolones.

Ampicillin does not penetrate well into sputum; however, it is an effective agent in the treatment of certain bacterial infections that cause acute exacerbations of chronic bronchitis. Fluoroquinolones penetrate well into bronchial tissue and have been demonstrated to be very effective in treating acute exacerbations of chronic bronchitis. Table 26-3 reviews antibiotic agents used for patients with chronic bronchitis and pneumonia.

Aminopenicillins

Aminopenicillins, such as ampicillin, inhibit the final step of bacterial cell wall synthesis by binding to one or more of the penicillin-binding proteins. They are safe for use in children, adults, and pregnant women. Table 26-3 reviews the dosages of aminopenicillins for chronic bronchitis.

Contraindications

Aminopenicillins should not be administered to patients with severe hypersensitivity reactions to these agents.

Adverse Events

Hypersensitivity reactions to aminopenicillins manifest as eosinophilia or rash (urticarial, erythematous, morbilliform). Angioedema, exfoliative dermatitis, or erythema multiforme have also been reported as hypersensitivity reactions to aminopenicillins. These reactions occur less frequently than

eosinophilia or rash. Rarely, Stevens-Johnson syndrome has been reported as a hypersensitivity reaction to aminopenicillins.

Nausea, vomiting, and diarrhea, however, are the most common adverse effects that occur with aminopenicillins. Pseudomembranous colitis may occur during or after the antibiotic treatment.

Interactions

Aminopenicillins may interrupt the enterohepatic circulation of estrogen by reducing the bacterial hydrolysis of conjugated estrogen in the gastrointestinal tract. Therefore, the efficacy of oral contraceptives is decreased. Probenecid may increase the effects of aminopenicillins by competing with renal tubular secretion. An increased risk for rash occurs with the coadministration of allopurinol (Xyloprim) and aminopenicillins; the exact mechanism of this interaction has not been established.

Cephalosporins

Cephalosporins consist of several agents, including cefaclor (Ceclor), cephalexin (Keflex), cefuroxime axetil (Ceftin), and cefpodoxime (Vantin), that are frequently used for the treatment of acute exacerbations of chronic bronchitis. Like penicillins, cephalosporins inhibit bacterial cell wall synthesis by binding to one or more of the penicillin-binding proteins. These drugs are safe for use by children and adults. The dosages of cephalosporins are listed in Table 26-3.

Contraindications

Cephalosporins are contraindicated in patients who have had hypersensitivity reactions to any member of the cephalosporin class of antimicrobial agents. There is a 5% to 7% cross-sensitivity reaction between cephalosporins and penicillins, and therefore cephalosporins should be avoided in patients who have had an anaphylactic reaction to penicillins.

Adverse Events

Nausea, diarrhea, and vomiting are common adverse effects with cephalosporins. Fungal infections and pseudomembranous colitis can also occur with the administration of cephalosporins.

Interactions

Probenecid increases the serum concentrations of cephalosporins by reducing their renal clearance.

Doxycycline

Doxycycline inhibits protein synthesis by binding with the 30S and possibly the 50S ribosomal subunits of susceptible microorganisms. The dosage of doxycycline is listed in Table 26-3.

Contraindications

Doxycycline is contraindicated in patients with severe hypersensitivity reactions to doxycycline or tetracycline. The drug should not be administered to children 8 years of age or younger; its use in infants has resulted in retardation of bone

Table 26.3

Overview of Selected Antibiotics for Bronchitis and Pneumonia

Generic (Trade) Name and Dosage	Selected Adverse Events	Contraindications	Special Considerations
Aminopenicillins			
ampicillin (Omnipen, Principen) Adults: 250–500 mg q6h Under 20 kg: 50–100 mg/d qid	Nausea, vomiting, diarrhea, rash, hypersensitivity reactions, gastritis	Hypersensitivity reactions to penicillin Pregnancy category B	High incidence of development of rash in patients with infectious mononucleosis. Ampicillin should be used with extreme caution in this patient population.
amoxicillin (Amoxil, Trimox) 250–1000 mg tid Adults: 500 mg q8h Children: 40 mg/kg/d in divided doses	Nausea, vomiting, diarrhea, gastritis, hypersensitivity reactions	Hypersensitivity reactions to penicillin. Pregnancy category B	High incidence of development of rash in patients with infectious mononucleosis. Amoxicillin should be used with extreme caution in this patient population. Take with or without food. Food may decrease GI symptoms. Interacts with warfarin and oral contraceptives; probenecid decreases renal excretion, and allopurinol increases the risk of rash. Safe for young children
amoxicillin–clavulanate Adults: (Augmentin) 500 mg/125 mg tid 875 mg bid Children: same as for amoxicillin	Nausea, vomiting, diarrhea, gastritis, hypersensitivity reactions, Stevens-Johnson syndrome, seizures (high doses)	Hypersensitivity reactions to penicillin, clavulanic acid Pregnancy category B	High incidence of development of rash in patients with infectious mononucleosis. Amoxicillin clavulanate should be used with extreme caution in this patient population. Take with or without food. Food may decrease GI symptoms. Interacts with warfarin and oral contraceptives; probenecid decreases renal excretion, and allopurinol increases the risk of rash. Safe for young children
Cephalosporins			
cefaclor (Ceclor) 250–500 q8h Not recommended in children <16 y	Nausea, vomiting, diarrhea, rash, hypersensitivity reactions, fungal infections Serious: pseudomembranous colitis	Hypersensitivity to cephalosporin. Not recommended in children <1 mo Pregnancy category B	Cephalosporins should be avoided in patients who have had an anaphylactic hypersensitivity reaction and should be used with caution in patients with a delayed type of reaction to other beta-lactam antibiotics. Take with or without food. Food may decrease GI symptoms. Probenecid decreases renal excretion.
cephalexin (Keflex) Adults: 500 mg qid Children: 25–50 mg/kg/d qid; max 100 mg/kg/d	Nausea, vomiting, diarrhea, rash, hypersensitivity reactions, fungal infections Serious: pseudomembranous colitis, seizures (high doses)	Hypersensitivity or allergy to cephalosporin antibiotics. Not recommended in children <1 mo	Avoid cephalosporins for patients who have had an anaphylactic hypersensitivity reaction. Use with caution in patients with a delayed type of reaction to other beta-lactam antibiotics. Take with or without food. Food may decrease GI symptoms. Probenecid decreases renal excretion.
cefuroxime axetil (Ceftin) Adults: 250–500 mg bid Children: 20 mg/kg/d in 2 divided doses	Same as above	Same as above	Same as above
cefpodoxime (Vantin) Adults: 200 mg q12h Children: 85 mg/kg q12h; max 200 mg	Same as above	Same as above	Same as above
Tetracyclines			
doxycycline (Vibramycin, Doryx, Vibra-tab, Monodox) 100 mg bid for 1 day then 100 mg qd	GI upset (nausea, vomiting, diarrhea, bulky, loose stools, anorexia), hypersensitivity reactions, photosensitivity reactions, superinfection, enterocolitis, rash, blood dyscrasias, hepatotoxicity	Hypersensitivity reactions to any tetracycline Pregnancy category D, breast-feeding Not recommended in children <8 y	Capsules or tablets should be administered with adequate amounts of fluid. Capsules or tablets should not be given to patients with esophageal obstruction or compression.

(continued)

Table 26.3

Overview of Selected Antibiotics for Bronchitis and Pneumonia (*Continued*)

Generic (Trade) Name and Dosage	Selected Adverse Events	Contraindications	Special Considerations
trimethoprim–sulfamethoxazole (Bactrim) Adults: 800 mg sulfamethoxazole/ 160 mg trimethoprim bid Children >2 mo: 8 mg/kg/d trimethoprim/40 mg/kg/d sulfamethoxazole		Allergy to sulfa Pregnancy	Antacids containing aluminum, calcium, or magnesium should be given 1 to 2 h before. Avoid sunlight or ultraviolet light. Use of drug during tooth development may cause dental discoloration.
Macrolides erythromycin (Eryc, PCE) Adults: 250–500 mg qid Children: 30–50 mg/kg qid (not to exceed 100 mg/kg/d)	Abdominal pain and cramping, nausea, vomiting, diarrhea, hepatic dysfunction, urticaria, fungal infection, skin eruptions, rash, ototoxicity	Allergy to erythromycin, hypersensitivity to macrolides, hepatic dysfunction or preexisting liver disease	Erythromycin inhibits the hepatic cytochrome P450 microsomal enzyme system. Thus, elevations of serum concentrations of the following agents can be seen: carbamazepine, cyclosporine, theophylline, zidovudine, digoxin, didanosine, ritonavir, midazolam, and warfarin. Take on empty stomach for better absorption 1 h before or 2 h after a meal.
clarithromycin (Biaxin) Adults: 500 mg bid or 1000 mg qd Children >6 mo: 7.5 mg/kg q12h	Diarrhea, nausea, abnormal taste, dyspepsia, abdominal discomfort, fungal infection, pseudomembranous colitis, hepatic dysfunction, headache, mild urticaria, mild skin eruptions	Hypersensitivity to macrolides, hepatic dysfunction or preexisting liver or renal disease, pregnancy or breast-feeding	Clarithromycin is an inhibitor of the hepatic cytochrome P450 microsomal enzyme system. Thus, elevations of serum concentrations of the following agents can be seen: carbamazepine, cyclosporine, theophylline, zidovudine, didanosine, ritonavir, midazolam, and warfarin.
azithromycin (Zithromax) Bronchitis: Adults: 500 mg qd for 1 day then 250 qd for 4 d CAP: 500 mg for 7–10 d Children >6 mo: 10 mg/kg for 1 d then 5 mg/kd/d for 4 d	Diarrhea, loose stools, nausea, abdominal pain, dizziness, headache, rash photosensitivity, fungal infection, dizziness, fatigue, palpitations	Hypersensitivity to macrolides Use with caution in hepatic disease. Safety not established in pregnancy, lactation, or in children <2 y.	Administer the suspension 1 h before or 2 h after a meal. Use of antacids with aluminum or magnesium decreases serum levels. Interactions: warfarin, pimozide, carbamazepine
Fluoroquinolones gatifloxacin (Tequin) 400 mg qd Not recommended for children <18 y	Nausea, diarrhea, vomiting, abdominal pain or discomfort, photosensitivity	Hypersensitivity to fluoroquinolones Under age 18 Pregnancy category C Breast-feeding	Antacids should be administered 2–4 h apart from fluoroquinolones because antacids, sucralfate, iron, and multivitamins with zinc can decrease absorption. (Elevations of digoxin plasma concentrations have occurred with gatifloxacin.)
levofloxacin (Levaquin) 500 mg qd Not recommended for children <18 y	Nausea, diarrhea, vomiting, abdominal pain or discomfort, photosensitivity	Same as above	Same as above
moxifloxacin (Avelox) 400 mg qd Not recommended for children <18 y	Same as above	Same as above	Same as above Should be administered 4 h before or 8 h after antacids, sucralfate, iron, or multivitamins with zinc.

GI, gastrointestinal.

growth. Doxycycline can localize in the enamel of developing teeth, resulting in enamel hypoplasia and permanent yellow-gray to brown discoloration of the teeth. Doxycycline is a pregnancy category D drug and should not be administered to pregnant or lactating women.

Adverse Events

Gastrointestinal adverse effects such as nausea, vomiting, diarrhea, and bulky, loose stools commonly occur with the administration of doxycycline. Superinfection, enterocolitis, blood dyscrasias, and hepatotoxicity have also been reported to occur with the administration of doxycycline.

Interactions

The administration of antacids, iron, and bismuth subsalicylate (Pepto-Bismol), which contain divalent or trivalent cations, reduces the efficacy of doxycycline by impairing its absorption because of chelation of the cation by doxycycline. Barbiturates, phenytoin (Dilantin), and carbamazepine (Tegretol) can reduce the serum concentration of doxycycline by induction of its hepatic metabolism. The effects of warfarin (Coumadin) can be potentiated when it is administered with doxycycline.

Doxycycline can decrease vitamin K production by gastrointestinal bacteria. The significance of this interaction is unknown, but patients should be monitored for signs of bleeding when anticoagulant drugs are used concomitantly with doxycycline.

Macrolides

The three macrolides—erythromycin, clarithromycin, and azithromycin—work by inhibiting RNA-dependent protein synthesis by binding to the 50S ribosomal subunit. The dosage regimens of the macrolides are listed in Table 26-3.

Contraindications

Macrolides are contraindicated in patients with known hypersensitivity reactions to erythromycin, clarithromycin, or azithromycin, and these products should not be administered to patients with hepatic impairment or preexisting liver disease. Clarithromycin and some formulations of erythromycin should not be administered to pregnant and lactating women because the safety of these agents has not been fully established.

Adverse Events

Abdominal pain, cramping, nausea, vomiting, diarrhea, and hepatic dysfunction commonly occur with the administration of macrolides. Skin rashes and pseudomembranous colitis have also been reported.

Interactions

Erythromycin and clarithromycin are inhibitors of the hepatic cytochrome P450 microsomal enzyme system. Elevations of carbamazepine, cyclosporine (Sandimmune), theophylline (SloPhyllin), zidovudine (Retrovir), didanosine (Videx), ritonavir (Norvir), midazolam (Versed), and warfarin can occur when these agents are administered concomitantly with erythromycin or clarithromycin. Antacids should not be administered with azithromycin because they inhibit its absorption.

Fluoroquinolones

Gatifloxacin (Tequin), levofloxacin (Levaquin), and moxifloxacin (Avelox) inhibit DNA gyrase and topoisomerase IV in susceptible microorganisms, thereby interfering with protein synthesis. The dosing regimens of the fluoroquinolones are listed in Table 26-3.

Contraindications

Fluoroquinolones are contraindicated in patients with known hypersensitivity reactions to any member of the fluoroquinolone class of antimicrobial agents. Fluoroquinolones generally should not be administered to patients younger than 18 years of age nor to pregnant or lactating women. Gatifloxacin, levofloxacin, and moxifloxacin should be used cautiously in patients with known prolongation of the QT interval, in patients with uncorrected hypokalemia, and in those receiving class IA (eg, quinidine [CinQuin], procainamide [Pronestyl]) or class III (eg, amiodarone [Cordarone], sotalol [Betapace]) antiarrhythmic agents. These agents should also be used cautiously in patients who are receiving other agents known to prolong the QT interval, such as erythromycin, antipsychotics, and tricyclic antidepressants.

Gatifloxacin and levofloxacin are eliminated through the kidneys; therefore, dosage adjustments are necessary in patients with renal impairment. Moxifloxacin, which is metabolized primarily through sulfate and glucuronide conjugation, is not recommended for use in patients with mild to severe hepatic impairment.

Adverse Events

Gastrointestinal adverse effects (eg, nausea, diarrhea, vomiting, and abdominal pain) have commonly been reported with the administration of fluoroquinolones. Central nervous system adverse effects such as headache, agitation, confusion, and restlessness have occurred after the administration of fluoroquinolones. Photosensitivity has been reported with the administration of some fluoroquinolones.

Interactions

Fluoroquinolones should not be administered concomitantly with antacids, calcium products, sucralfate (Carafate), iron, multivitamins with zinc, and didanosine-buffered tablets or pediatric powder. These products should be spaced at least 2 to 4 hours apart from the fluoroquinolone. The manufacturers of moxifloxacin recommend spacing at least 4 hours before or 8 hours after the administration of iron- or zinc-containing multivitamins, magnesium, calcium, or aluminum products, sucralfate, or didanosine-buffered tablets or pediatric powder.

Selecting the Most Appropriate Agent

For simple chronic bronchitis, treatment with an aminopenicillin (ampicillin or amoxicillin) is sufficient. In patients with complicated chronic bronchitis, therapy with a second- or third-generation cephalosporin, amoxicillin–clavulanate, a macrolide, or a fluoroquinolone is effective. For chronic bronchial infections, a fluoroquinolone is the agent of choice because gram-negative microorganisms, such as *Pseudomonas* species, need to be considered as potential pathogens (Table 26-4 and Fig. 26-2 provide more information about treatment choices).

Table 26.4

Recommended Order of Treatment for Chronic Bronchitis

Order	Agent	Comments
First line	Aminopenicillin (ampicillin or amoxicillin) for 10–14 d	Therapy typically used for simple chronic bronchitis
Second line	Fluoroquinolone (gatifloxacin, levofloxacin, or moxifloxacin) Penicillin plus beta-lactamase inhibitor (Augmentin), doxycycline Second- or third-generation cephalosporin Macrolide antibiotics (erythromycin, clarithromycin, azithromycin)	Therapy typically initiated for complicated chronic bronchitis
Third line	Fluoroquinolone	Effective for chronic bronchial infections

Special Population Considerations

Pediatric

Antimicrobials related to the tetracyclines (eg, doxycycline) may discolor dental enamel in fetuses and children while teeth are developing.

Women

Women who take antibiotics, especially the aminopenicillins, may experience secondary symptoms, such as vaginitis, that require treatment.

MONITORING PATIENT RESPONSE

Signs and symptoms of infection should improve within days of drug administration. If patients fail to improve, sputum culture and sensitivity analyses should be performed to evaluate the possibility of resistance.

The recommended duration of therapy for acute exacerbation of chronic bronchitis is 10 to 14 days. This decreases morbidity and increases the posttherapy infection-free period in patients. Some patients may require a longer duration of therapy or hospitalization with parenteral therapy. Because patients with chronic bronchitis are predisposed to recurrent infections, antimicrobial agents that were previously successful in eradicating the infection should be readministered.

Measures to prevent exacerbations of chronic bronchitis should be initiated by the clinician. One such method is annual administration of an influenza vaccine. This reduces the rate and severity of infections with the influenza virus in some patients with chronic bronchitis. Patients should also receive the pneumococcal vaccine, with readministration 6 years later. Sufficient data do not exist to support the theory that the pneumococcal vaccine may reduce the frequency or severity of exacerbations in patients with chronic bronchitis. However, this vaccine may potentially reduce the frequency of pneumococcal pneumonia.

PATIENT EDUCATION

Drug Information

The patient needs to understand that the entire course of antimicrobial therapy should be finished to ensure eradication of the causative microorganisms. Moreover, the patient should be cautioned to report adverse effects, such as diarrhea, immediately to the health care provider for further evaluation. Other adverse effects may include photosensitivity, and the patient needs to be advised to protect the skin from excessive exposure to sunlight or ultraviolet light, particularly when taking doxycycline. If sunburn-like reactions or skin eruptions occur, the patient should contact the prescriber immediately.

Additional patient counseling includes whether to take the drug with food or on an empty stomach. Absorption of ampicillin, for example, is decreased both by rate and extent when taken with food. Thus, ampicillin should be taken on an empty stomach (ie, 1 hour before or 2 hours after a meal). Storage instructions include whether the drug needs refrigeration, as do the oral suspensions of ampicillin and amoxicillin, which are stable for only 7 days at room temperature but for 14 days under refrigeration. The reconstituted oral suspension of amoxicillin–clavulanate should be kept in the refrigerator, as should oral cephalosporin suspensions.

Patients should be encouraged to take the macrolides with food to lessen the gastrointestinal adverse effects, except for the oral suspension of azithromycin, which must be taken on a empty stomach. The oral suspension of erythromycin should be refrigerated, but the oral suspension of clarithromycin should not be refrigerated because it is more palatable when taken at room temperature. The oral suspension of azithromycin can be refrigerated if the patient so desires.

Because fluoroquinolones may cause dizziness and light-headedness, patients need to be aware of this when operating an automobile or other potentially dangerous machinery or engaging in activities requiring mental alertness or coordination.

A Web source for patient information on updated information about bronchitis is www.nih.gov/medlineplus/bronchitis.html.

COMMUNITY-ACQUIRED PNEUMONIA

Community-acquired pneumonia (CAP) is an acute infection of the lower respiratory tract that is usually associated with the following:

- Some symptoms of acute infection, and
- Acute infiltrate detected by chest x-ray, or
- Auscultatory findings consistent with pneumonia on physical examination

New, potent antimicrobial agents and vaccines have helped enhance the fight against this infection; however, morbidity and mortality rates remain high. CAP accounts for at least 10 million physician visits, 1 million hospitalizations, and 45,000 deaths in the United States (Bartlett, 1998; Rhew et al., 1998). Approximately 258 cases/100,000 population and 962 cases/100,000 people 65 years of age or older require hospitalization due to CAP (Bartlett, 1998). The mortality rate in an outpatient setting remains low; however, the mortality rate is close to 25% in patients who are hospitalized (Khurana & Litaker, 2000). In the United States approximately $9 billion is spent for diagnosing and treating CAP annually (Halm & Teirstein, 2002).

The bacteriology and antibiotic choices for CAP have changed in the last decade. The elderly and patients with other coexistent illnesses such as COPD, diabetes mellitus, renal insufficiency, congestive heart failure, and chronic liver disease are at a high risk for acquiring pneumonia compared with other patient populations. New microorganisms have been identified as possible causes for bacterial infections in these patients. More potent antibiotics have been developed to treat CAP and decrease the likelihood of resistance.

CAUSES

Several pathogens are identified in CAP. Before the discovery of antibiotics, *S. pneumoniae* accounted for 80% of pneumonia cases (Bartlett, 1997). *S. pneumoniae* still emerges as the most commonly isolated pathogen in patients with CAP. Nearly 65% of all diagnosed CAP cases can be attributed to *S. pneumoniae*. Other pathogens that have been commonly isolated in patients with CAP are *H. influenzae* (12%), *Staphylococcus aureus* (2%), and gram-negative bacilli (1%). Less common pathogens that have been implicated in CAP are *M. catarrhalis*, *Streptococcus pyogenes*, *Chlamydia psittaci*, and *Neisseria meningitidis*. Atypical microorganisms, such as *Legionella* species, *M. pneumoniae*, and *C. pneumoniae*, account for 10% to 20% of cases of CAP. Between 2% and 15% of CAP cases are due to viral infections. The most common virus known to be associated with CAP is the influenza virus; however, parainfluenza virus, RSV, and adenovirus also have been isolated as CAP pathogens.

Certain microorganisms are associated with CAP based on age and coexistent illnesses. In outpatients 60 years of age or younger without any coexistent illnesses such as COPD, diabetes, congestive heart failure, or chronic liver disease (American Thoracic Society, 2001), the most common pathogens include *S. pneumoniae*, *M. pneumoniae*, *C. pneumoniae*, *H. influenzae*, and respiratory viruses. *Legionella* species, *S. aureus*, and gram-negative bacilli have also been implicated in causing CAP in this group. In patients older than 60 years of age with coexisting illness, the most likely microorganisms are *S. pneumoniae*, *H. influenzae*, aerobic gram-negative bacilli, *S. aureus*, and RSV. Less common pathogens include *M. catarrhalis* and *Legionella* species. A major difference between these age groups is the isolation of gram-negative bacilli and *M. catarrhalis*.

Coexisting illnesses from gram-negative microorganisms are associated with CAP. In patients who are hospitalized but not critically ill, *S. pneumoniae*, *H. influenzae*, gram-negative bacilli, *Legionella* species, *S. aureus*, *C. pneumoniae*, and

respiratory viruses have been known to cause CAP. In patients with severe CAP, *S. pneumoniae*, *Legionella* species, aerobic gram-negative bacilli, *M. pneumoniae*, *H. influenzae*, and respiratory tract viruses are frequently identified causes.

PATHOPHYSIOLOGY

Microorganisms gain access to the lower respiratory tract by inhalation as airborne particles, by way of the bloodstream to the lung from an extrapulmonary site of infection, or, most commonly, through aspiration of oropharyngeal contents. This is a common method of transmission of microorganisms into the lower respiratory tract for both healthy and ill people.

DIAGNOSTIC CRITERIA

Patients with pneumonia typically present with cough, fever, and sputum production. It is difficult to distinguish other respiratory tract infections such as bronchitis from pneumonia based on signs and symptoms (Fig. 26-3). A chest x-ray can help differentiate pneumonia from other infections and can also indicate whether coexisting conditions, such as COPD or pleural effusions, are present (American Thoracic Society, 2001).

The presence of infiltrates on chest x-ray usually indicates pneumonia, which necessitates treatment with an antibiotic. In general, chest x-rays cannot distinguish between bacterial and nonbacterial microorganisms. However, certain findings on the chest x-ray can guide the practitioner to a diagnosis. The severity of illness can also be detected by an x-ray; multilobar involvement typically indicates severe illness. Table 26-5 depicts common findings on chest x-rays in immunocompetent patients and suggests possible pneumonia-causing pathogens. Gram stain of the sputum specimen is useful in the initial evaluation of patients with pneumonia. The sensitivity and specificity of a Gram stain can vary; however, it can provide the practitioner with some clues to the causative microorganism. Bacterial cultures of sputum are useful when resistant microorganisms are suspected. Invasive diagnostic techniques such as transtracheal aspiration, bronchoscopy, bronchoalveolar lavage, and direct needle aspiration may be useful in patients with severe CAP.

It can be difficult to determine when an outpatient needs hospitalization for closer observation. Box 26-2 lists the indications for hospitalization in a patient with severe CAP. However, once patients are hospitalized, several routine tests must be performed to determine the severity of the illness, possible complications, the status of underlying conditions, and the most appropriate treatment choices. A WBC count is not useful for distinguishing between the various causative microorganisms; however, a WBC count greater than 12,000 cells/mm^3 typically suggests bacterial infection. A complete blood count can determine whether a patient has anemia, which can indicate *Mycoplasma* infections or complicated pneumonia. Pulse oximetry can help reflect the severity of the disease. An arterial oxygen saturation (SaO$_2$) of less than 90% on room air is a standard criterion for hospital admission.

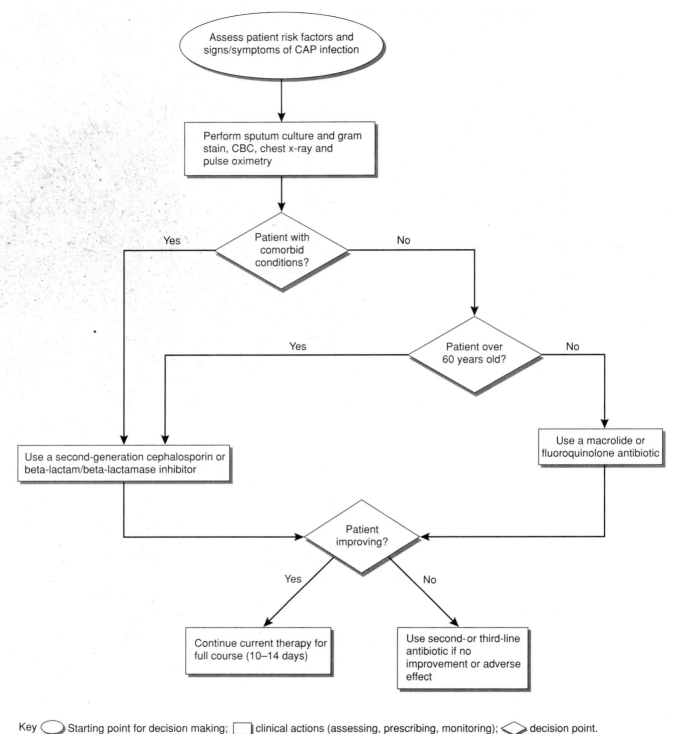

Key ⬭ Starting point for decision making; ▭ clinical actions (assessing, prescribing, monitoring); ◇ decision point.

Figure 26–3   Treatment algorithm for outpatient treatment of community-acquired pneumonia (CAP).

INITIATING DRUG THERAPY

General treatment approaches for pneumonia consist of providing adequate hydration (replacement of loss of water that may occur because of fever, poor intake, or vomiting), providing bronchodilators for dyspnea, and controlling fever with acetaminophen, ibuprofen, or aspirin. Early identification of the causative microorganism is optimal for proper management of CAP. However, diagnostic tests cannot always identify all potential pathogens, and therefore empiric therapy is often initiated by the clinician.

Goals of Drug Therapy

The goals of pharmacotherapy for pneumonia include eradication of the offending microorganism through the selection of appropriate antibiotic therapy and effecting a

Table 26.5

Differential Diagnosis of Pneumonia Based on Chest X-Ray in Immunocompetent Patients

X-ray Finding	Possible Pathogen
Focal opacity	*Streptococcus pneumoniae*
	Chlamydia pneumoniae
	Haemophilus influenzae
	Staphylococcus aureus
	Legionella
	Mycoplasma pneumoniae
Interstitial/miliary involvement	Viruses
	M. pneumoniae
Hilar adenopathy ± segmental or interstitial infiltrate	*Chlamydia psittaci*
	M. pneumoniae
Cavitation	Anaerobes

Adapted from Bartlett, J. G. (1997). *Management of respiratory infections*. Baltimore: Williams & Wilkins.

Table 26.6

Recommended Antimicrobial Treatment for Outpatients With CAP*

Agents	Comments
macrolides (erythromycin, azithromycin, clarithromycin)	Azithromycin is preferred if *Haemophilus influenzae* is the suspected cause of CAP.
fluoroquinolones (gatifloxacin, levofloxacin, moxifloxacin)	Preferred treatment if high-level penicillin-resistant *Streptococcus pneumoniae* is the suspected cause of CAP
doxycycline	Good agent to use in patients between 17 and 40 y old

*In CAP, the order of treatment of depends on the cause of CAP. If the cause remains unknown, the prescriber recommends empiric therapy and makes adjustments if needed depending on the patient's response.

complete clinical cure, as well as minimizing adverse effects of medications.

Antibiotics

Empiric antibiotic treatment for outpatients with pneumonia should always be active against *S. pneumoniae* because this pathogen is one of the most commonly identified causes of bacterial pneumonia. Aminopenicillins and cephalosporins are not recommended as agents of choice for treating pneumonia on an outpatient basis because of the increasing resistance of *S. pneumoniae* to these agents. A macrolide (ie, erythromycin, clarithromycin, and azithromycin), or doxycycline are the agents of choice for treating pneumonia on an outpatient basis. A fluoroquinolone (eg, gatifloxacin, levofloxacin, moxifloxacin) is recommended if a patient with CAP has received antibiotic therapy within the previous 10 to 14 days (Table 26-6).

Differences among these agents were discussed previously in the chronic bronchitis section, and must be considered when choosing antimicrobial therapy for CAP. Resistance patterns also should be considered when choosing an agent. For erythromycin and clarithromycin, resistance patterns to *S. pneumoniae* and *H. influenzae* have been documented in certain regions of the United States. *S. pneumoniae* and *H. influenzae* appear to be less resistant to azithromycin than to erythromycin and clarithromycin. If a *Legionella* species is suspected, erythromycin should be added to the regimen. Ciprofloxacin should not be used for treating pneumonia because of the high level of resistance that *S. pneumoniae* exhibits to this drug. A fluoroquinolone with good *S. pneumoniae* coverage should be used, such as gatifloxacin, levofloxacin, or moxifloxacin. In young adults between the ages of 17 and 40 years, doxycycline can be helpful.

If aspiration pneumonia is suspected, then the agent of choice is amoxicillin–clavulanate. If the prescriber suspects that the CAP is caused by a high level of penicillin-resistant *S. pneumoniae* (defined as a minimum inhibitory concentration ≤2 µg/mL), a fluoroquinolone is the agent of choice.

Hospitalized patients should receive a fluoroquinolone or a combination of a macrolide (azithromycin or clarithromycin) and β-lactam, such as cefotaxime (Claforan) or ceftriaxone (Rocephin) (Box 26-3). Patients hospitalized in the intensive care unit for pneumonia should receive the same therapy as other hospitalized patients, unless *Pseudomonas aeruginosa* is a concern. If the latter is true, then an antibiotic with broader gram-negative coverage (ie, piperacillin–tazobactam, cefepime) should be added.

BOX 26–2. INDICATIONS FOR HOSPITALIZATION

- Severe vital sign abnormality: pulse >140/min; systolic blood pressure <90 mm Hg; respiratory rate >30/min; temperature >38.3°C (101°F)
- Altered mental status (newly diagnosed): disorientation to person, place or time; stupor or coma
- Arterial hypoxemia: PO$_2$ <60 mm Hg on room air
- Suppurative pneumonia-related infection: empyema, septic arthritis, meningitis, endocarditis
- Severe electrolyte, hematologic, metabolic laboratory value not known to be chronic

Adapted from Bartlett, J. G. (1997). *Management of respiratory infections*. Baltimore; Williams & Wilkins.

Selecting the Most Appropriate Agent

Identification of the likely microorganism simplifies treatment for pneumonia. The reader is referred to the comprehensive references for appropriate antimicrobial agents that are commonly used once pathogens have been identified (American Thoracic Society, 2001; Mandell et al., 2003; also see Figure 26-3).

MONITORING PATIENT RESPONSE

The patient's response to therapy must be evaluated carefully. Response to treatment should be based on clinical illness, pathogen isolated, severity of illness, host, and chest

BOX 26–3. PREFERRED ANTIMICROBIAL CHOICES FOR PATIENTS HOSPITALIZED WITH PNEUMONIA

General Inpatient
- Beta-lactam antibiotic with or without a macrolide antibiotic
- Fluoroquinolone

Alternatives include cefuroxime with or without a macrolide antibiotic or azithromycin (alone).

Intensive Care
- Antipseudomonal cephalosporin (cefotaxime, ceftriaxone) plus a macrolide or fluoroquinolone
- Beta-lactam/beta-lactamase inhibitor (eg, ampicillin/sulbactam, ticarcillin/clavulanate, piperacillin/tazobactam

x-ray findings. Subjective symptoms usually respond within 3 to 5 days of initiating therapy. Objective findings such as fever, leukocytosis, and chest x-ray abnormalities resolve at different times. Fever lasts for 2 to 4 days in most cases of CAP; however, defervescence occurs more quickly with *S. pneumoniae* infection. Leukocytosis usually resolves by the fourth day of initiation of antimicrobial therapy. Chest x-rays indicate that signs of pneumonia last longer than symptoms.

Of course, this depends on many factors, such as the causative microorganism and underlying illness. The overall suggested chest x-ray follow-up is 7 to 12 weeks after initiation of therapy.

Duration of therapy for treating CAP depends on the severity of the illness and the antimicrobial agent that was used to treat the infection. Patients treated for mild episodes of CAP with azithromycin typically have a short duration of therapy. Because the half-life of azithromycin is 11 to 14 hours, it remains in the tissues longer than erythromycin or clarithromycin. Five days of azithromycin therapy is sufficient to treat mild CAP. Bacterial infection with *S. pneumoniae* is treated for 7 to 14 days. *M. pneumoniae* and *C. pneumoniae* infections usually require 10 to 14 days of therapy. Patients with Legionnaires disease who are immunocompetent typically receive 14 days of treatment.

PATIENT EDUCATION

The patient must take the full course of medication even though he or she may feel better within days of initiation of antibiotics. Early discontinuation of therapy can result in reinfection or the development of resistant microorganisms. If the patient continues to worsen despite several days of therapy, he or she should contact the prescriber immediately. The organism causing infection in the patient could be resistant to the antibiotic originally prescribed. Readers should refer to the chronic bronchitis section for further information on drug therapy.

■ Case Study

R. R., a 58-year-old man, presents to the clinic with complaints of increasing shortness of breath, chills, malaise, and cough productive of a yellowish-green sputum. His medical history is significant for hypertension and chronic lower back pain. He has a 35 pack-year history of cigarette smoking. Physical examination is significant for rales on auscultation of the chest. Clubbing of the fingernails is apparent. Vital signs are blood pressure, 138/88 mm Hg; pulse rate, 96 beats/min; respiration rate, 32 breaths/min; and temperature, 99.7°F. Laboratory test results and chest x-ray findings are pending.

Diagnosis: Pneumonia

1. List specific treatment goals for RR.
2. What drug therapy would you prescribe? Why?
3. What are the parameters for monitoring success of the therapy?
4. Describe specific patient based on the prescribed therapy.
5. List one or two adverse reactions for the selected agent that would cause you to change therapy.
6. What would be the choice for second-line therapy?
7. What dietary and lifestyle changes should be recommended for this patient?
8. Describe one or two drug–drug or drug–food interactions for the selected agent.

Bibliography

*Starred references are cited in the text.

*American Thoracic Society. (2001). Guidelines for the management of adults with community-acquired pneumonia. *American Journal of Respiratory and Critical Care Medicine, 163,* 1730–1754.

Balter, M. S., LaForge, J., Low, D. E., et al. (2003) Canadian guidelines for the management of acute exacerbations of chronic bronchitis. *Canadian Respiratory Journal, 10* (Suppl. B), 3B–32B.

*Bartlett, J. G. (1997). *Management of respiratory tract infections.* Baltimore: Williams & Wilkins.

*Bartlett, J. G. (1998). Community-acquired pneumonia in adults: Guidelines for management. *Clinical Infectious Diseases, 26,* 811–838.

*Grossman, R. F. (1997). Guidelines for the treatment of acute exacerbations of chronic bronchitis. *Chest, 112,* 310S–313S.

*Halm, E. A., & Teirstein, A.S. (2002) Management of community-acquired pneumonia. *New England Journal of Medicine, 347,* 2039–2045.

Heffelfinger, J. D. (2000). Management of community-acquired pneumonia in the era of pneumonococcal resistance. *Archives of Internal Medicine, 160,* 1399–1408.

*Hueston, W. J., & Mainous, A. G. (1998). Acute bronchitis. *American Family Physician, 57,* 1270–1276.

*Khurana, P. S., & Litaker, D. (2000). The dilemma of nosocomial pneumonia: What primary care physicians should know. *Cleveland Clinic of Medicine, 67,* 25–41.

*Mandell, L. A., Bartlett, J. G., Dowell, S. F., et al. (2003). Update of practice guidelines for the management of community-acquired pneumonia in immunocompetent adults. *Clinical Infectious Diseases, 37,* 1405–1433.

Niederman, M. S. (1998). Update on pulmonary medicine. *Annals of Internal Medicine, 128,* 208–215.

Pauwels, R. A., Buist, A. S., Calverly, P. M. A., et al. (2001). Global strategy for the diagnosis, management, and prevention of chronic obstructive pulmonary disease. *American Journal of Respiratory and Critical Care Medicine, 163,* 1256–1276.

*Rhew, D. C., Riedinger, M. S., Sandhu, M., et al. (1998). A prospective, multicenter study of pneumonia practice guidelines. *Chest, 114,* 115–119.

Visit the Connection web site for the most up-to-date drug information.

27

TUBERCULOSIS

■ JANIS KUBIS MILLER

Tuberculosis (TB) is a disease caused by *Mycobacterium tuberculosis*. TB most commonly affects the lungs but can affect almost any tissue or organ. TB infection may be detected by a positive response to a skin test in a person with no physical signs or symptoms on examination and a chest x-ray that reveals only granulomas or calcification in the lung or regional lymph nodes. Tuberculous disease is infection with presenting signs and symptoms or x-ray findings that confirm TB.

Nationwide, active TB cases reported to the Centers for Disease Control and Prevention (CDC) declined steadily from 84,000 cases in 1953 to 22,255 cases in 1984 (CDC, 1993). However, by 1991 the trend had reversed, resulting in an 18% rise in reported cases, which, when calculated, is 39,000 cases more than anticipated (assuming that the decline in incidence had continued).

Coincident with this rise in reported cases was the emergence and transmission of human immunodeficiency virus (HIV), a dramatic increase in the incidence of homelessness, and an increase in the rates of immigration to the United States. In addition, while the number of TB cases rose, there were no longer facilities dedicated solely to the containment and complete treatment of patients with diagnosed TB. Consequently, noncompliance with therapy became an issue, which resulted not only in perpetuation of the spread of disease, but in the development of drug-resistant strains of TB. Noncompliance and multidrug-resistant TB (MDR-TB) have serious implications for treatment failure in individual patients, as well as posing a threat to the public health.

Despite the problem with noncompliance and MDR-TB the number of reported cases of TB continues to decline. In 1996, there were 8 cases/100,000 population, or 21,337 actual cases, and in 2000, there were 5.8 cases/100,000 population, 16,377 actual cases. (CDC, 2003). The highest incidence is among first-generation immigrants from high-risk areas (eg, Asia and the former Soviet Union), Native Americans, the homeless, and residents of correctional facilities.

The ultimate responsibility for the successful treatment of TB lies with the public health department or private health provider. Directly observed therapy (DOT) is recommended for all patients taking antituberculosis medications. This strategy encourages observation of the patient taking each dose of medicine to maximize completion of a prescribed regimen. Intensive regimens that use DOT have higher rates of successful treatment than regimens that do not. Measures that facilitate adherence to regimens often include the involvement of various social agencies. These may include incentives for treatment and services that enable treatment such as assistance with transportation, housing, and treatment of substance abuse. Local public health departments are valuable and experienced resources for patients without access to medication and testing, as well as to recommend and intervene to enhance compliance.

PATHOPHYSIOLOGY

The tuberculin bacillus is a rod-shaped organism, spread by airborne droplet with nuclei varying in size from 1 to 5 μm. Its cell wall is waxy, which accounts for its resistance to acid stain decolorization, resulting in its classification as an acid-fast bacillus. Although many bacteria are rapid dividers, TB bacteria are slow, dividing only once every 18 to 24 hours. They require few nutrients for survival and are believed to achieve their virulence from the ability to secrete acidic lipids and ammonium ions, which enable the organisms to evade ingestion by host defense mechanisms.

The bacilli are inhaled in the form of droplets, some of which reach the level of the alveoli. In the alveoli, they are ingested by macrophages and remain and divide in the macrophage if they are not destroyed by it. They continue to replicate without producing any response to infection for approximately 4 to 8 weeks until a threshold number of bacilli is reached. A cellular immune reaction then occurs, which is accompanied by a spread of the bacilli through the blood and the lymphatic system. This also corresponds to the period required for development of skin reactivity, or a positive purified protein derivative (PPD) reaction. When this cell-mediated immune response occurs, granulomas are formed by the action of macrophages and activated T cells that clump together and surround the tubercule bacilli. The bacilli are usually grouped in the acidic center of the granuloma, which has become avascular and necrotic because of surrounding fibrosis. This is usually the final stage of primary infection in patients with intact immune systems. No symptoms are usually apparent at this stage, and although adequately surrounded to prevent dissemination of disease, a few of the bacilli remain alive in the granuloma.

An immunocompetent, untreated person carries a 10% risk for development of active infection at some time during his or her life from this initial infection. During this period, however, if a patient's immune system cannot arrest the primary infection by cell-mediated immunity, the infection progresses directly to active disease. Active disease may take the form of systemic illness, affecting the kidneys, bones, or meninges, but 80% to 85% of active disease affects the pulmonary structures. The incubation period from infection to positive skin test results is 2 to 12 weeks (median, 3–4 weeks). The risk for development of disease is highest during the 6 months after infection and remains high for 2 years. Most untreated disease lies dormant and never progresses to clinical disease in a healthy host.

DIAGNOSTIC CRITERIA

Symptoms of active TB disease include cough (initially non-productive) and fever, including night sweats (affecting more than half of patients with active TB). As the disease progresses, the cough becomes productive, and malaise and weight loss occur. Pleuritic chest pain associated with pleural effusions may occur, and in such cases, pleural fluid culture results may prove diagnostic.

Skin testing (Mantoux test) with the use of PPD is a valuable tool in the early identification of people exposed to or infected with TB. Individual risk factors for the development of TB must be considered when deciding which patients should undergo screening with PPD.

In the United States, widespread PPD screening programs are discouraged. Testing is considered appropriate in patients at high risk for latent tuberculosis infection (LTBI) and for developing TB who will benefit from treatment if the test result is positive. The American Thoracic Society (ATS) states that a decision to perform skin testing is a decision to treat the patient if the test is positive (ATS, 2000). Patients considered to be at high risk are those who have recently been infected or who have clinical conditions that put them at an increased risk of developing active TB if in fact they have LTBI. In this manner, *targeted tuberculin testing* will also eliminate needless extensive evaluations of false-positive tests in low-risk patients.

People considered to be high risk for whom the CDC and Advisory Council on the Elimination of Tuberculosis recommend skin testing are identified in Box 27-1. Patients who had a positive skin test in the past or who received bacillus Calmette-Guerin vaccine (BCG) may prove positive for life. Box 27-2 lists the guidelines for interpreting skin tests.

All patients with newly positive skin test results should have a chest x-ray to determine if active disease is present. Indicators of active disease include infiltrates, either nodular or nonnodular (especially in the middle and lower lobes), cavitation, adenopathy (commonly in the hilum), or pleural effusion. These indicators, if detected on chest x-ray, strongly suggest active TB, but further diagnostic evaluation is required.

The single most important tool in obtaining a diagnosis and following the progression of active disease is a sputum culture. A sputum culture is imperative if the patient has a positive skin test and abnormal chest x-ray findings, or if the patient has a negative chest x-ray study but is symptomatic. Three first-morning samples of sputum are ideal because they tend to contain the heaviest concentration of bacilli. If patients are unable to produce sputum, samples must be

---

BOX 27–1. PATIENTS FOR WHOM SKIN TESTING IS RECOMMENDED

The following groups of patients are considered to have risk factors for tuberculosis and are recommended to undergo skin testing:

- Patients with HIV infection or suspected HIV infection
- Close contacts (eg, coworkers and household members) of patients with known or suspected TB
- Health care providers and social workers who serve high-risk patients
- Patients who have immigrated within the last 5 years from countries with high incidence of TB (eg, Central or South American, Asia, and Africa)
- High-risk minority groups (ethnic or racial, locally defined)
- Patients with known or suspected drug abuse
- Residents and staff of long-term care facilities (eg, correctional and mental institutions, nursing homes)
- Patients who are immunosuppressed because of disease or medical therapy

---

induced by ultrasonic hypertonic saline solution. If sputum still is not produced, or samples are inadequate, bronchoscopy with bronchoalveolar lavage or needle biopsy may be used. The results of culture and sensitivity testing form the basis for proper pharmacotherapy and for evaluating the efficacy of treatment.

Various laboratories also offer nucleic acid amplification testing. When a sputum smear is positive for acid-fast bacilli, nucleic acid amplification can identify *M. tuberculosis* as the organism in 1 day. However, cultures must still be processed because sensitivity testing is imperative. Furthermore, some specimens contain an inhibitor that prevents detection by nucleic acid amplification. In addition, patients with previously treated TB will have a positive amplification test finding and a negative culture results because nucleic acids are still detectable in nonviable organisms.

A commercially available blood test is able to detect high concentrations of interferon gamma (IFN-γ) production by T cells in response to *M. tuberculosis*, and thus to help detect LTBI. Although false-positive results occur for numerous reasons, in patients who indeed have a positive PPD, the QuantiFERON-TB (QTB) test results correlate well with PPD reactivity. This test is currently considered a supplement to the diagnostic pool of tests, not a replacement for PPD testing. QTB testing is not performed by all laboratories, and serum samples must be processed within 12 hours of being drawn. Active tuberculous disease is associated with suppression of IFN-γ. Thus, QTB testing is not recommended in patients with suspected active TB, only for patients at high risk of LTBI. Further studies are being conducted to develop methods to detect antigenic proteins expressed only by *M. tuberculosis*. This would rapidly identify LTBI and active disease with a high degree of sensitivity and specificity.

BOX 27–2. INTERPRETATION OF TUBERCULIN SKIN TESTS

A reaction of 15 mm or more is considered positive in any patient. Skin reaction measures the area of induration, not erythema. Levels of reactivity are considered positive in the following patient groups:

≥10 mm	≥5 mm
Patients with coexisting medical conditions	Close contacts (eg, coworkers, cohabitators) of patients with infectious TB
Foreign-born patients from high-prevalence countries	
Patients of high-risk minority populations	Patients with known or suspected HIV infection
Indigent or medically underserved groups	
Intravenous drug users	Patients with radiographic evidence of healed TB lesions
Residents of long–term care facilities	
Health care workers	Patients receiving immunosuppressive therapy
Children and adolescents	

Diagnostic Criteria in Children

Diagnosis in special populations of patients warrants specific considerations. Children with active disease tend to have more fulminant presentations. Children and infants may have such enlarged regional lymph nodes that adjacent bronchi become compressed. Infants born of mothers with known or suspected disease should have skin testing and a chest x-ray study at 4 to 6 weeks of age and, if negative, again at 3, 4, and 6 months of age.

Diagnostic Criteria in Pregnant Women

PPD testing of pregnant women can be performed safely and routinely. Chest x-rays with the use of a protective shield and sputum samples are recommended in pregnant women with a newly positive skin test response exceeding 5 mm of induration.

Diagnostic Criteria in Immunocompromised Patients

Patients with HIV infection or immunocompromised host defense systems due to either medications or coexistent medical conditions present further considerations. HIV-infected patients may have false-negative PPD reactions despite having active disease because their ability to mount a delayed-type hypersensitivity (DTH) reaction may be impaired. This impaired DTH is directly correlated with a declining $CD4^+$ T-lymphocyte count. Patients with HIV infection have a higher incidence of TB because of altered immunity. They also have a much more rapid progression of TB compared with patients with intact immunity. In addition, active TB accelerates the replication of HIV and, consequently, accelerates the course of both diseases. Patients with advanced HIV disease may have trouble absorbing antituberculosis medications from the gastrointestinal (GI) tract, and difficulty tolerating them with their multiple anti-HIV medications.

Patients with HIV infection and a positive PPD carry approximately an 8% chance per year for development of active disease (ATS, 1994). As such, accurate assessment of PPD and TB status in HIV-infected patients is critical. In 1997, the CDC recommended that patients with HIV infection be skin tested for anergy (inability to mount a DTH response) to common antigens, such as mumps virus and *Candida*, at the time of PPD testing. Patients who do not have responses to common antigens are considered anergic and unable to mount a sufficient immune response to either the antigens or to PPD, even if infected with TB. Since these guidelines were instituted, various studies have challenged the usefulness of the assumptions behind anergy testing and demonstrated limitations to it as part of TB screening. It is now recommended that anergy testing not be used routinely with PPD testing for purposes of screening and preventive therapy. However, anergy testing may prove helpful with additional information, such as risk factors, laboratory findings, and current health status.

Patients in residential facilities such as nursing homes, mental health hospitals, and correctional facilities represent a population in whom transmission of disease may become widespread. As such, routine screening and prompt intervention are indicated. Although many doubt the reliability of negative test results in the elderly, numerous studies have demonstrated that most elderly patients with negative skin tests are indeed immunocompetent.

INITIATING DRUG THERAPY

Drug therapy is used to treat latent and active TB (Fig. 27-1). The term *prevention* is actually a misnomer because patients with positive skin tests and suspect chest x-ray findings are already infected. In 2000, the nomenclature was changed from preventive therapy to *treatment for latent tuberculosis infection* (LTBI). This term more accurately describes the intervention. The goal of treating LTBI is to prevent the development of active TB and to control the threat of spread to the community.

Because treatment of LTBI has potential side effects, the risk for development of active TB must be weighed against the likelihood of experiencing serious adverse reactions to medications. Box 27-3 identifies people for whom the ATS and CDC recommend treatment for LTBI based on skin test positivity and associated risk factors. All patients with active TB, regardless of the risk for adverse reactions to medications, must be started on a medication regimen immediately after (and sometimes even before, when active TB is highly suspected) a diagnosis is made. However, baseline testing is required before initiating drug therapy (Box 27-4).

Although drug therapy is essential in treating LTBI and active TB, smoking cessation, a nutritious diet, and exercise are nonpharmacologic ways that patients with active and inactive TB can manage and improve their own health. Smoking cessation is important in all disease management. It often is unsuccessful in patients undertaking and initiating complex and protracted courses of medication, as is the case for patients with TB. Occasionally, however, patients

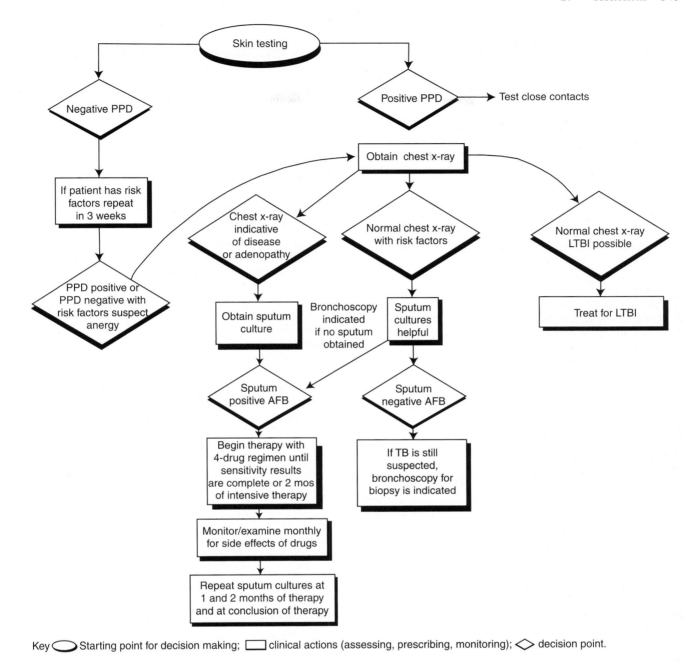

Figure 27–1 Treatment algorithm for tuberculosis (TB).

succeed in quitting when frightened by their diagnosis and motivated to improve their health.

Nutritional issues also must be addressed because patients may be somewhat malnourished by the disease course, fatigue, lack of ability or interest in meal preparation, and altered taste sensation from therapeutic regimens. Vitamin supplementation is warranted, particularly B_6 (see the discussion of isoniazid). Patients should be encouraged to remain physically active and to incorporate an exercise program into their daily routine.

Goals of Drug Therapy

Goals of therapy depend on whether the patient has LTBI or active disease. The goal of treating LTBI is to eliminate or significantly decrease the bacterial load in lesions that are seen on x-ray films and considered old, as well as those that are not visible on x-ray films but assumed to be present, thus preventing LTBI from becoming active TB disease.

Therapeutic goals for active TB are threefold:

- The patient will become symptom free and noninfectious to close contacts.
- The patient's sputum culture will be negative for *M. tuberculosis*, which is the best measure of regimen efficacy.
- At the conclusion of therapy, the patient's chest x-ray will show no active disease.

Other goals include preventing the development of MDR-TB and preventing death from complications of TB.

BOX 27–3. INDICATIONS FOR TREATMENT FOR LTBI

Patients with a Positive PPD

1. Foreign-born patients from high-prevalence countries (eg, Asia, Africa, and Central or South America)
2. Indigent or medically underserved groups (eg, homeless patients)
3. Patients of high-risk minority populations (eg, Asians, African Americans, and Latinos)
4. Residents and staff of long-term care facilities (eg, mental and correctional facilities and nursing homes)

Regardless of Age, Treatment for LTBI Is Indicated.

5. Close contacts of newly diagnosed patients (eg, coworkers or household members); in some cases, even if the close contact is PPD negative.
6. Patients with HIV infection and patients with unknown but suspected HIV infection. Patients in this group with negative PPD, but who are in a high-risk group, are candidates for preventive therapy.
7. Patients with recently converted PPD; specifically, all children <2 years of age with ≥10 mm reaction; ≥10 mm increase over a 2-year span in patients <35 years of age; ≥15 mm for patients ≥35 years of age.
8. Patients with coexistent medical conditions, specifically patients with:

   - Diabetes, especially poorly controlled type 1
   - Long-term or frequent courses of corticosteroids
   - Immunosuppressive therapy, such as posttransplantation patients
   - Hematologic diseases or malignaucies
   - IV drug users, regardless of HIV status
   - End-stage renal disease. Decision is based on previous skin test positivity because these patients are often anergic.
   - Rapid weight loss candidates (eg, malabsorption syndromes and intestinal bypass)

LTBI, latent tuberculosis infection

BOX 27–4. BASELINE STATUS TESTING

Because of the potential side effects and toxicities of the intensive treatment regimens, testing at the initiation of drug therapy is crucial. This not only establishes a patient's baseline status, but identifies patients in whom various medications are contraindicated or patients at higher risk for development of complications. Because initial therapies may be changed and unexpected regimens used, laboratory tests should be widespread and encompass an array of values.

- Serum tests should include a complete blood count with platelets; hepatic enzymes and bilirubin; and chemistries, including blood urea nitrogen, creatinine, and uric acid levels.
- Visual acuity and color blindness testing also are indicated, because ethambutol is part of most drug regimens.
- In cases of aminoglycoside use, patients require audiometric testing before and periodically throughout therapy.
- The American Thoracic Society does not recommend routine follow-up laboratory tests in asymptomatic patients with normal baseline values.
- Hepatic enzymes are frequently elevated during therapy, although patients are relatively symptom free.

Isoniazid

Isoniazid (INH), an antitubercular anti-infective, is an ideal agent for treating TB. It is inexpensive, easy to administer, and has a low adverse event profile (Table 27-1). It is the drug of choice in large residential treatment facilities.

Mechanism of Action

Isoniazid has bacteriostatic action that interferes with the biosynthesis of lipids and nucleic acid. It is highly effective against actively growing TB organisms. It also penetrates body tissues and cavities very well after GI absorption. Peak serum levels occur within the first 2 hours after ingestion. INH interferes with the synthesis of mycolic acids, which are integral components of the mycobacterial cell wall, and thus renders the cell unviable.

Adverse Events

Hepatitis and peripheral neuropathies are the most common adverse events associated with INH therapy. Hepatitis can be severe in some instances, especially in patients who consume large quantities of alcohol. Hepatitis, if it occurs, usually manifests early in therapy. The risk for development of hepatitis from INH appears to be related to advancing age; patients younger than 20 years of age have little or no risk, whereas those older than 50 years of age have a 2.3% likelihood for development of hepatitis (ATS, 1994).

Peripheral neuropathies, which are believed to result from INH interfering with the metabolism of pyridoxine (vitamin B_6), occur less commonly than hepatitis. Administration of pyridoxine is recommended for pregnant women and patients with coexisting medical problems associated with neuropathies.

Pyrazinamide

Mechanism of Action

Pyrazinamide (PZA), an antitubercular anti-infective, is also an excellent bactericidal agent against TB, although its

Table 27.1

Overview of Selected Drugs Used to Treat Tuberculosis

Generic (Trade) Name and Dosage	Selected Adverse Events	Contraindications	Special Considerations
isoniazid (INH) Daily dosing: Children: 10–20 mg/kg Adults: 5 mg/kg both to a maximum of 300 mg bid-tid Weekly dosing: Children: 20–40 mg/kg Adults: 15 mg/kg to a maximum of 900 mg/dose	Peripheral neuropathies Hepatitis (likelihood increased proportional to alcohol [ETOH] intake and advancing age) Nausea, vomiting, distress	Allergy to isoniazid, acute hepatic disease	Administer vitamin B_6, pyridoxine, to minimize neuropathies Obtain baseline liver function rests
pyrazinamide Daily dosing (children and adults): 15–30 mg/kg to maximum of 2 g bid-tid Weekly dosing: 50–70 mg/kg to maximum of 4 g for twice weekly, 3 g for 3 times weekly	Mild elevation of aminotransferases and uric acid levels; skin rashes, arthralgias, GI disturbances	Allergy to pyrazinamide; severe hepatic damage, acute gout	Not a first-line agent in pregnant women May be used in patients with MDR-TB, but becatogenicity data are insufficient
rifampin (Rifadin, Rimactane) Daily, twice and 3 times weekly dosing: Children: 10–20 mg/kg Adults: 10 mg/kg Both to maximum of 600 mg	GI upset, hepatitis, skin rashes, blood dyscrasias, headache, fatigue, dizziness	Allergy to any rifamycin; acute hepatic disease	Educate patients that all body fluids will be stained orange. Numerous drug interactions because it increases the rate of clearance of many medications Review all of patient's medications at each visit.
ethambutol (Myambutol) Adults and children same dose Daily: 15–25 mg/kg Twice weekly: 50 mg/kg Three times weekly: 25–30 mg/kg	Red-green color blindness, blurred vision, scotomas (all due to retrobulbar neuritis), GI disturbances	Use with extreme caution in patients with renal failure. Allergy to ethambutol Optic neuritis	Baseline and periodic visual acuity and color testing is necessary.
para-aminosalicylic acid (PAS) (Sodium PAS) ethionamide (ET) Trecator	Depression, browsiness, GI disturbances	Breast-feeding (PAS), pregnancy (ET) Allergy to aminosalicylate sodium, allergy to ethionamide	
streptomycin Twice to 3 times weekly dosing: 25–30 mg/kg to a maximum of 1-5 g/dose	Vertigo or hearing impairment due to eighth cranial nerve toxicity Nephrotoxicity	Pregnancy Careful administration in patients with borderline renal status	Usually not administered daily due to parenteral routes IM administration only; thus may be poorly absorbed in debilitated patients
ciprofloxacin (Cipro) 750 mg qd	Headache, nausea, diarrhea	Allergy to ciprofloxacin, allergy to fluoroquinolones	Not FDA approved for treating patients with TB, but commonly used in patients with MDR-TB.
ofloxacin (Floxin) 600 mg qd	Same as above	Same as above	Same as above
rifabutin (Mycobutin) Adults: 300 mg qd Not recommended for children	Rash, GI disturbances, headache, nausea, thrombocytopenia	Allergy to rifabutin or other rifamycins Patients with a WBC <1000/mm^3 or platelet count <50,000 mm^3 Use cautiously with breast-feeding	Rifabutin should never be administered as a single agent to patients with active TB because of the risk of rifabutin- and rifampin-resistant TB Educate patients that all body fluids will be stained reddish orange.
rifapentine (Priftin) dose: 600 mg twice weekly dosing, at least 72 h between doses	Hepatitis, rash, skin discoloration, GI disturbances, thrombocytopenia	History of any allergy to rifamycins Caution in patients with hepatic disease	Educate patients that all body fluids will be stained orange. Numerous drug interactions, especially with protease inhibitors

specific mechanism of action is unknown. Because it is stable and highly active in an acidic setting, its greatest efficacy is against TB organisms in macrophages, which are very acidic intracellularly. Like INH, PZA is well absorbed from the GI tract and reaches peak serum levels within a few hours. It also substantially penetrates tissues, including the cerebrospinal fluid (CSF).

Adverse Events

Hepatic function can be affected by PZA, but the drug does not appear to potentiate hepatitis when given along with INH and rifampin (Rifadin, Rimactane) during the first 2 months of therapy. Patients taking PZA frequently become hyperuricemic. Acute gout is uncommon in patients receiving PZA, but rashes, arthralgias, and GI disturbances sometimes occur.

Rifampin

Mechanism of Action

Rifampin (RIF), an antitubercular anti-infective, is also bactericidal against TB. It is a derivative of rifamycin. It is absorbed quickly and thoroughly after oral dosing, and peak serum levels are achieved within 2 hours. RIF penetrates cells, tissues, and inflamed meninges. RIF interferes with the activity of RNA polymerase in bacterial, but not mammalian, cells, suppressing RNA synthesis and thereby decreasing the ability of bacterial cells to reproduce. It is most active against rapidly growing cells.

Adverse Events

This drug has a wide range but low incidence of adverse effects, including GI upset, rashes, hepatitis, and blood dyscrasias. Because RIF is a hepatic enzyme inducer, it is likely to increase the clearance of many drugs that are metabolized hepatically. Thus, the compatibility and effectiveness of other drugs used during RIF therapy must be evaluated. Examples of medications that are likely to be affected include oral contraceptives, warfarin (Coumadin), theophylline (Slo-Phyllin), anticonvulsants, steroids, antiarrhythmics, antifungals, and oral hypoglycemics.

Chief among drugs whose serum concentrations are lowered substantially by RIF are the protease inhibitors and nonnucleoside reverse transcriptase inhibitors (NNRTIs). Serum concentrations of these drugs may be lowered to levels that are subtherapeutic.

Rifabutin

Mechanism of Action

Rifabutin (Mycobutin) is a derivative of RIF. It is an unclassified antimicrobial that demonstrates absorption and serum levels equal to those of RIF, and has a similar adverse event profile. RIF-resistant strains of TB are likely to be resistant to rifabutin as well. Rifabutin may be more effective in treating *Mycobacterium avium-intracellulare* complex, a mycobacterial opportunistic organism commonly infecting patients with acquired immunodeficiency syndrome (AIDS).

Adverse Events

Rifabutin has far less interaction with protease inhibitors and NNRTIs, but care must be taken because there are differences in interaction within classes of the antiviral medications. Rifabutin should never be administered as a single agent to patients with active TB because of the risk of rifabutin- and RIF-resistant TB.

Rifabutin has a low incidence, but varied type of adverse effects. Most commonly encountered are GI intolerance, skin rash, and neutropenia. As with RIF, all body fluids will be stained orange. Liver enzyme elevation is possible with all of the rifamycin compounds.

Rifapentine

Rifapentine (Priftin) is also an antibacterial derivative of rifamycin. Its mechanism of action is the same as RIF, with a similar range of antimicrobial activity. Taking rifapentine with food does not hinder absorption and may benefit patients who experience nausea with dosing. As a hepatic enzyme inducer, it alters the metabolism of various other medications, not as substantially as RIF does, but more substantially than rifabutin. Included among them are antiviral medications commonly used to treat patients with HIV.

Ethambutol

Ethambutol (Myambutol) is an antitubercular anti-infective. It is considered bacteriostatic, not bactericidal, at recommended doses. Although absorbed from the GI tract, the drug does not penetrate the CSF fully.

Mechanism of Action

The drug diffuses into mycobacteria that are actively growing, interferes with various metabolites, and consequently impairs the metabolism of the cell. No other strains of bacteria, fungi, or viruses are known to be susceptible to ethambutol. It is cleared by glomerular filtration and thus can accumulate in patients with renal disease.

Adverse Events

Dosing in patients with renal dysfunction can be difficult; the patients can receive a full dose of ethambutol at the conclusion of each dialysis treatment. Most of the toxic effects of ethambutol are related to vision. Retrobulbar neuritis is manifested by red-green color blindness, blurred vision, and, less commonly, scotomata.

Streptomycin

Streptomycin is an aminoglycoside antibiotic that is highly bactericidal in an alkaline environment. Globally, there has been an increased pattern of resistance to streptomycin. Although streptomycin has been demonstrated to have efficacy similar to ethambutol against TB, it is not recommended to be interchangeable with ethambutol in all countries.

Mechanism of Action

Streptomycin exerts its effect by interfering with normal protein synthesis in bacteria. It usually is administered intramuscularly to outpatients because it is not absorbed through the GI tract. It passes through inflamed meninges only.

Contraindications

Pregnancy is an absolute contraindication to the use of streptomycin, which is also contraindicated in patients with renal disease.

Adverse Events

Toxic effects can be severe. Ototoxicity results from damage to the eighth cranial nerve. Vertigo may occur in addition to hearing impairment. Nephrotoxicity occurs less commonly, but patients with borderline renal status and patients older than 60 years of age are at high risk for this adverse event.

Para-aminosalicylic Acid and Ethionamide

Para-aminosalicylic acid (PAS; Sodium P.A.S.) and ethionamide (Trecator) are antitubercular anti-infectives, with bacteriostatic activity against TB. They are used much less commonly since ethambutol became available in the 1960s. Both PAS and ethionamide have marked GI toxicity.

Because it is eliminated very quickly, PAS must be taken in high doses. PAS also is unstable in an acid medium. It is believed that PAS inhibits the synthesis of folic acid and possibly cell wall synthesis in *M. tuberculosis*. PAS is a pregnancy category C drug (having demonstrated occipital malformation in the rat fetus).

Ethionamide has been administered via rectal suppositories in an effort to decrease oral dosage and side effects, but such a regimen has unpleasant effects as well. Ethionamide is a teratogen and is used mainly if primary treatment fails. In many cases, adverse effects of concomitantly administered TB medications are intensified with the administration of ethionamide. Vitamin B_6 administration is recommended if ethionamide is used.

Ciprofloxacin and Ofloxacin

Ciprofloxacin (Cipro) and ofloxacin (Floxin) are fluoroquinolones that have demonstrated effectiveness against a number of gram-negative bacteria. Neither of these agents is approved by the U.S. Food and Drug Administration (FDA) for treating TB, but both have been used for MDR-TB. Both drugs exert their effects by disrupting the action of DNA gyrase, an enzyme that is the major catalyst in the transcription, duplication, and repair of DNA in bacterial cells. Both drugs are in pregnancy category C and have been detected in breast milk (see Chapter 8 for more information on ciprofloxacin and the fluoroquinolones).

Other Therapies

In addition to ethionamide and PAS, several drugs have FDA approval for use against TB, although they are not used commonly because of their adverse event profiles or lower efficacy. These include cycloserine (Seromycin) and capreomycin (Capastat Sulfate), antitubercular anti-infectives; amikacin (Amikacin) and kanamycin (Kantrex), aminoglycosides; and clofazimine (Lamprene), a leprostatic agent. In addition to ciprofloxacin and ofloxacin, numerous antimicrobials (eg, β-lactams, macrolides, and fluoroquinolones) not FDA approved for TB are used in cases of MDR-TB or intolerance to standard therapies. Such instances warrant referral to a pulmonologist or an infectious disease specialist to ensure adequacy of therapy.

Bacillus Calmette-Guerin Vaccine

Multiple vaccinations with BCG decrease the likelihood that a positive skin test result is due to infection, especially when chest x-ray findings are negative. BCG is a live vaccine prepared from attenuated strains of *Mycobacterium bovis*. The World Health Organization recommends administration at birth in certain instances to prevent disseminated and life-threatening diseases caused by *M. tuberculosis*.

BCG vaccine does not prevent TB infection, but it can be given in infancy and childhood to those who have negative skin test results and who are not infected with HIV. It may also be given to a child exposed to a person with contagious pulmonary TB that is resistant to INH or RIF, or TB that is untreated or ineffectively treated. It is given only if the child cannot be removed from the environment. BCG vaccine is administered between birth and 2 months of age with skin testing, but after that, the Mantoux text result must be negative.

Administration is contraindicated in skin infection, immunodeficiency, or pregnancy. Adverse events include a local reaction in 1% to 2% of patients, and abscesses and lymphadenopathy may ensue as well. There is usually skin test reactivity after immunization, but it is likely to persist at the size of 10 mm or more with *M. tuberculosis*. A reaction of 10 mm or more is unlikely more than 5 years after vaccination in infancy.

Selecting the Most Appropriate Agent for LTBI

First-Line Therapy

INH as a single daily dose is the recommended treatment for LTBI. In patients with HIV disease, 9 months of therapy are recommended. Six months is sufficient in patients who are immunocompetent. Drug regimens lasting for fewer than 6 months have been proven ineffective, whereas those lasting for more than 12 months do not seem to have greater efficacy. Patients who are less likely to be adherent to a daily regimen may take INH twice weekly only if DOT is used.

If patients are unlikely to adhere to the therapeutic plan and daily DOT is not logistically possible, regimens of 15 mg/kg administered twice weekly for 6 months have proved effective in children and adults. Pyridoxine (vitamin B_6), 10 to 25 mg/d, is given to patients who are taking anticonvulsants or who are pregnant, malnourished, or alcohol dependent. It is also given to patients with diabetes mellitus or chronic renal failure.

Second-Line Therapy

Four months of daily RIF is an acceptable alternative to daily INH. If patients are unlikely to adhere to either of these regimens, 2 months of daily RIF and PZA may be used. Close monitoring is essential because 21 cases of fatal and severe liver injuries occurred in the first 6 months in which this regimen was initially recommended (ATS, 2001). The RIF–PZA regimen should not be used in any patient with known liver disease or INH-induced hepatitis. It must be used cautiously in patients taking other medications that may cause hepatic injury, or in patients with alcoholism, even if the alcohol is stopped for the duration of treatment. RIF-based regimens are also useful in patients who are believed to have been infected by a patient with a known INH-resistant strain of TB.

Selecting the Most Appropriate Agent for Active Disease

To avoid the development of resistance to drug therapy, treatment must include more than one drug to which the

Table 27.2

Recommended Order of Treatment for Latent Tuberculosis Infection

		Comments
First line isoniazid 300 mg/d	Daily for 6–9 mo. Twice weekly dosing with DOT	9–12 mo in HIV patients. Add pyridoxine supplement.
Second line RIF and PZA	Daily for 2 mo. Twice weekly dosing for 2–3 mo with DOT	Offer to patient with known IHN-resistant, RIF-susceptible contact.
Third line RIF	Daily for 4 mo	Used in patients intolerant of PZA, with INH-resistant, RIF-susceptible contact.

organism is sensitive. Treatment must last long enough for eradication of the organisms.

First-Line Therapy

INH, RIF, PZA, and ethambutol are first-line drugs for treating active TB. Combinations of these first-line drugs (ie, combination regimens) are advised by the ATS and the CDC based on considerations for individual patient needs and capacities and, ultimately, on sputum culture and sensitivity test results. The use of a multidrug regimen is the single most important factor to consider when deciding on treatment. Single agents are absolutely contraindicated; even three-drug regimens may prove insufficient. Data from New York City demonstrated that 33% of reported TB cases were resistant to one drug, and 19% of the cases were resistant to both RIF and INH (CDC, 1993). Until culture and sensitivity testing is completed, it is recommended that patients receive four drugs regularly. Several first-line drug regimens are available (Table 27-3). Interventions to ensure therapeutic adherence may be necessary in some patients. These are described in Box 27-5.

The mainstays of therapy are INH and RIF. They are bactericidal to both rapidly growing and slowly replicating *M. tuberculosis* organisms. The cure rate is 95% when these two drugs are taken for only 9 months. Ethambutol is recommended to be added until sensitivity is documented. If the strain is sensitive to INH and RIF, ethambutol can be stopped. PZA kills rapidly growing organisms and is beneficial in the first 2 months of therapy. In the following 4 months, the drugs can be taken only twice a week. The regimen looks like one shown in Table 27-3. Pyridoxine 50 mg/d initially and 100 mg biweekly is recommended to decrease peripheral neuropathy.

Second-Line Therapy

Other drugs are used if the organisms are not sensitive to the first-line regimen. Before second-line therapy is selected, the patient should be referred to and monitored by a specialist. Pyridoxine (vitamin B_6) 50 mg/d or 100 mg biweekly is given to elderly patients with diabetes mellitus, chronic renal failure, or alcoholism. It is also given to patients receiving anticonvulsant therapy and those who are malnourished or pregnant.

Special Population Considerations

Women

Diagnosis of TB in a pregnant woman is not an indication for therapeutic abortion. However, treatment is mandated to protect the unborn, the mother, and family members. Treatment of LTBI in pregnant women with intact immune responses may be delayed until the postpartum period. Pregnancy itself has no impact on the progression of LTBI to active disease. If the pregnant patient has risk factors for progressing to active disease, then daily INH should be started immediately.

Because no teratogenic effects are associated with INH, RIF, and ethambutol, these drugs are considered safe for use during pregnancy. PZA may be used in pregnant women in whom drug resistance is suspected, but it is not a first-line agent in pregnancy because information regarding its possible teratogenicity is insufficient. As mentioned previously, streptomycin is contraindicated in pregnancy.

BOX 27–5. INTERVENTIONS TO ENSURE THERAPEUTIC COMPLIANCE

Patient-centered treatment strategies should always include and emphasize directly observed therapy (DOT). Any tactics or incentives that may help promote adherence to, and completion of, a regimen are worth investigating and discussing with the patient.

- DOT may be carried out by a relative or friend of the patient who is considered reliable and consistent. However, relatives with strong emotional connections may have difficulty enforcing administration of medications, creating additional family stress rather than relieving it. Ongoing family feedback is important.
- Social service agencies and public health outreach workers provide DOT with proven success.
- Twice or thrice weekly administration drug regimens are available for the convenience of the friend or relative performing DOT, as well as the patient.
- Public health facilities that provide medications free of charge and provide DOT are available.
- Another option is for the patient to come to the office or clinic on a set schedule for DOT.
- Patients also may meet the DOT contact at a location where they feel secure.
- Treatment completion is defined by the number of doses completed as well as the duration of therapy.

Table 27.3

Selected First-Line Treatment Regimens for TB in Order of Preference

Regimen 1	Regimen 2	Regimen 3	Regimen 4
INH, RIF, PZA and ETH daily for 2 mo. After INH and RIF sensitivities are established, INH and RIF or RPT alone daily or two to three times weekly for 4 mo.	Daily INH, RIF, PZA, and EMB for 2 wk. Then DOT twice weekly for 6 wk, then DOT for 16 wk of INH and RIF or RPT	Three times weekly DOT with INH, RIF, PZA, and EMB for 2 mo, then DOT for 18 wk of INH/RIF	INH/RIF/EMB daily for 2 mo Then INH/RIF daily or twice weekly for 8 mo

INH, isoniazid; RIF, rifampin; RPT, rifapentine; PZA, pyrazinamide; EMB, ethambutol; DOT, directly observed therapy.
All regimens must be continued for a minimum of 6 months, and *should continue* for 3 months after cultures becomes negative. If cultures remain positive after 3 months referral is indicated. Patients with HIV infection require a minimum of 9 months of therapy, and should continue for 6 months after cultures become negative.

Breast-feeding is not contraindicated during treatment of active or latent TB. All drugs will be present in small concentrations in breast milk. Toxic effects have not been reported; however, the concentrations in breast milk are not sufficient to be considered therapeutic to treat an infant. Pyridoxine supplementation is advised for infants of breast-feeding mothers taking INH.

The practitioner should advise mothers to take their TB medications after breast-feeding and to use a prepared bottle at the next feeding.

Patients With HIV Infection

Patients with HIV infection require a longer course of therapy. A minimum of 9 months of therapy is required for HIV$^+$ patients, including 6 months of therapy after the sputum cultures test negative for TB organisms. Rifabutin is used in patients with HIV receiving protease therapy because it decreases serum levels of protease inhibitors to a lesser extent than RIF or rifapentine.

MONITORING PATIENT RESPONSE

Sputum culture and sensitivity testing are essential for diagnosis and for evaluating therapeutic effectiveness. Quantitation of colonies is an excellent parameter to follow regarding the bacterial load of specimens. Sputum cultures should be repeated at 1-, 2-, 4-, and 6-month intervals throughout therapy. They should show a decrease in organism population. In approximately 50% of patients, sputum smears are negative for TB by 2 months of compliant therapy; 75% are negative for TB by 4 months; and by 6 months, culture results are negative for TB in more than 95% of patients. If the cultures are negative for TB at 2 months, the ATS suggests no further cultures until the completion of therapy. If the culture is still positive for TB at 2 months, sensitivities need to be re-evaluated and compared with the drug regimen being used and modifications made to the drug regimen if necessary.

Chest x-rays, although less significant than sputum culture, should demonstrate clinical improvement by 3 months of therapy, or an alternative diagnosis should be investigated while therapy continues. At the completion of a therapeutic regimen, all patients should have another chest x-ray study, which then serves as the new baseline for future comparison. Any residual scarring should be measured and its location well documented.

If the practitioner or patient notices any hint of toxicity, or if there is any clinical suspicion of toxicity, appropriate tests are warranted. If patients experience severe GI disturbances, all drugs suspected of causing these disturbances should be stopped and serologic testing performed. If no serum abnormalities are detected, drugs may be reinstituted at half of their previous dosage for several days, after which the full dosage schedule can resume. Hepatic aminotransferase levels are measured. If they are elevated, they are monitored until they return to normal levels, after which one drug should be restarted each week. Hepatic enzyme levels are monitored with the new start of each drug to determine which drug is responsible for elevated levels. If hepatic, renal, or pancreatic sources are the cause of GI disturbances, the patient should be referred for special treatment. For severe GI disturbances, patients may require hospitalization for parenteral hydration and nutrition.

PATIENT EDUCATION

Drug Information

The practitioner must educate patients and their families about drug therapy for TB. Patients taking INH or RIF need to know to take these drugs on an empty stomach 1 hour before or 2 hours after a meal. Ethambutol should be taken with food but not with aluminum-containing antacids.

The practitioner must educate patients and families about all signs and symptoms of toxicity and inquire about such findings at each visit with the patient. Patients need to be forewarned that RIF, rifabutin, and rifapentine stain all body fluids (including urine, tears, and perspiration) orange.

Health care providers save a great deal of time by educating patients in advance of expected side effects and those effects that are common but innocuous. RIF also increases the clearance rate of hepatically metabolized drugs. As a precaution, all medications that a patient takes should be reviewed at each office visit.

Patient education regarding vision-related adverse events is crucial to optimal therapy with ethambutol because dosing can be changed or discontinued before visual acuity is impaired.

To prevent the spread of the disease, patients are taught to take all drugs as prescribed; dispose of used tissues in a sealed plastic container; cover the mouth when sneezing, coughing, or laughing; and wash hands after they have been around the mouth and nose.

Patient-Oriented Information Services

Numerous resources are available for patients and providers. The CDC Web site www.CDC.gov has a plethora of information written in lay and scientific language. It provides links to scientific publications and to the ATS. Patients without access to computer and internet resources can obtain information from local health departments and by calling the American Lung Association.

Nutrition

Proper nutrition is often overlooked in the patient with TB. Many patients begin therapy in a poor nutritional state due to a variety of factors. Infection, cough, and fever place exceptional caloric demands on the body, and often lead to weight loss by the time of diagnosis. Additionally, fluid and electrolyte imbalances are possible due to fever and diaphoresis. Loss of appetite is common during the illness as well as from the medications to treat the infection or underlying illnesses. Altered taste sensation from medications may also contribute to anorexia. Fatigue and shortness of breath may dissuade patients from exerting effort to prepare nutritious meals. Cost of food with nutritional value is an inhibiting factor for many patients. Social service agencies may be helpful in providing food stamps or referrals to agencies that assist patients with meal acquisition and in some cases delivery of meals. Protein, fats, and carbohydrates are all essential for tissue growth/repair, calorie requirements, and energy sources, respectively. Consultation with a registered dietitian is warranted if patients fail to maintain weight or are unable to tolerate meals due to medications. Nutritive fluids are encouraged, but alcohol is strongly discouraged as it will, in most cases, accelerate hepatotoxicity. Vitamin B_6 supplementation is indicated if patients are taking INH.

Complementary and Alternative Medicines

TB as an infectious disease requires a proven, regimented, and protracted course of medications. No alternative therapies are approved for treatment of TB. Some symptoms that accompany TB may be alleviated by complimentary and alternative therapies, but risk is also incurred with oral preparations that may interfere with the absorption and distribution of required medications. Behavioral, cognitive, and relaxation therapies are often helpful in supplementing care. Yoga can be very therapeutic in relaxing and strengthening muscle groups that often weaken due to lack of use during illness. Physical activity should be encouraged as tolerated, but not to the point of fatigue.

■ Case Study

C. W. is a 59-year-old African American male social worker with a history of chronic bronchitis. He has been treated for numerous upper respiratory infections in the past with courses of Bactrim DS, macrolides, and fluoroquinolones. He is an unmarried heterosexual who quit smoking 20 years ago. He has had no recent hospitalizations nor has he traveled recently. He lives with his brother, who is well physically. He is allergic to penicillin.

He sought health care after 6 weeks of fever and a 10-lb weight loss. In the last 6 weeks, he has been treated with two courses of macrolides and a course of a fluoroquinolone. He continues to have fevers, night sweats, and a cough, which is usually dry but occasionally produces white sputum. Just 3 weeks before this visit, C. W. tested negative for HIV. He currently reports mild dyspnea for the last 2 days.

On physical examination, C. W. appears mildly ill and mildly dyspneic with conversation. He reports moderate dyspnea with exertion in the office setting. Other physical findings include temperature: 100.3°F; heart rate 96 and regular; blood pressure 132/84; and respiratory rate 24 at rest.

Lungs: upper lobes clear, fine crackles at the left base, crackles over lower third of the right lung. No "e to a" changes. Coughing occurs frequently during the examination. Pulse oximetry value is 94%.

Neck: no jugular vein distention, no carotid bruits or thyromegaly

Lymph nodes: no cervical, supraclavicular, or axillary nodes palpable

Clinical impression: TB highly suspected and a PPD test was performed on the patient's forearm. Because of his dyspnea and new findings on pulmonary auscultation, he was directly admitted to a medical-surgical floor bed in respiratory isolation to rule out TB.

Clinical course: Chest x-ray reveals a new, left upper-lobe infiltrate with possible cavitation. Sputum is induced by means of ultrasonic hypertonic saline using intermittent positive-pressure breathing. Numerous baseline clinical laboratory studies are conducted, including complete blood count with differential and blood chemistries, including hepatic and renal function tests. The HIV test is repeated.

All results are within normal limits and the patient is still HIV negative. Because acid-fast bacilli have been isolated from sputum specimens, the patient begins a four-drug regimen of isoniazid, ethambutol, pyrazinamide, and rifampin while awaiting sensitivity results. The PPD was reactive with an induration of 22 mm.

Diagnosis: Active TB

1. What treatment goals would you set for this patient? How does this person's lifestyle affect the goals?
2. How would you know the patient is taking the medication?
3. What are two or three key items you must discuss with this patient?
4. Describe one or two adverse reactions that may occur with your selected regiment that would cause you to change therapy.
5. How would you address the use of over-the-counter and/or alternative medications for this patient?
6. What dietary and lifestyle changes should be recommended for this patient?
7. Describe what you would do when the sensitivity results are known.
8. What would you monitor to determine success of the therapy and when would you do so?
9. Describe at least two drug–drug or drug–food interactions that might occur with this patient.

Bibliography

Starred references are cited in the text.

*American Thoracic Society. (1994). Treatment of tuberculosis and tuberculosis infection in adults and children. *American Journal of Respiratory and Critical Care Medicine, 149,* 1359–1374.

*American Thoracic Society. (2000). Targeted tuberculin testing and treatment of latent tuberculosis infection. *American Journal of Respiratory and Critical Care Medicine, 161,* S221–S247.

Anonymous. (1996). CDC issues recommendations for screening for tuberculosis in high-risk populations. *American Family Physician, 53,* 1433–1436.

Bates, J. H., & Stead, W. W. (1993). The history of tuberculosis as a global epidemic. *Medical Clinics of North America, 77,* 1205–1217.

Brost, B. C., & Newman, R. B. (1997). The maternal and fetal effects of tuberculosis therapy. *Obstetrics and Gynecology Clinics of North America, 24,* 659–671.

Centers for Disease Control. (1991). Purified protein derivative—tuberculin anergy and HIV infection: Guidelines for anergy testing and management of anergic persons at risk for tuberculosis. *Morbidity and Mortality Weekly Report, 40,* 27–33.

*Centers for Disease Control and Prevention. (1993). Initial therapy for tuberculosis in the era of multidrug resistance: Recommendations of the advisory council on the elimination of tuberculosis. *Morbidity and Mortality Weekly Report, Recommendations and Reports, 42,* 1–8.

Centers for Disease Control and Prevention. (1996). Tuberculosis morbidity—United States, 1996. *Morbidity and Mortality Weekly Report, 46,* 695–700.

Centers for Disease Control and Prevention (1997). Anergy skin testing and preventive therapy for HIV infected persons: Revised recommendations. *Morbidity and Mortality Weekly Report, Recommendations and Reports, 46,* 1–10.

Centers for Disease Control and Prevention. (2001). Update: Fatal and severe liver injuries associated with rifampin and pyrazinamide for latent tuberculosis infection, and revisions in American Thoracic Society/CDC recommendations–United States, 2001. *Morbidity and Mortality Weekly Review, 50,* 733–735.

*Centers for Disease Control and Prevention. (2003). Treatment of tuberculosis. *Morbidity and Mortality Weekly Report, Recommendations and Reports, 52,* 1–77.

Dunlap, N. E., & Briles, D. E. (1993). Immunology of tuberculosis. *Medical Clinics of North America, 77,* 1235–1251.

Kalafer, M. E. (1991). Tuberculosis: Epidemiology and prophylaxis. In R. A. Bordow & K. M. Moser (Eds.), *Manual of clinical problems in pulmonary medicine* (3rd ed., pp. 147–151). Boston: Little, Brown.

Knopf, S. A. (1914). Tuberculosis as a cause and result of poverty. *Journal of the American Medical Association, 63,* 1720–1725.

Mandell, G., Bennet, J., & Dobin, R. (1999). *Mandell, Douglass & Bennet's principles and practice of infectious disease* (5th ed., pp. 2586–2590). New York: Churchill Livingstone.

Mazurek, G., & Villarino, M. (2003). Guidelines for using the QuantiFERON-TB test for diagnosing latent *Mycobacterium tuberculosis* infection. *Morbidity and Mortality Weekly Report, Recommendations and Reports 52,* 15–18.

Peter, G. (Ed.). (2000). *The 2000 red book: Report of the Committee of Infectious Diseases* (24th ed.). Elk Grove Village, IL: American Academy of Pediatrics.

Pottumarthy, S., Morris, A. J., Harris, A. C., et al. (1999). Evaluation of the tuberculin gamma interferon assay: potential to replace the Mantoux skin test. *Journal of Clinical Microbiology, 37,* 3229–3232.

Rakel, R. (1999). *Conn's current therapy* (52nd ed.). Philadelphia: WB Saunders.

Rosenzweig, D. (1996). Tuberculosis and nontuberculosis mycobacterial diseases. In J. Noble (Ed.), *Primary care medicine* (2nd ed., pp. 1540–1551). St. Louis: Mosby.

Turkoski, B. B., Lance, B. R., & Janosik, M. F. (1999). *Drug information handbook for nursing 1998–99.* Cleveland, OH: Lexi-Comp.

Visit the Connection web site for the most up-to-date drug information.

NAUSEA AND VOMITING

■ JOLYNN KNOCHE AND VIRGINIA P. ARCANGELO

Nausea and vomiting are common complaints in humans. The severity of the event can range from a slight discomfort or queasiness to uncontrollable, forceful vomiting. Despite this range, all are perceived to be uncomfortable and troublesome and should be treated in a proper and timely manner. Patients may refer to this experience by many different names: *upchuck, urp, queasy, throw-up, puke*, to name a few. There are many different causes of nausea and vomiting, such as motion sickness, pregnancy, and medications. Likewise, many treatment options can be used to manage this complication. People of all ages experience emesis, although the etiology may be related to age-specific factors. Drugs are most frequently used for the treatment of nausea and vomiting, but alterations of nondrug factors may decrease the severity of emesis. This chapter reviews the pathophysiology and pharmacotherapy of specific types of nausea and vomiting.

CAUSES

There are multiple causes for nausea and vomiting; however, some of the most common are from the ingestion or administration of substances or drugs, gastrointestinal (GI) disorders, neurologic processes, and metabolic disorders. The presence of noxious stimuli is frequently a cause of nausea and vomiting. Supratherapeutic digoxin (Lanoxin) and theophylline (Theo-Dur or Slo-Phyllin) are known to produce emesis. Nausea and vomiting occur more frequently with high-dose chemotherapy than with moderate doses of the same drugs. Erythromycin and some penicillin derivatives are acknowledged for inducing uncomfortable GI complications. Emesis can also result from excessive ethanol intake. It is well known that other sensory experiences, such as pungent odors or gruesome sights, can induce nausea and vomiting. Box 28-1 presents specific etiologies for nausea and vomiting.

Patient-specific factors that increase susceptibility to nausea and vomiting include age, previous nausea and vomiting experiences, and sex. Most of the research identifying these characteristics was done in patients receiving chemotherapy. Poor control of nausea and vomiting with previous surgeries or chemotherapy predisposes a patient to subsequent episodes of emesis, also referred to as *anticipatory nausea and vomiting*. This form of emesis is often difficult to treat with standard antiemetics.

One study of patients with cancer reports a threefold increase in the incidence of emesis in patients previously treated with chemotherapy compared with chemotherapy-naive patients treated with identical chemotherapy regimens (Pisters & Kris, 1992).

Adult patients younger than 30 years of age have an increased incidence of emesis compared with their older counterparts. In addition, the younger patient population is more likely to experience extrapyramidal reactions from the drugs used to treat their nausea and vomiting. In patients who received the same chemotherapy and antiemetic premedications, women experienced more nausea and vomiting than men (Pisters & Kris, 1992).

Chronic ethanol intake exceeding 100 g/d (roughly five beers or mixed drinks per day) is associated with better emesis control and decreased incidence. A history of motion sickness may increase the risks of nausea and vomiting in another situation, such as with chemotherapy or surgery. Children in general experience nausea and vomiting more frequently than adults. Obesity and anxiety have also been associated with heightened emesis incidence.

The prevalence of nausea and vomiting may complicate 11% to 73% of surgical procedures. Prevalence is also increased by the use of certain inhalation agents (nitrous oxide, in particular) and by concomitant use of opiate medications; the use of propofol as an intravenous anesthetic agent lowers the risk of postoperative nausea and vomiting (PONV). PONV is more likely to occur after general than regional anesthesia, and its prevalence increases in parallel with the duration of surgery and anesthesia. PONV is especially common after gynecologic and middle ear surgery and also occurs more commonly with abdominal and orthopedic surgery than with laparoscopic or other extra-abdominal operations. PONV is also more likely in those with a history of PONV or motion sickness.

PATHOPHYSIOLOGY

The pathophysiology of nausea and vomiting is complex (Fig. 28-1) and involves the modulation of medullary sites and neurotransmitters. Many sensory centers accept noxious stimuli from the body, including the chemoreceptor trigger zone (CTZ), visceral afferent nerves, cerebral cortex, limbic system, vestibular system, and midbrain intracranial pressure receptors.

BOX 28–1. ETIOLOGIES OF NAUSEA AND VOMITING

Therapy-induced causes
  Chemotherapy
  Radiation therapy
  Opiates
  Anticonvulsants
  Ipecac
  Antibiotics
  Digitalis or digoxin toxicity
  Theophylline
  NSAIDs
  Hormonal therapies
Drug withdrawal
  Opiates
  Benzodiazepines
Metabolic disorders
  Addison disease
  Water intoxication
  Volume depletion
  Diabetic ketoacidosis
  Hypercalcemia
  Renal dysfunction–uremia
Gastrointestinal mechanisms
  Mechanical gastric outlet obstruction
    Peptic ulcer disease
    Gastric carcinoma
    Pancreatic disease
  Motility disorders
    Gastroparesis
    Drug-induced gastric stasis
    Irritable bowel syndrome
    Postgastric surgery
    Idiopathic gastric stasis
  Intra-abdominal emergencies
    Acute pancreatitis
    Acute pyelonephritis
    Acute cholecystitis

Acute cholangitis
Acute viral hepatitis
Intestinal obstruction
Acute gastroenteritis
  Viral gastroenteritis
  Salmonellosis
  Shigellosis
  Staphylococcal gastroenteritis (enterotoxins)
Cardiovascular disease
  Acute myocardial infarction
  Congestive heart failure
  Shock and circulatory collapse
Neurologic processes
  Cerebellar hemorrhage
  Increased intracranial pressure
    Hematoma
    Subdural effusion
    Tumor (benign or malignant)
    Hydrocephalus
    Reye syndrome
  Headache
    Migraine
    Severe hypertension
  Head trauma
  Vestibular disorders
Psychogenic causes
  Anorexia nervosa
  Anticipatory
Miscellaneous causes
  Pregnancy
  Noxious odors
  Ingestion of an irritant
  Operative procedures
  Septicemia
  Nicotine

Modulation of Nausea and Vomiting

These stimuli are transmitted to the vomiting center, also called the *emetic center*, which coordinates the sensory inputs and the act of vomiting. The vomiting center is the key component in the modulation of nausea and vomiting. Located in the lateral reticular formation of the medulla, it receives afferent impulses from the aforementioned sensory centers. On activation of the vomiting center, efferent impulses are sent to the nucleus tractus solitarius, an intertwined neural network that innervates the salivary, vasomotor, and respiratory centers and cranial nerves VIII and X. Efferent impulses are also sent to the stomach, abdominal muscles, diaphragm, and associated sphincters to execute the involuntary act of vomiting. Much like the sensory centers that stimulate it, the vomiting center is rich in dopamine, histamine, serotonin, and acetylcholine receptors and can also be affected by binding to opiate and benzodiazepine receptors. An intact vomiting center is essential for coordination of the vomiting act.

Stimulatory Centers

The CTZ is one of the most important chemosensory organs responsible for the detection of noxious stimuli. It is uniquely located in the area postrema in the floor of the fourth ventricle of the (medulla) brain and is exposed to both blood and cerebrospinal fluid (CSF). Thus, toxins in both the blood and CSF can stimulate a response by the CTZ. These toxins may be drugs (chemotherapy, opiates, digoxin), poisons, or substances found naturally in the body (excess calcium, hormones). The CTZ is rich in neurotransmitter receptors for dopamine, serotonin, histamine, and acetylcholine. An antiemetic effect is elicited when these receptors are blocked.

Gastrointestinal Tract

The GI tract and pharynx are sites of origin for the stimulation of nausea and vomiting. Visceral afferent nerves, also referred to as *splanchnic nerves*, from the pharynx and GI

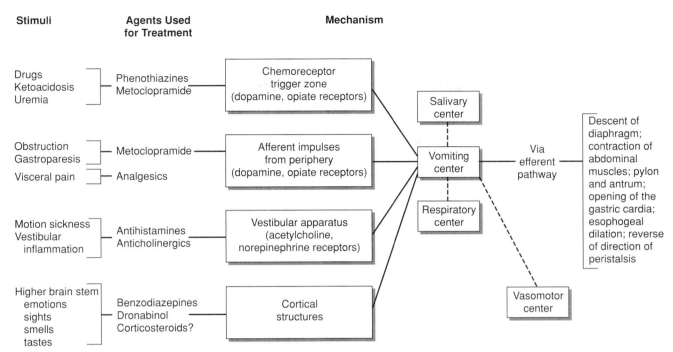

Figure 28–1 Pathophysiology of nausea and vomiting. (From Koda-Kimble, M. A., & Young, L. Y. [2004]. Nausea and vomiting. In: Koda-Kimble, M. A., Young, L. Y., & Guglielmo, B. J. [Eds.]. *Applied therapeutics: The clinical use of drugs* [8th ed.]. Philadelphia: Lippincott Williams & Wilkins.)

tract transmit impulses from local neuroreceptors along the vagus nerve to the vomiting center. The GI tract is rich in local dopamine, histamine, and serotonin receptors. The visceral afferent nerves are also responsible for transmitting stimuli from other peripheral sites such as the heart, lungs, and testes; hence, the vomiting response may occur when a person has been punched in the abdomen or kicked in the groin. Abdominal surgery is another example in which visceral afferent nerves are involved in nausea and vomiting.

Central Nervous System

Motion sickness is primarily a central nervous system (CNS) response mediated by the vestibular system. Acetylcholine and histamine receptors have been found in the vestibular center. Blockade of these receptors provides some degree of protection from emesis. The cerebral cortex, the largest portion of the brain, is responsible for the motor coordination of the body, sensory perception, learning, memory, and many other functions. Afferent impulses from specific sites of the cerebral cortex can result in emesis. The cerebellum is responsible for the regulation of balance, equilibrium, and coordination. Disruption of this portion of the brain can lead to temporary or chronic nausea and vomiting. These structures may also play a role in anticipatory emesis.

Limbic System

The limbic system and the midbrain intracranial pressure receptors can stimulate nausea and vomiting, although their mechanisms are not fully understood. In humans, the primary function of the limbic system is associated with the expression of mood, emotions, and feelings, as well as memory recall. Anxiety, fear, and other emotions may play

a role at this site in the perception of nausea and vomiting. Head trauma, intracranial bleeding, and mass effect from a benign or malignant tumor can produce increased pressure in the brain. This increased intracranial pressure can cause nausea and vomiting. The optimal treatment in these situations is a reduction in intracranial pressure through surgery or corticosteroids.

DIAGNOSTIC CRITERIA

The three identified phases of emesis are nausea, retching, and vomiting. Nausea is the unpleasant physical sensation of impending retching or vomiting. Nausea often occurs without the other two steps of emesis, although they are all treated with the same pharmacologic agents. Common symptoms accompanying nausea are flushing, pallor, tachycardia, and hypersalivation. Gastric stasis, decreased pyloric tone, mucosal blood flow, and contractions of the duodenum with reflux into the stomach are physiologic responses to nausea. Retching, the second phase of emesis, is the involuntary synchronized labored movement of abdominal and thoracic muscles before vomiting. Vomiting is the coordinated contractions of the abdominal and thoracic muscles to expel the gastric contents. The lower esophageal sphincter contracts, allowing GI retroperistalsis. The actual expulsion of gastric contents differentiates vomiting from retching.

The acuteness of the symptomatology is based on history and physical examination. Several issues need to be addressed such as whether this is an acute emergency, such as mechanical obstruction, perforation, or peritonitis, clinical clues that the problem is likely to be self-limited, such as would be expected with viral gastroenteritis or a potentially offending medication. The goal is to determine whether empiric treatment with an antiemetic, gastric acid-suppressing, or prokinetic agent would be beneficial or whether the patient should be admitted to the hospital to correct fluid and electrolyte imbalance.

Acute nausea and vomiting differs considerably from that of chronic nausea and vomiting so symptom duration is important. Acute onset of nausea and vomiting suggests gastroenteritis, pancreatitis, cholecystitis, or a drug-related side effect. When nausea and vomiting are associated with diarrhea, headache, and myalgias, the cause is viral gastroenteritis; in this instance, symptoms should resolve spontaneously within 5 days. A more insidious onset of nausea without vomiting is suspicious of gastroparesis, a medication-related side effect, metabolic disorders, pregnancy, or even gastroesophageal reflux disease. Nausea and vomiting are considered chronic when their duration is longer than 1 month.

Timing and description of the vomiting are important. Vomiting that occurs in the morning before breakfast is typical of that related to pregnancy, uremia, alcohol ingestion, and increased intracranial pressure. Projectile vomiting suggests intracranial disorders, especially those that result in increased intracranial pressure. In this case, vomiting may not be preceded by nausea.

The onset of vomiting caused by gastroparesis or gastric outlet obstruction tends to be delayed, usually by more than 1 hour, after meal ingestion. Vomiting may be suggestive of psychiatric disorders.

Associated symptoms, such as abdominal pain, fever, diarrhea, vertigo, or a history of a similar contemporaneous illness among family, friends, or associates are important data to gather.

Physical examination looks at vital signs for signs of dehydration. Jaundice, lymphadenopathy, abdominal masses, and occult blood in the stool may reveal features suggestive of thyrotoxicosis or Addison disease. The abdominal examination should look for distention, visible peristalsis, and abdominal or inguinal hernias. Areas of tenderness are important: tenderness in the midepigastrium suggests an ulcer; in the right upper quadrant, cholecystitis or biliary tract disease. Auscultation may demonstrate increased bowel sounds in obstruction or absent bowel sounds in ileus.

INITIATING THERAPY

The treatment of nausea, retching, or vomiting in any patient begins with an evaluation and correction of possible causes. Most sources of nausea and vomiting may be reversed or palliated by surgery or medical interventions. Infectious causes should be promptly treated with antibiotics, and metabolic disorders require medical management. Some drug toxicities may be treated with antidotes, such as digoxin toxicity reversed with digoxin immune Fab (Digibind). The following section discusses medications used to treat nausea and vomiting. They should be used with definitive treatments when possible.

Alterations in a patient's daily activities may aid in managing nausea and vomiting and decrease the resources used to control the problem. Nonpharmacologic management of nausea and vomiting should be tailored to the presumed etiology.

Changes in a patient's diet may affect the frequency or severity of nausea and vomiting, such as avoidance of spicy foods and excessive grease or oil, and decreased caffeine intake. Professional counseling or group therapy may prove favorable for patients with psychogenic nausea and vomiting.

Hypnosis, behavior modification, and imagery are beneficial tools in controlling nausea and vomiting that has an anxiety component, such as chemotherapy-related anticipatory emesis. However, prevention of anticipatory nausea and vomiting is the optimal form of management.

Goals of Drug Therapy

The goals of drug therapy are simple: to alleviate the subjective feeling of nausea and the objective act of vomiting and their associated complications (Box 28-2). It is important to rely on the patient's subjective response when evaluating the efficacy of a specific therapy for nausea. Secondary goals are to minimize drug toxicity/adverse events and contain costs. The prevention of nausea and vomiting is the goal in the setting of chemotherapy and certain surgical procedures. Control or improvement in nausea and vomiting should occur within 5 to 60 minutes of a pharmacologic intervention. If this does not ensue, another method should be used promptly. Table 28-1 reviews available antiemetic agents, dosages, comparable efficacy, and adverse effects. Pregnancy risk factors are included in the discussion of each drug class and in the pregnancy-related nausea and vomiting section.

BOX 28–2. COMPLICATIONS OF NAUSEA AND VOMITING

Metabolic abnormalities
- Dehydration
- Alkalosis
- Hypokalemia
- Hypomagnesemia
- Hyponatremia
- Hypochloremia
- Malnutrition

Structural damage
- Wound dehiscence
- Esophagogastric tears/Mallory-Weiss tears
- Increased bleeding under skin flaps
- Tension on suture lines

Patient dissatisfaction
- Noncompliance
- Poor oral intake; anticipatory nausea and vomiting
- Delayed ambulation after surgery/procedures
- Fatigue
- Depression

Increased use of resources
- Prolongation of hospital stay
- Unexpected hospital admission
- Alteration or additional therapy

Aspiration pneumonia

Venous hypertension

Table 28.1

Overview of Selected Antiemetic Agents

Generic (Trade) Name and Dosage	Selected Adverse Events	Contraindications	Special Considerations
Phenothiazines			
chlorpromazine (Thorazine) 10–25 mg q4–6 h prn PO 25–50 mg q4–6h prn IV, IM 50–100 mg q6–8h prn rectal	Sedation or drowsiness EPSs: agitation, insomnia, motor restlessness, spasms of facial muscles, protrusion of tongue, and mandibular tics Anticholinergic effects: dry mouth, urinary retention, blurred vision	Hypersensitivity Cautious use with other CNS depressants, Parkinson syndrome, poorly controlled seizure disorder, severe hepatic dysfunction	Increased incidence of autonomic response with IV administration Higher incidence of EPSs
fluphenazine (Prolixin) 0.5–5 mg q6–8h prn PO, IM	Same as above	Same as above	
perphenazine (Trilafon) 2–6 mg q4–6h prn PO 5–10 mg q6h prn IM	Same as above	Same as above	Higher incidence of EPSs compared with other phenothiazines
prochlorperazine (Compazine) 5–10 mg q4–6h prn PO, rectal, IM, IV 10–30 mg bid PO sustained-release capsule	Same as above	Same as above	Sustained-release capsule more expensive Higher incidence of EPSs compared with other phenothiazines
promazine (Sparine) 25–50 mg q4–6h prn PO, IM	Same as above	Same as above	
promethazine (Phenergan) 12.5–25 mg q4–6h prn PO, rectal, IM, IV	Same as above	Same as above	Less effective than prochlorperazine
thiethylperazine (Torecan) 10 mg q8–24h PO, rectal			Less effective than prochlorperazine
Antihistamines and Anticholinergics			
benzquinamide (Emete-con) 50 mg q3–4h prn IM 25 mg q3–4h prn IV	Sedation or drowsiness, confusion Anticholinergic effects: dry mouth, tachycardia, blurred vision, urinary retention, constipation	Hypersensitivity Caution in narrow-angle glaucoma, asthma, prostatic hypertrophy	IV preparation not recommended
buclizine (Bucladin-S) 50 mg q4–6h prn PO	Same as above	Same as above	
cyclizine (Marezine) 50 mg q4–6h prn PO, IM	Same as above	Same as above	Do not exceed 200 mg/d
dimenhydrinate (Dramimine) 50–100 mg q4–6h prn PO, IM, IV	Same as above	Same as above	Do not exceed 200 mg/d
diphenhydramine (Benadryl) 25–50 mg q6–8h prn PO 10–50 mg q2–4h prn IM, IV	Same as above	Same as above	Do not exceed 200 mg/d
hydroxyzine (Atarax, Vistaril) 25–100 mg q4–6h prn PO, IM	Same as above	Same as above	
meclizine (Antivert, Bonine) 25–50 mg q24h prn PO	Same as above	Same as above	
scopolomine (Transderm-Scop) 1.5 mg q3 days transdermal patch	Same as above	Same as above	
trimethobenzamide (Tigan) 250 mg q6–8h prn PO 200 mg q6–8h prn IM, rectal	Same as above	Same as above	
Benzodiazepines			
lorazepam (Ativan) 0.5–2 mg q4–8h prn PO, IM, IV	Drowsiness or fatigue, confusion, constipation	Same as above	Dose should be low in frail, elderly, or critically ill patients
diazepam (Valium) 2–5 mg bid–qid prn PO, IM, IV	Same as above	Same as above	Same as above
Serotonin Antagonists			
dolasetron (Anzemet) 100 mg PO 1 h before chemotherapy 100 mg IV 30 min before chemotherapy 12.5 mg IV 15 min before cessation of anesthesia 100 mg PO 2 h before surgery	Headache, diarrhea	Hypersensitivity Use with caution in patients with severe cardiac dysfunction	Very expensive (IV > PO) Use only when indicated
granisetron (Kytril) 10 µg/kg IV 30 min before chemotherapy 1 mg PO bid (q12h)—start before chemotherapy	Same as above	Same as above	Very expensive (IV > PO) Use only when indicated IV dose often rounded to 1- or 2-mg doses

(continued)

Table 28.1

Overview of Selected Antiemetic Agents *(Continued)*

Generic (Trade) Name and Dosage	Selected Adverse Events	Contraindications	Special Considerations
ondansetron (Zofran) 0.15 mg/kg IV 30 min before chemotherapy and at 4 and 8 h 8 mg PO bid (or tid)	Same as above	Same as above	Very expensive (IV > PO) Use only when indicated
Other Antiemetics			
dexamethasone (Decadron) 8–20 mg IV/PO before chemotherapy; 4–8 mg IV bid (delayed nausea and vomiting)	Hyperactivity, GI irritation, mood swings, depression, hyperglycemia, anxiety	Hypersensitivity Use with caution in diabetic patients, history of ulcers, young male patients	Give IV over 5–15 min Administer orally with food Avoid chronic administration
methylprednisolone (Solu-Medrol) 125–500 mg IV q6h	Same as above	Same as above	Same as above
dronabinol (Marinol) 5–15 mg/m² PO 1–3 h before chemotherapy and q4h × 6 2.5–10 mg PO bid	Sedation, confusion, dysphoria, increased appetite	Use with caution if patient is receiving other CNS depressants	Controlled substance
antacids 15–30 mL q2–4h prn	Diarrhea, constipation	Renal dysfunction	May decrease absorption of other drugs
metoclopramide (Reglan) 20–30 mg PO qid prn, 1–2 mg/kg IV before chemotherapy and q2–4h (high-dose)	EPSs Diarrhea Drowsiness		Side effects are dose dependent EPS reversible with diphenhydramine

Phenothiazines

Phenothiazines are the most commonly used class of drugs to treat nausea and vomiting. Prochlorperazine (Compazine), promethazine (Phenergan), and thiethylperazine (Torecan) are the most frequently used drugs in this class. Others include chlorpromazine (Thorazine), fluphenazine (Prolixin), perphenazine (Trilafon), and promazine (Sparine).

Mechanism of Action

Their mechanism of action presumably involves dopamine receptor blockade in the CTZ. Anticholinergic activity in the vomiting and vestibular centers of the brain may also contribute to the mechanism of action.

The phenothiazines may be used as monotherapy for mild to moderate nausea and vomiting or in combination with other antiemetics for more severe nausea and vomiting. A dose–response quality has been noted for this drug class; however, the incidence of adverse effects such as extrapyramidal effects and sedation can also be associated with higher doses. Promethazine has activities of an antihistamine antiemetic and could also be classified with the antihistamine–anticholinergic class of drugs. The phenothiazines are a viable and practical option for long-term treatment of nausea and vomiting. Products are available in oral, rectal, and injectable formulations. To improve tailoring of the drug regimen to the patient, oral preparations are available as tablets, sustained-release capsules, and liquids. Rectal suppositories are useful in patients who cannot retain oral medications and when intravenous (IV) access is not an option. Suppositories should be avoided in patients who are thrombocytopenic because of the increased risk of bleeding or hemorrhage.

Contraindications

Caution should be used in patients taking concomitant drugs that cause CNS depression, such as sedatives, hypnotics, and opiates, because further sedation may result. Phenothiazines may exacerbate the symptoms of Parkinson disease. The safety of phenothiazines during pregnancy is controversial; most studies find phenothiazines to be safe for the mother and fetus if used occasionally in low doses. Most phenothiazines are in pregnancy risk category C. Phenothiazines may decrease the seizure threshold and should be used cautiously in patients with seizure disorders.

Compared with other agents, prochlorperazine is slightly less effective than droperidol (Inapsine) and as effective as low-dose metoclopramide (Reglan). Prochlorperazine is more effective than promethazine and thiethylperazine. The phenothiazines are relatively inexpensive in relation to most of the other drug classes, with the exception of the sustained-release phenothiazine preparations, which tend to be costly.

Adverse Events

The most common adverse event of phenothiazine use is drowsiness or sedation. Phenothiazines also have the ability to evoke extrapyramidal symptoms (EPSs) by blocking the central dopaminergic receptors involved in motor function, particularly at higher doses. EPSs may present as dystonic reactions, feelings of motor restlessness, and parkinsonian signs and symptoms. Masklike face, drooling, tremor, cogwheel rigidity, pill-rolling motion, lack of ability to initiate voluntary movement, and gait abnormalities are all severe examples of parkinsonian presentations. Dystonic reactions may include spasm of the neck muscles or torticollis, extensor rigidity of back muscles, mandibular tics, difficulty swallowing or talking, and perioral spasms, often with protrusion of the tongue. Motor restlessness may consist of agitation, jitteriness, tapping of feet, and insomnia. Extrapyramidal reactions can be easily treated with the use of diphenhydramine (Benadryl) 25 mg orally or parenterally 3 to 4 times a day or benztropine (Cogentin) 1 to 4 mg orally or parenterally twice a day. Autonomic responses, such as hypotension and tachycardia, have been observed with IV phenothiazine use, particularly chlorpromazine. Hypotension and sedation are less likely to occur with prochlorperazine, thiethylperazine, and perphenazine, but these three agents are associated with a higher frequency of EPSs. Dry mouth, urinary retention, blurred vision, and other anticholinergic effects may occur with phenothiazine use. Reversible agranulocytosis is rarely associated (<1%) with phenothiazine therapy. This effect occurs more frequently in women and with chronic phenothiazine use. Cholestatic jaundice and photosensitivity are reactions that can occur rarely within the first few months of chronic phenothiazine use. These are more frequently observed in phenothiazine use for psychiatric conditions rather than emesis control.

Monitoring parameters include EPSs and parkinsonian symptoms. Doses may need to be decreased in severe hepatic dysfunction. Complete blood counts should be regularly monitored in chronic phenothiazine use, specifically prochlorperazine, chlorpromazine, fluphenazine, perphenazine, and thiethylperazine (see Table 28-1).

Interactions

These drugs potentiate CNS depression with alcohol and other CNS depressants. They potentiate the action of α blockers and levels of the drug can be increased with propranolol. Anticonvulsant drug doses may have to be adjusted. They may antagonize oral anticoagulants.

Antihistamines–Anticholinergics

A plethora of agents are available in the antihistamine–anticholinergic drug class. These agents are most useful for mild nausea, such as motion sickness. Hydroxyzine (Vistaril, Atarax), meclizine (Bonine, Antivert), dimenhydrinate (Dramamine), and scopolamine (Transderm Scop) are some of the more common agents of this class. Unlike most of the other classes of agents discussed in this chapter, some of the antihistamine–anticholinergic agents are available without a prescription.

Mechanism of Action

The mechanism of action appears to be interruption of visceral afferent pathways that are responsible for stimulating nausea and vomiting. These drugs are most frequently administered orally, but some can be given IV, intramuscularly, transdermally, or rectally.

The antihistamines are particularly useful for the treatment and prevention of motion sickness. For this indication, it is recommended that a dose be taken at least 30 to 60 minutes before the event (eg, boating, air flight, car ride) and then repeated at regular intervals several times a day. The scopolamine patch is a highly useful agent for the prevention of motion sickness. A patch should be applied to clean, dry skin 1 to 2 hours before the potentially emetogenic event, and a new patch may be reapplied every 3 days.

Many of the antihistamines and anticholinergics have been used for the treatment of nausea in pregnancy.

Contraindications

Animal studies have indicated teratogenic effects of antihistamines (buclizine [Bucladin] and cyclizine [Marezine]) in animals, but they appear not to have these effects in humans. Many of the manufacturers of these drugs, however, consider these agents to be contraindicated in early pregnancy because of lack of clinical data. They are not available in the U.S.

Adverse Events

Adverse effects limit the use of anticholinergics–antihistamines. Patients frequently experience sedation, drowsiness, or confusion. The anticholinergic effects are troublesome, including blurred vision, dry mouth, urinary retention, and tachycardia. These anticholinergic effects are also dose related and occur more frequently as the dose increases or the drug is given more often. Caution is warranted in patients with narrow-angle glaucoma, prostatic hypertrophy, and asthma because these patients are more prone to the anticholinergic effects of these drugs.

Anticholinergic effects may be managed by nondrug therapies. Chewing gum or sucking on ice chips or hard candy may refresh dry mouth. The intake of a high-fiber diet and adequate daily fluid consumption may curb constipation.

Monitoring for anticholinergic effects is of paramount importance. Severe effects may warrant discontinuation of drug. Symptoms of overdose may include dilated pupils, tachycardia, hypertension, CNS depression, flushed skin, or, more seriously, respiratory failure and circulatory collapse. Adverse effects occur more commonly in patients with renal or hepatic dysfunction.

Interactions

These drugs can potentiate CNS depression with alcohol, tranquilizers, and sedative–hypnotics.

Benzodiazepines

Often used for other indications, benzodiazepines offer useful qualities to the antiemetic armamentarium. Not only do these agents treat and prevent emesis, they can cause anxiolysis and amnesia. These latter effects are particularly beneficial in anticipatory nausea and vomiting associated with chemotherapy.

Lorazepam (Ativan) is the most frequently used benzodiazepine for nausea and vomiting. Its mechanism of action is not fully elucidated; however, it probably acts centrally to inhibit the vomiting center. Lorazepam has only moderate antiemetic properties and is usually used in combination with other agents to control chemotherapy-associated anticipatory nausea and vomiting and delayed chemotherapy-associated nausea and vomiting.

Dosage

Both oral and parenteral forms of lorazepam are available. Patient-specific variables should be considered when identifying an appropriate dose. Usual oral or IV doses range from 0.5 to 2 mg at least 30 minutes before start of chemotherapy. As needed (prn) antiemetic doses range from 0.5 to 3 mg IV or orally every 4 to 6 hours. To prevent oversedation, patients with poor performance status, the elderly, or frail individuals require low initial doses of lorazepam. Patients with compromised pulmonary or poor cardiac function should receive IV lorazepam with caution and have close monitoring of respiratory and cardiac status.

Contraindications

Lorazepam is not recommended for use in patients with hepatic or renal failure. Several studies have indicated that diazepam (Valium) may also cause fetal toxicity when administered to pregnant women, and thus should be avoided in this patient population. The benzodiazepines are in pregnancy risk category D.

Adverse Events

For benzodiazepines, CNS depression occurs most often, with drowsiness, fatigue, memory impairment, impaired coordination, and confusion occurring frequently. Lorazepam has an amnesic effect that for some patients is a benefit, whereas others may find it unacceptable. Paradoxical CNS stimulation resulting in restlessness, anxiety, nightmares, and increased muscle spasticity may occur. The drug should be discontinued if paradoxical stimulation occurs. Other adverse effects include constipation, headache, and increased or decreased appetite. Parenteral administration may cause hypotension, bradycardia, or apnea, particularly in the elderly and critically ill (see Table 28-1).

Monitoring parameters include cardiovascular and respiratory status for initial doses. Because the liver metabolizes the benzodiazepines, liver function tests should be assessed before dosing. Presence of adverse CNS effects should be evaluated with each clinic or hospital visit.

Interactions

These drugs potentiate CNS depression when used with other drugs that depress the CNS and alcohol.

Serotonin Antagonists

The serotonin antagonists are the most recent class of antiemetics to be introduced to the market. Ondansetron (Zofran), granisetron (Kytril), palonosetron (Aloxi) and dolasetron (Anzemet) are available in the United States.

Mechanism of Action

These agents work by antagonizing the type 3 serotonin ($5HT_3$) receptors centrally in the CTZ and also peripherally at the vagal and splanchnic afferent fibers from the enterochromaffin cells in the upper GI tract. The serotonin antagonists were initially indicated for the treatment and prevention of chemotherapy-induced nausea and vomiting. They have changed the way nausea and vomiting are treated and have greatly improved the quality of life for patients receiving highly emetogenic chemotherapy regimens. Radiation-induced nausea and vomiting and PONV are two other areas where the serotonin antagonists have been studied.

The unequivocal efficacy and lack of significant adverse effects make these agents ideal for select indications.

The serotonin antagonists are available orally as tablets and liquids and parenterally for IV use. Because these agents are used to prevent nausea and vomiting, oral administration in this situation is encouraged, even with highly emetogenic chemotherapy. There have been few data to support superior efficacy of one agent over another when used at recommended dosages. All of the serotonin antagonist preparations are costly and should be used conservatively and appropriately. Many institutions have created antiemetic guidelines to identify the approved indications of serotonin antagonists to optimize care and resources. The appropriateness of these agents in specific circumstances is discussed later.

Contraindications

There are inadequate human data for use in pregnancy; however, animal studies do not reveal evidence of harm to the fetus. Two case reports cite the efficacy of ondansetron in the treatment of hyperemesis gravidarum, without adverse sequelae to the fetus. The serotonin antagonists are in pregnancy risk category B. The serotonin antagonists should be used with caution in breast-feeding mothers; once again human data are lacking, but ondansetron is distributed into the milk of lactating rats.

Adverse Events

Mild to moderate headache can occur in approximately 20% to 25% of patients receiving oral or parenteral serotonin antagonists, followed in frequency by diarrhea in 8% to 16% of patients (Audhuy et al., 1996). A few patients experience severe headaches requiring discontinuation of the drug. Other adverse effects that occur in less than 10% of patients are abdominal or epigastric pain, increased serum hepatic enzyme levels on liver function tests, hypertension, malaise or fatigue, constipation, pruritus, and fever. Rare cardiovascular effects have been reported, although a definite causal relationship has not been established. All three of the agents can cause electrocardiographic (ECG) alterations (prolongation of the PR interval and QT interval and QRS complex widening). This is best documented in the studies of dolasetron, but these ECG changes were deemed to be clinically nonsignificant by the authors (Audhuy et al., 1996). Conservatively, in patients with severe cardiac dysfunctions such as arrhythmia and heart block, the serotonin antagonists should be used cautiously.

Important monitoring parameters for serotonin antagonists include baseline and follow-up liver function tests. Dosage reductions may be made for severe hepatic dysfunction. To avoid ECG-related complications, electrolyte assessment and correction of hypokalemia and hypomagnesemia are indicated (see Table 28-1).

Interactions

Caution is used when given with drugs that prolong cardiac conduction interval, diuretics, and cumulative high-dose anthracycline.

Metoclopramide and Other Antiemetics

Metoclopramide (Reglan) has been used to treat nausea and vomiting caused by several different stimuli. It is a highly useful agent in the treatment of diabetic gastric stasis, postsurgical gastric stasis, and gastroesophageal reflux, which may be associated with some degree of nausea.

Mechanism of Action

For these indications, metoclopramide enhances motility and gastric emptying by increasing the duration and extent of esophageal contractions, the resting tone of the lower esophageal sphincter, gastric contractions, and peristalsis of the duodenum and jejunum. Metoclopramide is also used in the prevention and treatment of chemotherapy-induced nausea and vomiting. Its mechanism of action is dopamine receptor inhibition in the CTZ. The central and peripheral actions of this agent make it efficacious in multiple clinical situations. Metoclopramide can be administered orally, IV, and intramuscularly. A sugar-free syrup exists for diabetic patients who cannot take the pills. Because metoclopramide is eliminated primarily by the kidneys, the dose of this drug should be decreased by 50% if the patient's creatinine clearance is less than 40 mL/min. Subsequent doses are based on the patient's clinical response. Periodic assessment of renal function is prudent. Patients should be informed of the sedative qualities of this agent and that use of other CNS depressants could potentiate this effect.

Adverse Events

The most clinically concerning adverse effects of metoclopramide are EPSs. Much like the effects seen with high doses of phenothiazines, facial spasms, rhythmic protrusions of the tongue, involuntary movements of limbs, motor restlessness, agitation, and other dystonic reactions can occur. These effects occur most commonly in children and young adults, in men more than women, and at high doses of metoclopramide. Twenty-five percent of adults 18 to 30 years of age experience dystonic reactions after receiving high-dose metoclopramide for treatment of chemotherapy-induced emesis. The EPSs occur within 24 to 48 hours of the initial dose and subside within 24 hours of drug discontinuation. High-dose metoclopramide is usually defined as 2 mg/kg per dose. EPSs can be prevented or treated with the addition of diphenhydramine 25 to 50 mg IV or orally. IV administration of diphenhydramine is preferred for serious presentations. Other reversal agents are benztropine and diazepam. Secondary to its actions in the intestinal tract, metoclopramide can cause diarrhea. Management of diarrhea includes discontinuation or dosage reduction of metoclopramide, increased fluid resuscitation, and electrolyte replacement. The use of metoclopramide may not be a prudent choice in a patient who already has diarrhea. Drowsiness and fatigue are noted in approximately 10% of patients. There are inadequate data for the use of metoclopramide in pregnancy; however, supratherapeutic doses in rats did not produce evidence of fetal harm. Metoclopramide is in pregnancy risk category B. Metoclopramide is known to be distributed into breast milk but does not appear to present a risk to the infant if the mother is taking 45 mg/d or less.

Interactions

A hypertensive crisis can occur when metoclopramide is used with monoamine oxidase inhibitors (MAOIs). Additive sedation can be seen when used with alcohol or other CNS depressants. These drugs are antagonized by anticholinergics and narcotics. They may diminish gastric and accelerate intestinal absorption of drugs and food.

Corticosteroids

Corticosteroids are usually reserved for chemotherapy-induced nausea and vomiting. Appreciation of the antiemetic properties of this class of agents occurred when clinicians observed decreased episodes of nausea and vomiting with Hodgkin disease protocols that included prednisone compared with protocols that did not include prednisone.

Mechanism of Action

The true mechanism of action in the relief of nausea and vomiting is unknown, but one postulated theory is the inhibition of prostaglandins. In nausea and vomiting secondary to increased intracranial pressure, corticosteroids provide relief by decreasing inflammation. Dexamethasone (Decadron) and methylprednisolone (Solu-Medrol) are the two most common corticosteroids used; however, the addition of prednisone (Deltasone) to lymphoma and leukemia chemotherapy regimens can provide heightened control of emesis. These corticosteroids are almost always used in combination with other agents in the control or prevention of emesis from highly emetogenic regimens.

Corticosteroids are available orally and parenterally. The oral form is beneficial for low doses or prolonged administration, but may cause significant GI toxicity. Patients should be encouraged to take oral corticosteroids with food to minimize GI irritation and complications. IV administration is ordinarily used in the prevention of nausea and vomiting, primarily to avoid GI complications. IV preparations should be infused over 5 to 15 minutes to prevent burning, flushing, and itching sensations associated with the phosphate salt dissociation. Of the corticosteroids studied, the utility of dexamethasone has been best defined. In clinical trials, single-agent dexamethasone was superior to prochlorperazine and comparable with high-dose metoclopramide when used for mildly to moderately emetogenic chemotherapy regimens. The combination of dexamethasone and high-dose metoclopramide was the standard of care for prevention of cisplatin-induced emesis until the introduction of the serotonin antagonists. IV doses of dexamethasone as a premedication range from 8 to 20 mg.

Corticosteroids should be used with caution in uncontrolled diabetic patients. Sliding-scale insulin or careful alterations of oral hypoglycemic agent regimens may be used for unacceptably high blood glucose levels.

Adverse Events

Although very useful, the corticosteroids are associated with many toxicities and adverse effects. Mental disturbances range from mood swings, depression, anxiety, and aggression to frank psychosis and personality changes. Men are particularly susceptible to this aggressive behavior. Headache, restlessness, and insomnia are not infrequent, particularly with higher doses of corticosteroids. Patients and family members and loved ones will benefit from knowing that these effects may occur with therapy. Sleep aids may be necessary for secondary insomnia. Temazepam (Restoril) or diphenhydramine are viable options. Variable increases in blood glucose and decreased glucose tolerance result from glucocorticoid use. Regular evaluations of blood glucose in diabetic patients is warranted. Glucocorticoids, especially in large or chronic doses, can increase the susceptibility to and mask the symptoms of infection, such as fever. Many consequences of long-term corticosteroid use can be detrimental. Muscle wasting, adrenocortical insufficiency, fluid and electrolyte disturbances, cataract formation, and atrophy of the protein matrix of bone resulting in osteoporosis, vertebral compression fractures, aseptic necrosis of femoral or humeral heads, and pathologic fractures are some of the most serious complications of chronic corticosteroid use. Whenever possible, chronic corticosteroid use should be curtailed.

Interactions

Glucocorticoids may decrease effects of barbiturates, hydantoins, rifampin, and ephedrine. Potassium levels should be monitored when glucocorticoids are used with potassium-depleting diuretics.

Cannabinoids

Cannabinoids are indicated only for nausea and vomiting associated with chemotherapy. In the 1970s, it was observed that patients on chemotherapy who smoked marijuana experienced a lower incidence of nausea and vomiting. Investigators then determined that tetrahydrocannabinol (THC) has antiemetic properties.

Mechanism of Action

The true mechanism of action of THC is unknown, but it is most likely related to effects on the vomiting center and the opiate receptors in the CNS and cerebral cortex, but probably does not involve the CTZ. The agents available in the United States is dronabinol (Marinol).

The cannabinoids can be used to treat and prevent chemotherapy-induced nausea and vomiting. Because it is necessary to reach therapeutic blood levels of THC before chemotherapy administration to prevent emesis, administration of the cannabinoids should occur at least 6 to 12 hours before chemotherapy. Emesis can be controlled from mildly to moderately emetogenic chemotherapy regimens, and cannabinoids may provide some relief to patients where other agents have failed. When used with mildly to moderately emetogenic regimens, THC has been found to be superior to placebo, prochlorperazine, low-dose metoclopramide, and haloperidol. These agents are seldom front-line therapy because of their incidence and severity of adverse effects.

Patients should be cautioned about the deleterious CNS effects and told not to drive or operate machinery. Dosages can be reduced if the patient is experiencing CNS toxicities. Patients should avoid alcohol and other CNS depressants.

Adverse Events

Most of the adverse effects of the cannabinoids are CNS related and include sedation, ataxia, and dysphoria. Dysphoria may be expressed as confusion, hallucinations, anxiety, fear, memory loss, time distortion, and other undesired occurrences. Orthostatic hypotension, blurred vision, and tachycardia have been observed with the use of these drugs. With repeated doses, the patients usually become tolerant to most of the CNS adverse effects, but not to the antiemetic activity. There is a correlation between antiemetic response and a psychological "high." Younger patients and patients who have had previous experiences with recreational cannabinoids appreciate greater antiemetic efficacy from this drug class. The side effects of the cannabinoids occur more frequently than with many of the other agents and are particularly distressing to older adults. One potentially beneficial adverse effect is appetite stimulation, which may prove useful in hematology and oncology patients. The cannabinoids are in pregnancy risk category D and should be avoided in pregnancy or lactation.

Antacids

Over-the-counter (OTC) antacid preparations may provide relief to patients experiencing mild nausea and vomiting. The general mechanism by which these agents exhibit their effects is by coating the stomach and neutralizing gastric acid. Most preparations contain one or several of the following: calcium carbonate, magnesium hydroxide, aluminum hydroxide, or aluminum carbonate. Between 15 and 30 mL orally of an antacid preparation may provide relief. Patients should be encouraged to seek medical attention if they experience continued nausea and vomiting, and the patient may need medical workup for more serious GI diseases.

Toxicities from OTC antacids are infrequent, but they do exist. The agents containing magnesium may cause diarrhea; conversely, the agents containing aluminum or calcium may cause constipation. These adverse effects are dose dependent. Calcium-containing antacids can cause phosphate depletion. Caution should be used in patients with renal dysfunction because aluminum and magnesium may accumulate. Antacids, by coating the GI tract, can decrease the absorption of many oral medications such as digoxin, some antibiotics, corticosteroids, and allopurinol (Zyloprim), which may lead to decreased efficacy of therapy. (For additional information on antacids, see Chapter 29.)

Selecting the Most Appropriate Agent

Nausea and Vomiting Not Chemotherapy-Induced

It is necessary for the practitioner to assess the etiology of the nausea and vomiting. If an organic cause can be determined, the cause should be corrected to alleviate the symptoms. For example, if the nausea and vomiting is a side effect of a medication, the medication is to be discontinued. If the cause is diabetic ketoacidosis, insulin is given. Figure 28-2 shows the treatment algorithm.

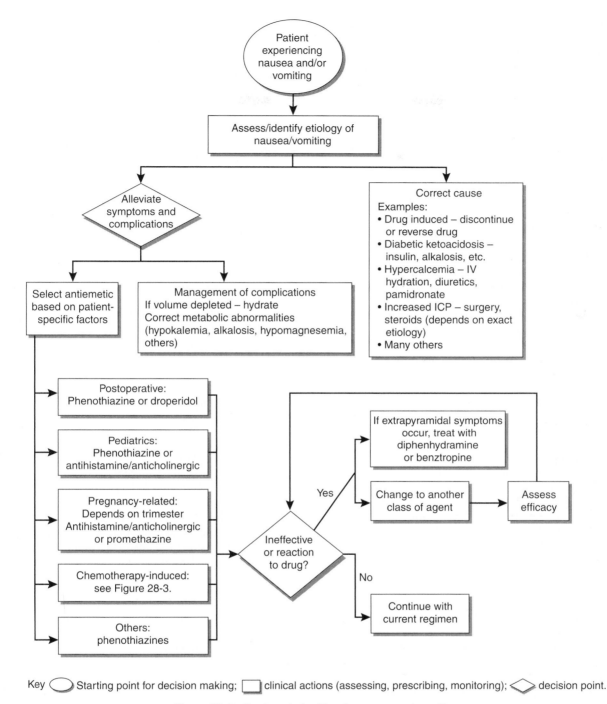

Figure 28–2 Treatment algorithm for nausea and vomiting.

First-Line Therapy

An antiemetic is selected based on patient-specific factors. Initially, a phenothiazine is used for mild to moderate nausea and vomiting. Promethazine and prochlorperazine are usually effective.

Second-Line Therapy

If the above treatment is not effective, an antihistamine or anticholinergic preparation can be used. These are usually not as effective as phenothiazines but may be useful in mild nausea.

Third-Line Therapy

If the first two therapies are not successful, the patient should be reevaluated for a physiological cause that has not been treated and therapy based on patient data.

Table 28-2 lists the recommended order of treatment for nausea and vomiting.

Chemotherapy-Induced Nausea and Vomiting

Nausea and vomiting are two of the toxicities of chemotherapy that patients fear most. Although not usually a life-threatening complication, uncontrolled nausea or vomiting

Table 28.2

Recommended Order of Treatment for Nausea and Vomiting

Order	Agents	Comments
First line	Phenothiazines	Most frequently used for mild to moderate nausea and vomiting Promethazine, prochlorperazine usually effective
Second line	Antihistamine Anticholinergic preparation	Usually not as efficacious as phenothiazines, but may be useful in mild nausea
Third line	Depends on response to other antiemetics	Tailor to patient-specific factors

*Consider patient-specific factors when choosing an antiemetic agent.

can greatly affect a patient's quality of life and attitude. Fortunately, new agents and combinations of agents make it possible to control emesis.

The severity of chemotherapy-induced emesis depends on numerous factors. Most significant is the intrinsic ability of the chemotherapy regimen to cause nausea and vomiting. Before the U.S. Food and Drug Administration approves a drug for use, phase 1 and 2 studies must be performed to prove efficacy and safety and identify adverse effects. The incidence and severity of nausea and vomiting are initially reported at this time, when the drug is given as a single agent. Each chemotherapy agent can be identified as having highly, moderately high, moderate, moderately low, and low emetogenic potential. Based on this information, antiemetic regimens can be tailored to the chemotherapy regimen to prevent emesis. Mechanisms to identify the emetogenicity of combination chemotherapy regimens are presented in this section. Other factors that may increase the incidence of chemotherapy-induced nausea and vomiting are previous exposure to chemotherapy, psychosocial factors such as anxiety and depression, poor performance status, and younger age (<30 years). A history of alcohol abuse and male sex may correlate with a decreased incidence or severity of nausea and vomiting. The classifications of chemotherapy-induced nausea and vomiting include acute, delayed, and anticipatory.

Acute Emesis

Acute emesis is vomiting occurring within 24 hours of treatment. The onset of acute emesis is usually within 1 to 2 hours after the start of chemotherapy. It peaks within 4 to 10 hours and resolves within 24 hours, but these factors vary from agent to agent. This most common type of chemotherapy-induced nausea and vomiting is associated with a higher frequency and severity than the other two classifications. Acute emesis is strongly related to the agent or agents administered and the doses given (Box 28-3 identifies the emetogenic potential of specific agents).

By definition, highly emetogenic chemotherapy agents induce emesis in greater than 90% of patients receiving that drug without antiemetic premedication. Chemotherapy agents that have moderately high emetogenicity cause emesis in 60% to 90% of patients receiving chemotherapy. Chemotherapy that is moderately emetogenic has an incidence of 30% to 60%, moderately low has a 10% to 30% incidence of emesis, and low emetogenicity is defined as an incidence of less than 10%.

All patients receiving single agents that are moderately to highly emetogenic should be adequately pretreated to prevent the incidence of nausea and vomiting for at least 24

hours or the expected duration of nausea or vomiting. The current standard of care of antiemetic prophylaxis is the combination of a serotonin antagonist and a corticosteroid, such as granisetron or ondansetron with dexamethasone, at least 30 minutes before chemotherapy administration. Repeated doses may need to be given to prevent and treat emesis for 24 hours, depending on the pharmacokinetics of the agents used. Some practitioners use once-daily administration of serotonin antagonists, claiming that once the receptors are blocked, duration of receptor binding is the functional component rather than the plasma half-life. Because the purpose of these agents is to prevent nausea and vomiting, and the patient is not actively experiencing these effects, it is often acceptable to administer antiemetics orally. Combination regimens containing drugs that are moderately to highly emetogenic are given prophylactically in similar fashion. Although the aforementioned antiemetic combination is not universally effective, an estimated 70% to 90% of patients experience sufficient control. Examples of difficult clinical situations that may prohibit the use of a corticosteroid include poorly controlled diabetes and uncontrolled hypertension.

Contraindications to serotonin antagonists include hypersensitivity or severe cardiac dysfunction. Alternative prophylactic antiemetics must be chosen for patients who have relative contraindications and are to receive emetogenic chemotherapy. High-dose metoclopramide with dexamethasone may be considered an option to a serotonin antagonist with dexamethasone because this was the gold standard for highly emetogenic regimens before the appearance of ondansetron. Once again, the antiemetic regimen should be tailored to the patient and the chemotherapy regimen.

Single-agent or combination chemotherapy regimens that are expected to be moderately low or low in emetogenic potential can be managed less aggressively. These drugs do not warrant the use of a serotonin antagonist. For some chemotherapy regimens and agents, such as the taxanes and fluorouracil, premedication frequently is not necessary; however, patients should be encouraged to use antiemetic medications as needed to control any nausea and vomiting after chemotherapy. Premedication with dexamethasone with or without a phenothiazine or metoclopramide may be used if a patient experiences nausea and vomiting from previous chemotherapy. All of these antiemetic drugs may be scheduled for a 24- to 36-hour period to prevent any nausea and vomiting. Patient-specific factors must be considered to identify an appropriate antiemetic regimen.

Regardless of the emetogenicity of a chemotherapy regimen or the use of premedications, antiemetics should be prescribed for prn or break-through use. Preferred prn chemotherapy antiemetic therapy (Box 28-4) are tremendously effective.

Delayed Emesis

Delayed nausea and vomiting is defined as emesis that begins or persists more than 24 hours after completion of chemotherapy. Some investigators suggest that because there is a "peak" in incidence at 18 hours after cisplatin-based chemotherapy, a revised definition of delayed emesis should include this timetable. The new-found, reliable control of acute emesis from highly to moderately emetogenic chemotherapy regimens has unveiled delayed nausea and vomiting as a more vexing problem. Many chemotherapy agents produce mild delayed nausea and vomiting, but cyclophosphamide, cisplatin, and the anthracyclines are particularly noted for their delayed emesis.

Delayed emesis usually is not as frequent or severe as acute emesis. The mechanism of delayed emesis is believed to be different from that of acute emesis. It is believed that delayed emesis is mediated by neurotransmitters, although serotonin does not play a major role. Combination antiemetic regimens have proven to be more effective than single-agent therapies. Single-agent serotonin antagonists were found to be equally as effective as metoclopramide or placebo and less effective than dexamethasone, unlike their efficacy in preventing acute emesis. Regimens identified as most effective for delayed emesis include metoclopramide 0.5 mg/kg orally four times a day for 4 days with dexamethasone 8 mg orally twice a day for 2 days, followed by dexamethasone 4 mg orally twice a day for 2 days.

The use of scheduled phenothiazines (including long-acting phenothiazines) with dexamethasone is another effective option

---

BOX 28-3. EMETOGENIC POTENTIAL OF CHEMOTHERAPY AGENTS

Highly emetogenic (>90%)
  Carmustine >250 mg/m^2
  Cisplatin >50 mg/m^2
  Cyclophosphamide >1500 mg/m^2
  Dacarbazine
  Lomustine
  Mechlorethamine
  Streptozocin
Moderately high (60%–90%)
  Carboplatin
  Carmustine ≤250 mg/m^2
  Cisplatin ≤50 mg/m^2
  Cyclophosphamide ≤1500 mg/m^2 or >750 mg/m^2
  Cytarabine >1000 mg/m^2
  Doxorubicin >60 mg/m^2
  Methotrexate >1000 mg/m^2
  Procarbazine oral
Moderate (30%–60%)
  Cyclophosphamide ≤750 mg/m^2
  Cyclophosphamide oral
  Doxorubicin 20–60 mg/m^2
  Idarubicin
  Ifosfamide
  Methotrexate 250–1000 mg/m^2
  Mitoxantrone
  Topotecan
Moderately low (10%–30%)
  Docetaxel
  Etoposide
  5-Fluorouracil
  Gemcitabine
  Methotrexate >50 mg/m^2 or <250 mg/m^2
  Mitomycin
  Paclitaxel
Low (<10%)
  Bleomycin
  Busulfan
  Chlorambucil oral
  Cladribine
  Fludarabine
  Hydroxyurea
  Melphalan oral
  Thioguanine oral
  Vinblastine
  Vincristine
  Vinorelbine

BOX 28-4. BASIC PRINCIPLES OF CHEMOTHERAPY ANTIEMETIC THERAPY

- Consider emetogenic potential of chemotherapy regimen.
- Give appropriate antiemetics to prevent nausea and vomiting at least 30 min before emetogenic chemotherapy.
- Schedule antiemetics throughout anticipated period of nausea and vomiting risk.
- Always prescribe as-needed (prn) antiemetics for breakthrough nausea and vomiting between scheduled doses.
- Use antiemetic combinations with nonoverlapping mechanisms of action and adverse effects, when possible.
- Consider patient-specific variables when choosing a regimen (eg, anxiety, performance status).
- Re-evaluate patients frequently during and between chemotherapy courses for efficacy and toxicity of antiemetic regimen.
- Consider nonpharmacologic interventions, especially in patients with anticipatory nausea and vomiting.

---

antiemetics, such as prochlorperazine or metoclopramide, are effective, inexpensive, and easily administered. These agents provide reliable, safe control of mild nausea. These agents may be used before meals to alleviate anorexia secondary to nausea. Patients should be counseled about the common adverse effects of these agents, and each patient should be encouraged to report ineffective control of nausea and vomiting. When adhered to, the basic principles of for the prevention of delayed nausea and vomiting. Addition of a benzodiazepine to the antiemetic regimen may prove useful for the control of emesis in anxious patients or patients with difficulty resting.

Anticipatory Emesis

Anticipatory nausea and vomiting occurs in up to 25% of patients receiving chemotherapy. It is usually associated with a history of uncontrolled nausea and vomiting with prior chemotherapy and is a conditioned response. Multiple factors can stimulate anticipatory nausea and vomiting, but most factors remind the patient of the previous unfavorable experience. For example, patients tell stories of becoming nauseated by the sight of their oncologist's office or by a smell that reminds them of receiving chemotherapy. Other triggers may be tastes, sounds, or thoughts of chemotherapy. Anticipatory nausea and vomiting most frequently occurs before the administration of chemotherapy, and it can lead to poorer control of nausea and vomiting with subsequent courses. The most effective treatment for delayed nausea and vomiting is prevention. It is crucial to premedicate adequately for highly to moderately emetogenic chemotherapy and to reassess control on a frequent and regular basis. This form of emesis is frequently refractory to standard antiemetic treatment; however, the benzodiazepines and butyrophenones may provide anxiolysis as well as antiemetogenicity. The addition of one of these agents is strongly encouraged for patients who have had previous unsatisfactory control of nausea and vomiting.

Many practice guidelines are available for the use of antiemetics in chemotherapy-induced nausea and vomiting (Antiemetic Subcommittee of the Multinational Association of Supportive Care in Cancer, 1998; Gandara et al., 1998; Gralla et al., 1999; Nolte et al., 1998). These guidelines are created by experts and are based on current literature (Table 28-3 and Fig. 28-3). To review treatment choices for other types of nausea and vomiting, see Table 28-2 and Figure 28-2.

Special Population Considerations

Pediatric

The treatment of nausea and vomiting in children differs from that in adults. It is particularly important in the pediatric population to focus on treating the cause of the problem. The etiology of emesis can vary with age (Box 28-5). Because they are smaller, children are predisposed to dehydration and electrolyte abnormalities caused by emesis.

Pediatric patients experience more extrapyramidal or neuromuscular reactions to phenothiazines, particularly when the drugs are administered during an acute viral illness such as chickenpox, measles, or gastroenteritis. Because of its antihistamine quality, promethazine may be a viable phenothiazine option. Also, on a milligram-per-kilogram basis, children experience more extrapyramidal reactions from metoclopramide, even at IV doses as low as 0.5 mg/kg 4 times a day.

Most antiemetic agents are dosed according to milligram-per-kilogram of body weight or the age of the child, and many of the available agents are not recommended for use in patients younger than 2 or 3 years. Some agents that are considered safe and effective in most situations are dimenhydrinate or oral or rectal trimethobenzamide (Tigan; IV not recommended). The phenothiazines are beneficial but should be used cautiously. For pediatric patients receiving chemotherapy, the prevention and treatment of emesis is similar to that in their adult counterparts, although specific pediatric dosing of the agents applies.

Women

Nausea and vomiting is experienced by more than 50% of pregnant women. A few women experience hyperemesis gravidarum, which can present as uncontrollable vomiting with inability to tolerate oral intake. These symptoms are most common in the first trimester of gestation but can occur at any time during pregnancy. Pregnancy-related emesis is believed to be modulated by CTZ stimulation.

Teratogenicity is the paramount concern when evaluating the safety of an agent in pregnant women. The first trimester of the pregnancy is when drugs or other exogenous substances can most affect embryonal development. Many of the studies performed to study the teratogenic effects of drugs encounter several difficulties. Most fetal malformations occur rarely, and frequently only a small sample size is obtained and reported. Mothers with underlying diseases, such as seizure disorder, hypertension, diabetes, and cancer, are known to have a higher incidence of infants with

---

Table 28.3

Recommended Order of Treatment for Chemotherapy-Induced Nausea and Vomiting

Order	Agents	Comments
Acute Prophylaxis for High, Moderately High, and Moderately Emetogenic Regimens		
First line	Serotonin antagonist + dexamethasone	May add other agents as needed
Second line	High-dose metoclopramide + dexamethasone	Prophylaxis for EPSs with metoclopramide
Third line	Depends on response to other antiemetics	Tailor to patient-specific factors
Acute Prophylaxis for Moderately Low and Low Emetogenic Regimens		
First line	No premedication or phenothiazine ± dexamethasone	Depends on chemotherapy regimen
Second line	Metoclopramide ± dexamethasone	Use low-dose metoclopramide
Third line	Depends on response to other antiemetics	Tailor to patient-specific factors
Delayed Nausea and Vomiting		
First line	Metoclopramide + dexamethasone	Continue 3–4 d after chemotherapy
Second line	Long-acting phenothiazine + dexamethasone	Monitor for EPSs
Third line	Depends on response to other antiemetics	Tailor to patient-specific factors

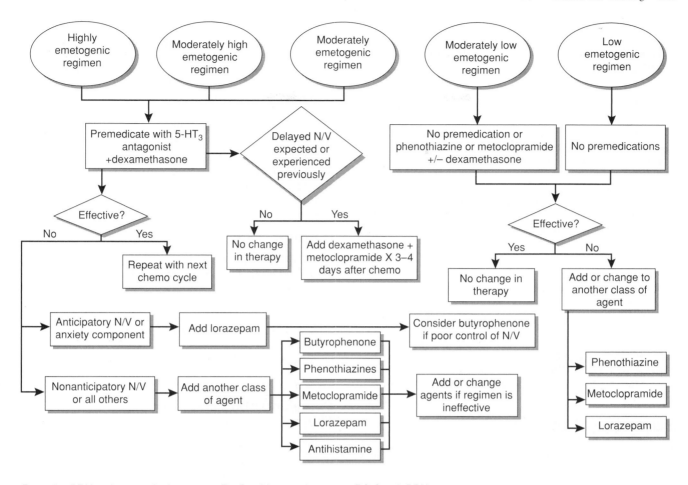

Prescribe PRN antiemetics for home use. Ex: Prochlorperazine 10 mg PO Q4-6h PRN.
Antiemetic regimen should be continued for the duration of emetic potential of the agent(s).

Key ⬭ Starting point for decision making; ▭ clinical actions (assessing, prescribing, monitoring); ◇ decision point.

Figure 28–3   Treatment algorithm for chemotherapy-induced nausea and vomiting.

malformation. In these patient populations, the role of drugs versus the role of the disease in fetal abnormalities is unclear. Recall bias may play a factor in teratogenicity studies as well. Ultimately, current evidence-based information on the safety and risk of drugs during pregnancy should be used to make clinical decisions.

Agents that are used for mild to moderate nausea and vomiting in pregnancy include the phenothiazines, antihistamine–anticholinergic agents, and metoclopramide. Antihistamine drugs are generally believed to be safe for the pregnant women and her fetus, although there are incidental findings of malformations in fetuses exposed to antihistamines. Anticholinergic drugs have been proven to cause neonatal meconium ileus. Conversely, some anticholinergic agents such as scopolamine have not been associated with consistent teratogenesis.

Phenothiazines readily cross the placenta, but the bulk of evidence indicates their use is safe in this population. Antacids, such as calcium carbonate, may provide safe and reliable relief from mild nausea. Antihistamines, phenothiazines, metoclopramide, haloperidol, droperidol, and ondansetron have all been used in hyperemesis gravidarum without adverse fetal sequelae. Drug classes that should be avoided in pregnant women are the benzodiazepines and cannabinoids. Increased rates of malformations and fetal complications have been associated with the use of these classes of agents; however, the use of other prescribed and illicit drugs by many of these mothers could cloud the picture. Corticosteroids are rarely used for the control of nausea and vomiting in pregnant women. The risks versus benefits of each drug and situation must be weighed carefully. Further studies to assess safety in this patient population are greatly needed.

MONITORING PATIENT RESPONSE

The best measure of nausea control is how the patient feels. To make evaluation of nausea more objective, nausea can be rated as none, mild, moderate, or severe. Another method is to ask the patient to rate the nausea on a scale from 0 to 10, with 0 equal to no nausea and 10 equal to severe nausea. These methods may help to compare nausea from day to day or week to week in the same patient. Vomiting is easily quantified by episodes per day and volume. If the volume of vomit exceeds 200 to 500 mL/d, the patient should be evaluated for electrolyte abnormalities.

BOX 28–5. DIFFERENTIAL DIAGNOSIS OF VOMITING BY AGE

Newborn
- Congenital obstructive GI malformations
  - Atresias or webs of esophagus or intestine
  - Meconium ileus or plug; Hirschsprung disease
- Inborn errors in metabolism

Infant
- Acquired or milder obstructive lesions
  - Pyloric stenosis
  - Malrotation and volvulus
  - Intussusception
- Metabolic diseases, milder inborn errors of metabolism
- Nutrient intolerances
- Functional disorders: gastroesophageal reflux
- Psychosocial disorders: rumination, injury due to child abuse

Child or Adolescent
- Please refer to adult etiologies (Box 28-1).

PATIENT EDUCATION

It is pivotal to identify the cause of the nausea and vomiting and to educate the patient about actions that need to be taken. Many cases of mild nausea and vomiting can be alleviated without additional medications.

Drug Information

Some drugs may be taken with food to avoid GI discomfort, and dietary adjustments may prove to be helpful for some cases of nausea. This knowledge gives patients more control over their own well-being. Anxiety or mental illness are components of some occurrences of nausea and vomiting; therefore, counseling and education are the key components in the treatment of nausea and vomiting of this type. Patients can also be educated about the nonprescription drugs available. Realistic goals of nausea control should be set and discussed with the patient. For example, many women have morning sickness with pregnancy; however, medications should be used as infrequently as possible at the lowest dose possible.

With antiemetics, as with any other drug therapy, usual or serious toxicities should be reviewed with the patient. EPSs are frightening and uncomfortable; consequently, patients need to be aware of this potential effect and how to reverse it if necessary (diphenhydramine). Sedation and anticholinergic effects are common with many antiemetics. For most antiemetics, encourage caution when using machinery or driving. Proper administration of the medication should be reviewed. Will the patient take this on a schedule or only as needed? All of this information ensures that the patient has optimal benefit from the prescribed medication.

Nutritional and Lifestyle Changes

Maintenance of proper hydration during all forms of vomiting is important and should be emphasized to patients predisposed to nausea and vomiting (eg, children, patients following surgery and chemotherapy, patients with GI disorders and infections). Rehydration with clear liquids is preferred over colas, milk, or caffeinated beverages. Patients should be educated on when to seek medical attention because of excessive vomiting or dehydration.

Complementary and Alternative Therapies

Patients suffering from nausea and vomiting of pregnancy (NVP) frequently do not receive therapy, in part because of fears of adverse effects of medications on the fetus. Several vitamin-based and herbal therapies have been shown to be effective and safe. Two randomized trials of vitamin B_6 have shown a benefit in reducing NVP. Women taking periconceptional multivitamins are less likely to have severe NVP. The combination of vitamin B_6 and doxylamine (previously marketed in the United States as Bendectin) has been shown to be safe for the fetus and effective in reducing NVP. Ginger was shown, in 2 studies, to reduce NVP. Vitamin B_1 (thiamine) deficiency can lead to Wernicke encephalopathy in women with severe NVP. Replacement is needed for all women with vomiting of more than 3 weeks' duration. Prophylaxis with multivitamins and therapy with B_6, with or without doxylamine, are safe and effective therapies for NVP.

■ Case Study

S. B. is a 57-year-old African American man with newly diagnosed late-stage small-cell lung cancer. He has undergone radiation therapy to the brain for his metastases and is to start chemotherapy next week. His past medical history includes hypertension. He has no known drug allergies. A combination chemotherapy regimen has been chosen: cisplatin 100 mg/m² for one dose on the first day and etoposide 100 mg/m² IV every day for 3 days. He has experienced nausea and vomiting.

Diagnosis: Chemotherapy-induced nausea and vomiting

1. List specific goals for treatment for S. B.

2. What drug therapy would you prescribe? Why?

3. What are the parameters for monitoring success of the therapy?

4. Discuss specific patient education based on the prescribed therapy.

5. List one or two adverse reactions for the selected agent that would cause you to change therapy.

6. What would be the choice for the second-line therapy?

7. What OTC and/or alternative medications would be appropriate for this patient?

8. What dietary and lifestyle changes should be recommended for this patient?

9. Describe one or two drug–drug or drug–food interactions for the selected agent.

Bibliography

Starred references are cited in the text.

*Antiemetic Subcommittee of the Multinational Association of Supportive Care in Cancer (MASCC). (1998). Prevention of chemotherapy and radiotherapy-induced emesis: Results of the Perugia Consensus Conference. *Annals of Oncology, 9,* 811–819.

Audhuy, B., Cappelaure, P., Martin, M., et al. (1996). A double-blind, randomised comparison of the antiemetic efficacy of two intravenous doses of dolasetron mesylate and granisetron in patients receiving high-dose cisplatin chemotherapy. *European Journal of Cancer, 32A,* 807–813.

Flake, Z. A, Scolly, R. D., & Bailey, A. G. (2004). Practical selection of antiemetics. *American Family Physician 69*(5), 1169–1174.

*Gandara, D. R., Roila, F., Warr, D., et al. (1998). Consensus proposal for 5HT3 antagonists in the prevention of acute emesis related to highly emetogenic chemotherapy. *Supportive Care in Cancer, 6,* 237–243.

Goodwin, T. M. (2002). Nausea and vomiting of pregnancy: An obstetric syndrome. *American Journal of Obstetrics & Gynecology 185* (5 Suppl understanding), S184–189.

*Gralla, R. J., Osoba, D., Kris, M. G., et al. (1999). Recommendations for the use of antiemetics: Evidence based, clinical practice guidelines. *Journal of Clinical Oncology, 7,* 2971–2994.

Hoechst Marion Roussel. (1997). *Anzemet package insert.* Kansas City, MO: Author.

Italian Group for Antiemetic Research. (1995). Dexamethasone, granisetron, or both for the prevention of nausea and vomiting during chemotherapy for cancer. *New England Journal of Medicine, 332,* 15.

Magee, L. A., Mozzatta, P., & Koren, G. (2002). Evidence-based view of safety and effectiveness of pharmacological treatment for nausea and vomiting of pregnancy. *American Journal of Obstetrics & Gynecology 185* (5 Suppl understanding), S256–261.

Neibyl, J. R., & Goodwin, T. M. (2002). Overview of nausea and vomiting of pregnancy with emphasis on vitamins and ginger. *American Journal of Obstetrics & Gynecology 185* (5 Suppl understanding), S253–255.

*Nolte, M. J., Berkery, R., Pizzo, B., et al. (1998). Assuring the optimal use of serotonin antagonist antiemetics: The process of development and implementation of institutional antiemetic guidelines at Memorial Sloan-Kettering Cancer Center. *Journal of Clinical Oncology, 16,* 771–778.

*Pisters, K. M. W., & Kris, M. G. (1992). Management of nausea and vomiting caused by anticancer drugs: State of the art. *Oncology, 6*(2, Suppl.), 99–104.

Quinley, E. M., Hasler, W. L., & Parkmen, H. P. (2001). AGA technical review on nausea and vomiting. *Gastroenterology, 120*(1), 263–286.

Valley, A. W., & Morris, A. K. (1995). Antiemetic therapy in the outpatient oncology setting. *Journal of Pharmacy Practice, 8,* 269–279.

Visit the Connection web site for the most up-to-date drug information.

29

GASTROESOPHAGEAL REFLUX DISEASE AND PEPTIC ULCER DISEASE

■ JANIS BONAT, CATHERINE J. DRAGON, AND VIRGINIA P. ARCANGELO

Two related disorders of the gastrointestinal (GI) tract can cause abdominal discomfort, gastroesophageal reflux disease (GERD) and peptic ulcer disease (PUD). They are both common reasons for patients to present in primary care. The treatment for these diseases is with many of the same drugs.

GASTROESOPHAGEAL REFLUX DISEASE

Gastroesophageal reflux disease (GERD) is a term used to describe signs or symptoms caused by reflux of stomach contents into the esophagus. It affects all segments of the population and is one of the most common conditions presenting in primary care. GERD refers to the abnormal exposure of the esophageal mucosa to retrograde gastric contents, resulting in symptoms or tissue damage. The concept of gastroesophageal reflux and its consequences was first described in a landmark article by Winkelstein (1935), who suggested that gastric secretions caused mucosal damage. In 1946, Allison used the term *reflux esophagitis* to identify the pathophysiologic process that results in inflammation of the esophagus through exposure to gastric refluxate. GERD is one of the most prevalent conditions in the GI tract, affecting approximately 360 individuals per 100,000 population (Shaheen & Provenzale, 2003). Over 60 million Americans have heartburn at least once a day. Of patients with GERD symptoms, 40% to 60% have reflux esophagitis and only 10% have erosive esophagitis. GERD accounts for 50% percent of noncardiac chest pain. Seventy-eight percent of patients with persistent hoarseness have GERD as do 82% of patients with asthma. Reflux is especially common during pregnancy. For most patients, GERD is a chronic disorder that significantly impairs quality of life and leads to high use of medical resources.

CAUSES

The cause of GERD is gastric contents entering and remaining in the lower esophagus because of transient relaxation of the lower esophageal sphincter (LES). Additional causes are an increase in intra-abdominal pressure, delayed gastric emptying, medication use, hiatal hernia, and poor esophageal acid clearance. The many risk factors for GERD are listed in Box 29-1.

PATHOPHYSIOLOGY

The fundamental abnormality of GERD is exposure of esophageal epithelium to gastric secretions, eliciting symptoms or resulting in histopathologic injury. Under normal circumstances, the LES, located at the gastroesophageal junction, provides an antireflux barrier. The mechanisms by which esophagogastric junction incompetence occur are:

- Transient LES relaxation
- Abdominal strain from increased gastric volume secondary to delayed gastric emptying
- Aggressive refluxate passing through the patulous LES
- Impaired esophageal epithelium defense mechanisms
- Motility abnormalities causing impaired clearance of refluxed materials
- Hiatal hernia

Transient LES relaxation is part of a normal reflex that permits gas to escape from the stomach to facilitate belching. Stress reflux and free reflux become increasingly likely as LES pressure decreases as a result of exposure to fatty foods, gastric distention, alcohol consumption, and smoking. In addition, many medications used to treat other common medical conditions have been associated with altered LES tone. They include nitrates, theophyllines, oral contraceptives, calcium channel blockers, especially nifedipine (Procardia), and others, as listed in Box 29-1.

The composition and volume of gastroesophageal refluxate are important factors in GERD. It has been demonstrated that a high degree of esophagus exposure to acid facilitates esophageal mucosal injury and increases the severity of the disease.

One of the distinguishing characteristics between patients with GERD and others is the effectiveness of the esophageal

---

BOX 29–1. RISK FACTORS FOR GERD

- Obesity
- Fatty foods
- Chocolate
- Peppermint
- Alcohol
- Nicotine
- Citrus juices
- Tomato products
- Caffeine
- Assuming recumbent position after eating
- Medications (anticholinergics, α-adrenergic agonists, β-adrenergic agonists, calcium channel blockers, dopaminergic agents, sedatives/tranquilizers, tricyclic antidepressants, theophylline, potassium chloride, ferrous sulfate, NSAIDs, alendronate)

Adapted from Levine, J. S. (1998). Treatment of gastroesophageal reflux disease (GERD). *Primary Care Case Reviews, 1,* 22–30.

BOX 29–2. SYMPTOMS OF GERD

Frequent Symptoms
- Heartburn
- Acid regurgitation
- Epigastric pain
- Belching
- Water brash

Atypical Symptoms
- Noncardiac chest pain
- Hoarseness
- Nausea
- Respiratory complications: asthma, nocturnal cough, wheezing, recurrent pneumonia, and lung abscesses

Alarm Symptoms
- Dysphagia
- Odynophagia
- Anemia
- Bleeding
- Weight loss

---

defense mechanisms. There are four main defensive forces against development of reflux esophagitis:

- A competent gastroesophageal junction, as previously discussed
- Effective clearance of refluxed material
- Neutralization of acid by salivary bicarbonate and secretion of bicarbonate by submucosal esophageal glands
- An intact diffusion barrier of the esophageal mucosa

The defense mechanism most commonly altered in patients with GERD is prolonged acid clearance time. Normally, most fluid is cleared from the esophagus, leaving only a small amount that is eventually neutralized by swallowed saliva. In patients with GERD, the main contributors to impaired acid clearance are peristaltic dysfunction of the esophagus and re-reflux that is associated with hiatal hernia.

DIAGNOSTIC CRITERIA

For the most part, GERD is a clinical diagnosis that may be objectively confirmed by a very good history and some diagnostic tests. The symptoms of GERD are varied and range from the classic heartburn or regurgitation to atypical presentation of chest pain, hoarseness, asthma, or cough. Heartburn and regurgitation are very sensitive and specific for diagnosing GERD. However, up to 50% of patients with endoscopic evidence of esophagitis present with atypical symptoms. Symptoms that may predict more severe disease and complications include dysphagia and odynophagia. For a breakdown of the symptoms, see Box 29-2.

GERD can be classified as mild, moderate, or severe. Characteristics of each category are listed in Box 29-3.

Patients complaining of atypical symptoms, with or without the classic symptoms of GERD, present a diagnostic dilemma. Hoarseness may be the only manifestation of

GERD. Asthma has been associated with GERD, especially when paroxysmal nocturnal exacerbations are reported.

The spectrum of endoscopic findings is varied as well. Approximately 50% of patients with GERD have a normal-appearing esophagus, whereas the other 50% have complications such as esophagitis, strictures, or Barrett esophagus.

The clinical diagnosis is made if symptoms are relieved with a therapeutic trial of antireflux therapy. Diagnostic testing includes barium x-rays, esophagoscopy, and pH monitoring.

BOX 29–3. CLINICAL STAGES OF GERD

Mild
Heartburn fewer than 3 times weekly
No symptoms suggesting complicated disease

Moderate
Heartburn 3 or more time weekly
No symptoms suggesting complicated disease

Severe
Moderate GERD that fails appropriate therapy
Strictures, erosive esophagitis, or Barrett esophagus detected by endoscopy
Alarm symptoms suggesting complications (dysphagia, odynophagia, unexplained weight loss, iron-deficiency anemia, melena, hematemesis, hoarseness, asthma, unexplained lung disease)

Adapted from Levin, J. S. (1998). Treatment of gastroesophageal reflux disease (GERD). *Primary Care Case Reviews, 1,* 23.

INITIATING DRUG THERAPY

The cornerstones of therapy are lifestyle modifications that include elevating of the head of the bed, decreasing fat intake, stopping smoking, and avoiding recumbency for 3 hours after meals. These modifications may be sufficient for symptom control in patients with mild disease. However, the clinical efficacy of lifestyle changes alone is limited, and symptoms usually continue. Therefore, drug therapy is usually required in addition to lifestyle modifications.

Goals of Drug Therapy

The goals of drug therapy are to:

- Relieve symptoms
- Heal the esophageal mucosa
- Prevent complications
- Maintain remission

An empirical trial of symptom-relieving medications may be the most expeditious way to diagnose GERD in those with classic symptoms. Those with classic symptoms are given 2 weeks of therapy with a histamine-2 receptor antagonist (H_2RA) or a proton pump inhibitor (PPI) 30 to 60 minutes before the first meal of the day. If the H_2RA twice a day does not relieve symptoms, the patient is switched to a PPI daily. If a PPI has been tried and the patient still has symptoms, the dose is increased or an additional dose is given 30 minutes before the evening meal. If there is response to therapy, the patient is continued on therapy for 8 to 12 weeks. The dosage is then tapered over 1 month to the lowest dose that gives the patient relief. If the symptoms recur, the patient is again given the initial effective medication and dose and further testing is recommended. If the initial therapy does not produce symptom relief, diagnostic testing is recommended.

GERD is a chronic, relapsing disease, so recurrence of reflux symptoms and esophagitis is frequently observed and is resolved only in a minority of patients once therapy is discontinued. Symptoms can recur quickly if therapy is stopped or the drug dose decreased. Long-term therapy is usually required. Drugs used to treat GERD act to decrease acid secretion and decrease or neutralize the acidity of gastric acid. They include

- Antacids, which raise the pH of refluxed gastric secretions and deactivate pepsin
- H_2RAs, which decrease gastric acid secretion by inhibiting stimulation of parietal cells by histamine
- PPIs, which suppress gastric acid

PEPTIC ULCER DISEASE

It has been estimated that 1 in 10 Americans or approximately 10% of the population of the United States have had peptic ulcer disease (PUD) at some time. It accounts for 1 million hospitalizations, 6500 deaths a year, and a cost of about $6 billion annually. Thus, PUD is a significant cause of morbidity in the United States, and appropriate diagnosis

and treatment can reduce medical expenditures associated with acute and chronic PUD and its complications.

CAUSES

Infection by the *Helicobacter pylori* bacterium and long-term use of nonsteroidal anti-inflammatory drugs (NSAIDs) are the major causes of PUD. Less common causes of PUD include cancer and other idiopathic or hypersecretory disorders such as Zollinger-Ellison syndrome.

Most cases of PUD can be linked to infection with *H. pylori*. The organism is present in approximately 10% to 20% of healthy adults younger than 40 years of age and approximately 50% to 80% of those older than 60 years. Although *H. pylori* is a common infection, most people have asymptomatic and chronic antral gastritis but do not progress to the development of ulcers. Only about 15% of those infected eventually have an ulcer. Patients who have duodenal and gastric ulcers are infected with *H. pylori* in more than 90%, and 60% to 90% of cases, respectively. *H. pylori* infection is also associated with increased risk of gastric cancer and lymphoid lymphoma, and therefore the absence of infection in a patient with PUD suggests a more serious etiology and the need for an additional workup. The reasons for this are not clear.

The most significant risk factor for *H. pylori* infection is the socioeconomic status of the family during childhood. Evidence supports various routes of transmission (eg, oral–oral, fecal–oral, iatrogenic), but no one route has been clearly identified as a more likely source. It appears alcohol consumption may be protective, coffee consumption may be associated with an increased prevalence, and smoking has no clear association with active *H. pylori* infection. One report also identified increasing age, lower income and education level, and musculoskeletal pain or headache as risk factors for recent active ulcers, whereas smoking more than one pack of cigarettes a day was a risk factor for chronic active ulcer disease.

NSAID-induced ulcerations are thought to occur in 10% to 30% of people taking the drugs. Serious complications of PUD, such as bleeding, occur in 2% to 4% of NSAID users. NSAIDs are one of the most commonly used prescription and nonprescription medications in the United States. NSAIDs are associated with the development of gastric ulcer twice as often as with duodenal ulcers.

Several factors increase the risk for development of GI complications from NSAIDs, including age (particularly age >75 years), history of PUD or ulcer bleeding, NSAID dosage and long duration of use, and concomitant drug therapy (eg, anticoagulants, glucocorticoids). These serious complications are associated with increased hospitalization, mortality rates, and use of health care resources. It has been estimated that 15% to 35% of all complications of peptic ulcers are caused by the use of NSAIDs.

PATHOPHYSIOLOGY

Defensive mechanisms that protect the gastric mucosa from injury include mucous and bicarbonate secretion, mucosal blood flow, epithelial cell restitution and growth, and prostaglandins. Mucus protects underlying cells by acting as a barrier between the gastric mucosa and its contents and by preventing the back-diffusion of H$^+$ ions from the gastric lumen into the mucosa. Gastric and duodenal epithelial cells secrete bicarbonate, which buffers the gastric mucosal surface. Mucosal blood flow in gastric and duodenal cells maintains the integrity of gastric mucosa by preventing ischemia. Rapid gastric epithelial cell turnover and epidermal growth factor aid in the restoration of damaged cells and wound healing, respectively. Prostaglandins play a key role in providing mucosal protection by stimulating and maintaining each of the aforementioned mucosal defense mechanisms.

When factors such as *H. pylori* and NSAIDs disrupt the normal mucosal physiology, peptic ulcers can form. It is likely that several factors, such as pathophysiologic abnormalities and environmental and genetic factors, act together to affect normal gastric and duodenal defense and healing mechanisms to result in ulcer formation.

H. pylori organisms are flagellated, spiral-shaped bacteria that burrow into the mucous layer of the gastric epithelium. The organism also produces urease, which neutralizes the hydrogen ions in gastric acid, making it uniquely protected against gastric acid and relatively inaccessible to antibiotics. Within 2 to 3 days after infection by *H. pylori*, an inflammatory response begins, acute gastritis ensues, and an antibody response is mounted. *H. pylori* induces ulcer formation as a result of increased gastrin secretion from the antral mucosa, increased acid secretion by the stomach, and increased acid load in the duodenum. The increased acid load, along with bacterial enzymes, toxins, and inflammatory mediators, is thought to weaken the protective mucous lining of the stomach or duodenum and result in ulcer formation. Immunoglobulin A (IgA) and IgG antibody titers can be used to detect infection by *H. pylori*, which is typically lifelong when left untreated. Humans are thought to be the principal carrier of *H. pylori* infection.

The NSAIDs induce gastroduodenal injury by two different mechanisms. NSAIDs cause a superficial irritation directly on the mucosa, as well as acting systemically by inhibiting the production of protective prostaglandins. NSAIDs inhibit cyclooxygenase (COX) in the arachidonic acid cascade, which in turn inhibits the production of mucosal prostaglandins. Recent data support the discovery of two subtypes of COX enzymes, COX-1 and COX-2. COX-1 plays an integral role in the maintenance of GI integrity and is found in the stomach, intestines, kidney, and platelets. COX-2 is inducible in areas of inflammation and is undetectable in most tissues. Until recently, all NSAIDs inhibited both COX enzymes. Newer NSAIDs selectively inhibit COX-2 to a great extent and have the potential for an improved GI side effect profile compared with older NSAIDs that inhibit both COX enzymes. Selective COX-2 inhibitors have comparable efficacy with older NSAIDs but may be associated with a lower risk for development of NSAID-induced ulcers. The basic understanding of topical versus systemic toxic effects of NSAIDs is still unclear. A considerable amount of debate continues in the literature regarding the relative roles each of these mechanisms play in the pathogenesis of NSAID-induced ulcers.

DIAGNOSTIC CRITERIA

Classically, PUD is characterized by symptoms of epigastric pain and dyspepsia. These are typical presenting symptoms that occur in approximately two thirds of patients with

duodenal and one third of patients with gastric ulcer. The symptomatology of PUD is considered to be relatively nonspecific and does not assist in the differentiation of duodenal versus gastric ulcer. In addition, pain does not correlate well with ulcer presence or healing. NSAID-induced ulcers are less likely to cause symptoms compared with PUD associated with *H. pylori* infection.

Numerous methods, both invasive and noninvasive, are available for diagnosing infection by *H. pylori*. Urease tests, culture, and polymerase chain reaction, performed after endoscopy and biopsy, are considered to be invasive tests, whereas serology, stool antigen, and the urea breath test are considered noninvasive. Endoscopy is the gold standard test that, although invasive and expensive, is appropriate for initial evaluation of patients older than 45 years of age who present with significant dyspeptic symptoms (eg, weight loss, poor appetite, vomiting) and no documented history of PUD. A follow-up endoscopy is neither cost effective nor practical for documenting eradication but may be useful to document refractory ulceration where recurrences are frequent. Culture is useful, particularly when it is suspected that antibiotic-resistant isolates are present or when retreatment is necessary after exposure to an antibiotic that fosters resistance, because sensitivity testing of *H. pylori* can be performed with selected antibiotics. Cultures, however, require an incubation period of up to 10 days. Enzyme-linked immunosorbent assay for IgA and IgG antibodies to *H. pylori* has been the most widely used noninvasive test for diagnosing *H. pylori* infection, but it is not reliable for documenting eradication because antibody titers fall slowly after antibiotic therapy. In addition, the results of serologic tests vary widely from one laboratory to the next. The more recently available noninvasive urea breath test is a reliable means of determining the presence of *H. pylori* as well as documenting eradication after treatment. This is a quick, simple test that is reported to have very high sensitivity and specificity, equal to those of endoscopy, for diagnosing *H. pylori* in adult patients. The stool antigen test has a sensitivity of about 94% and specificity of about 90%. This cannot be used to test for eradication until 6 to 8 weeks after therapy.

INITIATING DRUG THERAPY

Several pharmacologic options are available for treating PUD, depending on the etiology, symptoms, and diagnostic information (Table 29-1). A combination of antibiotics or antibiotic and antisecretory agents, antacids, H$_2$RAs, PPIs, misoprostol (Cytotec), and sucralfate (Carafate) can all be used appropriately for effective management of PUD. In the past, traditional antiulcer agents such as H$_2$RAs, PPIs, sucralfate, and antacids were used as empiric therapy for patients who presented with signs and symptoms of uncomplicated PUD. These agents are effective in healing ulcers if used appropriately, but relapses of PUD are common and can be prevented only by eradicating *H. pylori*.

The American Gastroenterological Association (AGA) cautions against empirical use of antisecretory agents for suspected PUD because such treatment may delay important diagnostic testing and appropriate long-term treatment. Nor does the AGA support treatment of *H. pylori*-induced ulcers

Table 29.1

Overview of Agents Used to Treat PUD and GERD

Generic (Trade) Name and Dosage	Selected Adverse Events	Contraindications	Special Considerations
Antibiotics			
amoxicillin (Amoxil) 500 mg qid	Diarrhea, nausea, hypersensitivity	Known allergy to penicillins, cephalosporins, or imipenem	Take without regard to meals.
clarithromycin (Biaxin) 500 mg bid–tid	Diarrhea, abnormal taste, nausea	Known allergy to macrolide antibiotics, concomitant use of astemisole, cisapride, or pimozide	Take without regard to meals. Consider avoiding use for retreatment if initial clarithromycin-containing regimen fails.
metronidazole (Flagyl) 250 mg qid	Peripheral neuropathy, metallic taste, nausea, disulfiram-like reaction if taken with alcohol	Known allergy to metronidazole	Avoid use of alcohol during therapy and for 1 d afterward. Available as Helidac (a patient-friendly kit containing bismuth subsalicylate, tetracycline) Take on an empty stomach with plenty of water and avoid ingestion of tetracycline simultaneously with dairy products, antacids, laxatives, or iron-containing products (these can be taken 2 h before or after tetracycline).
tetracycline (Sumycin) 500 mg qid	Diarrhea, esophageal ulcers, photosensitivity	Allergy Prescribe with caution in patients with renal or hepatic dysfunction.	May render oral contraceptives ineffective
H₂ Receptor Antagonists			
cimetidine (Tagamet) 300 mg qid, 400 mg bid, or 800 mg hs	Rarely, CNS side effects (eg, headache, fatigue, dizziness, confusion), gynecomastia, impotence	Hypersensitivity to cimetidine or other H₂ antagonists	Take without regard to meals. Stagger doses if taking antacids. Patients should inform health care providers of any other drugs that are taken concomitantly because of the possibility of drug interactions.
famotidine (Pepcid) 20 mg bid or 40 mg hs	Rarely, CNS side effects (eg, headache, fatigue, dizziness, confusion)	Hypersensitivity to famotidine or other H₂ antagonists	May be taken without regard to meals
nizatidine (Axid) 150 mg bid or 300 hs mg	Rarely, CNS side effects (eg, headache, fatigue, dizziness, confusion)	Hypersensitivity to famotidine or other H₂ antagonists	May be taken without regard to meals
ranitidine (Zantac) 150 mg bid or 300 mg hs	Rarely, CNS side effects (eg, headache, fatigue, dizziness, confusion)	Hypersensitivity to famotidine or other H₂ antagonists	May be taken without regard to meals, stagger doses if taking antacids
Proton Pump Inhibitors			
omeprazole (Prilosec) 40 mg qd or 20 mg bid	Diarrhea, headache	Hypersensitivity to omeprazole	Take before meals
lansoprazole (Prevacid) 30 mg bid–tid	Diarrhea, headache	Hypersensitivity to lansoprazole	Same as above
pantoprazole (Protonix) 40 mg qd	Diarrhea, headache, flatulence	Hypersensitivity to other proton pump inhibitors	Can be taken with antacids
Nexium (esomeprazole) 20–40 mg qd	Diarrhea, headache	As above	Take before meals
Other Agents Used in PUD			
antacids Widely variable, depends on product contents and formulation	Rebound hyperacidity, diarrhea with magnesium-containing antacids, constipation with aluminum-containing antacids	None significant	Use magnesium–aluminum combination products to avoid diarrhea or constipation Monitor for drug interactions between antacids and other drugs, such as fluoroquinilone antibiotics, tetracycline, ketoconazole, iron products.
sucralfate (Carafate) 1 g qid	Constipation	None significant	Take on an empty stomach (1 h before meals) Avoid antacids for 30 min before or after taking sucralfate.
misoprostol (Cytotec) 200 μg qid	Diarrhea, abdominal pain, nausea	Hypersensitivity to prostaglandins, pregnancy	Take with food. Reduce dose to 100 μg if diarrhea cannot be tolerated. Avoid use in pregnancy and in women trying to become pregnant.

without serologic or breath test results confirming *H. pylori*-induced infection.

When a treatment regimen is selected, it should be individualized based on a patient's age, comorbidities, concurrent medications, likelihood for adherence, and risk factors for complications from progressive ulcer disease and treatment.

Eradication of *H. pylori* facilitates ulcer healing, eliminates the need for maintenance therapy, and markedly reduces the risk of ulcer recurrence. Therefore, as suggested by a 1994 National Institutes of Health (NIH) consensus panel statement, antibiotic therapy is indicated for all patients with *H. pylori*-infected duodenal and gastric ulcers (NIH Consensus Panel, 1994). Available regimens are complex and expensive, have side effects, and require 7 to 14 days of at least three agents to achieve cure rates exceeding 80%. To complicate decision making, the study design and drug dosages and schedules, and thus eradication rates, of trials evaluating regimens for treatment of *H. pylori* vary greatly.

Goals of Drug Therapy

The therapeutic goals of treatment for PUD associated with *H. pylori* are to relieve ulcer pain and dyspepsia, heal existing ulcers and erosions, and eradicate *H. pylori* to reduce recurrence and cure PUD.

Although the goals for treating NSAID-induced PUD are similar, an additional consideration is identifying an alternative to the NSAID for pain management, if possible, or prophylaxis to prevent further ulceration if treatment with an NSAID continues. Prophylaxis could include changing to an enteric-coated NSAID that can be taken with meals, adding misoprostol to the therapeutic regimen, or switching to an NSAID with COX-2 selectivity that may be associated with less GI toxicity.

DRUGS USED IN TREATMENT OF GERD AND PUD

Antibiotics

The antibiotics used to treat PUD work in various ways (Table 29-2).

Clarithromycin

Clarithromycin (Biaxin) is a macrolide antibiotic that, like azithromycin (Zithromax), is more acid-stable than erythromycin (Eryc) and inhibits bacterial protein synthesis. The half-life of clarithromycin is 3 to 4 hours, twice that of erythromycin but significantly shorter than that of azithromycin. Clarithromycin has significant activity against *H. pylori* when used as the sole antibiotic and especially when used in combination with at least one additional antibiotic and antisecretory agent. However, resistance to clarithromycin develops rapidly, so it should not be used in subsequent regimens once a treatment failure has occurred. Clarithromycin is commonly used at a dose of 500 mg twice daily. Clarithromycin can inhibit cytochrome P450 3A4 isoenzymes and should not be given concurrently with nonsedating antihistamines, such as loratadine (Claritin).

Table 29.2

Oral Drug Regimens Used to Eradicate
***Helicobacter pylori*–Induced PUD**

Therapy	Duration
Triple Therapy	
Clarithromycin 500 mg bid +	7–14 d
Amoxicillin 1 g bid +	
A PPI	
Quadruple Therapy	
Bismuth subsalicylate 2 tablets (525 mg) or 30 mL qid +	14 d
Metronidazole 500 mg qid +	
Tetracycline 500 mg qid +	
A PPI	
Combination Products	
Helidac Therapy	
14 blister cards each with eight 262.4-mg bismuth subsalicylate tablets, four 250-mg metronidazole tablets and four 250-mg tetracycline tablets	14 d
Prevpac	
14 blister cards each containing two 30-mg lansoprazole capsules, four 500-mg amoxicillin tablets, two 500-mg clarithromycin tablets	14 d

Metronidazole

Metronidazole (Flagyl) is active against various anaerobic bacteria and protozoa and is the mainstay of many commonly used *H. pylori* treatment regimens. Metronidazole is thought to enter the cells of microorganisms that contain nitroreductase, where the nitro group in metronidazole is reduced, attaches to DNA, inhibits synthesis, and causes cell death. The effectiveness of metronidazole is not dependent on pH. *H. pylori* is highly sensitive to metronidazole in areas where metronidazole use is low; however, where use is pervasive, up to 80% of *H. pylori* isolates can be resistant (Saledo & Al-Kawas, 1998). In a study evaluating resistant *H. pylori* organisms, 21% of patients had primary resistance to metronidazole (Adamek et al., 1998). When used as a single agent, especially in areas where use is high, metronidazole results in very low eradication rates. Resistance is less likely to develop if metronidazole is used with bismuth or in combination with another antibiotic. It has been demonstrated that metronidazole-resistant *H. pylori* significantly affects the efficacy of quadruple therapy that includes metronidazole, colloidal bismuth subcitrate, tetracycline, and omeprazole (Prilosec). The half-life of metronidazole is 8 hours. Metronidazole is typically administered as 250 mg 4 times daily or 500 mg 3 times daily.

Amoxicillin

Amoxicillin (Amoxil) is an aminopenicillin that kills bacterial cells by interfering with cell wall synthesis. Although amoxicillin concentrations in gastric juices are high and *H. pylori* is highly sensitive to amoxicillin, monotherapy results in eradication rates of less than 20%. Amoxicillin is most active at a neutral pH, which may explain the low cure rate. When amoxicillin is used in combination with omeprazole, however, the concentration of amoxicillin in gastric juice increases substantially and results in a significantly higher eradication rate. Because amoxicillin has diminished activity at a low pH, the omeprazole-induced increase in gastric pH results in a substantial increase in bactericidal activity. Dual therapy with amoxicillin and omeprazole, however, has been associated with less-than-optimal eradication rates.

Amoxicillin is associated with higher eradication rates when it is used as one of three or four agents. In a nonrandomized study, one such regimen using omeprazole, amoxicillin, and metronidazole for 7 to 14 days was studied in over 300 British patients and resulted in a 90% eradication rate with few side effects (Bell et al., 1995). *H. pylori* does not typically develop resistance to amoxicillin, so it can be used again in subsequent treatment regimens. Amoxicillin is typically administered at a dose of 500 mg 4 times daily.

Tetracycline

Tetracycline inhibits bacterial protein synthesis and is used for a wide variety of gram-positive and gram-negative bacterial infections. Tetracycline is stable at a low pH and acts topically against *H. pylori*. Although *H. pylori* is very sensitive to tetracycline and bacterial resistance has not been reported, it must be used with at least one other agent that has activity against *H. pylori* to achieve eradication. With significant variations in dosages and administration schedules, a bismuth compound, metronidazole, and either amoxicillin or tetracycline are drugs commonly used in a classic triple-drug regimen to eradicate *H. pylori*.

Tetracycline is usually given 2 hours before or 2 hours after food to increase systemic absorption. It has been recommended that tetracycline be administered along with bismuth subsalicylate (BSS) to facilitate binding, decreasing systemic absorption and increasing local exposure of tetracycline to the gastric mucosa. One study (Healy et al., 1997), however, has determined that the tetracycline actually binds to a suspending agent called *veegum,* that is present only in the liquid form of BSS (Pepto-Bismol). The clinical significance of this interaction has yet to be determined in a clinical study. Because *H. pylori* resistance to tetracycline has not been reported, it may be used for retreatment, if necessary. The dose of tetracycline is usually 500 mg 4 times daily.

Bismuth Subsalicylate

The mechanism of action of bismuth against *H. pylori* is complex and involves inhibition of protein, cell wall, and adenosine triphosphate synthesis as well as a topical action to prevent adherence of *H. pylori* to gastric epithelial cells. With cure rates of approximately 10%, bismuth is not effective as a single agent for eradication. When used in combination with at least two additional antibiotics, however, significant eradication of *H. pylori* is achieved. In the United States, bismuth is formulated as BSS in chewable tablets and liquid and ranitidine bismuth citrate tablets (Tritec). Each BSS tablet and 15 mL of liquid contains 262 mg of bismuth, which is not absorbed, and 100 mg of salicylate, which is absorbed, similar to aspirin. Ranitidine bismuth citrate is available in 400-mg tablets and is approved by the Food and Drug Administration (FDA) for use with clarithromycin. In Europe, bismuth is available as colloidal bismuth subcitrate. Thus, many published studies conducted in countries other than the United States have involved administration of this compound to patients with PUD. The short half-life of bismuth results in the need for 3 to 4 times daily dosing of the product, although the ranitidine bismuth citrate dose is taken twice daily. Because *H. pylori* does not develop resistance to bismuth after repeated exposure, it may be used for retreatment, when necessary.

Histamine-2 Receptor Antagonists

All H_2RAs suppress gastric acid and pepsin secretion by competitively and reversibly occupying H_2 receptors. The H_2RAs differ in their relative potencies, with famotidine (Pepcid) being the most and cimetidine (Tagamet) being the least potent of the four. When administered in equipotent doses, the H_2RAs suppress gastric secretion equally. As a class, the H_2RAs are comparable in their volumes of distribution, serum half-lives, and clearance parameters. With the exception of nizatidine (Axid), the H_2RAs undergo extensive first-pass metabolism in the liver, and thus bioavailability is reduced to 30% to 80% of an administered dose. Although elimination occurs through both renal and hepatic routes, active renal tubular secretion is the primary mechanism of elimination for the H_2RAs; it therefore is recommended that doses be reduced in patients with severe renal impairment.

The H_2RAs achieve 70% to 95% healing rates in duodenal and gastric ulcers in 4 to 6 weeks when current dosing recommendations are followed. The published data are inconsistent in suggesting an advantage for any one H_2RA in producing initial healing. Multicenter, randomized, double-blinded, comparative studies of ranitidine (Zantac) with cimetidine, nizatidine, or famotidine have demonstrated equal efficacy and tolerability in treating and maintaining healed lesions in duodenal ulcers. Although the healing rates in gastric ulcers for the H_2RAs are relatively lower than in duodenal ulcers, the rates are very similar between the different agents used. As part of triple or quadruple therapy, the H_2RAs play an important role in treating PUD of an infectious origin. Symptom relief occurs more readily and efficacy rates may be higher when an antisecretory agent, such as an H_2RA, is added to a regimen.

The H_2RAs also may improve the activity of some antibiotics by increasing gastric pH. Ranitidine is the most widely studied H_2RA used in anti-*H. pylori* regimens and is available in combination with a bismuth compound as ranitidine bismuth citrate. The H_2RAs used in *H. pylori* regimens are usually dosed once or twice daily.

Adverse events associated with H_2RAs include thrombocytopenia, neutropenia, bradycardia, arrhythmias, confusion, depression, and gynecomastia. Cimetidine and ranitidine have been reported to cause dyskinesia, whereas famotidine and cimetidine can cause impotence, particularly at high doses.

Cimetidine is associated with more pharmacokinetic drug–drug interactions than the other H_2RAs, primarily because of its effect on drug-metabolizing enzymes. The interactions considered to be most important are those with cimetidine and warfarin (Coumadin), phenytoin (Dilantin), or theophylline (Slo-Phyllin). Other interactions, such as those with benzodiazepines and other drugs commonly used in elderly patients, can also problematic. Large doses of ranitidine may inhibit one of the cytochrome P450 isoenzymes and interfere with metabolism of other drugs.

Proton Pump Inhibitors

The PPIs bind to the proton pump of the parietal call, inhibiting secretion of the hydrogen ion into the gastric lumen. The binding results in a profound inhibition of both basal and stimulated acid secretion. PPIs relieve pain and heal peptic ulcers more rapidly than the H$_2$RAs.

The PPIs are used once a day 30 to 60 minutes before the first meal of the day for treatment of GERD and are used once or twice a day for treatment of PUD. Notably, as with many other agents used in regimens for eradication of *H. pylori*, the overall effectiveness of the PPI regimen can be significantly affected by the dose of the drug. It has been suggested that because these drugs are thought to have direct activity against *H. pylori*, the use of higher doses may result in better eradication rates. The most commonly reported treatment-related adverse event during maintenance therapy is diarrhea. Drug interactions with the PPIs usually are not clinically significant.

Other Agents

Antacids

The numerous antacids available consist primarily of sodium bicarbonate, calcium carbonate, aluminum salts, and magnesium salts. The inorganic salts of antacids dissolve in gastric acid and release anions that partially neutralize the hydrochloric acid in the stomach. In usual doses, by increasing the gastric pH above 4, antacids inhibit the activity of pepsin. Antacids are minimally absorbed, and their neutralizing action on acid is local rather than systemic. When used to treat PUD, antacids must be administered many times daily in large doses. This frequent administration is not practical and can potentially decrease the absorption of many drugs. Antacids are not used to heal ulcers, but may be helpful when used in combination with other antiulcer agents for intermediate, rapid relief of ulcer pain or dyspepsia.

The most frequent side effects associated with antacids are constipation or diarrhea. Sodium bicarbonate is limited to short-term use because of an increase in urinary sodium content as well as its potential to alter systemic pH. Calcium carbonate has been associated with hypercalcemia and acid production through the release of gastrin. Aluminum antacids may cause hyperaluminemia in patients with chronic renal failure. Similarly, hypermagnesemia, characterized by hypotension, nausea, vomiting, and electrocardiographic changes, may occur with continued administration of magnesium antacids in patients with renal impairment. Antacids may potentially cause drug interactions by altering the rate and the extent of absorption of concomitantly administered drugs.

Sucralfate

Sucralfate is a sulfated disaccharide compound with aluminum hydroxide that forms polyvalent bonds with damaged tissues as well as with normal GI mucosa. This complex adheres to an ulcer site, providing a barrier that prevents the penetration of acid, pepsin, and bile into gastric mucosa. Because sucralfate acts locally and is minimally absorbed

from the GI tract, it is mostly excreted in the stool. Sucralfate, at 4 g/d, is as effective as ranitidine or cimetidine in promoting healing of duodenal and gastric ulcers and in rapidly relieving symptoms. Systemic adverse effects are rarely observed for sucralfate because of its minimal absorption. Of these side effects, constipation is most frequently reported. There has been concern over aluminum retention when sucralfate is administered to patients with impaired renal function. In addition, the aluminum released may chelate other drugs that are administered simultaneously. Although sucralfate is approved by the FDA for the treatment and maintenance of duodenal ulcers and is commonly used for stress ulcer prophylaxis, there is no role for sucralfate in the eradication of *H. pylori*.

Misoprostol

Misoprostol, a prostaglandin E$_1$ analog, inhibits the secretion of gastric acid, both basally and in response to food, histamine, pentagastrin, and coffee, by a direct action on parietal cells. Misoprostol has cytoprotective effects on the integrity of the gastric mucosa exposed to noxious stimuli. Misoprostol is an effective healing agent for patients with duodenal ulcers. However, it has FDA approval only for preventing NSAID-induced gastric ulcers.

Several placebo-controlled studies have demonstrated that misoprostol significantly reduces duodenal ulcer development in patients taking NSAIDs. When used to treat duodenal ulcers, misoprostol is not more effective than the H$_2$RAs, and it has a worse adverse effect profile. The MUCOSA trial demonstrated that misoprostol was significantly more effective than placebo, however, in preventing NSAID-induced ulcer complications in high-risk patients (Simon et al., 1996).

Convincing data that misoprostol is effective in patients taking NSAIDs who have clinical ulcers are limited. These ulcers heal faster when the NSAID therapy is discontinued, but can be managed with an H$_2$RA or, ideally, with a PPI if the NSAID therapy continues.

Moreover, misoprostol does not relieve pain in patients with ulcers. Consensus panel recommendations suggest avoiding the use of NSAIDs in patients who develop ulcers while taking NSAIDs and misoprostol, although published data in this regard are limited. The dose of misoprostol does not need adjustment in patients with renal impairment.

The most frequently reported adverse event for misoprostol is diarrhea, which occurs in up to 40% of patients. The disorder can be severe enough to warrant the discontinuation of treatment. Studies indicate a dose–response relationship for diarrhea, ranging from 6% to 39% depending on the dosage regimen.

Misoprostol also may cause vaginal bleeding in postmenopausal women and should be avoided in women who are pregnant. Women taking misoprostol during childbearing years should be advised regarding appropriate use of contraception and should have a negative pregnancy test before beginning therapy.

Selecting the Most Appropriate Agent for GERD

Reflux esophagitis is a chronic disease that is likely to relapse, with 75% to 92% of patients reporting recurrence

Table 29.3

Recommended Order of Treatment for GERD

Order	Agents	Comments
First line	H₂ antagonists (cimetidine, ranitidine, famotidine, nizatidine)	For moderate GERD
Second line	Proton pump inhibitors (omeprazole, lansoprazole, rabeprazole, pantoprazole)	Rapid return of symptoms usually occurs if drug therapy stops. Works most effectively if given 2 times a day initially for 4–8 wk, then decreased to once a day.
Third line	Referral for endoscopic examination	

of symptoms 6 to 12 months after therapy is discontinued. Predictably, patients with more severe cases of GERD have higher relapse rates. Continued relapse puts the patient at risk for complications of esophagitis as well as deterioration of esophageal function; thus, maintenance acid-suppressive therapy is often necessary. Reducing the dosage of the medication or attempting maintenance with a less potent agent than used in healing also often results in recurrence.

Long-term suppression of acid secretion in patients infected with *H. pylori* appears to promote the proximal spread of the infection and the development of atrophic gastritis. This could in turn result in an increased risk of gastric cancer. Therefore, the European *Helicobacter pylori* Study Group (EHPSG; 1997) considered it *advisable* on the basis of *supportive evidence* that *H. pylori* should be eradicated when GERD requires long-term treatment with PPIs.

In patients with mild GERD (symptoms fewer than 3 times a week), lifestyle changes are often effective, although drug therapy may be indicated. In moderate to severe GERD, drug therapy (Table 29-3) is needed along with lifestyle changes (Fig. 29-1).

First-Line Therapy

H₂RAs are used as first-line therapy for mild GERD. The most effective treatment for initial therapy is twice-daily dosing, with the first dose in the morning and the second dose approximately 1 hour after the evening meal. If symptoms diminish by 90%, therapy is continued for 2 to 3 months. The dose is then tapered and the daily dose stopped. The drug may then be used on an as-needed basis.

Second-Line Therapy

If the patient has an inadequate response to the first line of therapy or if symptoms intensify, a PPI is substituted for an H₂RA. It is recommended that the PPI be given twice daily initially. These drugs provide more complete control of acid secretion than H₂RAs and are the most effective agents for treating GERD. Approximately 83% of patients report symptom relief. Treatment usually must continue with a once-daily dosing because there is a 75% to 92%

recurrence rate of symptoms if therapy is discontinued (DeVault, 1999).

Third-Line Therapy

If the first and second lines of therapy fail, the patient is referred to a gastroenterologist for endoscopy. In patients with esophagitis confirmed by endoscopy, PPI therapy begins immediately because of the superior healing rate associated with this drug class. If symptoms are eliminated, maintenance therapy is indicated at the lowest dosage necessary to prevent recurrence, continue healing, and eliminate the possibility of complications. In most cases, patients with erosive esophagitis cannot be weaned from acid suppression therapy because a rebound effect is common (see Table 29-3).

Special Population Considerations

Pediatric

Gastroesophageal reflux is common in healthy infants. These infants spit up or vomit after each feeding without discomfort. One half of infants outgrow this by age 6 months and the rest by age 18 months. Children with chronic gastroesophageal reflux exhibit poor growth, vomiting, hoarseness, coughing, and chronic sore throat. Treatment in infants is to thicken the formula or breast milk with 1 to 2 tablespoons of rice cereal per 2 ounces of liquid. The infant is burped after 1 to 2 ounces of formula or when changing the breast. The infant should be kept upright for 30 minutes after feeding. The head of the crib is raised 30 degrees.

Geriatric

Older patients often take drugs that decrease LES tone, causing symptoms of reflux. It is recommended that antacids containing sodium not be used in this population, nor are aluminum hydroxide-containing antacids recommended if the patient is constipated because their use can lead to hypophosphatemia, causing bone changes. Magnesium-containing antacids can be used if there is no renal disease present and may be helpful if the patient is also constipated.

Pantoprazole may have greater effect in elderly patients than in younger adults, and the dosage may have to be modified. In cases of liver disease, the dosage may also require adjustment because pantoprazole is metabolized and excreted by the hepatic system.

Women

Heartburn is a common occurrence in pregnancy. Antacids are in general safe when used in moderation; however, sodium bicarbonate is to be avoided because of the potential for alkalosis.

MONITORING PATIENT RESPONSE

Patients are seen 1 to 2 weeks after starting therapy to determine response. If the symptoms decrease, a full course of therapy continues for 8 weeks. After 8 weeks, the dosage is reduced to the lowest level that decreases symptoms and given once a day before meals. If symptoms continue after

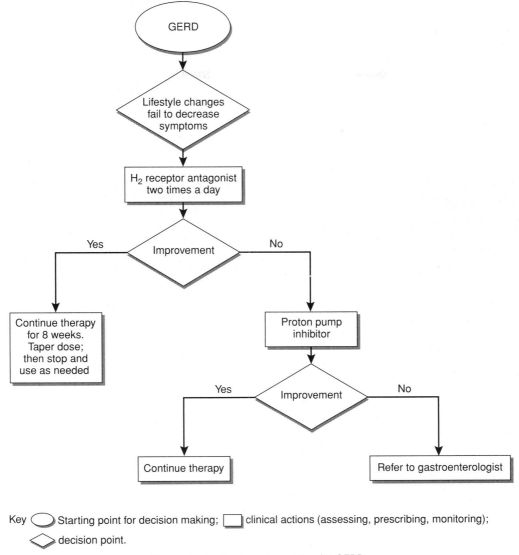

Figure 29–1 Treatment algorithm for GERD.

8 weeks, the patient continues on therapy and may be referred to a gastroenterologist.

Because some patients may achieve remission after a single course of therapy, it is reasonable to attempt to identify these patients by a therapeutic trial and discontinuation of therapy. In most, symptoms recur, and endoscopy can be used to stratify patients. Another approach would be to treat again, skipping endoscopy and following the patient's response. Patients who are started on empiric therapy without success, as well as those with atypical symptoms who respond poorly to therapy, should undergo endoscopy.

If symptom recurrence is frequent, the patient should be on a maintenance therapy regimen. Dosage should be titrated up to a level that eliminates symptoms, including increased or more frequent dosing of H_2RAs and twice-daily PPIs. It is rare for patients to continue to have symptoms despite high-dose acid suppression. Patients with continuing symptoms should be studied by 24-hour esophageal pH monitoring to confirm the GERD diagnosis. It may also be appropriate to suggest endoscopic surgery at this time.

PATIENT EDUCATION

Drug Information

Medication instruction should include the reason for taking antacids 1 to 2 hours after the H_2RA if these drugs are taken in combination. Reminders that antacids are not to be used for more than 2 weeks and that antacid tablets are not as potent as the liquid form are shared with the patient. If antacid tablets are taken, they should be thoroughly chewed and followed by a full glass of water. Effervescent tablets should be dissolved completely in water and drunk after the bubbles subside.

AstraZeneca has a Web site for patients with general information about GERD. It is www.gerd.com.

Nutritional and Lifestyle Changes

Lifestyle changes are as important as drug therapy in managing GERD. Discussion with the patient and family should cover the following important dietary changes: avoidance of excess alcohol and food intake; decreased amounts of chocolate and spicy, fried, or fatty foods eaten; and avoidance of the recumbent position for at least 3 hours after meals. Because these recommended changes involve many activities or foods that are pleasurable for the patient, they should occur gradually—one at a time. A nutritionist can be consulted to help the patient learn to choose and prepare less problematic foods.

Additional measures include teaching the patient to elevate the head of the bed approximately 4 to 6 inches (using blocks); to avoid tight, restrictive clothing; and to lose weight if necessary. Smoking cessation is another goal of patient education.

Complementary and Alternative Medicine

Peppermint is used by some for the treatment of GERD. It relaxes the sphincter of Oddi by reducing calcium influx and stimulates bile flow in animals by the choloretic action of its flavonoid components. The menthol has a direct spasmolytic effect on smooth muscle of the digestive tract.

Selecting the Most Appropriate Agent for PUD

For eradicating *H. pylori*, the ideal first-line regimen is one that is relatively cost effective and easily adhered to by patients (Fig. 29-2). The ideal second- and third-line regimens

are those that are relatively cost effective and easily followed by patients.

First-Line Therapy

Triple-therapy regimens offer good eradication rates (80%) as well as a relatively greater chance of compliance compared with quadruple-therapy regimens.

A recommendation has been published suggesting that triple therapy with metronidazole, omeprazole, and clarithromycin (MOC) be considered a regimen of first choice based on the eradication rate of 88% or higher, favorable tolerability, and need for only twice-daily dosing. The MOC regimen was the most cost-effective treatment regimen in another study, although it was neither the least expensive nor the most effective of four treatment strategies evaluated (Duggan et al., 1998). This regimen is administered twice daily for 10 to 14 days but is also efficacious when administered for as few as 7 days. Lansoprazole, clarithromycin, and amoxicillin is another effective triple-therapy regimen, although its eradication rate in one study was slightly less than 80%. Table 29-2 lists the regimens.

Second-Line Therapy

Regimens with fair to good eradication rates and likely compliance may be considered second-line choices.

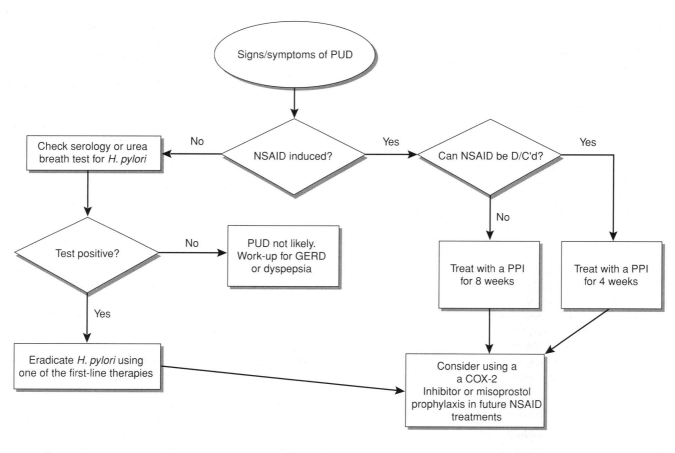

Key ⬭ Starting point for decision making; ▭ clinical actions (assessing, prescribing, monitoring); ◇ decision point.

Figure 29–2   Treatment algorithm for PUD.

Third-Line Therapy

Regimens with fair eradication rates may be considered third-line alternatives for eradication of *H. pylori*.

Preventive Therapy in NSAID-Induced PUD

Clinical data do not support the use of misoprostol or a PPI to prevent ulcers in all patients taking NSAIDs. According to published guidelines from the American College of Gastroenterology, people at high risk for NSAID-induced ulcer, bleeding, and perforation should receive prophylaxis with misoprostol if they must continue receiving NSAID therapy (Lanza, 1998).

The PPIs are acceptable alternatives for patients at risk for GI complications from NSAIDs. Factors that increase the risk for development of these complications include prior history of a GI event, age older than 60 years, use of a higher dose of NSAID, and concurrent corticosteroid or anticoagulant use.

The H$_2$RAs are not recommended for prophylaxis because of their low efficacy in preventing gastric versus duodenal ulcers. For treating an NSAID-related ulcer, any drug that has the ability effectively to heal gastric or duodenal ulcer can be used.

Published guidelines recommend a PPI as the preferred therapy when an NSAID-induced ulcer needs to be healed, particularly when the NSAID cannot be discontinued (Lanza, 1998).

Special Population Considerations

It is important for the prescribing practitioner to be aware of unique considerations when dealing with the special populations of children, older adults, and women.

Pediatric

Epidemiologic data suggest that acquisition of *H. pylori* infection occurs in childhood, most likely before the age of 5 years. It is thought that the tissue damage and disease caused by *H. pylori* is progressive. Despite this suggestion, as well as the lack of evidence that preventing or treating infections acquired in youth produces long-term health benefits, children are not routinely screened for *H. pylori*. According to results of the limited number of small studies conducted in pediatric patients, eradication of *H. pylori* in children has been effective in curing PUD. However, there are no consensus guidelines for managing this infection in children. Recently published guidelines apply to adults only. Two regimens—MOC and clarithromycin, amoxicillin, and omeprazole—have both produced eradication rates greater than 80%. Because of the potential for significant adverse effects on teeth and bones, tetracycline should not be used in children younger than 8 years of age.

Geriatric

The prevalence of *H. pylori* infection increases with age and eradication of *H. pylori* is necessary when gastric or duodenal ulcers are present in elderly patients. Age is a factor that significantly increases the risk for development of GI complications from NSAIDs. The presentation of PUD is often atypical in the elderly; hence, a high index of suspicion is necessary. Elderly patients are also at high risk for development of complications of PUD. Treatment of PUD in the elderly is similar to that in younger patients, although elderly patients are more likely to experience adverse effects and drug interactions from medications used to manage PUD. A heightened awareness and increased monitoring for these treatment-related complications are essential when treating the geriatric population.

Women

Women taking misoprostol during childbearing years should be advised regarding appropriate use of contraception and should have a negative pregnancy test before beginning therapy.

MONITORING PATIENT RESPONSE

Because the most common cause of PUD recurrence after treatment with antibiotics is failure to eradicate *H. pylori*, several issues should be considered in attempt to prevent treatment failures. Noncompliance is a common cause for failure to eradicate *H. pylori*; thus, a primary treatment goal is ensuring patient adherence to an effective regimen for 7 to 14 days. Initial therapies to eradicate *H. pylori* are typically prescribed for 7 to 10 days, but in situations where retreatment is necessary because of recurrent disease, a minimum of 14 days of therapy is often recommended. Adherence to a prescribed regimen is of paramount importance in achieving eradication rates quoted in the literature. Because many effective regimens are complex, some requiring up to 16 pills per day, it is important to individualize therapy as much as possible and to stress the importance of rigorous patient compliance and its link to successful eradication and thus treatment of PUD. Antibiotic resistance to metronidazole or clarithromycin can also lead to treatment failure. Finally, alterations in the dose or timing of administration of antibiotics can affect the success of an eradication regimen (eg, tetracycline with regard to meals).

In addition to pretreatment screening to diagnose active infection by *H. pylori*, it is sometimes desirable to conduct a diagnostic test to determine the presence or absence of *H. pylori* after treatment. The urea breath test is particularly useful as a follow-up test in the early posttreatment period. Patients can be tested 4 to 6 weeks after the completion of antibiotic therapy using this noninvasive, simple test that is specific for active *H. pylori* infection. A urea breath test is widely available in the United States. Serology testing of IgG titers alone does not distinguish current infection from past infection until 6 months to 1 year after completion of treatment.

The practice of obtaining serial IgA titers has proven useful. In this study, drops in serum IgA titers at 3 months were adequately able to confirm eradication. This approach, however, is based on relative changes from pretreatment titers, and because results of the particular assay used in this study can vary greatly, a major disadvantage is the need to run both samples in parallel to minimize variation.

When the NSAID is discontinued in a patient with an NSAID-induced ulcer and appropriate ulcer treatment is initiated, the ulcer should heal after 8 weeks. Patients with an NSAID-induced ulcer should also be screened for the presence of *H. pylori* because it needs to be determined whether the ulcer is from the NSAID or due to infection with *H. pylori*. If *H. pylori* is present, treatment with a three- or four-drug anti-*H. pylori* regimen should be initiated.

PATIENT EDUCATION

Drug Information

Antacids can be used along with other antiulcer drugs for more immediate relief of symptoms of dyspepsia. Also, it is important for patients to understand that *H. pylori* infection can be cured with the appropriate antibiotic therapy. The adverse effects of the therapy can be unpleasant but the patient is to be encouraged to finish the therapy to ensure eradication.

Information for patients about PUD can be found at *www.cdc.gov/ulcer/*.

Nutritional and Lifestyle Changes

Patients diagnosed with PUD should be encouraged to eliminate cigarette smoking, NSAID use (if possible), and excessive caffeine and alcohol intake. Taking an NSAID with food, reducing the dose of the NSAID, or switching to a potentially less toxic agent such as acetaminophen or a COX-2 inhibitor are possible options in patients taking an NSAID. Stress management initiatives may also aid in PUD symptom relief.

Complementary and Alternative Medicine

Licorice has been used for PUD because of its anecdotal use for gastric irritation. However, licorice can be dangerous if consumed in large amounts. Consumption of 30 to 40 g/d for extended periods has resulted in electrolyte imbalances.

■ Case Study

J.G. is a 42-year-old white man presenting with a 2-month history of intermittent mid-epigastric pain. The pain sometimes wakes him up at night and seems to get better after he eats a meal. J.G. informs you that he was told by his doctor 6 months ago that he had an infection in his stomach. He never followed up and has been taking over-the-counter Zantac for 2 weeks without relief. He is concerned because the pain is continuing. He has no other significant history except he is a 20 pack-year smoker and he drinks 5 cups of coffee a day. He eats late at night and goes to bed about 30 minutes after dinner. He also takes Motrin twice a day for shoulder pain. He is allergic to penicillin.

Diagnosis: PUD

→ 1. List the specific goals for treatment for J.C.

→ 2. What drug therapy would you prescribe for J.C.? Why?

→ 3. What tests would you prescribe to determine the success of the therapy?

→ 4. Discuss specific patient education based on the diagnosis and the prescribed therapy.

→ 5. List one or two adverse reactions to the therapy that J.C. might have.

→ 6. What would be the choice for second-line therapy?

→ 7. What dietary and lifestyle changes should be recommended for this patient?

→ 8. Describe one or two drug–drug or drug–food interactions for the selected therapy.

Bibliography

Starred references are cited in the text.

*Adamek, R. J., Suerbaum, S., Pfaffenbach, B., & Opfentuch, W. (1998). Primary and acquired *Helicobacter pylori* resistance to clarithromycin, metronidazole and amoxicillin. Influence on treatment outcome. *American Journal of Gastroenterology, 93*, 386–389.

*Allison, P. R. (1946). Peptic ulcer of the esophagus. *Journal of Thoracic Surgery, 15*, 308–317.

*Bell, J. D., Powell, K. U., Burridge, S. M., et al. (1995). Rapid eradication of *Helicobacter pylori* infection. *Alimentary Pharmacology and Therapeutics, 9*, 41–46.

Bolami, J., & Laippala, P. (1995). Prevalence of symptoms suggestive of gastro-oesophageal reflux disease in the adult population. *Annals of Medicine, 27*(1), 67–70.

*DeVault, K. (1999). Overview of medical therapy for gastroesophageal reflux disease. *Gastrointestinal Clinics, 28*, 831–845.

*Duggan, A. E., Tolley, K., Hawkey, C. J., et al. (1998). Varying efficacy of *Helicobacter pylori* eradication regimens: Cost effectiveness study using a decision analysis model. *British Medical Journal, 316,* 1648–1654.

*The European *Helicobacter pylori* Study Group (EHPSG). (1997). Current European concepts in the management of *H. pylori* infection: The Maastricht Consensus Report. *Gut, 41,* 8–13.

Fennerty, M. B., Castell, D., Fendrick, A.M., et al. (1996). The diagnosis and treatment of gastroesophageal reflux disease in a managed care environment. *Archives of Internal Medicine, 156,* 477–484.

Gerson, L. B., Robbins, A. S., Garber, A., et al. (2000). A cost-effective analysis of prescription strategies in the management of gastroesophageal reflux disease. *American Journal of Gastroenterology, 95,* 395–407.

Hatelbakk, J. G., Katz, P. O., & Castel, D. O. (1999). Medical therapy in management of the refractory patient. *Gastrointestinal Clinics of North America, 28,* 847–860.

*Healy, D. P., Danserau, R. J., Dunn, A. B., et al. (1997). Reduced tetracycline bioavailability caused by magnesium aluminum salicylate in liquid formulations of bismuth subsalicylate. *Annals of Pharmacotherapy, 31,* 1460–1464.

Howden, C. W., & Hunt, R. H. (1998). Guidelines for the management of *Helicobacter pylori* infection. *American Journal of Gastroenterology, 93,* 2330–2338.

Katz, P. O. (1998). Gastroesophageal reflux disease. *Journal of the American Geriatrics Society, 46,* 1558–1565.

Klinkenberg-Knol, E. C., Festen, P. M., & Jansen, J. B. (1994). Long-term treatment with omeprazole for refractory reflux esophagitis: Efficacy and safety. *Annals of Internal Medicine, 121,* 161–167.

Kuipers, E. J., Lundell, L., Klinkenberg-Knol, E. C., et al. (1996). Atrophic gastritis and *Helicobacter pylori* infection in patients with reflux esophagitis treated with omeprazole or fundoplication. *New England Journal of Medicine, 334,* 1018–1022.

*Lanza, F. L. (1998). A guideline for the treatment and prevention of NSAID-induced ulcers. *American Journal of Gastroenterology, 93,* 2037–2046.

Lee, J. M., & O'Morain, C.A. (1998). Trends in the management of gastro-oesophageal reflux disease. *Postgraduate Medical Journal, 74*(869), 145–150.

*Levine, J. S. (1998). Treatment of gastroesophageal reflux disease (GERD). *Primary Care Case Reviews, 1,* 22–30.

Locke, G. R., Talley, N. J., Fett, S. L., et al. (1997). Prevalence and clinical spectrum of gastroesophageal reflux: A population-based study in Olmstead County, Minnesota. *Gastroenterology, 112,* 5–12.

McColl, K. E., el-Omar, E. M., & Gillen, D. (1997). The role of *H. pylori* in the pathophysiology of duodenal ulcer disease. *Journal of Physiology and Pharmacology, 48,* 287–295.

McDougall, N. I., Johnston, B. T., Kee, F., et al. (1996). Natural history of reflux oesophagitis: A 10 year follow up of its effect on patient symptomatology and quality of life. *Gut, 38,* 481–486.

Meurer, L. N., & Bower, D. J. (2002). *Helicobacter pylori* infection. *American Family Physician, 65*(7), 1327–1336.

*National Institutes of Health (NIH) Consensus Development Panel. (1994). *Helicobacter pylori* in peptic ulcer disease. *Journal of the American Medical Association, 272,* 65–69.

Nebel, O. T., Fornes, M. F., & Castell, D. O. (1976). Symptomatic gastroesophageal reflux: Incidence and precipitating factors. *American Journal of Digestive Disease, 21,* 953–956.

Pinson, J. B., & Weart, W. (1996). Acid-peptic products. In *Handbook of nonprescription drugs* (11th ed.). Washington, DC: American Pharmaceutical Association.

Ramirez, B., & Richter, J. E. (1993). Review article: Promotility drugs and the treatment of gastro-oesophageal reflux disease. *Alimentary Pharmacology and Therapeutics, 7,* 5–20.

Robinson, M., Sahba, B., Avner, D., et al. (1995). A comparison of lansoprazole and ranitidine in the treatment of erosive esophagitis. *Alimentary Pharmacology and Therapeutics, 9,* 25–31.

*Saledo, J. A., & Al-Kawas, F. (1998). Treatment of *Helicobacter pylori* infection. *Archives of Internal Medicine, 158,* 842–851.

Schwartz, H., Krause, R., & Sabha, B. (1998). Triple versus dual therapy for eradicating *Helicobacter pylori* and preventing ulcer recurrence: A randomized, double-blind, multicenter study of lansoprazole, clarithromycin and/or amoxicillin in different dosing regimens. *American Journal of Gastroenterology, 93,* 584–590.

*Shaheen, N., & Provenzale, D. (2003). The epidemiology of gastroesophageal reflux disease. *American Journal of Medicine Science, 326*(5), 264–273.

Shiotoni, A., & Graham, D.Y. (2002). Pathogenesis and therapy of gastric and duodenal ulcers. *Medical Clinics of North America, 86*(6), 1447–1466.

*Simon, L. S., Hatoum, H. T., Bittman, R. M., et al. (1996). Risk factors for serious nonsteroidal-induced gastrointestinal complications: Regression analysis of the MUCOSA trial. *Family Medicine, 28,* 204–210.

Smoot, D. T., Go, M. F., & Cryer, B. (2001). Peptic ulcer disease. *Primary Care, 28*(3), 487–503.

Sonnenberg, A., Inodorni, J. M., & Becker, L. A. (1999). Economic analysis of step-wise treatment of gastroesophageal reflux disease. *Alimentary Pharmacology and Therapeutics, 13,* 1003–1013.

Thijs, J. S., van Zwet, A. A., Thijs, W. J., et al. (1996). Diagnostic tests for *Helicobacter pylori*: A prospective evaluation of their accuracy, without selecting a single test as the gold standard. *American Journal of Gastroenterology, 91*(10), 2125–2129.

van Veldhuyzen, Z., Sander, J. O., Sherman, P. M., et al. (1997). *Helicobacter pylori*: New developments and treatments. *Canadian Medical Association Journal, 156,* 1565–1574.

Vanderhoff, B. T., & Tahboub, R. M. (2002). Proton pump inhibitors: an update. *American Family Physician, 66*(2), 273–280.

*Winkelstein, A. (1935). Peptic esophagitis: A new clinical entity. *Journal of the American Medical Association, 104,* 906–909.

Visit the Connection web site for the most up-to-date drug information.

30

CONSTIPATION, DIARRHEA, AND IRRITABLE BOWEL SYNDROME

■ VERONICA WILBUR AND TIM BRISCOE

Functional bowel disorders of the lower gastrointestinal (GI) tract can include symptoms of hypogastric cramping abdominal pain, diarrhea, or constipation. Constipation and diarrhea can be self-limiting. Temporary dysfunctions of the bowel can include common GI upsets that can cause diarrhea or short-lived episodes of constipation. One of the most puzzling functional bowel disorders is irritable bowel syndrome (IBS). IBS typically presents with vague, crampy hypogastric pains and can be accompanied by alternating constipation and diarrhea. Similar pharmacologic agents are used to treat these symptoms, whether self-limited or chronic.

CONSTIPATION

Constipation is a common GI symptom that is defined as infrequent or difficult evacuation of stool. Every individual affected by constipation defines it differently, but normal defecation can vary from daily to three times a day or to every 3 days. Constipation can be a consequence of multiple factors, including diet, lifestyle, medications, and many disease states. In a systematic review of the epidemiology of constipation in North America by Higgins and Johanson (2004), the mean prevalence of constipation in the general population was found to be 12% to 19%. Constipation affects 2.2 females to 1 male and the incidence increases with age, especially in those over 65 years. Dietary and lifestyle modifications are the preferred therapy for constipation, but many patients use over-the-counter (OTC) laxatives for relief. Americans spend over $1 billion for more than 150 types of OTC and prescription laxatives (Smith et al., 2002; Stessman, 2003). Most of these laxatives are considered safe and effective, but overuse or abuse may have serious consequences.

CAUSES

Constipation may be initially diagnosed based on a thorough history and physical examination. If an identifiable cause is present, constipation is then classified as a secondary symp-

tom. However, constipation may be a symptom of an underlying disease state (Box 30-1). The patient's lifestyle (eg, diet, inactivity) or concomitant medications (Box 30-2) may also contribute to constipation. When no cause can be found for the symptoms of constipation, the disorder is categorized as idiopathic. Idiopathic constipation is usually caused by a reduction in the propulsive capacity of the colon (slow transit constipation) or a functional outlet. Although constipation is often a benign condition, it can be a symptom of a more serious problem. If left untreated in an elderly patient, constipation may lead to impaction, stercoral ulceration, anal fissures, megacolon, volvulus, and possibly carcinoma of the colon.

PATHOPHYSIOLOGY

The absorptive capacity and motility of the colon are major factors of bowel function. Approximately 9 L of fluid enters the small intestine daily from ingestion or intestinal secretions. Approximately 80% of this fluid load is absorbed by the small intestine, which is approximately half of its capacity. The colon absorbs the remainder, with the exception of approximately 0.1 L of water that is passed in the stool. If absorption of the small intestine is reduced, the fluid load adds to the burden of the colon, which is capable of absorbing 4 to 5 L of fluid per day. Fluid in excess of this amount results in diarrhea. Likewise, excessive reabsorption of water results in constipation.

The colon can be divided into three distinctive functional areas: (1) the cecum and proximal colon, (2) the transverse colon, and (3) the distal colon and rectum. Each area performs different roles in preparing the chyme for expulsion. The variation in the neurogenic tone of each area affects the capacity of the colon to retain or release the fecal material.

The motility of the bowel is affected by the flow of chyme from the coloileal reflex and its visceral hypersensitivity can contribute to the sense of urgency and tenesmus of proximal colonic transit. The neurogenic aspects of colon motility are poorly understood and need further study. Some of the stimuli thought to affect colonic activity are awakening from sleep or rest, ingestion of a high-calorie meal, and the sight or smell of food.

BOX 30–1. DISORDERS ASSOCIATED WITH CONSTIPATION

Bowel obstruction	Irritable bowel syndrome
Colonic tumors	Megacolon
Depression	Parkinsonism
Diabetes	Spinal injury
Diverticulitis	Stroke
Hypercalcemia	Uremia
Hypothyroidism	

DIAGNOSTIC CRITERIA

The definition of constipation varies widely between health care providers and patients. Constipation can be idiopathic and is functionally defined as infrequent bowel movements accompanied by straining. Feces are hard, leading to straining and a feeling of incomplete evacuation of the rectum. An important distinction between chronic constipation and IBS is the absence of abdominal pain associated with the bowel pattern.

The diagnosis of constipation stems primarily from the history. A careful history (Box 30-3) can help the provider decide which diagnostic tests may be appropriate. Abrupt onset of constipation or onset in patients 45 to 50 years old suggests an organic cause and requires immediate attention (Dosh, 2002; Schiller, 2001; Stessman, 2003).

INITIATING DRUG THERAPY

Lifestyle modifications are preferred over pharmacologic therapy for treating constipation. Diet, exercise, and bowel habit training are usually targeted. However, research is inconclusive as to the value of increasing fluid intake and exercise. According to the National Center for Health Statistics, Americans eat 5 to 14 grams of fiber daily, far short of the recommended 20 to 35 grams recommended by the American Dietetic Association (Dosh, 2002). Increased dietary fiber can be recommended for most patients without fear of colon obstruction. Fiber should be both soluble and insoluble

BOX 30–2. SELECTED MEDICATION ASSOCIATED WITH CONSTIPATION

Activated charcoal	Diuretics
Antacids (aluminum- or magnesium-containing)	Ferrous salts
	HMG-CoA reductase inhibitors (ie, "statins")
Anticholinergics	Narcotic analgesics
Antihistamines (sedating)	Sodium polystyrene sulfonate
Antipsychotics	Sucralfate
Bile acid sequestrants	Tricyclic antidepressants
Calcium supplements	Verapamil
Clonidine	

BOX 30–3. HISTORY AND PHYSICAL EXAMINATION FOR CHRONIC CONSTIPATION

Important history questions:
Onset and duration of symptoms
Patient's definition of constipation
Presence of abdominal cramping relieved by defecation (*if yes, think irritable bowel syndrome*)
Presence of blood in the stool
Important aspects of the physical examination:
Evaluation of the perianal area for scars, fistulas, fissures, and external hemorrhoids
Observe the perineum at rest and while patient is bearing down.
Digital rectal examination—check for fecal impaction, stricture, or rectal masses.

in the form of fruits, vegetables, and whole grains, which cannot be digested by the body. Fiber should be slowly increased to 20 to 25 grams per day over a 1- to 2-week period to improve compliance with therapy. Dietary fiber increases stool weight and shortens intestinal transit time. However, fiber therapy may not be effective for all patients. Fiber accelerates right colon transit, but there are few treatments for patients where the transit problem is the left colon.

One additional lifestyle modification includes establishing a regular pattern for bathroom visits. Patients should also be counseled not to ignore the urge to defecate, because this delay increases the time for absorption of fluid from the stool. Biofeedback, a method of retraining the pelvic floor muscles to relax during defecation, may be effective in selected patients.

Goals of Drug Therapy

An adequate trial of lifestyle modification should be attempted first. If this fails, pharmacologic management with laxatives may be appropriate. Laxatives should be used for the shortest time possible because the patient may become dependent on the drug to defecate.

The goal of therapy for constipation is to increase the water content of the feces and increase motility of the intestines to promote comfortable defecation, using the lowest effective dose of a laxative for the least amount of time possible. This conservative approach helps avoid the complications and side effects that can occur with overuse or abuse of some laxatives. Responses to laxatives vary and depend on the patient as well as the preparation. Several classes of laxatives are available for the symptomatic treatment of constipation: bulk-forming agents, saline laxatives, lubricant laxatives, surfactants (emollients), hyperosmotic laxatives, and stimulant laxatives. Proper selection of a laxative should be based on the individual clinical situation (Table 30-1).

Bulk-Forming Laxatives

Bulk forming laxatives work by binding to the fecal contents and pulling water into the stool. This ultimately softens and

Table 30.1

Overview of Selected Laxatives

Generic (Trade) Name and Dosage	Selected Adverse Events	Contraindications	Special Considerations
Bulk-Forming Laxatives			
methylcellulose (Citrucel) 2–6 g/d	Flatulence, stomach upset, fullness	GI obstruction	Take with plenty of water. Avoid in patients with GI ulceration.
psyllium (Metamucil) 3.4–10.2 g/d	Same as above	Same as above	Same as above
polycarbophil (FiberCon) 1–6 g/d	Same as above	Same as above	Same as above Calcium content may interact with tetracycline or quinolone antibiotics.
malt soup extract (Maltsupex) 12–64 g/d	Same as above	Same as above	Same as above
Lubricants and Surfactants			
mineral oil 5–45 mL/d	Rectal seepage, irritation	Do not use with surfactants.	Impairs absorption of fat-soluble vitamins Caution in elderly and very young due to potential for development of lipid pneumonia
docusate sodium (Colace) 50–500 mg/d	Stomach upset	Do not use with mineral oil.	Most effective at preventing "straining" in high-risk patients (see text)
docusate calcium (Surfak) 50–240 mg	Same as above	Same as above	Same as above
docusate potassium (Dialose) 100–300 mg	Same as above	Same as above	Same as above
Saline Agents			
sodium phosphate enema (Fleet) 118 mL/d	Alterations in fluid/electrolyte balance, diarrhea	Caution in patients with CHF, hypertension, edema, and renal dysfunction	Care should be taken in the elderly and those with existing electrolyte disturbances.
sodium phosphate (Fleet Phospho-soda) 20–30 mL in water/d	Alterations in fluid electrolyte balance, dehydration, diarrhea	Same as above	Same as above Caution in renal dysfunction and the elderly
magnesium citrate 240 mL/d	GI upset, diarrhea	Caution in renal dysfunction	Stagger administration times of tetracycline and quinolone antibiotics.
magnesium hydroxide (Phillips Milk of Magnesia) 30–60 mL/d	GI upset diarrhea	Same as above	Caution in renal dysfunction and the elderly Stagger administration times of tetracycline and quinolone antibiotics.
magnesium sulfate (Epsom salt) 1–2 tsp in ½ glass water	GI upset, diarrhea	Same as above	Caution in renal dysfunction and the elderly Stagger administration times of tetracycline and quinolone antibiotics.
Hyperosmotic Agents			
lactulose (Chronulac, Constilac, Duphalac) 15–60 mL	GI upset, diarrhea, flatulence	Caution in diabetic patients	Use lactulose with caution in patients with diabetes. Avoid combination of antacids with lactulose.
sorbitol 130–150 mL	GI upset, diarrhea, flatulence	Same as above	Caution in diabetic patients
Stimulants			
senna (Senakot) Tabs: 2–8/d Supp: 1 qhs Granules: 1–4 tsp/d	Griping, diarrhea, gas, discoloration of urine	GI obstruction	Caution: laxative abuse, cathartic colon
bisacodyl (Dulcolax) Tabs: 1–3/d Supp: 1 pr qd	Griping, diarrhea, gas	GI obstruction	Do not crush or chew tablets. Avoid concomitant administration of antacids and pH-lowering agents.
castor oil 15–60 mL/d	Stomach upset, diarrhea, colic	GI obstruction	Too potent for routine use

lubricates the stool, eases its passage, and reduces straining. Water is reabsorbed from fecal masses that stay in the colon for extended periods, and the result is dry stools. Bulk-forming agents hold water in the stool or swell and increase stool bulk. The bulk stimulates the movement of the intestines and facilitates the passage of intestinal contents. Bulk-forming laxatives generally consist of psyllium seed husk, methylcellulose, and polycarbophil and are made of poly-saccharides or cellulose derivatives such as methylcellulose (Citrucel) or psyllium (Metamucil). Polycarbophil (FiberCon) has significant water-absorptive properties and also is used as an antidiarrheal. Like all other bulk-forming agents used for constipation, polycarbophil should be taken with plenty of fluid (8 ounces) to increase efficacy. Malt soup extract (Maltsupex) made from barley malt reduces fecal pH. This may contribute to its laxative effect. Traditionally, these products have been marketed only as powders, which must be dissolved in water. Now a variety of OTC fiber products are available in powder, wafer, and caplet forms. Patients may need to try several before finding one that works for them. Brand names include Metamucil, FiberCon, and Citrucel. Psyllium (Metamucil) is the preferred agent because it is the safest and most physiologic. Sugar-free methylcellulose and psyllium products are available for patients with diabetes.

Contraindications to the use of bulking agents are symptoms of an acute surgical abdomen, intestinal obstruction or perforation, or inability to drink an adequate amount of fluid.

Action for all agents may begin in 12 to 24 hours, but a full effect is not usually seen for up to 3 days.

A half-cup to one bowl daily of wheat bran can provide adequate fiber supplementation, but synthetic forms of fiber are often better absorbed than food. Other foods can also add fiber to the diet and should be reviewed with the patient. The patient should be encouraged to drink adequate amounts of fluid throughout the day; if not contraindicated, up to 2,500 mL is preferred. These agents are more likely to be used as preventive measures. However given, they can take effect within 12 to 24 hours, and some acute relief of symptoms is possible.

Adverse Events

Overall, these agents are usually well tolerated, but compliance can be a problem because the most common side effect is increased flatulence, and some bloating can occur. With severe constipation, all agents can cause abdominal fullness and cramping. If these agents are used excessively, nausea and vomiting may occur.

Contraindications

Because bulk-forming laxatives have the most physiologic effect and are not systemically absorbed, they are the preferred agents for symptomatic treatment of constipation. However, these agents are not completely benign and should be avoided in patients with strictures of the esophagus, GI ulcerations, or stenosis secondary to the possibility of obstruction from increased bulk of intestinal contents. In addition, some bulk-forming agents may contain as much as 20 g carbohydrates per dose. Sugar-free bulk-forming agents are available and are recommended for diabetic patients.

Interactions

The sugar-free preparations may contain aspartame, which is metabolized to phenylalanine and should be used cautiously with patients who must restrict their phenylalanine intake. Extensive long-term use of bulking agents can lead to laxative dependence. Concomitant administration of calcium-containing bulk laxatives may reduce the effectiveness of quinolone or tetracycline, so patients should separate the administration time of these agents.

Hyperosmotic Laxatives

Glycerin, lactulose (Cephulac), sorbitol, and polyethylene glycol/electrolyte solution (PEG-ES) (CoLyte) are examples of hyperosmotic laxatives. These agents serve as or are metabolized to solutes in the intestinal tract. The increased concentration of solutes creates osmotic pressure by drawing fluid from a less concentrated gradient to the more concentrated gradient inside the GI tract. This increase in osmotic pressure stimulates intestinal motility and propulsion of fecal contents.

In addition to its osmotic effect, glycerin also has a local irritant effect in the suppository form. The irritant action adds to the osmotic action to stimulate bowel movement.

Lactulose is a disaccharide analog that is metabolized by bacteria to acids that increase osmotic pressure and acidify the contents of the colon. The result is increased intestinal motility and secretion.

In addition to its use for the symptomatic treatment of constipation, sorbitol is also used to prevent constipation in combination with activated charcoal for poisoning. Sodium polystyrene sulfonate (Kayexalate), a cation exchange resin used for treating hyperkalemia, is often combined with sorbitol to reduce the potential for constipation from the resin.

PEG-ES is a nonabsorbable solution that acts as an osmotic agent. It is usually used to evacuate the bowel before a GI examination such as a flexible sigmoidoscopy or colonoscopy. The solution is reconstituted with 1 gallon of tap water and should be chilled before consumption to increase palatability. The patient should begin drinking the solution at 4 PM the day before the procedure. One glass (8 ounces) of the reconstituted solution should be consumed every 10 minutes over 3 hours until all 4 L are consumed. The patient should fast for 4 hours before ingesting the solution, and only clear liquids are allowed after ingestion.

Contraindications

Lactulose syrup should be used with caution in diabetic patients because it contains lactose and galactose. Lactose is also contraindicated in patients with appendicitis, acute surgical abdomen, fecal impaction, or intestinal obstruction. Caution must be used in diabetic patients because of sugar content.

Other osmotic agents such as magnesium hydroxide (Milk of Magnesia) or magnesium citrate (Citroma) can be used to promote defecation. Approximately 15% to 30% of the magnesium in these agents may be absorbed systemically; therefore, caution is needed in patients who have renal failure and decreased ability to excrete magnesium.

In addition, sorbitol as a caloric sweetener has the potential to affect blood glucose levels and should be used with caution in diabetic patients. PEG-ES is not recommended in patients with gastric obstruction, bowel perforation, or colitis.

Adverse Reactions

Glycerin is among the safest laxative preparations available and is often used in infants and children. Rectal irritation is the most common side effect of glycerin suppositories. The most common side effects associated with lactulose and sorbitol include GI upset and diarrhea. PEG-ES rapidly cleanses the bowel and often causes nausea, abdominal fullness, cramps, and bloating.

Interactions

There are few documented interactions with the osmotic laxatives. However, because antacids may neutralize the acids produced from lactulose and interfere with its mechanism of action, concomitant administration of antacids should be avoided with lactulose. No other medications should be given within 1 hour of consumption of PEG-ES because the medication will likely be flushed from the GI tract.

Contraindications

When taken appropriately, these agents are well tolerated. The most common adverse events are abdominal cramping or nausea. Extensive, long-term use of these agents can lead to laxative dependence.

Saline Laxatives

Like hyperosmotic laxatives, saline laxatives draw water into the intestine through osmosis. This creates an increase in intraluminal pressure and a resultant increase in intestinal motility. Magnesium citrate (Citrate of Magnesia), magnesium hydroxide (Phillips Milk of Magnesia), magnesium sulfate (Epsom salt), sodium phosphate, and sodium biphosphate (Fleet Phospho-soda) are examples of saline laxatives. Magnesium citrate and sodium phosphate and biphosphate are used as bowel evacuants for endoscopic examinations such as flexible sigmoidoscopy. A typical dose is one bottle of magnesium citrate at 4 PM the day before the test and two Fleet enemas 1 hour before leaving home the morning of the test.

Contraindications

Caution should be used when administering sodium phosphate salts to patients on sodium-restricted diets (eg, hypertension, congestive heart failure, edema). In addition, phosphates can accumulate in patients with renal dysfunction, leading to serious complications such as hyperphosphatemia, hypokalemia, hypocalcemia, hypernatremia, metabolic acidosis, and coma.

Magnesium hydroxide and magnesium sulfate are commonly used for the symptomatic treatment of constipation. Because the kidneys eliminate magnesium, magnesium-containing laxatives should be used with caution in the elderly and in patients with decreased renal function. Excessive magnesium levels can result in central nervous system depression (drowsiness), muscle weakness, decreased blood pressure, and electrocardiographic changes.

Adverse Events

Dehydration is a concern with the use of saline laxatives, and these agents must be used with caution in patients who cannot tolerate excessive fluid loss and dehydration.

Interactions

Because Milk of Magnesia also has antacid properties and can increase the pH of the intestines, it should not be administered at the same time with agents that require an acidic environment to be absorbed. The most common example of this type of interaction is with the antifungals itraconazole (Sporanox) and ketoconazole (Nizoral). Therefore, administration of any antacid should be separated from administration of ketoconazole or itraconazole by at least 2 hours. In addition, the magnesium found in magnesium hydroxide and magnesium sulfate can bind with tetracycline and quinolone antibiotics to form a nonabsorbable complex that may reduce the effectiveness of the antibiotics. Administration of quinolones and tetracyclines should be separated from administration of magnesium-containing compounds.

Stimulant Laxatives

These laxatives vary in effects but act by increasing peristalsis through direct effects on the smooth muscle of the intestines and simultaneously promoting fluid accumulation in the colon and small intestine. Because of the irritating effect of the agents on the musculature, these agents should be avoided in long-term treatment. Stimulant laxatives include bisacodyl (Dulcolax) and senna concentrates (Senokot, Senokot S).

Contraindications

As with other laxatives, stimulants are contraindicated in patients with appendicitis, acute surgical abdomen, fecal impaction, or intestinal obstruction. Rectal fissures and hemorrhoids can be exacerbated by stimulation of defecation. Action begins 6 to 10 hours after oral administration and 15 minutes to 2 hours after rectal administration.

Adverse Events

These agents are not as well tolerated as the osmotic laxatives or bulking agents because of their side effects, which include nausea, vomiting, and abdominal cramping. These side effects can be more severe with cases of severe constipation. Long-term or excessive use can lead to laxative dependence.

Surfactant Laxatives

This class of laxatives reduces the surface tension of the liquid contents of the bowel. Ultimately, this promotes incorporation of additional liquid into the stool, forming a softer mass, and promotes easier defecation. Examples of this class include docusate sodium (Colace) and docusate calcium (Surfak). This is the laxative of choice for patients who should not strain during defecation. Emollient laxatives only prevent constipation; they do not treat it. Combining these agents with fiber products helps promote defecation. Administration of emollient laxatives concomitantly with mineral oil is contraindicated because of increased absorption of the mineral oil. Action with these agents usually occurs between 1 and 3 days.

Contraindications

Docusate calcium or docusate potassium may be recommended for patients on sodium-restricted diets (eg, hypertension, congestive heart failure). The sodium content of Colace (docusate sodium) is quite small (5.2 mg per capsule) and is likely insignificant.

Adverse Events

These agents are extremely well tolerated when used to prevent constipation. The most common side effect is stomach upset; other side effects, such as mild abdominal cramping, diarrhea, and throat irritation, are infrequent. Patients should take surfactants with plenty of water to improve effectiveness.

Interactions

Docusate, as a surfactant emollient laxative, may increase the absorption of mineral oil and potentially increase the risk for liver toxicity; therefore, this combination should be avoided.

Lubricant Laxatives

Mineral oil coats and softens the stool and prevents reabsorption of water from the stool by the colon. Lubricant laxatives are effective at preventing straining in high-risk patients (eg, rectal surgery, labor and delivery, stroke, hemorrhoids, hernia, myocardial infarction).

Contraindications

Mineral oil may be aspirated and cause lipid pneumonia when administered to young, elderly, or bedridden patients. With the availability of safer laxative preparations, mineral oil should probably be avoided in these populations. If mineral oil is chosen, it should not be administered to patients before bedtime or when they are reclining to prevent aspiration.

Adverse Events

Mineral oil has an unpleasant taste, and because it is not absorbed, large single doses can seep through the anal sphincter and cause irritation. Dividing doses may prevent this.

Interactions

Mineral oil can impair the absorption of fat-soluble vitamins A, D, E, and K. Because warfarin (Coumadin) interferes with the synthesis of vitamin K–dependent clotting factors, a reduction in absorption of vitamin K may increase the effects of the anticoagulant. Although no direct interactions with oral anticoagulants have been reported, prothrombin levels may decrease. The docusates, as surfactant emollient laxatives, may increase the absorption of mineral oil and potentially increase the risk for liver toxicity; therefore, this combination should be avoided.

Selecting the Most Appropriate Agent

If lifestyle modification fails to reverse constipation, then selection of an appropriate laxative is necessary. The choice of laxative agent depends on several factors, including medical history, goal of therapy, concomitant medications, potential for side effects, age, and personal preference. Table 30-2 describes first-, second-, and third-line therapies (Fig. 30-1).

Table 30.2

Recommended Order of Treatment for Constipation

Order	Agents	Comments
First line	Bulk-forming agents (methylcellulose, psyllium, polycarbophil, malt soup extract)	Avoid in patients with GI obstruction or ulceration. Take with plenty of water.
	Docusate derivatives	Most effective at preventing straining at stool in high-risk patients (see text)
	Glycerin	Used most often in infants and small children
Second line	Milk of magnesia, magnesium sulfate	Caution in renal dysfunction and the elderly
	Lactulose, sorbitol	Use with caution in diabetic patients.
Third line	Stimulant laxatives (senna, cascara sagrada, casanthranol, bisacodyl)	Caution: laxative abuse, cathartic colon
	Mineral oil	Impairs absorption of fat-soluble vitamins; used with caution in elderly and very young (lipid pneumonia)
	Sodium biphosphates	Use with caution in congestive heart failure, hypertension, edema, and renal dysfunction.
	Magnesium citrate	Used as a bowel evacuant for endoscopic examinations
	Castor oil	Too potent to be used routinely for constipation

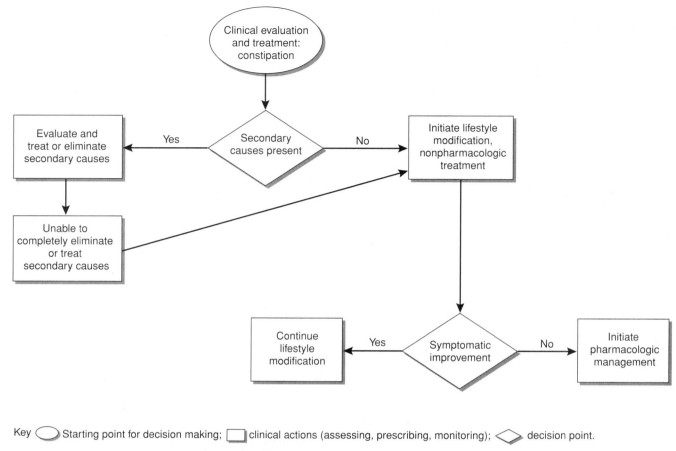

Key ⬭ Starting point for decision making; ☐ clinical actions (assessing, prescribing, monitoring); ◇ decision point.

Figure 30–1 Treatment algorithm for constipation.

First-Line Therapy

Provided no contraindications exist, a bulk-forming laxative is usually chosen as first-line therapy for constipation. Bulk-forming laxatives are not systemically absorbed. In addition, their pharmacologic effect is the most physiologic, meaning they have an effect similar to that of the natural effect of fiber from food on the GI tract. Their side effects are usually mild, and if necessary they can be administered safely for longer durations than other classes of laxatives such as the stimulants.

When hard or dry stools are the chief complaint or in situations where straining should be avoided (eg, hernia, cardiovascular disease), a stool softener such as docusate is considered first-line therapy. Stool softeners also are not systemically absorbed and their side effects are usually minimal.

Glycerin suppositories have a local irritant effect on the rectum and are probably the safest of all preparations. This is preferred as first-line therapy in infants.

Second-Line Therapy

If a more rapid onset of action is desired, magnesium hydroxide may be chosen. Although it has a faster onset of action, dehydration from excessive use is a concern, particularly in patients unable to tolerate excessive fluid loss. In addition, magnesium-containing preparations should be avoided in patients with renal insufficiency or the elderly.

If the bulk-forming agents and magnesium hydroxide are ineffective or contraindicated, an osmotic laxative such as lactulose or sorbitol may be chosen. However, flatulence and the sweet taste limit compliance. In addition, lactulose and sorbitol should be used with caution in patients with diabetes.

Third-Line Therapy

If bulk-forming or osmotic diuretics fail to work, a stimulant laxative may be chosen. Stimulant laxatives are very effective but have the highest potential for abuse. This high potential for abuse can cause serious complications. Therefore, stimulant laxatives should be reserved as third-line agents after other agents have failed or are contraindicated.

Mineral oil is effective as a lubricant laxative and may be an option in patients who should avoid straining. However, although mineral oil would seem safe, its ability to impair absorption of necessary vitamins and cause aspiration pneumonitis limits its use. In addition, seepage is an inconvenient side effect that likely limits compliance. If an agent is necessary to soften the stool to prevent straining, docusate is a safer alternative.

Sodium biphosphate as an oral solution or enema is another option. These agents have the potential to cause fluid and electrolyte abnormalities and exacerbate concomitant disease states such as hypertension and congestive heart failure. Therefore, these agents should be used only after safer agents have failed. Because sodium biphosphate enemas and magnesium citrate solutions have a rapid onset of action, these agents are often preferred and are usually reserved for endoscopic procedures.

Castor oil is a potent cathartic that should not be used routinely for treating constipation.

Special Populations

Pediatrics

Constipation can be distressing for children, particularly young children. Stress over potty training or painful stools secondary to acute constipation can result in avoidance of defecation by the child. This in turn can result in larger, harder, and more painful stools, which eventually leads to soiling. Constipation and encopresis, a condition where soft stool is involuntarily lost, are often combined. Parents usually pay little attention to their child's bowel frequency unless incontinence occurs. The parents may become angry with the child, leading to further stress. To avoid constipation that may result in soiling, parents should be cognizant of their child's bowel habits.

Constipation may also result in urinary incontinence and urinary tract infections in children, particularly girls. Overflow incontinence may occur when the distended rectum presses on the bladder wall, causing bladder outflow obstruction. Fecal soiling in the external urethral opening predisposes constipated girls to infection. Treatment of constipation can reduce infection and incontinence.

Treatment with pharmacologic agents in children is controversial, and few well-designed placebo-controlled trials have been conducted on the use of osmotic laxatives, fiber, formula-switching, sorbitol-containing juices, rectal stimulation by thermometer, or glycerin suppositories. The use of sodium phosphate enemas in children under 2 years of age has been associated with electrolyte disturbances, dehydration, and cardiac arrest.

For infants, malt soup extract or corn syrup (Karo) may be used at a dosage of 5 to 10 mL twice daily. For children older than 6 months of age, milk of magnesia, lactulose, or sorbitol at a dosage of 1 to 3 mL/kg/day given in one to two doses may be used. Senna syrup at a dosage of 5 to 10 mL/day for children from 1 to 5 years of age and 10 to 20 mL/day for children 5 to 15 years of age is another option.

Geriatric

The choice of a laxative preparation may depend on the patient's attitude or beliefs about normal bowel habits. Normal bowel frequency can range from two or three bowel movements per day to two or three per week. However, many people think that less than one bowel movement per day is abnormal. These patients may seek an OTC laxative to keep them "regular." This concern about regular bowel movements is particularly common in the elderly. The self-reported incidence of constipation increases with advancing age, but the actual bowel movement frequency usually does not decline.

The overuse of laxatives in the elderly can be of particular concern because this population is more intolerant to the fluid and electrolyte abnormalities that accompany laxative

abuse. In addition, many of the laxatives should be used with caution in elderly persons because they are more likely to have the disease states that some laxatives can exacerbate (eg, heart failure, hypertension). Elderly patients are also more likely to take medications that may cause constipation, such as antipsychotics, tricyclic antidepressants, calcium supplements, and certain blood pressure medications.

Elderly patients should be carefully assessed to determine the cause of the constipation, and causative factors should be eliminated. Careful selection and judicious use of laxatives are necessary to avoid complications in this population.

Women

Girls and women with bulimia or anorexia nervosa may abuse laxatives as a means of reducing nutrient absorption to cause weight loss. Bulimia is 10 times more common in women than in men; it affects up to 3% of young women.

For the pregnant woman, the use of laxatives that are not absorbed into the systemic circulation, such as docusate and bulk-forming agents, should be considered as first-line therapy. Docusate sodium has not been found to be associated with fetal malformations and may be safe to use during pregnancy. Lactulose and sorbitol have not been found to be teratogenic in animals and may be safe to administer to pregnant women. Stimulant laxatives should be used only occasionally, if necessary. Cascara sagrada may cause loose stools in breast-fed infants. Castor oil should be avoided in pregnant women because of the risk of stimulation of uterine contractions. Mineral oil should be avoided because its use can reduce the absorption of necessary vitamins by the mother, which may result in deficiencies for the neonate.

MONITORING PATIENT RESPONSE

Monitoring the patient's response to laxative therapy usually is accomplished by asking the patient whether he or she has regained normal bowel patterns after using the laxative. Different patients have different perceptions of what "normal" bowel habits are. Patients should be informed that the reason for treating with a laxative is not to increase the frequency of defecation but to promote comfortable defecation. Any misunderstanding by the patient on the goal of therapy may lead to chronic abuse of laxatives.

PATIENT EDUCATION

In most cases, the occasional use of laxatives poses no major problems for the patient. Laxatives are relatively safe when used in moderation. However, the fact that many laxatives are available OTC may give consumers the false impression that these agents are not dangerous and can be used routinely.

Health care providers should warn patients of the potential complications of laxatives. OTC laxatives carry a warning for the consumer not to use them for more than 7 days. For chronic constipation, use of a bulk-forming laxative may be a safer alternative, provided no contraindications exist. However, patients should be counseled that bulk-forming laxatives take time to work (up to 3 days). Because patients are usually looking for an immediate response, they may draw the conclusion that these agents are not effective if a bowel movement has not occurred within the first day. The next step taken by the patient is usually to look for a more potent agent such as a stimulant laxative, which may lead to chronic use and abuse.

Patient-Oriented Information Sources

Providing patients with information about constipation can help them understand constipation and their role in treatment. Patient education items are readily available on the Internet through the National Digestive Diseases Information Clearinghouse (NDDIC), which provides information to consumers on a wide variety of GI topics.

Nutrition/Lifestyle Changes

Patients should be educated on the lifestyle modifications discussed previously to reduce the need for a laxative. An increase in fluid intake improves the efficacy of most laxatives. Patients should also be educated on the potential for side effects of the laxative chosen as well as the appropriate method to administer the laxative.

Complementary and Alternative Medications

Senna is used as a laxative. It increases peristaltic activity in the lower bowel; it also has anti-absorptive properties and stimulates secretions.

DIARRHEA

True diarrhea is an increase in frequency of loose, watery stools (three or more daily), usually over a period of 24 to 48 hours. It is a relatively common disorder of the GI tract that is experienced occasionally by most people. The organisms that cause diarrhea are easily transferred from person to person through food and water. Globalization and industrialization of the world has increased the ability of these organisms to spread. The Centers for Disease Control and Prevention estimates that 211 million people experience acute diarrhea every year; an average of 16 million seek medical attention, resulting in 1.2 million hospitalizations and 600 deaths (Bushen & Gurerrant, 2003). Children, the elderly, and those who are immunocompromised are most susceptible to the complications of diarrhea, and serious dehydration can result from the disorder. Proper hydration and symptomatic treatment as well as elimination of causative factors are necessary to prevent these complications. Ultimately, diarrhea can have a profound impact on public health, and proper diagnosis and treatment can prevent an epidemic.

CAUSES

Diarrhea may be caused by a host of different medications (Box 30-4), infective organisms (Box 30-5), or disease states or procedures (Box 30-6). Prompt attention to causative factors, as well as rehydration, prevents complications.

BOX 30–4. MEDICATIONS COMMONLY CAUSING DIARRHEA

Antacids (magnesium-containing)
Antibiotics
Antidepressants (selective serotonin reuptake inhibitors)
Cholinergic agents
Colchicine
Digoxin
Gastrointestinal stimulants (metoclopramide)
Laxatives
Metformin
Prostaglandins (dinoprostone)
Prostaglandin analog (misoprostil)
Quinidine

Medications

Antibiotics may cause diarrhea by direct irritation of the intestinal tract or disruption of the normal intestinal flora. The poor absorption of erythromycin (E-mycin) lends itself to irritation of the GI tract. Clarithromycin (Biaxin) and azithromycin (Zithromax) may cause less diarrhea than erythromycin. The clavulanic acid component of the combination of amoxicillin–clavulanic acid (Augmentin) is also a GI irritant, and diarrhea is a common side effect. Tetracycline and ceftriaxone (Rocephin) cause diarrhea by disrupting the normal balance of the gut flora.

Clostridium difficile, a normal part of the flora of the colon in up to 20% of hospitalized patients, normally does not cause disease unless chemotherapeutic medications or antibiotics trigger its toxins. Only certain antibiotics have been implicated in *C. difficile*–associated diarrhea. Less common causes of

---

BOX 30–5. INFECTIVE ORGANISMS ASSOCIATED WITH DIARRHEA

Aeromonas species
Bacillus cereus
Campylobacter
Chlamydia trachomatis
Clostridium difficile
Cryptosporidium
Escherichia coli
Entamoeba histolytica
Giardia
Mycobacterium avium-intracellulare
Salmonella
Shigella
Staphylococcus aureus
Viral agents
Yersinia

BOX 30–6. DISORDERS AND PROCEDURES ASSOCIATED WITH DIARRHEA

Acquired immunodeficiency syndrome
Bowel resection
Colon cancer
Diverticulitis
Enteral feedings
Gastroenteritis
Hyperthyroidism
Inflammatory bowel disease
Irritable bowel syndrome
Lactose intolerance
Malabsorption
Pheochromocytoma

C. difficile diarrhea are vancomycin (Vancocin), erythromycin, tetracyclines, trimethoprim–sulfamethoxazole (TMP-SMZ), quinolones, and aztreonam (Azactam). The antibiotics most likely to cause *C. difficile* diarrhea are beta-lactam antibiotics (penicillins, cephalosporins, carbapenems) and clindamycin (Cleocin). Box 30-7 gives more information.

BOX 30–7. TREATING *CLOSTRIDIUM DIFFICILE* DIARRHEA

Clostridium difficile diarrhea may occur weeks after stopping antimicrobial therapy. The diarrhea may progress to colitis if left untreated. While awaiting the results of *C. difficile* toxin assay of the stool specimen, empiric therapy with metronidazole (Flagyl) 250 mg PO qid or vancomycin 125 to 250 mg PO qid for 5 to 7 days should be initiated. Clinical improvement should be seen within 3 days (Cunha, 1998).

Because routine use of vancomycin (Vancocin) may contribute to the emergence of vancomycin-resistant *Enterococcus* species and oral vancomycin is more costly than oral metronidazole, it has been suggested that oral vancomycin be reserved for the more severe, life-threatening forms of the disorder, for cases that fail to respond to oral metronidazole, or for patients who are not able to tolerate oral metronidazole.

For *C. difficile* diarrhea advancing to colitis, the preferred agent is intravenous metronidazole 1 g every 24 hours with oral vancomycin for 10 days or until colitis has resolved on computed tomography scan. Patients should not be given bowel antispasmodics because this may reduce the elimination of the toxins from the body (Cunha, 1998).

Infectious Organisms

Patients traveling to a developing region may contract diarrhea from bacterial organisms. *Giardia* should be suspected if the patient travels to mountainous areas, recreational waters, or Russia. Pathogens transmitted by the fecal-to-oral route should be suspected in homosexual men (*Shigella, Salmonella, Campylobacter,* and intestinal protozoa) and in patients exposed to daycare centers (*Shigella, Giardia, Cryptosporidium*).

Traveler's diarrhea is usually a self-limiting, non–life-threatening illness; it affects 20% to 50% of people visiting developing countries. The cause is ingestion of fecally contaminated food products or water. High-risk areas include Latin America, Africa, Asia, and the Middle East. The typical duration is 2 to 3 days; symptoms include nausea and vomiting, cramps, and bloody stools. The most common pathogen is *Escherichia coli*; *Salmonella, Shigella,* and *Campylobacter* are the culprits less frequently.

Dietary restrictions are the main prevention for traveler's diarrhea. Travelers should avoid foods and beverages that are not steaming hot, raw vegetables, unpeeled fruit, tap water, and ice.

PATHOPHYSIOLOGY

Diarrhea may be classified by duration and category. Acute diarrhea lasts 1 to 14 days and is considered self-limiting. Persistent diarrhea lasts longer than 14 days but less than 30 days, and chronic diarrhea last more than 30 days. Diarrhea may also be categorized as osmotic, secretory, or exudative (inflammatory), or the diarrhea may be related to altered intestinal motility (transit). Some diarrheal illnesses involve more than one of these mechanisms. Diarrhea may also be a defense mechanism against toxins and invading organisms.

Osmotic Diarrhea

Osmotic diarrhea occurs when nonabsorbed solutes are retained in the lumen of the intestinal tract. The result is a hyperosmolar state that pulls water and ions into the intestinal lumen. Poorly absorbed salts (magnesium sulfate), lactose (in lactase deficiency), and large amounts of sugar substitutes (sorbitol) found in candy or chewing gum, diet foods, and soft drinks draw fluid into the intestinal tract, resulting in an overload of the colon.

Secretory Diarrhea

In secretory diarrhea, colonic absorption of fluid is secondary to active transport of Na^+ through Na^+-K^+-adenosine triphosphatase activity in the colonic epithelium. The colon absorbs chloride by exchanging it for HCO_3^2 and by uptake of sodium chloride. Any agent that increases concentrations of cyclic adenosine 3,5-monophosphate in the cells of the colon inhibits sodium chloride uptake and causes secretion of chloride. This results in secretion of fluid in the colon. Prostaglandins E2 and I2 and vasoactive intestinal peptide stimulate adenyl cyclase activity. Cholinergic agents and cholinesterase inhibitors cause secretion of sodium chloride and water. Secretory diarrhea can be classified as pure (eg, cholera) or a part of a complex disease process (eg, celiac disease, Crohn disease). Other stimuli that can cause secretory diarrhea include bacterial endotoxins, hormones from endocrine neoplasms, dihydroxy bile acids, hydroxylated fatty acids, and inflammatory mediators. Certain laxatives (senna, castor oil) and bile acids may also induce secretory diarrhea.

Exudative Diarrhea

Exudative (inflammatory) diarrhea may result from inflammatory diseases of the mucosa. Inflammation occurs due to the compromise of the tight junctions of the epithelial cells in the intestine. These diseases may cause an increase of blood, mucus, pus, and serum proteins that increase fluid and overload the colon, resulting in diarrhea. Enteritis, ulcerative colitis, and carcinoma are examples of inflammatory conditions that may result in exudative diarrhea.

Altered Intestinal Motility

Intestinal contents need to have sufficient time to be in contact with the lining of the intestinal tract for fluid, electrolytes, and nutrients to be absorbed adequately. Any factor that increases or decreases the motility of the intestinal tract may result in decreased absorption of fluid and electrolytes. Resection of the bowels, vagotomy, and certain agents (serotonin, laxatives, prostaglandins, prokinetic agents) can increase intestinal motility. Decreases in motility can result from autonomic injury or smooth muscle injury to the intestine and result in bacterial overgrowth, subsequently leading to diarrhea.

DIAGNOSTIC CRITERIA

A careful travel and social history is important to identify and treat specific causes, such as infection. Use of empiric antibiotic therapy is not recommended due to increasing resistance of many strains of bacteria. Selective testing of stool will be cost-effective while helping to guide the clinician in the use of specific therapy. According to the guidelines of the Infectious Disease Society of America (Guerrant et al., 2001), diarrhea can be divided into three categories: community-acquired or traveler's diarrhea, nosocomial diarrhea, or persistent diarrhea. Each category can be specifically evaluated, leading to more precise therapy.

The fecal leukocyte, lactoferrin, or Hemoccult blood test is useful in patients with moderate to severe cases of acute infectious diarrhea because it supports the use of empiric antibiotic therapy in the febrile patient. However, measuring fecal leukocytes can be unreliable if specimens are transported, refrigerated, or frozen. Fecal lactoferrin, as a measure of polymorphonuclear neutrophils, has an advantage over fecal leukocytes as a highly sensitive and specific testing method for intestinal inflammation. Stool cultures have traditionally been used to identify the pathology of diarrhea, but the positive yields are very poor and incur high costs. Controversy exists regarding when to obtain stool cultures. The absence of vomiting with persistent diarrhea may also indicate the need for stool cultures. Hypotension, tachycardia, orthostasis, bloody stool, and abdominal pain and tenderness were not found to be good predictors of a positive stool culture.

Laboratory evaluation for ova and parasites should be performed in the following:

- A person not previously treated with empiric antiparasitic therapy
- A person with persistent diarrhea for more than 7 days
- A person who recently traveled to mountainous regions, Russia, or Nepal
- A person who was exposed to infants at daycare centers or who was exposed through a community water-borne outbreak
- A person with bloody diarrhea with few or no fecal leukocytes
- Homosexual men or patients with AIDS

For food- or water-borne pathogens, the incubation period and clinical features can give clues as to the source of infection.

Diarrhea and vomiting 6 hours after exposure to a food item suggests exposure to *Staphylococcus aureus* or *Bacillus cereus*. An incubation period of 8 to 14 hours suggests *Clostridium perfringens*. With an incubation period greater than 14 hours, with vomiting as the predominant feature, viral agents are suspected. In patients with fever greater than 101.3°F plus leukocyte-, lactoferrin-, or Hemoccult-positive stools, or acute dysentery (grossly bloody stools), the most common pathogens identified by normal stool culture are *Shigella*, *Salmonella*, *Campylobacter*, *Aeromonas*, and *Yersinia*. Additionally, patients with grossly bloody stools should be tested for *E. coli* O157 or HUS.

INITIATING DRUG THERAPY

Most cases of diarrhea are self-limiting and can be self-treated. However, patients with profuse, watery diarrhea with dehydration, passage of blood and mucus, and fever exceeding 101.3°F should be evaluated for an inflammation-producing pathogen. These patients may benefit from antimicrobial therapy. In addition, a good history helps to determine the cause of illness. In diarrhea caused by infectious organisms, the pathogen should be identified so that therapy may be initiated to eradicate the organism and to prevent exposure to unnecessary antibiotics.

For traveler's diarrhea, prophylactic agents may be given to patients who should not, cannot, or will not comply with dietary restrictions. Chemoprophylaxis of traveler's diarrhea is controversial and usually is not recommended for patients unless the patient has an underlying illness (AIDS, prior gastric surgery), the purpose of the trip is particularly important (politicians, honeymoon), or the patient cannot or will not comply with dietary restrictions. In such cases, the use of bismuth subsalicylate (BSS) (Pepto-Bismol), 2 tablets with meals and at bedtime, is recommended unless the reason for prophylaxis is a serious underlying illness. In these cases, a quinolone antibiotic should be used.

If prophylactic therapy is not prescribed, empiric therapy with a quinolone antibiotic at the first symptoms of diarrhea is recommended (Table 30-3). Patients should be properly hydrated, and BSS may be used to treat symptoms. Loperamide (Imodium) is a more effective option than BSS, but loperamide should be used with caution in the presence of fever or bloody stools because the antimotility effects of the

Table 30.3

Indications for Empiric and Specific Antimicrobial Therapy in Infectious Diarrhea

Indication for Antimicrobial Therapy	Suggested Antimicrobial Therapy
Fever (oral temperature >38.5°C or 101.3°F) together with one of the following: dysentery (grossly bloody stools) or those with leukocyte-, lactoferrin-, or Hemoccult-positive stools	Quinolone:* NF 400 mg, CF 500 mg, OF 300 mg bid for 3–5 d
Moderate to severe traveler's diarrhea	Quinolone:* NF 400 mg, CF 500 mg, OF 300 mg bid for 1–5 d
Persistent diarrhea (possible *Giardia* infection)	Metronidazole 250 mg qid for 7 d
Shigellosis	If acquired in the U.S., give TMP-SMX 160/800 mg bid for 3 d; if acquired during international travel, treat as febrile dysentery (above); check to be certain of susceptibility to drug used.
Intestinal salmonellosis	If healthy host with mild or moderate symptoms, no therapy; for severe disease or that associated with fever and systemic toxicity or other important underlying condition, use TMP-SMX 160 mg/800 mg or quinolone:* NF 400 mg, CF 500 mg, OF mg bid for 5–7 d depending on speed of response
Campylobacteriosis	Erythromycin stearate 500 mg bid for 5 d
Enteropathogenic *Escherichia coli* diarrhea (EPEC)	Treat as febrile dysentery
Enterotoxigenic *E. coli* diarrhea (ETEC)	Treat as moderate to severe traveler's diarrhea
Enteroinvasive *E. coli* diarrhea (EIEC)	Treat as shigellosis
Enterohemorrhagic *E. coli* diarrhea (EHEC)	Antimicrobials are usually withheld except in particularly severe cases, in which usefulness of these drugs is uncertain.
Aeromonas diarrhea	Treat as febrile dysentery
Noncholera *Vibrio* diarrhea	Treat as febrile dysentery
Yersiniosis	For most cases, treat as febrile dysentery; for severe cases, give ceftriaxone 1 g qd IV for 5 d.
Giardiasis	Metronidazole 250 mg qid for 7 d or (if available) tinidazole 2 g in a single dose or quinacine 100 mg tid for 7 d
Intestinal amebiasis	Metronidazole 750 mg tid for 5–10 d plus a drug to treat cysts to prevent relapses: diiodohydroxyquin 650 mg tid for 20 d or paromomycin 500 mg tid for 10 d or diloxanide furoate 500 mg tid for 10 d
Cryptosporidium diarrhea	None; for severe cases, consider paromomycin 500 mg tid for 7 d
Isospora diarrhea	TMP-SMX 160 mg/800 mg bid for 7 d
Cyclospora diarrhea	TMP-SMX 160 mg/800 mg bid for 7 d

TMP-SMX, trimethoprim–sulfamethoxazole.
*Fluoroquinolones include norfloxacin (NF), ciprofloxacin (CF), and ofloxacin (OF).
Reproduced with permission of DuPont, H. L., and the Practice Parameters Committee of the American College of Gastroenterology. (1997). Guidelines on acute infectious diarrhea in adults. *American Journal of Gastroenterology, 92,* 1962–1975.

drug may prolong disease by reducing the elimination of possible infectious pathogens. If an antidiarrheal medication is necessary, selection should be based on patient-specific variables, including potential side effects, convenience, efficacy, and the patient's symptoms. For patients with moderate or severe traveler's diarrhea, empiric antimicrobial therapy with a quinolone antibiotic may be given (see Table 30-3). Patients with persistent diarrhea lasting 2 to 4 weeks without systemic symptoms or dysentery may be studied for the cause and treated, or given metronidazole (Flagyl) for empiric anti-*Giardia* therapy.

Goals of Drug Therapy

The goals of drug therapy are to reduce the symptoms of diarrhea and to make the patient as comfortable as possible. Causative factors should be identified and eradicated. Fluid and electrolyte replacement is particularly important to avoid serious complications from dehydration. Rehydration is discussed later in this chapter.

Antidiarrheal Agents

Several types of drugs are used for the symptomatic relief of diarrhea; they include antimotility agents, adsorbents and absorbents, and the atypical antisecretory agent BSS.

Table 30-4 provides an overview of these drugs, and Table 30-5 covers the recommended order of prescription.

Antimotility Agents

The antimotility agent loperamide is a congener of the narcotic analgesic meperidine (Demerol). It is not well absorbed and does not provide analgesic or euphoric effects. Loperamide slows GI motility by direct effects on circular and longitudinal muscles in the intestines. Another meperidine congener, diphenoxylate with atropine (Lomotil), is a controlled substance (Class V).

Contraindications

The antimotility effects may exacerbate infectious diarrhea by preventing the excretion of the infecting organism, allowing the organism more contact time in the intestines. Caution should be observed in using loperamide in patients with fever, bloody stools, or fecal leukocytes. In nondysenteric forms of diarrhea caused by invasive pathogens, loperamide can be used, provided antimicrobial therapy is administered.

Because loperamide undergoes extensive first-pass metabolism, caution should be used in patients with hepatic dysfunction because excessive side effects (central nervous system toxicity) may occur in these patients.

Table 30.4

Overview of Selected Antidiarrheals

Generic (Trade) Name and Dosage	Selected Adverse Events	Contraindications	Special Considerations
Antimotility Agents			
diphenoxylate (Lomotil) 2.5–5 mg qid	Dry mouth, dry eyes, urinary retention, blurred vision, drowsiness, dizziness	Caution in patients with liver disease, fever, bloody stool, or fecal leukocytes	Drug Enforcement Administration Class V controlled substance
loperamide (Imodium) 4–16 mg/d in divided doses	Abdominal discomfort, constipation, drowsiness, dry mouth	Caution in patients with fever, bloody stools, or fecal leukocytes	May induce drowsiness; warn patients about driving or performing activities that require alertness.
Selected Antisecretory Agents			
bismuth subsalicylate (Pepto-Bismol) Start: 2 tablets or 30 mL Range: 2 tablets or 30 mL every 30 min to 1 h up to 8 doses	Black stools, darkening of tongue, tinnitus	Caution in patients who are aspirin sensitive or are taking medications that interact with warfarin. Caution in children and teenagers with the flu or chickenpox	
polycarbophil (Fiber-Con) 1–6 g/d	Stomach upset, bloating, gas	Caution: Potential for drug interactions with tetracycline or quinolones	
kaolin, pectin, and attapulgite (Kaopectate) Start: 30–120 mL of liquid or 2 tablets after each bowel movement Range: Up to 7 doses a day	Constipation, feeling of fullness, stomach bloating, gas		May adsorb nutrients and medications. Separate administration time of adsorbents and other medications.

Because of the antimotility effects of diphenoxylate, it should be used with caution in patients with infectious diarrhea associated with fever or bloody stools. Diphenoxylate provides euphoric and analgesic effects at high doses, but not at therapeutic doses. For this reason, diphenoxylate is combined with atropine to discourage abuse. Diphenoxylate should be used with caution in patients with liver impairment because the liver extensively metabolizes it.

Adverse Events

Adverse effects of loperamide include abdominal discomfort, constipation, and dry mouth. Although loperamide does not cross the blood–brain barrier, it may still induce drowsiness in some patients. Patients should be warned of the potential for drowsiness before driving or performing activities that require alertness. Although loperamide is usually well tolerated, it is not recommended in children younger than 4 years of age because shock, enterocolitis, fatal intestinal obstruction, and central nervous system toxicity have occurred.

Atropine has anticholinergic effects such as dry mouth, dry eyes, urinary retention, constipation, blurred vision, and tachycardia. Diphenoxylate may cause drowsiness or dizziness, and patients should be warned of these effects and should avoid activities that require alertness. The liquid formulation is recommended in children because the dose needs to be carefully tailored to the child based on age and weight. Diphenoxylate with atropine can cause respiratory depression in infants and young children and should be avoided in children younger than 4 years of age.

Interactions

Diphenoxylate may potentiate the action of depressants such as alcohol, barbiturates, or benzodiazepines. In addition, atropine may potentiate the effects of other agents with anticholinergic properties such as tricyclic antidepressants,

Table 30.5

Recommended Order of Treatment for Diarrhea

Order	Agents	Comments
First line	Loperamide	Easy to use, tablet or liquid
Second line	Adsorbents or antisecretory agent	Selection based on drug–drug interactions or allergies (eg, aspirin sensitivity and bismuth subsalicylate)
Third line	Diphenoxylate	Side effect profile, especially with atropine added, lowers the utility of this agent.

antipsychotics, and antihistamines. Diphenoxylate has a structure similar to that of meperidine, and when used concomitantly with monoamine oxidase inhibitors can induce a hypertensive crisis.

Atypical Antidiarrheal

BSS has antisecretory, antimicrobial, and adsorbent properties, making it a reasonably useful agent for traveler's diarrhea.

Contraindications

BSS is broken down in the intestinal tract to salicylate; therefore, it should be used with caution in patients taking aspirin therapy or those hypersensitive to aspirin. In addition, caution should be used in children and adolescents with the flu or chickenpox because this population is at risk for aspirin-induced Reye syndrome.

Adverse Effects

Side effects of BSS include black stools, darkening of the tongue, and tinnitus, which can be a potential sign of salicylate toxicity.

Interactions

Because BSS has a salicylate component, it may interact with other medications that interact with aspirin (eg, warfarin).

Adsorbents and Absorbents

Mechanism of Action

Kaolin, pectin, and attapulgite (Donnagel, Kaopectate) are all examples of adsorbents used alone or in combination in antidiarrheal preparations. These agents adsorb water and help to solidify loose stools. Adsorbents are usually given after each bowel movement until diarrhea is relieved or a maximum dose is reached. Dosages of different products and product combinations vary, but the dose of most adsorbents usually ranges from 30 to 120 mL or 2 tablets after each bowel movement up to six or seven doses per day for adults.

Polycarbophil (FiberCon, Fiberall), an absorbent, absorbs water in the GI tract and is used as an antidiarrheal. Its fiber content also makes it useful as a bulk-forming laxative when taken with plenty of water.

Adverse Events

The most common side effects of the adsorbents are constipation and a feeling of fullness. Absorbents may also produce upset stomach, bloating, and gas. Adsorbents and absorbents are generally considered safe because the medication works locally and is not absorbed systemically. However, adsorbents may not be as effective as antimotility agents at reducing the symptoms of diarrhea.

Interactions

Adsorbents are not selective and may adsorb nutrients and medications. This interaction must be taken into consideration because several doses may be necessary each day. Separating administration times of adsorbents and other medications is advised. Polycarbophil contains calcium and may interact with fluoroquinolone and tetracycline antibiotics.

Selecting the Most Appropriate Agent

The choice of antidiarrheal agent should be based on several factors, including the patient's history, potential side effects of the medication, potential for drug interactions, and efficacy of the available agents (see Table 30-5; Fig. 30-2).

First-Line Therapy

Although the adsorbents are not absorbed into the systemic circulation and are usually safe and well tolerated, they are not as effective at controlling diarrhea as loperamide. Therefore, loperamide may be considered as first-line therapy secondary to its efficacy. Loperamide is also reasonably well tolerated and has few drug interactions. However, patients should be warned about the potential for loperamide to cause drowsiness (particularly patients who must stay alert).

Because loperamide is an antimotility agent, it should be used with caution in patients with fever or bloody stools to avoid exacerbation of infectious diarrhea. In addition, caution should be used in patients with liver failure.

Second-Line Therapy

For patients who cannot tolerate loperamide or for those with contraindications, an adsorbent or antisecretory agent may be chosen.

Antisecretory agents such as BSS should be used with caution in patients taking warfarin and should be avoided in children or adolescents with the flu. Antisecretory agents should also be avoided in patients with a documented hypersensitivity to salicylates. Black stools, darkening of the tongue, and tinnitus are side effects that may be disturbing to the patient. BSS may be useful for prophylaxis against traveler's diarrhea and may be preferable over the adsorbants in a patient who also has indigestion or stomach upset that accompanies the diarrhea.

Although adsorbents may inhibit the absorption of nutrients from the diet and can cause some abdominal cramping, they are usually well tolerated.

Third-Line Therapy

Although diphenoxylate with atropine is an effective agent for treating diarrhea, the atropine component can cause significant anticholinergic effects that may exacerbate certain conditions and interact with other agents with anticholinergic activity. In addition, diphenoxylate is a Drug Enforcement Administration Schedule V drug, and its potential for abuse limits this agent to third-line therapy.

Special Populations

Pediatrics

The Provisional Committee on Quality Improvement, Subcommittee on Acute Gastroenteritis (1996), published recommendations on the use of antidiarrheals in children. Their

400

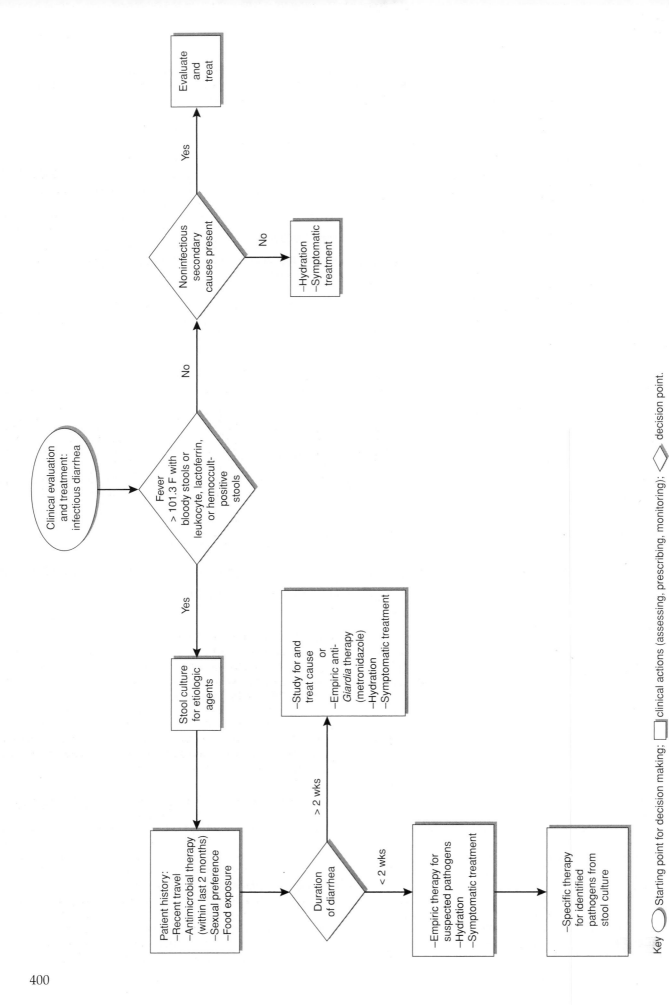

Figure 30-2 Treatment algorithm for diarrhea.

Key: ◯ Starting point for decision making; ▢ clinical actions (assessing, prescribing, monitoring); ◇ decision point.

recommendations apply to children 1 month to 5 years of age who have no previously diagnosed disorders. They suggested that opiate and atropine combination drugs such as diphenoxylate with atropine be avoided in acute diarrhea in children because of the potential for side effects and the limited scientific evidence for efficacy. The committee also stated that loperamide and BSS are not recommended based on limited scientific evidence. Adsorbents are also not recommended based on limited evidence. The committee recognized that major toxic effects from adsorbents are in general not a concern, but the potential for poor absorption of nutrients and antibiotics is a potential disadvantage. The committee concluded that oral rehydration is most important and that routine use of antidiarrheal agents is not recommended based on lack of evidence or the potential for side effects.

If the health care provider still decides to choose diphenoxylate with atropine, the liquid formulation should be used because specific dosing is required based on the child's weight and age. In addition, diphenoxylate with atropine is contraindicated in children younger than 2 years of age.

Geriatrics

As with the pediatric population, rehydration is of paramount importance in the geriatric population. Elderly patients are likely to have multiple disease states that cause them to be intolerant of dehydration (eg, congestive heart failure, diabetes, renal insufficiency). In addition, the antidiarrheal preparations may interact with agents that are commonly prescribed in the geriatric population. Diphenoxylate and loperamide may increase the sedative potential of benzodiazepines, antidepressants, anticholinergics, and antipsychotics. Adsorbents can reduce the absorption not only of important nutrients, but also of other medications. BSS should be used with caution in elderly patients taking aspirin and agents that interact with aspirin.

Women

As with constipation, antidiarrheals such as the adsorbents that are not absorbed systemically should be considered as first-line therapy for pregnant women with diarrhea. However, adsorbents can inhibit the absorption of important nutrients. Iron supplementation may be particularly important in pregnant women taking adsorbents for diarrhea. Loperamide has not been shown to be teratogenic in animals but has been inadequately studied in humans; therefore, the routine use of loperamide is not recommended. Diphenoxylate with atropine should be avoided because it has been shown to be teratogenic in animals. In addition, malformations in infants after first-trimester exposure have been reported. Both Lomotil and loperamide are excreted in breast milk. Salicylates have been shown to be teratogenic in animals. Therefore, use of BSS in the pregnant woman should be avoided.

MONITORING PATIENT RESPONSE

For most cases of diarrhea, the major concern is dehydration. Fluid and electrolyte depletion can lead to hypotension, tachycardia, and vascular collapse. Vascular collapse may occur quickly in the very old or the very young. Severe dehydration may result in decreased plasma volume and a decrease in perfusion, which may be of clinical significance, particularly in patients with congestive heart failure or chronic renal disease. Bicarbonate loss from excessive diarrhea may result in metabolic acidosis. This may be of particular concern in patients with type 1 diabetes mellitus who may be prone to ketoacidosis.

Patients should be monitored for signs of dehydration, such as orthostatic hypotension and poor skin turgor. The body weight of an infant is mostly water, and therefore infants may be weighed to determine significant fluid loss and dehydration from severe diarrhea. Monitoring of serum electrolytes as well as the patient's intake of fluid and output of stools benefits patients who are hospitalized secondary to dehydration.

As stated earlier, the goal of therapy is not only to prevent dehydration but also to make the patient as comfortable as possible. Monitoring the effectiveness of an antidiarrheal preparation requires interviewing the patient to ensure a decrease in stool frequency and improved formation. Frequency and formation of stools vary from patient to patient, and determination of relief is subjective on the patient's part.

PATIENT EDUCATION

To avoid complications, patients should be educated about appropriate rehydration. In most cases, simple replacement of fluid and electrolytes with sports drinks, fruit juices, soft drinks, soda crackers, broths, and soups is all that is necessary in the nondehydrated adult with diarrhea. In the elderly or immunocompromised patient, solutions with sodium content in the range of 45 to 75 mEq/L are recommended. Boiled potatoes, noodles, rice, cereals, crackers, bananas, yogurt, soup, and boiled vegetables are recommended during the acute phase of diarrhea. The diet may return to normal as stools become formed.

Infants and children are particularly susceptible to dehydration with diarrhea. Oral replacement therapy is the preferred treatment to replace fluids and electrolytes in children with mild to moderate dehydration because it is less expensive than intravenous therapy and can be administered in many settings, including the home. Oral glucose–electrolyte solutions available in the United States (Table 30-6) are based on physiologic principles and should be recommended over commonly used nonphysiologic solutions such as colas, apple juice, chicken broth, and sports beverages.

The Provisional Committee (1996) Practice Parameter includes recommendations for rehydration in children 1 month to 5 years of age. For children with mild diarrhea, supplemental oral replacement solutions (ORS) may not be necessary, provided age-appropriate feeding is continued and fluids are encouraged. For children with mild dehydration (3% to 5% loss of total body weight), 50 mL/kg of ORS is recommended plus 10 mL/kg for each loose stool to replace continuing losses of fluid. For moderate dehydration (loss of 6% to 8% total body weight), 100 mL/kg of ORS is recommended plus replacement of continuing losses from stool. Severe dehydration (loss of 10% total body weight) can result in shock and is a medical emergency requiring intravenous therapy with normal saline or lactated Ringer's solution. In all situations, age-appropriate feeding should begin after dehydration is corrected.

Table 30.6

Commercially Available Oral Rehydration Solutions

Product	Carbohydrate (g/L)	Na⁺ (mEq/L)	K⁺ (mEq/L)	Cl⁻ (mEq/L)	Base (mEq/L)	Calories (kcal)
Infalyte* (Mead-Johnson)	30 (rice syrup solids)	50	25	45	34 (citrate)	126
Pedialyte† (Ross Laboratories)	25 (dextrose)	45	20	35	30 (citrate)	100
Rehydralyte (Ross Laboratories)	25 (dextrose)	75‡	20	65	30 (citrate)	100
WHO Solution§ (Ianas Bros. Packaging Co.)	20 (glucose)	90‡	20	80	10 (citrate)	80

*Available in hospitals as 6-ounce nursing bottle.
†Available in hospitals as 8-ounce nursing bottle.
‡The American Academy of Pediatrics recommends these solutions with sodium contents of 75–90 mEq/L for replacement of deficit during initial rehydration (*Pediatrics, 75,* 358, 1985).
§Must be mixed with 1 L of boiled or treated water; packets available in stores or pharmacies in all developing countries.
   Source: Manufacturer's product information.
   Reproduced with permission from American Journal of Gastroenterology. (1997). Commercially available oral rehydration solutions. *American Journal of Gastroenterology, 92,* 1962–1975.

Drug Information

Patients need to be aware of the potential side effects of antidiarrheal medications. Constipation can occur if these agents are taken for too long. Antidiarrheal agents taken in the setting of infectious diseases can prolong or worsen the disease. It is always best to contact a health care provider if diarrhea lasts more than 2 days.

Patient-Oriented Information Sources

Providing patients with information about acute diarrhea and what to expect can help them understand diarrhea and their role in the treatment. Patient education items are readily available on the Internet through the National Digestive Diseases Information Clearinghouse (NDDIC), which provides information to consumers on a wide variety of GI topics. The Centers for Disease Control and Prevention also has a wide array of patient information about diarrhea.

Nutrition/Lifestyle Changes

The widely held approach is to hold food until the gut can adequately absorb nutrients. However, in a fasting state, the enterocyte renewal of the gut is slowed.

Complementary and Alternative Medications

Acidophilus is used to treat diarrhea resulting from antibiotic use. It restores the natural flora to the bowel. One to 10 billion viable organisms per day in three or four divided doses is appropriate.

IRRITABLE BOWEL SYNDROME

Irritable bowel syndrome (IBS) is a functional bowel disorder that presents with abdominal discomfort and an alteration in bowel pattern. The disorder is an international health problem that can be one of the most perplexing

chronic abdominal complaints reported to primary care providers and gastroenterologists. Epidemiologic studies in North America suggest a prevalence of 10% to 15%, with a 4:1 female predominance (Ringel, Sperber, & Drossman, 2001)

Once thought to be associated primarily with psychological problems and stress, research is changing to an emphasis on motility of the gut, autonomic system imbalances, and increased visceral hypersensitivity. A syndrome in childhood known as recurrent abdominal pain can be a hallmark of adult IBS. The majority of patients seeking care are between 20 and 50 years old, and symptoms can wax and wane over a lifetime.

CAUSES

For many years, the chief cause of IBS was thought to be primarily psychological. Now, however, research has identified physiologic causes that are accentuated by psychological stress. Symptoms are experienced when a dysregulation occurs between the brain and the gut. Typically, the symptoms can be worse during times of physical and emotional stress, including sexual or physical abuse. In addition, some patients can identify foods that exacerbate the condition (eg, lactose, caffeine, and fatty or spicy foods). Depending on the severity of the illness, pharmacotherapy may not be required and symptoms may respond solely to lifestyle changes. These lifestyle changes need to become incorporated into the patient's daily routines. Pharmacologic interventions may be required only intermittently to maintain symptom control.

PATHOPHYSIOLOGY

In general, the syndrome is believed to have the components of motility and sensory abnormalities. This leads to dysregulation of the bowel as modulated by the central nervous system (CNS). Many neuroimmune and neuroendocrine modulators, such as serotonin (5-HT), substance P, CCK, neurotensin, cytokines, and others, contribute to the increase in visceral sensitivity, central mechanisms controlling pain and dysregulation of the brain–gut axis. Local reflex mechanisms can also be responsible for mechanical distention of the gut in response to short chain fatty acids, affecting the emptying rate of the proximal colon. The prevailing theory is that the emptying rate of the proximal colon may be the key determination of overall colon function. The GI tract is innervated intrinsically and extrinsically by various neurohormonal agents from local or distant sources. Intrinsic factors include the neurons found in the enteric nervous system, which function similarly to the CNS. Bowel motor dysfunction can be associated with inflammation as well as changes in neurotransmitters, such as 5-hydroxytryptamine (5-HT3; serotonin). This neurotransmitter is found in the GI tract, and blocking it pharmacologically can decrease visceral pain, colonic transit, and GI secretions. External factors that can alter colonic activity are eating and drinking, stress, and endogenous hormones. Increased motility and abnormal contractions of the intestinal tract can result in either diarrhea or constipation-predominant IBS, due to either accelerated whole-gut transit times or delays in colonic transit. The IBS patient's sensory perception of colonic activity in response to balloon dilatation is more sensitive than that of patients with normal colonic activity. Sensory perception is also accentuated by external factors that lead to enhanced sensations that differ from those of healthy patients. However, evidence is increasing that IBS is not a psychological illness. This is supported by the fact that IBS exists in about 12% to 20% of the general adult population.

DIAGNOSTIC CRITERIA

The hallmark symptom of IBS is abdominal pain associated with a change in the consistency of stools that is relieved by defecation. Symptoms are usually first noticed in young adulthood and can be persistent or intermittent. Weight loss, rectal bleeding, fever, acute onset, and onset after the age of 50 years are unusual in IBS and should raise suspicion of organic causes, not IBS. Diagnosis can be predominantly based on symptoms and appropriate treatment initiated, with reassessment in 3 to 6 weeks.

In 1978 the original Manning criteria proposed identifying IBS based on the presence of four symptoms: abdominal distention, pain relief with bowel action, more frequent stools with the onset of pain, and looser stools with the onset of pain. These criteria led to the establishment of an international group called the Multinational National Working Teams for Diagnosis of Functional GI Disorders. This team identified key criteria for IBS, leading to the establishment of the Rome criteria (Box 30-8), currently in the second revision, with a third revision planned for release in 2006.

For IBS to be considered as a diagnosis, the presenting clinical features may be sporadic, intermittent, or continuous but should be present for an extended period, as defined by the Rome II criteria (see Box 30-8). The chief complaint most patients report is abdominal discomfort that can be relieved with defecation; however, symptom relief is often short-lived. Patients can also report abnormal bowel habits that alternate between diarrhea and constipation or are predominantly diarrhea or constipation; it is much more common to have bowel habits that are predominantly one type. Associated components can be abdominal distention, bloat-

BOX 30–8. ROME II CRITERIA FOR IRRITABLE BOWEL SYNDROME (1999)

Symptom duration:
- Twelve weeks out of 12 months
- Symptoms required only for 1 out of 7 days
- Not required to be consecutive weeks
Symptoms include:
- Abdominal pain or discomfort
- Relief with defecation
- Change in frequency of stool

ing, and gassiness. Extreme urgency after a meal can be common and can result in an "explosive" bowel movement that relieves the overall discomfort.

Organic symptoms of abdominal pain that do not suggest IBS are those that awaken the patient from sleep, initial onset in the elderly years, a change in abdominal pain that is not associated with bowel movements, significant weight loss, rectal bleeding, steatorrhea, and fever. Also, steadily worsening symptoms should be considered atypical. These symptoms would suggest the need for additional studies. However, compared to the general population, IBS patients are not more likely to have organic causes for disease.

A key component of IBS treatment is a thorough history of symptoms, psychosocial stress, medications (because of GI symptoms from many drugs), and dietary habits (to identify nutritional patterns, gaps, and intolerances). Even in the general population, stress can result in GI symptoms. However, in the patient with IBS, these symptoms can become more pronounced. The relationship between psychological distress and GI symptoms has been well researched. Chronic and acute life stresses, including a history of verbal or sexual abuse, especially in childhood, may preclude early symptoms of IBS. These chronic stresses can contribute later in life to IBS symptoms.

Physical examination findings are often normal except for a slight diffuse abdominal tenderness with palpation, especially in the left lower quadrant near the sigmoid colon. Mild abdominal distention may also be present.

The American College of Gastroenterology Task Force (2002), in an evidence-based position paper on the management of IBS in North America, recommended minimal testing. Current treatments were evaluated and the conclusion was reached that care is often based on non-randomized, non–placebo-controlled trials. The best available data show that only 1% of IBS patients have alarming symptoms signifying serious organic disease. The minimal recommended diagnostic studies are complete blood count (CBC), chemical analysis, thyroid function testing, and stool testing for occult blood, ova, and parasites. Patients with significant diarrhea should be routinely tested for celiac sprue disease. Patients with persistent diarrhea should also have their stools tested for ova and parasites, *Giardia*-specific antigen, and *Clostridium difficile*. Other studies such as abdominal ultrasound, flexible sigmoidoscopy, barium enema, or colonoscopy do not lead to any change in the proposed treatment. Additional testing may be indicated for patients with the key symptoms previously identified or if the patient is older than 50.

Types of IBS

Mild IBS usually shows a sporadic pattern. Symptoms are worsened by stress and dietary factors. There is no alteration in the patient's daily activities because of the symptoms.

In *intermittent* IBS, the symptoms are worse and begin to affect the patient's daily life. It is more difficult to relate symptoms to specific precipitants, and a psychological component to the syndrome may be developing.

In *continuous* IBS, the symptoms affect every aspect of the patient's daily routines. An inability to pinpoint precipitants still exists, and there is a definite psychological component to the syndrome.

INITIATING DRUG THERAPY

Initial therapy is focused on establishing a therapeutic relationship and mapping out a long-term strategy. This provides the patient with knowledge regarding the disease process and lets the patient know that improvement may be a slow process, taking many months.

Patients with mild symptoms may be responsive to dietary and lifestyle changes (Box 30-9). Assessing the diet for potentially offending substances and removing those substances may improve symptoms. These substances may be lactose, caffeine, beans, cabbage, fatty foods, or alcohol. In a 1998 study, Vesa and colleagues showed a positive correlation between IBS and lactose intolerance, female sex, and abdominal pain in childhood. A 2-week trial of a lactose-free diet is worth pursuing. Aspartame, an artificial sweetener found in many soft drinks and diet foods, may also provoke diarrhea. Trial elimination may also be worthwhile, especially in diarrhea-predominant IBS. However, with most IBS therapies the placebo effect is often just as successful as the therapy itself.

Maintaining a daily diary of food intake, bowel patterns, and emotional stressors can be helpful in the treatment of IBS. It serves to identify factors that can be addressed and evaluates the effectiveness of treatment. Lifestyle modification requires the patient to understand the stressors in his or her life and the effect these stressors have on physiologic functions. Identifying ways to reduce stress can be critical to improving IBS symptoms. Biofeedback can be used to decrease gut

---

BOX 30–9. DIETARY AND LIFESTYLE CHANGES

Avoid foods that exacerbate the symptoms (eg, lactose, caffeine, fatty or spicy foods).
Incorporate routine exercise into daily activities.
Explore the life stressors that aggravate the symptoms.
Learn ways to deal with stress, such as meditation, counseling, and biofeedback.

---

sensitivity, along with relaxation tapes to decrease stressors. Verne and Cerda (1997) showed some benefit of regular exercise in reducing stress and improving bowel transit. However, as previously discussed in the section on constipation, exercise has little benefit on bowel transit time.

Goals of Drug Therapy

The pharmacologic agents used for IBS are the same as those discussed in the constipation and diarrhea sections of this chapter. The goal of pharmacotherapy for IBS is to alleviate or control the specific symptoms. Generally, clinical trials have been inadequate to establish a definite link between administration of specific drugs and relief of symptoms. In patients with IBS, between 50% and 75% still have symptoms after 5 years. Response rates to a placebo can be as high as 70% (Carlson, 1998; Mertz, 2003).

Bulk-Forming Laxatives

Previously, administration of dietary fiber in the form of a bulking agent was commonly the first agent prescribed in IBS (Table 30-7). However, administration of fiber to patients with IBS has become controversial. While the hypothesis exists that fiber increases colonic transit time and therefore lessens colon wall tension and ultimately abdominal pain, clinical trials on the use of fiber in IBS have had small sample sizes and have been short in duration. Also, fiber can exacerbate the diarrhea component of IBS. This led the American Gastroenterology Task Force in 2002 to conclude that fiber is no more effective than placebo and is not recommended for the treatment of IBS.

Hyperosmotic Laxatives

When the patient requires a laxative, it is preferable to administer one that is osmotic (see Table 30-7). These agents can work either as a disaccharide sugar, which produces an osmotic effect in the colon, resulting in colonic distention and promotion of peristalsis, or by an osmotic effect in the small intestine, drawing water into the lumen and softening the stool. Lactulose or sorbitol, disaccharide sugars, can be used for patients with predominant constipation. Polyethylene glycol 3350 (Miralax) is a glycolated laxative that can be safely used for a long period without adverse pharmacologic effects.

Contraindications

The same contraindications exist as when using these agents to treat chronic constipation. Lactulose is contraindicated in patients who must restrict their galactose intake and in patients with appendicitis, acute surgical abdomen, fecal impaction, or intestinal obstruction. Caution must be used with administration to diabetic patients because of sugar content.

Other osmotic agents such as magnesium hydroxide (Milk of Magnesia) or magnesium citrate (Citroma) can be used to promote defecation. Approximately 15% to 30% of the magnesium in these agents may be absorbed systemically; therefore, caution needs to be used in patients who have renal failure and a decreased ability to excrete magnesium.

Table 30.7

Overview of Selected Agents Used to Treat Irritable Bowel Syndrome

Generic (Trade) Name and Dosage	Selected Adverse Events	Contraindications	Special Considerations
Selected Bulk-Forming Laxatives			
psyllium (Konsyl, Metamucil, Perdiem) Start: 1 tsp in 8 oz liquid bid–tid Range: 1–2 tsp in 8 oz liquid bid–tid	Abdominal fullness, increased flatus	Symptoms of acute surgical abdomen, intestinal obstruction, or perforation Inability to drink adequate amounts of water	Comes in granules, powder, or wafers Takes 12 h to 3 d to work
calcium polycarbophil (Equalactin, FiberCon, Mitrolan) Start: 500 mg tablets qd Range: 500–1000 mg qid	Abdominal fullness, increased flatus	Same as above	Takes 12 h to 3 d to work
methylcellulose (Citrucel) Start: 1 tsp in 8 oz liquid bid–tid Range: 1–2 tsp in 8 oz liquid bid or tid	Nausea, abdominal cramps	Same as above	Takes 12 h to 3 d to work
Hyperosmotic Laxatives			
lactulose (Duphalac) syrup Start: 15–30 mL PO daily Range: 15–60 mg/d	Flatulence, intestinal cramps, diarrhea, nausea, vomiting, electrolyte imbalances	Galactose-restricted diets, appendicitis, acute surgical abdomen, fecal impaction, or intestinal obstruction Use with caution in diabetic patients.	
magnesium citrate (Citroma) oral solution Start: 5 oz qhs Range: 5–10 oz qhs	Abdominal cramping, nausea	End-stage renal disease	Can cause increased magnesium levels in patients with end-stage renal disease
magnesium hydroxide (Milk of Magnesia/M.O.M.) Start: 15 mL qhs Range: 15–60 mL qhs	Abdominal cramping, nausea	End-stage renal disease	Same as above
Stimulant Laxatives			
bisacodyl (Dulcolax) Start: 10 mg PO in evening or before breakfast Range: 10–15 mg	Abdominal cramping, nausea, vomiting, burning sensation in rectum with suppositories		Oral: 6–8 h Rectal: 15–60 min
senna concentrates (Senokot) Start: 2 tabs or 1 level tsp at hs Range: 2–4 tabs or 1–2 tsp qhs	Abdominal cramping, nausea	Signs and symptoms of appendicitis, abdominal pain, nausea, vomiting	Elderly or debilitated, halve the dose
Surfactant Laxatives			
docusate calcium (Surfak) Start: 240 mg/d Range: 240 mg/d	None	None	May increase the systemic absorption of mineral oil
docusate sodium (Colace) Start: 50 mg/d Range: 50–200 mg/d	Bitter taste, throat irritation, nausea, rash	Signs and symptoms of appendicitis	Onset: 1–3 days Not to be used for acute relief of constipation
Antidiarrheal Agents			
diphenoxylate HCl with atropine sulfate (Lomotil) Start: 5 mg qid Range: 5–10 mg qid; maintenance may be 10 mg qd	Sedation, dizziness, dry mouth, paralytic ileus	Pseudomembranous enterocolitis, obstructive jaundice, diarrhea caused by organisms that penetrate intestinal mucosa Under 2 y of age Pregnancy category C	Onset 45–60 min
loperamide HCl (Imodium) Start: 4 mg after first loose stool then 2 mg after each following stool Range: 4–16 mg/d	Constipation	Acute dysentery	Peak levels 2.5 h after liquid and 5 h after capsule
Selected Antispasmodics (Anticholinergic Agents)			
belladonna alkaloids (Donnatal) Start: 1 tab or capsule tid or qid Range: 1–2 tabs/capsules tid or qid	Drowsiness, anticholinergic effects, paradoxical excitement	Glaucoma, unstable coronary artery disease, GI or GU obstruction, paralytic ileus, severe ulcerative colitis	Antacids may inhibit absorption. Additive anticholinergic effects with other anticholinergics, antihistamines, narcotics, tricyclic antidepressants

(continued)

Table 30.7

Overview of Selected Agents Used to Treat Irritable Bowel Syndrome (*Continued*)

Generic (Trade) Name and Dosage	Selected Adverse Events	Contraindications	Special Considerations
dicyclomine HCl (Bentyl) Start: 20 mg qid Range: 20–40 mg qid if tolerated	Same as above	Same as above	Same as above
clidinium (Librax) Start: 1 capsule qid—ac and qhs Range: 1–2 capsules qid—ac and qhs	Drowsiness, anticholinergic effects, paradoxical excitement, ataxia, confusion, jaundice	Glaucoma, GI or GU obstruction	Same as above
hyoscyamine sulfate (Levsin, Levabid, Levsin SL) *Levsin* Start: 1 tab q4h prn Range: 1–2 tabs q4h prn; max 12 tabs/d *Levabid* Start: 1 tab q12h Range: 1–2 tabs q12h; max 4 tabs/d *Levsin SL* Start: 1 tab swallowed or chewed q4h prn Range: max 12 tabs/d	Same as above	Same as above	Same as above
Serotonin-3 Receptor Antagonist Alesotron (Lotronex) 1 mg po qd–bid	Severe constipation, ischemic colitis	Constipation-predominant IBS, intestinal obstruction	Access restricted to approved providers only
Serotonin-4 Agonist Tegaserod (Zelnorm) 6 mg po bid	Serious diarrhea, cholecystitis	Severe renal dysfunction or liver disease, moderate to severe bowel obstruction	Approved for use 4–6 weeks; may repeat × 1

Adverse Events

When taken appropriately, these agents are well tolerated. The most common adverse events are abdominal cramping or nausea. Extensive, long-term use of these agents can lead to laxative dependence.

Stimulant Laxatives

These laxatives vary in effects but act by increasing peristalsis through a direct effect on the smooth muscle of the intestines and by simultaneously promoting fluid accumulation in the colon and small intestine. Because of the irritating effect of the agents on the musculature, these agents should be avoided in long-term treatment. Stimulant laxatives include bisacodyl (Dulcolax) and senna concentrates (Senokot, Senokot S). As with other laxatives, stimulants are contraindicated in patients with appendicitis, acute surgical abdomen, fecal impaction, or intestinal obstruction. Rectal fissures and hemorrhoids can be exacerbated by stimulation of defecation. Action begins 6 to 10 hours after oral administration and 15 minutes to 2 hours after rectal administration (see Table 30-7).

These agents are not as well tolerated as osmotic laxatives or bulking agents because of their side effects, which include nausea, vomiting, and abdominal cramping. These side effects can be more severe with cases of severe constipation. Long-term or excessive use can lead to laxative dependence. Several OTC products use the brand name of Dulcolax. One has the main ingredient of bisacodyl and another is docusate sodium, which is a stool softener. This could be important, especially when the patient has been instructed to use the drug as bowel preparation for a GI study.

Surfactant Laxatives

This class of laxatives reduces the surface tension of the liquid contents of the bowel. Ultimately, this promotes incorporation of additional liquid into the stool, forming a softer mass, and promotes easier defecation. Examples of this class include docusate sodium (Colace, Dulcolax) and docusate calcium (Surfak). This is the laxative of choice for patients who should not strain during defecation. However, emollient laxatives only prevent constipation; they do not treat it. Administration of emollient laxatives concomitantly with mineral oil is contraindicated because of increased absorption of the mineral oil. Action with these agents usually occurs in 1 to 3 days. The practitioner should consider this class for prevention purposes, not for acute treatment (see Table 30-7). These agents are extremely well tolerated when used to prevent constipation. Side effects include mild abdominal cramping, diarrhea, and throat irritation, but these are infrequent.

Antidiarrheal Agents

Antidiarrheal agents for patients with IBS with predominant diarrhea can be used on an occasional basis (see Table 30-7). Loperamide HCl (Imodium) inhibits peristaltic activity, thereby prolonging transit time, and it can increase anal sphincter tone. Approximately 40% of the drug is absorbed from the GI tract and 75% is metabolized in the hepatic system; excretion is primarily in the feces. As previously discussed, the drug does not cross the blood–brain barrier into the CNS. Because of these properties, it is the preferred agent for treating diarrhea. Conversely, diphenoxylate HCl with atropine (Lomotil) is an opiate similar to meperidine that increases smooth muscle tone in the GI tract, inhibits motility and propulsion, and diminishes gut secretions. It is absorbed orally and extensively metabolized by the liver. It can affect the CNS, and atropine has been added to discourage abuse.

Neither of these antidiarrheal agents should be used in a patient suspected of having diarrhea from pseudomembranous colitis or ulcerative colitis, or diarrhea resulting from poisoning or microbial infection. Diphenoxylate HCl is contraindicated in patients who are hypersensitive to atropine or meperidine and patients with hepatic impairment. The atropine in Lomotil may aggravate glaucoma in patients with this disease. For additional discussion of contraindications and adverse events, see the diarrhea section.

Antispasmodic Agents

Treatment for patients with postprandial abdominal pain may require the use of antispasmodics (see Table 30-7). However, the efficacy of these medications remains unproven in controlled studies. The presumed desired action is by direct relaxation of the smooth muscle component of the GI tract. These agents competitively block the effects of acetylcholine at muscarinic cholinergic receptors that mediate the effects of parasympathetic postganglionic impulses. Examples of commonly used anticholinergics are dicyclomine HCl (Bentyl) and hyoscyamine sulfate (Levbid, Levsin SL). Less commonly used are the belladonna alkaloids (Donnatal) and clidinium (Librax). Dosing of the anticholinergics is variable and general side effects are associated with the anticholinergic actions.

Contraindications

These agents are contraindicated in patients who have glaucoma, stenosing peptic ulcer, chronic obstructive pulmonary disease, cardiac arrhythmias, impaired liver or kidney function, and myasthenia gravis. Caution should be used in patients with hypertension, hyperthyroidism, and benign prostatic hyperplasia.

Adverse Events

Side effects include dry mouth, altered taste perception, nausea, vomiting, dysphagia, blurred vision, palpitations, and urinary hesitancy and retention. Anticholinergic side effects can be used as a measure of titration to achieve the desired pharmacologic end. It is important to monitor for signs of drug toxicity: CNS signs resembling psychosis, accompanied by peripheral effects that include dilated, nonreactive pupils; blurred vision; hot, dry, flushed skin; dry mucous membranes; dysphagia; decreased or absent bowel sounds; urinary retention; hyperthermia; tachycardia; hypertension; and increased respiration.

Antidepressants

Antidepressants as a class have also been used in the treatment of IBS. It is not clear whether these agents work by improving a concomitant depression or by improving the anxiety and stress often associated with IBS. Initial work was done with use of the tricyclic agents such as imipramine (Tofranil), desipramine (Norpramin), and amitriptyline (Elavil) in patients with severe symptoms. Careful monitoring is important when tricyclic antidepressants are given to patients with IBS in which constipation predominates, because these agents can cause constipation. Newer agents in the selective serotonin reuptake inhibitor (SSRI) class may also prove beneficial. It has been suggested based on current investigations that antidepressants alter perceived pain thresholds, which are often abnormal in patients with IBS. See Chapter 44 for further discussion of these drugs.

Serotonin-3 Receptor Antagonist and Serotonin-4 Agonist

A newer class of drugs has evolved to address the brain–gut–neurotransmitter (5-HT3 and 5-HT4) connection with regard to colonic transit time. Currently there is only one drug in each class.

5-HT3 Antagonist

The serotonin-3 receptor antagonist in animal models has been shown to decrease abdominal pain, slow colonic transit time, increase rectal compliance, and improve stool consistency. Alosetron (Lovenex) was initially marketed in 1999 but pulled from the market in November 2000 by the FDA due to concerns regarding ischemic colitis and severe constipation. Alosetron is available only through providers who have officially signed with the pharmaceutical company (CDC, June 2002) and is indicated for patients who have diarrhea and no constipation.

5-HT4 Agonist

The serotonin-3 receptor antagonist is a prokinetic drug and a partial agonist of the serotonin-4 receptor. Tegaserod (Zelnorm) is an agent that acts on the neurotransmitters that stimulate the peristaltic reflex and intestinal secretions, along with inhibiting visceral sensitivity. The dosage is 6 mg twice a day; it is approved for use up to 12 weeks in women who have constipation-predominant IBS. The efficacy of this agent has been studied in four randomized placebo-controlled trials and appears superior to placebo.

Contraindications

Tegaserod is contraindicated in patients with severe renal impairment, moderate or severe hepatic impairment, a history of bowel obstruction, symptomatic gallbladder disease, and suspected sphincter of Oddi dysfunction or abdominal adhesions. Patients with gallbladder disease were more likely to need a cholecystectomy (0.17%) than those given placebo (0.06%) (FDA Talk Paper, 2002).

Adverse Events

Patients who experience worsening of abdominal pain or diarrhea while taking Tegaserod should immediately discontinue the drug. In postmarketing surveillance rare but serious cases of severe diarrhea have been reported (FDA Talk Paper, 2004). Severe diarrhea can cause hypovolemia, hypotension, and syncope. Intestinal ischemia and colitis can also occur with the use of Tegaserod; this has not been established as a causal relationship, but precautions should be taken if the patient develops rectal bleeding, bloody diarrhea, or new or worsening abdominal pain.

Interactions

Tegaserod has not been shown to interact with theophylline, digoxin, warfarin, or oral contraceptives.

Selecting the Most Appropriate Agent

The emphasis in the care of patients with IBS should be multidimensional. IBS can present in many stages: mild, moderate, or severe. Selection of the most appropriate drug therapy should be based on the presenting symptoms. Each case needs to be evaluated, and treatment should be individualized (Fig. 30-3 and Table 30-8).

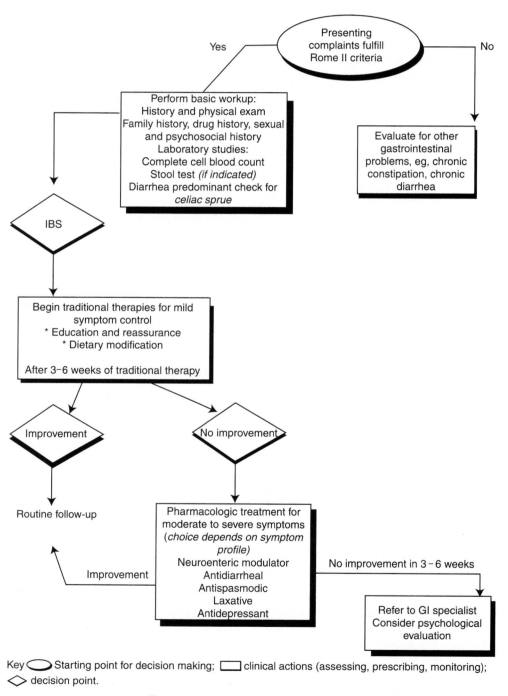

Figure 30-3 Treatment algorithm for IBS.

Table 30.8

Recommended Order for Treatment for Irritable Bowel Syndrome

Order	Agents	Comments
First Line		
Predominant constipation	Osmotic laxative—lactulose syrup, magnesium citrate, magnesium hydroxide	Milk of Magnesia is less expensive than citrate. Use magnesium products cautiously in patients with renal impairment. Use lactulose cautiously in diabetic patients.
Predominant diarrhea	Antidiarrheal—loperamide HCl (Imodium)	May cause constipation
Abdominal bloating/gas	Antispasmodics—dicyclomine HCL (Bentyl)	Caution about drowsiness; may have a dry mouth
Psychological symptoms	Antidepressants—selective serotonin reuptake inhibitors	Generally, as a class, these agents may be helpful with chronic syndromes. Cost may be an issue.
Second Line		
Predominant constipation	Continue osmotic laxatives.	
Predominant diarrhea	Antidiarrheal—diphenoxylate HCl (Lomotil)	Generalized central nervous system effects
Abdominal bloating/gas	Antispasmodics—hyoscyamine sulfate (Levsin, Levobid, Levsin SL)	Monitor for anticholinergic effects.
Psychological symptoms	Antidepressants—tricyclic agents (imipramine, desipramine, amtriptyline (Tofranil, Norpramin, Elavil)	Onset of action and steady states vary with each drug. Caution with cardiac patients
Third Line		
Predominant constipation	Laxatives—bisacodyl (Dulcolax), senna concentrates (Senakot), emollient laxatives, docusate sodium (Colace), docusate calcium (Surfak), alosetron (Lovenex)	Can aggrevate abdominal cramping Use only as additive to keep stools soft. Only approved providers can prescribe this drug.
Abdominal bloating/gas	Antispasmodics—belladonna alkaloids (Donnatal), clidinium (Librax)	More severe generalized anticholinergic effects

First-Line Therapy

First-line therapy is selected based on the presenting symptoms. Qualitatively, patients often feel the burden of this disease but believe this is not appreciated by primary care providers and specialists. Pharmacologic agents need to be considered only when an exacerbation of the disease occurs. Constipation-predominant IBS can be treated with an osmotic laxative on a long-term basis without adverse effects. Antidiarrheal agents are preferred in patients with diarrhea-predominant IBS. Loperamide is the preferred agent because it causes the least CNS activity and has the added benefit of improving anal sphincter tone. As with any chronic syndrome, use of low-level antidepressants may be helpful for symptom control.

With the additional problems of pain, gas, and abdominal bloating, a trial of an antispasmodic may relieve symptoms. Dicyclomine is the agent of first choice because of its shorter half-life, which may minimize the anticholinergic side effects of the class. Psychological symptoms associated with IBS may be treated by antidepressants. Selection of an antidepressant should be based on the specific symptoms of depression, stress, or anxiety. The SSRIs are the most commonly selected agents because of their safety profile and efficacy.

Second-Line Therapy

Unresolved complaints of predominant diarrhea can be treated with diphenoxylate HCl, which has a longer duration of action but can be addictive because of its opioid properties and should be reserved for short-term use. For postprandial abdominal pain, gas, and abdominal bloating, longer-acting antispasmodics such as hyoscyamine sulfate can be considered. The second-line choice for psychological symptoms is the tricyclic antidepressants; these agents have more side effects than SSRIs.

Third-Line Therapy

The use of stimulant laxatives in cases of constipation-predominant IBS should be reserved for more resistant cases, but these agents should be used with caution. They should not be used for long periods, and they can aggravate abdominal cramping. The older anticholinergics such as the belladonna alkaloids and clidinium should be used very sparingly for postprandial abdominal pain, gas, and abdominal bloating because they produce more intense anticholinergic side effects.

Special Considerations

Pediatrics

Children with crampy abdominal pain, constipation, or diarrhea present a challenge to the practitioner. Although these symptoms sound like IBS, there are no established criteria for children. As previously discussed, some experts think that these children may acquire IBS later in life. Treatment for these symptoms can include some of the same approaches of increasing fiber and use of antidiarrheal agents and the newer antispasmodics. Close follow-up is an important aspect of care.

Geriatrics

Initial presentation of IBS in people older than 50 years of age is rare, and abdominal pain in older patients should be considered a more ominous symptom unless they have been previously diagnosed with IBS or spastic colon, a version of colitis. Older patients may report a long-standing history of bowel trouble with any of these diagnoses.

Women

In Western society, women are more likely to have IBS and to seek care. A history of verbal or sexual abuse may also contribute to IBS. Women have surgery more often when the origins of abdominal pains are unclear.

MONITORING PATIENT RESPONSE

Monitoring the patient's response to therapy should take place within 3 to 6 weeks of the initial evaluation. For patients with mild symptoms, the initial treatment includes working with the patient regarding dietary and lifestyle changes, education about the disease process, and reassurance about lack of organic causes. Patients with intermittent symptoms require the same initial approach, but addition of pharmacologic therapy can prove helpful, if only for the placebo effect of the drugs. Psychological counseling may also be helpful with these patients. Severe IBS requires all of these interventions and the addition of intensive psychotherapy. Patients with mild to intermittent symptoms can easily be managed in the primary care office with close monitoring initially, every 3 to 6 weeks, and then more routine care.

IBS is a disease of exacerbations and remissions, but up to 70% of patients respond to treatment within 12 to 18 months. Those with a shorter duration of symptoms and fewer psychological symptoms have a better prognosis. Referral to a specialist should occur when there is no relief with any therapies, or when the patient has atypical symptomatology. Some patients do not respond. Continued symptoms rarely need a reappraisal of the diagnosis, but appropriate testing should be performed.

PATIENT EDUCATION

Patient education needs to cover dietary modifications, psychological stresses, and lifestyle changes. Begin by acknowledging the patient's fears and concerns and show that you take them seriously. According to current evidence-based research, patients can be reassured of the absence of organic disease based on the history and physical examination. The patient should be informed that this is a chronic disease and that IBS does not lead to cancer, colitis, or an altered life expectancy. Making the necessary dietary changes can be crucial for symptom relief, especially with mild symptoms. A multidisciplinary approach is often the best method of care, using the services of a dietitian and psychological counselor.

Drug Information

A variety of drugs are available to help control symptoms, and most have minimal side effects. However, the drugs need to be used in conjunction with stress relief techniques, identification of influencing factors, and education about the disease to help provide an improved quality of life.

Patient-Oriented Information Sources

Many resources exist for patients with IBS. One of the most comprehensive resources is the American College of Gastroenterology, which covers many topics on GI health. The International Foundation of Functional Bowel Disorders also has a comprehensive website with resources for both patients and health care providers (Box 30-10).

Nutrition/Lifestyle Changes

A major focus of caring for patients with IBS is helping them assess their diet, making adjustments as necessary. A trial of removing lactose foods from the diet poses no risks to the patient and may have a benefit if it relieves symptoms.

BOX 30–10. PATIENT RESOURCES FOR IRRITABLE BOWEL SYNDROME

http://www.gastro.org/generalPublic.html
http://www.aboutibs.org/
http://www.iffgd.org/index.html

■ Case Study 1

C.J. is a 71-year-old woman who presents for follow-up. She complains of hard, dry stools over the past week. She remembers reading an educational brochure she picked up in her pharmacy that suggested increasing her fiber and fluid intake, but this has not alleviated her problem. C.J.'s past medical conditions include hypertension and chronic renal insufficiency. She had a stroke 1 year ago with little or no residual. Her medications include verapamil SR 240 mg daily, lisinopril 10 mg orally once daily, calcium carbonate 1,250 mg twice daily orally, and aspirin 325 mg orally once daily.

Diagnosis: Constipation

1. List specific goals of treatment for this patient.
2. What drug therapy would you prescribe? Why?
3. What are the parameters for monitoring the success of the therapy?
4. Discuss specific patient education based on the prescribed therapy.
5. List one or two adverse reactions for the selected agent that would cause you to change therapy.
6. What would be the choice for second-line therapy?
7. What OTC or alternative medications would be appropriate for this patient?
8. What dietary and lifestyle changes should be recommended for this patient?
9. Describe one or two drug/drug or drug/food interactions for this patient.

■ Case Study 2

J.T. is a 34-year-old white man who presents with diarrhea of 2 days' duration. His other symptoms are nausea with vomiting and bloody stools for 1 day. The history reveals that the patient has just returned from a 3-day honeymoon in Mexico. He was careful to eat steaming hot foods and beverages but did have a frozen drink the last night of the trip.

Diagnosis: Traveler's diarrhea

1. List specific goals of treatment for this patient.
2. What drug therapy would you prescribe?
3. What are the parameters for monitoring the success of the therapy?
4. Discuss specific patient education based on the prescribed therapy.
5. List one or two adverse reactions for the selected agent that would cause you to change therapy.
6. What would be the choice for second-line therapy?
7. What OTC or alternative medications would be appropriate for this patient?
8. What dietary and lifestyle changes should be recommended for this patient?
9. Describe one or two drug/drug or drug/food interactions for this patient.

■ Case Study 3

S.C. is a 38-year-old woman who presents with intermittent diarrhea with cramping that is relieved by defecation. The diarrhea is not bloody or accompanied by nausea and vomiting. Review of past medical history includes some childhood "problems with my stomach," hypertension, and a recent cholecystectomy. She works as a housekeeper in a local inn and does not drink alcohol or smoke cigarettes.

Diagnosis: Irritable bowel syndrome

1. List specific goals of treatment for this patient.
2. What drug therapy would you prescribe?
3. What are the parameters for monitoring the success of the therapy?
4. Discuss specific patient education based on the prescribed therapy.
5. List one or two adverse reactions for the selected agent that would cause you to change therapy.
6. What would be the choice for second-line therapy?
7. What OTC or alternative medications would be appropriate for this patient?
8. What dietary and lifestyle changes should be recommended for this patient?
9. Describe one or two drug/drug or drug/food interactions for this patient.

Bibliography

Starred references are cited in the text.

Abyad, A., & Mourad, F. (1996). Constipation: Common-sense care of the older patient. *Geriatrics, 51*(12), 28–36.

Alaimo, K., McDowell, M. A., Briefel, R. R., Bischof, A. M., Caughman, C. R., Loria, C. M., & Johnson, C. L. (1994). *Dietary intake of vitamins, minerals and fiber of persons ages 2 months and over in the United States: Third National Health and Nutrition Examination Survey, Phase 1, 1988–91.* Hyattsville, MD: National Center for Health Statistics; Advance data from vital and health statistics: No 258.

American Academy of Pediatrics. (1996). Guidelines for the management of acute gastroenteritis in young children. *Pediatrics, 97*(3). Retrieved July 11, 2004, from www.aap.org/policy/gastro.htm.

*American College of Gastroenterology Functional Gastrointestinal Disorders Task Force. (2002). Evidence-based position statement on the management of irritable bowel syndrome in North America. *American Journal of Gastroenterology, 97(11),* S1.

American Dietetic Association. (1997). Health implications of dietary fiber–Position of ADA. *Journal of American Dietetic Association, 97,* 1157.

Annelis, M., & Koch, T. (2003). Constipation and the preached trio: diet, fluid, intake, exercise. *International Journal of Nursing Studies, 40,* 843. Abstract obtained from Medline.

Baig, M., Zhao, R., Woodhouse, S., Abramson, S., Singh, J., Weiss, E., Nogueras, J., & Wexner, S. (2002). Variability in serotonin and enterochromaffin cells in patients with colonic inertia and idiopathic diarrhea as compared to normal controls. *Colorectal Disease, 4,* 348.

Baker, S. S., Liptak, G. S., Colletti, R. B., Croffie, J. M., Di Lorenzo, C., Ector, W., & Nurko, S. (1999). Constipation in infants and children: evaluation and treatment. A medical position statement of the North American Society for Pediatric Gastroenterology and Nutrition. *Journal of Pediatric Gastroenterology and Nutrition, 29*(5), 612.

Barry, M. (2004). Review of the book *Travelers' Diarrhea. New England Journal of Medicine, 350,* 1801.

Bertram, S., Kurland, M., Lydick, E., Locke, R., & Yawn, B. (2001). The patient's perspective of irritable bowel syndrome. *Journal of Family Practice, 50*(6), 521.

Besedovsky, A., & Bu, L. (2004). Across the developmental continuum of irritable bowel syndrome: Clinical and pathophysiologic considerations. *Current Gastroenterology Reports, 6*(3), 247. Abstract obtained from Medline.

Bonapace, E. S., & Fischer, R. S. (1998). Constipation and diarrhea in pregnancy. *Gastroenterology Clinics of North America, 27,* 197.

Bouhnik, Y., Neut, C., Raskine, L., Michel, C., Riottot, M., Andrieux, C., Guillernot, F., Dyard, F., & Flourie, B. (2004). Prospective randomized, parallel-group trial to evaluate the effects of lactulose and polyethylene glycol-4000 on colonic flora in chronic idiopathic constipation. *Alimentary Pharmacology & Therapeutics, 19,* 889. Abstract obtained from http://ejournals.ebsoco.com. Retrieved on May 11, 2004.

Brandt, L. J., Bjorkman, D., Fennerty, M. B., Locke, G. R., Olden, K., Peterson, W., Quigley, E., Schoenfeld, P., Schuster, M., & Talley, N. (2002). Systematic review on the management of irritable bowel syndrome in North America. *American Journal of Gastroenterology, 97*(11), S7.

*Bushen, O., & Guerrant, R. (2003). Acute infectious diarrhea: approach and management in the emergency department. *Topics in Emergency Medicine, 25,* 139.

Camilleri, M. (1999). Therapeutic approach to the patient with irritable bowel syndrome. *American Journal of Medicine, 107*(5A), 27S.

Camilleri, M., & Ford, M. (1998). Review article: colonic sensorimotor physiology in health, and its alteration in constipation and diarrhoeal disorders. *Alimentary Pharmacology & Therapeutics, 12,* 287.

Camilleri, M., Mayer, E. A., Drossman, D. A., Health, A., Dukes, G. E., McSorley, D., Kong, S., Mangel, A. W., & Northcutt, A. R. (1999). Improvement in pain and bowel function in female irritable bowel patients with alosetron, a 5-HT$_3$ receptor agonist. *Alimentary Pharmacology & Therapeutics, 13,* 1149.

*Carlson, E. (1998). Irritable bowel syndrome. *Nurse Practitioner, 23*(1), 82–93.

Centers for Disease Control and Prevention. (1992). The management of acute diarrhea in children: oral rehydration, maintenance, and nutritional therapy. *MMWR, 41* (No. RR-16).

Chaussade, S., & Minic, M. (2003). Comparison of efficacy and safety of two doses of two different polyethylene glycol-based laxatives in the treatment of constipation. *Alimentary Pharmacologic Therapeutics, 17,* 165.

Chen, B., Knowles, C., Scott, M., Anand, P., Williams, S., Milbrandt, J., & Tam, P. (2002). Idiopathic slow transit constipation and megacolon are not associated with neurturin mutations. *Neurogastroenterology Motility, 14,* 513.

*Cunha, B. A. (1998). Nosocomial diarrhea. *Critical Care Clinics, 14,* 329–338.

Dalton, C., & Drossman, D. (1997). Diagnosis and treatment of irritable bowel syndrome. *American Family Physician, 55*(3), 875.

DePontini, F., & Tonini, M. (2001). Irritable bowel syndrome: new agents targeting serotonin receptor subtypes. *Drugs, 61*(3), 317.

DeYoung, G. R. (2004). Tegaserod (Zelnorm) for irritable bowel syndrome. *American Family Physician, 69,* 363.

*Dosh, S. (2002). Evaluation and treatment of constipation. *Journal of Family Practice, 51.* Retrieved from http://www.jpoline.com/content/2002/06/jfp_0602_0555c.asp on June 30, 2004.

Drossman, D., & Thompson, W. G. (1992). The irritable bowel syndrome: review and a graduated multicomponent treatment approach. *Annals of Internal Medicine, 116*(12), 1009.

DuPont, H. I., and the Practice Parameters Committee of the American College of Gastroenterology. (1997). Guidelines on acute infectious diarrhea in adults. *American Journal of Gastroenterology, 92,* 1962.

Ellis, M., & Meadows, S. (2002). What is the best therapy for constipation in infants? *Journal of Family Practice, 51,* 708. Retrieved from http://www.jpoline.com/content/2002/08/jfp_0802_0708c.asp on June 30, 2004.

El-Salhy, M., & Spangeus, A. (2002). Gastric emptying in animal models of human diabetes: correlation to blood glucose level and gut neuroendocrine peptide content. *Upsala Journal of Medical Science, 107,* 89.

*FDA Talk Paper (2002). FDA approves first treatment for women with constipation-predominant irritable bowel syndrome. Retrieved from http://www.fda.gov/bbs/topics/ANSWERS/2002/ANSO1160.html on May 23, 2004.

*FDA Talk Paper (2004). FDA updates Zelnorm labeling with new risk information. Retrieved from http://www.fda.gov/bbs/topics/ANSWERS/2004/ANSO1285.html on May 23, 2004.

Field, M. (2003). Intestinal ion transport and the pathophysiology of diarrhea. *Journal of Clinical Investigation, 111,* 931.

Fleming, K. A., Zimmerman, H., & Shubik, P. (1998). Granulomas in the livers of humans and Fischer rates associated with ingestion of mineral hydrocarbons: A comparison. *Regulatory Toxicology and Pharmacology, 27,* 75.

Gallagher, C. (2003). A guideline-based approach for managing acute gastroenteritis in children. *JSPN, 8*(3),107.

Gattuso, J. M., & Kamm, M. A. (1994). Adverse effects of drugs used in the management of constipation and diarrhea. *Drug Safety, 10*(1), 47.

Greenberg, M., Amitrone, H., & Galiczynski, E. (2002). A contemporary review of irritable bowel syndrome. *Physician Assistant, 26*(8), 26.

*Guerrant, R., Van Gilden, T., Steines, T., Thielman, N., Slutsker, L., Tauxe, R., Hennessy, T., Griffin, P., DuPont, H., Sack, R. B., Tart, P., Neill, M., Nachamkin, I., Reller, L. B., Osterholm, M.,

Bennish, M., & Pickering, L. (2001). Practice guidelines for the management of infectious diarrhea. *Clinical Infectious Disease, 32,* 331.

Guthrie, E., & Thompson, D. (2002). ABC of psychological medicine: Abdominal pain and functional gastrointestinal disorders. *British Medical Journal, 325,* 701.

Hagemann, T. M. (1998). Gastrointestinal medications and breast-feeding. *Journal of Human Lactation, 14,* 259–262.

Hatari, D., Gurwitz, J. H., Avorn, J., Bohn, R., & Minaker, K. L. (1996). Bowel habit in relation to age and gender: Findings from the National Health Interview survey and clinical implications. *Archives of Internal Medicine, 156,* 315.

Hatari, D., Gurwitz, J. H., Avorn, J., Bohn, R., & Minaker, K.L. (1997). How do older persons define constipation? Implications for therapeutic management. *Journal of General Internal Medicine, 12,* 63–66.

*Higgins, P. D., & Johanson, J. F. (2004). Epidemiology of constipation in North America: a systematic review. *American Journal of Gastroenterology, 4,* 750–759. Abstract obtained from PubMed.

Holten, K. (2003). Irritable bowel syndrome: minimize testing, let symptoms guide treatment. *Journal of Family Practice, 52*(12), 942.

Jancin, B. (2002). New evidenced-based guidelines target IBS: Diagnostic work-up simplified. *OB/GYN News, Dec. 1.* Retrieved from http://www.findarticles.com/cf_ds/mOCYD/23_37/95514144/print.jhtml on Feb. 6, 2004.

Kellow, J. E., Delvaux, M. M., Azpiroz, F., Camilleri, M., Quigley, E. M. M., & Thompson, D. G. (2000). Principles of applied neurogastroenterology: Motility/sensation. In D. A.Drossman, E. Corazziari, N. J. Talley, W. G. Thompson, & W. E. Whitehead (Eds.), *Rome II: The functional gastrointestinal disorders* (2nd ed., pp. 91–156). Lawrence, KS: Allen Press.

Larson, S. C. (1997). Traveler's diarrhea. *Emergency Medicine Clinics of North America, 15,* 179.

Lembo, A., & Camilleri, M. (2003). Current concepts: chronic constipation. *New England Journal of Medicine, 345,* 1360.

Levron, J. C., Moing, L., & Chwetzoff, E. (1996). Example of active therapeutic follow-up: Itraconazole. *Therapie, 51,* 502–506.

Loening-Bauke, V., Miele, E., & Staiano, A. (2004). Fiber (glucomannan) is beneficial in the treatment of childhood constipation. *Pediatrics, 113,* 259.

Loening-Bauke, V. (1996). Encopresis and soiling. *Pediatric Clinics of North America, 43,* 279.

Loening-Bauke, V. (1997). Urinary incontinence and urinary tract infection and their resolution with treatment of chronic constipation of childhood. *Pediatrics, 100,* 228.

McGilley, B. M., & Pryor, T. L. (1998). Assessment and treatment of bulimia nervosa. *American Family Physician, 57,* 2743.

*Mertz, H. (2003). Irritable bowel syndrome. *New England Journal of Medicine, 349,* 2136.

Montgomery, L., & Scoville, C. (2002). What is the best way to evaluate diarrhea? *Journal of Family Practice, 51,* 575. Retrieved from http://www.jpoline.com/content/2002/06/jfp_0602_0575c.asp on June 30, 2004.

Moser, R. (1986). Irritable bowel syndrome: A misunderstood psychophysiological affliction. *Journal of Counseling and Development, 65,* 108.

National Digestive Diseases Information Clearinghouse (2003). *What I need to know about constipation* [Brochure] (NIH publication No. 03-2754).

National Digestive Diseases Information Clearinghouse (2004). *Constipation in children* [Brochure] (NIH publication No. 04-4633).

O'Sullivan, G. C. (2001). Probiotics. *British Journal of Surgery, 88,* 161.

*Ringel, Y., Sperber, A. D., & Drossman, D. A. (2001). Irritable bowel syndrome. *Annual Review of Medicine, 52,* 319.

*Schiller, L. (2001). Constipation. *Best Practice of Medicine, Oct. 22.* Retrieved from http://merck.praxis.md on Feb. 6, 2004.

Schmulson, M., & Chang, L. (1999). Diagnostic approach to the patient with irritable bowel syndrome. *American Journal of Medicine, 107*(5A), 20S.

Shafik, A. (2003). Anorectal motility in patients with achalasia of the esophagus: recognition of an esophagorectal syndrome. *BMC Gastroenterology, 3,* 28. Retrieved from http://www.biomedcenteral.com/1471-230X/3/28.

Shafik, A., Shafik, A.A., & Ahmend, I. (2003). Effect of colonic distention on ileal motor activity with evidence of coloileal reflex. *Journal of Gastrointestinal Surgery, 7,* 701.

Sloots, C. E. J., & Felt-Bersma, R. J. F. (2003). Rectal sensorimotor characteristics in female patients with idiopathic constipation with or without paradoxical sphincter contraction. *Neurogastrology and Motility, 15,* 187.

*Smith, C., Hellebusch, S., & Mandel, K. (2002). Patient and physician evaluation of a new bulk fiber laxative tablet. *Gastroenterology Nursing, 26,* 31.

Steffen, R., DuPont, H., Heusser, R., Helminger, A., Witassek, F., Manhart, M., & Shar, M. (1986). Prevention of diarrhea by the tablet form of bismuth subsalicylate. *Antimicrobial Agents and Chemotherapy, April,* 625.

*Stessman, M. (2003). Biofeedback: its role in treatment of chronic constipation. *Gastroenterology Nursing, 26,* 251.

Talley, N. J., Jones, M., Nuyts, G., & Dubois, D. (2003) Risk factors for chronic constipation. *98*(5), 1107. Abstract obtained from MedLine.

Thielman, N., & Guerrant, R. (2004). Acute infectious diarrhea. *New England Journal of Medicine, 350,* 38.

Toner, B., Emmott, S., Myran, D., & Drossman, D. (1999). *Cognitive-behavioral treatment of irritable bowel syndrome: The brain-gut connection.* New York: Guilford Press.

Tucker, M. (2000). First evidence-based guideline on constipation. *Family Practice News, Jan. 15.* Retrieved from http://www.find-articles.com/cf_dis/mOBJI/2_30/59616045/print.jhtml on Feb. 6, 2004.

U.S. Food and Drug Administration Center for Drug Evaluation and Research. (2002). *Medication guide for Lotronex tablets.* Retrieved from http://www.fda.gov/cder/drug/infopage/lotronex/medguide060502.htm.

*Verne, N., & Cerda, J. (1997). Irritable bowel syndrome: Streamlining the diagnosis. *Postgraduate Medicine, 102*(3), 197.

*Versa, T., Seppo, L., Marteau, P., et al. (1998). Relief of irritable bowel syndrome in subjective lactose intolerance. *American Journal of Clinical Nutrition, 67,* 710–715.

Visit the Connection web site for the most up-to-date drug information.

31

INFLAMMATORY BOWEL DISEASE

■ LIZA TAKIYA

Inflammatory bowel disease (IBD) is a generic term used to describe two main chronic inflammatory conditions of the gastrointestinal (GI) tract: Crohn's disease (CD) and ulcerative colitis (UC). Although these conditions are similar in clinical presentation, CD is a chronic inflammatory disease characterized by transmural lesions located at any point on the GI tract, whereas UC is a chronic disease consisting of mucosal inflammation limited to the colon. IBD affects approximately 1 million Americans. The prevalence of CD is estimated to be approximately 133 cases per 100,000; the prevalence of UC is estimated to be 229 cases per 100,000 (American Gastroenterological Association [AGA], 2001). Both conditions are more common in whites than in blacks, Asians, or Native Americans, and those of Jewish descent have a three- to sixfold greater incidence than the non-Jewish population. IBD shows no gender predilection and is usually first diagnosed in men or women between the ages of 15 and 25 years (AGA, 2001). Although the mortality rate is low for the disease, it significantly affects the patient's overall mental status, physical health, and quality of life. The most common emotional issues surrounding uncontrolled IBD appear to be anger, frustration, depression, and low self-esteem. These issues usually stem from the patient's inability to participate in routine activities, leading to a decreased quality of life. The disease has a negative impact on social interactions and daily functional status, leading to decreased productivity and attendance at work or school, decreased social engagements, and loss of independence. Health-related issues mirror those related to poor GI absorption, including nutritional deficiencies, electrolyte abnormalities, dehydration, cachexia, and iron deficiency anemia. Fatigue and lack of sleep are also common in patients with IBD. All of these may result in frequent hospitalizations, altered lifestyle, and poor general health. Overall, in 2000, IBD had an estimated financial burden of $105 million in indirect healthcare costs and over $1 billion dollars in direct costs (AGA, 2001).

CAUSES

The etiology of CD and UC is related to the stimulation of immunologic mechanisms. The inflammatory nature of the condition has led researchers to believe that an infection or autoimmune mechanism may predispose patients to IBD. A defect in the GI mucosal barrier that results in enhanced permeability and increased uptake of proinflammatory molecules and infectious agents is associated with its development. Tissue biopsy of the GI mucosal lining of patients with IBD reveals a high proportion of immunologic cytokines, including tumor necrosis factor, leukotrienes, and interleukin-1. A few bacterial and viral organisms have been associated with disease progression, including *Mycobacterium paratuberculosis*, measles virus, and *Listeria monocytogenes*; however, none has been definitively correlated with IBD.

Many other factors such as genetics, psychological factors, and the environment may contribute to the development and exacerbation of IBD. The high incidence of IBD in the Jewish population supports a genetic component of the etiology of CD and UC. A study comparing relatives of patients with IBD with the general population found a 10-fold increase in risk for development of IBD in those with familial occurrence (Orholm, Munkholm, Langholz, et al., 1991). Although the relationship between genetic factors and IBD is being studied aggressively, no specific genetic mutation or marker has been identified.

Psychological factors such as depression, anger, anxiety, or mental stress are associated with exacerbations of CD and UC, although these factors do not have a predictable effect over a large population. Various studies have associated isolated mental instability or stressful events with IBD exacerbations, but a positive correlation between psychiatric illness and IBD is unsupported.

Environmental factors, including geographic location, dietary habits, oral contraceptive use, and smoking status, are all theorized to affect CD and UC. IBD is more prevalent in the northern parts of the United States as well as in England and Scandinavian countries rather than the Mediterranean countries, suggesting that temperature or weather patterns may have an impact on CD or UC. Various dietary habits such as high sucrose consumption have been identified as exacerbating CD or UC, but no one particular food or group of foods seems to have a reliable effect in a large population. Oral contraceptive use and cigarette smoking have variable effects on CD versus UC; oral contraceptives and nicotine have been found to exacerbate CD, but not UC.

PATHOPHYSIOLOGY

Differentiating CD from UC is difficult because of their similar clinical presentation. Hallmark symptoms of IBD are bloody diarrhea, weight loss, and fever. Generally, CD can be distinguished from UC based only on fiberoptic findings. The GI mucosal lining in CD is usually characterized by discontinuous, narrowed, thick, edematous, leathery patches with the presence of lesions, ulcerations, fissures, strictures, granulomas, and fibrosis. Fistulas and abscess formation occur most commonly in patients with deep transmural lesions. UC usually affects the rectum and areas proximal, possibly extending throughout the entire large intestine with continuous, superficial uniform inflammation and ulceration. Other pathologic findings are rare in UC but may occur in patients with chronic, long-standing inflammation. Granulomas and fistulas usually occur exclusively in patients with CD (Table 31-1).

Extraintestinal complications, including skin malformations, liver disease, joint deformities, and ocular manifestations, may also occur, although they typically occur more often in CD than UC because of a higher incidence of malabsorption of nutrients (see Table 31-1). Because the complications affect a variety of organ systems and result in nonspecific complaints, it is difficult to associate the complaints with CD or UC; however, it is important to be aware of the complications because their presence indicates poorly controlled disease.

DIAGNOSTIC CRITERIA

Because the clinical presentation of patients with CD or UC is highly nonspecific, definitive diagnosis relies on fiberoptic or radiologic studies. Visualization techniques must be used to differentiate CD from UC because of their similar clinical presentations. Usually, fiberoptic techniques are preferred over radioactive isotopes because they permit direct visualization of the mucosal lining with increased specificity as to the extent of lesions, ulcerations, and inflammation, as well as providing the opportunity to obtain mucosal specimens for biopsy and further evaluation. The risk of mucosal perforation, however, may limit the use of fiberoptic technology in patients with severely active disease.

Sigmoidoscopy is preferred as a first-line diagnostic procedure over endogastroduodenoscopy (EGD)/colonoscopy because it is conveniently used in office settings and is less expensive than EGD. EGD may be used if the sigmoidoscopy findings are negative or to visualize damage to the upper GI tract. Colonoscopic examination may be used rather than EGD if lower GI tract involvement is suspected. Radiologic studies, including either an upper GI series or barium enema, may be preferred in patients with severely active symptoms to decrease the risk of mucosal perforation.

Antibody tests are sometimes helpful in determining the diagnosis of CD or UC. The perinuclear antineutrophil cytoplasmic antibody (pANCA) and/or the anti-*Saccharomyces cerevisiae* antibody (ASCA) tests maybe positive in patients with IBD, but there is a significant rate of false-negative results, since only 60% to 70% of patients with CD or UC are actually antibody positive (Kornbluth & Sachar, 2004). The combination of a positive pANCA and a negative ASCA may indicate the presence of UC, whereas the opposite may indicate CD; however, the combined result still has a significant percentage of false negatives. Therefore, these tests are not used routinely to diagnose IBD.

INITIATING DRUG THERAPY

CD and UC share many clinical characteristics with pseudomembranous colitis, irritable bowel disease, peptic ulcer disease (PUD), traveler's diarrhea, colon cancer, and hemorrhoids. Evaluation of patients with suspected IBD must include a complete history focusing on recent use of antibiotics, recent international travel, diet history, use of laxatives or antidiarrheals, frequency and quality of daily bowel movements, history of PUD, family history of IBD, and smoking status to rule out similar presenting conditions.

Physical examination should include assessment of vital signs and weight loss, a thorough abdominal examination, and special attention to extraintestinal complications. Guaiac testing and stool cultures may be helpful in ruling out PUD or infectious causes. Although there are no reliable surrogate laboratory markers that may indicate the presence of CD or UC, baseline laboratory studies, including electrolytes, liver panel, complete blood count (CBC), and hematology panel, are important in assessing the severity of the condition.

Initiation of proper drug therapy is based on the severity and extent of disease. The Working Definitions of Crohn's Disease Activity or the Criteria for Severity of Ulcerative Colitis may be used as a guide to determine severity (Tables 31-2 and 31-3). Each scale highlights specific subjective and objective parameters that should be evaluated when assessing the progression of disease. Both scales highlight certain key features when predicting the severity of the condition,

Table 31.1

Common Signs and Symptoms of Crohn's Disease Versus Ulcerative Colitis

	Ulcerative Colitis	Crohn's Disease
Signs		
Abdominal mass	0	++
Fistulas	+/−	++
Strictures	+	++
Small bowel involvement	+/−	++
Rectal involvement	++	+/++
Extraintestinal disease		
Arthritis/arthralgia	++	++
Erythema nodosum	+/−	+/−
Abnormal liver function		
test values	++	++
Iritis/uveitis	+/−	+/−
Ankylosing spondylitis	+	+
Growth retardation	+	+
Toxic megacolon	+	+/−
Recurrence after colectomy	0	+
Malignancy	+	+/−
Symptoms		
Fever	+	++
Diarrhea	++	++
Weight loss	++	++
Rectal bleeding	++	+
Abdominal pain	+	++

Key: +, common; ++, very common; +/−, possible; 0, rare.

Table 31.2

Working Definitions of Crohn's Disease Activity

Mild to Moderate
- Ambulatory patients
- Able to tolerate oral alimentation
- No evidence of:
  - Dehydration
  - High fevers
  - Rigors
  - Prostration
  - Abdominal tenderness
  - Painful mass
  - Abdominal obstruction
- <10% weight loss

Moderate to Severe
- Failed treatment for mild to moderate disease OR
- Have
  - High fever
  - >10% weight loss
  - Abdominal pain/tenderness
  - Intermittent nausea or vomiting (without obstructive findings)
  - Significant anemia

Severe–Fulminant
- Persistent symptoms despite outpatient steroid therapy OR
- Have
  - High fever
  - Persistent vomiting
  - Intestinal obstruction
  - Rebound tenderness
  - Cachexia
  - Abscess

Remission
- Asymptomatic without inflammatory sequelae
- Not dependent on steroids

Table 31.3

Criteria for Severity of Ulcerative Colitis

Mild UC
- <4 stools daily (with or without blood)
- No presence of anemia, fever, or tachycardia
- Normal erythrocyte sedimentation rate (ESR)

Moderate UC
- >4 stools daily
- Minimal anemia, fever, or tachycardia

Severe UC
- >6 bloody stools daily
- Positive fever, tachycardia, anemia, or elevated ESR

Fulminant UC
- >10 stools daily
- Continuous bleeding
- Abdominal tenderness and distention
- Anemia requiring blood transfusion
- Colonic dilation

such as the frequency of stools per day and the presence of abdominal pain, fever, and anemia.

Treatment for IBD consists of aminosalicylates, corticosteroids, immunosuppressive agents, antibiotics, and biological agents. The decision to use one or a combination of these agents is based on the presence of CD versus UC, the severity of the disease, and whether treatment is targeted at active disease or maintenance of remission. In general, aminosalicylates, corticosteroids, and intravenous cyclosporine are used for treating acute exacerbations of IBD, although aminosalicylates and immunosuppressive agents are also used for maintaining remission. Antibiotics are reserved for treating and maintaining remission for mild CD, whereas tumor necrosis factor inhibitors are reserved for treating and maintaining remission of severe CD only (Table 31-4).

Goals of Drug Therapy

Because no pharmacologic cure is available for CD or UC, the goals of treatment focus on symptom management and quality-of-life issues. With proper treatment, the patient should be able to:

- Resume normal daily activities
- Restore general physical and mental well-being
- Attain appropriate nutritional status
- Maintain remission of disease
- Decrease the number and frequency of exacerbations

- Decrease side effects related to medications
- Increase life expectancy

Ideally, patients should expect to recover from an acute exacerbation within 1 to 2 weeks, have minimal exacerbations throughout the year, and participate in any desired activity.

Aminosalicylates

Aminosalicylates remain the gold standard for the treatment of CD and UC. Although the exact mechanism of action is unknown, these drugs decrease inflammation in the GI tract by inhibiting prostaglandin synthesis, which results in a decrease in various immune mediators, including interleukin-1, cyclooxygenase, and thromboxane synthase. Therapy with these agents may improve symptoms within 1 week of initiating therapy or dosage adjustment. However, patients may need to take these agents over the long term to prevent exacerbations. Although they are safe for use in most patients, aminosalicylates are contraindicated in patients with aspirin allergy or glucose-6-phosphate dehydrogenase deficiency. Sulfasalazine is also contraindicated in patients who are hypersensitive to sulfa products (see Table 31-4). All of these agents must be used at maximum doses for maximum therapeutic benefit, although the incidence of side effects also increases with increased doses.

Sulfasalazine

Sulfasalazine (Azulfidine, Azulfidine EN) is efficacious and cost-effective for CD and UC therapy, but it has a limited role because of its unfavorable side effect profile. Sulfasalazine is a combination product that is cleaved in the proximal colon by bacterial azo-reductases to release sulfapyridine and mesalamine. The mesalamine compound is responsible for virtually all of the therapeutic effect, whereas sulfapyridine is responsible for many of the side effects associated with sulfasalazine. Sulfasalazine may be administered up to four times a day; the most effective and maximum daily dosage is approximately 8 g daily.

Table 31.4

Overview of Agents Used to Treat Inflammatory Bowel Disease

Generic (Trade) Name and Dosage	Selected Adverse Events	Contraindications	Special Considerations
Aminosalicylates			
sulfasalazine (Azulfidine, Azulfidine EN) Start: 500 mg bid Range: 1–8 g	Stevens-Johnson syndrome, rash, photosensitivity, nausea, vomiting, skin discoloration, agranulocytosis, crystalluria, hepatitis	Sulfa allergy, aspirin allergy, G6PD deficiency	Most efficacious at high doses Drug released in the proximal colon Available in enteric-coated tablets Dosage increases may occur as frequently as every other day.
oral mesalamine (Asacol, Pentasa) Start: 500–800 bid Range: 1–3 g	Nausea, headache, malaise, abdominal pain, diarrhea	Aspirin allergy, G6PD deficiency	Asacol released in ileum, Pentasa released in duodenum May increase dose as frequently as every other day
rectal mesalamine (Rowasa Suppository) Start: 500 bid Range: 1–2 g Enema Start: 4 g HS Range: 1–4 g	Malaise, abdominal pain	Aspirin allergy, G6PD deficiency	Only for distal ulcerative colitis, proctitis, left-sided disease Suppository most effective in sigmoid colon, and enema may treat distal and sigmoid colon
olsalazine (Dipentum) Start: 500 mg bid Range: 1–2 g	Nausea, headache, malaise, abdominal pain, diarrhea	Aspirin allergy, G6PD deficiency	Drug released in proximal colon May increase dose as frequently as every other day High incidence of diarrhea
balsalazide (Colazide) Start: 1.5 g PO bid Range: 1.5–6.75 g	Headache, abdominal pain, diarrhea	Aspirin allergy, G6PD deficiency	Only approved for treatment of mild to moderate ulcerative colitis
Selected Corticosteroids			
prednisone (Orasone, Deltasone) Start: 40–60 mg qd Range: 10–100 mg	Hyperglycemia, increased appetite, insomnia, anxiety, tremors, hypertension, fluid retention, electrolyte imbalances	Active GI bleeding	Taper patient off steroids within 1–2 mo of initiation to decrease risk of long-term side effects.
oral methylprednisolone (Medrol) Start: 20–50 mg qd Range: 10–100 mg	Same as above	Same as above	Same as above
IV methylprednisolone (Solu-Medrol) Start: 5–10 mg q6h Range: 10–50 mg	Same as above	Same as above	IV treatment used for severe exacerbations Treatment duration should be a maximum of 7–14 d, then switch to oral therapy.
oral hydrocortisone (Cortef) Start: 160–240 mg qd Range: 50–300 mg	Same as above	Same as above	Has higher incidence of fluid and sodium retention than others Taper patient off steroids within 1–2 mo of initiation to decrease risk of long-term side effects.
rectal hydrocortisone suppositories (Anusol-HC) Start: 25 mg bid Range: 25–100 mg Enema (Cortenema) Start: 100 mg hs Range: 100 mg	Same as above		Used only for distal ulcerative colitis treatment Enema is more effective than suppositories for distal colitis.
IV hydrocortisone (Solu-Cortef) Start: 50–100 bid Range: 25–150 bid	Same as above	Active GI bleeding	IV treatment used for severe exacerbations Treatment duration should be a maximum of 7–14 d, then switch to oral therapy.
dexamethasone (Decadron) Start: 5–15 mg qd Range: 2–20 mg	Same as above	Same as above	Has longer onset of action than other agents
Oral budesonide (Entocort EC) Start: 9 mg bid	Minimal nausea	Same as above	Minimal sytemic absorption Taper after 8 weeks of therapy
Selected immunosuppressives			
azathioprine (Imuran) Start: 50 mg qd Range: 2–2.5 mg/kg	Pancreatitis, fever, arthralgias, nausea, rash, agranulocytosis, diarrhea, malaise, hepatotoxicity	Pregnancy, active liver disease, bone marrow suppression	Decrease dose for patients with severe renal dysfunction
6-mercaptopurine (Purinethol) Start: 50 mg qd Range: 1–2.5 mg/kg	Same as above	Same as above	Same as above

Table 31.4

Overview of Agents Used to Treat Inflammatory Bowel Disease (*Continued*)

Generic (Trade) Name and Dosage	Selected Adverse Events	Contraindications	Special Considerations

oral methotrexate (Rheumatrex)
    Start: 5 mg TIW
    Range: 5–7.5 mg TIW
	Hepatic cirrhosis and fibrosis, neutropenia, pneumonitis, skin rash, nausea, diarrhea	Same as above	Same as above

IV cyclosporine Start: 4–8 mg/kg/day	Hypertension, nephrotoxicity, superinfection, hypomagnesemia	Renal failure, hepatic failure	Only used for severely acute ulcerative colitis that is refractory to steroids. Total duration of therapy 7–10 d; has many drug interactions

Selected Antibiotics
metronidazole (Flagyl)
    Start: 20 mg/kg
    Range: 10–20 mg/kg
	Nausea, diarrhea, disulfiram reaction, metallic taste, peripheral paresthesias, dizziness	Liver failure, renal failure, first trimester of pregnancy, uncontrolled seizure disorder	Should not be used with alcohol
			Most efficacious if used chronically >3 mo

ciprofloxacin (Cipro)
    Start: 500 mg bid
    Range: 500–2000 mg
	Dizziness, nausea, diarrhea, photosensitivity	Children <12 y, pregnancy, uncontrolled seizure disorder	May cause arthropathies in patients <12 y
			Must be administered 2 h before or after divalent and trivalent cations

Tumor Necrosis Factor Inhibitor
IV infliximab (Remicade)
    Start: 5 mg/kg
    Range: 5–10 mg/kg/day
	Fatigue, malaise	Hypersensitivity to murine products	For severe CD
			Is administered over 2 h as a single infusion

G6PD, glucose-6-phosphate dehydrogenase.

Mesalamine

Mesalamine (Asacol, Rowasa, Pentasa) is available in various formulations, including oral tablets, oral capsules, enemas, and rectal suppositories. Each formulation is released in various areas of the GI tract, allowing for targeted drug therapy; however, in clinical trials the capsules and tablets had similar efficacy at equivalent doses. The oral tablets (Asacol) are formulated with an acrylic resin coating that disintegrates at pH 7, allowing the active ingredient to be released in the distal ileum and colon. The sustained-released capsules (Pentasa) have ethylcellulose-coated granules that allow for the slow release of the drug beginning in the proximal small intestine and continuing throughout the colon. The rectal suppositories are used primarily for UC-associated proctitis, whereas the enema delivers mesalamine to the distal and sigmoid colon. The enema is typically given at bedtime to allow for direct contact of the drug with the mucosa for at least 8 hours. The capsules may be taken up to four times a day, the tablets three times a day, and the suppositories twice daily.

Olsalazine

Olsalazine (Dipentum), the third aminosalicylate preparation, consists of two mesalamine molecules joined by an azo-bond. As with sulfasalazine, the azo-bond is cleaved by bacterial azo-reductases, allowing the drug to be released in the proximal colon. It is administered twice daily, with patients taking up to 8 capsules per day for a total dosage of 2 g/day. Although each tablet of olsalazine has twice as much active ingredient as the mesalamine capsules, the efficacy is minimally enhanced.

Balsalazide

The newest aminosalicylate product on the market is balsalazide (Colazide). Balsalazide is a combination product consisting of 5-aminosalicylic acid (mesalamine), the therapeutically active portion of the molecule, and 4-aminobenzoyl-alanine, an inert moiety. The product is cleaved by bacterial azo-reductases in the colon to release the active compound. Each capsule contains granules of balsalazide that are insoluble in acid and designed to be delivered to the colon intact. It is administered three times a day, up to 9 capsules per day, for a total dosage of 6.75 g/day, equaling 2.4 g/day of pure mesalamine. Currently it has been studied only for use in mild to moderate ulcerative colitis. Side effects and contraindications are similar to those of mesalamine.

Adverse Events

Mesalamine, olsalazine, and balsalazide are poorly absorbed from the GI tract and thus are considered primarily topical agents, with limited systemic side effects and drug interactions. The major side effects of mesalamine include headache, malaise, abdominal pain, and diarrhea. Olsalazine has a similar side effect profile but has a higher incidence of diarrhea than mesalamine. Initially, diarrhea may not be easily distinguished from IBD exacerbation, and therefore close monitoring of improvement of symptoms is essential. Sulfapyridine is absorbed systemically, accounting for many of the side effects and drug interactions incurred by sulfasalazine. Common adverse effects include nausea, vomiting, photosensitivity, oligospermia, and skin discoloration, which may be tolerable for most patients. Severe adverse reactions associated with sulfasalazine include Stevens-Johnson syndrome, agranulocytosis, crystalluria, pancreatitis, and hepatitis, which may necessitate discontinuation of therapy. Sulfasalazine is known to decrease folate levels, so patients taking sulfasalazine should be supplemented with folic acid. Although drug interactions with sulfasalazine are limited, it may significantly decrease the effect of warfarin (Coumadin), and therefore close INR monitoring is essential.

Corticosteroids

Corticosteroids are used intermittently to treat acute IBD exacerbations only. Corticosteroids allow for added immunosuppression and prostaglandin inhibition when the disease fails to respond to aminosalicylate therapy. Corticosteroids may be used in conjunction with aminosalicylates or as monotherapy to treat acute exacerbations.

Dosage

Corticosteroids with relatively quick onset of action and high glucocorticoid activity such as prednisone (Orasone, Deltasone) and methylprednisolone (Medrol) are desirable in the treatment of CD or UC. Recently, oral budesonide (Entocort EC) was specifically approved for the treatment of IBD. Budesonide is unique due to its limited absorption from the GI tract, thus theoretically leading to a localized effect in the GI lumen with minimal systemic side effects. A rectal corticosteroid formulation used for distal UC is available only as hydrocortisone base. Doses equivalent to prednisone 40 to 60 mg/day are used in patients with mild, moderate, or severe exacerbations of CD or UC. A beneficial effect is usually seen with 7 to 10 days of therapy. Patients with mild to moderate exacerbations are usually treated with oral or rectal corticosteroids for approximately 4 to 8 weeks, after which drug dosages are tapered. In severe exacerbations, patients should receive 7 to 10 days of intravenous therapy and then switch to oral corticosteroid therapy for the remainder of the treatment period (see Table 31-4).

Adverse Events

Short-term corticosteroid use (less than 3 months) is associated with increased glucose levels, increased appetite, insomnia, anxiety, tremors, and increased fluid retention, leading to increases in blood pressure and electrolyte imbalances. Although discontinuation of therapy is not recommended with short-term corticosteroid treatment, routine monitoring is necessary.

Long-term corticosteroid use is associated with decreased bone density, leading to osteoporosis; fat redistribution, leading to the characteristic "buffalo hump"; decreased prostaglandin synthesis, resulting in gastric and duodenal ulcers; hypertriglyceridemia; cataracts; and hirsutism. Therefore, long-term treatment with corticosteroids is not recommended.

Interactions

Many corticosteroids are substrates of the cytochrome P450 isoenzyme 3A4, including prednisone, prednisolone, methylprednisolone, and budesonide. Therefore, agents that inhibit or induce this enzyme system, such as ketoconazole, clarithromycin, phenytoin, and pioglitazone, may alter the efficacy of the corticosteroid. Budesonide requires an acidic environment (pH < 5.5) to be released, so agents that inhibit acid production or neutralize acid in the GI tract (ie, H2 antagonists, proton pump inhibitors, antacids) may limit the effectiveness of budesonide. Corticosteroids may also decrease the effectiveness of antidiabetic and antihypertensive agents due to their ability to increase blood glucose levels and blood pressure.

Immunosuppressive Agents

Immunosuppressive agents are used in IBD as adjunctive treatment with aminosalicylates to induce and maintain remission if exacerbations occur while the patient is being tapered off corticosteroid therapy or if frequent exacerbations occur with maximum dosages of aminosalicylates. Cyclosporine is the exception: it is solely used to treat severe, acute exacerbations when the patient is refractory to corticosteroids.

Azathioprine and 6-Mercaptopurine

Azathioprine (Imuran) and 6-mercaptopurine (Purinethol) are antimetabolites that act as purine antagonists to inhibit the synthesis of protein, RNA, and DNA. By doing so, azathioprine and 6-mercaptopurine decrease the production of various inflammatory mediators. Because 6-mercaptopurine is the active metabolite of azathioprine, these agents are similar in efficacy, side effect profile, and dosing frequency (see Table 31-4). Although these agents have a short plasma half-life of approximately 1 to 2 hours, both have active metabolites with long half-lives of 3 to 13 days, resulting in optimal therapeutic effects within 10 to 15 weeks of initiation of therapy.

These agents should be initiated during an acute exacerbation once the patient can tolerate oral medications to induce and maintain remission. Because of their slow onset of action, however, these agents are not effective for treating an acute exacerbation. The initial dosage of these agents is 50 mg/day in one dose; the dosage is increased every 2 weeks to a target dosage of 1 to 2 mg/kg/day for 6-mercaptopurine and 2 to 2.5 mg/kg/day for azathioprine. Because these agents are cleared by the renal system, dosages must be decreased in patients with creatinine clearance values under 50 mL/minute. The dose for azathioprine and 6-mercaptopurine is usually decreased by 50% if the patient's creatinine clearance value falls below 50 mL/minute to decrease the risk of accumulation and unwanted effects. Although these agents have the potential to cause significant adverse events, they are in general well tolerated. These agents should not be used in pregnancy or in patients with active liver disease.

Methotrexate

Methotrexate (Rheumatrex) has a therapeutic effect similar to that of azathioprine and 6-mercaptopurine; however, it inhibits intracellular dihydrofolate reductase, which results in inhibition of purine synthesis and suppression of interleukin-1 production. Both the intramuscular and oral preparations of methotrexate are efficacious in the induction and maintenance of CD remission, but similar efficacy has not been shown for UC. Doses of 25 mg/week injected intramuscularly or 5 mg orally three times a week have been effective in inducing remission in patients with steroid-dependent CD after 12 to 16 weeks of therapy. At low doses, methotrexate is nearly completely absorbed when administered orally; therefore, there is no foreseen benefit in using the intramuscular preparation over the oral formulation during normal GI function.

Methotrexate dosages must be adjusted based on renal function. Patients with creatinine clearance values less than 50 mL/minute should receive 50% of the normal dose. Methotrexate should not be prescribed to patients with active liver disease or pregnant women.

Cyclosporine

Cyclosporine (Sandimmune, Neoral) is reserved for the acute treatment of severe, steroid-refractory exacerbations of UC. Cyclosporine is a lipophilic, fungus-derived polypeptide that suppresses cell-mediated immunity by predominantly inhibiting interleukin-2 synthesis and release. Therapeutic effect is correlated with appropriate dosing. Intravenous infusion of cyclosporine has been found effective at dosages of 4 to 8 mg/kg/day for UC. The use of cyclosporine in acute CD exacerbations is reported to have variable results. Because of poor systemic absorption, oral cyclosporine should not be used. Improvement of symptoms with intravenous therapy usually occurs within 2 to 3 days, and the duration of therapy is usually 7 to 10 days.

Adverse Events

Although azathioprine and 6-mercaptopurine are usually well tolerated, significant side effects may occur. These agents are associated with both allergic- and nonallergic-type side effects. Allergic-type side effects include pancreatitis, fever, rash, arthralgias, malaise, nausea, and diarrhea, which may occur regardless of dose. The main nonallergic-type side effects include bone marrow suppression and hepatotoxicity, which appear to be dose dependent. Pancreatitis warrants discontinuation of therapy; hematologic and hepatic abnormalities may be managed by decreasing the dose.

Side effects of methotrexate include hepatic cirrhosis and fibrosis, bone marrow suppression, pneumonitis, folic acid deficiency, and rash. Nausea and diarrhea are also reported, but they occur more frequently with the oral formulation. Bone marrow suppression and liver dysfunction are dose dependent, and doses should be decreased in patients with these disorders. Folic acid should be administered concomitantly to limit folic acid deficiency.

Cyclosporine is most associated with nephrotoxicity, hypomagnesemia, and hypertension. Risk factors for nephrotoxicity are high-dose treatment, long-term treatment, and advanced age. Discontinuation of cyclosporine may restore renal function within 2 weeks. Other side effects of cyclosporine include nausea, vomiting, opportunistic infections, paresthesias, tremor, and seizures. Opportunistic infections occur because of the drug's immunosuppressive effects and may be managed by appropriate antibiotic therapy.

Interactions

Cyclosporine significantly interacts with various agents because of its metabolism through the cytochrome P450 3A4 isoenzyme system. Enzyme inhibitors, such as erythromycin (Eryc) and ketoconazole (Nizoral), increase blood levels of cyclosporine by inhibiting its metabolism, whereas enzyme inducers, such as phenytoin (Dilantin), carbamazepine (Tegretol), and rifampin (Rifadin), decrease cyclosporine blood levels. Grapefruit juice increases blood levels of cyclosporine, which may increase the incidence of side effects.

Antibiotics

The association between IBD and infectious causes has led to the treatment of IBD with antibiotics. Because the exact organism has not been isolated, it is difficult to determine which antibiotics are most appropriate for treatment. In general, an antibiotic that acts against gram-negative and *Mycobacterium* organisms with a low side effect profile and poor systemic absorption is desirable. Many agents have been studied, including broad-spectrum antibiotics, metronidazole (Flagyl), fluoroquinolones, antituberculars, and macrolides. However, based on the scarce published, controlled trials, mild to moderately active CD appears to respond only to metronidazole and ciprofloxacin (Cipro), and possibly clarithromycin (Biaxin) (see Table 31-4). Beneficial effects of antibiotic therapy have not been replicated in patients with UC.

Metronidazole was first found effective in treating perianal CD. Since then, however, many studies have found beneficial effects of metronidazole in the treatment of mild to moderately active CD when used in combination with aminosalicylates or alone. The mechanism by which metronidazole alone exerts its beneficial effects in CD is unknown, although it is thought that the immune-modulating effects are more prominent than the antibacterial effects in IBD treatment.

The normal dosage for treatment of mild to moderately active CD is 20 mg/kg/day. Once remission is attained, the dosage is titrated to 10 mg/kg/day for maintenance. The usual duration of therapy is up to 12 months, although remission is usually attained within 1 to 2 months. Although exacerbations of CD have been reported with the discontinuation of metronidazole, long-term use is associated with significant side effects.

Ciprofloxacin is emerging as the antibiotic of choice for CD because of its similar efficacy to metronidazole and decreased side effects. Ciprofloxacin is excellent for treating gram-negative organisms and *Mycobacterium* species, as well as some gram-positive organisms, and is usually well tolerated. Along with inhibiting DNA gyrase, which is its main antibacterial mechanism of action, ciprofloxacin also is reported to have immunosuppressive properties. A dosage of oral ciprofloxacin of 500 mg, twice daily, has proved as efficacious as 4 g of mesalamine daily in preliminary trials. Remission is attained after approximately 6 weeks of therapy. Ciprofloxacin is contraindicated in children and pregnant women.

Clarithromycin has been studied at dosages of 500 mg orally twice daily for patients with active CD, although the studies have been small, with varied results. Clarithromycin is associated with activity against *Mycobacterium*, indicating a possible role for it in managing CD.

Adverse Events

Short-term metronidazole therapy is associated with fairly benign side effects, including dry mouth, metallic taste, nausea, and vomiting. Abdominal distress, including cramping and diarrhea, may also occur, but these effects are difficult to distinguish from IBD symptoms. Long-term use of metronidazole is associated with neurotoxic effects such as peripheral paresthesias, dizziness, pruritus, and vertigo that may warrant discontinuation of therapy.

Ciprofloxacin is usually well tolerated. The most common side effects include nausea, diarrhea, dizziness, and rashes secondary to photosensitivity. Clarithromycin causes metallic taste, nausea, and vomiting that may resolve if the medication is taken with food.

Interactions

Metronidazole is associated with severe nausea and vomiting (disulfiram effect) if taken concurrently with alcohol. Ciprofloxacin inhibits theophylline (Slo-Phyllin) metabolism, so theophylline serum levels may need to be monitored with chronic ciprofloxacin use. Any divalent or trivalent cation, such as calcium or iron, may interfere with the absorption of ciprofloxacin, so at least a 4-hour dosing interval should be maintained between these agents. Because clarithromycin is metabolized through the cytochrome P450 3A4 isoenzyme system, concomitant administration with agents that are inducers or inhibitors of the enzyme system such as ketoconazole, phenytoin, or cyclosporine should be avoided to prevent significant adverse effects.

Biological Agents

Many biological agents are being investigated for the treatment of IBD, including tumor necrosis factor inhibitors, growth factors, lymphocyte inhibitors, and transcription inhibitors. Currently infliximab (Remicade), a tumor necrosis factor inhibitor, is the only biological agent approved for the treatment and maintenance of CD. The GI mucosal tissues of patients with active CD are found to overexpress numerous immunologic cytokines, including tumor necrosis factor. Infliximab is a synthetically derived monoclonal antibody consisting of 25% murine antibodies and 75% human antibodies (see Table 31-4). It neutralizes soluble forms of tumor necrosis factor and competitively inhibits its binding. Infliximab is indicated for treating moderate to severe CD refractory to conventional therapy as well as for inducing and maintaining remission of CD.

Infliximab is available only as an intravenous solution, and it is administered at a dosage of 5 mg/kg over 2 hours. A single infusion dose is used for the treatment of an acute exacerbation; a series of three infusions or infusions every 8 weeks is used to maintain remission. However, adverse events may worsen with repeated doses due to the murine component, and infliximab therapy may be limited because of its significant expense. Infliximab has not been adequately studied in pregnant women, so caution should be used when prescribing it in pregnancy as well as in patients with heart failure. The primary side effects associated with infliximab are transient hypersensitivity reactions and fever, possibly secondary to the murine products. Less common but significant side effects include the development of heart failure, tuberculosis, vasculitis, and pancytopenia. Although routine laboratory monitoring is not indicated currently, a heightened awareness of symptoms of heart failure and vasculitis is warranted. Extensive drug interaction studies have not been performed to date, but due to its ability to alter the immunologic response, infliximab should not be administered along with live vaccines. No significant drug interactions have been reported when infliximab is given with conventional IBD therapy.

Selecting the Most Appropriate Agent

For many diseases and disorders, there are drug treatment protocols that make clear distinctions between first-line, second-line, and third-line therapies. However, in IBD, the decision to use one therapeutic modality over another is based on the location of the inflammation, the severity and extent of disease, the patient's tolerance of the therapy, patient compliance, and cost (Table 31-5). The American

Table 31.5

Recommended Treatment Options for Crohn's Disease and Ulcerative Colitis

Severity of Disease	Distal UC	Extensive UC	CD
Mild	Oral/rectal aminosalicylate OR Rectal corticosteroid	Oral aminosalicylate	Oral aminosalicylate WITH/WITHOUT Antibiotic therapy
Moderate	Oral aminosalicylate AND Rectal aminosalicylate Oral/rectal steroid	Oral aminosalicylate AND Oral steroid	Oral aminosalicylate AND Oral steroid
Severe	IV corticosteroid AND/OR IV cyclosporine	IV corticosteroid AND/OR IV cyclosporine	IV corticosteroid AND/OR IV infliximab
Fulminant	IV corticosteroids AND/OR IV cyclosporine	IV corticosteroid AND/OR IV cyclosporine	IV corticosteroid AND/OR IV infliximab
Remission	Oral/rectal aminosalicylate WITH/WITHOUT Oral immunosuppressive	Oral aminosalicylate WITH/WITHOUT Oral immunosuppressive	Oral aminosalicylate WITH/WITHOUT Oral immunosuppressive/ IV infliximab

College of Gastroenterology has developed guidelines for managing CD and UC (Hanauer, Sandborn, et al., 2001; Kornbluth & Sachar, 2004).

Crohn's Disease

Mild to moderate CD is typically treated with oral aminosalicylates alone or in combination with antibiotic therapy. Oral agents are chosen over rectal agents because of the random presence of CD along the entire GI tract. Patients may be maintained on aminosalicylates or antibiotic therapy for months to years, but the goal is to taper the patient off the medication as soon as possible once remission is attained.

Treatment of moderate to severe CD usually consists of combination therapy with aminosalicylates and corticosteroids. Corticosteroid therapy is used acutely on a short-term basis for patients with moderate to severe disease to attain remission. Because of their high side effect profile, steroids are not used chronically to maintain remission. Oral agents may be used for patients with moderate to severe disease, and intravenous agents are used for severe to fulminant exacerbations. The typical duration of therapy is 4 to 12 weeks at the full dose, and then doses are tapered by 5 to 10 mg weekly until discontinued.

Severe to fulminant disease requires not only definitive drug therapy but also substantial supportive care measures due to their poor oral absorption and rapid GI transit time. Oral therapy, including aminosalicylates, should not be administered until the patient can tolerate oral alimentation. Intravenous corticosteroids are indicated to decrease inflammation. For patients with moderate to severe or severe to fulminant disease whose disease is refractory to corticosteroids (either oral or intravenous), intravenous infliximab is an option. Supportive care measures such as intravenous fluids, bowel rest, and parenteral nutrition should also be considered.

Therapy to maintain remission should be considered in patients who have frequent exacerbations or who are "steroid-dependent." Immunosuppressive agents, including azathioprine, 6-mercaptopurine, methotrexate, and infliximab, may be used with aminosalicylates to maintain remission in patients whose disease is refractory to aminosalicylate monotherapy. The agents may take effect after 8 to 12 weeks. Patients may be maintained on these agents for months to years, but the goal is to taper the patient off the medication as soon as possible due to the significant side effects. Antibiotics, specifically metronidazole and ciprofloxacin, have proved beneficial in maintaining remission of CD with long-term use (Fig. 31-1).

Ulcerative Colitis

For UC, guidelines specify various treatment approaches depending on the severity and location of disease. Distal colitis, identified as lesions below the splenic flexure, may be treated with oral, rectal, or intravenous agents. Rectal agents should not be used in patients with extensive colitis due to the location of disease. The decision to use systemic or local preparations for distal colitis largely depends on patient preference; however, topical products allow for less systemic absorption, less frequent dosing, and a quicker onset of effect (Fig. 31-2). Treatment of mild UC is best achieved with the use of aminosalicylates. The combination of oral and rectal aminosalicylates is more effective than either therapy alone. Corticosteroids may be used concurrently with aminosalicylates for moderate UC exacerbations. Depending on the severity of the exacerbation and the location of the lesions, either rectal or oral preparations may be appropriate. Severe exacerbations may require hospitalization. Discontinuation of oral and topical therapy due to rapid GI transit time and the initiation of intravenous corticosteroid therapy are standard. If improvement in the condition is not seen in 7 to 10 days with intravenous corticosteroids, intravenous cyclosporine may be considered. Surgery may be considered in patients whose disease fails to respond to drug therapy. The management of fulminant exacerbations is very similar to that of severe exacerbations, but the decision to perform a colectomy is considered at a much earlier stage for fulminant exacerbations. Along with definitive therapy, supportive measures including bowel rest, intravenous fluids, and adequate nutrition should be considered for those with severe and fulminant exacerbations. For those with frequent exacerbations or steroid dependence, immunosuppressive agents such as 6-mercaptopurine and azathioprine should be considered to induce and maintain remission. Typically, immunosuppressive agents are initiated after the patient can tolerate oral medications and are initiated along with aminosalicylate and corticosteroid therapy. The goal is to taper the corticosteroid and continue the aminosalicylate along with the immunosuppressive therapy for maintenance of remission.

Methotrexate has not been adequately studied in patients with UC and therefore is not recommended. Antibiotic therapy and infliximab have not been shown to improve UC symptoms.

Drug Selection

Sulfasalazine is considered the first-line aminosalicylate because of its remarkable efficacy, low cost, and availability in oral liquid and tablet preparations; however, it must be taken four times a day and causes significant adverse drug reactions. For maximum therapeutic benefit, 4 to 8 g/day is necessary, so patients must take up to 16 tablets or 32 teaspoonfuls daily. In addition, immediate-release sulfasalazine has activity limited to the colon, making it less effective in conditions affecting the upper GI tract.

Mesalamine has emerged as the aminosalicylate of choice because of its availability in many formulations, the dosing frequency, and its low side effect profile, but it is more expensive than sulfasalazine. Depending on the oral formulation and the severity of the disease, patients may need to take 6 to 16 pills daily to attain maximum therapeutic benefit. Normal dosages of oral mesalamine are 2 to 4 g/day. Olsalazine and balsalazide are rarely used because of their added cost without any significant clinical benefit.

The ideal corticosteroid for treating IBD would have high glucocorticoid activity, a low side effect profile, and targeted delivery to the diseased site and would be poorly absorbed from the GI tract, allowing for localized activity. Oral budesonide (Entocort) is approved specifically for the acute treatment of IBD due to its ideal characteristics, but any corticosteroid is an option to treat an acute exacerbation. The choice of steroid depends on the route of administration,

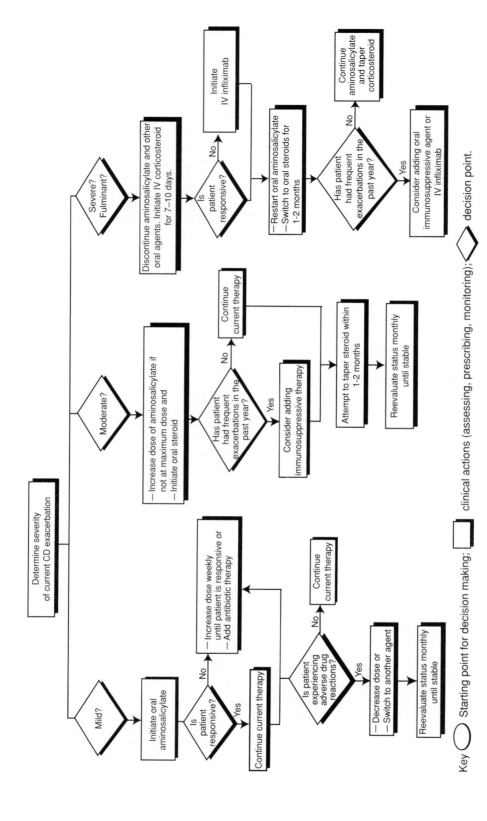

Figure 31–1 Treatment algorithm for active Crohn's disease.

Key ◯ Starting point for decision making; ▭ clinical actions (assessing, prescribing, monitoring); ◇ decision point.

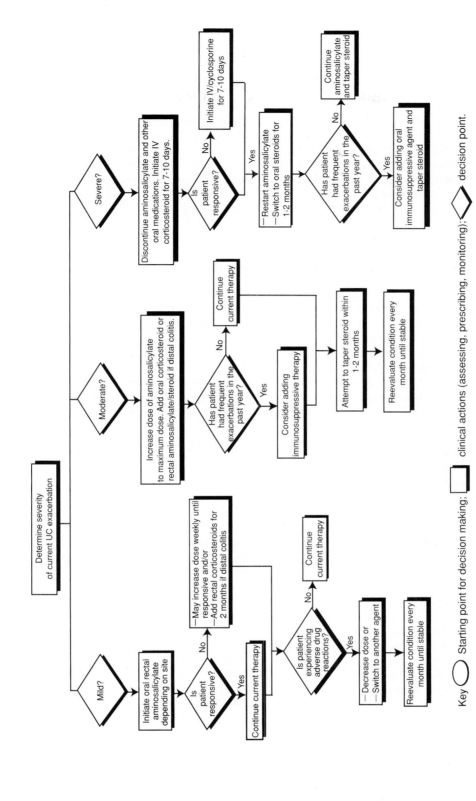

Figure 31-2 Treatment algorithm for active ulcerative colitis.

Key ◯ Starting point for decision making; ▭ clinical actions (assessing, prescribing, monitoring); ◇ decision point.

425

onset of action, and glucocorticoid versus mineralocorticoid potency. In general, agents with more glucocorticoid activity are preferred over mineralocorticoid steroids because they have better anti-inflammatory action. Oral agents are used primarily in patients with localized or generalized disease with mild to moderate exacerbations, rectal formulations are reserved for patients with mild to moderate exacerbations of distal disease, and intravenous treatment may be initiated in patients with severe exacerbations of CD or UC.

The use of immunosuppressive agents varies based on the type of IBD and the severity of disease. Cyclosporine is reserved for the acute treatment of severe UC exacerbations because of the high cost of therapy, ineffectiveness of the oral formulation, and high incidence of severe side effects. Because of a lack of comparative trials of methotrexate and azathioprine or 6-mercaptopurine, it is difficult to determine which agent would be considered first line; however, there are more data to support the use of azathioprine or 6-mercaptopurine than methotrexate for CD and UC. Azathioprine and 6-mercaptopurine are equally efficacious, with similar pharmacokinetic, adverse drug reaction, and cost profiles, so no great distinction can be made between the two.

The main distinction between methotrexate and the other two agents is its availability as an intramuscular injection and its dosing schedule. The infrequent dosing schedule of oral and intramuscular methotrexate may promote either compliance or noncompliance with the medication, depending on the patient. Combining these agents for the induction and maintenance of remission is not recommended because of overlapping side effect profiles and lack of efficacy data.

If antibiotic therapy is warranted, metronidazole or ciprofloxacin is an acceptable agent, depending on patient-specific factors. Because of the lack of consistent data on clarithromycin, it currently is not considered for treating CD.

Special Population Considerations

Pediatrics

IBD is typically diagnosed early in life, usually during the second or third decade, leading to significant implications of IBD in the pediatric population. Treatment must be aggressive to limit the potential for nutritional deficiencies leading to stunted growth, malnutrition, and anemias. However, many of the medications lead to untoward effects or are not well studied in pediatrics. The use of long-term corticosteroids may lead to growth abnormalities, whereas ciprofloxacin use is contraindicated in children because it can cause arthropathy, resulting in poor bone formation. Infliximab is not well studied in the pediatric population, so its use should be limited. Supplemental therapy including proper nutrition, iron therapy, and adequate hydration should also be considered to maintain growth and general health. Treating IBD in children involves aggressively managing the condition with the limited options available.

Pregnancy

The fertility rate in women with IBD is similar to the general population, but spontaneous abortions, stillbirths, and developmental defects are more common in pregnant women with active disease. Therefore, IBD should be treated aggressively in pregnant women to limit dehydration, anemia, and nutritional deficiencies that could adversely affect the fetus. However, treatment options are limited for pregnant women due to the risk of teratogenicity or unwanted effects on the fetus. Methotrexate is absolutely contraindicated in pregnancy and lactation due to its potential for spontaneous abortions and teratogenicity. Data are controversial regarding the use of mercaptopurine and azathioprine during pregnancy. If either of these agents is necessary during pregnancy, an azathioprine dosage of 2 mg/kg/day or less is recommended to limit pancytopenia in the fetus. Azathioprine and mercaptopurine are contraindicated during nursing due to the potential of fetal immunosuppression. The use of cyclosporine should be reserved for severe refractory cases because it can cause growth retardation. Ciprofloxacin and metronidazole should also be avoided in pregnancy and lactation because they can cause fetal malformations. Corticosteroids may be used at the lowest doses possible to induce remission for the shortest period of time to limit adrenal suppression of the fetus. Women taking sulfasalazine should be given higher dosages of folate (2 mg/day) because sulfasalazine interferes with folate absorption. Preconception counseling is imperative to discuss the condition, lifestyle changes, and treatment options with the patient. Special attention should be given to maintaining body weight before conception and preventing exacerbations during pregnancy.

MONITORING PATIENT RESPONSE

Various parameters must be monitored to detect efficacy and toxicity associated with therapy. Efficacy parameters include signs and symptoms of CD and UC, which are well defined in the Working Definition of Crohn's Disease Activity and Criteria for Severity of Ulcerative Colitis. Nutritional parameters such as weight, albumin, vitamin B_{12} levels, iron levels, and transferrin saturation should also be followed. Mental status and quality-of-life issues such as frequency of social interactions, attendance at work, and completion of activities of daily living all may indicate effectiveness of therapy. Although there are no definitive guidelines for the frequency of monitoring, it is important to monitor these end points when adjustments are made in drug therapy or exacerbations of disease occur. Due to the increased risk of developing colon cancer, routine colonoscopy is recommended for patients with IBD. The frequency of colorectal screening depends on the extent and duration of disease and the family history of colon cancer.

Specific monitoring of drug toxicities is imperative for all pharmacologic agents. Complete blood counts and liver function tests should be performed periodically to detect asymptomatic undesired reactions in patients taking sulfasalazine.

Corticosteroid treatment is associated with significant drug toxicities, but most occur with long-term use. In general, short-term corticosteroid treatment does not require intense monitoring. However, patients who have uncontrolled hypertension or who are glucose intolerant must have their blood pressure or fasting blood glucose level monitored periodically while taking corticosteroids. For patients taking corticosteroids on a long-term basis, baseline tests including a lipid panel, electrolytes, and fasting blood glucose studies should be performed every 6 to 12 months. A baseline bone density scan may be judicious and may be repeated yearly.

Azathioprine and 6-mercaptopurine are both associated with significant side effects, so it is important to acquire a baseline complete blood count with differential and serum creatinine, amylase, and liver function tests. The complete blood count should be monitored every 1 to 2 weeks for the first 3 months and then every 2 to 3 months for the duration of therapy. Liver function tests should be monitored every 3 months for the first year or until a stable dosage has been achieved, then every 4 to 6 months for the duration of treatment. Creatinine clearance is an important value in guiding the dosing regimen of azathioprine or 6-mercaptopurine, so serum creatinine and creatinine clearance should be monitored annually if renal function is stable, and more often if fluctuations in dosages or renal function occur. Amylase is not routinely ordered, but it may be checked upon patient complaints.

During the initial phase of methotrexate therapy, complete blood count and liver function tests should be performed every 2 to 4 weeks. If methotrexate therapy is continued beyond 16 weeks, complete blood count and liver function tests should be monitored every 4 to 8 weeks for the duration of therapy. Dosage adjustments must be made based on creatinine clearance, so serum creatinine must be monitored at baseline and at every dosage change. If renal function is stable, serum creatinine should be monitored annually at a minimum. Liver biopsies may be obtained once yearly if the patient is taking methotrexate, although formal recommendations have not been made.

Intravenous cyclosporine therapy requires daily monitoring of cyclosporine blood levels (200 to 400 ng/mL), blood urea nitrogen, serum creatinine, and blood pressure. Although cyclosporine is extensively metabolized by the liver, it is eliminated by the kidneys and is highly associated with permanent renal dysfunction; therefore, renal function must be monitored closely. Dosages should be adjusted daily based on renal function and cyclosporine blood levels. Opportunistic infections may occur with high-dose cyclosporine use, so complete blood count, signs of infection, and temperature should also be monitored daily.

Metronidazole and ciprofloxacin do not require significant drug monitoring, but long-term antibiotic treatment may lead to superinfection, so signs and symptoms of infection should be noted and treated. Patients receiving metronidazole therapy should also be monitored for peripheral paresthesias.

PATIENT EDUCATION

Drug Information

Patients and caregivers need to understand that uncontrolled IBD may affect quality of life, psychological well-being, and general physical health, so adherence to medication therapy is imperative.

Patients should swallow the enteric-coated sulfasalazine or mesalamine tablets and capsules whole so that the dosage form can penetrate the affected area. Sulfasalazine can discolor body fluids (eg, urine and tears), which may stain clothing and contact lenses. When taking metronidazole,

patients must abstain from alcohol to avoid the disulfiram reaction.

Often patients request chronic corticosteroid therapy because of its beneficial results, but these patients need to be informed of the long-term complications of corticosteroids and should be advised regarding other medications that may be more appropriate for chronic therapy.

Patient-Oriented Information Sources

Along with their health care professionals, there are many other resources available for patients who are seeking information on IBD. A local support group may be a good resource for patients having trouble dealing with the illness. Many local hospitals as well as the Crohn's and Colitis Foundation of America organize support groups for patients with IBD. For general medical information regarding IBD, the following websites offer helpful patient-specific information:

- American Gastroenterologic Association: www.gastro.org
- American College of Gastroenterology: www.acg.gi.org
- National Institute of Diabetes, Digestive, and Kidney Diseases: www.niddk.nih.gov
- MedlinePlus: www.nlm.nih.gov/medlineplus/
- Crohn's and Colitis Foundation of America: www.ccfa.org

Nutrition and Lifestyle Changes

Nutritional status is a significant issue for patients with active IBD and those with surgical resections. Patients with IBD are at risk for stunted growth, malnutrition, weight loss, iron deficiency anemia, macrocytic anemia, osteopenia, and other conditions. Nutrient deficiencies of iron, vitamin B_{12}, zinc, folate, calcium, and vitamin D may result from decreased oral intake, malabsorption, excessive losses, hypermetabolism due to infection, or drug-induced side effects. Concurrent administration of folate with methotrexate and sulfasalazine and administration of calcium and vitamin D with corticosteroids are recommended to limit the potential for nutritional deficiencies. Also, due to folate deficiencies, patients with IBD are at risk of hyperhomocystinemia, resulting in an elevated potential for thrombosis. Vitamin B_6 and vitamin B_{12} supplementation is recommended to decrease homocysteine levels.

Many special dietary agents have been studied in patients with IBD with varying results. Diets high in short-chain fatty acids are associated with a small decrease in disease severity, potentially due to an anti-inflammatory effect. Fish oils, also with potential anti-inflammatory properties, have been associated with a decreased frequency of exacerbations. An area of new research interest is the role of probiotics such as Lactobacillus and Saccharomyces in the treatment of IBD. By altering the GI flora, it is theorized that probiotic agents may control IBD exacerbations.

Enteral and parenteral routes of nutrition have been routinely used to improve the nutritional status of IBD patients. In general, enteral nutrition is preferred due to the complications of infection, thrombosis, and pancreatitis associated with parenteral nutrition. Along with correcting nutritional deficiencies, enteral nutrition has also been studied as a primary treatment measure in combination with aminosalicylates. Parenteral nutrition, however, is advocated in severe exacerbations when bowel rest is in order for proper healing of the IBD.

In general, nutritional supplementation plays a large role in the management of IBD. Depending on the severity of weight loss and general health status of the patient, a combination of vitamin and mineral supplementation along with either enteral or parenteral nutrition should be advocated.

Complementary and Alternative Therapies

Alternative therapies are used by many patients with IBD: according to one study, 47% of patients with IBD had used alternative therapies for their condition. The most common alternative therapies used were Acidophilus and flaxseed, along with massage therapy, even though data are limited regarding the efficacy of these agents in IBD. Omega-3 fatty acids have also been studied for use in IBD. The National Institutes of Health reported variable results with the use of omega-3 fatty acids for IBD, so widespread use cannot be endorsed at this time (Agency for Healthcare Research and Quality, 2004).

Surgical options are considered in patients who are at risk for a further decline in physical health and quality of life resulting from frequent exacerbations that are unresponsive to conventional therapy. Surgical options include procto-colectomy for UC and a variety of ostomy procedures for

Table 31.6

Surgical Interventions

Procedure	Area of Resection
Sigmoid colostomy	Distal end of large intestine
Descending colostomy	Descending colon and rectum
Transverse colostomy	Small portion of transverse colon
Proctocolectomy/ileostomy	Entire rectum and large intestine

patients with CD, depending on the location of disease (Table 31-6). Proctocolectomy, the removal of the entire colon and rectum, is a curative intervention for UC. However, surgical procedures for CD are not curative because exacerbations may recur in existing areas of the GI tract, and surgery is used only to maintain remission.

For patients who have undergone surgery, the practitioner must pay close attention to general drug therapy issues. Because of the resection of the GI tract, these patients have issues similar to those of patients with short bowel syndrome. Rectally administered agents such as suppositories and enemas are ineffective in patients with any type of lower GI resection. Depending on the site of resection, sustained-released agents and medications targeted to specific areas of the GI tract also are ineffective in general.

■ Case Study

B.F., age 28, presents with diarrhea and abdominal pain. He says he feels weak and feverish. His symptoms have persisted for 5 days. He tells you he has 8 to 10 bowel movements each day, although the volume of stool is only about "half a cupful." Each stool is watery and contains bright-red blood. Before this episode, he had noticed a gradual increase in the frequency of his bowel movements, which he attributed to a new vitamin regimen. He has not traveled anywhere in the past 4 months and has taken no antibiotics recently. His medical history is significant for UC; his most recent exacerbation was 2 years ago. He is taking no medications except vitamins.

Examination findings include a tender, slightly distended abdomen. His BP is 122/84 sitting, 110/78 standing; HR 96 bpm; and temperature 100°F. Otherwise, physical findings are unremarkable. Laboratory study results reveal hemoglobin, 12 g/dL; hematocrit, 38%; white blood cell count, 12,000/mm^3; platelet count, 242 k; sodium, 132; potassium, 3.6. All other study results are within normal limits. The most recent colonoscopy findings (4 years ago) revealed granular, edematous, friable mucosa with continuous ulcerations extending throughout the descending colon.

Diagnosis: Exacerbation of ulcerative colitis

1. List specific goals of treatment for B.F.

2. What drug therapy would you prescribe? Why?

3. What are the parameters for monitoring success of the therapy?

4. Discuss specific patient education based on the prescribed therapy.

5. List one or two adverse reactions for the selected agent that would cause you to change therapy.

6. What would be the choice for the second-line therapy?

7. What over-the-counter and/or alternative therapies might be appropriate for B.F.?

8. What lifestyle changes would you recommend to B.F.?

9. Describe one or two drug/drug or drug/food interactions for the selected agent.

Bibliography

Starred references are cited in the text.

*Agency for Healthcare Research and Quality. (2004) *Effects of omega-3 fatty acids on lipids and glycemic control in type 2 diabetes and the metabolic syndrome, and on inflammatory bowel disease, rheumatoid arthritis, renal disease, systemic erythematous lupus, and osteoporosis.* Publication no. 04-E012-1. (URL: http://www.ahrq.gov/clinic/epcsums/o3lipidsum.htm).

*American Gastroenterological Association. (2001). *The burden of gastrointestinal diseases.* Bethesda, MD: AGA.

Cabre, E., & Gassull, M. A. (2003) Nutritional and metabolic issues in inflammatory bowel disease. *Current Opinions in Clinical Nutrition and Metabolic Care, 6,* 563–576.

Colombel, J. F., Lemann, M., Cassagnou, M., et al. (1999). A controlled trial comparing ciprofloxacin with mesalamine for the treatment of active Crohn's disease. *American Journal of Gastroenterology, 94,* 674–678.

Connell, W., & Miller, A. (1999) Treating inflammatory bowel disease during pregnancy: risks and safety of drug therapy. *Drug Safety, 21*(4), 311–323.

Friedman, S., & Regueiro, M. D. (2002). Pregnancy and nursing in inflammatory bowel disease. *Gastroenterology Clinics of North America, 31,* 265–273.

Friend, D. R. (1998). Review article: issues in oral administration of locally acting glucocorticosteroids for treatment of inflammatory bowel disease. *Alimentary Pharmacology and Therapeutics, 12,* 591–603.

Gassull, M. A. (2003) Nutrition and inflammatory bowel disease: its relation to pathophysiology, outcome, and therapy. *Digestive Disorders, 211,* 220–227.

Graham, T. O., & Kandil, H. M. (2002) Nutritional factors in inflammatory bowel disease. *Gastroenterology Clinics of North America, 31,* 203–218.

*Hanauer, S. B., Sandborn, W., et al. (2001) Management of Crohn's disease in adults. *American Journal of Gastroenterology, 96*(3), 635–643.

Hanauer, S. (1996). Drug therapy: inflammatory bowel disease. *New England Journal of Medicine, 334,* 841–848.

Irvine, E. J. (1997). Quality of life issues in patients with inflammatory bowel disease. *American Journal of Gastroenterology, 92,* 18S–24S.

Klotz, U. (2000). The role of aminosalicylates at the beginning of the new millennium in the treatment of chronic inflammatory bowel disease. *European Journal of Clinical Pharmacology, 56,* 353–362.

*Kornbluth, A., & Sachar, D. B. (2004) Ulcerative colitis practice guidelines in adults (update): American College of Gastroenterology, Practice Parameters Committee. *American Journal of Gastroenterology, 99,* 1371–1385.

Lee, S. D., & Cohen, R. D. (2002). Endoscopy in inflammatory bowel disease. *Gastroenterology Clinics of North America, 31,* 119–132.

Lesko, S. M., Kaufman, D. W., Rosenberg, L., et al. (1985). Evidence for an increased risk of Crohn's disease in oral contraceptive users. *Gastroenterology, 89,* 1046–1049.

Liu, Y., van Kruiningen, H. J., West, A. B., et al. (1995). Immunocytochemical evidence of *Listeria, Escherichia coli,* and *Streptococcus* antigens in Crohn's disease. *Gastroenterology, 108,* 1396–1404.

Murray, A., Oliaro, J., & Schlup, M. (1995). *Mycobacterium paratuberculosis* and inflammatory bowel disease: frequency distribution in serial colonoscopic biopsies using the polymerase chain reaction. *Microbios, 83,* 217–228.

*Orholm, M., Munkholm, P., Langholz, E., et al. (1991). Familiar occurrence of inflammatory bowel disease. *New England Journal of Medicine, 324,* 84–88.

Pullan, R. D., Rhodes, J., Ganesh, S., et al. (1994). Transdermal nicotine for active ulcerative colitis. *New England Journal of Medicine, 330,* 811–815.

Rubin, D. T., & Hanauer, S. B. (2000). Smoking and inflammatory bowel disease. *European Journal of Gastroenterology and Hepatology, 12,* 855–862.

Sandborn, W. J., & Targan, S. R. (2002). Biologic therapy of inflammatory bowel disease. *Gastroenterology, 122,* 1592–1608.

Sands, B. E. (2000). Therapy of inflammatory bowel disease. *Gastroenterology, 118,* S68–82.

Sonnenberg, A., McCarty, D. J., & Jacobsen, S. J. (1991). Geographic variation of inflammatory bowel disease within the United States. *Gastroenterology, 100,* 143–149.

Stein, R. B., & Hanauer, S. B. (1999). Medical therapy for inflammatory bowel disease. *Gastroenterology Clinics of North America, 28*(2), 297–321.

Thompson, N. P., Montgomery, S. M., Pounder, R. E., et al. (1995). Is measles vaccination a risk factor for inflammatory bowel disease? *Lancet, 345,* 1071–1074.

Ursing, B., Alm, T., Barany, F., et al. (1982). A comparative study of metronidazole and sulfasalazine for active Crohn's disease: the Cooperative Crohn's Disease Study in Sweden. II: Results. *Gastroenterology, 83,* 550–562.

Walker, E. A., Roy-Byrne, P. P., Katon, W. J., et al. (1990). Psychiatric illness and irritable bowel syndrome: a comparison with inflammatory bowel disease. *American Journal of Psychiatry, 147,* 1656–1661.

Visit the Connection web site for the most up-to-date drug information.

PARASITIC INFECTIONS

■ SAMANTHA VENABLE AND ANDREW M. PETERSON

The parasitic diseases are commonly grouped into protozoan infections, helminthic infections, and arthropodal infections. The protozoan infections malaria, amebiasis, and giardiasis are discussed in this chapter; *Pneumocystis carinii* pneumonia and trichomoniasis are discussed in other chapters. Among the common helminthic (worm) infections are hookworm, roundworm, tapeworm, and pinworm infections.

The third type of parasitic infection is caused by arthropods, which are the vectors of disease. These vectors include ticks, mosquitoes, biting flies, and ectoparasites, such as mites, chiggers, lice, and fleas, which infect external body surfaces. Common arthropodal infections include scabies and pediculosis.

Parasitic diseases are caused by close personal contact. This contact may involve vectors, as in malaria; ingestion, as in giardiasis; inhalation; or direct contact, as in scabies and lice. Pharmacologic intervention for parasites must be specific to not only the type of parasite, but also the stage of its life cycle. Some parasites have a simple life cycle and others have extremely complex ones. Thus, many parasitic diseases are treated with a combination of drugs to eradicate all stages of the parasite.

MALARIA

Malaria causes the most morbidity and mortality of all the parasitic diseases. The World Health Organization estimates that 300 million people worldwide are affected by malaria and between 1 and 1.5 million people die from it every year. In the United States, malaria is confined to people who have visited areas around the world such as Africa, Asia, and Latin America, where malaria is endemic.

Untreated malaria may lead to coma, renal failure, pulmonary edema, and death. Another potential complication is cerebral malaria. Once that occurs, the prognosis is poor, even with treatment, and residual neurologic deficits are possible.

In endemic areas outside the United States, especially areas of Africa, the mortality rate is high. This is related to drug resistance due to massive and continuous exposure to malaria and lack of sufficient medical care. In the United States, the prognosis is good if the patient receives appropriate therapy. In general, each type of malaria may recur once or more, then spontaneously terminate. Poor outcomes are usually related to noncompliance with drug therapy or with follow-up care.

CAUSES

Malaria is caused by protozoan parasites of the genus *Plasmodium*. There are four species of plasmodia that produce disease in humans: *Plasmodium falciparum*, *Plasmodium vivax*, *Plasmodium ovale*, and *Plasmodium malaria*. *P. falciparum* is the most widespread and dangerous of the four.

PATHOPHYSIOLOGY

Malaria begins when a female *Anopheles* mosquito bites a human whose blood contains the sexual forms of the malaria parasite (gametocytes). In the now infected mosquito, the gametocyte completes a maturation process and becomes a sporozoite, which is stored in the salivary glands. When the mosquito next feeds, the sporozoites inoculate another human host.

Plasmodia enter the human host as sporozoites. Once in the human host, the asexual life cycle begins. The first stage of asexual development, the exoerythrocytic phase, occurs in the liver. During this phase, the plasmodium is called a tissue schizont. At the end of the phase, the plasmodia, now called merozoites, are released from the liver into the bloodstream.

The second stage of asexual development, the erythrocytic phase, begins when the merozoites are released into the bloodstream. The merozoites invade the erythrocytes and develop into erythrocytic schizonts. They, in turn, create more merozoites in the red blood cells. At the end of the phase, the erythrocytes rupture, releasing the merozoites, along with pyrogenic substances, into the bloodstream to invade new red blood cells. The release of merozoites into the bloodstream initiates symptoms of fever, shivering, joint pain, and headache. With *P. vivax* and *P. ovale*, merozoites may reinvade the liver tissue and enter a dormant hepatic stage (hypnozoite) that is responsible for subsequent relapses.

The cycle of invasion, multiplication, and blood cell rupture is repeated many times. After a few cycles, some of the asexual parasites develop into sexual forms (gametocytes) that remain in the bloodstream. When a mosquito bites a human with gametocytes in the blood, the cycle begins again (Fig. 32-1). Because of the complex life cycle of the

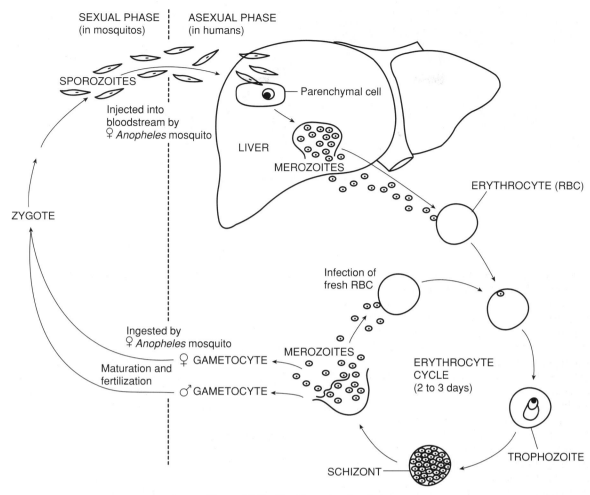

SEXUAL PHASE
(in mosquitos)

ASEXUAL PHASE
(in humans)

SPOROZOITES

Injected into
bloodstream by
♀ *Anopheles* mosquito

Parenchymal cell

LIVER

MEROZOITES

ERYTHROCYTE (RBC)

ZYGOTE

Infection of
fresh RBC

Ingested by
♀ *Anopheles* mosquito

Maturation and
fertilization

MEROZOITES

♀ GAMETOCYTE

♂ GAMETOCYTE

ERYTHROCYTE
CYCLE
(2 to 3 days)

TROPHOZOITE

SCHIZONT

Figure 32–1 The life cycle of malaria.

plasmodial parasites, malaria is usually treated with combination drug therapy.

DIAGNOSTIC CRITERIA

Signs and symptoms of malaria vary, but most patients experience fever. In addition to fever, common associated symptoms include headache, back pain, chills, sweats, myalgias, nausea, vomiting, diarrhea, and cough. The diagnosis of malaria should be considered for any person who has these symptoms and who has traveled to an area associated with malaria transmission. The gold standard for diagnosis is demonstration of malarial parasites in the blood.

INITIATING DRUG THERAPY

Practitioners always emphasize prevention because there is no nonpharmacologic therapy for active malaria. Clinicians should teach patients to avoid malaria by preventing mosquito bites (see the Patient Education section for more information).

Goals of Drug Therapy

The goal of therapy is to eradicate the parasite in both its erythrocytic and exoerythrocytic forms. Plasmodia are killed most easily in the erythrocytic stage. Exoerythrocytic

plasmodia are more difficult to eradicate, but it can be done. Sporozoites do not respond to current drug therapy. Because of these differences, there are three separate goals of therapy:

1. Prophylaxis (suppressive therapy)
2. Treatment of an acute attack (clinical cure)
3. Prevention of relapse (radical cure)

Suppression

Appropriate pharmacotherapy begins with the prescription of suppressive drugs before the patient travels to an area where malaria is a health hazard. Suppressive therapy cannot prevent primary infection of the liver because drug therapy does not affect sporozoites. Suppressive therapy does prevent the erythrocytic infection, which causes the symptoms of malaria. However, once the liver has a primary infection, the patient can have an acute attack when he or she is no longer taking the suppressive drugs.

Selection of suppressive drug therapy depends on which region the patient intends to visit (Fig. 32-2). In chloroquine-sensitive areas, chloroquine (Aralen) is the drug of choice for suppressive therapy. In chloroquine-resistant areas, mefloquine (Lariam) is the preferred suppressive agent. Alternative agents include hydroxychloroquine (Plaquenil), doxycycline

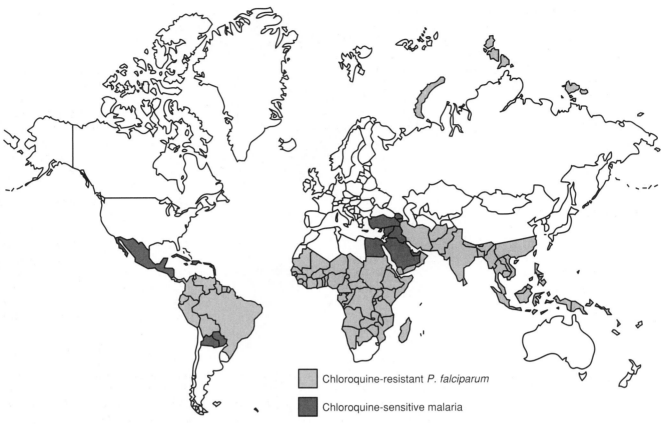

Figure 32–2 Distribution of *Plasmodium falciparum*.

(Vibramycin), and a pyrimethamine/sulfadoxine combination (Fansidar). Table 32-1 summarizes the drugs used for therapy.

Treatment of Acute Attack

Drugs that eradicate plasmodia in the erythrocytic stage of replication are used to treat an acute attack. These drugs include chloroquine, hydroxychloroquine, mefloquine, primaquine, pyrimethamine (Daraprim), and quinine. The choice of drugs depends on the type of malaria identified by blood analysis.

Prevention of Relapse

A radical cure for malaria is necessary for strains of *P. vivax* because the infection is harbored in the liver. The radical cure is postponed until the patient leaves the endemic malarial area because reinfection with continued bites is almost a certainty. The drug of choice for radical cure is primaquine.

Chloroquine and Derivatives

To treat chloroquine-sensitive plasmodia, chloroquine is the drug of choice. Chloroquine may also be used for treating amebiasis and rheumatoid arthritis.

Chloroquine, a 4-aminoquinoline, is classified as a blood schizonticide. In treating malaria, chloroquine is taken up by digestive vacuoles of plasmodia residing in the erythrocytes. Chloroquine is thought to increase the pH and upset phos-

pholipid metabolism, resulting in an interruption in RNA and DNA synthesis.

Chloroquine is rapidly and completely absorbed from the gastrointestinal (GI) tract. The drug concentrates in erythrocytes, liver, spleen, kidney, lung, heart, and brain as well as melanin-containing tissues, such as the retina and epidermis. It penetrates the central nervous system (CNS) and crosses the placenta and enters breast milk. Although chloroquine peaks rapidly, its half-life is between 1 and 2 months. Approximately 70% of chloroquine is excreted unchanged by the kidneys, and any unabsorbed drug is excreted in the feces. Small amounts of chloroquine have been detected in urine months and even years after treatment.

Contraindications

Chloroquine is contraindicated in patients with a hypersensitivity to any 4-aminoquinoline, such as hydroxychloroquine. Chloroquine is also contraindicated in patients with preexisting ocular disease. The drug should be used with caution in many patients with preexisting diseases; for instance, psoriasis and porphyria are exacerbated by chloroquine.

Adverse Events

Chloroquine can cause corneal opacities, keratopathy, or retinopathy. Retinopathy can lead to blindness and can progress even after the drug is discontinued. Infrequent, but important, potential sensory adverse effects include blurred

Table 32.1

Overview of Selected Antiparasitic Agents Used to Treat Protozoan Infections

Generic (Trade) Name and Dosage	Selected Adverse Events	Contraindications	Special Considerations
Chloroquine Derivatives for Malaria			
chloroquine phosphate (Aralen) **Suppression** *Adult:* 300 mg base (500 mg salt) PO, once/week *Child:* 5 mg/kg base (8.3 mg/kg salt) PO, once/week, up to maximum adult dose of 300 mg base **Acute disease** *Adult:* PO: 600 mg base initially; then 300 mg 6 h later and on days 2 and 3 IM: 160–200 mg base initially and 6 h later as needed *Child:* PO: 10 mg base/kg initially, then 5 mg base/kg 6 h later and on days 2 and 3 IM: 5 mg/kg base initially and 6 h later as needed	Hypotension, ECG changes, nausea/vomiting/diarrhea, abdominal pain; blurring of vision, difficulty focusing, changes in accommodation, irreversible retinal damage; tinnitus, reduced hearing in patients with pre-existing auditory damage; headaches or psychic stimulation, convulsive seizures, neuromyopathy; blood dyscrasias, exacerbation of porphyria, pruritus, skin discoloration, skin eruption, hair bleaching or loss	Hypersensitivity to any 4-aminoquinoline Pre-existing ocular disease	Schedule same-day weekly therapy. Arrange for periodic ophthalmologic examinations during long-term therapy. Monitor for hearing loss or change. Calculate pediatric doses carefully.
hydroxychloroquine sulfate (Plaquenil) **Suppression** *Adult:* 310 mg base (400 mg salt) PO, once/week *Child:* 5 mg/kg base (6.5 mg/kg salt) PO, once/week, up to maximum adult dose **Acute disease** *Adult and child >15 y:* Initially, 800 mg (620 mg base) PO, then 400 mg (310 mg base) after 6–8 h, then 400 mg (310 mg base) PO once daily on days 2 and 3 *Child <15 y:* Initially, 13 mg/kg of body weight (10 mg base/kg, single dose not to exceed 620 mg base) PO, then 6.5 mg/kg (5 mg base/kg, single dose not to exceed 310 mg base) PO after 6 h, then 6.5 mg/kg (5 mg base/kg) PO after an additional 18 h, then 6.5 mg/kg (5 mg base/kg) PO after a further 24 h	Same as chloroquine	Same as chloroquine	Same as chloroquine
mefloquine (Lariam) **Suppression** *Adult:* 228 mg base (250 mg salt) PO, once/week *Child:* <15 kg: 4.6 mg (base); 5 mg (salt)/kg/wk 15–19 kg: 1/4 tab/wk 20–30 kg: 1/2 tab/wk 31–45 kg: 3/4 tab/wk >45 kg: 1 tab/wk **Acute disease** *Adult:* 5 tablets (1250 mg) as a single PO dose with at least 240 mL of water	Dizziness, vomiting, syncope, extrasystoles Acute malaria: nausea, vomiting, fever, headache, myalgias, chills, diarrhea, skin rash, abdominal pain, fatigue, loss of appetite, tinnitus, alopecia, sinus bradycardia and ECG changes, vertigo, visual disturbances, psychotic manifestations	Hypersensitivity Seizure disorder Pregnancy Overwhelming infection	Obtain cultures to ensure mefloquine sensitivity. Arrange for concomitant administration of primaquine for exoerythrocytic parasites. Delay administration at least 12 h after last dose of quinine or quinidine to avoid cardiac toxicity or convulsions. Arrange for periodic ophthalmologic examinations during long-term therapy.

(continued)

Table 32.1

Overview of Selected Antiparasitic Agents Used to Treat Protozoan Infections *(Continued)*

Generic (Trade) Name and Dosage	Selected Adverse Events	Contraindications	Special Considerations
Child: 16.5 mg/kg PO as a single dose, with at least 240 mL water.			
primaquine **Active disease** *Adult:* 26.3 mg (15 mg base) PO once daily for 14 d. Alternatively, a dose of 79 mg (45 mg base) may be given once weekly for 8 wk. To eliminate gametocytes of *P. falciparum*, a single dose of 79 mg (45 mg base) may be given. Some strains of *P. vivax* (especially those from southeast Asia) may require 39.4–52.6 mg (22.5–30 mg base) daily for 14 d for a radical cure. *Child:* 0.5 mg/kg/day (0.3 mg base/kg/day) PO given once a day for 14 d. Alternatively, a dose of 1.5 mg/kg (0.9 mg/kg base) may be given once a week for 8 wk.	Nausea, vomiting, epigastric discomfort, leukopenia, hemolytic anemia in patients with G6PD deficiency	Hypersensitivity to primaquine or iodoquinol Actue illness with systemic disease and hematologic depression	Schedule same-day weekly therapy. Administer with chloroquine. Monitor CBC. Monitor for signs of hemolytic anemia and methemoglobinemia.
Other Antimalarials pyrimethamine (Daraprim) Adults and children >10 y: 25 mg PO weekly Children 4–10 y: 12.5 mg PO weekly Children <4 y: 6.25 mg weekly	Anorexia, vomiting, megaloblastic anemia, leukopenia, thrombocytopenia, pancytopenia	Allergy, G6PD deficiency Prescribe with caution in pregnancy and lactation.	Used to prevent malaria
doxycycline **Suppression** *Adult:* 100 mg PO; qd *Child:* >8 years of age: 2 mg/kg of body weight orally/day up to adult dose of 100 mg/day	Nausea, vomiting, diarrhea, abdominal pain, glossitis, dysphagia, damage to developing teeth, blood dyscrasias, photosensitivity	Hypersensitivity to tetracycline or tartrazine Pregnancy and lactation Children <8 y	Ensure pregnancy status before prescribing. Advise to take on an empty stomach. Monitor for severe GI complaints.
quinine sulfate *Adult:* *Chloroquine-resistant malaria:* 650 mg q8h PO for 5–7 d *Chloroquine-sensitive malaria:* 600 mg q8h PO for 5–7 d *Child:* *Chloroquine-resistant malaria:* 25 mg/kg/d q8h for 5–7 d *Chloroquine-sensitive malaria:* 10 mg/kg PO q8h 5–7 d	Vision disturbances, nausea, vomiting, diarrhea, and other GI complaints, blood dyscrasias, rashes, cinchonism	Allergy, G6PD deficiency, optic neuritis, tinnitus, history of blackwater fever Pregnancy category X, lactation Prescribe cautiously to patients with cardiac dysrhythmias.	Increases effects of anticoagulants and neuromuscular blocking agents; raises digoxin levels Take drug with food or meals to decrease GI upset. Teratogenic drug Report severe ringing in ears, headache, vision changes, bleeding, bruising, fever, chills.
Amebicides iodoquinol (Yodoxin) *Adult:* 650 mg tid PO after meals for 20 d *Child:* 40 mg/kg/d PO in 3 divided doses for 20 d, maximum dose 650 mg/dose	Blurred vision, weakness, fatigue, nausea, vomiting, diarrhea, anorexia, rash, pruritus, fever, chills	Hepatic failure, allergy to iodine or 8-hydroxyquinolines Use cautiously with pregnancy and lactation and thyroid disease.	Take drug after meals. Schedule periodic eye examinations.
paromomycin (Humatin) *Adults and children:* 25–35 mg/kg/d in three divided doses for 5–10 d	Vertigo, headache, nausea, vomiting, abdominal cramps, diarrhea, decreased urine output, superinfection	Allergy to drug, intestinal obstruction Prescribe with caution in pregnancy and lactation.	May cause malabsorption of sucrose and fats

Table 32.1

Overview of Selected Antiparasitic Agents Used to Treat Protozoan Infections (Continued)

Generic (Trade) Name and Dosage	Selected Adverse Events	Contraindications	Special Considerations
metronidazole (Flagyl) *Amebiasis:* Adult: 750 mg tid PO for 5–10 d Child: 35–50 mg/kg/d PO in 3 doses for 10 d *Giardiasis:* Adult: 250 mg tid PO for 7 d	Headache, dizziness, ataxia, metallic taste, anorexia, nausea, vomiting, diarrhea, cramps, darkened urine, disulfiram-like interactions with alcohol, rash	Hypersensitivity, pregnancy Prescribe cautiously in CNS disease, blood dyscrasias, lactation.	Take with food.
furazolidone (Furoxone) *Adults:* 100 mg qid for 7 d *Children >1 mo:* 5–8 mg/kg/d in four divided doses for 7 d	Discoloration of urine, headache, abdominal pain, nausea, vomiting, diarrhea, orthostatic hypotension, hypoglycemia	Hypersensitivity to drug Alcohol (ETOH) use G6PD deficiency Do not give to children <1 mo.	Avoid alcohol during drug therapy. Avoid amine-rich foods; the drug–food interaction may increase blood pressure, leading to hypertensive crisis.

vision, difficulty focusing, changes in accommodation, and irreversible retinal damage.

Chloroquine concentrates in the liver and can produce toxic effects in patients with hepatic disease, alcoholism, or concurrent use of hepatotoxic drugs. Chloroquine can cause gastric irritation and exacerbate preexisting GI disease. Chloroquine concentrates in the blood cells and can exacerbate blood dyscrasias or anemia. Potential hematologic adverse effects include agranulocytosis, aplastic anemia, pancytopenia, neutropenia, and thrombocytopenia. In addition, chloroquine can cause myelosuppression, resulting in an increased risk of infection, especially in patients with preexisting dental disease. Chloroquine may also cause polyneuritis, ototoxicity, seizures, or neuromyopathy, especially in patients with preexisting neurologic disease.

Despite the risks associated with chloroquine, patients taking the drug usually experience few adverse effects. The most frequent reported effects are hypotension, nausea, vomiting, diarrhea, and abdominal pain. Patients taking chloroquine for acute malaria or other diseases that require prolonged administration or high dosages may experience more severe adverse effects.

Patients should be monitored for changes in muscle strength and deep tendon reflexes, especially knee and ankle reflexes. Potential integumentary effects are pruritus, skin discoloration, skin eruption, and hair bleaching or loss. Close monitoring is mandatory with children and breast-feeding mothers because children and infants are extremely susceptible to chloroquine toxicity. Fatalities have occurred with relatively small doses.

Interactions

Chloroquine may interact with cimetidine (Tagamet), digoxin (Lanoxin), penicillamine (Cuprimine), rabies vaccine, and antacids or kaolin. Chloroquine may increase the serum levels of digoxin and penicillamine, resulting in potential toxicity of these drugs or increasing the risk of adverse effects. Cimetidine may decrease the metabolism of chloroquine, resulting in chloroquine toxicity. Co-administration of chloroquine and rabies vaccine may decrease the antibody response to the rabies vaccine when the vaccine is administered intradermally. Mean serum titers of rabies anti-body may be lower than expected. The intramuscular route is unaffected by this interaction. There is also a decreased absorption of chloroquine with kaolin and antacids containing magnesium.

Hydroxychloroquine

Like chloroquine, hydroxychloroquine may be used to treat malaria, although it is more commonly used to treat rheumatoid arthritis and systemic lupus erythematosus.

Mechanism of Action

The pharmacokinetics and pharmacodynamics of hydroxychloroquine are the same as those of chloroquine, except it is unknown whether the drug enters breast milk. Because the drugs are so similar and chloroquine does enter breast milk, the safest course is to refrain from its use in patients who are breast-feeding.

Hydroxychloroquine is rapidly and almost completely absorbed from the GI tract. Bioavailability is roughly 74%. Peak plasma concentrations are achieved in approximately 3 hours. The drug is widely distributed into body tissues, with higher concentrations in the liver, kidneys, spleen, lungs, heart, and brain than in plasma. Hydroxychloroquine is partially metabolized in the liver. The major metabolite is desethylhydroxychloroquine, which also may have some antiplasmodial activity. Excretion is mainly, but very slowly, through the urine; the drug can be detected for several months, or even years, after treatment is discontinued. Elimination appears to take place in a biphasic manner, and the terminal half-life is approximately 50 days in blood and 32 days in plasma. Unabsorbed drug is excreted in the feces.

Adverse Events

The most common adverse effects of hydroxychloroquine involve the GI tract. Patients should take hydroxychloroquine with food to minimize these effects. Hydroxychloroquine has the same extensive adverse effects profile as chloroquine. The adverse effects are a greater concern with long-term treatment.

Interactions

Hydroxychloroquine used concurrently with penicillamine can increase penicillamine plasma concentrations, possibly causing serious adverse hematologic, renal, or skin reactions.

When used concurrently with digoxin, hydroxychloroquine can increase serum digoxin levels, resulting in digoxin toxicity. Its absorption can be affected by concurrent use of magnesium trisilicate or kaolin products.

Mefloquine

Mefloquine, a 4-quinolinemethanol derivative, is chemically related to quinine. In chloroquine-resistant areas, mefloquine is the drug of choice. As a blood schizonticide, it prevents the replication of erythrocytic parasites but has no action on exoerythrocytic parasites. Its mechanism of action is unknown, but it may work by raising the intravascular pH in parasite acid vesicles, causing death.

Despite its variable absorption, mefloquine is given orally because it is so irritating to tissues. It is widely distributed, crosses the placenta, and may enter breast milk. It is highly bound to plasma proteins and concentrates in erythrocytes. Drug clearance is hepatic, but its route of excretion is unknown.

Mefloquine is well absorbed from the GI tract, with a bioavailability greater than 85%. The rate of absorption is usually relatively rapid, but it may be prolonged in some patients. Absorption may be incomplete in seriously ill patients, such as those with cerebral malaria. The drug is distributed to the blood, urine, cerebrospinal fluid, and tissues and concentrated in erythrocytes. It is also distributed to breast milk in low concentrations. Mefloquine is partially metabolized by the liver, primarily to the carboxylic acid metabolite. Mefloquine is eliminated very slowly, mainly through bile into the feces; subtherapeutic concentrations may persist in the blood for several months or more. Approximately 5% of an oral dose is excreted unchanged in the urine. The elimination half-life ranges from 13 to 33 days.

Contraindications

Mefloquine is contraindicated in patients with known hypersensitivity and in cases of overwhelming acute *P. falciparum* infection. Patients should receive intravenous antimalarial treatment initially, followed by oral mefloquine treatment. Mefloquine is contraindicated for use in patients with seizure disorders or psychiatric disturbances. It is also contraindicated during pregnancy because of its potential teratogenic and embryotoxic effects.

Adverse Events

The most common adverse effects of mefloquine used in suppressive therapy are vomiting, dizziness, syncope, and extrasystole. When used for acute malaria, mefloquine is associated with symptoms similar to the disease itself: nausea, vomiting, fever, headache, myalgias, and chills. Additional adverse effects include diarrhea, rash, abdominal pain, fatigue, loss of appetite, tinnitus, alopecia, sinus bradycardia, and electrocardiographic (ECG) changes. Neuropsychiatric adverse effects include vertigo, visual disturbances,

and psychotic manifestations such as hallucinations, nightmares, confusion, anxiety, severe mood swings, and depression. Further, suicidal ideation has been reported in people taking this medication. Development of these symptoms warrants discontinuation of the drug.

Interactions

There are several significant drug–drug interactions with mefloquine. Concurrent use of beta blockers or quinine can result in ECG abnormalities or cardiac arrest. Co-administration with chloroquine or quinine increases the risk for seizure activity. Concurrent use with valproic acid (Depakote) may decrease valproic acid concentrations, resulting in loss of seizure control. Although it is not available in the United States, halofantrine (Halfan), in combination with mefloquine, may induce potentially fatal cardiac conduction abnormalities, including prolongation of the QT interval, ventricular dysrhythmias, and atrioventricular conduction disorders. The practitioner must remember to explore any previous use of halofantrine before prescribing mefloquine.

Primaquine

Primaquine, an 8-aminoquinoline, is classified as a tissue schizonticide. Its exact mechanism of action is uncertain, although it is believed to interfere with the function of plasmodial DNA. Primaquine is the only tissue schizonticide available for the radical cure of *P. vivax* and *P. ovale* infection. In addition to the destruction of exoerythrocytic (tissue) forms, primaquine prevents the development of erythrocytic (blood) forms, which cause relapses in *P. vivax* infection. Primaquine is also gametocidal for all four plasmodial species. It is not used as a first-line drug, with the exception of chloroquine-resistant malaria, because of its toxicity.

Primaquine is administered orally and is rapidly absorbed from the GI tract. Oral bioavailability is roughly 96%, with peak plasma levels achieved in approximately 3 hours. It is widely distributed throughout the body, but there is no accumulation in erythrocytes. Primaquine crosses the placenta, but it is not known whether it is excreted into breast milk. Metabolism produces three identifiable metabolites. The major metabolite is carboxyprimaquine, which greatly exceeds plasma concentrations of primaquine. The other two metabolites have hemolytic activity in vitro. Carboxyprimaquine is eliminated more slowly than primaquine, and multiple dosing results in accumulation. The drug is almost undetectable after 24 hours.

Contraindications

Primaquine is contraindicated in patients with known sensitivity. Patients with iodoquinol (Yodoxin) hypersensitivity may have cross-sensitivity to primaquine. Because of its association with hematologic problems, the drug should be prescribed cautiously to African Americans and ethnic groups from the eastern Mediterranean region, where glucose-6-phosphate dehydrogenase (G6PD) deficiency is most prevalent. Patients with preexisting hematologic conditions are at risk for development of hemolytic anemia and methemoglobinemia.

Adverse Events

Symptoms such as dark-colored urine, anorexia, pallor, unusual fatigue or weakness, and back, leg, or abdominal pain may indicate the development of hemolytic anemia. Bluish fingernails, lips, or skin, dizziness, breathing difficulty, or unusual fatigue or weakness may indicate methemoglobinemia. These occur most frequently with high-dose therapy. Immediate discontinuation of primaquine is necessary if any of these adverse reactions occur.

Nausea, vomiting, and abdominal pain or cramps are common adverse effects with primaquine. Taking the medication with meals may reduce these symptoms.

Interactions

Toxicity may occur when primaquine is given concurrently with other antimalarial drugs such as quinacrine. Hematologic adverse effects may occur when primaquine is given concurrently with drugs that cause bone marrow depression.

Pyrimethamine

Pyrimethamine is a folic acid antagonist that blocks the protozoal enzyme dihydrofolate reductase. This results in a blockage of folic acid metabolism. Like chloroquine and hydroxychloroquine, pyrimethamine is a blood schizonticide with some tissue schizonticidal activity. However, its blood schizonticidal activity is slower that that of the 4-aminoquinoline compounds.

Pyrimethamine is used prophylactically for susceptible strains of plasmodia. It may be used concurrently with fast-acting antimalarials such as chloroquine for transmission control and suppressive care; it should not be used alone for an acute attack. In treating malaria, pyrimethamine is combined with sulfadoxine (Fansidar, Daraprim). This combination drug product contains 25 mg pyrimethamine and 500 mg sulfadoxine.

Pyrimethamine is orally administered. Peak plasma levels occur in 2 to 6 hours. Distribution is mainly into the kidneys, lungs, liver, and spleen, with concentrations in blood erythrocytes. Suppressive concentrations may persist for up to 2 weeks. The drug crosses the placenta and enters breast milk. Metabolism occurs in the liver and produces several unidentified metabolites that are all excreted in the urine. The apparent elimination half-life of pyrimethamine ranges from 54 to 148 hours; that of sulfadoxine ranges from 100 to 231 hours. Urinary excretion can persist for up to 30 days.

Contraindications

Pyrimethamine should be used cautiously in patients with anemia, folate deficiency, and bone marrow suppression. It is prescribed cautiously for patients with preexisting anemia because folic acid antagonism can potentiate anemias, especially megaloblastic anemia. Bone marrow suppression may result in myelosuppression, leading to leukopenia, agranulocytosis, or thrombocytopenia. Some practitioners routinely prescribe folinic acid when treating toxoplasmosis because higher doses of pyrimethamine are necessary. Routine complete blood counts (CBCs) are also prudent. High doses of pyrimethamine may precipitate seizures.

Pyrimethamine should be used with extreme caution during the first 14 to 16 weeks of pregnancy. Possible interference with folic acid metabolism could cause birth defects. If its use cannot be avoided, concurrent use of folinic acid is recommended. Use during breast-feeding should be avoided because it may interfere with the infant's folic acid metabolism.

Adverse Events

Common GI complaints with pyrimethamine include anorexia, nausea, vomiting, abdominal pain, and diarrhea. As with other antimalarials, taking the medication with food may decrease these symptoms.

Potential dermatologic reactions include urticaria, toxic epidermal necrolysis, exfoliative dermatitis, and Stevens-Johnson syndrome. Pyrimethamine should be discontinued at the first sign of rash.

CNS effects related to pyrimethamine therapy include weakness, ataxia, tremor, and rarely respiratory failure. In patients with preexisting seizure disorders, pyrimethamine may precipitate seizures, especially in patients receiving high-dose therapy.

Interactions

Drug–drug interactions include other bone marrow depressants or folate antagonists because of the potential for the development of blood dyscrasias. Bone marrow depression may be more likely with sulfonamide combination therapy. Other drugs that can interact with pyrimethamine in this manner include carbamazepine (Tegretol), clozapine (Clozaril), chloramphenicol (Chloromycetin), phenothiazines, procainamide (Pronestyl), antiretroviral agents, antineoplastic agents, or antithyroid agents. Folic acid (vitamin B$_9$) can interfere with the action of pyrimethamine and therefore should not be used concomitantly with pyrimethamine.

Quinine Sulfate

Quinine sulfate has been used for malaria treatment for 170 years. Quinine is significantly more toxic than chloroquine. It is active against the asexual erythrocytic forms of plasmodial organisms. Adjunctive therapy with other drugs such as tetracycline (Sumycin), pyrimethamine–sulfadoxine, or clindamycin (Cleocin) is required because quinine does not affect the exoerythrocytic forms of Plasmodium.

Mechanism of Action

Although the exact mechanism of action is unknown, quinine elevates the pH of parasitic acid vesicles and may upset molecular transport and phospholipase activity. Quinine is administered orally, achieving peak plasma levels within 3 hours. It distributes widely into the liver, lungs, kidneys, and spleen, with some distribution into the cerebrospinal fluid. It has a half-life of about 4 to 5 hours. It crosses the placenta and enters breast milk, although the American Academy of Pediatrics considers quinine to be compatible with breast-feeding. It is hepatically metabolized into several metabolites and renally excreted.

Contraindications

Quinine should not be used in patients with a known allergy to quinidine (Cardioquin). Quinidine is not a frequently used drug in the management of malaria; it is used only for life-threatening events. Patients with quinidine hypersensitivity may have cross-sensitivity to quinine. According to the drug manufacturer, quinine is in pregnancy category X; it can cause congenital malformation and has been associated with stillbirths. Large doses may be oxytocic, and quinine has been used as an abortifacient. For these reasons, most practitioners believe the risks of use during pregnancy clearly outweigh any potential benefits.

Quinine stimulates the release of insulin and should not be used in patients with hypoglycemia. *P. falciparum* malarial attacks also can induce hypoglycemia, and pregnant women and children are more susceptible.

Quinine should not be used in patients with optic neuritis or tinnitus because it can exacerbate these conditions. Even at therapeutic dosages, quinine may cause cinchonism (tinnitus, headache, nausea, vertigo, and vision impairment).

Quinine should be used cautiously in patients with G6PD deficiency, myasthenia gravis, and cardiac arrhythmias. Patients with G6PD deficiency have a higher risk for development of hemolytic anemia. Quinine produces neuromuscular blockade, exacerbating muscular weakness, and can cause respiratory distress and dysphagia in myasthenic patients. Patients with cardiac arrhythmias may be at risk for development of quinine-induced dysrhythmias. Patients treated with quinine have shown prolonged QT intervals.

Interactions

Quinine is associated with several important drug–drug interactions. It interacts with digitalis preparations, flecainide (Tambocor), warfarin (Coumadin), rifampin (Rifadin), quinidine, and mefloquine. High doses of quinine can affect the clearance of digitalis glycosides; dosage adjustments are needed to avoid digoxin toxicity. Lower doses may have no effect on digitalis clearance.

Flecainide clearance is inhibited by quinine. This increases flecainide serum concentrations and the risk for adverse effects. In combination, ECG changes have been noted, but the etiology of the changes is uncertain. Until further data are available, the concurrent use of these drugs should be avoided.

Alkalinization of the urine by acetazolamide (Diamox) can decrease the renal clearance of quinine. Increased plasma levels of quinine due to reduced clearance can increase the risk of toxicity.

Quinine can increase the hypoprothrombinemic effects of warfarin. Dosage adjustment of the anticoagulant may be necessary during quinine therapy. The possibility of cinchonism is increased if quinine and quinidine are administered concomitantly. In addition, rifampin is a potent inducer of hepatic metabolism. Rifampin significantly accelerates quinine clearance and reduces its half-life. Higher doses of quinine may be required in patients receiving rifampin.

Quinine should not be used concomitantly with mefloquine because additive cardiac effects can produce arrhythmias and seizures. It is important to remember that mefloquine has a long half-life.

Doxycycline

Doxycycline (Vibramycin) is a long-acting tetracycline with many clinical uses. Although it is not used in treating acute malaria, it is an alternative prophylactic regimen for patients who cannot tolerate mefloquine. Doxycycline is contraindicated in pregnant or breast-feeding women and children younger than 8 years of age because of its effects on bone and tooth formation. Doxycycline also is associated with photosensitivity, which is a particular problem in most malarial endemic areas because of bright sunlight.

Selecting the Most Appropriate Agent

First-Line Therapy

Chloroquine is the preferred therapy for *P. vivax*, *P. ovale*, *P. malariae*, and chloroquine-sensitive *P. falciparum* infection. Mefloquine is the drug of choice for chloroquine-resistant *P. vivax* and *P. falciparum*. See Table 32-2 for a summary.

Second-Line Therapy

Hydroxychloroquine is given for *P. vivax*, *P. ovale*, or *P. malariae* infection. Primaquine is used for prevention of relapse in *P. vivax* or *P. ovale* disease.

Third-Line Therapy

Quinine (oral) or quinidine (intravenous) is used for chloroquine-resistant *P. falciparum* disease. Fansidar

---

Table 32.2

Recommended Order of Treatment for Malaria

Order	Agents	Comments
First line	chloroquine	Chloroquine treats *Plasmodium vivax*, *P. ovale*, *P. malariae*.
	or	
	mefloquine	Mefloquine treats chloroquine-resistant *P. vivax* and *P. falciparum*.
Second line	hydroxychloroquine	Hydroxychloroquine treats *P. vivax*, *P. ovale*, or *P. malariae*.
	or	
	primaquine	Primaquine treats *P. vivax* or *P. ovale* to prevent relapse.
Third line	quinine (PO) or quinidine (IV)	IV quinidine is for *life-threatening* chloroquine-resistant *P. falciparum*.
	or	
	combination pyrimethamine–sulfadoxine	Pyrimethamine may be used for some chloroquine-resistant *P. falciparum*.

(pyrimethamine–sulfadoxine) may be used for some chloroquine-resistant strains of *P. falciparum*.

Special Population Considerations

Pediatric

Continued exposure to malaria can impede a child's educational and physical development. Further, children under 5 years of age are the most likely to die from malaria. The period just after a mother's immunity wears off, typically 6 months of age, and before the child's immunity fully develops, is the most vulnerable period (WHO Expert Report, 2000). Infants and children are susceptible to chloroquine toxicity and must be monitored closely.

Geriatric

Elderly patients may have preexisting health conditions that make them susceptible to the many adverse effects of chloroquine and hydroxychloroquine. A complete physical assessment needs to be performed as a baseline before prescribing drug therapy. Subsequent assessment and close attention to patient reports are required during drug therapy.

Women

As noted previously, none of the pharmacotherapies for malaria is approved by the manufacturer for administration during pregnancy. Continued pharmacotherapy during pregnancy is controversial. According to Phillips-Howard and Wood (1996) and Parke and Rothfield (1996), there is no evidence that antimalarials (with the exception of doxycycline and quinine) are teratogenic. Although not considered teratogenic, primaquine is not recommended because of the potential risk of hemolytic effects on the fetus.

The push for protecting pregnant women from infection is being lead by the Roll Back Malaria Global Partnership (RBMGP). Their push is to use insecticide-treated mosquito nets and intermittent preventive treatment (IPT). IPT involves giving antimalarial treatment to women during their antenatal care visits. The results reported by the RBMGP indicate a 9% absolute reduction in placental infection and a 13% decrease in low-birthweight children secondary to IPT (http://www.rbm.who.int).

MONITORING PATIENT RESPONSE

When treating patients for malaria suppression, therapeutic monitoring is unnecessary. However, frequent follow-up is required for patients taking antimalarial drugs to treat the disease itself.

Patients taking chloroquine or hydroxychloroquine should have a baseline CBC, liver and renal function tests, blood pressure measurement, and neurologic examination, including muscle strength and deep tendon reflexes. Chloroquine may affect the eyes; therefore, a complete baseline ophthalmologic examination including visual acuity and slit-lamp, funduscopic, and visual field tests should be done. The patient should be evaluated monthly for adverse effects. Serial laboratory and ophthalmologic examinations should be conducted every 6 months.

Patients receiving primaquine or pyrimethamine should have serial CBCs throughout therapy. In addition to CBCs, patients receiving quinine should have serial blood glucose monitoring, ECGs, and ophthalmologic examinations at a frequency similar to that for patients receiving chloroquine or hydroxychloroquine. The ECG of patients receiving mefloquine should also be monitored routinely.

PATIENT EDUCATION

Patients with malaria should take their medications at the same time of day with food and as directed. They need to learn to recognize signs and symptoms of serious adverse effects and to report them to the practitioner.

In addition to learning how to take prophylactic drugs to suppress malaria, patients who travel may be advised to carry a supply of the combination drug pyrimethamine–sulfadoxine and to treat any fever during travel, if professional care is not available within 24 hours. This is a presumptive self-treatment and considered only a temporary measure until health care is obtained.

Many pharmaceutical companies are actively testing malaria vaccines. Many of these vaccines have been field tested on humans. The results have been sporadically immunogenic. At this time, none has been approved for use in the United States.

Drug Information

There are a variety of sources of information about the drugs. Readily available sources include the manufacturer (through the website or via the package insert) as well as other published secondary sources like "Drug Facts and Comparisons." There are several malaria-related websites such as Malaria Foundation International (http://www.malaria.org). and the Centers for Disease Control and Prevention (CDC). The patient taking Lariam (mefloquine) should also be directed to review the FDA Medication Guide (http://www.fda.gov/cder/foi/label/2003/19591s19lbl_Lariam.pdf) for information on identifying and dealing with the serious psychiatric reactions that may occur with this drug.

Other information is available from the World Health Organization (http://www.who.int/en/). Within this website is a link to the Roll Back Malaria website, a global partnership designed to halve the world's malaria burden by 2010. This partnership was founded in 1998 by the World Health Organization, the World Bank, the United Nations Development Programme, and the United Nations Children's Fund. The website is a repository of information from countries all over the world. There is information on grants and research in progress as well as reports on progress in reducing the malaria burden throughout the world.

Patient-Oriented Information Sources

The CDC has a patient information website dedicated to malaria (http://www.cdc.gov/travel/malinfo.htm). Links also exist informing patients of the steps they need to take before embarking on travel outside the United States. They also provide a toll-free number (1-877-FYI-TRIP) about international travel as well as regional travel. Patients may obtain the information from the website or can have material faxed to them using the toll-free number.

Nutrition/Lifestyle Changes

To prevent malaria, patients should learn ways to avoid mosquito bites by protecting themselves with intact mosquito netting, sleeping in screened areas, spraying the screened area with permethrin-containing insecticide before the sun sets, wearing protective clothing, using DEET (N,N-diethyl meta-toluamide, 30 mL in 250 mL water) to impregnate cotton garments, minimizing nocturnal exposure by wearing long-sleeved clothing and long pants out of doors after sunset, and applying DEET insect repellents to exposed skin. Refined lemon eucalyptus oil may also be used on the skin.

Complementary and Alternative Medications

Patients should be informed about halofantrine, the oral antimalarial agent used throughout the world but not commercially available in the United States or Canada, and atremisinin. Atremisinin and its derivatives are renowned for their potent activity for both suppression and treatment of malaria. Atremisinin (qinghaosu) is derived from a plant that has been used in Chinese herbal medicine for thousands of years. The atremisinin derivatives have an unusual mode of action involving the iron-catalyzed generation of a carbon-centered free radical followed by the alkylation of malaria-specific proteins. Atremisinin is an extremely efficacious drug with complete eradication of parasitemia within 48 hours. To prevent recrudescence, treatment is extended beyond the disappearance of parasites as a monotherapy or in combination with other antimalarial agents.

AMEBIASIS

Amebiasis is present worldwide, but it is most common in tropical areas where crowded living conditions and poor sanitation exist. Africa, Latin America, Southeast Asia, and India have significant health problems associated with this disease. In the United States, amebiasis is seen with increasing frequency among homosexual men.

CAUSES

Amebic disease is most often caused by the microorganism *Entamoeba histolytica*. *E. histolytica* is transmitted host to host by ingestion of fecally contaminated food or water or is vector-borne by flies.

PATHOPHYSIOLOGY

The microorganism is ingested in cyst form. The cyst has a double cystic membrane and can resist the action of stomach acids. In the intestine, the cysts assume a sexually active form called a trophozoite, which produces the active disease. Trophozoites do not have a double cystic membrane and they disintegrate rapidly after expulsion into the exter-

nal environment. The active disease may remain in the intestine (intestinal amebiasis) or the trophozoites may penetrate the intestinal wall, in which case abscesses develop in other tissues and organs (extraintestinal amebiasis).

DIAGNOSTIC CRITERIA

Symptoms range from mild to severe. Mild symptoms include mucoid diarrhea, flatulence, fatigue, weight loss, and colicky abdominal pain. Severe disease may present with frequent odoriferous stool with mucus and blood, fever to 105°F, tenesmus, generalized abdominal tenderness, and vomiting.

INITIATING DRUG THERAPY

As with malaria, the only nonpharmacologic therapy is prevention. Thorough hand washing is the best way to prevent the spread of infectious diseases of the intestinal tract. Good hand-washing habits are especially important after going to the bathroom, before preparing meals, and before eating. Patients with infants should wash their hands before and after changing diapers.

Children who attend daycare centers should be kept at home if they have diarrhea. If household members or other contacts have symptoms, they should be tested for amebiasis also.

Goals of Drug Therapy

The goal of therapy is to eradicate the pathogen with the fewest adverse effects, coupled with a decrease in or elimination of symptoms. See Table 32-1 for a review of drugs used to treat amebiasis.

Iodoquinol

Iodoquinol, an oral amebicide used for treating intestinal amebiasis, exerts its action directly on the large intestine, although the exact mechanism of action is unknown. Iodoquinol is active against both the trophozoite and encysted forms of the parasite. It can be used alone in patients with mild cases or in asymptomatic carriers. In more severe cases, it should be used in combination with other amebicidal drugs. Iodoquinol is poorly absorbed from the GI tract. It reaches high concentrations in the intestinal lumen and produces its effects precisely at the site of infection without significant systemic absorption.

Hypersensitivity is the only contraindication to iodoquinol. Safety for use during pregnancy and lactation has not been established.

Adverse effects associated with iodoquinol include mild GI disturbances, skin disorders, discoloration of hair and nails, thyroid enlargement, fever, chills, headache, vertigo, and malaise. Caution should be used in patients with optic neuritis, optic atrophy, and peripheral neuropathy because these are potential adverse effects that have occurred after prolonged high-dose therapy.

Although there are no significant drug–drug interactions with iodoquinol, it may affect the results of thyroid function tests. These effects may persist for as long as 6 months after discontinuing therapy.

Paromomycin

Paromomycin (Humatin) is an oral aminoglycoside amebicide used to treat amebiasis and hepatic coma. It also has been used for cestodiasis, although it is not the drug of choice because it can cause release of viable eggs from the tapeworm. Paromomycin also has been beneficial in treating *Cryptosporidium parvum* infection in patients with human immunodeficiency virus (HIV) infection. This agent is not effective in extraintestinal amebiasis.

Paromomycin is poorly absorbed and has only local effects in the intestine. It is not prescribed for patients with renal impairment or intestinal obstruction. Patients with ulcerative intestinal lesions can inadvertently absorb the drug.

Potential adverse effects include nephrotoxicity, ototoxicity, neuromuscular blocking effects, hypocholesterolemia, malabsorptive effects, rash, headache, vertigo, eosinophilia, exanthema, and unexplained hematuria.

A reduced rate and extent of digoxin (Lanoxin) absorption can occur when digoxin is given concurrently with paromomycin. The combination of paromomycin and succinylcholine (Anectine) in patients with renal impairment can lead to a potentiation of the neuromuscular effects.

Diloxanide Furoate

Diloxanide furoate is an orphan drug available from the CDC or one of the two compounding pharmacies (see Drug Information section below). It is used for treating asymptomatic amebiasis or in extremely mild symptomatic amebiasis in combination with other drugs. The mechanism of action of the drug is unknown.

If the initial course of treatment is unsuccessful, another course may be given; however, no more than three courses should be administered in any 12-month period.

Orally administered diloxanide furoate is hydrolyzed by intestinal esterases and absorbed as diloxanide, which is excreted mainly in urine. Diloxanide is contraindicated for use during pregnancy and in children younger than 24 months.

Adverse effects are usually mild and restricted to GI symptoms such as excessive flatulence, vomiting, persistent or recurrent diarrhea, cramping, and esophagitis. Rarely, the drug induces paresthesias and urticaria. There are no significant drug–drug interactions.

Dehydroemetine

Dehydroemetine is a parenteral amebicide reserved for extraintestinal amebiasis in patients who do not respond to or who cannot take metronidazole (Flagyl). Like diloxanide, dehydroemetine is available through the CDC or the manufacturer, Hoffman LaRoche. Dehydroemetine is believed to exert its effects by inhibiting protein synthesis. The drug should be used cautiously in patients with congestive heart failure, recent myocardial infarction, cardiomyopathy, or primary muscular or neurologic disorders. Dehydroemetine has not been approved for use in pregnant or breast-feeding women.

Dehydroemetine may precipitate cardiac failure in patients with impending cardiac failure and may induce conduction defects and arrhythmias in susceptible patients. It can prolong the QT and PR intervals, the QRS complex, and the ST segment. Hypotension may occur in up to 25% of patients. CNS adverse effects include polyneuritis with transient paralysis that may persist for up to 2 months. Other adverse effects include injection site reactions, diarrhea, and nausea. There are no significant drug–drug interactions.

Selecting the Most Appropriate Agent

In amebiasis treatment, the drug of choice depends on the presentation of the disease. Metronidazole (see Chapter 37) is indicated for amebiasis that infects the intestine, liver, and all other sites. Iodoquinol is used for asymptomatic intestinal amebiasis. Other antiparasitic drugs, such as paromomycin, chloroquine, dehydroemetine, and diloxanide furoate, are reserved for later use if needed. For a summary, see Table 32-3.

First-Line Therapy

Metronidazole is the drug of choice for systemic or symptomatic amebiasis. In patients with asymptomatic amebiasis, the drug of choice is iodoquinol. For symptomatic disease, a course of iodoquinol (at asymptomatic disease dosages) should be given after completing the metronidazole treatment.

Second-Line Therapy

Because of the serious side effects and monitoring needs associated with paromomycin, this drug is a second choice for treating amebiasis. As with first-line therapy, treatment with paromomycin for symptomatic disease should be followed by a course of iodoquinol at asymptomatic disease dosages.

Third-Line Therapy

The orphan drugs dehydroemetine and diloxanide furoate are the last choices for treating amebiasis.

Table 32.3

Recommended Order of Treatment for Amebiasis

Order	Agents	Comments
First line	metronidazole	Metronidazole treats both systemic and symptomatic amebiasis.
	or	
	iodoquinol	Iodoquinol treats asymptomatic amebiasis.
Second line	paromomycin	Associated with serious toxicities; monitoring is essential
Third line	dehydroemetine or diloxanide furoate	Orphan drugs available only through CDC

MONITORING PATIENT RESPONSE

Because amebiasis may not cause symptoms in people who are carriers of the disease, therapy needs to continue until laboratory test results are negative for the parasite. Beginning 2 to 4 weeks after completion of treatment, at least three stools should be examined at 2- to 3-day intervals. Follow-up stool specimens should be obtained at 1, 3, and 6 months to validate eradication of the disease.

Complications of amebiasis include peritonitis, hepatitis or liver abscess, lung abscess, and pericardial infection. Ameboma (a solid mass of granulation tissue) may also occur, resulting in a colon obstruction. The mortality rate for untreated hepatic abscess or ameboma is high. The prognosis for amebiasis with appropriate drug therapy is excellent.

PATIENT EDUCATION

The spread of amebiasis can be prevented with proper handwashing techniques and safe food handling and preparation. Cooking kills amebic cysts. In areas where amebiasis is endemic, travelers should avoid fresh, uncooked vegetables or fruits that are not peeled. In countries with poor sanitation, it is advisable to drink water from sources known to be free of sewage contamination. Infected food handlers should not work before treatment concludes.

Drug Information

Diloxanide furoate is not commercially available but can be compounded by Panorama Compounding in Nan Nuys, California (800-247-9767), or Medical Center Pharmacy, New Haven, Connecticut (203-688-6816).

Dehydroemetine should be used only in patients in whom metronidazole has failed; it is available only as an investigational agent through the manufacturer, Hoffman LaRoche.

Patient-Oriented Information Sources

The CDC's Division of Parasitic Disease is an excellent source of patient information regarding amebiasis (http://www.cdc.gov/ncidod/dpd/parasites/amebiasis/factsht_amebiasis.htm). Also, the National Institutes of Health (NIH) Medline Plus service contains useful information. Neither of these sites, though, goes into much drug detail, but the NIH also has a site specific for drug information where patients can find information about antiamebic agents.

Nutrition/Lifestyle Changes

There are no major lifestyle changes except for the handwashing recommendations noted earlier. Travelers should avoid drinking unsanitary water in countries with poor sanitation.

Complementary and Alternative Medications

There appears to be no study of complementary or alternative medications for the treatment of amebiasis. However, there has been a single report in which colonic irrigation caused amebiasis (Anon., 1981). The practitioner should be aware of a potential link between colonic irrigation and amebiasis.

GIARDIASIS

Giardiasis, a common parasitic disease, is more prevalent in children than in adults, possibly because many people seem to acquire a lasting immunity after infection. The disease is common in daycare centers, especially those in which diapering is done. This disease also affects many homosexual men, both HIV-positive and HIV-negative; this is presumed to be due to sexual transmission.

CAUSES

Giardiasis is a common disease caused by a flagellated protozoan, *Giardia lamblia*. It is transmitted by fecal contamination. Hikers who drink unfiltered water or travelers to foreign countries where the water supply is impure are most susceptible to this disease.

PATHOPHYSIOLOGY

Giardiasis affects the intestinal system, resulting in acute or chronic diarrhea and possibly malabsorption syndrome. The acute phase may last days to weeks; the chronic phase may last years.

DIAGNOSTIC CRITERIA

Symptoms include diarrheal, soft, or steatorrheal stools with mucus but without blood. Abdominal cramps, vomiting, flatulence, and weight loss also may occur. Diagnosis can be made by identifying the causative organism in the stool specimen by microscopy, nucleic acid amplification, or antigen assay.

INITIATING DRUG THERAPY

Prevention is the only nonpharmacologic therapy for giardiasis. Treatment is usually begun after the organism is identified.

Goals of Drug Therapy

The goals of drug therapy are eradication of the disease-causing organism, prevention of further transmission, and relief of symptoms (see Table 32-1 for more information).

Metronidazole

The drug of choice for giardiasis is metronidazole. Metronidazole, which is extremely efficacious, is discussed in Chapter 37. Quinacrine, the former drug of choice, is more effective than metronidazole but is no longer available in the United States.

Furazolidone

Furazolidone (Furoxone) is an oral anti-infective agent. It is used to treat bacterial or protozoal diarrhea and enteritis. Furazolidone may be useful in treating traveler's diarrhea, cholera, and bacteremic salmonellosis. Furazolidone exerts its bactericidal action by interfering with several bacterial enzyme systems. It is also structurally similar to the monoamine oxidase inhibitors (MAOIs) and has MAOI activity.

The drug is slowly metabolized and slowly excreted. It may be detected in the urine up to 2 months after therapy has been discontinued. It is contraindicated in patients with hypersensitivity to the drug, those with G6PD deficiency, pregnant or lactating patients, or patients taking MAOIs.

Adverse effects of furazolidone include hypotension, urticaria, fever, arthralgia, colitis, proctitis, anal pruritus, nausea or vomiting or both, headache, malaise, a disulfiram (Antabuse)-like reaction, and hemolysis in G6PD deficiency. Urine may be colored orange or brown.

Furazolidone may induce a disulfiram-like reaction when taken concurrently with alcohol. It may increase the efficacy and adverse effects of levodopa (Dopar). When furazolidone is taken with meperidine (Demerol), the patient may experience agitation, seizures, diaphoresis, fever, coma, or apnea. Furazolidone inhibits MAO. Increased pressor effects are expected when it is administered with sympathomimetic drugs because sympathomimetics cause the release of large amounts of norepinephrine. Concurrent use with tricyclic antidepressants can produce hypertension, hyperpyrexia, seizures, tachycardia, and acute psychosis.

Nitazoxanide

Nitazoxanide, an orphan drug manufactured by Romark Laboratories, is thought to interfere with the pyruvate/ferredoxin oxidoreductase (PFOR) enzyme-dependent reaction in the protozoa. This reaction is thought to be essential to anaerobic energy metabolism. It appears to be well absorbed, with peak plasma concentrations occurring within 1 to 4 hours after oral administration. Alinia is available in an oral suspension of 100 mg/5 mL. Once in the body, it is 99% protein-bound. Nitazoxanide is hydrolyzed to the active metabolite, tizoxanide. Tizoxanide then undergoes conjugation, primarily by glucuronidation. This metabolite is found in the urine and bile.

The typical dosage is 100 mg BID for children 24 to 47 months of age or 200 mg BID for children 2 to 11 years old. The duration of therapy for giardiasis is 3 days. Adverse effects are mild and transient and include abdominal pain, nausea, vomiting, and headache.

Selecting the Most Appropriate Agent

First-Line Therapy

Metronidazole is indicated for all patients except those with metronidazole hypersensitivity (Table 32-4).

Second-Line Therapy

For patients with metronidazole hypersensitivity or when metronidazole is contraindicated, furazolidone is the second choice.

Third-Line Therapy

Paromomycin can be used in case of failure, adverse reaction, or intolerance to either the first- or second-line agent.

Special Population Considerations

Pediatrics

The Food and Drug Administration (FDA) has approved Alinia (nitazoxanide) oral suspension for the treatment of diarrhea caused by giardiasis in children ages 1 through 11 years. The manufacturer, Romark Laboratories, is also seeking FDA approval for a tablet form.

MONITORING PATIENT RESPONSE

Resolution of giardiasis is monitored by serial stool culture. A stool specimen should be obtained for culture every week beginning 2 weeks after completion of therapy until the result is negative for *G. lamblia*.

Metronidazole is extremely efficacious in giardiasis treatment. Approximately 40% of those who are diagnosed with giardiasis demonstrate disaccharide intolerance during detectable infection and up to 6 months after the infection can no longer be detected. Lactose intolerance may be observed. Chronic infections lead to a malabsorption syndrome and severe weight loss. Chronic cases of giardiasis in immunodeficient patients are frequently refractory to drug treatment. In some immunodeficient patients, giardiasis may shorten the life span.

PATIENT EDUCATION

Teaching points include food and water handling and preparation, hand washing and bathroom hygiene, and, for new mothers and caregivers for infants, diapering instructions related to hygiene and hand washing.

Patient-Oriented Information Sources

The traveler should be directed to the CDC website for travelers (http://www.cdc.gov/travel/food-drink-risks.htm) for education regarding avoidance of contaminated food or water.

Nutrition/Lifestyle Changes

Hikers and travelers can protect themselves by boiling drinking water for 1 minute, filtering the drinking water (the filter's pore size must be less than 5 microns), or using a few drops of bleach or tincture of iodine per liter of water.

Table 32.4

Recommended Order of Treatment for Giardiasis

Order	Agents	Comments
First line	metronidazole	Treatment of choice for all
Second line	furazolidone	Treatment for patients who cannot take metronidazole
Third line	paromomycin	Used when other treatments fail

However, the cysts that cause giardiasis are very resistant to chemical treatment, so boiling is preferred.

Complementary and Alternative Medications

There are no natural remedies or complementary therapies appropriate to this condition, but dietary advice can help.

HELMINTHIC INFECTIONS

The incidence of helminthic (worm) infections is rapidly growing in the United States. This may be related to the increased incidence of travel and immigration. Helminths are grouped into three categories: nematodes (roundworms), trematodes (flukes), and cestodes (tapeworms).

INTESTINAL NEMATODES

Ascariasis, caused by *Ascaris lumbricoides* (giant roundworm), is one of the most common intestinal helminth infections in the United States. It is endemic in areas where hygiene and sanitation are poor or where human feces are used as fertilizer. Transmission is by the ingestion of fecally contaminated food or fluids. There is no human-to-human transmission. Once ingested, the giant roundworm eggs migrate to the small bowel, where they hatch. The motile larvae thus released migrate from the small bowel to the heart and lungs, then to the esophagus and back to the small bowel. They can survive for up to 5 years and may grow as long as 30 cm. Symptoms of ascariasis include low-grade fever, nonproductive cough, blood-tinged sputum, wheezing, dyspnea, and substernal pain. Heavy infestation of adult worms in the intestine may produce peptic ulcer–like symptoms. Masses of worms may cause intestinal obstruction, volvulus, or intussusception. Rarely, larvae lodge in the brain, kidney, eye, and spinal cord, causing symptoms related to those organs. Reports of lung abscess or laryngeal obstruction with suffocation are rare.

Enterobiasis, caused by *Enterobius vermicularis* (pinworm), is the most common helminthic infection in the United States. Children are infected more frequently than adults. Transmission occurs from contact with ova in food or water or on bed linens. Adult worms inhabit the cecum and adjacent bowel areas. Female pinworms migrate through the anus to the perianal skin and deposit large numbers of eggs, especially at night. The eggs become infective in a matter of a few hours and can be transmitted to others or be autoinfective. The most common symptoms are pruritus ani (rectal itching) and pruritus vulvae (vulvar itching).

Strongyloidiasis is caused by infection with *Strongyloides stercoralis* (threadworm). This is a potentially serious infection in an adult because the worm has the ability to multiply in the host. When the parasite is in its filariform larval cycle, transmission occurs as the larvae penetrate the skin from soil, enter the bloodstream, and are carried to the lungs. From the lungs, they escape from the alveoli and ascend the bronchial tree to the glottis. The larvae are then swallowed and carried to the small intestine, where they mature into adults. The mature worm embeds itself in the mucosa, where

eggs are laid and hatched. The larvae disseminate into the lungs and most other tissues and may cause local inflammation and formation of granulomas. Symptoms include skin reactions such as inflammation, petechiae, and urticaria. Intestinal symptoms include diarrhea, abdominal pain, and flatulence. Pulmonary symptoms include dry cough, throat irritation, dyspnea, wheezing, and hemoptysis. Hyperinfection syndrome caused by intense dissemination of larvae to the lungs and other tissues can result in complications such as pleural effusion, pericarditis, and myocarditis. There also may be perforation of the colon and peritonitis, gram-negative septicemia, and shock, leading to death.

Trichuriasis infection is acquired by ingestion of an infective egg of *Trichuris trichiura* (whipworm). Human-to-human transmission is not possible. Whipworms attach to the mucosa of the large intestine by means of their anterior whiplike end. Symptoms include abdominal cramps, tenesmus, diarrhea, flatulence, nausea, vomiting, and weight loss. Potential complications include rectal prolapse and hematochezia or chronic occult blood loss. These complications may occur with heavy infections. Invasion of the appendix resulting in appendicitis is rare.

Trichinosis is caused by *Trichinella spiralis* (pork roundworm). The disease is acquired by ingesting encysted larvae in inadequately cooked meat, especially pork. Gastric juices liberate the encysted larvae, which migrate to the intestines, where they mature, mate, and produce eggs that hatch into new larvae. These larvae are transported throughout the body and enter skeletal muscle tissues, producing an inflammatory response. Eventually the larvae are re-encysted and remain within the tissues without symptoms. Initial symptoms include diarrhea, cramps, and malaise. As the infection progresses, patients may experience muscle pain, tenderness, fever, periorbital and facial edema, and conjunctivitis. Potential complications include granulomatous pneumonitis, encephalitis, and cardiac failure.

BLOOD AND TISSUE NEMATODES

Filariasis infections are among the more serious and debilitating helminthiases. There are two forms of filarial infections. The first type is caused by the microbes *Wuchereria bancrofti* and *Brugia malayi*. Mosquito vectors transmit both microbes. Bancroftian filariasis is also called elephantiasis because the helminths migrate to the lymphatic system, causing lymphadenopathy with resultant extremity edema. Brugian filariasis, which also affects the lymphatic system, produces microfilariae that circulate in the bloodstream. The second type of filariasis, also known as onchocerciasis or river blindness, is caused by *Onchocerca volvulus*. The adult helminth resides in subcutaneous nodules and migrates to the eye, causing ocular lesions and eventual loss of vision.

CESTODE INFECTIONS

Taeniasis or tapeworm infection is transmitted by the ingestion of contaminated, raw, or improperly cooked fish (*Diphyllobothrium latum*), beef (*Taenia saginata*), and pork (*Taenia solium*). The adult tapeworm consists of a head (scolex), which attaches to the intestinal wall, and segments called proglottids. The proglottids contain tapeworm eggs and are expelled in the feces. Beef and fish tapeworms do not cause serious illness; however, pork tapeworms produce larvae that enter the bloodstream and invade other body tissues. Symptoms include nausea, vomiting, and diarrhea as well as fatigue, hunger, and dizziness. Because the worm competes with the human host for vitamin B_{12}, deficiency is a potential complication.

TREMATODE INFECTIONS

Schistosomiasis is the second leading cause of morbidity and mortality in parasitic diseases. The vector of this disease is a specific snail. There are three major types of schistosome. Each migrates to a specific part of the human host and produces specific clinical symptoms. Adult helminths generate a granulomatous response in human tissues. The disease is divided into the acute and chronic phases. In the acute phase, symptoms are abdominal pain, weight loss, headache, malaise, chills, fever, myalgia, diarrhea, dry mouth, hepatomegaly, and eosinophilia. Symptoms of the chronic phase of *Schistosoma mansoni* or *Schistosoma japonicum* infection can include a syndrome of diarrhea, abdominal pain, bloody stool, hepatomegaly or hepatosplenomegaly, and bleeding from esophageal varices. Symptoms of *Schistosoma haematobium* infection include terminal hematuria, urinary frequency, and urethral and bladder pain.

DIAGNOSTIC CRITERIA

Around the world, helminthiasis is not always treated. Many parasitic worms do not reproduce in the human host, and therefore the infection may subside spontaneously as the adult worms die. In the United States, medication is readily available and recognized infection is treated.

INITIATING DRUG THERAPY

Identification of the type of infestation is essential in treating helminthiasis. Worms can be isolated and identified in stool specimens. A common pinworm infection can be identified by the "Scotch-tape" test in which a piece of transparent tape is placed over the anal meatus at bedtime. During the night, the pinworms exit the anus and are found attached to the tape in the morning.

Goals of Drug Therapy

The goal of drug therapy is to eradicate the helminth and avoid its transmission to others.

Choices for pharmacotherapy depend on the type of helminth. With appropriate diagnosis and treatment, helminth infections do not usually pose a great threat to most people. Patients from countries with endemic helminthic infections or travelers to these countries have a high risk for these infections. Immunocompromised patients have the greatest risk of all for poor outcomes.

Table 32-5 highlights the efficacy of selected anthelmintic agents, Table 32-6 identifies current preferred agents and dosages, and Table 32-7 gives the recommended order of treatments.

Mebendazole

Mebendazole (Vermox) is a broad-spectrum anthelmintic used for treating roundworm, hookworm, whipworm, threadworm, and pinworm infections. It selectively damages cytoplasmic microtubules in the absorptive and intestinal cells of helminths, but not the host. This microtubular deterioration is irreversible and leads to disruption of the absorptive and

Table 32.5

Efficacy of Selected Anthelmintics

	mebendazole	albendazole	diethylcarbamazine	ivermectin	praziquantel
Nematode Infections					
Ascariasis	++	++	−	++	−
Trichuriasis	++	+	−	±	−
Hookworm	+	++	−	−	−
Strongyloidiasis	±	+	−	++	−
Enterobiasis	++	++	−	+	−
Trichinellosis	±	±	−	−	−
Intestinal capillariasis	+	+	−	−	−
Cutaneous larva migrans	−	+	−	−	−
Visceral larva migrans	+	+	+	−	−
Lymphatic filariasis	−	−	++	++	−
Onchocerciasis	−	−	++	++	−
Loiasis	−	−	++	++	−
Cestode and Trematode Infections					
Taeniasis	±	+	?	?	++
Hymenolepis nana	−	−	?	?	++
Cysticercosis	±	+	?	?	+
Echinococcosis	+	+	?	?	±
Schistosoma mansoni	±	−	?	?	++
Schistosoma haematobium	±	−	?	?	±
Fascioliasis	−	−	?	?	++
Fasciolopsiasis	−	−	?	?	+
Clonorchiasis	−	±	?	?	+
Opisthorchiasis	−	±	?	?	+
Paragonimiasis	−	−	?	?	++

Table 32.6

Overview of Selected Anthelmintic Agents

Generic (Trade) Name and Dosage	Selected Adverse Events	Contraindications	Special Considerations
mebendazole (Vermox) *Adult:* 1 tablet PO morning and evening on 3 consecutive days	Transient abdominal pain, diarrhea	Hypersensitivity, lactation, pregnancy	Can be crushed or mixed with food Treat whole family.
thiabendazole (Mintezol) <150 lb: 10 mg/lb per dose PO >150 lb: 1.5 g/dose PO Maximum daily dose is 3 g *For strongyloidiasis and ascariasis:* 2 doses/d for 2 successive days or single dose of 20 mg/lb *For enterobiasis (pinworm):* 2 doses/d for 1 d; repeat in 7 d to reduce risk of reinfection	Dizziness, drowsiness, headache, anorexia, nausea, GI complaints, hypotension, foul-smelling urine, rash	Hypersensitivity, pregnancy Prescribe cautiously in renal or hepatic dysfunction, anemia.	Interacts with xanthines, so monitor serum xanthine levels as appropriate and adjust dosage accordingly. Take drug with food. Tablets should be chewed and then swallowed. Treat all family members. Disinfect linens, towels, night clothing, underwear, and toilet facilities.
pyrantel pamoate (Antiminth, Pin-X) *Adult:* 11 mg/kg, PO, as single oral dose; maximum 1 g *Child:* Safety and efficacy not established in child <24 mo	Headache, dizziness, drowsiness, abdominal cramps, diarrhea, anorexia, nausea, vomiting, rash	Hypersensitivity Lactation, pregnancy Hepatic disease	Avoid concomitant use with piperazine. Take entire dose at once. Treat all family members. Disinfect linens, towels, night clothing, underwear, and toilet facilities.
praziquantel (Biltricide) *Adult:* 3 doses of 20 mg/kg PO as a 1 d treatment (dose interval, 4–6 h)	Headache, dizziness, GI discomfort, drowsiness, rash, weakness	Hypersensitivity Lactation, pregnancy Optical cysticercosis	Take drug with food. Bitter tasting; swallow tablet whole.
ivermectin (Stromectol) *Adult:* 200 μg/kg, single PO dose for strongyloidosis	Dizziness, tremors, GI complaints, rash, fatigue, abdominal pain	Hypersensitivity Lactation, pregnancy Prescribe with caution in patients with eye conditions.	Avoid breast-feeding on treatment day and for 3 full days after.

secretory functions of the cells that are essential to the helminths' survival.

Mebendazole is primarily eliminated by the liver and can accumulate in patients with hepatic impairment, increasing the risk of adverse effects. It is not known whether mebendazole is excreted in human milk; therefore, it should be prescribed with caution to breast-feeding mothers. It has not been evaluated for use in children younger than 24 months.

Mebendazole is a chewable tablet that is minimally absorbed from the GI tract because significant first-pass hepatic metabolism transforms mebendazole to an inactive metabolite. Approximately 10% of the drug is excreted unchanged in the urine; the remainder is excreted in the feces.

Contraindications

Mebendazole is contraindicated in people who have shown hypersensitivity to the drug. Mebendazole is used with caution in patients who are pregnant, especially in the first trimester, or who have inflammatory bowel disease and hepatic disease. Patients with Crohn's disease or ulcerative colitis may have increased absorption, resulting in an increased risk of toxicity.

Adverse Events

Because of its poor absorption, mebendazole rarely causes systemic toxicity except in patients with diseases that increase absorption of drugs from the bowel. Transient abdominal pain, diarrhea, dizziness, headache, and fever are common. However, this reaction may be a response to the expulsion of worms after therapy rather than to the drug itself. Other reported adverse effects include hematologic effects such as leukopenia, thrombocytopenia, and eosinophilia. Integumentary effects include pruritus, rash, and flushing. In the renal system, hematuria and crystalluria are possible. Mebendazole may elevate serum liver enzyme levels.

Interactions

Mebendazole may interact with carbamazepine and hydantoins, although the mechanism of interaction is unknown. Pharmacologic effects of mebendazole may be decreased, leading to failure to eradicate the helminth. However, no special precautions appear necessary. If an interaction is suspected, the dosage of mebendazole may need to be increased.

Thiabendazole

Thiabendazole (Mintezol) is a vermicidal agent structurally related to mebendazole. It has more limited usefulness than mebendazole because of its potential toxicity. The precise mechanism of action is not clear. It is known to inhibit specific enzymes in the helminth. Thiabendazole is used for pinworm, roundworm, threadworm, and hookworm infestation. It is the drug of choice for strongyloidiasis.

Thiabendazole may be administered orally or topically. After oral administration, thiabendazole is rapidly absorbed

Table 32.7

Recommended Order of Treatment for Worm Infections

Order	Agents	Comments
Nematodes		
ROUNDWORM		
First line	mebendazole	Repeat after 3 wk if first dose was not curative. Chew or crush tablet and mix with food.
Second line	pyrantel pamoate	Available OTC. Administer without regard to food or time of day.
Third line	albendazole	Take with food.
PINWORM		
First line	pyrantel pamoate	Same as above
Second line	mebendazole	Same as above
Third line	albendazole	Repeat after 2 wk. Take with food.
WHIPWORM		
First line	mebendazole	Same as above
Second line	albendazole	Same as above
HOOKWORM		
First line	pyrantel pamoate	Same as above
Second line	mebendazole	Same as above
THREADWORM		
First line	thiabendazole	Take with food. Chew tablets before swallowing.
Second line	ivermectin	Take tablets with water.
TRICHINOSIS		
First line	thiabendazole	Indicated during invasive phase. Limited clinical experience in children weighing <30 lb. Take with food and chew tablets before swallowing.
Second line	mebendazole	Used in addition to steroids for severe symptoms.
FILARIASIS		
First line	diethylcarbamazine	Take immediately after meals. Available from manufacturer without charge for compassionate use.
Onchocerciasis		
First line	ivermectin	Take tablets with water.
Second line	diethylcarbamazine	Take immediately after meals. Available from manufacturer without charge for compassionate use.
Trematodes		
Schistosomiasis	praziquantel	Take with liquids during meals. Do not chew tablets.
Cestodes		
Tapeworm or cestodiasis	praziquantel	Same as above

from the GI tract. Peak plasma levels are attained within 1 to 2 hours. The half-life of thiabendazole is roughly 1.2 hours. Approximately 90% of an oral dose is excreted in the urine as metabolites, and approximately 5% is excreted in feces within 48 hours.

Contraindications

Thiabendazole is contraindicated in patients with known hypersensitivity to the drug. It is used cautiously in patients with hepatic disease because it undergoes extensive hepatic metabolism. The drug is prescribed with caution in children weighing less than 15 kg, in patients with hepatic or renal dysfunction, and in patients with severe dehydration, malnutrition, or anemia.

Adverse Events

Because thiabendazole is better absorbed from the bowel, adverse effects are more common than with mebendazole. Adverse effects include GI disturbances and CNS symptoms such as dizziness and headache. Seizures and psychiatric disturbances have also been reported. Other potential adverse effects include hypotension, hyperglycemia, transient leukope-

nia, and sensory disturbances such as tinnitus, blurred vision, and xanthopsia.

Thiabendazole can also interfere with the metabolism of xanthine derivatives such as theophylline (Slo-Phyllin), reducing their clearance by up to 50%. Toxic serum concentrations of theophylline can result. Reduction of the theophylline dosage may be necessary during concomitant treatment.

Pyrantel Pamoate

Like mebendazole, pyrantel pamoate (Antiminth, Pin-X) is indicated for use in pinworm, hookworm, and roundworm infections. By stimulating the release of acetylcholine, inhibiting cholinesterase, and stimulating ganglionic neurons, the drug acts as a depolarizing neuromuscular blocking agent in helminths. These actions cause extensive depolarization of the helminth muscle membrane, producing tension in the helminths' muscles, which causes paralysis and releases their hold on the intestinal wall.

Pyrantel is administered orally and has poor and incomplete absorption from the GI tract. Peak plasma levels occur within 1 to 3 hours. The absorbed drug is partially metabolized in the liver, with approximately 7% being excreted in the urine as unaltered drug and metabolites, and more than 50% of each dose is excreted unchanged in the feces.

Pyrantel is used with caution in patients with liver dysfunction, malnutrition, dehydration, and anemia. It has not been approved for use during pregnancy or for patients younger than 24 months. Pyrantel and piperazine are mutually antagonistic and should not be given together.

Diethylcarbamazine

Diethylcarbamazine is a piperazine derivative used in filariasis treatment. It works in two ways. First, it decreases muscular activity and causes eventual paralysis of the microfilariae. It also causes changes in the parasite's surface membrane, which make the parasite susceptible to the host's immune system defenses. Diethylcarbamazine is the only agent currently used for the suppression and cure of bancroftian and brugian filariasis. Diethylcarbamazine is absorbed readily. It undergoes rapid and extensive metabolism. Metabolites are excreted in the urine.

Common adverse effects include nausea and vomiting, anorexia, and headache. Another type of reaction, caused by the dying microfilariae, is called the Mazzotti reaction. This reaction consists of severe itching, papular rash, tachycardia, and an intense headache. Rapid drug-induced death of *O. volvulus* microfilariae in the eye can result in permanent loss of vision. Hypersensitivity is the only contraindication.

Praziquantel

Praziquantel (Biltricide) is used in treating schistosomes, flukes, and tapeworms. Praziquantel works by increasing the cell membrane permeability in susceptible worms, causing vacuolization and disintegration of the schistosome. Praziquantel is rapidly absorbed from the GI tract. It undergoes extensive hepatic metabolism and is excreted in the urine.

Adverse reactions are minimal; the most frequent are malaise, headache, dizziness, and abdominal discomfort. Patients should be warned not to drive a car or operate machinery on the day of treatment and the following day. In extensive animal trials, praziquantel has not proved mutagenic, carcinogenic, or teratogenic. However, providers advise women who are breast-feeding to refrain from nursing on the day of treatment and for the subsequent 72 hours.

Ivermectin

Ivermectin (Stromectol) is an oral antiparasitic agent used in the treatment of onchocerciasis and strongyloidiasis. Its parasitic action involves increasing the permeability of the parasite membrane to chloride ion, which hyperpolarizes nerve and muscle and causes paralysis. Ivermectin is rapidly absorbed from the GI tract. It undergoes hepatic metabolism and is excreted in the urine.

The most common adverse effects in patients being treated for strongyloidiasis are diarrhea, nausea, dizziness, and pruritus. In patients being treated for onchocerciasis, the most common adverse reactions are related to allergic and inflammatory responses to the death of the microfilariae. They include arthralgia; axillary, cervical, inguinal, and other lymph node enlargement and tenderness; pruritus; peripheral edema; papular and pustular or urticarial rash; and fever. Myalgia, abdominal pain, and headache have also been reported.

Albendazole

Albendazole (Albenza) is not routinely available in the United States. It can be requested without charge from Lederle Laboratories for the treatment of hydatid disease and neurocysticercosis. It can also be used to treat ascariasis, trichuriasis, enterobiasis, and strongyloidiasis, although it is not approved for these helminthic infections. Albendazole selectively damages cytoplasmic microtubules in the absorptive and intestinal cells of nematodes but not of the host. This microtubular deterioration is irreversible and leads to disruption of absorptive and secretory functions of the cells, which are essential to the worm's survival.

After oral administration, albendazole is absorbed and completely metabolized. The half-life of albendazole in the plasma is 8.5 hours. The metabolite is essentially eliminated through the urine. Albendazole is best taken with meals, especially with food containing fat, to help absorption. Tablets may be chewed, swallowed whole with a small amount of liquid, or crushed and mixed with food.

Like mebendazole, albendazole is teratogenic and has not been tested for use in children. In most clinical trials, it has been more efficacious than mebendazole for treating intestinal and systemic nematodes. In limited trials, it has been effective against systemic cestode infections, which historically have been refractory to chemotherapy.

MONITORING PATIENT RESPONSE

Monitoring of drug therapy usually is not warranted. In cases of prolonged or recurrent infections, the patient should be monitored for adverse effects of the individual agents.

PATIENT EDUCATION

Families and other close contacts of the infected person should be treated at the same time because of the easy communicability of helminths. Hands should be washed before preparing, handling, or eating food. Fingernails should be kept short and scrubbed with a nailbrush. Children with intestinal helminths should wear underpants under their pajamas to prevent the transmission of eggs to their fingers if they scratch during sleep. The anal area should be washed in the morning to remove any eggs laid overnight. Clothing and bedding should be washed in hot water or dry-cleaned.

ECTOPARASITIC INFECTIONS

Scabies is a dermatitis caused by infestation with *Sarcoptes scabiei*. The mite is barely visible to the naked eye. Transmission is acquired by sleeping with an infected person, by sleeping in infested bedding, or by other close contact. The lesions consist of generalized excoriations with small pruritic vesicles, pustules, and burrows. The infestations occur on the sides of the fingers and the palms, wrists, elbows and around the axillae. The head and neck are usually spared in adults. Diagnosis is made by identification of the parasite, ova, or feces on a slide under a microscope.

Pediculosis (lice) infections occur on the scalp (pediculosis capitis), trunk (pediculosis corporis), or pubic areas (pediculosis pubis). For both head lice and body lice, transmission can occur during direct contact with an infected person. Head lice cannot jump or fly, but they can be transmitted by head-to-head contact or by sharing items of clothing, combs, brushes, hats, or headphones. Shared surfaces such as pillows, mattresses, sleeping bags, car seats, or upholstered furniture can also contribute to transmission of head lice. Although other means are possible, pediculosis pubis is most often transmitted through sexual contact.

DIAGNOSTIC CRITERIA

Pediculosis is an infestation of the hairy parts of the body or clothing with eggs, larvae, or adult lice. The crawling stages of this insect feed on human blood, which can result in severe itching. Head lice can be found anywhere on the scalp, but infestation is heaviest behind the ears and just above the hairline along the nape of the neck. Pubic lice are found in the pubic area and along seams of clothing, from which they travel to the skin to feed. They are more commonly found in sexually active young adults. Pubic lice are rarely found on the head. Body lice, similar to pubic lice, are found in clothing that is in direct contact with the body, such as underwear, in the armpits of shirts, or the crotch of trousers. These type of lice are more commonly seen in colder climates, where people may change their clothes less frequently.

INITIATING DRUG THERAPY

School-age children have the highest risk for ectoparasitic infections and should be taught to prevent lice infestation by not sharing brushes, combs, barrettes, or other personal items. Good hand washing also limits the spread of ectoparasites. Because both types of ectoparasites are easily communicable, laundering bed linens, towels, and clothing in hot water is important and should be a part of the treatment procedure.

Goals of Drug Therapy

The goal of drug therapy is eradication of the ectoparasite. Lindane (Kwell, Scabene) is a powerful pesticide used in treating pediculosis and scabies. Another treatment for pediculosis is permethrin (Elimite, Nix), and an additional treatment for scabies is crotamiton (Eurax).

Lindane

Lindane is available in both lotion and shampoo form. It is slowly and incompletely absorbed through intact skin, through the GI tract when ingested, and through mucous membranes when inhaled. After topical administration, some lindane is systemically absorbed. Absorption is greater through damaged skin. The drug is stored in body fats, metabolized in the liver, and excreted in urine and feces. If absorbed systemically, lindane is a CNS stimulant, producing adverse effects similar to those produced by DDT, a potent insecticide that has been banned from use in the United States for almost 30 years.

Lindane is a topical scabicide that is absorbed through the exoskeleton of parasites, presumably causing excessive CNS stimulation that results in convulsions and death. Lindane is a topical application and systemic absorption occurs only when it is placed on open or damaged skin.

Lindane is contraindicated in patients with seizure disorders and known hypersensitivity. CNS toxicity may precipitate

seizures. Lindane should not be used where there is a skin rash, abrasion, or inflammation because systemic absorption may be enhanced, which increases the possibility of CNS toxicity. Lindane is also contraindicated in children younger than 24 months; children of this age have more permeable skin and there may be significant systemic absorption. Caution should be used with children between 2 and 10 years of age because of an increased risk of toxicity. Use of lindane during pregnancy is questionable because of the potential for serious adverse CNS effects. Lindane is not recommended for use while breast-feeding because it is secreted into breast milk; an alternative form of feeding should be used for at least 2 days. For more information, see Table 32-8.

Permethrin

Permethrin, a synthetic agent, is active against lice, ticks, mites, and fleas. It acts on the nerve cell membrane to disrupt the sodium channel current. The result is paralysis of the pests. It is used for treating head lice and their nits. If live lice are observed after 7 days, a second treatment may be given. Infection with head lice is often accompanied by pruritus, erythema, and edema, which may be temporarily exacerbated with permethrin treatment. Hypersensitivity is the only contraindication to permethrin use. Patients using permethrin should be advised to towel-dry their hair after washing and rinsing it.

Crotamiton

Crotamiton is a scabicidal and antipruritic agent used for treating *S. scabiei* infestation (scabies) and for symptomatic treatment of pruritic skin. Crotamiton should be applied from the chin to the toes after taking a bath or shower. A second application is advisable 24 hours later. Clothing and bed linens should be changed the second day. Contaminated clothing and bed linen may be dry-cleaned or washed in the hot cycle of the washing machine. A cleansing bath should be taken 48 hours after the last application. The only contraindication to crotamiton use is hypersensitivity, and it should be used with caution in pregnancy. Pediatric safety has not been established. Crotamiton should not be applied to the eyes or mouth because it may cause irritation. It should not be applied to acutely inflamed skin or raw or weeping surfaces until the acute inflammation has resolved. The only reported adverse reaction is the potential for rash.

Selecting the Most Appropriate Agent

For a brief review of treatment options for lice and scabies infestations, see Table 32-9. Some practitioners recommend lindane as a last choice because it is associated with the most adverse effects, but in general the most appropriate agent is the product preferred by the practitioner.

MONITORING PATIENT RESPONSE

Sexual contacts should be treated simultaneously. Patients should avoid using medications on open cuts and extensive excoriations. Although many patients exhibit persistent pruritus after treatment, this is rarely a sign of treatment failure and is not an indication for retreatment unless living mites can be demonstrated.

Table 32.8

Overview of Selected Antiectoparasitic Agents

Generic (Trade) Name and Dosage	Selected Adverse Events	Contraindications	Special Considerations
lindane (Kwell, Scabene) *Adults and children, scabies and pediculosis:* For application of cream: • Clean and dry the skin well. • Apply the cream from the neck to the toes and rub in well. • Leave on skin for 8–12 h, then wash the skin well. For application of shampoo: • Wash and dry the hair and allow to cool. • Apply shampoo to dry hair and rub into the scalp. • Allow shampoo to remain in place for 4 min. • Add enough water to work up a good lather. • Rinse thoroughly and towel dry. • Use fine-tooth comb when hair is thoroughly dry.	Nausea, vomiting (with oral or prolonged/treatment), rash, tingling	Neonates, pregnancy and lactation	Associated with seizures in young children; insomnia, irritability also seen with prolonged treatment or excessive dosing
crotamiton (Eurax) *Scabies:* Same as above *Pediculosis:* Same as above	Irritation	Allergy to crotamiton—caution in patients with inflamed or raw skin	Pruritus may persist even after treatment.
Permethrin (Elimite, Nix) *Scabies:* Same as above *Pediculosis:* Same as above	Pruritus, erythema, numbness, tingling, and rash	Allergy to permethrin or chrysanthemums	As effective as lindane, without the neurotoxicity

Patients who have a history of seizure disorders and who use lindane should be monitored for signs of seizure activity. Patients undergoing recurrent treatment should also be monitored for signs of neurologic toxicity. Patients receiving crotamiton or permethrin need to be monitored for efficacy of treatment only.

PATIENT EDUCATION

The patient should be informed of the consequences of no treatment, or inadequate treatment. In most cases, the lack of treatment may lead to nuisance syndromes, such as malaise and a general feeling of illness. Only the body louse is a vector for transmitting bacterial diseases. For example, louse-borne typhus fever comes from the *Rickettsia prowazekii* organism and louse-borne relapsing fever comes from *Borrelia recurrentis*. Infection with these organisms is rare, but the consequences of non-treatment may be severe. The

Rickettsia-borne fever has occurred on all continents except Australia; if not treated, it may be fatal in 10% to 40% of the cases. The Borrelia-borne infection is characterized by 2 to 9 days of fever alternating with 2 to 4 afebrile days. Typically, only 2% to 4% of patients with this infection die.

Drug Information

It is important to give explicit instructions to parents for using scabicides such as lindane. When given appropriately, lindane is safe, but when it is given on a serial basis or left on the patient for a long time, adverse neurologic effects may ensue. The practitioner needs to be sure the caregiver understands that the treatment is for one time only; the caregiver should also know the appropriate length of time to leave the lotion or shampoo in place before rinsing the area thoroughly. The philosophy "if some is good, then more is better" is not appropriate in this situation. The only nonpharmacologic treatment

Table 32.9

Recommended Order of Treatment for Pediculosis and Scabies

Order	Agents	Comments
First line	lindane	Safe when used as directed for lice and scabies infections (*Note:* Some practitioners believe that lindane is too dangerous a chemical to be used in children.)
Second line	permethrin	An alternative to lindane treatment for lice Permethrin does not kill the lice; rather, it paralyzes them.
	crotamiton	Like permethrin, crotamiton is a safer alternative to lindane treatment for scabies.

for pediculosis is manual removal with an appropriate comb, such as the LiceMeister comb.

Patient-Oriented Information Sources

WHO offers information for both professionals and the lay public. Its website, http://www.who.int/docstore/water_sanitation_health/vectcontrol/ch25.htm, contains good information, with the basics of transmission, treatment, and removal presented both textually and graphically.

Nutrition/Lifestyle Changes

The primary lifestyle change that needs to be implemented is regular hand washing and combing of hair. Individuals should be encouraged not to share combs, brushes, or hair-related items. Shaving of hairy areas (head shaving for boys) was previously recommended but has since been replaced by effective medications (eg, lindane). Washing clothing in hot water (>60°C) is required to eliminate infestation.

Complementary and Alternative Medications

While there are reports of using kerosene baths or laundry detergent baths to eliminate the exoparasitic organism, these often make it worse and should not be used. There are no complementary or alternative medications that have good evidence of efficacy.

■ Case Study

L.A., a 38-year-old man, arrives at the clinic today with a chief complaint of loose stools for the past 3 weeks and uncontrollable diarrhea for the last 48 hours. He states that he decided to come to the clinic because he now has a fever. He reports abdominal cramps as well but denies other symptoms. He has no history of medical disorders or surgeries. L.A. is a football coach. He is married with three children younger than 6 years of age; two children attend preschool, and one is in kindergarten. L.A.'s wife does not work outside the home, and she has no symptoms at this time. L.A. is a nonsmoker and a nondrinker. He has not been out of the country for the past 3 years. He enjoys hiking in the mountains, which he did as recently as 3 weeks ago.

On physical examination, L.A. appears tired. His skin is hot to the touch. Vital signs include temperature, 101.4°F; pulse rate, 110; respiratory rate, 20; and blood pressure, 100/60. He has mild tenting to the chest. Other findings include the following:

- HEENT unremarkable
- Chest CTA
- Cor: RRR, no MRG
- Abdomen: flat, hyperactive bowel sounds in all four quadrants. Diffusely tender across abdomen, but no hepatosplenomegaly. Perirectal area bright red, small external hemorrhoid noted. Firm sphincter tone. No feces in vault, but green mucoid material recovered on glove. Guaiac test negative for occult blood.

Diagnosis: probable giardiasis

→ 1. Given the presenting symptoms and probable diagnosis of giardiasis, what are the therapeutic goals for L.A.?

→ 2. Given his age and symptoms, what drug therapy would be your first-line choice for L.A.?

→ 3. How and when would you monitor the outcome of this drug therapy?

→ 4. What specific patient education would you give to L.A. regarding this drug therapy?

→ 5. Describe one or two primary adverse reactions that you would monitor for, and what you would do if one occurred.

→ 6. What would be your choice for second-line drug therapy?

→ 7. What over-the-counter and/or alternative medications would be appropriate for L.A.?

→ 8. What dietary and lifestyle changes should L.A. put into practice?

→ 9. Describe one or two drug–drug or drug–food interactions for the first- and second-line agents you chose.

Bibliography

*Starred references are cited in the text.

*Anon. (1981). Amebiasis associated with colonic irrigation: Colorado. *MMWR Morbidity Mortality Weekly Report, 30*(9), 101–102.

Anon. (April 2002). Drugs for parasitic infections. *The Medical Letter on Drugs and Therapeutics*, April, 1–12.

Burnham, G. (1995). Malaria, an unclear but present danger. *Maryland Medical Journal, 44*, 1035–1038.

DeVries, P. J., & Dien, T. K. (1996). Clinical pharmacology and therapeutic potential of atremisinin and its derivatives in the treatment of malaria. *Drugs, 52*, 818–836.

Drug facts and comparisons. (2003). St. Louis: Facts and Comparisons Division, J. B. Lippincott.

Frayha, G. J., Smyth, J. D., Bobert, J. G., & Savel, J. (1997). The mechanisms of action of antiprotozoal and anthelminthic drugs in man. *Gen Pharmacology, 28*(2), 273–299.

Hardman, J. G., Limbird, L. E., Molinof, P. B., Ruddon, R. W., & Gilman, A. (Eds.). (1997). *Goodman and Gilman's the pharmacological basis of therapeutics* (9th ed.). New York: McGraw-Hill.

Nosten, F., & Price, R. N. (1995). New antimalarials: A risk-benefit analysis. *Drug Safety, 12*, 264–273.

*Parke, A. L., & Rothfield, N. F. (1996). Antimalarial drugs in pregnancy: The North American experience. *Lupus, 5*(Suppl. 1), S67–S69.

Pellegrini, M., & Ruff, T. A. (1999). Malaria: The latest in advice for travelers. *Australian Family Physician, 28*, 683–688.

*Phillips-Howard, P. A., & Wood, D. (1996). The safety of antimalarial drugs in pregnancy. *Drug Safety, 14*(3), 131–145.

Porth, C. (1998). *Pathophysiology: Concepts of altered health states* (2nd ed.). Philadelphia: Lippincott Williams & Wilkins.

*Roll Back Malaria Global Partnership. What is malaria? http://www.rbm.who.int Accessed Feb. 3, 2004.

*Products (Alinia®). http://romark.com/index/products. Romark Laboratories. Accessed Feb. 10, 2004.

Shuster, H., & Chiodini, P. L. (2001). Parasitic infections of the intestine. *Current Opinion in Infectious Diseases, 14*, 587–591.

Stephenson, L., & Wiselka, M. (2000). Drug treatment of tropical parasitic infections: Recent achievements and developments. *Drugs, 60*(5), 985–995.

Touze, J. E., et al. (1997). Is halofantrine still advisable in malaria attacks? *Annals of Tropical Medicine and Parasitology, 91*, 867–873.

VandeWaa, E. A., et al. (1998). Common helminth infections: Battling wormlike parasites in primary care. *Clinician Reviews, 8*(5), 75–92.

*World Health Organization (2004). Malaria. Fact Sheet No. 94. http://www.who.int.en Accessed Feb. 3, 2004.

*World Health Organization (2000). WHO Expert Committee on Malaria. Available at http://www.whoe.int.en. Accessed Feb. 3, 2004.

van Vugt, M., & White, N. J. (1999). The treatment of chloroquine-resistant malaria. *Tropical Doctor, 29*, 176–179.

Visit the Connection web site for the most up-to-date drug information.

VII

Pharmacotherapy for Genitourinary Tract Disorders

33

URINARY TRACT INFECTION

■ VIRGINIA ARCANGELO AND ANNE NICHOLS

Urinary tract infection (UTI) is a broad term used to describe inflammation of the urethra, bladder, and kidney. Bacteria, yeast, or chemical irritants can cause inflammation in the urinary tract. UTIs are a common problem encountered in health care. UTIs occurs across the life span, with nearly 50% of all American women experiencing a UTI at some time in their life, including 25% to 35% of women between the ages of 20 and 40 years. Three percent of girls and 1% of boys will have a UTI by age 11 (Schaeffer, 2002). Approximately 7 million ambulatory care visits and 1 million emergency room visits for UTI and 250,000 cases of acute pyelonephritis are reported yearly. There are countless phone calls to health care providers annually as a result of symptoms of UTIs. The annual cost of UTIs exceeds $1.5 billion (Foxman, 2002; Foxman & Brown, 2003).

CAUSES

Women contract UTIs in a 30:1 ratio to men because of their short urethra and its proximity to the rectum. Sexual intercourse is a contributing factor. With intercourse, periurethral and urethral bacteria may ascend into the bladder. After 65 years of age, the ratio of UTIs in women to men becomes closer to 1. Risk factors for UTIs in men include homosexuality, intercourse with an infected partner, and an uncircumcised penis.

Normal urine is sterile. Infection occurs when microorganisms, usually bacteria from the digestive tract, cling to the opening of the urethra and multiply. *Escherichia coli* is the causative pathogen in 70% to 95% of community-acquired UTIs. *Staphylococcus saprophyticus* accounts for approximately 5% to 20% of UTIs in young women.

Bacterial growth is decreased by dilute urine and a low urine pH. Glucose in urine is an enhanced medium for the growth of *E. coli*. The urine from pregnant women has a more suitable pH for growth of *E. coli*. Diaphragm and spermicide use (nonoxynol-9), estrogen deficiency, and constipation also are risk factors for UTIs. Inefficient bladder emptying causes UTIs because of stagnating urine. Underlying conditions that predispose to UTI are listed in Box 33-1.

PATHOPHYSIOLOGY

The development of a UTI depends on the virulence of the organism, the inoculum size, and the adequacy of the host's defense mechanisms. In general, the urinary tract is resistant to invading bacteria and rapidly eliminates organisms that reach the bladder. When bacteria enter the bladder, there is increased micturition and diuresis to empty the bladder.

Most pathogens enter the urinary tract and ascend the urethra to the bladder. Most of the microorganisms are from fecal flora, but the vagina is an important source of infecting organisms. Bacteria that cause UTIs originate in the fecal flora, colonize the vagina and periurethral introitus, and ascend to the urethra and bladder. In the bladder, the bacteria multiply and travel up the urethra to the renal pelvis and parenchyma, especially if there is vesicoureteral reflux. With cystitis, there is silent involvement of the kidneys in approximately 50% of cases.

The longer urethra in men increases the distance between the rectum and the urethral meatus, and the drier environment around the urethra and the antibacterial activity of prostatic fluid also decrease the risk of UTIs in men.

DIAGNOSTIC CRITERIA

In women of childbearing age, the most frequent presentation of cystitis is the classic triad of urinary urgency, frequency, and dysuria, with symptoms of abrupt onset. There may also be pressure or fullness in the suprapubic area and back pain. Pyelonephritis presents with flank pain, nausea and vomiting, and temperature greater than 38°C with or without symptoms of cystitis.

Differentiation must be made between complicated and uncomplicated UTI before progressing with diagnostic evaluation. An uncomplicated UTI is defined as occurring in a premenopausal, sexually active, nonpregnant women who has not recently had a UTI. A complicated UTI is one that occurs in a man, a postmenopausal or pregnant woman, or a patient with urinary structural defects, neurologic lesions, or a catheter. A UTI also is considered complicated if symptoms have persisted for more than 7 days. In sexually active men with symptoms of cystitis, urethritis must be ruled out.

BOX 33–1. UNDERLYING CONDITIONS THAT PREDISPOSE INDIVIDUALS TO URINARY TRACT INFECTIONS

- Female sex
- Pregnancy
- Diabetes
- Chronic degenerative neurologic conditions
- Paralysis
- Recurrent UTI
- Ineffective bladder emptying
- Estrogen deficiency
- Constipation
- Delayed postcoital micturition
- History of recurrent childhood UTI
- Sickle cell disease
- Polycystic kidney disease
- Structural defects of the urinary system
- Renal transplant

Pyelonephritis presents with recurrent fevers, chills, flank pain, and a positive urine culture.

The diagnosis of UTI is made after a careful history, physical examination, and limited laboratory studies. Because UTI is the most common infection for which adults receive antibiotics, its evaluation and management must be cost effective. Cultures are not performed if the criteria for an uncomplicated UTI are met, because antimicrobial susceptibility profiles are predictable and culture results do not return until after the symptoms have resolved.

The leukocyte dipstick test is 75% to 95% sensitive in detecting pyuria. Examination of spun or unspun urine that does not show leukocytes should suggest a diagnosis other than UTI. Hematuria occurs in approximately half of all acute UTIs. Pretreatment and posttreatment cultures should be performed for male patients. Pretreatment cultures are ordered in suspected pyelonephritis; posttreatment cultures are performed only if symptoms recur within 2 weeks or if the symptoms do not resolve with treatment initially.

INITIATING DRUG THERAPY

A urine culture with 10^5/mL organisms or greater is a diagnostic indicator of UTI with or without symptoms. A patient who has symptoms and a culture with 10^2/mL organisms or greater is treated.

Although most UTIs resolve spontaneously if not treated, they are treated for symptom relief. The treatment for UTI is antibiotics. The choice of antibiotic and the length of treatment depend on whether the infection is uncomplicated or complicated and on the sex and age of the patient.

A short course of treatment increases compliance and decreases cost and side effects. There is no benefit to treatment exceeding 3 days in uncomplicated UTIs in women unless nitrofurantoin is used; the length of treatment for this drug is 5 to 7 days.

Goals of Therapy

The goals of therapy for UTIs are to destroy the offending organism, relieve symptoms, and prevent complications.

Antibiotics

Antibiotics are discussed in detail in Chapter 9. Those used for treatment of UTIs are listed in Table 33-1.

Urinary Analgesics

This class of drugs is used for the symptomatic relief of pain, urgency, burning, frequency, and discomfort associated with trauma to the lower urinary tract mucosa. They are used in infection, trauma, surgery, endoscopic procedures, and catheterization. They should not be used for more than 2 days and are not used for treatment of a UTI per se, but for symptom relief.

The azo dye in this class is excreted in the urine and exerts a rapid topical analgesic effect on the mucosa of the urinary tract. The urinary analgesics are used with caution in pregnancy and lactation and are contraindicated in renal insufficiency. For additional information, see Table 33-1.

Selecting the Most Appropriate Agent

Cystitis and pyelonephritis are treated with the same antibiotic, but the treatment course for pyelonephritis is longer. The most desirable antibiotic is one that is low in cost with an infrequent dosing schedule, lack of resistance in local pathogens, long duration in the urinary tract, and the potential to decrease the number of E. coli in the vaginal and fecal reservoirs. The antibiotic selected should spare the protective, natural bacterial flora of the vagina and gastrointestinal tract, and there should be a low side effect profile. Nonpregnant women with uncomplicated cystitis may be treated with a 3-day course of antibiotics (except with nitrofurantoin, which is 5 to 7 days). Postmenopausal women should be treated for 7 days (Fig. 33-1 and Tables 33-2 and 33-3). Men also require a 7-day treatment because of the increased chance of a complicated infection and prostatic infection.

There has been shown to be a 33% rate of in vitro resistance to amoxicillin and sulfonamides, a 1% to 2% resistance rate to nitrofurantoin, a 5% to 15% resistance to trimethoprim–sulfamethoxazole (TMP-SMZ), and a 1% to 3% resistance rate to fluoroquinolones (Nicolle, 2002).

First-Line Therapy

The first-line choice for cystitis is TMP-SMZ (Bactrim). This drug combination has little impact on normal vaginal flora but decreases the number of E. coli in vaginal and fecal reservoirs, decreasing the chance of reinfection. Amoxicillin (Amoxil) and the first-generation cephalosporins adversely affect vaginal and fecal flora and increase the chance of reinfection. The cure rate of amoxicillin is low because of the high resistance of E. coli to it. Trimethoprim appears to be similar in efficacy but with fewer side effects; it can also be used in patients with sulfa allergies. The sulfa ingredient may be more important for complicated cystitis and pyelonephritis.

Table 33.1

Overview of Selected Agents for Urinary Tract Infection

Generic (Trade) Name and Dosage	Selected Adverse Events	Contraindications	Special Considerations
Antibiotics			
trimethoprim-sulfamethoxazole (Bactrim) Children: 5 mg/kg/d in divided doses for 10 d Adults: 1 DS q12h for 10 d	Nausea/vomiting, anorexia, megaloblastic anemia, hallucinations, depression, seizures	Megaloblastic anemia Pregnancy (category C) Breast-feeding mother Not recommended for children <2 mo G6PD deficiency	May consider newer macrolide antibiotics, such as clarithromycin and azithromycin
trimethoprim (Trimpex) 100 mg q12h for 3 days	Same as above	Megaloblastic anemia Pregnancy (category C) Breast-feeding mother Sulfa allergy	G6PD-deficient patients can have hemolysis. May cause falsely elevated creatinine Increase fluid intake.
nitrofurantoin (Macrobid, Macrodantin) Macrobid—100 mg q12h for 7 d Macrodantin—100 mg qid for 7 d	Nausea, pulmonary allergic reaction, dizziness, hemolytic anemia	Anuria Oliguria Pregnancy at term Nursing mother	Take with food to increase absorption.
ciprofloxacin (Cipro) 100–250 mg q12h for 3 d for uncomplicated cystitis and 7 d for complicated cystitis, and 500 mg for 10–14 d for uncomplicated pyelonephritis	Nausea, diarrhea, altered taste, dizziness, drowsiness, headache, insomnia, agitation, confusion Serious: pseudomembranous colitis, Stevens-Johnson syndrome	Allergy to fluoroquinolones Avoid in patients <18 y Pregnancy Use with caution in renal disease, CNS disease, breast-feeding (safety not established)	Raises serum level of theophylline Avoid taking with aluminum- or magnesium-containing antacids. Food slows absorption. Drug interacts with antacids, theophylline, warfarin, probenecid, digoxin, foscarnet, glucocorticoids.
ofloxacin (Floxin) 200 mg q12h for 3 d for uncomplicated cystitis and 7 d for complicated cystitis, and 200–300 mg for 10–14 d for uncomplicated pyelonephritis	Nausea, diarrhea, headache, insomnia, photosensitivity	Pregnancy (category C) Breast-feeding Not recommended in children	Take at least 30 min before or 2 h after meal. Not to be taken with aluminum- or magnesium-containing antacids or sucralfate, iron, and multivitamins with zinc because these can decrease absorption Increase fluid intake significantly.
lomefloxacin (Maxaquin) 400 mg qd for 3 d for uncomplicated cystitis and 7 d for complicated cystitis, and 400 mg qd for 10–14 d for uncomplicated pyelonephritis	Photosensitivity, CNS stimulation, dizziness, GI upset, headache, tendinitis/tendon rupture	Not recommended in patients <18 y Pregnancy (category C) Breast-feeding	Avoid taking with aluminum- or magnesium-containing antacids or sucralfate, iron, and multivitamins with zinc because these can decrease absorption. Force fluids. NSAIDs may increase risk of seizures. May potentiate oral anticoagulants
levofloxacin (Levaquin) 250 mg qd for 3 d for uncomplicated cystitis and 7 d for complicated cystitis, and 10–14 d for uncomplicated pyelonephritis	Nausea, diarrhea, photosensitivity	Same as above	Increase fluid intake significantly. Avoid taking with aluminum- or magnesium-containing antacids or sucralfate, iron, and multivitamins with zinc because these can decrease absorption.
norfloxacin (Noroxin) 400 mg q12h for 3 d for uncomplicated cystitis and 7 d for complicated cystitis and 10–14 d for uncomplicated pyelonephritis	Seizures, dizziness, nausea, headache, tendinitis/tendon rupture	Same as above	Same as above
sparfloxacin (Zagam) 400 mg qd for day 1 then 200 mg/d for 2 d for uncomplicated cystitis and 7 d for complicated cystitis, and 400 mg day 1 then 200 mg/d for 13 d for uncomplicated pyelonephritis	Same as above	Same as above	Same as above
amoxicillin (Amoxil) 500 mg q12h for 3 d	GI upset, rash, Stevens-Johnson syndrome, pseudomembranous colitis	Allergy to penicillin	May produce false-positive Clinitest; potentiated by probenecid
cefadroxil (Duricef) 1000 mg qd for 3 d for uncomplicated cystitis 1000 mg bid for 10 d for complicated cystitis	GI upset, rash	Allergy to penicillin	As above

(continued)

Table 33.1

Overview of Selected Agents for Urinary Tract Infection (*Continued*)

Generic (Trade) Name and Dosage	Selected Adverse Events	Contraindications	Special Considerations
cefixime (Suprax) 400 mg qd for 3 d for uncomplicated cystitis and 7 d for complicated cystitis, and 10–14 days for uncomplicated pyelonephritis	Diarrhea GI upset, rash, drug fever, pruritus, headache, dizziness, vaginitis	Known allergy to cephalosporins Use with caution in penicillin-allergic patients. Use with caution in patients with renal impairment, continuous ambulatory peritoneal dialysis, dialysis, GI disease.	Pregnancy category B
cefpodoxime (Vantin) 100 mg q12h for 3 d for uncomplicated cystitis and 7 d for complicated cystitis, and 200 mg for 10–14 d for uncomplicated pyelonephritis	Diarrhea, nausea/vomiting, abdominal pain, vaginitis and fungal infections, headache Serious: pseudomembranous colitis, seizures (high doses)	Use with caution in patients allergic to penicillin.	Antacids, H₂ antagonists, and oral anticholinergics may decrease efficacy. Avoid use with diuretics.
fosfomycin (Monurol) 3 g (1 package) one time	Abdominal cramps, vaginitis, nausea, headache, dyspepsia, rash, back pain	Not recommended in patients <18 y Breast-feeding	Lower efficacy with drugs that increase GI motility
Urinary Analgesics			
methenamine (Urised) 2 tabs qid	Rash, anticholinergic effects, xerostomia, flushing, difficulty in urinating, acute urinary retention with benign prostatic hyperplasia, tachycardia, dizziness, blurry vision, urine or fecal discoloration	Glaucoma Not recommended in patients <6 y Pregnancy (category C) Breast-feeding Bowel obstruction Urinary obstruction Cardiospasm	May cause blue-green discoloration of urine or feces Is not antibacterial
phenazopyridine (Pyridium) 200 mg tid	Headache, rash, GI upset, hemolytic anemia	Renal insufficiency	Discolors urine and clothes (red-orange) Is not antibacterial Take after meals.
flavoxate (Urispas) 100–200 mg tid–qid	Nausea and vomiting, anticholinergic side effects, vertigo, headache, drowsiness, urticaria, confusion, tachycardia	GI obstruction Obstructive uropathies Glaucoma	Reduce dose on improvement.

G6PD, glucose-6-phosphate dehydrogenase.

One-day therapy is effective with fosfomycin (Monurol; Box 33-2). Three-day therapy is acceptable with TMP-SMZ, cefadroxil (Duricef), and amoxicillin. In general, 5-day regimens with beta-lactams are more effective than 3-day treatments. Nitrofurantoin (Macrobid, Macrodantin) should be given for 5 to 7 days. In a comparison of 3-day regimens of TMP-SMZ 160 to 800 mg twice a day, cefadroxil 500 mg twice a day, nitrofurantoin macrocrystals 100 mg four times a day, and amoxicillin 500 mg three times a day, the highest cure rate was found with TMP-SMZ. There were increased treatment failures with the use of nitrofurantoin (Hooton, Winter, Tiu, et al., 1995).

Patients with cystitis can also be given urinary tract analgesics. This group includes methenamine (Urised), phenazopyridine (Pyridium, Uristat), or flavoxate (Urispas).

Uncomplicated pyelonephritis is usually treated in the outpatient setting because of the available oral antibiotics. The patient with pyelonephritis is admitted to the hospital only if he or she cannot take oral fluids or oral antibiotics, has a high fever or marked debility, or has a social situation incompatible with outpatient treatment. First-line therapy for pyelonephritis is an antibiotic, as mentioned previously, for 10 to 14 days. Fluoroquinolones are usually given first if culture results are not available because of their broad spectrum of activity. No follow-up is required if the symptoms resolve.

Second-Line Therapy

If symptoms of cystitis do not resolve after 3 days of therapy, a 7-day course of antibiotics is recommended. Fluoroquinolones are not recommended as first-line agents for uncomplicated cystitis because of the increased cost and concerns over development of quinolone resistance. They should be reserved for treatment of UTIs in men and postmenopausal women and for patients with complicated UTIs and pyelonephritis.

In pyelonephritis, a culture is obtained after treatment. If the urine is not free of bacteria after initial therapy, 4 to 6 more weeks of therapy is prescribed.

Third-Line Therapy

The recurrence rate for UTIs is approximately 20%. At this point, a urine culture is done and treatment is based on the culture results. If the patient has fewer than two UTIs a year, treatment can be based on the previous culture results. If the patient has more than three recurrences a year and they

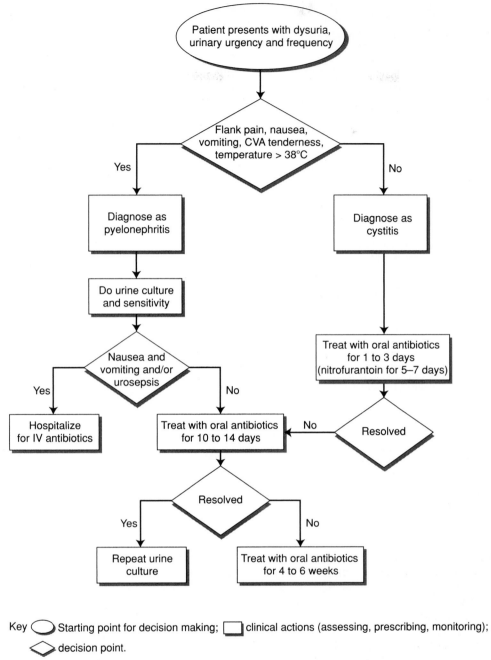

Figure 33–1   Treatment algorithm for urinary tract infection (UTI).

appear to be associated with coitus, postcoital treatment with antibiotics (TMP-SMZ, cephalexin, or nitrofurantoin) can be used. If reinfection is not associated with coitus, daily prophylaxis for 6 months with TMP-SMZ, nitrofurantoin, norfloxacin (Noroxin), or cephalexin is used.

Special Population Considerations

Geriatric

In elderly patients, UTIs are commonly asymptomatic. Postmenopausal women are more prone to UTIs because there is a uropathogen-dominant vaginal flora with the loss of estrogen. Lactobacilli diminish and pH increases.

Elderly patients are at increased risk for UTIs. Approximately 10% to 20% of the population older than 65 years of age has bacteriuria related to factors such as fecal incontinence, incomplete bladder emptying, malnutrition, and increased urine pH. Any UTI in a man is considered complicated. *E. coli* and *Enterobacter* species are the usual organisms. In elderly men, *Proteus, Klebsiella, Serratia, Pseudomonas,* and *Enterococcus* species are also responsible for UTIs. UTIs in men are most often seen in conjunction with prostatic hyperplasia with partial obstruction or persistent prostatitis.

Nitrofurantoin is not recommended in the elderly because it requires a creatinine clearance of 40 mL/min. Treatment is

Table 33.2

Recommended Order of Treatment for Uncomplicated Cystitis

Order	Agent	Comments
First line	Three-day oral therapy of • TMP-SMZ May also use 3-day oral therapy of: • ciprofloxacin • levofloxacin • ofloxacin • norfloxacin • lomefloxacin • sparfloxacin • cefixime • cefpodoxime proxetil *or* One-time therapy of fosfomycin or 7-day therapy of nitrofurantoin	Drink at least 8 glasses of fluids. Initiate 7-d therapy in postmenopausal women and in men. May use urinary analgesics in combination with antibiotics Higher incidence of treatment failure with nitrofurantoin for 3 d, so 7-d use is recommended
Second line	Seven-day oral therapy of • TMP-SMZ May also use 7-day oral therapy of: • ciprofloxacin • levofloxacin • ofloxacin • norfloxacin • lomefloxacin • enoxacin • sparfloxacin • cefixime • cefpodoxime proxetil	
Third line	Culture and sensitivity/testing, then treat based on results	

for 7 to 10 days in women and 10 to 14 days in men with uncomplicated UTIs.

Women

Asymptomatic bacteriuria occurs in approximately 7% of pregnant women. Of these, pyelonephritis develops in 30% if the bacteriuria is not treated. Untreated UTIs can contribute to prematurity or stillbirth. Amoxicillin is effective in approximately two thirds of UTIs in pregnant women and is safe for the fetus. Also safe are cephalexin and nitrofurantoin. Sulfonamides are safe except in the last trimester. In pregnancy, the urine is cultured 1 week after treatment and every 4 to 6 weeks during the pregnancy.

Physiologic changes in pregnancy increase the risk for pyelonephritis. The ureters become obstructed because of blockage from the enlarged uterus. In addition, increased progesterone relaxes the smooth muscles of the ureter and bladder.

In 5% to 10% of women with UTI, there are no symptoms. Pregnant women should be screened for UTIs, and

Table 33.3

Recommended Order of Treatment for Uncomplicated Pyelonephritis

Order	Agents	Comments
First line	Oral for 10–14 d: • ciprofloxacin • levofloxacin • enoxacin • norfloxacin • ofloxacin • sparfloxacin • TMP-SMZ • cefixime • cefpodoxime proxetil	Urine culture and sensitivity testing should be performed before treatment.
Second line	Oral therapy for 2–6 wk	
Third line	Hospitalization for IV therapy	For severe illness or possible urosepsis

BOX 33–2. RESEARCH COMPARISON OF SELECTED URINARY TRACT INFECTION THERAPIES

A study was done comparing a 5-day course of trimethoprim and a one-time dose of fosfomycin (Monuril) in uncomplicated urinary tract infection in women. There was an 83.3% cure rate in the trimethoprim-treated group and an 83% cure rate in the Fosfomycin-treated group. Fosfomycin has an antibacterial effect that lasts for 3½ days. Trimethoprim resistance was more often seen with *Escherichia coli* and fosfomycin resistance with *Staphylococcus saprophyticus* (Minassian, Lewis, & Chattopadhyay, 1998).

they must be treated regardless of whether they are symptomatic. Bacteriuria in pregnancy has been associated with a 20% to 30% incidence of pyelonephritis and premature delivery, intrauterine growth retardation, increased risk for death in the perinatal period, and congenital anomalies.

Children

UTIs in children may indicate a genitourinary anomaly. Accurate diagnosis usually requires invasive collection of urine, especially in very young children. It is important to start treatment quickly, especially in young children, because there is an increased risk of renal scarring in children under 5 from UTIs. UTIs recur in 32% to 40% of children. Renal/bladder ultrasounds are recommended by the American Academy of Pediatrics in children under 2 with a UTI. The American Academy of Pediatrics recommends 7 to 14 days of treatment for UTI in children.

MONITORING PATIENT RESPONSE

Cystitis that does not resolve or that recurs within a week after treatment requires culture and sensitivity testing and treatment with a fluoroquinolone for 7 days. UTIs recur within a year in approximately half of all women, although there is a very low incidence of pyelonephritis that develops as a result.

If pyelonephritis recurs within 2 weeks after treatment, a urine culture and sensitivity test and renal ultrasound or computed tomography scan should be performed to determine whether there is a urologic abnormality. If the organism is the same as the first, a 4- to 6-week course of antibiotics is recommended.

Patients who have three or more UTIs a year should be given prophylaxis, either continuous or postcoital. Continuous prophylaxis usually consists of TMP-SMZ 40 to 200 mg daily or three times a week. Postcoital therapy is indicated in women who identify intercourse as the cause of infection; the selected therapy is taken after intercourse. The use of estrogen replacement therapy in postmenopausal women decreases the number of recurrent UTIs. In cases of true relapse, the culture is repeated and therapy is prescribed for 2 to 4 weeks.

In pyelonephritis, a culture is repeated 1 to 2 weeks after completion of therapy. If there is a recurrence, therapy is recommended for 6 to 12 months.

PATIENT EDUCATION

Drug Information

Patients can get information about UTIs at http://kidney.niddk .nih.gov (National Institute of Diabetes and Digestive and Kidney Diseases); http://urinary-tract-infections.com; and http://www.urologychannel.com/uti.

Lifestyle Changes

Various behavioral factors, such as voiding after intercourse, the direction of toilet paper use after bowel movements, type of menstrual protection used, and method of contraception, have been investigated to assess their impact on the frequency of UTIs. The use of spermicides changes the vaginal flora, increasing the colonization of *E. coli* and the frequency of UTIs. Women with recurrent UTIs should use a method of birth control that does not involve spermicides.

Other preventive measures include urinating before and after sexual intercourse and avoiding bubble baths and "feminine hygiene" products. Changing position while voiding helps to empty the bladder fully. Drinking six to eight glasses of water daily helps prevent UTIs. Urinating every 2 hours, taking the time to empty the bladder completely, also helps prevent UTIs. Foods that irritate the bladder should be avoided, including tea, coffee, alcohol, cola, chocolate, and spicy foods.

Complementary and Alternative Medicine

Cranberry juice concentrate or cranberry concentrate capsules have been recognized as alternatives to antibiotics or for prevention of UTIs. Cranberry is believed to have antiadherence properties in the urinary tract and acidifies urine. One 300- to 400-mg capsule is taken two times a day with a glass of water, or 8 to 16 ounces of preparations with at least 30% cranberry juice can be taken. Vitamin C, 500 mg every 4 hours for the duration of the UTI, has been suggested, with 1,000 to 1,500 mg/day for prevention of UTIs.

Probiotics may decrease UTIs by restoring normal vaginal flora. Lactobacillus is thought to prevent colonization with *E. coli.*

■ Case Study

J.S., a 65-year-old woman with diabetes, seeks treatment for dysuria, frequent urination, flank pain, and costovertebral angle tenderness. She has a temperature of 102°F, and under the microscope her spun urine contains a large number of leukocytes.

Diagnosis: Cystitis with possible pyelonephritis

→   1. List specific goals for treatment for J.S.

→   2. What drug therapy would you prescribe? Why?

(Continued)

■ Case Study *(Continued)*

➤ 3. What are the parameters for monitoring success of the therapy?

➤ 4. Discuss specific patient education based on the prescribed therapy.

➤ 5. List one or two adverse reactions for the selected agent that would cause you to change therapy.

➤ 6. What would be the choice for second-line therapy?

➤ 7. What over-the-counter and/or alternative medications would be appropriate for J.S.?

➤ 8. What lifestyle changes would you recommend to J.S.?

➤ 9. Describe one or two drug/drug or drug/food interactions for the selected agent.

Bibliography

Starred references are cited in the text.

Bass, P. F., Jarvis, J. W., & Mitchell, C. K. (2003). Urinary tract infections. *Primary Care, 30*(1), 41–61.

*Foxman, B. (2002). Epidemiology of urinary tract infections: incidence, morbidity and economic costs. *American Journal of Medicine, 113*(Suppl 1A), 5S–13S.

*Foxman, B., & Brown, P. (2003). Epidemiology of urinary tract infections: transmission and risk factors, incidence and costs. *Infectious Disease Clinics of North America, 17*(2), 227–241.

*Hooton, T. M., Winter, C., Jui, F., et al. (1999). Randomized comparative trial and analysis of three-day antimicrobial regimens for treatment of acute cystitis in women. *Journal of the American Medical Association, 273*, 41–45.

Layton, K. (2003). Diagnosis and management of pediatric urinary tract infections. *Clinics in Family Practice, 5*(2), 367–375.

*Minassian, M. A., Lewis, D. A., & Chattopadhyay, D. (1998). A comparison between single-dose fosfomycin trometomal (Monuril) and a 5-day course of trimethoprim in the treatment of uncomplicated lower urinary tract infections in women. *International Journal of Antimicrobial Agents and Chemotherapy, 40*, 2200–2201.

*Nicolle, M. E. (2002). Urinary tract infections: traditional pharmacological therapies. *American Journal of Medicine, 113*(suppl. 1A), 35S–44S.

O'Donnell, J., Gelone, S., & Abrutyne, E. (2002). Selecting drug regimen for urinary tract infections: current recommendations. *Infectious Medicine, 19*, 14–22.

Reid, J., & Bruce, A. W. (2003). Urogenital infections in women: can probiotics help? *Postgraduate Medicine, 79*, 428–432.

Schaeffer, N. J. (2002). New concepts in the pathogenesis of urinary tract infections. *Urology Clinics of North America, 29* (1), 241–250.

Stapleton, A. (2003). Novel approaches to the prevention of urinary tract infections. *Infectious Disease Clinics of North America, 17*(2), 457–471.

Visit the Connection web site for the most up-to-date drug information.

PROSTATIC DISORDERS AND ERECTILE DYSFUNCTION

■ SHERRY RATAJCZAK AND VIRGINIA P. ARCANGELO

Disorders of the prostate appear as part of the normal aging process and also as abnormalities distinct from normal aging. Often it is not until 40 years of age that a man begins to show some form of noncancerous prostatic disorder, whereas prostate cancer usually is found after age 50 years. The incidence of prostatic disorders increases with age. It is estimated that 50% to 75% of all men older than 50 years of age have benign prostatic hyperplasia (BPH), often with symptoms. African-American men have prostate cancer twice as frequently as men of other races; Hispanic and Asian-American men have the lowest incidence of prostate cancer and a lower incidence of morbidity than their African-American counterparts (Bullock & Henze, 2000). Prostate disorders are diagnosed through clinical manifestations and screening procedures to detect or rule out prostate cancer. Lack of knowledge about prostate cancer and lack of available screening procedures are the major deterrents to accurate and timely diagnosis of prostate cancer.

Treatment of prostatic disorders itself may result in some untoward side effects, which must then also be managed. Often the man postpones seeking medical intervention and blames aging for many of the manifestations, thus delaying treatment. Some difficulties in seeking treatment can relate to the man's culture; sexuality—specifically, masculinity—can be perceived as synonymous with virility. For this reason, a man may choose not to discuss (even with a health care worker) clinical manifestations.

Prostatic disorders occur because of inflammation or infection (prostatitis), BPH, and prostatic cancer; prostatitis can involve the bladder neck, thus becoming prostatocystitis. A bacterial infection is often the cause of prostatitis, although some nonbacterial forms of prostatitis do exist; inflammation can be chronic or acute.

Adenocarcinoma is the most common type of prostate cancer. Metastasis can follow slowly or quickly, and often the symptoms of metastasis are what lead the man to seek medical intervention.

Presenting manifestations of prostatic disorders are usually specific to the urinary tract and include difficulty in onset of urine flow with or without a low flow of urine, frequency or urgency in voiding, incontinence, distention of the bladder, and hematuria. Management of prostatic disorders is specific to the particular disorder (cancerous vs. noncancerous), with some overlap in treatment.

PROSTATITIS

CAUSES

Prostatitis is caused primarily by bacterial invasion, but some nonbacterial forms occur as well. This disorder can be acute or chronic. With acute bacterial prostatitis, the chief organisms involved are gram-negative *Pseudomonas* species, although strains of staphylococci or streptococci also are seen. Chronic bacterial prostatitis is associated with not only *Pseudomonas* but also *Escherichia coli, Proteus mirabilis, Klebsiella pneumoniae*, and *Enterococcus* species, particularly *Enterococcus faecalis*. Nonbacterial prostatitis is essentially an inflammatory disorder.

PATHOPHYSIOLOGY

Often chronic, nonbacterial prostatitis is nonetheless problematic for the patient. Primary etiologies of this condition include two predominant patterns of inflammation. The first is that of an allergic condition and is associated with eosinophil infiltration. The second is a nonspecific form in which granulomatous inflammation by peculiar, large, pale macrophages is found.

In acute bacterial prostatitis, as with any type of bacterial invasion, the prostate becomes overwhelmed by the bacteria, leading to inflammatory response activation. Usually, acute bacterial prostatitis is seen as an infection ascending up the urinary tract, and younger men, 30 to 50 years of age, can be affected with this illness.

DIAGNOSTIC CRITERIA

Symptom manifestation revolves around urinary tract signs. There is pain in the lower abdomen, difficulty in bladder emptying with or without a small stream during urination, nocturia, and fever to 104°F. Along with the febrile state, as with other infections, general arthralgia and malaise can occur.

On examination and interview, the man often admits to painful ejaculation and pain in the rectal or perineal areas. All the symptoms are due to the edema associated with acute inflammation of the prostate. Because of the risk of generalized septicemia, pharmacotherapeutics are urgently warranted.

Culture isolation of prostatic urine is the most accurate method of diagnosis. Prostatic urine is defined as the third and fourth (urine) secretion specimens of four serial urine sample because prostatic fluid is at a significantly higher concentration in these last two of four serial voids. The four urine samples are obtained sequentially, beginning with the initial void, followed by a midstream urine specimen, prostatic massage secretion, and finally the urine voided after the prostatic massage. Standard laboratory culture techniques are applied to establish the causative organism.

Nonbacterial prostatitis is confirmed by negative prostatic urine cultures with a positive elevated white blood cell count and the presence of inflammatory cells in prostatic secretions. This condition and another nonbacterial type of prostatitis known as *prostatodynia* have the same symptoms as bacterial prostatitis. Treatment of the nonbacterial forms usually consists of symptom management without the use of antibiotics.

INITIATING DRUG THERAPY

Antibiotics are the required pharmacotherapy (see Chapter 8). Given that causative organisms are usually gram negative and, less commonly, gram positive, appropriate antibiotics are needed. The overall course of antibiotic therapy is of longer duration than that used to treat other systemic infections. Usually antibiotics are given for 3 to 4 weeks, but up to 12 weeks of therapy may be necessary.

Chronic prostatitis can be recalcitrant to treatment. A once-daily dose of trimethoprim–sulfamethoxazole (TMP-SMZ [Septra, Bactrim]) can be effective in preventing upper genitourinary tract infection. However, for the older patient, transurethral retrograde prostatectomy (TURP) may be warranted.

Adjunctive therapies that may be beneficial include the use of sitz baths, analgesics, stool softeners, and antipyretics, along with rest. Prostatic massage, voiding in a warm bath (to relax pelvic muscles), and discontinuation of alcohol and caffeinated beverages can also help to relieve symptoms. If possible, withdrawal from antidepressants, anticholinergics, or sedatives may also help bladder function.

Goals of Drug Therapy

The goal of pharmacotherapy for prostatitis is to eradicate the causative organism and restore the prostate to health. Allergies to TMP-SMZ may preclude its use as a first-line agent, in which case one of the second-line agents should be used. Prostatitis often becomes chronic, and therefore repeated trials with antibiotics or prolonged dosage schedules may be warranted.

ANTI-INFECTIVES

Table 34-1 depicts dosage information, adverse events, contraindications, and special considerations for the anti-infective management of bacterial prostatitis.

Trimethoprim–Sulfamethoxazole

This drug is a bacteriostatic combination product and is considered to be more powerful than its two components given separately. Also, when given as the combined form, resistance on the part of the causative organism arises less frequently. This agent ultimately adversely affects the production of proteins and nucleic acids of bacteria at the target (prostate) site. TMP-SMZ further inhibits growth of bacteria because of its antimetabolite property toward PABA (*para*-aminobenzoic acid). Drug–drug interactions can present when the patient is also taking phenytoin (Dilantin), oral hypoglycemics, or warfarin (Coumadin). Close monitoring of the seizure threshold, serum glucose level, or partial

Table 34.1

Overview of Selected Antibiotics Used to Treat Acute Bacterial Prostatitis

Generic (Trade) Name and Dosage	Selected Adverse Events	Contraindications	Special Considerations
trimethoprim-sulfamethoxazole (TMP-SMZ, Septra, Bactrim) 160 mg of TMP with 800 mg SMZ PO q12h	GI distress, rash	Allergy to sulfa and sulfa products	May prolong the INR for patients on oral anticoagulants
Fluoroquinolones ciprofloxacin (Cipro) 500 mg BID norofloxacin (Noroxin) 400 mg bid levofloxacin (Levaquin) 250 mg daily	Headache, diarrhea, nausea, drowsiness, altered taste, insomnia, agitation, confusion Serious: pseudomembranous colitis, Stevens-Johnson syndrome	Allergy to macrolides Pregnancy and lactation Use with caution in severe hepatic or renal disease.	May interfere with theophylline metabolism
doxycycline (Vibramycin) 200 mg PO as first dose, thereafter 100–200 mg PO q12h	GI distress, potential acute hepatotoxicity, potential for nephrotoxicity	Hypersensitivity to any of the tetracyclines Pregnancy and lactation	Decreased effectiveness with food and dairy products, so do not take with food unless side effects are significant. Can lead to diabetes insipidus because of antagonistic effect with antidiuretic hormone

thromboplastin time is important in the patient on TMP-SMZ who is also taking these other agents.

Fluoroquinolones

Fluoroquinolones are also effective for bacterial prostatitis. Effective against gram-negative anaerobes and some gram-positive bacteria, these agents decrease the growth and replication of bacteria by inhibiting bacterial DNA during synthesis. These agents may be the first choice for someone sensitive or allergic to TMP-SMZ.

The absorption of fluoroquinolones is reduced by milk, antacids (aluminum- or magnesium-based), iron or zinc salts, and sucralfate. For the patient who is also taking any of these medications, the dose should be taken either 2 hours after or 4 hours before the other medication.

Fluoroquinolones also affect the use of theophylline and warfarin. Elevated levels can occur, and thus a lower dosage of theophylline or warfarin may be necessary.

Doxycycline

A long-acting tetracycline, doxycycline (Vibramycin) has had a significant impact on the management of Lyme disease. As with its sibling tetracyclines, this medication acts by inhibiting protein synthesis: binding of tRNA is blocked at ribosomal mRNA.

Many of the metal ions—aluminum, calcium, iron, magnesium, and zinc—can interfere by creating chelates with doxycycline. Thus, if these metals are given (and they often are as components of antacids), at least 2 hours should separate their use from the ingestion of doxycycline.

Amoxicillin

Amoxicillin (Amoxil) is a penicillin-based drug that is further classified as an aminopenicillin. This subclassification moves it out of the narrow-spectrum range seen with penicillin and into the broad-spectrum range. Amoxicillin is effective against gram-positive aerobes and some gram-negative organisms. As with other penicillins, the agent weakens the bacterial cell well by inhibiting the transpeptidases, which causes autolysis. The primary contraindication is penicillin allergy. Amoxicillin, however, also may not be effective against the patient's invading organism.

Drug–drug interactions with amoxicillin do exist. The patient is primarily at risk for an interaction if he is also taking an anti-gout medication, potassium-sparing diuretics, rifampin (Rifadin), anticoagulants, and aminoglycosides.

Selecting the Most Appropriate Agent

Oral antibiotics are the treatment agents of choice.

First-Line Therapy

The primary choice for first-line antibiotic therapy is TMP-SMZ (Table 34-2). However, based on patient response or patient allergies, the practitioner may prescribe a second-line agent as primary therapy rather than TMP-SMZ. There is some concern over TMP-SMZ because it is ineffective against enterococci. Therapy lasts 4 weeks. See Figure 34-1 for more information.

Table 34.2

Recommended Order of Treatment for Prostatitis

Order	Agents	Comments
First line	trimethoprim–sulfamethoxazole (TMP-SMZ)	Ineffective against enterococci
Second line	fluoroquinolones doxycycline amoxicillin	

Second-Line Therapy

Doxycycline, fluoroquinolones, and amoxicillin are second-line agents. They are used when TMP-SMZ cannot be used because of sulfa allergies. If the infection is not resolved with 3 to 4 weeks of drug treatment, therapy can be continued for up to 12 weeks.

Special Population Considerations

In older men who are taking fluoroquinolones, creatinine clearance must be monitored.

MONITORING PATIENT RESPONSE

As a group, anti-infective agents should begin to elicit results after the first week of therapy. Subjective response from the patient indicating alleviation of symptoms is helpful in monitoring the effectiveness of these medications. Some patients may not notice symptom resolution until after 2 weeks; they should be told this and encouraged to continue taking the medication. Ultimately, 4 to 6 weeks of therapy may be required. Follow-up cultures may be obtained at the practitioner's discretion. Further diagnostic criteria may also be recommended for ongoing symptom manifestation.

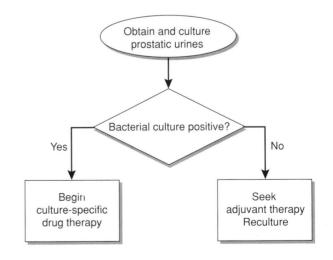

Figure 34–1 Treatment algorithm for prostatitis.

PATIENT EDUCATION

The patient should understand potential side effects, interactions, and appropriate use of the medications. Literature can provide patients with a guide for such potential concerns as well as dosing information. With a prepared and knowledgeable patient, these medications are effective against prostatitis. Cost also can be a factor of concern to the patient. The practitioner should be aware of any financial constraints the patient may have, because compliance with medication is important for effective treatment of bacterial prostatitis.

BENIGN PROSTATIC HYPERPLASIA (BPH)

BPH is the most common prostate problem in men over 50 years of age; the disease rarely causes symptoms before age 40. As life expectancy rises, so does the occurrence of BPH—an estimated 6.3 million men have BPH. In the United States alone, the disease accounts for 6.4 million doctor visits and more than 400,000 hospitalizations annually. Approximately 90% of men 80 years of age and older have histologic evidence of BPH, and more than 80% have BPH-related symptoms. Approximately 25% of men older than 55 years and 50% of men older than 75 years of age experience decreased urinary flow.

CAUSES

The cause of BPH is not well understood. It has been observed that BPH does not develop in men whose testes were removed before puberty. For this reason, some researchers believe that factors related to aging and the testes may spur the development of BPH. Men produce both testosterone and small amounts of estrogen. As men age, the amount of active testosterone in the blood decreases, leaving a higher proportion of estrogen. Studies performed on animals have suggested that BPH may occur because the higher amount of estrogen within the gland increases the activity of substances that promote cell growth. Another theory focuses on dihydrotestosterone (DHT), a substance derived from testosterone in the prostate, which may help control its growth. Some research has indicated that even with a drop in the blood's testosterone level, older men continue to produce and accumulate high levels of DHT in the prostate. This accumulation of DHT may encourage the growth of cells. Researchers have also noted that men who do not produce DHT do not develop BPH.

PATHOPHYSIOLOGY

The underlying pathophysiologic process of BPH is the formation of large, nonmalignant lesions at the periurethral region of the prostate gland. Prostatic hyperplasia is an overgrowth of normal cells in the stromal and epithelial tissues of the prostate gland. The hyperplasia originates in the transition zone of the prostate, which surrounds the prostatic urethra between the bladder and the anus. The etiology of the hyperplastic process is unknown, but it has been speculated that it is hormone-related because it occurs only in older men. The male aging process involves a decrease in testosterone production with a concomitant increase in estrogen; estrogen may be a sensitizer for the escalating hyperplasia.

Bladder control involves reflex activity of the peripheral autonomic nervous system (ANS). The reflex for normal micturition is housed in the brain stem and supported by descending and ascending pathways from the spinal cord. Both the external sphincter and the detrusor muscle are needed for bladder control. Reflex micturition is innervated at the S2 to S4 and T1 to L1 levels in the spinal cord. The cortical center of the brain appears to be important for inhibition or control of the micturition center to modulate contractile, filling, and expulsion activity.

Parasympathetic and sympathetic innervation is crucial to the role of the ANS in voiding. Parasympathetic interplay allows for the detrusor muscle to maintain tone and to contract, whereas sympathetic interplay allows for the bladder to expand and maintain a large filling capacity. It is for this reason that pharmacologic intervention is so effective in managing BPH—the ANS can be effectively manipulated by pharmacotherapy.

Disease manifests as urinary tract symptoms. Obstructed urine outflow, the predominant pattern, includes diminished force of the urine stream, an urgent need for nocturnal voiding, residual urine with or without overflow incontinence, and even a feeling of pressure in the abdomen. These manifestations result from either partial or complete compression of the urethra by the hyperplastic prostate. Bladder wall hypertrophy occurs, and herniation into the bladder can occur. Ultimately, if treatment is not initiated, a postrenal cause of renal failure can develop because of back-pressure on the renal system (ie, the ureters) and the onset of hydronephrosis.

DIAGNOSTIC CRITERIA

Diagnosis of BPH usually begins with the patient seeking medical intervention because of the annoying symptoms. Along with a complete social history and physical examination, a digital rectal examination (DRE) is performed to palpate the prostate. The degree of prostate enlargement has not been found to correlate with the severity of symptoms; rather, the location of the enlargement is what leads to symptom manifestation.

The American Urological Association (AUA) has created a Symptom Index Scale (Table 34-3) to correlate symptom severity with prostate size. In this numeric scale symptoms are scored as mild (0 to 7 points), moderate (8 to 19 points), or severe (20 to 35 points). The AUA recommends that this scale be used on initial assessment and then for following the course of illness by periodic ongoing assessment of the patient. Such follow-up management enables the practitioner to initiate more acute or intensive therapy when the score increases. Patients with severe BPH symptoms should not be managed by this scale.

Postvoid catheterization is performed to ascertain the degree of urine retention; any amount of residual urine beyond 100 mL is considered significant. Uroflowmetry provides information about the force of the urine stream. Urodynamics can also be assessed using noninvasive pneumatic technology. Other diagnostic tools include x-ray films, digital ultrasound, computed tomography (CT) scans, magnetic resonance imaging (MRI), and radionuclide scans. Biopsies can be added to the diagnostic workup for further clinical

Table 34.3

AUA Symptom Index

Questions To Be Answered	AUA Symptom Score (Circle 1 Number on Each Line)					
	Not At All	Less Than 1 Time in 5	Less Than Half the Time	About Half the Time	More Than Half the Time	Almost Always
1. Over the past month, how often have you had a sensation of not emptying your bladder completely after you finished urinating?	0	1	2	3	4	5
2. Over the past month, how often have you had to urinate again less than 2 hours after you finished urinating?	0	1	2	3	4	5
3. Over the past month, how often have you found you stopped and started again several times when you urinated?	0	1	2	3	4	5
4. Over the past month, how often have you found it difficult to postpone urination?	0	1	2	3	4	5
5. Over the past month, how often have you had a weak urinary stream?	0	1	2	3	4	5
6. Over the past month, how often have you had to push or strain to begin urination?	0	1	2	3	4	5
7. Over the past month, how many times did you most typically get up to urinate from the time you went to bed at night until the time you got up in the morning?	0 (None)	1 (1 time)	2 (2 times)	3 (3 times)	4 (4 times)	5 (5 times or more)

Sum of 7 circled numbers (AUA Symptom Score): mild (0–7 points); moderate (8–19 points); severe (20–35 points).

assessment of any hardened prostatic areas found by DRE. Laboratory monitoring of creatinine and blood urea nitrogen should be incorporated to determine whether renal involvement exists, and if so, to what degree. Prostate-specific antigen (PSA) levels can be elevated in patients with BPH.

Many symptoms of BPH stem from obstruction of the urethra and gradual loss of bladder function, which results in incomplete emptying of the bladder. The symptoms of BPH vary, but the most common ones involve changes or problems with urination, including a hesitant, interrupted, or weak stream; urgency, dribbling, or urinary retention; more frequent urination, especially at night; painful urination; and incontinence.

It is extremely important to evaluate men at risk for these symptoms. In 8 out of 10 cases, these symptoms suggest BPH, but they also can signal more serious conditions, such as prostate cancer.

INITIATING DRUG THERAPY

Management of BPH can include medical, surgical, and a combination of medical and surgical intervention. Pharmacotherapy is prescribed with both medical and surgical approaches to care. The progression of BPH is unique to the individual; the man often will "watch and wait" before proceeding further into active therapy because the process of hyperplasia can be slow. This is acceptable as long as the AUA score is 19 or less.

The Medical Therapy of Prostatic Symptoms (MTOPS) trial tested whether finasteride (Proscar), doxazosin (Cardura), or a combination of the drugs could prevent progression of BPH and the need for surgery or other invasive treatments. Physicians at 17 MTOPS medical centers treated 3,047 men with BPH for an average of 4.5 years. Participants were randomly assigned to receive doxazosin, finasteride, combination therapy, or placebo. Vital signs, urinary symptoms, urinary flow, adverse effects, and medication use were assessed every 3 months. DRE, serum PSA level, and urinalysis were performed yearly. Prostate size was measured by ultrasound at the beginning and end of the study. Progression of disease was defined by one of the following: a 4-point rise in the AUA score, urinary retention, recurrent urinary tract infection, or urinary incontinence.

Finasteride, a 5-alpha-reductase inhibitor, and doxazosin, an alpha-1 receptor blocker, together reduced the overall risk of BPH progression by 66% compared with placebo. The combined drugs also provided the greatest symptom relief and improvement in urinary flow rate. Doxazosin alone reduced the overall risk of progression by 39% and finasteride alone by 34% relative to placebo.

The combination treatment and finasteride alone significantly reduced the risk of invasive therapy by 67% and 64%, respectively. Doxazosin did not reduce the long-term risk of invasive therapy.

The MTOPS trial also found that combination therapy was especially effective in men at highest risk for BPH progression—those with prostates larger than 40 mg (30% of participants) or serum PSAs above 4 ng/mL (20% of participants).

Progression of BPH occurred in only 5% of men (49) receiving combination therapy, in 10% of men (85) taking doxazosin, in 10% of men (89) taking finasteride, and in 17% of men (128) taking placebo. Events signaling disease progression mostly included worsening symptoms (78%) but also included acute urinary retention (12%) and incontinence (9%).

The risk of urinary retention was reduced 81% with combination therapy and 68% with finasteride alone. Doxazosin alone did not reduce the risk of urinary retention. The risk of incontinence was reduced 65% with combination therapy. Only five men developed urinary tract or blood infections. No patients developed impaired kidney function related to BPH.

Twenty-seven percent of men taking doxazosin, 24% of men taking finasteride, and 18% of men taking combination therapy stopped treatment early, primarily because of adverse effects. The most common adverse effects included sexual dysfunction in men treated with finasteride and dizziness and fatigue in men treated with doxazosin.

Goals of Therapy

The goals of therapy include reduced bladder outlet obstruction, improved quality of life, fewer symptoms, and decreased residual urine volume.

The mainstay of medical management is pharmacotherapy. Pharmacotherapy is used for both controlling hyperplasia and managing annoying side effects, either as primary therapy or as an adjunct to surgical intervention. Management of hyperplasia is based on the premise that there are hormonal changes related to aging and that alpha-adrenergic receptors are present in prostate tissue, specifically smooth muscle. Pharmacotherapeutic interventions consist of hormonal manipulation and blocking effects achieved by alpha-adrenergic blockers. For dosage, adverse events, contraindications, and special considerations of drugs used for BPH, see Table 34-4.

5-Alpha-Reductase Inhibitors

Finasteride (Proscar) and dutasteride (Avodart), androgen hormone inhibitors, are used for managing the symptoms of BPH. They aid in the inhibition of androgen transformation from their steroid precursors.

Mechanism of Action

5-alpha-reductase inhibitors act by specifically blocking 5-alpha-reductase, the enzyme that activates testosterone in the prostate. It impairs prostate growth by inhibiting the conversion of testosterone to dihydrotestosterone (DHT), and causes changes in the epithelial cells of the transition zone. By preventing testosterone activation, 5-alpha-reductase inhibitors lessen or prevent urinary system symptoms. They also decrease prostatic volume and prevent the progression of the disease in men with a significantly enlarged prostate. There is a slow reduction of 80% to 90% in the serum DHT level. As a result, prostatic volume decreases by about 20% over 3 to 6 months of treatment. Dutasteride blocks both types 1 and 2 5-alpha-reductase.

Studies have been done to determine the efficacy of finasteride and placebo. The larger Proscar Safety Plus Efficacy Canadian Two-Year Study (PROSPECT) found that treatment with finasteride led to significant improvements in urinary symptoms and flow rates (Nickel et al., 1996). However, in the PROSPECT study, the improvements with finasteride were significantly less than those with any alpha blocker or surgery.

5-alpha-reductase inhibitors decrease PSA levels by 40% to 50%. In a patient taking finasteride who has PSA screening, PSA levels should be doubled and then compared in the usual fashion to age-related norms.

Dosage

The dosage for finasteride is 5 mg/day; that for dutasteride is 0.5 mg/day. These dosages are recommended for use as long-term therapy; studies have shown benefit beyond the usual 2-year period, with beneficial effects in the third year.

Adverse Events

Adverse events include decreased libido, impotence, ejaculatory failure, and gynecomastia. Finasteride can also falsify the PSA level after 6 months of therapy.

Alpha-Adrenergic Blockers

Alpha-adrenergic blockers include terazosin (Hytrin), doxazosin (Cardura), prazosin (Minipress), and tamsulosin (Flomax).

Table 34.4

Overview of Selected Agents Used to Treat Benign Prostatic Hyperplasia

Generic (Trade) Name and Dosage	Selected Adverse Events	Contraindications	Special Considerations
α-Adrenergic Blockers			
terazosin (Hytrin) 1–20 mg PO qd	Orthostatic hypotension, somnolence, dizziness	Hypersensitivity to terbutaline Tachyarrhythmias, hypertension, pregnancy, lactation Use with caution in cardiac insufficiency.	Take at bedtime to avoid hypotension.
doxazosin (Cardura) 4–8 mg PO qd	Dizziness, headache, fatigue, malaise	Lactation Use with caution in CHF, renal failure, hepatic impairment.	May have secondary benefit to client with cardiac disease Avoid combination with alcohol, nitrates, or other antihypertensive drugs.
tamsulosin HCl (Flomax) 0.4 mg/d PO qd; increase to 0.8 mg/d PO qd	Orthostasis, headache, problems with ejaculation	Allergy to tamsulosin Prostatic cancer, pregnancy, lactation	Ejaculatory problems more common in higher dosage (0.8 mg/d) Interaction with cimetidine decreases clearance of tamsulosin.
5α-Reductase Inhibitor			
finasteride (Proscar) 5 mg daily dutasteride (Avodart) 0.5 mg daily	Impotence, decreased libido, smaller ejaculate volume	Not to be handled by pregnant women	Inform patient that effective outcome of therapy may take up to 6 mo.

Mechanism of Action

As a pharmacologic classification, alpha-adrenergic blockers are functional antihypertensives with potential effects on glomerular filtration rate, renal perfusion, and heart rate. They are strongly linked with fluid retention. They relax the smooth muscle of the prostate and bladder neck without interfering with bladder contractility, thereby decreasing bladder resistance to urinary outflow. In general, weeks to months may pass before benefits from these medications are noted. However, benefits may last for up to 2 years, in some cases longer.

Adverse Events

Side effects can be a major concern, especially considering the potential for hypotension, specifically orthostatic hypotension, and fluid retention. However, cardiac output can actually improve, thus preventing heart failure. Of the four agents, prazosin has more potential for causing orthostatic hypotension than the others.

Side effects such as dizziness, postural hypotension, fatigue, and asthenia affect 7% to 9% of patients treated with nonselective alpha blockers. Side effects can be minimized by bedtime administration and slow titration of the dosage.

Tamsulosin (Flomax) is a highly selective alpha$_{1A}$-adrenergic antagonist that was developed to avoid the side effects of nonselective agents. Some patients who do not respond to nonselective alpha blockers may respond to tamsulosin and, because of the selectivity, may have fewer side effects.

Selecting the Most Appropriate Agent

The most appropriate agent is the one that achieves symptom control and produces the fewest adverse effects (Table 34-5 and Fig. 34-2).

First-Line Therapy

If symptoms are mild (AUA score < 7), no medical treatment is recommended. The man should limit his fluid intake after dinner, avoid decongestants, massage the prostate after intercourse, and void frequently.

Second-Line Therapy

Pharmacotherapy is initiated when the AUA score is more than 7. An alpha-adrenergic blocker or a 5-alpha-reductase inhibitor can be prescribed. To limit the number of daily drugs, it may be prudent to use an alpha-adrenergic blocker in the patient who is also hypertensive. A 5-alpha-reductase

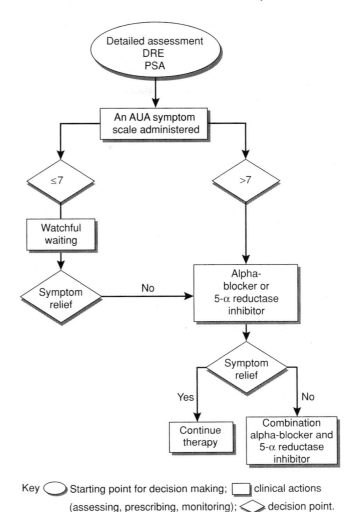

Figure 34–2 Treatment algorithm for benign prostatic hyperplasia (BPH).

inhibitor may be prescribed if the prostate is enlarged to 40 g or more.

Analyzed together, the results of multiple studies suggest that 5-alpha-reductase inhibitors may work best in men with a large gland, whereas alpha blockers are effective across the range of prostate sizes.

Third-Line Therapy

Combination therapy with a 5-alpha-reductase inhibitors and alpha blocker may show greater improvement.

Table 34.5

Recommended Order of Treatment for Benign Prostatic Hyperplasia

Order	Agents	Comments
First line	If AUA score is 7 or less, watchful waiting	
Second line	Alpha-adrenergic blocker or 5-alpha reductase inhibitor	Alpha-adrenergic blocker can be prescribed for patients with hypertension; 5-alpha reductase inhibitor is recommended if prostate enlargement exceeds 40 g.
Third line	Combination alpha-blocker and 5-alpha-reductase inhibitor	

Fourth-Line Therapy

Referral to a urologist for possible surgery is recommended if other therapy fails.

The prevailing surgical intervention is prostatic resection or prostatectomy. Transurethral resection of the prostate (TURP) is the most common surgical intervention. Regardless of the surgical technique used (ie, retrograde, perineal, or suprapubic approach), removal of the prostate is not without potential complications. The primary side effect, which can be permanent, is impotence from nerve damage. Incontinence is rare and usually only temporary; retrograde ejaculation can occur. Prostatectomy using laser technique is also an option, as is balloon dilatation or urethral stent implantation. Laser surgery requires only an overnight stay; stent insertion is recommended for the man with cardiac or pulmonary morbidities, although it does not address the underlying problem of BPH itself.

Transurethral microwave thermotherapy is performed on an outpatient basis. Although anesthesia is not required, use of a local or general antianxiety agent may be helpful because the procedure is performed by catheter insertion into the prostate, through the urethra. This procedure uses heat derived from microwave energy (approximately 45°C) to remove or destroy excess cells of the prostate while cool water is circulated to preserve surrounding tissue.

MONITORING PATIENT RESPONSE

As noted previously, the AUA symptom score can be used to monitor men with mild or even moderate BPH. Abatement of symptoms is used to evaluate the success of pharmacotherapy. If side effects become evident with a chosen agent, a different agent can be tried. The patient's blood pressure should be monitored frequently during the first 2 weeks of treatment to observe for an untoward hypotensive response. In addition, the practitioner should not pass off subjective complaints related to sexual health, because it could lead to medication noncompliance.

PATIENT EDUCATION

Drug Information

With terazosin use, an improvement in urine flow may begin within 1 to 2 weeks; thus, the patient must be informed that urine flow improvement will not occur overnight. The man should rise slowly from a sitting or standing position and quickly sit down or recline if abrupt vertigo occurs.

Lifestyle Changes

Patients with BPH can obtain symptomatic relief with regular, relaxed, and frequent voiding, decreasing fluid intake several hours before bedtime, and avoiding diuretics and alcohol. Other medications to avoid include anticholinergics, antihistamines, and antidepressants.

Alternative Therapies for BPH

Many men are using herbal and nutritional therapies to support prostate health. Men are encouraged to lose weight if overweight, to eat a low-fat, high-fiber diet, and to drink

Table 34.6
Alternative Therapies for Benign Prostatic Hyperplasia

Agent	Dosage
Saw palmetto	Doses vary based on manufacturer.
Pygeum	50–100 mg PO bid
Zinc	150 mg PO qd for 2 mo, 50–100 mg qd thereafter

a minimum of 2 quarts of water daily. Supplements to maintain prostate health include saw palmetto, pygeum, and zinc (Table 34-6). Because these are not found in standard pharmacologic compendiums, dosages for saw palmetto and pygeum should follow the manufacturer's recommendations.

Saw palmetto, an herb derived from the dark berries of a palm tree native to the southern United States, is reported to have been in use since the 1700s. Purportedly, it is useful for the management of prostate inflammation by a threefold mechanism. First, it inhibits testosterone conversion to DHT, resulting in the prevention of prostate enlargement. Second, it stops DHT binding to receptor sites; third, it has a general inhibitory effect on both estrogen and androgen receptors. There is no evidence of deleterious effects on PSA levels with the use of saw palmetto. Saw palmetto is available in capsule, liquid, or softgel form and as a tea; the tea is not believed to be effective for BPH. Saw palmetto often is used in combination with pygeum (http://www.sawpalmetto.com).

Pygeum is the ground and powdered bark of the pygeum tree, an evergreen of southern Africa. It is prepared as a tea for easing complaints related to the genitourinary system. Widely used in Europe for symptom relief in BPH and thus postponement of surgery or the use of stronger medications, the efficacy of pygeum is being researched at the University of Southern California. Dosage recommendations are 50 to 100 mg twice daily; gastrointestinal irritation is a rare side effect (http://www.mothernature.com).

Zinc also plays a role in BPH, improving general prostate health by preventing or even decreasing prostate enlargement. Research has supported that doses of zinc sulfate lead to the inhibition of 5-alpha-reductase, the enzyme for conversion of testosterone to DHT. The recommended dosage for zinc sulfate is 150 mg/day for 2 months followed by a maintenance dose of 50 to 100 mg/day.

PROSTATE CANCER

Prostate cancer is the most common type of cancer affecting men and the second leading cause of cancer death in men (of the cancers, lung cancer remains the top killer of men). In the decade from 1980 and 1990, the incidence of prostate cancer increased by 50%, although this is actually perceived as a positive development, indicating enhanced screenings rather than a truly increased incidence of disease. This disease is more common in African-American men than in white men and, in general, in men from North, Central, and South America, Africa, and the Near East.

Ironically, in African-American men, prostate cancer develops at a significantly higher rate than in their native African counterparts. Men of Asian heritage have a low incidence of prostate cancer and low death rates from the disease. Once again, Asian-American men have a slightly higher incidence of prostate cancer than their native Asian counterparts.

Incidence reports estimate that 1 of every 11 men will have cancer of the prostate; as the man ages, the risk for development of prostate cancer also increases. Greater than 80% of the diagnosed prostate cancers have been in men aged 65 or older (Bullock & Henze, 2000).

CAUSES

The disease seems to be closely aligned with the aging process; the exact cause is not well understood, although a genetic predisposition has been found. Thus, sons of men who have had prostate cancer are at higher risk for developing prostate cancer themselves. No link between prostate cancer and BPH has been uncovered. From an environmental and occupational perspective, association with cadmium in the workplace is correlated with the later onset of prostate cancer.

Essentially 95% of prostate cancers are adenocarcinomas, with most occurring at the prostate's periphery. How aggressive the neoplasm becomes seems to be more highly correlated with the degree of anaplasia, or lack of differentiation, of the cancer cells as opposed to tumor size. Progression of the cancer begins with local extension, but metastasis to distant sites occurs through blood and lymphatic vessels. Given the anatomic location of the prostate, it is easily understood how progression to the pelvis and rectum, lumbar and thoracic spine and ribs, and femur can ensue.

PATHOPHYSIOLOGY

In many cases, symptoms present only with advanced disease. As with BPH, bladder-associated problems occur first—slow urine stream, inadequate emptying of bladder, painful urination, frequency, and nocturia. However, with prostate cancer, unlike BPH, there is no remission from these symptoms. Difficulty in defecation, and even obstruction of the large bowel, can also occur depending on how the tumor is spreading, but again this is usually seen with advanced disease.

DIAGNOSTIC CRITERIA

Early detection of prostate cancer is crucial. Enhanced screening has alerted many men to seek medical intervention for prostate cancer well before symptom manifestation. African-American men are still diagnosed at a more advanced stage, and their rate of survival is poorer than among whites. Thus, public education targeting African-American men is of paramount importance.

Three screening methods are commonly used. The first is the DRE; the second is the serum level of PSA. When either result is abnormal, an ultrasound study is performed transrectally. The man should be cautioned to avoid ejaculation for 48 hours before obtaining a PSA because false-positive results may be obtained. The diagnostic yield rises dramatically when ultrasound is incorporated with DRE and PSA. It is recommended that all men over 40 years of age undergo an annual DRE, and all men over 50 years of age also have their PSA level tested annually in addition to the DRE. Normal PSA values should be less than 2.7 in men under age 40 and 4.0 or less in men over age 40.

However, for confirmation of cancer, and with suspect findings, further diagnostic investigation is warranted. This includes a biopsy to confirm the diagnosis and identify the cancer's histologic type, after which MRI and CT scans are necessary to determine the extent of metastasis.

Treatment options include surgery, chemotherapy, and radiation, either alone or in combination. Regardless of the treatment modality, loss of physiologic function can occur. This loss of function varies from temporary loss of urinary control to permanent incontinence. In addition to loss of urinary control, fecal incontinence can also result. Sexual dysfunction frequently occurs and involves the ability to attain an erection or have emission or ejaculation. Return to normal physiologic function often occurs over time, but some permanent dysfunction can result.

INITIATING DRUG THERAPY

Pharmacologic intervention can also help the patient return to normal physiologic function after other treatments, such as partial or radical prostatectomy, which are options based on the cancer's histologic type and the extent of metastasis. Often, surgery is performed after a period of radiation or chemotherapy. A main postoperative concern is that bladder dysfunction will persist; this manifests as incomplete emptying, incontinence, decreased force of stream, and urinary scarring.

Bilateral orchiectomy has also been used for advanced disease to decrease the risk of complications and spread of prostate cancer, but it is not considered curative in the setting of metastasis or advanced disease. Bilateral orchiectomy is radical surgery used to extend the man's life; it provides relief from symptoms. There is minimal morbidity and mortality associated with the surgery, but it may have a negative impact on the man's self-esteem and sense of identity. Postsurgical pharmacologic management is crucial to promoting the man's self-esteem and correcting, as much as possible, the altered physiologic function. Chemotherapy is discussed in Chapter 56.

ERECTILE DYSFUNCTION

Erectile dysfunction (ED) is the repeated inability to achieve or maintain an erection that is firm enough for sexual intercourse. ED can be a total inability to achieve erection, an inconsistent ability to do so, or a tendency to sustain only brief erections. The incidence of ED increases with age: about 5% of men age 40 experience ED, compared with 15% to 25% of men age 65. However, ED is not an inevitable part of aging.

It is estimated that at least 10 to 20 million American men suffer from ED. Laumann and colleagues (1999) showed that the prevalence of male sexual dysfunction approached 31% in a population survey of approximately 1,400 men aged 18 to 59.

CAUSES

An erection requires a precise sequence of events, and ED can occur when any of the events are disrupted. The sequence includes nerve impulses in the brain, the spinal column, and the area around the penis and response in muscles, fibrous tissues, veins, and arteries in and near the corpora cavernosa. Damage to nerves, arteries, smooth muscles, and fibrous tissues (often as a result of disease) is the most common cause of ED. Chronic diseases such as diabetes, kidney disease, chronic alcoholism, multiple sclerosis, atherosclerosis, vascular disease, and neurologic disease account for about 70% of ED cases. Between 35% and 50% of men with diabetes experience ED.

Surgery (especially radical prostate surgery for cancer) can injure nerves and arteries near the penis, thus causing ED. Injury to the penis, spinal cord, prostate, bladder, and pelvis can lead to ED by harming nerves, smooth muscles, arteries, and fibrous tissues of the corpora cavernosa.

Many common drugs such as antihypertensives, antihistamines, antidepressants, tranquilizers, appetite suppressants, and cimetidine can have ED as an adverse event. Psychological factors such as stress, anxiety, guilt, depression, low self-esteem, and fear of sexual failure cause 10% to 20% of ED cases. Other possible causes of ED include smoking, which affects blood flow in veins and arteries, and hormonal abnormalities, such as low testosterone levels.

PATHOPHYSIOLOGY

The penis is innervated by both autonomic and somatic nerves. Sympathetic and parasympathetic fibers in the cavernous nerves regulate blood flow into the corpus cavernosum during erection and detumescence. Erection, at the level of the penis, begins with transmission of impulses from parasympathetic nerves and nonadrenergic, noncholinergic nerves. This neural stimulus leads to the release of nitric oxide from the nonadrenergic, noncholinergic nerves and possibly the endothelial cells. Nitric oxide increases intracellular levels of cyclic guanosine monophosphate (cGMP) in the cavernosal smooth muscle, which acts to relax cavernosal tissue, perhaps by activating protein kinase G and stimulating phosphorylation of the proteins that regulate corporal smooth muscle tone. The actions of the parasympathetic nervous system, nitric oxide, and cGMP permit rapid blood flow into the penis and the development of an erection. As pressure within the corporal body increases, small emissary veins traversing the tunica albuginea are occluded, trapping blood in the corpus cavernosum. The erection is maintained until ejaculation, which usually leads to detumescence.

Phosphodiesterases (PDEs) are hydrolytic enzymes that play a critical role in regulating physiologic processes by terminating signal transduction through their hydrolytic action on cyclic nucleotides. They play a key role in the physiology of erection.

Significant changes in penile structure occur with aging. Collagen and elastic fibers in the tunica albuginea are key structures that permit increases in the girth and length of the penis during tumescence, and ultrastructural analysis of penile biopsies has shown that the concentration of elastic fibers decreases with age. This decrease results in a reduction in elasticity, which could contribute

to ED in elderly men. Additionally, there is a decrease of up to 35% in the smooth muscle content of the penis in men older than 60 years. Decreases in the ratio between corpus cavernosum smooth muscle and connective tissue has been associated with increased likelihood of diffuse venous leak that may contribute to ED. It has also been noted that the concentration of type III collagen decreases and that of type I collagen increases in the aging penis. It has been suggested that this change makes the corpus cavernosum less compliant, reduces filling of vascular spaces, and also contributes to veno-occlusive dysfunction. It has also been hypothesized that changes in the collagen content of the penis may result in chronic ischemia that leads to loss of smooth muscle cells. Any condition, disease, medication, or injury or surgery that affects the ability to initiate erections or to fill the lacunar space or store blood may cause ED.

ED involves multiple organic and psychogenic factors, which often coexist. Psychogenic factors are the most common causes of intermittent ED in younger men, but these are usually secondary to or may coexist with organic factors in older men. Other factors contributing to ED include vasculogenic, neurogenic, endocrinologic, structural (traumatic), and pharmacologic causes and lifestyle factors, such as obesity, a sedentary lifestyle, and alcohol and tobacco use. Many of the conditions that contribute to ED are chronic and systemic, involving multiple avenues of damage. These conditions include cardiovascular disease, hypertension, diabetes mellitus, and depression. Many of the diseases linked to ED involve endothelial dysfunction.

DIAGNOSTIC CRITERIA

A thorough history is paramount to diagnosing ED. Every male patient should be asked about medical conditions and sexual function. Testosterone levels can yield information about problems with the endocrine system and is indicated especially in patients with decreased sexual desire.

INITIATING DRUG THERAPY

ED can be very traumatic to men. There are now drugs that can assist with achieving and maintaining an erection that is firm enough for sexual intercourse. Testosterone levels should be determined and a complete cardiac history and evaluation should be done to determine whether there are contraindications to these medications.

Goals of Drug Therapy

The goals of drug therapy for ED are to enable the patient to achieve sexual satisfaction and to achieve and maintain an erection.

Phosphodiesterase-5 Inhibitors

Phosphodiesterase-5 (PDE5) inhibitors promote penile erection by inhibiting the breakdown of one of the messengers involved in the erectile response. The PDE5 is the main cGMP-catalyzing enzyme in human trabecular smooth muscle. It is also expressed in vascular smooth muscle, lung, platelets, and a wide variety of other tissues but is not present in cardiac muscle cells. Human corpus cavernosum also contains PDE types 2, 3, and 4 enzymes. PDE5 inhibitors are contingent on the presence of cGMP in the smooth muscle cell. In the presence of sexual stimulation, the PDE inhibitors reinforce the normal cellular signals that increase cyclic nucleotide concentrations by blocking cyclic nucleotide hydrolysis, thereby facilitating the initiation and maintenance of an erection.

Dosage

The recommended dosage of sildenafil is 50 mg 30 to 60 minutes before intercourse, but doses range from 25 to 100 mg. The maximum is one dose a day. Food can delay absorption.

The recommended dose of tadalafil is 10 mg, but doses range from 5 to 20 mg. Tadalafil can be taken without restriction on food or alcohol intake.

The recommended dose of vardenafil is 10 mg, but doses range from 2.5 to 20 mg. It is taken 60 minutes before intercourse. Food can delay absorption.

Time Frame for Response

Sildenafil and vardenafil are rapidly absorbed, reaching maximum plasma concentrations within 30 to 120 minutes (median 60 minutes) of oral dosing in the fasted state; a high-fat meal has been found to reduce the rate of absorption. The elimination half-life is approximately 4 hours, and no more than one dose should be taken per 24-hour period.

Tadalafil has an onset of action of 30 minutes and allows intercourse for at least 30 hours. This is significant because it may eliminate the need for planning sexual activity.

Contraindications

PDE5 inhibitors can potentiate the vasodilatory properties of nitrates, so their administration in patients who use nitrates in any form is contraindicated. In an emergency situation, nitrates can be used 24 hours after administration of sildenafil and vardenafil and 48 hours after tadalafil.

PDE5 inhibitors are contraindicated in patients with unstable angina, hypotension with a systolic blood pressure below 90, uncontrolled hypertension of more than 170/110, history of recent stroke, life-threatening arrhythmia, myocardial infarction within 6 months, and severe

cardiac failure. They are also contraindicated in patients with severe hepatic impairment or end-stage renal disease requiring dialysis.

Sildenafil has a relative contraindication with the concomitant use of alpha-blockers and should not be taken within 4 hours of an alpha blocker and at a dose no greater than 25 mg. Tadalafil should not be taken with an alpha blocker other than tamsulosin, 0.4 mg once a day. Vardenafil is contraindicated with any alpha blocker.

Adverse Events

Most adverse events are vasodilatory, including headache, flushing, and nasal congestion. Dyspepsia has also been reported. With sildenafil abnormal color vision has been reported.

Interactions

Potent CYP3A4 inhibitors can cause increased levels of PDE5 inhibitors. They may also be affected by amlodipine, beta blockers, cimetidine, diuretics, and erythromycin.

Selecting the Most Appropriate Agent

It is important to include the significant other in counseling about ED. A complete cardiac history must be taken. If there is any question as to the stability of the cardiac status, further testing must be done. Testosterone, serum glucose (or alternatively glycosylated hemoglobin), and serum lipid levels must be determined in all cases of ED. Depending on patient history and physical examination findings, more extensive laboratory tests may be necessary. If testosterone levels are abnormal, testosterone replacement is needed. See Table 34-7 for selected agents.

The patient with the following factors is considered at low risk for a cardiac event with the use of PDE5 inhibitors: fewer than three risk factors for coronary artery disease, controlled hypertension, mild, stable angina, uncomplicated myocardial infarction more than 8 weeks previously, mild valvular disease, and heart failure NYHA class 1. See Box 34-1 and Figure 34-3.

First-Line Therapy

The first-line therapy for ED is a PDE5 inhibitor (Table 34-8).

Table 34.7

Overview of Selected Agents Used to Treat Erectile Dysfunction

Generic (Trade) Name and Dosage	Selected Adverse Events	Contraindications	Special Considerations
Tadalafil (Cialis) 5–20 mg per day	Headache, flushing, GI disturbance, nasal congestion, rash, priapism	Nitrates and alpha blockers except tamsulosin 0.4 mg once a day	Food and alcohol make no difference in absorption. May remain in system for 36 hours.
Vardenafil (Levitra) 5–20 mg per day	As above	Nitrates and alpha blockers	High-fat meal delays absorption.
Sildenafil (Viagra) 25–100 mg per day	As above and color disturbances	Nitrates and within 4 hours of an alpha blocker and at a dose no greater than 25 mg	As above

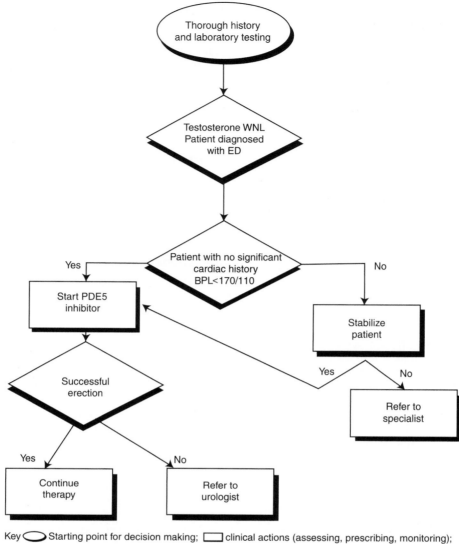

Figure 34–3 Treatment algorithm for erectile dysfunction.

Second-Line Therapy

If PDE5 inhibitors are not successful in treating ED, the patient should be referred to a urologist. Alternative therapies include penile intracavernosal injection therapy, a medical intraurethral system for erections, a vacuum erection device, and penile prostheses.

MONITORING PATIENT RESPONSE

The patient should be followed in 6 months to determine the effectiveness of therapy and to reevaluate his cardiac status. If the patient does not meet the criteria for low risk, the PDE5 inhibitors are discontinued.

PATIENT EDUCATION

Drug Information

With sildenafil and vardenafil, a high-fat meal has been found to reduce the rate of absorption. Food and alcohol have no effect on the absorption of tadalafil.

Sildenafil has a relative contraindication with the concomitant use of alpha-blockers and should not be taken within 4 hours of an alpha blocker and at a dose no greater than 25 mg. Tadalafil should not be taken with an alpha blocker other than tamsulosin 0.4 mg once a day. Vardenafil is contraindicated with any alpha blocker.

Complementary and Alternative Medicine

Yohimbine, an agent derived from the bark of the African yohimbe tree, has been found to be beneficial in some cases of ED. It is reported to act by both peripheral and central mechanisms, acting peripherally as a presynaptic stimulant at parasympathetic NANC nerves and presynaptically as an adrenergic depressant at sympathetic alpha$_1$-adrenoceptors, both mechanisms augmenting penile blood flow. It also appears to have CNS activity, with blockade of the erection-suppressing alpha$_2$-adrenoceptors; several studies have reported a more favorable response with yohimbine compared with placebo in ED of psychogenic origin.

BOX 34–1. LOW-RISK FACTORS FOR CARDIAC EVENTS FROM PDE5 INHIBITORS

Less than three risk factors for coronary artery disease
Controlled hypertension
Stable angina
Uncomplicated myocardial infarction more than 8 weeks previously
Mild valvular disease
Heart failure NYHA Class 1 (see Chapter 21)

Table 34.8

Recommended Order of Treatment for Erectile Dysfunction

Order	Agent	Comment
First line	Phosphodiesterase-5 inhibitors	Contraindicated if on nitrates, unstable hypertension, unstable cardiac condition
Second line	Referral to urologist	Procedures available include penile intracavernosal injection therapy, medical intraurethral system for erections, vacuum erection device, penile prostheses.

■ Case Study

M.P., age 45, works as an accountant in a busy firm. He is of African-American descent. He and his wife have been married for 25 years and have two children, aged 21 and 18 years. His father is alive and well at age 68 years but was diagnosed with BPH 5 years ago. M.P. considers himself to be in good health and has no allergies; he is approximately 15% overweight. His wife insisted that he seek medical intervention because of urinary symptomatology: he has difficulty starting his stream of urine, burning on urination, nocturia, and lower back and pelvic discomfort. The result of a PSA test, his first in over 2 years, is 3.1.

Diagnosis: BPH

1. List specific goals for treatment for M.P.
2. What drug therapy would you prescribe? Why?
3. What are the parameters for monitoring the success of the therapy?
4. Discuss specific patient education based on the prescribed therapy.
5. List one or two adverse reactions for the selected agent that would cause you to change therapy.
6. What would be the choice for second-line therapy?
7. What OTC and/or alternative medications would be appropriate for this patient?
8. What dietary and lifestyle changes should be recommended for this patient?
9. Describe one or two drug/drug or drug/food interactions for the selected agent.

Bibliography

Starred references are cited in the text.

Ahmad, K. (2004). New therapy for prostatic hyperplasia? *Lancet Oncology, 5*(2), 72.

*Bullock, B. A., & Henze, R. L. (2000). *Focus on pathophysiology.* Philadelphia: Lippincott Williams & Wilkins.

Cohon, P., & Koreman, S. G. (2001). Erectile dysfunction. *Journal of Clinical Endocrinology and Metabolism, 86*(6), 2391–2394.

Fagelman, E. (2002). Herbal medicines to treat benign prostatic hyperplasia. *Urology Clinics of North America, 29*(1), 23–29.

Hua, V. N. (2004). Acute and chronic prostatitis. *Medical Clinics of North America, 88*(2), 483–494.

*Laumann, E., Paik, A. & Rosen, R. C. (1999). Sexual dysfunction in the United States: Prevalence and predictor. *Journal of the American Medical Association, 281*(6), 537–544.

Lam, J. S., Cooper, K. L., & Kaplan, S. A. (2004). Changing aspects in evaluation and treatment of the patient with benign prostatic hyperplasia. *Medical Clinics of North America, 88*(2), 281–308.

Morales, A. (2001). Erectile dysfunction: An overview. *Clinical Geriatric Medicine, 19*(3), 529–538.

*Nickel, J. C., Fradet, Y., Boake, R., et al. (1996). Efficacy and safety of finasteride therapy for benign prostatic hyperplasia: Results of a 2-year randomized controlled trial (the PROSPECT study). *Canadian Medical Journal, 155*(9), 1251–1259.

Ramsey, E. W., Elhilali, M., Goldenberg, S. L., et al. (2000). Practice patterns of Canadian urologists in benign prostatic hyperplasia and prostate cancer. *Journal of Urology, 163*(2), 499–502.

Rosen, R. C. (2003). Overview of phosphiodiesterase 5 inhibition in erectile dysfunction. *American Journal of Cardiology, 92*(9A), 9M–18M.

Stefel, A. D. (2004). Erectile dysfunction: Etiology, evaluation and treatment options. *Medical Clinics of North America, 88*(2), 387–416.

Tarig, S. H., Omran, M. L., Kaiser, F. E., et al. (2003). Erectile dysfunction: Etiology and treatment in young and old patients. *Clinical Geriatric Medicine, 19*(3), 539–551.

Visit the Connection web site for the most up-to-date drug information.

INCONTINENCE

■ VIRGINIA P. ARCANGELO

Urinary incontinence is defined as an uncontrolled loss of urine severe enough to be a problem for the patient or family. Approximately 13 million Americans have urinary incontinence. This problem can be easily identified and treated. In people between 15 and 64 years of age, the prevalence is 10% to 30% in women and 1.5% to 5% in men. The highest prevalence occurs in the women and the elderly. The anatomy of the urinary system of women places them at greater risk than men.

In the population older than 60 years of age, the prevalence of urinary incontinence is 15% to 35%, with women affected twice as much as men. Approximately half of all institutionalized elderly patients have urinary incontinence. This problem is related to immobility, fecal incontinence, and dementia. The total cost of urinary incontinence is estimated at $26.3 billion annually.

Urinary incontinence causes psychosocial problems, including dependency and decreased social interaction. The four types of incontinence are stress, urge, mixed, and overflow (Box 35-1).

Urge incontinence is a contributing factor for falls and hip fractures among elderly women because they rush to the toilet to avoid spilling of urine. It also contributes to skin problems in the elderly, especially when a pad or containment device is used.

CAUSES

The causes of urinary incontinence are anatomic, physiologic, and pathologic factors affecting the urinary tract. Factors outside the genitourinary tract also may contribute. Many of the conditions outside the genitourinary tract are reversible, and their management can promote resolution or decreased severity of urinary incontinence. For example, discontinuation of a diuretic may resolve urinary incontinence. Box 35-2 lists risk factors for urinary incontinence, which include urinary tract infection, atrophic vaginitis, pregnancy, and prostatectomy. Hyperglycemia, volume overload, and excess fluid intake are also risk factors.

Incontinence may be a side effect of drugs such as caffeine, alpha-adrenergic blockers, alcohol, and others. If a patient presents with incontinence and is taking an alpha-adrenergic blocker for hypertension, then the practitioner should change the medication to an angiotensin-converting enzyme inhibitor or another class of drug used for hypertension. Medications with alpha-adrenergic blocking properties are listed in Box 35-3.

PATHOPHYSIOLOGY

Physiologic changes related to aging sometimes account for urinary incontinence. As a person ages, changes in the urinary tract include decreased bladder capacity, detrusor instability, and decreased bladder elasticity. Decreased elasticity can lead to incomplete emptying. In the younger woman, estrogen receptors are present in the urethra and bladder. As the woman ages and estrogen decreases, accompanying atrophy of the bladder's epithelial lining results in diminished sphincter effectiveness. For this reason, postmenopausal women are at greatest risk for all types of urinary incontinence.

Stress incontinence results from urethral hypermobility due to anatomic changes or defects. Increased periods of intra-abdominal pressure cause urethral hypermobility or displacement of the urethra and bladder neck. The result is loss of urine during coughing, sneezing, laughing, or other activities that increase intra-abdominal pressure without a detrusor contraction or overdistended bladder.

Urge incontinence results from involuntary detrusor contractions, detrusor hyperactivity with malfunctioning bladder contractility, or involuntary sphincter relaxation. An involuntary loss of urine is associated with a strong desire to urinate.

Mixed incontinence is a combination of both stress incontinence and urge incontinence. A fourth type of urinary incontinence is overflow incontinence. The cause of overflow incontinence is an acontractile or underactive detrusor due to use of drugs, fecal impaction, diabetes, lower spinal cord injury, or disruption of motor innervation of the detrusor muscle.

In men, the most common pathophysiologic cause of urinary incontinence is an enlarged prostate. Treatment for this condition is discussed in Chapter 34.

DIAGNOSTIC CRITERIA

Urinary incontinence can be diagnosed using a simple cystometry test or cystometrography. The practitioner often makes a diagnosis simply according to the patient's self-report.

BOX 35–1. TYPES OF URINARY INCONTINENCE

Stress Incontinence
Loss of urine from sudden increase in intra-abdominal pressure without detrusor muscle contraction (eg, from sneezing, coughing, or laughing). Often the leak is continuous or occurs with minimal exertion.

Urge Incontinence
Involuntary loss of urine associated with strong desire to void as bladder contracts, usually as a result of detrusor instability. The patient must strain to empty the bladder, but emptying is incomplete.

Mixed Incontinence
Symptoms of both stress and urge incontinence. One symptom is usually most bothersome.

Overflow Incontinence
Involuntary loss of urine associated with overdistention of the bladder from an underactive or acontractile detrusor or outlet obstruction. In men, the condition often results from benign prostatic hyperplasia.

INITIATING DRUG THERAPY

Before initiating intervention for urinary incontinence, the practitioner must determine the cause of the incontinence. If the cause is a reversible condition such as a fecal impaction or a side effect of a medication, the condition should be corrected. If the urinary incontinence continues, the practitioner should initiate further treatment.

There are three methods of treating urinary incontinence: behavior modification, pharmacologic intervention, and surgery. The patient and the practitioner must work together to develop a plan of care that works best for the patient. Behavior modification includes pelvic muscle rehabilitation, bladder training, toileting assistance (scheduled toileting), and fluid management (restriction).

Pelvic muscle rehabilitation involves pelvic muscle exercises such as Kegel exercises and pelvic floor exercises. These exercises strengthen the periurethral and perivaginal muscles that aid in the closing of the urethra and support the pelvic visceral structures. Pelvic muscle rehabilitation is successful for patients with stress incontinence, urge incontinence, and mixed incontinence. Instructions for Kegel exercises are found in Box 35-4.

Biofeedback, which uses instruments to relay information about physiologic activity to patients, has proven useful in treating urinary incontinence. Through biofeedback, the patient learns to change the physiologic responses that control bladder function. This therapy is successful for patients with stress incontinence, urge incontinence, and mixed incontinence.

Before introducing pharmacologic therapy, the practitioner must determine which type of urinary incontinence exists, because different drugs are more effective with different conditions. Surgical intervention is considered when other therapies have failed.

BOX 35–2. RISK FACTORS FOR URINARY INCONTINENCE

- Immobility
- Impaired cognition
- Medications and substances
  - Diuretics
  - Caffeine
  - Anticholinergics (urinary retention, overflow incontinence, fecal impaction)
  - Psychotropics (anticholinergic actions, sedation, delirium)
  - Narcotic analgesics (urinary retention, fecal impaction, delirium, sedation)
  - Alpha-adrenergic blockers (urethral relaxation)
  - Beta-adrenergic agonists (urinary retention)
  - Calcium channel blockers (urinary retention)
  - Alcohol
- Morbid obesity
- Smoking
- Fecal impaction
- Delirium
- Low fluid intake
- Environmental barriers
- High-impact physical activities
- Diabetes
- Stroke
- Menopause
- Pelvic muscle weakness
- Childhood nocturnal enuresis
- Pregnancy, vaginal delivery, episiotomy

Goals of Drug Therapy

The goal of drug therapy is to promote continence for as long as therapy is effective and tolerated. An overview of the drugs used for incontinence is given in Table 35-1.

Alpha-Adrenergic Agonists

The sympathetic and parasympathetic nervous systems innervate the bladder neck and proximal urethra. Pseudoephedrine

BOX 35–3. MEDICATIONS WITH ALPHA-ADRENERGIC BLOCKING PROPERTIES

prazosin (Minipress)
terazosin (Hytrin)
doxazosin (Cardura)
labetalol (Normodyne, Trandate)
phenoxybenzamine (Dibenzyline)
methyldopa (Aldomet)
clonidine (Catapres)
guanfacine (Tenex)
guanadrel (Hylorel)

BOX 35–4. HOW TO PERFORM KEGEL EXERCISES

- Draw up the pelvic floor (as though trying to suck water into the vagina) and hold for 3 to 10 seconds while breathing normally.
- Relax the muscles for 5 seconds and then repeat.

Begin with a set of 10 of these 4 times a day. Increase the number by 5 each time every week, and do the exercises 4 times a day.

is most effective in stress incontinence. It was shown to reduce stress incontinence by 20% to 60% (Alhasso, Glazener, Pickard & N'Dow, 2003).

Mechanism of Action

Alpha-adrenergic receptors regulate sympathetic innervation of the neck of the bladder. The alpha-adrenergic agonists stimulate the alpha receptors to contract and to strengthen the proximal urethra, causing increased outlet resistance.

Dosage

The alpha-adrenergic agonist available is pseudoephedrine (Sudafed), 15 to 30 mg three times a day.

Contraindications

Alpha-adrenergic agonists are contraindicated in patients with severe hypertension and coronary artery disease. They must be used with caution in patients with hypertension, hyperthyroidism, diabetes mellitus, increased intraocular pressure, and prostatic hypertrophy.

Adverse Events

Adverse events include nausea, xerostomia, insomnia, rash, itching, headache, anxiety, dizziness, and hypertension.

Interactions

These drugs decrease the antihypertensive effects of methyl-dopa (Aldomet). Increased hypertension may result if the patient takes an alpha-adrenergic agonist with guanethidine (Ismelin).

Estrogen

Estrogen is an adjunct therapy in stress incontinence. Estrogen increases urethral coaptation, vascularity, and tone and enhances the alpha-adrenergic responsiveness of the urethral muscle in postmenopausal women. Prescribers must combine estrogen with progesterone in women with intact uteri to prevent endometrial cancer. However, in light of recent findings about the potential dangers of estrogen, it is not recommended as a first-line agent.

Oral estrogen cannot be recommended as first-line therapy, but local vaginal estrogen may be helpful. Vaginal creams and a ring impregnated with estrogen that is changed every 3 months may be helpful.

Tricyclic Antidepressants

The tricyclic antidepressant (TCA) imipramine is effective for nocturnal and mixed incontinence.

Mechanism of Action

Imipramine has dual alpha-agonist and anticholinergic activity. It increases urethral outlet resistance through adrenergic stimulation of the smooth muscle of the neck of the

---

Table 35.1

Overview of Selected Drugs Used to Treat Urinary Incontinence

Generic (Trade) Name and Dosage	Selected Adverse Events	Contraindications	Special Considerations
Alpha-Adrenergic Agonists pseudoephedrine (Sudafed) 15–30 mg tid	Palpitations, headaches, increased BP, dizziness, GI upset, tremor	Hypertension, coronary artery disease, prostatic disorders	Give at least 2 h before bedtime; do not crush, break, or chew tablets.
Tricyclic Antidepressants imipramine (Tofranil) 10–25 mg qd–tid	Drowsiness, orthostatic hypotension, restlessness, insomnia, xerostomia, nausea, constipation, headache	Acute post-MI	Imipramine is best taken at bedtime because of its sedative effect.
Anticholinergics oxybutynin (Ditropan) 5 mg 2 to 3 times a day (max 20 mg/d) (Ditropan XL) 5–30 mg qd Transdermal oxybutynin (Oxytrol)— apply twice a week	Dry skin, xerostomia, nausea, constipation, blurred vision, changes in mental status	Narrow-angle glaucoma Intestinal obstruction Paralytic ileus Severe colitis Myasthenia gravis Unstable cardiovascular disease	Use with care in activities that require mental alertness. May increase CNS side effects if the patient has pre-existing cognitive impairment Use with care in elderly and cognitively impaired. Increased symptoms of angina may occur if coronary artery disease exists.
tolterodine (Detrol) 1–2 mg bid (Detrol LA) 2–4 mg qd	Same as above	Same as above	Same as above

bladder and proximal urethra and assists in urine storage by decreasing bladder contractility.

Dosage

Imipramine has sedating effects, so patients tolerate it best at bedtime. Combining a TCA at bedtime with an anticholinergic, antispasmodic agent such as oxybutynin (Ditropan) during the day decreases bladder contractility. However, there may be additional anticholinergic side effects. The dosage of imipramine is 10 to 25 mg, one to three times a day.

Contraindications

Imipramine is contraindicated in patients taking monoamine oxidase inhibitors (MAOIs) or within 14 days of the use of MAOIs—that is, the patient should discontinue MAOI therapy at least 2 weeks before starting imipramine. Death can result when TCAs are used with MAOIs.

Adverse Events

Adverse events include drowsiness, orthostatic hypotension, restlessness, insomnia, gastrointestinal symptoms, anticholinergic effects, and photosensitivity. In addition, TCAs may produce changes in electrocardiographic recordings.

Interactions

Imipramine potentiates alcohol and other central nervous system depressants. Barbiturates, carbamazepine (Tegretol), and phenytoin (Dilantin) are antagonists.

Anticholinergics

The recommended anticholinergics for urinary incontinence are oxybutynin (Ditropan) and tolterodine (Detrol), an anticholinergic drug that has proven successful in treating urge incontinence. Both intermediate-release preparations reduce incontinence by about 45% to 50% (Anderson, Mobley, Blank, et al., 1999; Appell, 1997). Extended-release tolterodine reduces incontinence by about 71% and extended-release oxybutynin by about 83% (Diokno, Appell, Sand, et al., 2003). Transdermal oxybutynin (Oxytrol) is available.

Mechanism of Action

Oxybutynin acts directly to relax smooth muscle and inhibits the effects of acetylcholine at muscarinic receptors. Tolterodine is selective for the bladder receptors rather than the salivary gland receptors, so xerostomia is less of a problem.

Dosage

The dosage of oxybutynin is 5 mg two or three times a day, with a maximum of 20 mg/day. Oxybutynin extended release (Ditropan XL) is started at 5 mg once a day and can be increased weekly in 5-mg increments to a maximum of 30 mg/day. The patient must swallow the tablet whole (the tablet cannot be crushed or chewed). A transdermal oxybutynin patch is applied twice a week; it releases 3.9 mg over 24

hours. The dosage for tolterodine is 1 to 2 mg twice a day. Practitioners also may prescribe propantheline (Pro-Banthine) 7.5 to 30 mg three to five times a day.

Contraindications

Anticholinergics are contraindicated in patients with bowel obstruction, colitis, ileus, glaucoma, and myasthenia gravis. They should be used cautiously in patients with hepatic and renal impairment.

Anticholinergics are in pregnancy category B. Patients may have central nervous system side effects, especially if preexisting cognitive impairment is present. These medications must be used with care in elderly and cognitively impaired patients.

Adverse Events

In a patient with symptomatic coronary artery disease, the anticholinergic effects may increase the heart rate, leading to increased symptoms of angina. Adverse events with oxybutynin include drowsiness, headache, dry skin, xerostomia, nausea, constipation, blurred vision, change in mental status, tachycardia, and decreased sweating. Because of the symptom of dry mouth, elderly patients may greatly increase their fluid intake, predisposing them to hyponatremia. Extended-release formulations appear to diminish the adverse events.

Interactions

Cytochrome P450-34A inhibitors may increase plasma levels of tolterodine.

Selecting the Most Appropriate Agent

To prescribe the most appropriate agent (Fig. 35-1 and Table 35-2), the practitioner needs to determine which type of incontinence exists.

First-Line Therapy

The most effective drugs for use in *stress incontinence* are alpha-adrenergic agonists, which increase bladder outlet resistance.

Urge incontinence is the most difficult type to treat. It affects both men and women, and its incidence increases with advancing age. The most successful drug therapies for urge incontinence are anticholinergics. Anticholinergics are used as first-line therapy; they antagonize the muscarinic receptors of the bladder, increasing the bladder capacity, decreasing the amplitude of the contraction, and increasing the volume before the bladder contracts.

In *mixed incontinence*, one symptom is usually more bothersome than another, and that symptom is the one targeted for treatment.

Overflow incontinence resulting from an acontractile detrusor is usually treated by catheterization rather than medications.

Second-Line Therapy

The TCAs are second-line therapy for stress incontinence and urge incontinence. These agents facilitate urine storage,

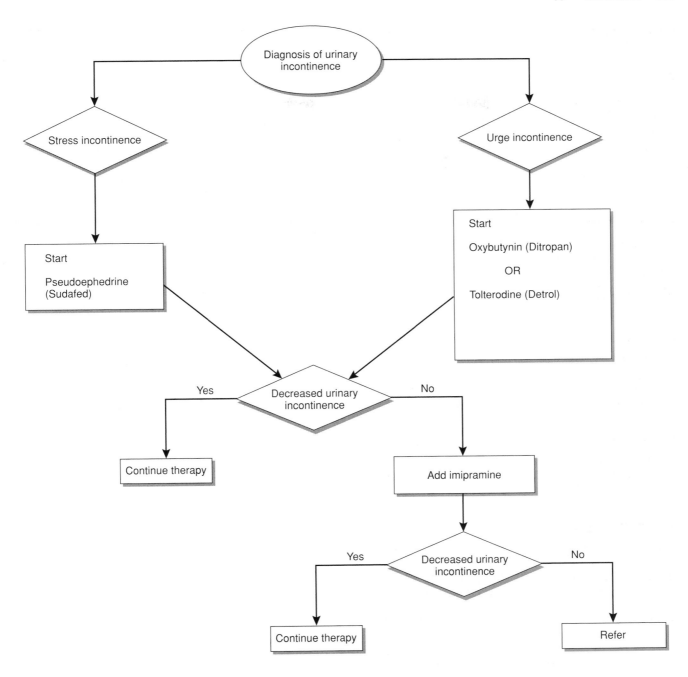

Key ⬭ Starting point for decision making; ▭ clinical actions (assessing, prescribing, monitoring); ◇ decision point.

Figure 35–1 Treatment algorithm for urinary incontinence.

and prescribers can add them to the first-line regimen, although the anticholinergic effects may be additive and intolerable.

Third-Line Therapy

If, after a trial of drug therapy, there is still no success or the side effects of drugs are intolerable, referral to an urologist is recommended and surgery or another treatment is considered.

Newer treatments include instillation of vanilloids capsaicin and resiniferatoxin directly into the bladder. These preparations selectively inhibit reflex bladder contractions and are most effective in urge incontinence from spinal cord lesions, multiple sclerosis, or Parkinson's disease.

Another form of treatment is botulinum toxin injected directly into the urethral and bladder skeletal and smooth muscle, causing irreversible chemical denervation.

The InterStim system, another therapy, involves surgical placement of a lead into the S3 nerve root attached to a neurostimulator implanted under the skin on the back and controlled by a handheld programmer that can be adjusted to increase or decrease bladder contractions.

Table 35.2

Recommended Order of Treatment for Urinary Incontinence

Order	Agents	Comments
First line		First-line drug therapy depends on the type of incontinence.
Stress incontinence	Alpha-adrenergic agonists	Pharmacotherapy is not used to treat overflow incontinence;
Urge incontinence	Anticholinergics	catheterization is the usual intervention.
Mixed incontinence	Agent that best treats predominant symptom	
Second line	Tricyclic antidepressants	
Third line	Referral to urologist	

MONITORING PATIENT RESPONSE

Monitoring of therapy is by the patient's self-report and office follow-up. Postvoid measurements of residual urine can be done.

PATIENT EDUCATION

Drug Information

Medications for urinary incontinence may produce dry mouth, causing increased fluid intake. This can result in water intoxication in the elderly. Intake should be carefully monitored.

Lifestyle/Nutritional Modifications

Patients may learn Kegel exercises to strengthen pelvic muscles (see Box 35-4). In addition, the practitioner may recommend scheduled voiding, in which the patient delays voiding as long as possible to build up bladder capacity. The patient should avoid dietary irritants such as alcohol and caffeine. He or she should drink six to eight glasses of fluid a day but drink nothing after 7 PM to avoid nocturia. Changing the position on the toilet may also help the patient to empty the bladder more completely.

Disposable garments are available to avoid embarrassment with incontinence.

Complementary and Alternative Medicine

Behavioral training including biofeedback, verbal feedback, and physical therapy/pelvic floor muscle training focuses on altering the physiologic responses of the bladder and pelvic floor muscles. These approaches require a commitment by the provider and the patient. They are not curative but can reduce symptoms.

■ Case Study

C. J. is a 55-year-old postmenopausal woman presenting with a 2-year history of incontinence. She reports that she often cannot get to the bathroom in time when she feels the urge to urinate. She also wets herself when she laughs or sneezes. She is very embarrassed about this problem and has decreased her excursions from the house because of it. She drinks six cups of coffee a day and takes hydrochlorothiazide for hypertension.

Diagnosis: Stress incontinence

1. List specific goals for treatment for C. J.

2. What drug therapy would you prescribe? Why?

3. What are the parameters for monitoring the success of the therapy?

4. Discuss specific patient education based on the prescribed therapy.

5. List one or two adverse reactions for the selected agent that would cause you to change therapy.

6. What would be the choice for second-line therapy?

7. What OTC and/or alternative medications would be appropriate for this patient?

8. What dietary and lifestyle changes should be recommended for this patient?

9. Describe one or two drug/drug or drug/food interactions for the selected agent.

Bibliography

Starred references are cited in the text.

Agency for Health Care Policy and Research (AHCPR). (1996). *Urinary incontinence in adults: Acute and chronic management.* Bethesda, MD: U.S. Department of Health and Human Services.

*Alhasso, A., Glazener, C. M., Pickard, R., & N'Dow, J. (2003). Adrenergic drugs for urinary incontinence in adults. *Cochrane Database System Review 2,* CD001842.

*Anderson, R. U., Mobley, D., Blank, B., et al. (1999). Once-daily controlled versus immediate-release oxybutynin chloride for urge urinary incontinence. OROS Oxybutynin Study Group. *Journal of Urology, 161,* 1809–1812.

*Appell, R. A. (1997). Clinical efficacy and safety of tolterodine in the treatment of overactive bladder; a pooled analysis. *Urology, 50(Suppl 6A),* 90–96.

Bump, R. C., & Norton, P. A. (1998). Epidemiology and natural history of pelvic floor dysfunction. *Obstetrics and Gynecology Clinics of North America, 25,* 723–746.

Chutka, D. S., Fleming, K. C., Evans, M. P., et al. (1996). Urinary incontinence in the elderly population. *Mayo Clinic Proceedings, 71(1),* 93–101.

*Diokno, A. C., Appell, R. A., Sand, P. K., et al. (2003). Prospective, randomized, double-blind study of the efficacy and tolerability of extended-release formulations of oxybutynin and tolterodine for overactive bladder: Results of the OPERA Trial. *Mayo Clinic Proceedings, 78,* 687–699.

Gray, M. (2003). The importance of screening, assessing and managing urinary incontinence in primary care. *Journal of the American Academy of Nurse Practitioners, 15(3),* 102–107.

Office on Women's Health of the US Department of health and Human Services (2003). The public health implications of urogenital disease; a focus on overactive bladder. *Clinician, 21(4),* 1–21.

Robinson, D. (1998). Pathophysiology of female lower urinary tract dysfunction. *Obstetrics and Gynecology Clinics of North America, 25,* 747–756.

Wyman, J. F. (2003). Treatment of urinary incontinence in men and older women. *American Journal of Nursing, 3(Suppl),* 36–45.

Visit the Connection web site for the most up-to-date drug information.

36

SEXUALLY TRANSMITTED INFECTIONS

■ NANCY TOMASELLI AND VIRGINIA P. ARCANGELO

Sexually transmitted infections (STIs) are among the most common illnesses in the world. They have far-reaching health, social, and economic consequences. Our knowledge about the global prevalence and incidence of these infections is limited by the quality and quantity of data available from throughout the world.

In 2002, the Centers for Disease Control and Prevention (CDC) updated the guidelines for treating STIs (Table 36-1). Available from the CDC, these guidelines are one of the most widely used documents published by that organization. The guidelines emphasize the development of management strategies that are adaptable to the managed care environment. Because the guidelines are considered the gold standard for treating STIs, most of the information in this chapter is based on them. The goals of therapy for all STIs are to eradicate the causative organism and prevent complications.

CHLAMYDIAL INFECTION

Chlamydial infection is the most prevalent STI in the United States, with 3 to 4 million cases reported annually. The detection and treatment of this disease is important because the complications can be serious.

CAUSES

Chlamydial infection is caused by *Chlamydia trachomatis*, which shares properties of both bacteria and viruses. The organism is transmitted sexually or perinatally. Repeated infections are common.

In infants, perinatal exposure to the mother's cervix causes the infection. The prevalence is greater than 5% regardless of race, ethnicity, or socioeconomic status. In preadolescent children, sexual abuse must be considered as a causative factor for chlamydial infection; infection of the nasopharynx, urogenital tract, and rectum may persist for greater than 1 year. Because criminal investigation is always a possibility, cultures should be confirmed by microscopic fluoroscopy, which can detect conjugated monoclonal antibodies specific for *C. trachomatis*.

Chlamydial infections occur most frequently in women less than 25 years old. All adolescents and young women should be screened for chlamydia yearly, as should any woman who has a new or multiple sex partners.

PATHOPHYSIOLOGY

Chlamydial organisms are like viruses in that they are obligate intracellular parasites. They resemble bacteria by containing both DNA and RNA, by dividing by binary fission, and by having cell walls that resemble those of gram-negative bacteria. Species of chlamydial organisms include *C. psittaci* and *C. trachomatis*, the latter of which has a number of serotypes. These species cause numerous diseases, including lymphogranuloma venereum, blinding trachoma, conjunctivitis, nongonococcal urethritis, cervicitis, salpingitis, proctitis, epididymitis, and newborn pneumonia.

DIAGNOSTIC CRITERIA

The infection may be silent: more than half of infected patients have no clinical signs or symptoms. In symptomatic women, the clinical presentation includes vaginal discharge, mucopurulent cervicitis with edema and friability, urethral syndrome or urethritis, pelvic inflammatory disease, ectopic pregnancy, infertility, and endometritis. Men may report a thin, clear discharge and dysuria. Chlamydial organisms are the major causes of nongonococcal urethritis and epididymitis in young men.

In infants 1 to 3 months of age, chlamydial infection presents in the mucous membranes of the eye, oropharynx, urogenital tract, and rectum and as subacute, afebrile pneumonia; in neonates, it presents as an asymptomatic infection of the oropharynx, genital tract, and rectum. However, chlamydial infection most commonly presents as conjunctivitis 5 to 12 days after birth and is the most frequent identifiable infectious cause of ophthalmia neonatorum. Therefore, for all infants with conjunctivitis who are no older than 30 days, a chlamydial etiology should be considered.

Diagnostic tests for chlamydial ophthalmia neonatorum include tissue cultures and nonculture tests. Ocular exudate should also be tested for *Neisseria gonorrhoeae*.

Chlamydial infection is diagnosed by examination, culture, and antigen detection methods, including direct fluorescent monoclonal antibody staining, enzyme-linked immunosorbent assay, DNA probe assay, and polymerase chain reaction.

Table 36.1

Pharmacotherapy for Sexually Transmitted Infections

Infection	Treatment	Comments

Chlamydial infection	azithromycin 1 g PO once *or*
	 doxycycline 100 mg PO bid for 7 d
	 Alternative
	    erythromycin base 500 mg PO qid for 7 d *or*
	    erythromycin ethylsuccinate 800 mg PO qid for 7 d
	    or ofloxacin 300 mg bid for 7 d *or*
	    levofloxacin 500 mg PO for 7 days
		Use amoxicillin, erythromycin, *or* azithromycin in pregnancy.

Gonorrhea	cefixime 400 mg PO once *or*
	 ceftriaxone 125 mg IM once *or*
	 ciprofloxacin 500 mg PO once *or*
	 levofloxacin 250 mg PO once *or*
	 ofloxacin 400 mg PO once plus azithromycin
	    1 g PO once *or*
	 doxycycline 100 mg PO bid for 7 d
	 Alternative
	    spectinomycin 2 g IM once	

Pelvic inflammatory disease	ofloxacin 400 mg PO bid *or* levofloxacin 500 mg daily *and* metronidazole 500 mg PO bid for 14 d *or* ceftriaxone 250 mg IM once *or* cefoxitin 2 g IM *and* probenecid 1 g PO once *and* doxycycline 100 mg PO bid for 14 d	

Genital herpes	*Initial episode treatment* for 7–10 d
	    acyclovir 400 mg PO tid *or*
	    acyclovir 200 mg PO 5 times a day *or*
	    famciclovir 250 mg PO tid *or*
	    valacyclovir 1 g PO bid
	 Recurrent treatment for 5 d
	    acyclovir 400 mg PO *or*
	    acyclovir 200 mg PO 5 times a day *or*
	    acyclovir 800 mg bid *or*
	    famciclovir 125 mg PO bid *or*
	    valacyclovir 500 mg PO bid *or*
	    valacyclovir 1 g once a day
	 Suppressive treatment
	    acyclovir 400 mg bid *or*
	    famciclovir 250 mg bid *or*
	    valacyclovir 500 mg or 1000 mg qd
		Treatment can be extended if healing is not complete after 10 d.

Human papilloma virus	*Patient applied*
	    podofilox 0.5% solution or gel for 3 d, then 4 d of
	    no therapy
	    imiquimod 5% cream 3 times a week up to 16 wk
	 Provider applied
	    podophyllin resin 10%–25% in compound of
	    tincture of benzoin weekly as needed
	    trichloroacetic acid or bichloroacetic acid
	    80%–90% weekly as needed
		Solution applied with cotton swab and gel with finger to visible warts. This is done for 3 d, then 4 d with no therapy, and may be repeated four times.
		 Area should be washed with mild soap and water 6–10 h after application.
		
		 Allow to air dry. Wash off 1–4 h after application.
		 Apply only to warts and let dry; white "frosting" appears; powder with talc or sodium bicarbonate to remove unreacted acid.

Syphilis	*Early primary, secondary, or latent syphilis <1 y*
	    Adult: benzathine penicillin G 2.4 million U, IM
	    single dose
	    Child: 50,000 U/kg, IM, single dose up to
	    2.4 mil unit
	 Latent disease >1 y or unknown duration
	    Adult: benzathine penicillin G 2.4 million U, IM,
	    for 3 doses at 1-wk intervals
	    Child: 500,000 U/kg, IM, for 3 doses at 1-wk
	    intervals
	 Allergic to penicillin and not pregnant
	    doxycycline 100 mg PO bid for 14 d *or*
	    tetracycline 500 mg PO bid for 14 d
	 Allergic to penicillin and pregnant
	    Desensitization followed by treatment with
	    penicillin	

Centers for Disease Control and Prevention. (2002). Guidelines for treatment of sexually transmitted diseases. *Morbidity and Mortality Weekly Reports, 51*(RR-6), 20–98.

INITIATING DRUG THERAPY

Treatment for all STIs consists of antimicrobial therapy followed by preventive education.

Goals of Drug Therapy

Patients are treated to eradicate the organism and prevent transmission to sex partners or to a newborn during birth. Because chlamydial infections often are accompanied by gonococcal infections, patients may be treated for both infections.

Antibiotic Therapy

Antibiotic treatments are prescribed to cure infection and usually relieve symptoms (CDC, 2002). Azithromycin (Zithromax) and erythromycin (E-mycin), macrolide antibiotics; doxycycline (Vibramycin), a tetracycline antibiotic; and ofloxacin (Floxin), a fluoroquinolone, are drugs of choice for chlamydial infections.

If therapeutic compliance is in question, azithromycin should be available for treatment because it is prepared as a single-dose drug. Doxycycline, however, has been used more extensively and is less expensive. Erythromycin is less efficacious and has gastrointestinal side effects. Ofloxacin is as efficacious as doxycycline and azithromycin but is more expensive and has no advantage with regard to dosing regimen. Other fluoroquinolones are not effective or have not been adequately tested (Table 36-2).

In infants, erythromycin base treatment has an efficacy of 80%. A second course of therapy may be required, and follow-up of the infant is recommended.

Mechanism of Action

Azithromycin and erythromycin bind to bacterial ribosomes to block protein synthesis. The drugs are also bactericidal,

Table 36.2

Overview of Drugs Used to Treat Chlamydial Infections*

Generic (Trade) Name and Dosage	Selected Adverse Events	Contraindications	Special Considerations
azithromycin (Zithromax) Adult: 1 g PO single dose Pregnancy: 1 g PO in a single dose Child (≥45 kg, <8 y): 1 g PO in a single dose Child (≥8 y): 1 g PO in a single dose (or doxycycline as below)	GI upset, abdominal pain, pseudomembranous colitis, angioedema, cholestatic jaundice	Hypersensitivity to azithromycin, erythromycin, or any macrolide antibiotic Use with caution with impaired hepatic or renal function.	Do not take with aluminum- or magnesium-containing antacids.
doxycycline (Vibramycin) Adult: 100 mg bid for 7 d Child (≥8 y): 100 mg PO bid for 7 d	Superinfection, photosensitivity, GI upset, enterocolitis, rash, blood dyscrasias, hepatotoxicity	Pregnancy, lactation, hypersensitivity to any of the tetracyclines	Monitor blood, renal, and hepatic function in long-term use. Use of drug during tooth development may discolor teeth. Advise patient to avoid excessive sunlight or ultraviolet light. Caution patient that drug absorption is reduced when taken with food or bismuth subsalicylate.
amoxicillin (Augmentin) Pregnancy: 500 mg tid for 7 d	Hypersensitivity reactions, pseudomembranous colitis, GI upset, rash, urticaria, vaginitis	History of Augmentin-associated cholestatic jaundice, hepatic dysfunction, or allergic reactions to any penicillin	Monitor blood, renal, and hepatic function in long-term use.
ofloxacin (Floxin) 300 mg bid for 7 d	Rash, hives, rapid heartbeat, difficulty swallowing or breathing, photosensitivity, angioedema, dizziness, lightheadedness	Pregnancy, hypersensitivity to ofloxacin or quinolones Use with caution with hepatic or renal insufficiency.	Do not take with food. Drink fluids liberally.
levofloxacin (Levaquin) 500 mg daily for erythromycin base (E-mycin) Adult: 500 mg qid for 7 d Pregnancy: 500 mg qid for 7 d or 250 mg qid for 14 d Children: 50 mg/kg/d PO divided into 4 doses daily for 10–14 d erythromycin gluceptate (Ilotycin) Topical: 0.5–1 cm in each conjunctival sac	Same as above GI upset, pseudomembranous colitis, hepatic dysfunction, cardiac dysrhythmias, CNS disturbances, urticaria, skin eruptions, hearing loss, superinfection and local irritation	Same as above Known hypersensitivity to erythromycin Prescribe with caution for patients with impaired hepatic function and children who weigh <45 kg.	Same as above Effectiveness of treatment is approximately 80%; a second course of therapy may be required. Use for prophylaxis of ophthalmia neonatorum and infant pneumonia.
erythromycin ethylsuccinate (E.E.S.) Adult: 800 mg qid for 7 d Pregnancy: 800 mg qid for 7 d or 400 mg qid for 14 d	Same as above	Same as above	Same as above

*In adults, pregnant women, children, ophthalmia neonatorum, and infant pneumonia.

depending on their concentration. (For more information on antibiotic actions, see Chapter 8.) Doxycycline is thought to act in a similar way, whereas ofloxacin kills bacteria by blocking DNA gyrase and inhibiting DNA synthesis.

Dosages

A single 1-g dose of azithromycin or 100 mg of doxycycline twice a day for 7 days is the usual initial therapy.

Contraindications

Sensitivity to erythromycin or other macrolides is the main contraindication to therapy.

The safety and efficacy of azithromycin in pregnant and lactating women are not known. Doxycycline and ofloxacin are contraindicated in pregnant women.

Adverse Events

In some patients, gastrointestinal side effects (nausea, vomiting, diarrhea, abdominal discomfort) cause them to discontinue therapy.

Selecting the Most Appropriate Agent

The most appropriate therapy is the one that best matches the needs of the patient in different situations or stages of life. Figure 36-1 and Tables 36-1 and 36-2 summarize treatment options.

Special Population Considerations

Pediatric

To prevent chlamydial infection among neonates, prenatal screening is recommended. In general, patients appropriate for screening include pregnant women younger than 25 years of age with new or multiple sex partners.

C. trachomatis infection of neonates results from perinatal exposure to the mother's infected cervix. The prevalence of *C. trachomatis* infection among pregnant women does not vary by race/ethnicity or socioeconomic status. Neonatal ocular prophylaxis with silver nitrate solution or antibiotic ointments does not prevent perinatal transmission of *C. trachomatis* from mother to infant. However, ocular prophylaxis with those agents does prevent gonococcal ophthalmia and therefore should be continued.

Initial *C. trachomatis* perinatal infection involves mucous membranes of the eye, oropharynx, urogenital tract, and rectum. *C. trachomatis* infection in neonates is most often recognized by conjunctivitis that develops 5 to 12 days after birth. Chlamydia is the most frequent identifiable infectious cause of ophthalmia neonatorum. *C. trachomatis* also is a common cause of subacute, afebrile pneumonia with onset from 1 to 3 months of age. Asymptomatic infections also can occur in the oropharynx, genital tract, and rectum of neonates.

A chlamydial etiology should be considered for all infants aged 30 days or less who have conjunctivitis.

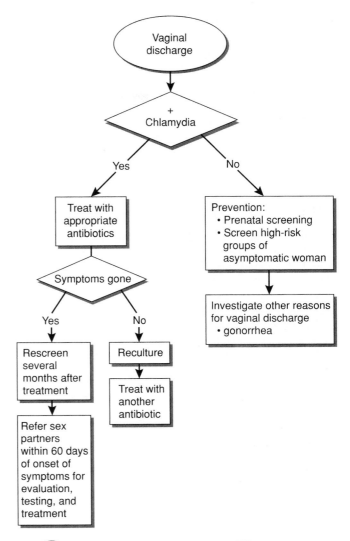

Key ⬭ Starting point for decision making; ▭ clinical actions (assessing, prescribing, monitoring); ◇ decision point.

Figure 36–1   Treatment algorithm for chlamydial infection.

Pregnancy

The recommended regimen for pregnancy is erythromycin base 500 mg orally four times a day for 7 days or amoxicillin 500 mg orally three times daily for 7 days.

Alternative regimens are erythromycin base 250 mg orally four times a day for 14 days; erythromycin ethylsuccinate 800 mg orally four times a day for 7 days or 400 mg orally four times a day for 14 days; or azithromycin 1 g orally, single dose. Erythromycin estolate is contraindicated during pregnancy because of drug-related hepatotoxicity.

MONITORING PATIENT RESPONSE

Because therapy with azithromycin or doxycycline is highly efficacious, patients do not need to be retested after treatment is completed. However, 3 weeks after completion of treatment with erythromycin (or amoxicillin–clavulanate), a test of cure may be considered because the drugs are not highly efficacious and the frequent side effects may discourage patient adherence. (Women retested after several months of treatment showed high rates of infection, presumed to be a result of reinfection. Therefore, rescreening women several months after treatment may help to detect further morbidity.)

Screening for *C. trachomatis* should be performed in high-risk groups when the practitioner performs a pelvic examination. High-risk groups include sexually active adolescents and women aged 20 to 24 years, particularly those who have new or multiple sex partners, those attending family planning clinics, prenatal clinics, or abortion facilities, or those in juvenile detention centers. Screening for high-risk men should be considered when they seek health care.

Patients do not need to be retested for chlamydia after completing treatment with doxycycline or azithromycin unless symptoms persist or reinfection is suspected. A test of cure may be considered 3 weeks after completion of treatment with erythromycin.

Sex partners should be evaluated, tested, and treated if they had sexual contact with the patient during the 60 days preceding onset of symptoms in the patient or diagnosis of chlamydia. The most recent sex partner should be evaluated and treated even if the time of the last sexual contact was more than 60 days before symptom onset or diagnosis.

PATIENT EDUCATION

The patient's sex partner must be treated. Patients should abstain from sexual intercourse for 7 days after single-dose therapy or until the 7-day regimen is completed. Abstinence should also continue until the patient's sex partner has been treated, to prevent reinfection. Sex partners should be treated if they have had sexual contact with the patient during the 60 days preceding onset of symptoms in the patient or the diagnosis of chlamydial infection. The most recent sex partner should be treated even if the time of the last sexual contact was greater than 60 days before onset or diagnosis.

GONORRHEA

Approximately 1 million new infections with *Neisseria gonorrhoeae* occur each year in the United States. They are the major causes of pelvic inflammatory disease, tubal scarring, infertility, ectopic pregnancy, and chronic pelvic pain in the United States. Most men seek treatment before serious complications develop, but not soon enough to prevent transmission to others. In women, symptoms may not develop until complications such as pelvic inflammatory disease occur. Screening of men and women at high risk for STIs is an important component of gonorrhea control (CDC, 2002).

CAUSES

Gonorrhea is caused by *N. gonorrhoeae*, a gram-negative diplococcal bacterium. It is transmitted by sexual contact, and the rate of male-to-female transmission is higher than female-to-male or male-to-male. Women with gonorrhea have a high

prevalence of other STIs, including chlamydial infection, trichomoniasis, bacterial vaginosis, and herpes genitalis.

Uncomplicated anogenital gonorrhea in women can involve the endocervix, urethra, Skene's glands, Bartholin's glands, and anus. The endocervix is the most common site of infection. Pharyngeal infection can also occur and is usually asymptomatic.

PATHOPHYSIOLOGY

Several strains of gonorrhea have been identified. Gonococcal sensitivity and resistance to antibiotics is clinically significant. Certain strains of the organism are resistant to sulfonamides. Penicillinase-producing *N. gonorrhoeae* and chromosomal-resistant *N. gonorrhoeae* are resistant to penicillin, and tetracycline-resistant *N. gonorrhoeae* is resistant to tetracycline.

DIAGNOSTIC CRITERIA

In the United States, an estimated 600,000 new *N. gonorrhoeae* infections occur each year. Most infections among men produce symptoms that cause them to seek curative treatment soon enough to prevent serious sequelae, but this may not be soon enough to prevent transmission to others. Among women, many infections do not produce recognizable symptoms until complications such as pelvic inflammatory disease have occurred. Up to 30% of women with gonorrheal infection have symptoms. Signs and symptoms include purulent or mucopurulent cervical discharge, dysuria, anal bleeding, menorrhagia, and pelvic discomfort. Men may have discharge and regional lymphadenopathy.

Gonorrhea is diagnosed by examination and culture for *N. gonorrhoeae*. Diagnosis is confirmed by identification of the organism on culture, positive oxidase reaction, and gram-negative diplococcal morphology on Gram's stain.

INITIATING DRUG THERAPY

Preventive education is always offered. Sex partners should be referred for evaluation and treatment of *N. gonorrhoeae* and *C. trachomatis* infection if their last contact with the patient was within 60 days before onset of symptoms or diagnosis of infection. The patient's most recent sex partner should be treated even if the patient's last sexual intercourse was more than 60 days before onset of the symptoms or diagnosis. All patients diagnosed with gonorrhea should be tested for syphilis.

Patients treated for gonococcal infection are also treated for chlamydial infection because patients with gonorrhea are commonly coinfected with *C. trachomatis*. The occurrence of fluoroquinolone-resistant *N. gonorrhoeae* in the United States is rare. Patients with treatment failure should undergo culture and susceptibility testing, and the local health department should be notified (CDC, 2002).

Goals of Drug Therapy

The goal of drug therapy is to eradicate disease and prevent complications and spread of infection to others.

Table 36.3

Overview of Selected Drugs Used to Treat Uncomplicated Gonococcal Infections in Adults and Children*

Generic (Trade) Name and Dosage	Selected Adverse Events	Contraindications	Special Considerations
ceftriaxone (Rocephin) Adult: 125 mg IM in a single dose Child. ophthalmia neonatorum: 25–50 mg/kg IV or IM in a single dose, not to exceed 125 mg Child: 125 mg IM in a single dose or 50 mg/kg (maximum dose 1 g) IM or IV in a single dose daily for 7 d or 50 mg/kg (maximum dose 2 g) IM or IV in a single dose daily for 10–14 d Child (<45 kg with bacteremia or arthritis): 50 mg/kg: max 1 g IM or IV in a single daily dose for 7 d Child (>45 kg with bacteremia or arthritis): 50 mg/kg, max 2 g, IM or IV in a single daily dose for 10–14 d	Pseudomembranous colitis, rash, GI upset, hematologic abnormalities	Known allergy to cephalosporins Prescribe with caution to penicillin-sensitive patients. Prescribe with caution to hyperbilirubinemic infants, especially premature infants.	Use for uncomplicated gonococcal infection of the pharynx. Prescribe prophylactically in infants whose mothers have gonococcal infection.
cefixime (Suprax) 400 mg PO in a single dose	Pseudomembranous colitis, GI upset, skin rash, headache, dizziness	Known allergy to cephalosporins Prescribe with caution to penicillin-sensitive patients and patients with renal impairment or GI disease. Prescribe with caution in patients on hemodialysis or continuous ambulatory peritoneal dialysis.	
ciprofloxacin (Cipro) 500 mg PO in a single dose	Pseudomembranous colitis, photosensitivity, dizziness, lightheadedness, restlessness, GI upset	Hypersensitivity to ciprofloxacin or fluoroquinolones	Advise patient to take 2 h after meals, drink fluids liberally, and avoid taking antacids, which interfere with absorption. Prescribe for uncomplicated gonococcal infection of the pharynx.
ofloxacin (Floxin) 400 mg PO in a single dose	Rash, hives, rapid heartbeat, difficulty swallowing and breathing, photosensitivity, angioedema, dizziness, lightheadedness	Pregnancy Hypersensitivity to ofloxacin or fluoroquinolones Prescribe with caution in patients with hepatic or renal insufficiency.	Advise patient to take drug on empty stomach and drink fluids liberally. Prescribe for uncomplicated gonococcal infection of the pharynx.
levofloxacin (Levaquin) 250 mg in a single dose spectinomycin (Trobicin) Adult: 2 g IM in a single dose Child: 40 mg/kg (max dose 2 g) IM in a single dose	Same as above Pain at injection site, urticaria, transient rash, pruritus, dizziness, headache, GI upset, chills, fever, nervousness, insomnia, rare anaphylaxis, low Hg, high BUN and ALT levels	Same as above Hypersensitivity to spectinomycin Administer with caution in patients with hypersensitivity or allergies.	Same as above Prescribe for patients who cannot tolerate cephalosporins or fluoroquinolones. Unreliable against pharyngeal infections Unreliable for treating pharyngeal infections in children Perform follow-up culture after treatment.
ceftizoxime (Cefizox) 500 mg IM	Eosinophilia, thrombocytosis; high AST, ALT, alkaline phosphatase, and BUN levels; GI upset, pseudomembranous colitis, headache, dizziness, tinnitus	Known allergy to ceftizoxime Prescribe with caution for patient with hypersensitivity to penicillin or allergies or GI disease.	Monitor renal function.
cefotaxime (Claforan) 500 mg IM	Pseudomembranous colitis, rash, pruritus, fever, GI upset	Hypersensitivity to cefotaxime or cephalosporins Prescribe with caution to penicillin-sensitive patients and those with GI disease and renal impairment.	
cefotetan (Cefotan) 1 g IM	Pseudomembranous colitis, GI upset, hypersensitivity reactions	Known allergy to cephalosporins	Avoid drinking alcohol during therapy.

(Continued)

Table 36.3

Overview of Selected Drugs Used to Treat Uncomplicated Gonococcal Infections in Adults and Children* *(Continued)*

Generic (Trade) Name and Dosage	Selected Adverse Events	Contraindications	Special Considerations
cefoxitin (Mefoxin) with probenecid (Benemid) 2 g IM: 1 g PO	*cefoxitin:* Pseudomembranous colitis, thrombophlebitis, rash, pruritus, eosinophilia, fever, dyspnea, hypotension, GI upset *probenecid:* Headache, dizziness, GI upset, hypersensitivity, acute gouty arthritis, nephrotic syndrome, uric acid stones	Prescribe with caution to penicillin-sensitive patients and those with GI disease. *cefoxitin:* Hypersensitivity to cefoxitin or cephalosporins Prescribe with caution to penicillin-sensitive patients and those with GI disease. *probenecid:* Hypersensitivity to probenecid Children <2 y, blood dyscrasias, uric acid kidney stones Prescribe with caution to patients with peptic ulcer.	
enoxacin (Penetrex) 400 mg PO in a single dose	Pseudomembranous colitis, GI upset, hypersensitivity, headache, dizziness	Hypersensitivity to enoxacin, tendinitis or tendon rupture associated with use of enoxacin or fluoroquinolones	Do not take antacids, bismuth subsalicylate, iron, or multivitamins with zinc for 8 h before or 2 h after taking drug. Avoid caffeine. Drink fluids liberally.
lomefloxacin (Maxaquin) 400 mg PO in a single dose	Severe photosensitivity, pseudomembranous colitis, dizziness, lightheadedness, hypersensitivity	Hypersensitivity to lomefloxacin or fluoroquinolones	Advise patient to drink fluids liberally, avoid mineral supplements or vitamins with iron 2 h before or after taking drug. Avoid sucralfate or antacids 4 h before or 2 h after taking drug.
norfloxacin (Noroxin) 800 mg PO in a single dose	Pseudomembranous colitis, dizziness, lightheadedness, photosensitivity, hypersensitivity, headache, GI upset	Hypersensitivity to norfloxacin, tendinitis or tendon rupture associated with the use of the drug or fluoroquinolones	Take 1 h before or 2 h after a meal or milk ingestion; drink fluids liberally; avoid multivitamins, antacids, iron, or zinc 2 h before or after taking the drug.
azithromycin (Zithromax) 2 g PO Uncomplicated gonococcal infection of the pharynx: 1 g PO in a single dose	GI upset, abdominal pain, pseudomembranous colitis, angioedema, cholestatic jaundice	Hypersensitivity to azithromycin, erythromycin, or any macrolide antibiotic Prescribe with caution in patients with impaired hepatic or renal function.	Take 1 h before or 2 h after meals for greatest absorption. Avoid taking with aluminum- or magnesium-containing antacids. Comes in powder form
doxycycline (Vibramycin) 100 mg PO bid for 7 d	Superinfection, photosensitivity, GI upset, enterocolitis, rash, blood dyscrasias, hepatotoxicity	Pregnancy, lactation, hypersensitivity to any of the tetracyclines	Monitor blood, renal, and hepatic function in long-term use. Because of photosensitivity, patient should avoid sunlight or UV light. Use of drug during tooth development may discolor teeth. Absorption is reduced when drug is taken with food or bismuth subsalicylate (Pepto-Bismol). Prescribe for uncomplicated gonococcal infection of the pharynx.

*Infections of the cervix, urethra, and rectum; uncomplicated gonococcal infection of the pharynx, ophthalmia neonatorum, and gonococcal infection in children.

Antibiotics

The CDC describes recommended regimens for uncomplicated gonococcal infections of the cervix, urethra, and rectum (Table 36-3).

Cefixime

Cefixime (Suprax) covers an antimicrobial spectrum similar to that of ceftriaxone (Rocephin), but cefixime 125 mg intramuscularly (IM) provides a higher and more sustained bacterial level than the 400-mg oral dose of cefixime. The advantage of cefixime is that it can be administered orally, and clinical trials have shown a 97.1% cure rate for uncomplicated urogenital and anorectal gonococcal infections.

Ceftriaxone

A single injection of 125 mg of ceftriaxone provides sustained, high antibacterial levels in the blood. Extensive clinical experience shows that the drug is safe and effective for treating uncomplicated gonorrhea at all sites, with a cure rate of 99.1% in clinical trials for uncomplicated urogenital and anorectal infections.

Fluoroquinolones

Ciprofloxacin (Cipro) is safe and relatively inexpensive, can be administered orally, and is effective against most strains of *N. gonorrhoeae*. A 500-mg single dose provides sustained antibacterial levels in the blood. It has a cure rate of 99.8% in clinical trials of uncomplicated urogenital and anorectal infections.

Ofloxacin is also effective against most strains of *N. gonorrhoeae*. Clinical trials show the 400-mg dose to be effective for treating uncomplicated urogenital and anorectal infections, with a cure rate of 98.4%.

Levofloxacin 250 mg in a single dose is also effective.

Other

The CDC also recommends several alternative treatments. Spectinomycin (Trobicin) has been effective for uncomplicated urogenital and anorectal gonococcal infections, curing 98.2% in clinical trials. However, the drug is expensive and must be injected IM in a 2-g single dose. It is used for patients who cannot tolerate cephalosporins and quinolones.

Safe and highly effective single-dose cephalosporins for uncomplicated urogenital and anorectal gonococcal infections include ceftizoxime (Cefizox) 500 mg IM, cefotaxime (Claforan) 500 mg IM, cefotetan (Cefotan) 1 g IM, and cefoxitin (Mefoxin) 2 g IM with probenecid (Benemid) 1 g orally. Clinical experience with these regimens is limited, however, and none offers an advantage over ceftriaxone.

Single-dose fluoroquinolone regimens are safe and effective for uncomplicated gonorrhea, but data are limited regarding their use. These include enoxacin (Penetrex) 400 mg orally, lomefloxacin (Maxaquin) 400 mg orally, and norfloxacin (Noroxin) 800 mg orally. None of the drugs offers advantages over ciprofloxacin 500 mg or ofloxacin 400 mg.

The CDC also recognizes other antimicrobials for use against *N. gonorrhoeae*. A single dose of azithromycin (Zithromax) 2 g orally is effective for uncomplicated gonococcal infection, but it is expensive and causes gastrointestinal distress. Doxycycline 100 mg twice daily for 7 days is also effective.

The regimen recommended by the CDC for uncomplicated gonococcal infections of the pharynx is summarized in Table 36-1 and Figure 36-2. These infections are more difficult to treat than urogenital and anorectal infections. Few drugs can reliably cure these infections more than 90% of the time. Treatment for gonorrhea and chlamydial infection is suggested, even though chlamydial coinfection of the pharynx is unusual.

Selecting the Most Appropriate Agent

Therapy for uncomplicated gonococcal infections includes a cephalosporin or fluoroquinolone, as follows:

- Single-dose cefixime 400 mg orally, or
- Single-dose ceftriaxone 125 mg IM, or
- Single-dose ciprofloxacin, 500 mg, or

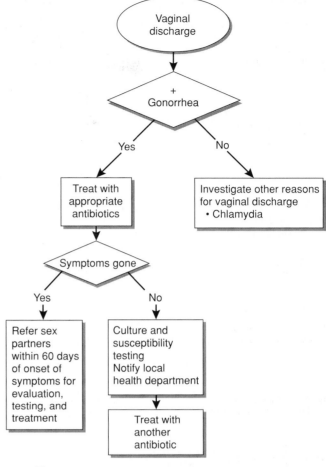

Figure 36–2 Treatment algorithm for gonorrheal infection.

- Single-dose ofloxacin 400 mg, or
- Single-dose levofloxacin 250 mg

PLUS

- Single-dose azithromycin 1 g, or
- Doxycycline 100 mg orally twice daily for 7 days

The choice is based on the practitioner's assessment of the patient's reliability, allergies, and preferences. If there is a question regarding the patient's reliability, ceftriaxone IM may be the treatment of choice because it is administered in the office.

Special Population Considerations

Pediatric

Gonococcal infection may be transmitted to infants exposed to infected cervical exudate at birth. The infection presents as an acute illness 2 to 5 days after birth. The prevalence in infants depends on the prevalence of infection in pregnant women, whether pregnant women are screened for gonorrhea, and whether newborns receive prophylactic treatment. Manifestations of the infection in newborns include ophthalmia neonatorum, which may result in perforation of the ocular globe and blindness, sepsis with arthritis, and meningitis, rhinitis, vaginitis, urethritis, and inflammation at fetal monitoring sites. Cultures should be taken when typical gram-negative diplococci are identified in conjunctival exudate, and testing for chlamydial organisms should be done in all cases of neonatal conjunctivitis. Presumptive treatment can be given for newborns who are at increased risk for gonococcal ophthalmia or who have conjunctivitis but no gonococci in a Gram-stained smear of conjunctival exudate. Infants with gonococcal ophthalmia should be hospitalized and monitored for signs of disseminated infection. Many physicians prefer to continue therapy until cultures are negative for gonococcal organisms at 48 to 72 hours.

To prevent ophthalmia neonatorum, prophylactic agents, including silver nitrate, erythromycin, and tetracycline, are recommended for instillation in the eyes; this is required by law in most states, regardless of whether delivery was vaginal or cesarean (Table 36-4).

In preadolescent children, sexual abuse is the most frequent cause of gonococcal infection. Vaginitis is the most common manifestation, followed by anorectal and pharyngeal infections, which are commonly asymptomatic. Standard culture procedures should be used to diagnose the infection, and non-culture gonococcal tests should not be used alone.

Follow-up cultures are not needed if ceftriaxone is used. Only parenteral cephalosporins are recommended for use in children. Quinolones are not approved for use in children because of concerns regarding toxicity. A follow-up culture is needed to ensure that treatment was effective if spectinomycin is used. All children with gonococcal infections should be evaluated for syphilis and chlamydial coinfection.

Women

Women who are pregnant should not be treated with fluoroquinolones or tetracycline. An alternate cephalosporin can be used, and if the patient cannot tolerate a cephalosporin, a single 2-g dose of spectinomycin IM can be substituted. For presumptive or diagnosed *C. trachomatis* infection, erythromycin or amoxicillin–clavulanate can be used.

MONITORING PATIENT RESPONSE

Patients who have had uncomplicated gonorrhea and who were treated with any of the recommended regimens do not need to return for test of cure. If symptoms persist after treatment, the patient is evaluated by culture for *N. gonorrhoeae*, and isolated gonococci should be tested for antimicrobial susceptibility. If infection is identified, its source is usually reinfection rather than treatment failure. In patients treated with spectinomycin for pharyngeal infection, culture should be performed 3 to 5 days after treatment because spectinomycin is not highly effective against these infections.

PATIENT EDUCATION

Patient education concentrates on prevention. All patients should be encouraged to adopt meticulous hygiene and practice safe sex, to insist that partners seek treatment, and to schedule and keep follow-up health care appointments.

SYPHILIS

In the 1990s, syphilis reemerged in endemic forms in the United States, with a significant increase in the incidence of primary, secondary, and congenital syphilis. The increase has been attributed to greater use of illicit drugs, most notably crack cocaine, and high-risk sexual behavior related to drug use. Approximately 120,000 cases of primary and secondary syphilis occur annually in the United States (CDC, 2002).

CAUSES

Syphilis is a chronic, infectious disease caused by the spirochete *Treponema pallidum*. Infection may be active, and characterized by symptoms, or inactive (latent). The latent stage has no clinical symptoms. During the latent stage, infections can be detected by serologic testing. Early latent syphilis is defined as latent syphilis acquired within the preceding year. Any other cases of latent syphilis are either late latent syphilis or syphilis of unknown duration (CDC, 2002).

Table 36.4

Prophylaxis for Ophthalmia Neonatorum

Topical Agent	Adverse Events	Contraindications	Special Considerations
silver nitrate 1% aqueous solution in a single application	Mild chemical conjunctivitis With repeated applications, cauterization of the cornea and blindness may occur.	Hypersensitivity to silver nitrate	Instill one of these preparations into both eyes of the neonate as soon as possible after birth. Use single-use tubes of the agent. Preparation is caustic and irritating to skin and mucous membranes.
erythromycin (Ilotycin) 0.5% ophthalmic ointment in a single application	Sensitivity reactions	Hypersensitivity to erythromycin	Same as above
tetracycline (Achromycin) 1% ophthalmic ointment in a single application	Dermatitis, increased lacrimation, transient stinging or burning, foreign body sensation	Hypersensitivity to tetracycline	Same as above

PATHOPHYSIOLOGY

T. pallidum is considered a bacterium because of its cell wall and response to antibiotic therapy. *T. pallidum* is not readily grown in vitro and cannot be seen by light microscopy.

DIAGNOSTIC CRITERIA

Patients who contract syphilis may seek treatment for signs or symptoms of primary infection, which include an ulcer or chancre at the infection site. The chancre erupts approximately 3 weeks after exposure. Signs and symptoms of secondary syphilis are low-grade fever, malaise, sore throat, hoarseness, headache, anorexia, rash, mucocutaneous lesions, alopecia, and adenopathy. Signs and symptoms of tertiary infection include cardiac, neurologic, ophthalmic, auditory, or gummatous lesions. Definitive methods for diagnosing early syphilis include dark-field examination and direct fluorescent antibody study of the chancre's exudate or tissue. The serologic tests used to confirm the syphilis diagnosis are nontreponemal and treponemal. The nontreponemal tests are the Venereal Disease Research Laboratory (VDRL) test and the rapid plasma reagin test. The treponemal tests include the fluorescent treponemal antibody absorption test and the microhemagglutination assay for antibody to *T. pallidum*. The two serologic tests are necessary because false-positive nontreponemal test results occur on occasion secondary to certain medical conditions. Treponemal test antibody titers do not correlate accurately with disease activity and should not be used to assess treatment response.

A single test cannot be used to diagnose all cases of neurosyphilis. The diagnosis is made using a combination of tests, including combinations of reactive serologic test results; abnormalities of cerebrospinal fluid (CSF) cell count or protein; or reactive VDRL-CSF with or without clinical manifestations (CDC, 2002).

INITIATING DRUG THERAPY

Although sexual transmission occurs only when mucocutaneous syphilitic lesions, including the rash, are present, people exposed in any stage should be evaluated clinically and serologically. Treatment should be given to those who were exposed within 90 days preceding the diagnosis of primary, secondary, or early latent syphilis in a sex partner, because the partner might be infected even if he or she is seronegative. Treatment should also be given to those who were exposed more than 90 days before the diagnosis of primary, secondary, or early latent syphilis in a sex partner if serologic test results are unavailable and follow-up tests and treatments are uncertain. Patients who have syphilis of unknown duration and who have high nontreponemal serologic test titers are considered to have early syphilis. Sex partners should be notified and treated. Long-term partners of patients with late syphilis should have a clinical and serologic evaluation and should be treated based on the findings.

For all stages of syphilis, penicillin is the preferred treatment. The stage and clinical manifestations of the disease determine the preparation used as well as the dosage and duration of treatment. However, no adequate trials have been performed to determine the optimal penicillin regimen. The only therapy with documented efficacy for syphilis during pregnancy or neurosyphilis is parenteral penicillin G benzathine. Penicillin G has been used for the past five decades to achieve a local cure and to prevent late sequelae.

Goals of Drug Therapy

The goal of treatment for primary and secondary syphilis is cure. The goal of treatment for latent syphilis is to prevent occurrence or progression of late complications. There is limited evidence supporting specific regimens for penicillin, even though clinical experience has shown the effectiveness of penicillin in achieving these goals.

Antibiotics

Penicillin

Adults with primary or secondary syphilis should be treated with penicillin G benzathine (Bicillin). Other choices for unusual situations include doxycycline, tetracycline (Achromycin), ceftriaxone, and erythromycin (Table 36-5).

Mechanism of Action

Penicillins are bactericidal. They disrupt synthesis of the bacterial cell wall and bind to enzyme proteins, interfering with the biosynthesis of mucopeptides and preventing the structural components of the cell wall from leaking out. As such, the bacteria cannot lay protein cross-links in the cell wall. In addition, autolytic enzymes, which promote lysis of bacteria, are activated.

Contraindications

Penicillin is contraindicated in patients with allergies to penicillin, cephalosporin, or imipenem (Primaxin).

Adverse Events

Hypersensitivity, urticaria, laryngeal edema, fever, eosinophilia, anaphylaxis, hemolytic anemia, leukopenia, thrombocytopenia, neuropathy, and nephropathy are some of the adverse effects of the penicillins.

Interactions

Penicillin decreases the effect of oral contraceptives. Hyperkalemia can result from concurrent use of potassium-sparing diuretics, angiotensin-converting enzyme inhibitors, and potassium supplements with parenteral penicillin G.

Doxycycline, Tetracycline, and Others

Nonpregnant patients with latent syphilis who are allergic to penicillin should be treated with doxycycline or tetracycline. Both drugs should be given for 2 weeks if the infection is of less than 1 year's duration; otherwise they should be given for 4 weeks. Patients who are not pregnant but who are allergic to penicillin and who have primary or secondary syphilis should be treated with doxycycline or tetracycline. For patients who cannot tolerate these, ceftriaxone is recommended. Although erythromycin is less effective than other regimens, it can be

Table 36.5

Overview of Selected Drugs Used to Treat Syphilis

Generic (Trade) Name and Dosage	Selected Adverse Events	Contraindications	Special Considerations
Nonallergic Adults penicillin G benzathine (Bicillin) *Primary, secondary, and early latent infection:* 2.4 million U IM single dose *Late latent infection, infection of unknown duration, or tertiary infection:* 7.2 million U; total 3 doses of 2.4 million U IM each at 1-wk intervals	Hypersensitivity, urticaria, laryngeal edema, fever, eosinophilia, serum sickness–like reactions, anaphylaxis, hemolytic anemia, leukopenia, thrombocytopenia, neuropathy, nephropathy	Hypersensitivity to any penicillin or procaine	Use with caution with patients with allergies or asthma. Do not inject into or near an artery or nerve.
Nonallergic Children *Primary, secondary, and early latent infection:* 50,000 U/kg IM up to adult dose of 2.4 million U in a single dose *Late latent infection, infection of unknown duration:* 50,000 U/kg IM up to adult dose of 2.4 million U administered as 3 doses at 1-wk intervals (total 150,000 U/kg up to adult dose of 7.2 million U)	Same as above	Same as above	Same as above
Nonpregnant, Penicillin-Allergic Patients doxycycline (Vibramycin) 100 mg PO bid for 2 wk *Latent syphilis:* 100 mg PO bid for 4 wk (if infection is <1 y, give for 2 wk)	Superinfection, photosensitivity, GI upset, enterocolitis, rash, blood dyscrasias, hepatotoxicity	Pregnancy, lactation Hypersensitivity to any of the tetracyclines	Monitor blood, renal, and hepatic function in long-term use. Avoid sunlight or UV light. Use of drug during tooth development may cause dental discoloration. Absorption is reduced when taken with food or bismuth subsalicylate.
tetracycline (Achromycin) 500 mg PO qid for 2 wk *Latent syphilis:* 500 mg PO qid for 4 wk (if infection is <1 y, give for 2 wk)	Photosensitivity, GI upset, glossitis, dysphasia, enterocolitis, pancreatitis, anogenital lesions, elevated hepatic enzymes, hepatic toxicity, rash, hypersensitivity, dizziness, tinnitus, visual disturbances	Hypersensitivity to any tetracyclines	Use of drug during tooth development may cause dental discoloration. Use of tetracycline may render oral contraceptives less effective.
ceftriaxone (Rocephin) 1 g PO qd for 8–10 d	Pseudomembranous colitis, rash, GI upset, hepatologic abnormalities	Known allergy to cephalosporins	Prescribe with caution to penicillin-sensitive patients.
erythromycin (Ilosone) 500 mg PO qid for 2 wk	GI upset, abdominal pain, anorexia, hepatic dysfunction, rash, superinfection, pseudomembranous colitis	Hypersensitivity to erythromycin Hepatic disease	Prescribe with caution in patients with hepatic disease or myasthenia gravis, or patients who are breast-feeding.

used for nonpregnant, compliant patients. Patients whose compliance is questionable or pregnant patients who are allergic to penicillin should be desensitized and treated with penicillin. For more information, see Chapter 8.

Selecting the Most Appropriate Agent

Penicillin G therapy is the first and usually only choice for patients who have syphilis and who are not allergic to penicillin. For patients who are allergic to penicillin and who are not pregnant, first-line therapy relies on doxycycline or tetracycline. There are no proven alternative drugs for pregnant women who have syphilis and who are allergic to penicillin. These women should be desensitized and then treated with penicillin (Fig. 36-3).

Special Population Considerations

Pediatric

Children with syphilis should have a CSF examination for asymptomatic neurosyphilis. To assess for congenital or acquired syphilis, birth and maternal records should be reviewed. Children who have primary or secondary syphilis should have an evaluation, consultation with child protection services, and treatment with a pediatric regimen.

Women

Pregnant women should be screened and treated for syphilis to protect the fetus and the newborn from exposure to syphilis. Screening is performed at the time pregnancy is

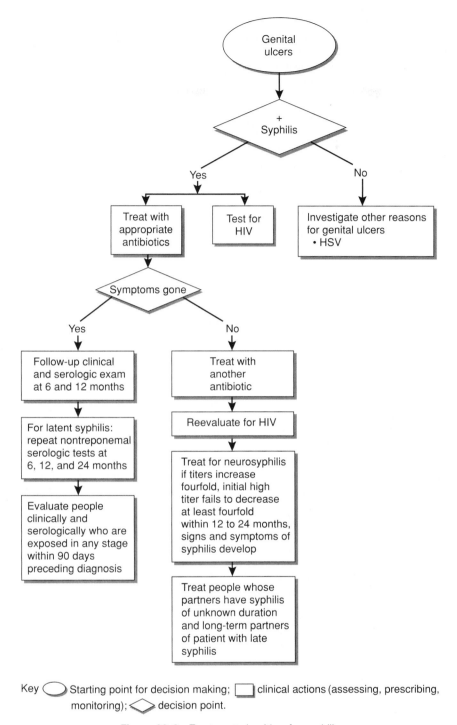

Figure 36–3 Treatment algorithm for syphilis.

confirmed. If the patient is in a high-risk group, testing should also occur at 28 weeks and at delivery. Pregnant patients who are allergic to penicillin should be desensitized and treated with penicillin.

At-Risk Populations

All patients with syphilis should be tested for human immunodeficiency virus (HIV) infection. In areas where the prevalence of HIV is high, patients with primary syphilis should be retested for HIV after 3 months if the first HIV result was negative.

MONITORING PATIENT RESPONSE

Patients should have a clinical and serologic examination at 6 and 12 months, or more frequently if follow-up results are uncertain. Those who fail to respond to treatment or who were reinfected, those who have signs that persist or recur, or those who have a sustained fourfold increase in nontreponemal test titer values within 6 months after treatment for primary or secondary syphilis should be retreated after evaluation for HIV infection. Treatment with three weekly injections of penicillin G benzathine is recommended if additional follow-up results are uncertain, unless CSF examination identifies neurosyphilis.

Patients with latent syphilis should be evaluated for tertiary disease. All patients with latent syphilis should have quantitative nontreponemal serologic tests repeated at 6, 12, and 24 months.

Patients should be evaluated for neurosyphilis and treated if titer values increase fourfold, an initially high titer fails to decrease at least fourfold within 12 to 24 months, or signs and symptoms related to syphilis develop. Patients with symptoms of neurologic or ophthalmic disease should be evaluated for neurosyphilis and syphilitic eye disease and treated appropriately according to the results (Table 36-6).

PATIENT EDUCATION

Teaching patients about preventive strategies is important in deterring the transmission of disease. All patients with a diagnosis of syphilis should be advised to undergo HIV testing as well.

GENITAL HERPES SIMPLEX VIRUS INFECTION

In the United States, genital herpes is the most prevalent genital ulcer disease. It is associated with a higher risk for HIV infection. This infection has been diagnosed by serologic tests in at least 45 million people in the United States. More than 500,000 new cases occur each year. Most infected people remain undiagnosed. They have mild or unrecognized infections that shed the virus in the genital tract intermittently. Although some first episodes of genital herpes may be characterized by severe disease requiring hospitalization, many people are unaware they have the infection or are asymptomatic when transmission occurs (CDC, 2002). The disease can be controlled, not cured. It recurs periodically.

CAUSES

Genital herpes simplex is caused by the herpes simplex virus (HSV), which has two serotypes: HSV-1 and HSV-2. The infection is transmitted by contact with an infected person by kissing or sexual intercourse, or during vaginal birth. Recurrent outbreaks may be triggered by injury to the infected area, an illness that alters immune status, emotional stress, or menses.

PATHOPHYSIOLOGY

Recurrent genital herpes is usually caused by HSV-2. After the virus enters the body through a susceptible mucosal surface, it resides and remains dormant in the cells of the nervous system until activated later. Exacerbations of varying frequency may or may not occur. In general, recurrent outbreaks are less severe than the initial episode.

DIAGNOSTIC CRITERIA

A diagnostic evaluation for herpes includes a health history and physical examination. In addition to serologic testing for HSV, patients should have a serologic test for syphilis. HIV testing should be considered as well. Specific tests for genital herpes include culture or antigen test for HSV. In addition, a POCkit-HSV-2 test can be performed.

The patient seeking treatment may report any one of three genital HSV syndromes. The first is primary infection, which is the first infection with genital HSV characterized by no preexisting antibodies to either HSV-1 or HSV-2. Symptoms include genital pain, vesicles, fever, malaise, regional adenopathy, and, in women, lesions on the cervix. The second syndrome is nonprimary first episode infection, which is the first clinically evident infection in women who have had a previous infection with the heterologous strains. The symptoms include fewer lesions, few constitutional symptoms, and a shorter, milder course. The third syndrome is recurrent infection, which usually has no constitutional symptoms, a shorter duration of viral shedding, and a shorter healing time.

Table 36.6

Overview of Drugs Used to Treat Neurosyphilis

Generic (Trade) Name and Dosage	Selected Adverse Events	Contraindications	Special Considerations
aqueous crystalline penicillin G 18–24 million U/d, give as 3–4 million U IV q4h for 10–14 d	Similar to penicillins	Hypersensitivity to penicillin	This penicillin preparation is the drug of first choice in treating neurosyphilis; second-line therapy is procaine penicillin.
procaine penicillin (Bicillin with probenecid, Benemid) 2.4 million U IM/d, plus probenecid 500 mg PO qid, both for 10–14 d	Similar to other penicillins *Probenecid:* Headache, dizziness, GI upset, hypersensitivity reactions, acute gouty arthritis, nephrotic syndrome, uric acid stones	Hypersensitivity to penicillin or probenecid Children <2 y, blood dyscrasias, uric acid kidney stones	If compliance can be ensured, avoid IV, intravascular, or intra-arterial administration. *Probenecid:* Use caution in prescribing for patients with peptic ulcer.

INITIATING DRUG THERAPY

The only effective therapy for genital herpes is drug therapy. Patient education is an important measure for preventing spread of the disease.

Goals of Drug Therapy

Treatment goals for first clinical episodes, recurrent episodes, and daily suppressive therapy aim to control the symptoms of the herpes episodes. The drugs do not eradicate the latent virus, and once discontinued they do not affect the risk, frequency, or severity of recurrences. Treatment trials show acyclovir (Zovirax), valacyclovir (Valtrex), and famciclovir (Famvir) to be beneficial for treating genital herpes. The use of topical acyclovir is discouraged because it is substantially less effective than the systemic drug. The recommended acyclovir dosing regimens have been approved by the U.S. Food and Drug Administration and reflect substantial clinical experience and expert opinion for initial and recurrent episodes (Table 36-7).

Antivirals: Acyclovir, Famciclovir, and Valacyclovir

The three first-line systemic agents used to control genital herpes infections are acyclovir, famciclovir, and valacyclovir. These drugs inhibit viral DNA replication and are highly effective.

Acyclovir, which has low bioavailability, works only in the cells infected by HSV. Famciclovir, a prodrug of penciclovir, is well absorbed. It is converted to penciclovir by first-pass metabolism. Valacyclovir, a prodrug of acyclovir, is converted rapidly by first-pass metabolism to acyclovir. It has a 50% bioavailability; it also deactivates viral DNA polymerase.

Because antiviral medications are excreted by the renal system, caution should be used in patients with renal disease. They should also be prescribed cautiously for pregnant patients, and are contraindicated in breast-feeding patients. These antivirals interact with probenecid, which increases the effect of the antiviral agent, and with zidovudine (Retrovir), which may cause drowsiness. For a detailed discussion of the role acyclovir, famciclovir, and valacyclovir play in controlling HSV-1 and HSV-2, see Chapter 12.

Selecting the Most Appropriate Agent

Therapy progresses from selecting treatment for the first clinical episode of infection to prescribing an antiviral agent for suppressive therapy (Fig. 36-4).

First-Line Therapy

Treatment for the first clinical episode of genital herpes includes antiviral therapy and counseling about the natural history of the virus, sexual and perinatal transmission, and methods to reduce transmission. Antiviral therapy for the initial outbreak includes the following:

- 7 to 10 days of acyclovir 400 mg three times daily, or
- Acyclovir 200 mg five times a day, or
- Famciclovir 250 mg three times a day, or
- Valacyclovir 1.0 g two times a day

Table 36.7

Overview of Selected Drugs to Treat Genital Herpes

Generic (Trade) Name and Dosage	Selected Adverse Events	Contraindications	Special Considerations
acyclovir (Zovirax) *First clinical episode:* 400 mg tid for 7–10 d or 200 g 5 times a day for 7–10 d *Recurrence:* 400 mg tid for 5 d or 200 mg 5 times a day for 5 d or 800 mg bid for 5 d *Daily suppressive therapy:* 400 mg bid *Severe disease:* 5–10 mg/kg IV q8h for 5–7 d or until clinical resolution occurs	GI upset (nausea, vomiting), headache, CNS disturbances, rash, malaise, vertigo, arthralgia, fatigue, viral resistance	Hypersensitivity to acyclovir Use with caution with renal impairment, pregnancy, breast-feeding mothers.	Do not exceed maximum dose.
famciclovir (Famvir) *First clinical episode:* 250 mg tid for 7–10 d *Recurrence:* 125 mg bid for 5 d *Daily suppressive therapy:* 250 mg bid	Headache, fatigue, GI upset With chronic use: pruritus, rash, laboratory test abnormalities, paresthesias	Hypersensitivity to famciclovir Pregnancy, lactation Use with caution in patients with renal dysfunction.	Easy to administer for prolonged treatment May be affected by drugs metabolized by aldehyde oxidase
valacyclovir (Valtrex) *First clinical episode:* 1 g PO bid for 7–10 d *Recurrent episodic infection:* 500 mg PO bid for 5 d *Daily suppressive therapy:* 500 mg PO qd (<9 episodes a year) or 1000 mg PO qd	GI upset, headache, dizziness, abdominal pain	Hypersensitivity to valacyclovir Do not use in children Use with caution with renal impairment, pregnancy, lactation.	Valacyclovir 500 mg qd is less effective than other valacyclovir regimens in patients with ≥10 episodes yearly. Be alert for renal or CNS toxicity in patients taking other nephrotoxic drugs.

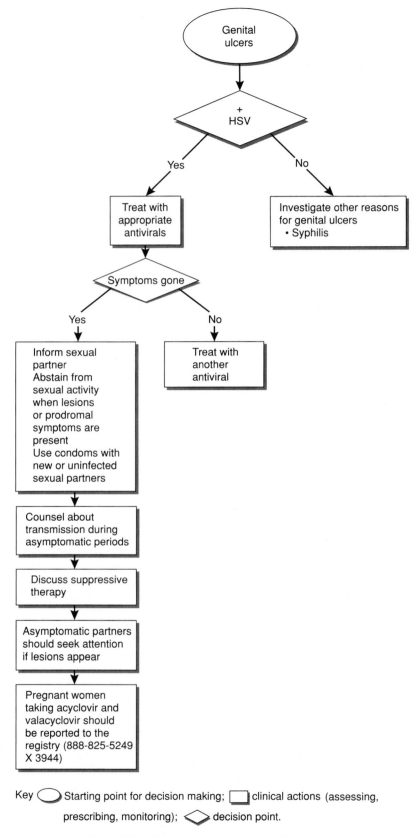

Figure 36–4   Treatment algorithm for genital herpes.

The choice is based on the cost of medication, patient preference, or scheduling issues.

Second-Line Therapy (Recurrent Episodes)

Most patients with genital herpes infection have recurrent episodes of genital lesions. Episodic or suppressive antiviral therapy may shorten the duration of lesions or prevent recurrences. Episodic therapy is beneficial for recurrent disease if the treatment is started during the prodromal phase or within 1 day after onset of the lesions. When given episodic treatment, the patient should also be given additional antiviral therapy so the treatment can be initiated at the first sign of prodrome or genital lesions. Recurrent episodes are treated for 5 days with:

- Acyclovir 400 mg three times a day, or
- Acyclovir 200 mg five times a day, or
- Acyclovir 800 mg two times a day, or
- Famciclovir 125 mg two times a day, or
- Valacyclovir 500 mg two times a day, or
- Valacyclovir 1.0 g once a day

Third-Line Therapy (Suppressive Therapy)

Third-line therapy is also known as suppressive therapy for HSV. The frequency of recurrent symptoms, or outbreaks, can be reduced by 75% or more with daily suppressive therapy, although suppressive therapy does not eliminate subclinical viral shedding. This therapy is used for patients with more than six episodes a year. Acyclovir has documented safety and efficacy for use for as long as 6 years, valacyclovir and famciclovir for 1 year. Discontinuation of therapy should be discussed with the patient after 1 year of continuous suppressive therapy to determine the rate of recurrence and the patient's psychological adjustment. In many patients, the frequency of recurrence decreases over time.

Asymptomatic viral shedding is reduced but not eliminated with suppressive treatment with acyclovir. Therapy is not discontinued in patients who are HIV positive.

Suppressive therapy is:

- Acyclovir 400 mg two times a day, or
- Famciclovir 250 mg two times a day, or
- Valacyclovir 500 or 1,000 mg once a day

Severe or Complicated Disease

For patients with severe disease or complications requiring hospitalization, intravenous (IV) therapy is indicated. The recommended regimen is acyclovir 5 to 10 mg/kg body weight IV every 8 hours for 5 to 7 days or until clinical resolution is attained.

Special Population Considerations

Pediatric

The risk for HSV infection in the neonate is not completely eliminated with cesarean delivery. Infants exposed to HSV during birth should be followed carefully. Before clinical signs develop, the CDC recommends that the infant have surveillance cultures of mucosal surfaces to detect HSV infection.

Infants born to women who acquired genital herpes near term should receive acyclovir therapy. Infants with neonatal herpes should be treated with acyclovir 30 to 60 mg/kg/day for 10 to 21 days.

Women

During pregnancy, the first clinical episode of genital herpes may be treated with oral acyclovir. IV administration of acyclovir is indicated for life-threatening maternal HSV infection. Acyclovir is not recommended for routine administration in pregnant women who have a history of recurrent genital herpes. The safety of systemic acyclovir and valacyclovir in pregnant women is unknown.

Women who acquire genital herpes close to the time of delivery (30% to 50%) are at high risk for transmitting the disease to the neonate. Those who have recurrent herpes at term or those who acquire genital HSV during the first half of pregnancy (3%) are at low risk for transmitting the disease to the neonate.

Sex partners who are symptomatic should have an evaluation and treatment similar to patients who have genital lesions. Most people who have genital HSV infection have no history of genital lesions. Therefore, asymptomatic sex partners of patients with newly diagnosed genital herpes should be interviewed regarding histories of typical and atypical genital lesions and encouraged to perform examinations and seek medical attention immediately if lesions appear.

MONITORING PATIENT RESPONSE

Response to therapy is monitored by symptom relief and resolution of lesions.

PATIENT EDUCATION

Patients should inform their sex partners that they have genital herpes and should abstain from sexual activity when lesions or prodromal symptoms are present. The practitioner can also discuss use of condoms with sex partners. Patients should also be counseled about transmission of HSV during asymptomatic periods.

The risk for neonatal infection should be discussed with both sexes, and women who are pregnant should advise their health care providers about the infection. Patients should also be advised that episodic antiviral therapy may shorten the duration of lesions during recurrent episodes and that recurrent outbreaks can be ameliorated or prevented with suppressive antiviral therapy . Prevention of neonatal herpes should be emphasized during late pregnancy and counseling provided regarding unprotected genital and oral sexual contact at this time.

Patients who have genital herpes should be educated about the natural history of the disease, with emphasis on the potential for recurrent episodes, asymptomatic viral shedding, and the attendant risks of sexual transmission. All persons with genital HSV infection should be encouraged to inform their current sex partners that they have genital herpes and to inform future partners before initiating a sexual relationship. Persons with genital herpes should be informed that sexual transmission of HSV can occur during asymptomatic periods.

Asymptomatic viral shedding is more frequent in genital HSV-2 infection than genital HSV-1 infection and is most frequent in the first 12 months of acquiring HSV-2.

PELVIC INFLAMMATORY DISEASE

It is estimated that pelvic inflammatory disease (PID) affects 1 million women each year. Approximately 250,000 of these women are hospitalized and more than 150,000 major surgical procedures are performed. The disease is associated with significant long-term consequences, including tubal-factor infertility, ectopic pregnancy, and chronic pelvic pain. Risk factors for PID include previous episodes of PID, presence of *N. gonorrhoeae*, *C. trachomatis*, or bacterial vaginosis in the lower genital tract, multiple sex partners, use of an intrauterine contraceptive device, adolescence, sexual intercourse during the last menstrual period, douching, and cigarette smoking. Oral contraceptives are thought to afford some protection against PID.

CAUSES

The most common etiologic agents for PID are *N. gonorrhoeae* and *C. trachomatis*. Other microorganisms that are part of the vaginal flora can also cause PID, as well as *Mycobacterium hominis* and *Ureaplasma urealyticum*.

PATHOPHYSIOLOGY

PID consists of several inflammatory disorders of the upper female genital tract that include any combination of endometritis, salpingitis, tubo-ovarian abscess, and pelvic peritonitis. It is an ascending infection that spreads from the lower genital tract to the endometrium, to the fallopian tubes, and to the peritoneal cavity.

DIAGNOSTIC CRITERIA

In all settings, no single historical, physical, or laboratory finding is sensitive and specific enough to make the diagnosis of acute PID. Many cases of PID are not recognized because they are asymptomatic or because the patient or health care provider fails to recognize mild or nonspecific symptoms.

The following diagnostic criteria are from the CDC (2002) guidelines. Empiric treatment of PID should be given to sexually active young women and others who are at risk for STIs if all of the following minimum criteria are present with no other causes for the illness: lower abdominal tenderness, adnexal tenderness, and cervical motion tenderness. Additional criteria may be used to enhance the specificity of the minimum criteria, including oral temperature exceeding 101°F, abnormal cervical or vaginal discharge, elevated erythrocyte sedimentation rate, elevated C-reactive protein, and laboratory documentation of cervical infection with *N. gonorrhoeae* or *C. trachomatis*. In selected cases, the following definitive criteria for diagnosing PID are warranted: histopathologic evidence of endometritis on endometrial biopsy; transvaginal sonography or other imaging techniques showing thickening, fluid-filled tubes with or without free pelvic fluid or tubo-ovarian complex; and laparoscopic abnormalities consistent with PID.

INITIATING DRUG THERAPY

Treatment for PID is prescribed when the patient's signs and symptoms meet the diagnostic criteria. Treatment includes empiric, broad-spectrum coverage of likely pathogens, including *N. gonorrhoeae*, *C. trachomatis*, anaerobes, gram-negative facultative bacteria, and streptococci. The CDC (2002) recommends patients be hospitalized when surgical emergencies cannot be excluded and when the patient is pregnant; does not respond clinically to oral antimicrobials; cannot tolerate an outpatient oral regimen; has severe illness, nausea and vomiting, or high fever; has a tubo-ovarian abscess; or is immunodeficient. There are no efficacy data that compare parenteral with oral regimens, and clinical experience should guide the decision to switch from parenteral to oral therapy, which may occur within 24 hours of clinical improvement.

Goals of Drug Therapy

In addition to ameliorating infection or preventing the progression of disease, the goal of drug therapy is to preserve the patient's reproductive health or at least minimize the effects of infection. Treatment should begin as promptly as possible because prevention of long-term sequelae has a direct correlation with immediate antibiotic coverage. Factors to consider in selecting treatment include drug availability and cost, patient acceptance, and antimicrobial susceptibility.

Antimicrobials and Appropriate Treatment Choices

For the most part, antimicrobial regimens for PID are those used for patients with chlamydial and gonorrheal infections. Refer to the sections on chlamydial infection and gonorrhea in this chapter, and also see Table 36-8 for an overview of drug therapy in PID and Figure 36-5 for a synopsis of the treatment.

Special Population Considerations

So that the mother and fetus can be closely monitored, pregnant women with suspected PID should be hospitalized and treated with parenteral antibiotics.

MONITORING PATIENT RESPONSE

Patients treated with oral or parenteral therapy should demonstrate substantial clinical improvement within 3 days after therapy has been initiated. Those who do not improve in this period usually require additional diagnostic tests or surgical intervention. The patient should be seen after 1 week of antibiotic therapy to check for residual pelvic abnormalities. Outpatient oral or parenteral therapy also requires a follow-up examination performed within 72 hours, using the criteria for clinical improvement.

PATIENT EDUCATION

If *N. gonorrhoeae* or *C. trachomatis* is present, the practitioner needs to explain to patients with PID that their sex partners should be examined and treated if they have had sexual contact with the patient during the 60 days before the onset of the patient's symptoms. Male partners of women

Table 36.8

Overview of Selected Drugs to Treat Pelvic Inflammatory Disease

Generic (Trade) Name and Dosage	Selected Adverse Events	Contraindications	Special Considerations
cefoxitin (Mefoxin) Mefoxin plus probenecid (Benemid) 2 g IV q6h Mefoxin plus doxycycline (Vibramycin) 100 mg PO for 14 d	*cefoxitin:* Pseudomembranous colitis, thrombophlebitis, rash, pruritus, eosinophilia, fever, dyspnea, hypotension, GI upset *doxycycline:* Superinfection, photosensitivity, GI upset, enterocolitis, rash, blood dyscrasias, hepatotoxicity	Hypersensitivity to cefoxitin or cephalosporins Pregnancy, lactation, hypersensitivity to any of the tetracyclines	Prescribe with caution to penicillin-sensitive patients and those with GI disease. Monitor, blood, renal, and hepatic function in long-term use. Avoid sunlight or UV light. Use of drug during tooth development may cause dental discoloration. Absorption is reduced when taken with food or bismuth subsalicylate.
doxycycline (Vibramycin) 100 mg PO bid for 14 d or clindamycin (Cleocin) 450 mg PO qid for 14 d	Same as above	Same as above	Parenteral therapy may be discontinued 24 h after patient improves clinically. Clindamycin is used with tuboovarian abscess rather than doxycycline.
ofloxacin (Floxin) 400 mg PO bid for 14 d	Rash, hives, rapid heartbeat, difficulty swallowing or breathing, photosensitivity, angioedema, dizziness, lightheadedness	Pregnancy Hypersensitivity to ofloxacin or fluoroquinolones	Use with caution with hepatic or renal insufficiency. Do not take with food.
metronidazole (Flagyl) 500 mg PO bid for 14 d	CNS stimulation, phototoxicity, GI upset, insomnia, headache, dizziness, tendinitis or tendon rupture, local reactions	Hypersensitivity to metronidazole Pregnancy, lactation	Take on empty stomach with full glass of water and maintain adequate hydration throughout therapy. Avoid excessive sunlight or UV light. Monitor blood, renal and hepatic function in long-term use. Use with caution with CNS disorders that increase seizure risk, and in renal or hepatic impairment.
ceftriaxone (Rocephin) 250 mg IM once	Pseudomembranous colitis, rash, GI upset, hematologic abnormalities	Known allergy to cephalosporins	Prescribe with caution to penicillin-sensitive patients.

with PID caused by *C. trachomatis* or *N. gonorrhoeae* are often asymptomatic and should be treated empirically with regimens that are effective against both infections.

HUMAN PAPILLOMA VIRUS INFECTION

The detection of human papilloma virus (HPV) infection has increased in frequency in the genital tracts of men and women. Genital warts, known as *condylomata acuminata*, have been detected with widely increasing frequency as well.

CAUSES

More than 30 HPVs are associated with infection of the genital tract. The sexual transmission of HPV is well documented, with the highest prevalence in young, sexually active adolescents and adults. Risk factors include the presence of other STIs, an increased number of sex partners, and use of oral contraceptives without other protection.

PATHOPHYSIOLOGY

Most HPVs cause no symptoms, are subclinical, or remain unrecognized. Warts that are visible in the genital tract are usually caused by HPV types 6 or 11, which also cause warts (that cannot be seen externally) on the uterine cervix and in the vagina, urethra, and anus. These viruses, which can produce symptoms, have also been associated with conjunctival, nasal, oral, and laryngeal warts. They are rarely associated with invasive squamous cell carcinoma of the external genitalia. Genital warts can be painful, friable, or pruritic, depending on their size and anatomic location.

Cervical dysplasia has been strongly associated with other HPV types in the anogenital region, including types 16, 18, 31, 33, and 35. These are found occasionally in visible genital warts and have been associated with external genital squamous intraepithelial neoplasia and vaginal, anal, and cervical intraepithelial dysplasia and squamous cell carcinoma. Visible genital warts can be infected simultaneously with multiple HPV types.

DIAGNOSTIC CRITERIA

Genital warts are diagnosed definitively by biopsy, which is needed only if the diagnosis is uncertain, if the lesions do not respond to standard therapy, if the disease worsens during therapy, if the patient is immunocompromised, or if the warts are pigmented, indurated, fixed, and ulcerated. The literature does not support HPV nucleic acid tests for use in the routine diagnosis or management of visible genital warts. For women who have exophytic cervical warts, high-grade squamous intraepithelial lesions must be ruled out before initiating treatment for genital warts (CDC, 2002).

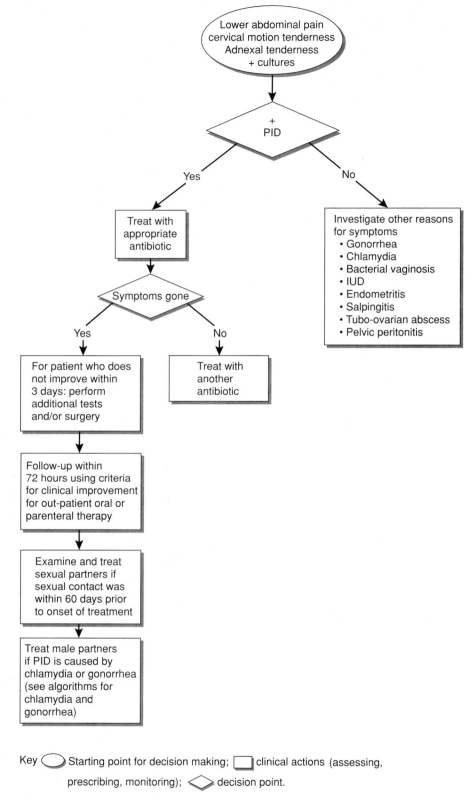

Figure 36–5   Treatment algorithm for pelvic inflammatory disease (PID).

INITIATING DRUG THERAPY

There is no evidence that current treatments eradicate or affect the natural history of HPV infection or the development of cervical cancer. Removal of warts may or may not decrease infectivity. Warts that are not treated may resolve on their own, remain unchanged, or increase in number and size. Treatment is guided by patient preference, cost of treatment and available resources, the experience of the health care practitioner, wart size and number, anatomic location of wart, wart morphology, convenience, and adverse effects. No single treatment is ideal for all patients, nor is one superior to another.

Visible genital warts may be self-treated by the patient if they are accessible, or by the health care practitioner. Non-pharmacologic therapies include surgery or laser therapy. Carbon dioxide laser is used for extensive warts or intraurethral warts and for patients who do not respond to other treatments. Pharmacotherapy may include podophyllin resin (Podofin), imiquimod (Aldara), trichloroacetic acid (TCA), bichloroacetic acid (BCA), or intralesional interferon (Intron A).

Goals of Drug Therapy

The primary goal in treating visible genital warts is the removal of symptomatic warts and prevention of HPV transmission. Removal can induce wart-free periods in most patients. Often, genital warts are asymptomatic. Pharmacologic therapy may include podofilox (Condylox), imiquimod, TCA, and BCA (Table 36-9).

Podofilox and Podophyllin Resin

Visible genital warts can be self-treated by the patient with podofilox. The patient must be able to identify and reach the warts to be treated. Podofilox in 0.5% solution or gel is safe, inexpensive, easy to use, and efficacious on mucosal surfaces.

A stronger preparation for application only by the health care provider is podophyllin resin, which may be administered at a 10% to 25% concentration in a compound with tincture of benzoin. The CDC does not recommend use of podophyllin by the patient because of rare but potential toxicity involving systemic absorption, bone marrow suppression, or serious gastrointestinal upset. The preparation is applied weekly as needed. Again, to guard against potential toxicities, the CDC recommends washing the preparation from the application site 1 to 4 hours after application. The most common adverse effect, which indicates the preparation is working, is local irritation. The preparation has not been established as safe for use during pregnancy.

Table 36.9

Overview of Selected Drugs and Procedures Used to Treat Genital Warts

Generic (Trade) Name and Dosage	Selected Adverse Events	Contraindications	Special Considerations
Patient Applied			
podofilox solution or gel (Condylox) 0.5% bid for 3 d followed by 4 d of no therapy; repeat cycle as needed for a total of 4 cycles	Mild or moderate pain or local irritation	The safety of podofilox during pregnancy has not been established.	Apply solution with cotton swab or apply gel with finger. Total wart area should not exceed 10 cm², and total volume of podofilox should not exceed 0.5 mL/d.
imiquimod cream (Aldara) 5% cream applied 3 times a week for up to 16 wk	Mild to moderate local inflammatory reactions	The safety of imiquimod during pregnancy has not been established.	Apply with finger at bedtime. Wash area with mild soap and water 6 to 10 h after application of cream. May clear area of warts in 8 to 10 wk or sooner
Practitioner Applied			
Cryotherapy	Pain, necrosis, blistering	Use of cryoprobe in the vagina is not recommended because of risk for vaginal perforation and fistula formation.	Repeat applications every 1–2 wk. Use local anesthetic. Indicated for urethral meatus warts, anal warts, oral warts
podophyllin or resin in compound tincture of benzoin 10% to 25% (Podofin)	Local irritation	The safety of podophyllin during pregnancy has not been established. Use with caution vaginally because of potential systemic absorption.	Apply small amount to each wart and allow site to air dry. Limit to ≤0.5 mL of podophyllin or ≤10 cm² of warts per therapy session. Wash off preparation 4 h after application to reduce local irritation. Repeat application weekly if necessary. With vaginal warts, allow to dry before removing speculum and treat with ≤2 cm² per session. For warts on the urethral meatus, treatment area must be dry before preparation comes in contact with normal mucosa.
trichloracetic acid or bichloroacetic acid 80%–90%	Can spread rapidly and damage adjacent tissue; pain		Apply small amount only to warts and allow site to dry. White "frosting" will develop. Use talc with baking soda to remove unreacted acid if an excess amount is applied. Repeat treatment weekly as needed. Indicated for vaginal warts

Imiquimod

Like podofilox, imiquimod may be self-administered by the patient. This antimitotic preparation enhances the immune response to HPV. Imiquimod can be topically applied three times weekly for 3 to 4 months. As with podophyllin, the imiquimod site should be washed with mild soap and water 6 to 10 hours after application. Warts should disappear in 8 to 10 weeks. During imiquimod therapy, sexual contact should be avoided to prevent viral transmission. Adverse effects include a local inflammatory reaction. The safety of use during pregnancy has not been established.

TCA and BCA

TCA and BCA are applied by the health care provider. These are strong, 80% to 90% acids that flow onto the wart site quickly, and the fluid can spread equally quickly. Application requires particular care and skill. The acid is applied only to the warts and left to air-dry. A white "frosting"

appears at the site. The practitioner can use talc or sodium bicarbonate powders to neutralize acid that falls on healthy tissue. TCA and BCA can be used effectively on keratinized areas and are safe for use during pregnancy. They are associated with low systemic toxicity.

Intralesional Interferon

Interferon is ineffective when used systemically. However, the use of intralesional interferon appears to be effective, and recurrence rates after therapy are comparable to those with other treatment modalities. Intralesional therapy appears to be effective because of interferon's antiviral or immunostimulating effects.

Selecting the Most Appropriate Agent

Treatment of genital warts should be guided by the preference of the patient, the available resources, and the experience of the health care provider. No definitive evidence suggests that

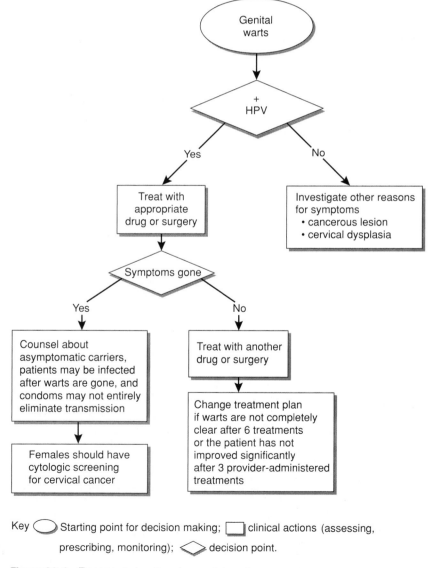

Figure 36–6 Treatment algorithm for genital warts.

any one of the available treatments is superior to the others, and no single treatment is ideal for all patients or all warts. Most patients have 10 or fewer genital warts. These warts respond to most treatment modalities. Factors that may influence selection of treatment include wart size, wart number, anatomic site of wart, wart morphology, patient preference, cost of treatment, convenience, adverse effects, and provider experience. Many patients require a course of therapy rather than a single treatment. In general, warts located on moist surfaces or in intertriginous areas respond better to topical treatment than do warts on drier surfaces. Figure 36-6 outlines the most appropriate patient- or practitioner-applied drug therapies in the most appropriate order.

Special Population Considerations

Pediatric

Laryngeal papillomatoses in infants and children are caused by HPV 6 and 11. The prevention value of cesarean section is unknown, and the route of transmission is not completely understood.

Women

Many experts recommend removing warts during pregnancy because they can proliferate and become friable.

MONITORING PATIENT RESPONSE

If the warts are not completely clear after six treatments or the patient has not improved significantly after three practitioner-administered treatments, the treatment plan should be changed. Evaluation of the risk/benefit ratio of treatment should occur throughout the course of therapy to avoid overtreatment. Women with genital warts should have cytologic screening for cervical cancer.

Once warts are eradicated, follow-up evaluations are not mandatory. Patients should monitor for recurrences, especially in the first 3 months. Patients who have concerns regarding recurrences can have a follow-up evaluation 3 months after treatment. Earlier follow-up visits may help to verify a wart-free state and monitor or treat complications, and can be used for patient education and counseling.

PATIENT EDUCATION

The practitioner needs to provide precise instruction and guidance for applying topical antimitotic preparations, such as by showing how to apply podofilox solution with a cotton swab and the gel with a finger to visible warts. Patients should also be informed that HPV organisms persist despite resolution of lesions. Sex partners do not need to be examined because reinfection is most likely minimal and treatment to reduce transmission is not realistic in the absence of curative therapy. However, partners should be counseled about having a partner with genital warts and should be informed that the patient may remain infectious even when the warts are gone. The use of condoms may not eliminate the risk for transmission.

Patients should be warned that ablative therapies may cause scarring in the form of persistent hypopigmentation or hyperpigmentation. Depressed or hypertrophic scars rarely occur. Disabling chronic pain syndromes can also occur, but are rare.

■ Case Study

J.R. is a 36-year-old white, middle-class woman who has been sexually active with one partner for the past 2 years. She and her partner have no history of STIs, but her partner has a history of fever blisters. She reports genital pain, genital vesicles and ulcers, and fever and malaise for the last 3 days. Examination reveals adenopathy and vaginal and cervical lesions.

Diagnosis: Genital herpes

   1. List specific goals for treatment for J.R.

   2. What drug therapy would you prescribe? Why?

   3. What are the parameters for monitoring the success of the therapy?

   4. Discuss specific education for J.R. based on the diagnosis and prescribed therapy.

   5. List one or two adverse reactions for the selected agent that would cause you to change therapy.

   6. What, if any, would be the choice for second-line therapy?

   7. What OTC or alternative medicines would you recommend?

   8. What dietary and lifestyle changes should be recommended for this patient?

   9. Describe one or two drug/drug or drug/food interactions for the selected agent.

Bibliography

Starred references are cited in the text.

Braverman, P. K. (2003). Sexually transmitted diseases in adolescents. *Clinical Pediatric Emergency Medicine, 4*(1), 21–36.

*Centers for Disease Control and Prevention. (2002). Guidelines for treatment of sexually transmitted diseases. *Morbidity and Mortality Weekly Reports, 51*(RR-6), 20–98.

Hollier, L. M., & Workowski, K. (2003). Treatment for sexually transmitted diseases in women. *Obstetric-Gynecology Clinics of North America, 30*(4), 751–775.

McKinzie, J. (2001). Sexually transmitted diseases. *Emergency Medicine Clinics of North America, 19*(3), 723–743.

Miller, K. E., Ruiz, D. E., & Graves, J. C. (2003). Update in prevention and treatment of sexually transmitted diseases. *American Family Physician, 67*(9), 1915–1922.

Zeger, W. (2003). Gynecological infections. *Emergency Medicine Clinics of North America, 21*(3), 631–648.

Visit the Connection web site for the most up-to-date drug information.

37

VAGINITIS

■ ANDREA WOLF

Vaginitis is one of the most common gynecologic complaints. Although infections account for most complaints, vaginitis may result from other inflammatory processes affecting the vagina.

The most common vaginal infections are candidiasis, a yeast infection; trichomoniasis, a protozoan infection; and bacterial vaginosis (formerly called *nonspecific vaginitis*). Other causes of vaginal irritation or inflammation include allergic reactions and atrophic changes in the vaginal mucosa.

CAUSES

Candidiasis

Most vaginal yeast infections are caused by *Candida albicans*, although other organisms, such as *Candida tropicalis* and *Candida glabrata*, are increasingly implicated, especially in recurrent candidiasis affecting both the vagina and the vulva. Colonization of *Candida* at other sites, such as the oral mucosa and the gastrointestinal tract, may be associated with recurrent vaginitis, but this mechanism is not fully understood. Candidal vaginitis is often accompanied by vulvitis, and thus the term *vulvovaginal candidiasis* (VVC) may better describe this disorder.

Trichomoniasis

Trichomonas vaginalis, an anaerobic protozoan, is one of the most commonly sexually transmitted organisms. Practitioners have long recognized that some asymptomatic women may harbor the organism. The organism, which can apparently survive in the environment for several hours, may be transmitted by contact, particularly with moist objects (eg, underclothing).

Bacterial Vaginosis

Bacteria, such as *Gardnerella vaginalis*, *Prevotella* species, *Mobiluncus* species, and *Mycoplasma hominis*, are responsible for the kind of vaginitis known as *bacterial vaginosis*. Although the cause of BV is not well understood, some studies suggest that other causes may include complications of pregnancy and infections associated with gynecologic procedures, pelvic inflammatory disease, and cervical intraepithelial neoplasia. It is unclear whether BV is only sexually transmitted. While infection is rare in women who have never been sexually active, treatment of male sex partners has not proven to be beneficial in preventing recurrence.

Allergies and Irritants

Conditions or products that irritate the vulva or the vaginal epithelium or local allergic reactions may produce symptoms similar to those of infectious vaginitis. Examples of irritants include vaginal lubricants, condoms, spermicides, and feminine hygiene products. Women who have other atopic skin conditions may experience vaginal and vulvar manifestations as well.

Atrophy

Low levels of estrogen in a postmenopausal woman may lead to atrophy of the vaginal epithelium and subsequent irritation and inflammation, which also may predispose the woman to vaginitis.

PATHOPHYSIOLOGY

A review of the normal physiology of the vaginal environment forms the basis for understanding the possible causes and pathophysiology of vaginitis. In postpubertal women, both anaerobic and aerobic bacteria make up the normal vaginal flora. These include potential pathogens, such as *Staphylococcus, Streptococcus*, and *Bacteroides* species, and nonpathogens, such as lactobacilli and diphtheroids. *C. albicans* is a saprophytic fungus that is a normal vaginal inhabitant in 15% to 25% of women.

One of the most important factors in the defense against infection is an acidic vaginal pH, which may be influenced by the acidic by-products produced by the normal vaginal flora. Hydrogen peroxide–producing strains of lactobacilli in vaginal secretions have been associated with protection against some vaginal infections as well. Therefore, variables that alter the vaginal pH or destroy lactobacilli may predispose a woman to vaginal infection. Among these variables are pregnancy, diabetes, sexual activity, hormonal changes, antibiotic therapy, and the use of feminine hygiene products. The thickness of the vaginal epithelium may also influence antimicrobial defenses.

507

DIAGNOSTIC CRITERIA

Candidiasis (VVC)

Symptoms of VVC include intense pruritus and erythema, dysuria, and a thick, white, curdlike vaginal discharge that tends to adhere to the vaginal walls. Diagnosis is made on the basis of presenting complaints, physical findings, and observation of pseudohyphae on potassium hydroxide (KOH) wet mount slide. Gram's stain and culture of the vaginal discharge are other methods that may be employed in the diagnosis of VVC. Vaginal cultures can confirm the diagnosis and identify the species of *Candida* causing infection. Since 10% to 20% of women harbor *Candida* in the vagina, it is not recommended that asymptomatic women be treated (CDC, 2002). If the vaginal pH is tested, the value in candidiasis is usually less than 4.5. *Candida* may also be identified on Papanicolaou (Pap) smears of symptomatic or asymptomatic women. VVC may be classified as complicated or uncomplicated (Box 37-1).

Trichomoniasis

Patients with vaginitis caused by *Trichomonas* organisms report a profuse, frothy, yellowish vaginal discharge, vaginal and vulvar irritation, dysuria, and dyspareunia. Microscopic identification of the motile organism on a wet-mount slide usually confirms the diagnosis. *Trichomonas* organisms may also be identified on a Pap smear. Because the organism may be recovered from male partners of infected women, this form of vaginitis is considered to be sexually transmitted.

Bacterial Vaginosis

Characteristics of BV are a "fishy" odor (especially after intercourse) and a thin, grayish, homogeneous discharge. The vaginal epithelium usually does not appear inflamed.

BOX 37–1. CDC CLASSIFICATION OF VULVOVAGINAL CANDIDIASIS (VVC)

Uncomplicated VVC	Complicated VVC
Sporadic or infrequent vulvovaginal candidiasis	Recurrent vulvovaginal candidiasis
or	*or*
Mild to moderate vulvovaginal candidiasis	Severe vulvovaginal candidiasis
or	*or*
Likely to be *C. albicans*	Non-*albicans* candidiasis
or	*or*
Non-immunocompromised women	Women with uncontrolled diabetes, debilitation, or immunosuppression, or those who are pregnant

CDC, 2002.

BOX 37–2. DIAGNOSTIC TESTS FOR BACTERIAL VAGINOSIS

Affirm VPIII	Becton-Dickinson, Sparks, Maryland
FemExam test card	Cooper Surgical, Shelton, Connecticut
Pip Activity TestCard	Litmus Concepts, Inc., Santa Clara, California

CDC, 2002.

Microscopic examination of the vaginal discharge discloses "clue cells" (epithelial cells that have been invaded by the offending organisms) but no lactobacilli or white blood cells. Three of the following clinical criteria are required for a diagnosis of BV (CDC, 2002):

1. Homogeneous, white, noninflammatory discharge
2. Clue cells on microscopic examination
3. pH of vaginal discharge greater than 4.5
4. Fishy odor before or after application of KOH to the vaginal discharge (called the *positive whiff test*)

While Pap tests have limited utility in the diagnosis of BV due to low sensitivity, other commercially available tests may be employed for a more accurate diagnosis (CDC, 2002). See Box 37-2 for a list of currently available products.

Allergic Vaginitis

Vaginitis resulting from allergy or irritants may be characterized by pruritus, discharge, and dyspareunia. The diagnosis often relies on exclusion. Although vaginal discharge may be increased, the secretions, when examined microscopically, do not harbor candidal organisms, trichomonads, or clue cells.

Atrophic Vaginitis

Vaginitis associated with atrophy of the vaginal walls produces pruritus, discharge, dryness, and dyspareunia. Physical examination reveals thinning of the vaginal walls with a characteristic shiny-smooth appearance. Introduction of the speculum into the vaginal introitus may cause bleeding. Microscopic examination reveals no candidal organisms, trichomonads, or clue cells.

INITIATING DRUG THERAPY

When considering pharmacotherapy for vaginitis, the practitioner explores lifestyle choices that may predispose the patient to infection or inflammation. Questions to ask regard the use of douches or other feminine hygiene products, sexual practices and partners, the possible relationship between sexual activity and appearance of symptoms, and recent antibiotic or oral contraceptive use. The practitioner should perform a thorough assessment to identify other possible irritants or complaints.

Before choosing a plan of therapy, the practitioner and patient also need to consider the issue of recurrent infection. In the case of recurrent VVC (four or more symptomatic episodes annually), the practitioner should be alert to the possibility of diabetes, and the need for screening should be discussed. In the case of recurrent trichomonal infection, sex partners should be examined and treated if they are found to be transmitting the organisms. It also is not uncommon for BV to recur.

Goals of Therapy

The primary goal of therapy in treating infectious vaginitis is eradication of the offending organism. The primary goals of therapy for allergic vaginitis include reducing inflammation and avoiding irritants. Addressing the hypoestrogenic state of postmenopausal women with hormone replacement therapy alleviates the symptoms of atrophic vaginitis. (Refer to Chapter 59 for a discussion of these treatment options.)

Another important goal of therapy is relief of symptoms. Vaginitis can cause considerable discomfort, both physically and emotionally. Women with vaginitis often experience embarrassment and even fear, particularly of the implications of a sexually transmitted disease. The frustration associated with recurrent infection may lead women to repeated attempts to self-treat, which delays proper evaluation by their primary care provider. For more information on self-treatment, see Box 37-3.

In the treatment of BV, additional goals of therapy include reduction of the risk of complications following gynecological procedures (eg, abortion and hysterectomy) and reduction in the risk of acquiring other sexually transmitted infections. Adverse pregnancy outcomes have been associated with both BV and trichomoniasis. The treatment of asymptomatic women with BV is not recommended, but some specialists recommend that women at high risk for preterm delivery be screened and treated for BV during the first prenatal visit.

Topical Azole Antifungals

Topical vaginal preparations for treating VVC include the following azoles: clotrimazole (FemCare, Mycelex G, Gyne-Lotrimin), butoconazole (Femstat), tioconazole (Vagistat), miconazole (Monistat), and Terconazole (Terazol). Treatment duration with these agents varies from 1 to 3 to 7 days. Response to treatment varies according to the duration of therapy. Types of topical preparations include creams, ointments, tablets, and suppositories.

Time Frame for Response

The cure rates for topically applied azoles have long been established at between 80% and 90%. It can take up to 3 days to see the effect of the medications. These preparations are considered to be more effective than the antifungal nystatin (Mycostatin). Table 37-1 lists the azole drugs currently available by prescription or without a prescription. In the case of VVC, only women who were previously diagnosed with this form of vaginitis should choose to self-treat with an OTC medication. Practitioners should advise women whose symptoms persist or recur within 2 months of self-treatment to seek medical care (CDC, 2002). In general, the only contraindication to the topical antifungals is hypersensitivity to the azole or components of the cream or gel.

Adverse Events

Topical azoles seldom cause systemic adverse events, although they may cause local irritation. Unfortunately, these effects may be difficult to distinguish from the conditions for which they are being used. Less common events may include penile irritation of the sex partner, abdominal cramps, or headache.

Interactions

Since these preparations are oil-based, they may weaken latex condoms and diaphragms.

Oral Azole Antifungal Agents

Fluconazole (Diflucan), the only oral azole to be recommended by the CDC for treating uncomplicated VVC, is available by prescription in a single 150-mg dose. It is as effective as the topical azoles. The findings of a study evaluating the acceptance of single-dose oral fluconazole by patients and physicians showed that most participants believed the drug to be effective in relieving or alleviating the symptoms of VVC. Ketoconazole (Nizoral; 100 mg once daily) and itraconazole (Sporanox; 400 mg once monthly or 100 mg once daily) have been recommended for maintenance therapy in recurrent VVC (CDC, 2002).

BOX 37–3. SELF-DIAGNOSIS AND SELF-TREATMENT OF VAGINITIS

Studies assessing the accuracy of self-diagnosis of vaginal symptoms found the incidence of misdiagnosis to be high (Ferris, Dekle, & Litaker, 1996; Njirjesy, Weitz, Grody, & Lorber, 1997). In both studies, women were self-treating symptoms that they attributed to vulvovaginal candidiasis with OTC antifungals (Ferris et al., 1996; Njirjesy et al., 1997) and other OTC alternative medicines (Njirjesy et al., 1997).

Although misuse of these pharmaceuticals rarely causes adverse reactions, a delay in diagnosis of infections such as pelvic inflammatory disease, bacterial vaginosis, or urinary tract infections could have significant consequences. Furthermore, repeated use of these medications unsuccessfully by women before their visit to the provider can make accurate assessment of the symptoms and physical findings difficult.

Table 37.1

Overview of Antifungal Agents

Generic (Trade) Name and Dosage	Selected Adverse Events	Contraindications	Special Considerations
OTC Preparations			
butoconazole 2% cream (Femstat) 1 applicatorful intravag. qhs for 3 d	Vaginal irritation, skin rash, hives	Allergy	Oil-based; might weaken latex condoms and diaphragms
butoconazole 2% cream	(Sustained-release)	1 applicatorful hs × 3d	Refer to product labeling for more information.
clotrimazole 1% cream (Gyne-Lotrimin, Mycelex-G) 1 applicatorful intravag. qhs for 7–14 d	Same as above	Same as above	Same as above
clotrimazole 100-mg tablets (Gyne-Lotrimin, Mycelex-G) 1 tab intravag. qhs for 7 d or 2 tabs intravag. qhs for 3 d	Same as above	Same as above	Same as above
clotrimazole 500-mg tablets (Gyne-Lotrimin) 1 tab intravag. hs single dose	Same as above	Same as above	Same as above
miconazole 2% cream (Monistat 7) 1 applicatorful intravag. qhs for 7 d	Same as above	Same as above	Same as above
miconazole 200-mg suppository (Monistat 3) 1 suppository intravag. qhs for 3 d	Same as above	Same as above	Same as above
miconazole 100-mg suppository (Monistat 7) 1 suppository intravag. qhs for 7 d	Same as above	Same as above	Same as above
tioconazole 6.5% ointment (Vagistat) 1 applicatorful intravag. qhs, single dose	Same as above	Same as above	Same as above
Prescription Preparations			
terconazole 0.4% cream (Terazol 7) 1 applicatorful intravag. qhs for 7 d	Same as above	Same as above	Same as above
terconazole 0.8% cream (Terazol 3) 1 applicatorful intravag. qhs for 3 d	Same as above	Same as above	Same as above
terconazole 80 mg suppositories (Terazol 3) 1 suppository intravag. qhs for 3 d	Same as above	Same as above	Same as above
nystatin 100,000-U tablet (Nilstat, Mycostatin) 1 tablet intravag. qhs for 14 d	Same as above	Same as above	None
fluconazole 150-mg tablet (Diflucan) 1 tablet orally, single dose	Headache, abdominal pain, nausea Rare: hepatic injury	Same as above	May interact with oral hypoglycemics, anticoagulants, cyclosporine, rifampin, theophylline, calcium channel antagonists, cisapride, astemizole, phenytoin, protease inhibitors, tacrolimus, terfenadine, trimetreate

CDC recommendations, 2002.

While the CDC recommends that maintenance therapy for recurrent VVC should be extended for 6 months, caution should be used with long-term ketoconazole therapy since hepatotoxicity may occur.

Contraindications

Contraindications to oral azole antifungals include known hypersensitivity to these azoles and the concomitant use of drugs with which they interact.

Time Frame for Response

Because patients treated with oral antifungals may not obtain relief of symptoms for 2 or 3 days, they may need to use an OTC antifungal cream for a few days. Failure to respond necessitates reevaluation.

Adverse Events

The most commonly reported adverse events noted in patients treated with oral fluconazole are headache, nausea, and abdominal pain. Ketoconazole and itraconazole can cause gastrointestinal disorders, headache, and pruritus. Hepatotoxicity may also occur, especially with ketoconazole. Liver enzyme levels may need to be monitored, especially with long-term use. Adverse effects tend to be dose-related. Interactions may occur because oral azoles are cytochrome P450 inhibitors.

Antibacterials/Antibiotics

Metronidazole (Flagyl) may be used orally or intravaginally for treating BV. Oral metronidazole 500 mg twice daily for 7 days is the standard treatment for BV, and only the oral form is effective in treating trichomonal infection (see Table 37-2 for specific dosages). Topical clindamycin cream 2% (Cleocin) should be used in patients who are allergic to metronidazole. Clindamycin 300 mg twice daily may also be used orally for a 7-day course. It is contraindicated in patients with a hypersensitivity to it or to other preparations containing lincomycin. Cleocin Ovules intravaginally are also effective if inserted at bedtime for 3 nights.

Contraindications

Metronidazole is no longer thought to be teratogenic, and therefore it is not contraindicated in the first trimester of pregnancy. It is contraindicated, however, in patients with a known hypersensitivity to it or other nitroimidazoles.

Adverse Events

Metallic taste, headache, and gastrointestinal distress are common side effects of metronidazole. To avoid the disulfiram-like effect of nausea and vomiting, patients must not consume alcohol during treatment and for 24 hours after treatment stops.

Interactions

Metronidazole may potentiate the anticoagulant effect of warfarin (Coumadin) and other oral anticoagulants. Although some animal studies have linked metronidazole to cancer, no current evidence indicates that the drug has a similar effect on humans.

Estrogens

Treatment of atrophic vaginitis consists of systemic estrogen replacement or topical estrogen creams administered externally or intravaginally. Refer to Chapter 59 for a complete discussion of these therapies.

Anti-inflammatories

Mild topical steroid preparations can be used on a short-term or episodic basis. Careful monitoring of the patient's response is advised.

Selecting the Most Appropriate Agent

First-Line Therapy: Candidiasis

In an attempt to guide therapeutic options, the CDC classifies VVC as either uncomplicated or complicated. Uncomplicated VVC is characterized as mild to moderate in severity, nonrecurrent, and caused by normally susceptible *C. albicans*. Complicated VVC encompasses conditions such as immunocompromise, recurrent infections, severe local infection, or infection

---

Table 37.2

CDC* Recommendations for Treating Bacterial Vaginosis

Generic (Trade) Name and Dosage	Selected Adverse Events	Contraindications	Special Considerations
Recommended Regimens metronidazole 500 mg tablets (Flagyl) 1 tab PO bid for 7 d	Metallic taste, headache, GI distress	Allergy (No longer contraindicated in pregnancy)	Avoid alcohol during therapy and for 24 h after stopping (will cause nausea and vomiting) May potentiate the anticoagulant effects of warfarin and other anticoagulants
clindamycin 2% cream (Cleocin) 1 applicatorful intravag. qhs for 7 d	Vaginal irritation, skin rash, hives	Allergy	Oil-based; may weaken latex condoms and diaphragms Refer to product labeling for more information.
metronidazole gel 0.75%. (Metrogel) 1 applicatorful intravag. bid for 5 d	Vaginal irritation, skin rash, metallic taste, GI distress	Same as above	Although blood levels are lower than with the use of oral metronidazole, alcohol still should be avoided.
Alternative Regimens metronidazole 2-g tablets (Flagyl) 1 tablet orally, single dose	Same as above	Same as above	See above. Lower efficacy for BV, but may increase compliance
clindamycin 300 mg tablets (Cleocin) 1 tablet orally bid for 7 d	GI distress	Same as above	None

*CDC recommendations as of 2002.
Clindamycin ovules 100 g intravaginally once hs for 3 d

Table 37.3

Recommended Order of Treatment for Vulvovaginal Candidiasis

Order	Agents	Comments
First line	OTC topical antifungals *or* Single-dose oral antifungal	Patients may self-treat before visit with practitioner.
Second line	Single-dose oral antifungal *or* Extend course of therapy of topical or oral antifungal *or* Maintenance therapy with an oral or topical antifungal *or* Boric acid suppositories	If not used as first line Vaginal cultures to determine presence of non-*albicans* candidiasis

with identifiably less susceptible strains of *Candida* (eg, *C. glabrata*).

OTC topical antifungals are typical first-line therapy of uncomplicated VVC and can be used before the patient seeks professional treatment. Women experiencing typical symptoms such as pruritus and vaginal discharge can obtain relief of symptoms promptly without the expense of a visit to the practitioner. Appropriate therapy consists of 1 to 7 days of treatment with the topical antifungals. It is recommended that self-treatment with OTC antifungals be reserved for women who have been previously diagnosed with VVC and who have not experienced a recurrence within 2 months.

Single-dose oral antifungals are an alternative first-line therapy in uncomplicated VVC, especially because the ease of administration may ensure therapeutic adherence. Fluconazole is the oral azole of choice and is recommended by the CDC for first-line therapy (CDC, 2002). The patient's sex partners need not be treated because candidiasis is not sexually transmitted. However, consideration may be given to treating male sex partners of women with recurrent infection. Male sex partners who have symptoms of balanitis may benefit from the use of topical antifungals. See Figure 37-1 and Table 37-3 for an overview of VVC treatment.

Second-Line Therapy: Candidiasis

If symptoms persist beyond the recommended course of therapy with first-line agents, second-line therapy involves assessing for possible recurrent VVC or infection with non-*albicans Candida,* such as *C. glabrata.* Vaginal cultures should be obtained to confirm the diagnosis and identify the species of *Candida* involved.

If an oral antifungal was not the first-line therapy, the practitioner may opt to treat with oral fluconazole as second-line therapy or extend the course of topical or oral therapy. It has been suggested that 7- to 14-day treatment with topical agents or a 150-mg dose of oral fluconazole repeated 3 days later may achieve remission in patients with recurrent VVC. Maintenance regimens are recommended for patients with recurrent VVC and include clotrimazole (500-mg suppositories once weekly), ketoconazole (100-mg dose once daily), fluconazole (100- to 150-mg dose once weekly), or itraconazole (400-mg dose once monthly or 100-mg dose once daily). These maintenance therapies should be continued for

6 months. Hepatotoxicity may occur in long-term treatment with ketoconazole, and these patients should be monitored accordingly.

Second-line therapy for patients with non-*albicans* VVC consists of 7- to 14-day treatment with a non-fluconazole azole drug followed by boric acid suppositories (600 mg in a gelatin capsule intravaginally once daily for 14 days), if the infection recurs. The CDC (2002) also includes topical flucytosine 4% and nystatin 100,000-unit vaginal suppositories as additional options in the treatment of non-*albicans* VVC. However, consultation with a specialist is recommended. Women who are immunocompromised also benefit from the prolonged therapy (7 to 14 days) with either topical or oral agents.

First-Line Therapy: Bacterial Vaginosis

Oral metronidazole (500 mg twice daily) 7-day therapy has long been considered standard first-line treatment for BV. However, the CDC (2002) also recommends topical clindamycin cream 2% (intravaginally for 7 days) and metronidazole gel 0.75% (intravaginally for 5 days) as acceptable first-line therapy. Alternative regimens for first-line therapy include metronidazole 2 g orally in a single dose, clindamycin 300 mg twice daily orally for a 7-day course, or clindamycin ovules 100 g intravaginally at bedtime for 3 days. Once-daily dosing with metronidazole 750-mg extended-release tablets has been approved by the U.S. Food and Drug Administration for the treatment of BV, but data are not available regarding the efficacy of this regimen (CDC, 2002). Treatment of sex partners is not recommended because clinical trials have not shown a relationship between treatment of partners and recurrence of BV (CDC, 2002). See Figure 37-2 and Table 37-4 for an overview of treatment.

Second-Line Therapy: Bacterial Vaginosis

Generally, treatment of recurrent BV consists of choosing a different treatment than that previously used. Although little data exist on efficacy, some studies have suggested that extending the duration of treatment with first-line agents to

Table 37.4

Recommended Order of Treatment for Bacterial Vaginosis

Order	Agents	Comments
First line	Oral metronidazole *or* clindamycin cream 2% *or* metronidazole gel 0.75% *or* metronidazole in single oral dose *or* clindamycin orally *or* clindamycin ovules	Traditionally used as first line
Second line	Extend duration of above agents *or* povidone–iodine gel suppositories *or* choose different Agent	*May* be effective

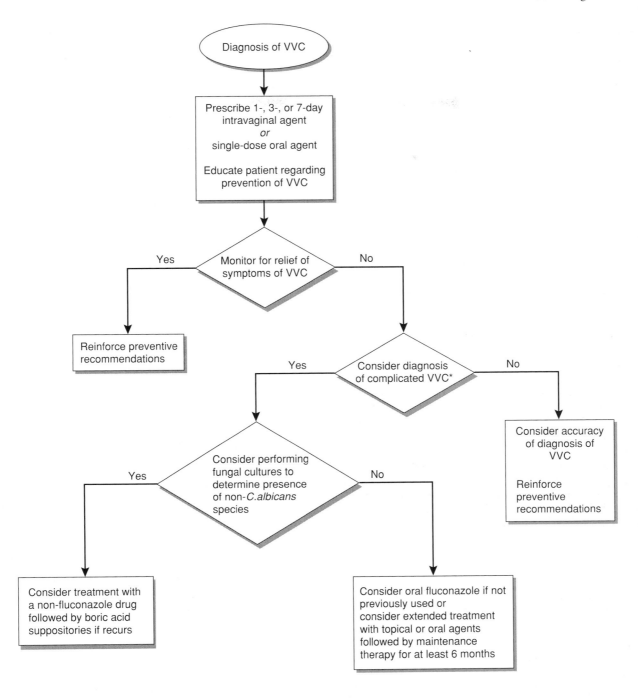

Key ⬭ Starting point for decision making; ▢ clinical actions (assessing, prescribing, monitoring); ◇ decision point.

*Complicated VVC is defined by the CDC as recurrent infections (4 or more symptomatic episodes of VVC per year), immunocompromised patient, severe infection, non-*C. albicans* species.

Figure 37–1 Treatment algorithm for vaginitis known as vulvovaginal candidiasis (VVC).

14 days or using povidone–iodine gel suppositories (5 g twice daily for 14 to 28 days) may be useful therapy for recurrent or resistant cases of BV. These alternatives are not listed as recommendations of the CDC (2002). Long-term maintenance is not currently recommended.

First-Line Therapy: Trichomoniasis

The CDC recommendations for treating trichomoniasis have not changed recently. Only one treatment regimen is considered to be clinically efficacious: metronidazole given as a single 2-g dose or as 500 mg twice daily for 7 days. A study

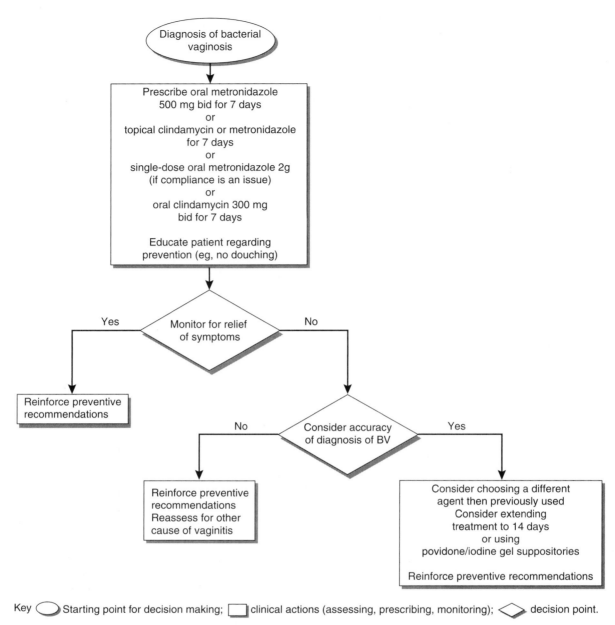

Key ⬭ Starting point for decision making; ▢ clinical actions (assessing, prescribing, monitoring); ◇ decision point.

Figure 37–2   Treatment of bacterial vaginosis (BV).

conducted by Spence, Harwell, Davies, and Smith (1997) found that a single 1.5-g dose is as effective as the 2-g dose; however, this dosage is not currently recognized by the CDC. Topical metronidazole, although effective in treating BV, does not achieve appropriate levels in the urethra and perivaginal glands and therefore is not recommended. Treatment of male sex partners (who are usually asymptomatic) is recommended, and patients and their partners should avoid intercourse until they have completed therapy and are symptom-free. Patients should be cautioned to avoid alcohol, as previously described. See Figure 37-3 and Table 37-5 for an overview of treatment.

Second-Line Therapy: Trichomoniasis

If treatment failure occurs, the patient should be treated with metronidazole 500 mg twice daily for 7 days. If treatment

failure occurs repeatedly, the CDC (2002) recommends a single 2-g dose of metronidazole once daily for 3 to 5 days. The CDC recommends consultation with a specialist if the infection continues to be refractory to these treatments. Acetic acid vaginal wash (3% or 10% solution) and povidone–iodine

Table 37.5

Recommended Order of Treatment for Trichomonal Infection

Order	Agents	Comments
First line	Metronidazole Single dose or 7-day therapy	A 1.5-g dose may be effective.
Second line	Extend the course of metronidazole *or*	
	Acetic acid vaginal wash or povidone–iodine solutions	*May* be effective

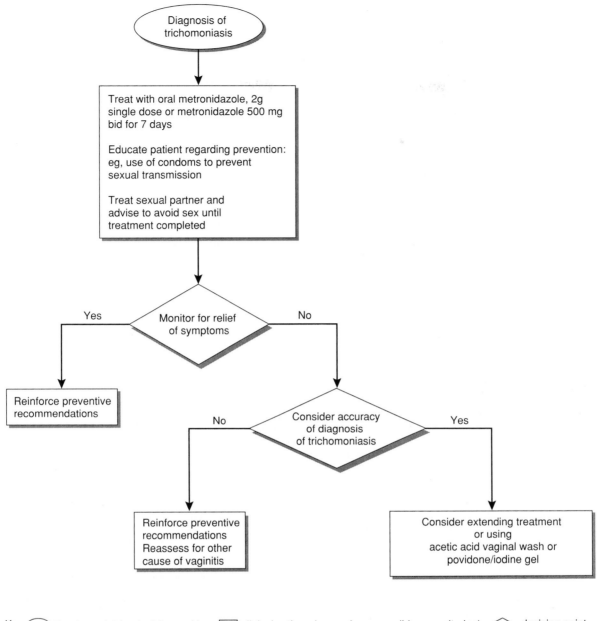

Figure 37–3 Treatment of vaginitis resulting from *Trichomonas* organisms.

solutions have been suggested for recurrent or resistant cases of trichomoniasis, but these treatments are not included in the current CDC recommendations.

Special Population Considerations

Pediatric

Before menarche, when estrogen levels are low, the vaginal epithelium is thin and the vaginal pH tends to be between 6.0 and 7.0. These conditions create a vaginal environment that is more susceptible to invading anaerobic bacteria if the child is exposed. Infections may be sexually transmitted or caused by contamination with fecal flora, and the possibility of sexual abuse must be considered. Poor hygiene and the use of vaginal irritants such as bubble baths and other products may also contribute to infections in the prepubertal

child. Because of the high vaginal pH of the prepubertal child, candidiasis usually does not occur.

Postmenopausal Women

The decline in estrogen levels that occurs in the postmenopausal woman produces conditions similar to those in prepubertal children, and these conditions predispose the woman to infection and atrophy. As noted previously, the practitioner needs to be aware that atrophic vaginitis is a common cause of vaginal symptoms, and accurate diagnosis is essential.

Pregnant Women

Because vaginitis may occur during pregnancy, therapeutic goals include relieving symptoms and avoiding complications.

BOX 37–4. CDC RECOMMENDATIONS FOR TREATMENT OF VAGINITIS IN PREGNANCY

Vulvovaginal Candidiasis
Topical azole therapies, *only*, for 7 d (most effective: butoconazole, clotrimazole, miconazole, terconazole)

Bacterial Vaginosis
Recommended: metronidazole 250 mg PO tid for 7 d *or* clindamycin 300 mg PO bid for 7 d

Trichomoniasis
Metronidazole 2 g orally single dose

Data are current for 2002.

Depending on the cause of vaginitis, therapy aims to achieve one or both of these goals. Refer to Box 37-4 for the CDC recommendations for the treatment of vaginitis in pregnancy.

Physiologic conditions of pregnancy increase the risk for VVC. For treatment of VVC during pregnancy, the CDC (2002) recommends that only topical azoles be used for a 7-day course of therapy. The most effective agents are butoconazole, clotrimazole, miconazole, and terconazole.

Because adverse pregnancy outcomes have been reported in patients with BV, it is recommended that women who are at high risk (ie, those who have previously delivered a premature infant) and who are asymptomatic should be treated. Symptomatic BV in women at low risk (no history of premature delivery) should be treated to relieve symptoms. Oral metronidazole and clindamycin may be used in both groups (see Table 37-3).

The use of topicals is not recommended because of reports of adverse events, such as premature birth. Although the use of oral metronidazole in pregnancy had long been controversial, multiple studies have found no relationship between birth defects and the use of metronidazole during pregnancy. Follow-up of high-risk pregnant women who have been treated for BV is recommended 1 month after completion of treatment to ensure a successful response.

The CDC (2002) advises that trichomoniasis may be associated with adverse pregnancy outcomes such as premature rupture of membranes and premature delivery. Studies are needed to assess these adverse outcomes. Symptomatic pregnant patients should be treated with a 2-g single oral dose of metronidazole to relieve symptoms.

MONITORING PATIENT RESPONSE

Diagnosis and management of vaginitis can be frustrating for both the patient and the practitioner, especially in patients with chronic symptoms and recurrent infections. Symptoms may recur or persist despite adherence to prescribed therapy. The practitioner should consult an expert if the patient fails to respond to current treatment recommendations.

The use of fungal cultures to assess response to therapy and to identify the offending candidal species is beneficial in assessing and treating patients with recurrent VVC. Fungal cultures play a role in detecting non-*albicans* candidal infections that may require second-line therapy.

Practitioners need to individualize the plan of care with each patient. They also need to maintain current knowledge of research regarding alternative therapies and to inform patients of findings. In many situations, yogurt and similar products may cause no harm and may provide patients with a perception of control over a frustrating condition.

Preventing the complications of BV has been the subject of much research. Several studies have identified an association between BV and the development of pelvic inflammatory disease (PID). One study showed that treatment of BV lowered the incidence of postabortion PID by 8.7% (Larsson et al., 1991). Although it is well documented that cervical intraepithelial neoplasia (CIN) and cervical cancer are strongly associated with human papilloma virus, a link between BV and CIN has been suggested. In a study using the retrospective identification of clue cells on Pap smears, it was determined that there was a significantly higher incidence of BV in women with CIN (Platz-Christensen et al., 1994). The CDC has made no formal recommendation regarding treatment of asymptomatic BV in these groups of women but does encourage that consideration be given to screening and treatment of women undergoing surgical abortion procedures or hysterectomy and in pregnant women who are at high risk for preterm delivery. Routine treatment of sex partners is not recommended because studies have shown that treatment of partners does not reduce the incidence of recurrence or relapse (CDC, 2002).

PATIENT EDUCATION

Drug Information

Metronidazole can cause nausea and vomiting if alcohol is ingested during therapy and up to 24 hours after therapy stops. Patients should be instructed to adhere to the directions included with the product. In patients taking oral azole and oral antibiotic medications, the practitioner should reinforce the importance of following directions carefully and completing the full course of antibiotic therapy even if symptoms subside earlier.

Lifestyle Changes

The patient should avoid tight-fitting clothing, should wear undergarments that allow adequate vaginal ventilation, and should avoid douches and other feminine hygiene products that may alter the normal vaginal pH. The possibility that sexual activity may be associated with the onset of symptoms should be discussed, and the patient should be instructed to monitor these patterns. The patient should use condoms to protect against sexually transmitted disease. Because the use of antibiotics and oral contraceptives may be factors that predispose patients to vaginitis, other treatment options should be explored.

Complementary and Alternative Medicine

Ingesting yogurt (or other commercially available products containing *Lactobacillus acidophilus*) to promote vaginal recolonization may be effective in preventing VVC. The true benefit of colonization with lactobacilli as protection against VVC or BV, however, has not been established. According to the CDC (2002), more data are needed to determine the efficacy of vaginal lactobacilli suppositories for the treatment of BV. The treatment of BV with non-vaginal lactobacilli or douching has not been shown to be effective.

■ Case Study

R.S. is a 32-year-old woman who seeks treatment for a vaginal discharge that she has had for the past month. She is sexually active and has had the same partner for the past 6 months. She reports noticing an odor, especially after sexual intercourse. Her history reveals that she has been using a commercial douche on a biweekly basis during the past year for hygienic purposes in an attempt to prevent vaginal infections. She denies any other associated symptoms. The physical examination reveals a white vaginal discharge. Microscopic examination of the vaginal discharge shows clue cells, and the pH is 5.5.

Diagnosis: Bacterial vaginosis

→ 1. List specific goals of treatment for this patient.

→ 2. What drug therapy would you prescribe? Why?

→ 3. What are the parameters for monitoring the success of the therapy?

→ 4. Discuss specific patient education based on the prescribed therapy.

→ 5. List one or two adverse reactions for the selected agent that would cause you to change therapy.

→ 6. What would be the choice for second-line therapy?

→ 7. What OTC or alternative medications would be appropriate for this patient?

→ 8. What dietary or lifestyle changes should be recommended?

→ 9. Describe one or two drug/drug or drug/food interaction for the selected agent.

Bibliography

Starred references are cited in the text.

*Centers for Disease Control and Prevention. (2002). 2002 guidelines for treatment of sexually transmitted diseases. *Morbidity and Mortality Weekly Reports, 51*(RR-6).

Eshenbach, D. (1993). Bacterial vaginosis and anaerobes in obstetric-gynecologic infection. *Clinical Infectious Diseases, 16*(Suppl. 4), S282–S287.

Kaplan, B., Rabinerson, D., & Gibor, Y. (1997). Single-dose systemic oral fluconazole for the treatment of vaginal candidiasis. *International Journal of Gynecology and Obstetrics, 57,* 281–286.

*Larsson, P. G., Platz-Christensen, J. J., Thejls, H., Frosum, U., & Pahlson, C. (1991). Incidence of pelvic inflammatory disease after first-trimester legal abortion in women with bacterial vaginosis after treatment with metronidazole: A double-blind, randomized study. *American Journal of Obstetrics and Gynecology, 66,* 100–103.

Nasraty, S. (2003). Infections of the female genital tract. *Primary Care, 30*(1), 193–203.

Nyirjesy, P. (2001). Vaginovulvar candidiasis. *American Family Physician, 63*(4), 697–702.

Paavonen, J., Mangione, C., Martin, M. A., et al. (2001). Bacterial vaginosis cure rates were similar with clindamycin vaginal ovules for 3 days and oral metronidazole for 7 days. *Evidence-Based Ob/Gyn, 3*(2), 86–87.

*Platz-Christensen, J. J., Sundstrom, E., & Larsson, P. G. (1994). Bacterial vaginosis and cervical intraepithelial neoplasia. *Acta Obstetricia et Gynecologica Scandinavica, 73,* 586–588.

Sweet, R. (1995). Role of bacterial vaginosis in pelvic inflammatory disease. *Clinical Infectious Diseases, 20*(Suppl. 2), S271.

*Spence, M. R., Harwell, T. S., Davies, M. C., & Smith, J. L. (1997). The minimum single oral metronidazole dose for treating trichomonas: A randomized, blinded study. *Obstetrics and Gynecology, 89,* 699–703.

Zeger, W. (2003). Gynecological infections. *Emergency Medicine Clinics of North America, 21*(3), 631–648.

Visit the Connection web site for the most up-to-date drug information.

VIII

Pharmacotherapy for Musculoskeletal Disorders

OSTEOARTHRITIS AND RHEUMATOID ARTHRITIS

■ CAROL GULLO MEST AND ANDREW M. PETERSON

The term *arthritis* is used to describe more than 100 conditions that affect the bones, joints, and muscles. It is often used as a generic, catch-all term that is rarely differentiated to a specific condition. This is unfortunate, because it means that many patients will experience pain, lack of function, and disability because of the lack of a concrete diagnosis coupled with appropriate treatment (Marlowe, 1998).

Although arthritis once was accepted as an expected part of the aging process, research has discovered treatments that can be prescribed to patients of all ages. However, many of these therapies are specific to one arthritis condition and do little good for another type of arthritis. Two of the major arthritis conditions, osteoarthritis (OA) and rheumatoid arthritis (RA), are discussed in this chapter.

OSTEOARTHRITIS

Osteoarthritis, formerly known as *degenerative joint disease*, is the most common joint problem in the United States. A chronic condition, it is the most prevalent cause of disability in the elderly. OA affects approximately 20% of people over 65 years of age. On x-ray studies, more than one third of adults show changes consistent with OA of the weight-bearing joints. However, the incidence of OA is severely underreported because clinical signs and symptoms are often attributed to the normal aging process.

OA is a progressive disease that, when it occurs in weight-bearing joints, results in chronic pain, restricted range of motion, and muscle weakness. The joints commonly affected by OA include the knees, hips, cervical and lumbar spine, distal interphalangeal (DIP) joints, and the carpometacarpal joint at the base of the thumb.

Obesity is the greatest risk factor for development of OA of the knees and hips, especially in women. This is due to mechanical stress on weight-bearing joints. There may also be a metabolic effect of excess fat on articular cartilage that may account for some of the significance of obesity as a systemic risk factor.

The incidence of OA varies across sex, age, and racial lines. The onset of OA occurs in men at an earlier age, with women eventually exceeding men in incidence by middle age. OA of the DIP and carpometacarpal joints is more common in white women; OA of the knees occurs more frequently in African-American women. In addition, certain recreational activities, sports, and occupations are associated with an increased early incidence of OA.

CAUSES

There are two forms of OA. *Primary*, or idiopathic, OA arises from physiologic changes that occur with normal aging. *Secondary* OA usually results from traumatic injuries or inherited conditions and may present as hemochromatosis, chondrodystrophy, or inflammatory OA.

PATHOPHYSIOLOGY

OA must be differentiated from other forms of arthritis because the physiologic changes specific to the condition dictate management. Although most forms of arthritis, including OA, result in degeneration of articular cartilage, the subsequent formation of new bone is a change specific to OA.

The physiologic changes associated with OA begin with deterioration of the articular cartilage. The articular cartilage is responsible for reducing joint friction during movement by diffusing mechanical stress to the underlying bone. Normal articular cartilage is smooth and is supported by subchondral bone. The subchondral bone serves as a flexible base to absorb mechanical force.

Articular cartilage consists of chondrocytes, connective tissue cells that are embedded in an extracellular matrix. The matrix is made up of collagen, water, and proteoglycans (macromolecules). The proteoglycans are responsible for providing elasticity and flexibility to the matrix, which allows the articular cartilage to resist direct pressure. In OA, there is a reduction in proteoglycans in the extracellular matrix, leading to a decrease in resiliency to mechanical stress. In time, the articular cartilage becomes friable. The underlying subchondral bone responds to this change through a process termed *remodeling*. Remodeling involves the production of new bone that is thicker than the original bone. If remodeling occurs at the joint margins, an osteophyte (bone spur) may develop. The adjacent cortical bone becomes fortified with new bone, resulting in an irregular narrowing of the joint space. Sclerosing and cyst formation may ensue.

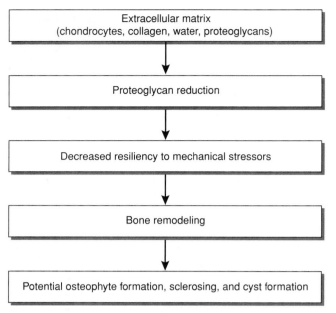

Figure 38–1 Destruction of cartilage in osteoarthritis.

In addition to cartilaginous changes, concomitant changes in the synovial fluid must be considered. Synovial fluid, the main lubricant of joints, is produced and excreted from the cartilage. Destruction of the proteoglycans in OA renders the mechanism of synovial release ineffective, thereby further impairing the smooth mechanical operation of the joint. Figure 38-1 demonstrates the mechanism of cartilage destruction.

DIAGNOSTIC CRITERIA

A thorough history and physical examination provide enough data to diagnose OA. The most common symptom is joint pain; the patient in an early stage of OA usually describes the pain as insidious, intermittent, and mild. As the disease progresses, the patient may describe the pain as more constant and more disabling. Most patients report remittance of pain with rest and exacerbation of pain with joint movement.

Although the symptoms of OA are localized, associated pain may be referred. For example, it is common for OA of the hip to be referred to the medial knee. Another symptom associated with OA is crepitus, a painless "crackling" in the joint. Crepitus most commonly affects the knee, but it may be heard in other joints affected by OA as well. As the OA progresses to the later stages of articular damage, deformity of the joint may be observed. The deformity usually appears as an enlargement of the joint, which may result from either increased bone production or synovitis. Other deformities resulting from OA of the knee include varus and valgus deformities of the lower extremities.

OA of the cervical spine may present with pain that radiates to the supraclavicular or upper trapezius areas. Depending on the level of nerve involvement, symptoms may progress to include pain in the distal upper extremities. OA of the lumbar spine may produce symptoms of neurogenic claudication.

On physical examination, decreased range of motion is the most common finding. This finding may be absent in the early stages of the disease but gradually progresses as the condition worsens. In later stages of the disease, joint contractures may occur, resulting in varus and valgus deformities. Patients with severe OA of the hip may present with gait disturbances.

Because OA is a progressive disease, complications such as joint effusion and enlargement may occur as the disease progresses. Occasionally, radicular problems may occur secondary to changes in the cervical vertebrae.

Joint enlargement due to the formation of osteophytes may be observed. Osteophyte formation in the DIP joint is called *Heberden's nodes*; in the proximal interphalangeal joint it is referred to as *Bouchard's nodes*.

Radiologic findings in OA may be used to confirm the suspected diagnosis. Narrow joint spaces with osteophyte formation are common radiologic findings.

Typical laboratory data are unaffected by OA, which is not a systemic disease, though there is promising information regarding a new biochemical marker, the collagen fragment CTX-II. This marker may be a valuable tool for diagnosing and monitoring the progression of OA. CTX-II is a type II collagen peptide fragment associated with cartilage destruction. In a controlled study, researchers found that patients with elevated CTX-II levels were more likely to be diagnosed with OA. These findings were independent of age, sex, and body mass index. Changes that occur in CTX-II with treatment have not yet been studied.

INITIATING DRUG THERAPY

Before initiating drug therapy, the practitioner should recommend appropriate physical activity or physical therapy. The goals of physical therapy are to reduce pain, improve motion, and maintain functional ability (Box 38-1).

In advanced OA, surgical intervention may be required. The most common surgical interventions include joint debridement, removal of free cartilage fragments, osteotomy, and joint replacement. Arthroscopic surgery of the knee is beneficial in removing loose foreign bodies. Patients who are likely to respond to this intervention are those who have the sensation of knee locking and who demonstrate tenacious joint effusions. Patients with advanced radiographic changes benefit from total joint replacement.

BOX 38–1. PHYSICAL THERAPIES FOR OSTEOARTHRITIS

- Moist heat to help diminish muscle spasm and relieve stiffness
- Weight loss if the patient is overweight
- Exercises to strengthen the muscles surrounding the involved joint(s) and a fitness program to maintain flexibility of the involved joint through swimming, walking, cycling, and isometric exercises
- Use of assistive devices to help with ambulation and activities of daily living

The goals of pharmacotherapy for OA are to maintain function, prevent further joint damage, and diminish associated pain. The degree of joint involvement and the severity of the symptoms usually dictate proper interventions for individual patients.

Analgesics

First-line pharmacotherapy for OA is geared toward analgesia. Usually, the first recommendation is acetaminophen (Tylenol) 650 to 1,000 mg every 4 to 6 hours. This is a cost-effective, safe approach to the early treatment of OA symptoms. Acetaminophen offers solely analgesia; it possesses no anti-inflammatory properties.

The recommended dose of up to 4 g/day is safe for patients with normal liver function. Higher doses have been associated with hepatotoxicity. Patients with a history of liver disease should not take more than 1,800 to 2,000 mg/day.

Another effective first-line agent for treating OA is tramadol (Ultram), an inhibitor of norepinephrine and serotonin. The therapeutic dose range is generally 50 to 100 mg/day. Unlike the nonsteroidal anti-inflammatory drugs (NSAIDs), tramadol does not produce serious gastrointestinal (GI) side effects, nor does it aggravate existing hypertension, congestive heart failure, or renal disease. The most common side effects of tramadol include nausea, dizziness, drowsiness, and sweating.

Other analgesics used for OA include the narcotic analgesics codeine and propoxyphene (Darvon). These drugs should be prescribed for a limited time because of potential dependence and withdrawal symptoms.

Nonsteroidal Anti-inflammatory Drugs

Second-line therapy for OA includes NSAIDs, the most commonly used class of drugs in the world. NSAIDs are further classified according to their chemical structure (Table 38-1). Although these classes have subtle differences, they all basically act by inhibiting cyclooxygenase (COX). These drugs may be prescribed if patients do not respond well to acetaminophen therapy or if an inflammatory process has begun.

Mechanism of Action

There are two mechanisms by which NSAIDs exert their anti-inflammatory action (Fig. 38-2). One is by inhibiting the conversion of arachidonic acid to prostaglandin, prostacyclin, and thromboxanes—all of which are mediators of pain and inflammation. The other is by interfering with protein kinase activation (especially when taken at higher doses).

COX is the enzyme that converts arachidonic acid to prostaglandin G_2 (PGG_2). The COX enzyme is present in two forms, COX-1 and COX-2. COX-1 enzymes are found in the GI tract and kidney. Because COX-1 produces protective prostaglandins for the GI tract and kidney, most research is focusing on preserving the activity of COX-1 in the GI tract. COX-2 is produced at nonspecific sites of inflammation. Inhibition of COX-2 produces anti-inflammatory and analgesic effects without the risk of dangerous GI side effects seen with nonselective COX inhibitors. There is evidence that COX-2 also plays a role in the maintenance of renal protective prostaglandins, and inhibition of this may compromise renal function as well.

The first COX-2 inhibitor approved for use in the United States is celecoxib (Celebrex). This drug is approved for treating both OA and RA. Celecoxib is available in 100- and 200-mg capsules. Typical dosage for OA is 100 mg twice daily or 200 mg once daily. Side effects include abdominal pain, diarrhea, dyspepsia, and headache. Because the drug is eliminated primarily through hepatic metabolism, patients with symptoms suggesting liver dysfunction should be monitored carefully. Valdecoxib, a newer COX-2 inhibitor, has similar efficacy and side effects to celecoxib. Both agents have sulfa moiety that can precipitate allergic reactions in susceptible individuals.

Dosage

Dosing of NSAIDs is variable. The drugs are classified into short-, intermediate-, and long-acting categories. NSAIDs require five half-lives to reach peak therapeutic levels and five half-lives to be fully excreted. Categories with a longer half-life require longer periods to reach therapeutic levels.

Some common agents used to treat OA are ibuprofen, diclofenac, or the COX-2 inhibitors celecoxib and valdecoxib. Diclofenac is given at 50 mg twice daily and ibuprofen is usually given at 400 mg four times. The daily dose of ibuprofen must not exceed 1,600 mg for the treatment of OA. The typical dosage of celecoxib is 100 mg twice daily or 200 mg once daily. For valdecoxib, the dosage is 10 mg daily. Patients should be encouraged to use the NSAID consistently for 2 to 3 weeks to determine its effectiveness. Table 38-1 gives information about other agents and dosing considerations.

Time Frame for Response

Patient responses to NSAIDs are quite variable. Patients who do not respond to one NSAID may respond to another, even one of the same class. This response variability is also seen in the side effect profile of NSAIDs. The practitioner should be familiar with several of the NSAIDs from each

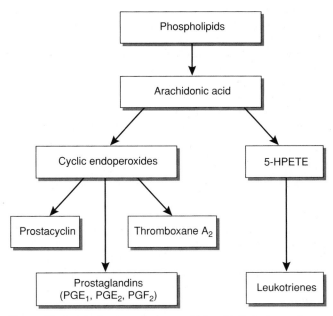

Figure 38–2 Mechanism of nonsteroidal anti-inflammatory drug action.

Table 38.1

Overview of Selected Anti-inflammatory Agents Used to Treat Osteoarthritis and Rheumatoid Arthritis

Generic (Trade) Name and Dosage	Selected Adverse Events	Contraindications	Special Considerations
Nonsteroidal Anti-inflammatory Drugs (NSAIDs)			
acetaminophen (Tylenol) 650–1000 mg q4–6h			
Short-Acting NSAIDs*			
ibuprofen (Motrin) OA and RA: 1200–3200 mg/d PO; individualize dosage	Headache, dizziness, sleepiness or insomnia, nausea, GI discomfort, flatulence, constipation, blood dyscrasias, renal impairment, rash, peripheral edema	Allergy to the drug, salicylates, or other NSAIDs Pregnancy, lactation Use cautiously with impaired hepatic or renal function.	Therapeutic response may occur over several weeks.
fenoprofen (Nalfon) OA and RA: 800–3200 mg/d PO in divided doses; do not exceed 3200 mg/d	Same as above	Same as above	Patient should have ophthalmic examination periodically during long-term therapy.
indomethacin (Indocin) OA and RA: 50–200 mg/d in divided doses	Same as above	Same as above, and also GI bleeding with history of proctitis or rectal bleeding	Increased toxic effects if taken concomitantly with lithium; decreased diuretic effect with loop diuretics; and potential decreased antihypertensive effect with beta-adrenergic blockers, such as captopril
tolmetin (Tolectin) OA and RA: 600–2000 mg/d in 3–4 doses	Same as above	Pregnancy, lactation Use cautiously with allergies, renal, hepatic, CV, and GI conditions.	May affect results (false positive) of proteinuria tests using acid precipitation tests Patient should have ophthalmic examination periodically during long-term therapy.
meclofenamate (Meclomen)[†] RA: 200–400 mg/d PO in 3 or 4 equal doses	Same as above	Same as above	Patient should have ophthalmic examination periodically during long-term therapy. May be taken with food or milk to reduce GI upset
diclofenac sodium (Voltaren) OA: 100–150 mg/d PO in divided doses RA: 100–200 mg/d PO in divided doses	Same as above	Significant renal impairment, pregnancy, lactation Use cautiously with impaired hearing; allergies; hepatic, CV and GI conditions.	
diclofenac potassium (Cataflam) OA: 50 mg PO bid–tid RA: 50 mg PO bid–tid	Same as above	Significant renal impairment, pregnancy, lactation Use cautiously with impaired hearing; allergies; hepatic, CV and GI conditions.	Increases serum levels of lithium and risk of lithium toxicity
Intermediate-Acting NSAIDs*			
acetylsalicylic acid (aspirin; Bayer, others)	Nausea, GI upset, bleeding, hypersensitivity reaction, bronchospasm, dizziness, tinnitus	Allergy to salicylates, other NSAIDs, tartrazine, hemophilia and other bleeding disorders, pregnancy (possibly teratogenic), and more Do not use in children after illness because of association with Reye's syndrome.	Increased risk of bleeding when taken concomitantly with anticoagulants and other NSAIDs Consult package insert for extensive list of interacting drugs and effects.
celecoxib (Celebrex) Initially, 100 mg PO bid, may increase to 200 mg/d PO bid as needed	Abdominal pain, diarrhea, dyspepsia, headache	Allergy to the drug or to sulfonamides, NSAIDs or aspirin Significant renal impairment Pregnancy, lactation	Elimination of the drug occurs primarily through hepatic metabolism; therefore, patients with symptoms suggesting liver dysfunction should be carefully monitored.
naproxen (Naprosyn) OA and RA: 500–1500 mg/d PO in divided doses	Headache, dizziness, sleepiness or insomnia, nausea, GI discomfort, flatulence, constipation, blood dyscrasias, renal impairment, rash, peripheral edema	Allergy to naproxen, salicylates, other NSAIDs Pregnancy, lactation Use cautiously in patients with asthma, chronic urticaria, CV dysfunction, hypertension, GI bleeding, peptic ulcer, impaired hepatic or renal function.	May take with meals if GI upset occurs Patient should have ophthalmic examination periodically during long-term therapy. Increased serum levels of lithium and risk of lithium toxicity

Table 38.1

Overview of Selected Anti-inflammatory Agents Used to Treat Osteoarthritis and Rheumatoid Arthritis (*Continued*)

Generic (Trade) Name and Dosage	Selected Adverse Events	Contraindications	Special Considerations
sulindac (Clinoril) OA and RA: 150 mg PO bid initially; individualize dosage thereafter	Same as above	Same as above	Same as above
oxaprozin (DayPro) 1.2 g/d		Significant renal impairment Pregnancy, lactation Use cautiously with impaired hearing, allergies, hepatic, CV and GI conditions.	
*Long-Acting NSAIDs**			
nabumetone (Relafen) 750–2000 mg PO qd	Headache, dizziness, sleepiness or insomnia, nausea, GI discomfort, flatulence, constipation, blood dyscrasias, renal impairment, rash, peripheral edema	Same as above	May be taken in divided dose May be taken with or without food
piroxicam (Feldene) 20 mg PO qd	Same as above	Pregnancy and lactation Use cautiously with allergies, renal, hepatic, CV and GI conditions.	Because therapeutic response progresses over several weeks, evaluate response after 2 wk.
diflunisal (Dolobid) 250–500 mg bid etodolac (Lodine) 600 mg–1 g/d in 2 or 3 divided doses			
valdecoxib (Bextia) 10 mg daily	GI disturbances, headache	Sulfa allergy, advanced renal disease	May be taken with food

*Drugs in the short-acting group have serum half-lives of approximately 1–4 h, in the intermediate-acting group approximately 10–20 h (dose dependent), and in the long-acting group approximately 45 h for piroxicam and 72 h for phenylbutazone.
†Available in Canada.

class and should try to individualize the therapy based on symptom management and side effects.

Contraindications

The NSAIDs are contraindicated in patients allergic to aspirin, in patients with alcohol dependence, or in pregnant patients. Further, specific agents such as celecoxib and valdecoxib are contraindicated in patients with sulfa allergy. Caution should be used when prescribing an NSAID to patients with renal or hepatic impairment or in the elderly. The inhibition of the COX enzymes will hamper the production of the renal protective prostaglandin, reducing renal function.

Adverse Events

The NSAIDs have gained a reputation as innocuous agents because of their over-the-counter availability and widespread use. However, this class of drugs is far from benign, and patient education materials should highlight potential adverse reactions. The side effect profile of NSAIDs is quite extensive.

Visual changes, weight gain, headache, dizziness, nervousness, photosensitivity, weakness, tinnitus, easy bruising or bleeding, and fluid retention are side effects that have been associated with use of NSAIDs. Again, cautious use and frequent monitoring, particularly of elderly patients, is of paramount importance for safe NSAID use. The most common side effects of NSAIDs occur in the GI and renal systems.

Adverse GI events may run the gamut from minor GI irritation to ulcers, GI bleeding, perforation, and gastric outlet obstruction. These GI effects are why NSAIDs remain a second-line approach to OA treatment. Concomitant use of misoprostol (Cytotec) has been shown to decrease the incidence of ulcer disease and GI complications. Misoprostol, a prostaglandin analog, is given at 200 mg four times daily. Its use should be limited to patients at high risk for GI complications (the elderly and those with a history of congestive heart failure, ulcer, or GI bleeding).

Studies of the treatment of GI effects of NSAIDs have compared the efficacy of proton pump inhibitors and histamine-2 (H_2) receptor antagonists. Yeomans et al. (1998) determined that omeprazole (Prilosec), a proton pump inhibitor, healed existing ulcers and prevented further ulcer development more effectively than ranitidine (Zantac), an H_2 receptor antagonist. Similarly, Hawkey et al. (1998) found omeprazole and misoprostol equally successful at treating ulcers and other GI symptoms associated with NSAID use. However, omeprazole was better tolerated and also was associated with an improved relapse rate.

Patients with renal disease, congestive heart failure, cirrhosis, and volume depletion may experience renal aberrations, particularly related to renal blood flow. These side effects underscore the need for frequent monitoring of patients on long-term NSAID therapy.

Nonacetylated Salicylates

The nonacetylated salicylates (Box 38-2) are especially beneficial in patients who are sensitive to the GI irritation caused by long-term aspirin use. Diflunisal (Dolobid), the most

BOX 38–2. NONACETYLATED SALICYLATES

- diflunisal
- sodium salicylate
- choline salicylate
- magnesium salicylate
- choline magnesium trisalicylate
- salsalate

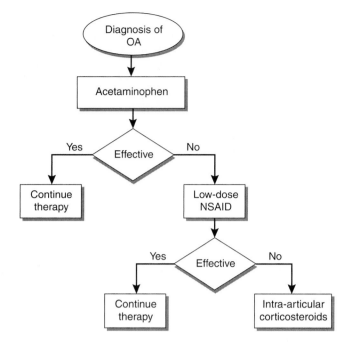

Key ⬭ Starting point for decision making; ▭ clinical actions (assessing, prescribing, monitoring); ◇ decision point.

Figure 38–3 Treatment algorithm for osteoarthritis (OA).

commonly used nonacetylated salicylate, is an effective COX-1 inhibitor with anti-inflammatory and analgesic properties, but its antipyretic activities are weak. In terms of symptom relief, the nonacetylated salicylates are probably as effective as aspirin in treating inflammatory disorders.

Corticosteroids

If symptoms of OA are restricted to one or two joints that have not responded to first- or second-line treatment, intra-articular corticosteroids may be helpful. Aseptic technique and a local anesthetic are required. The amount of drug injected depends on the size of the joint. Careful technique that avoids the surrounding soft tissues is imperative to avoid tissue atrophy. The side effect of localized pain may be treated with an NSAID or another appropriate analgesic. Injection of corticosteroids usually produces symptom relief within a few days, and the relief may last up to several months. Because of the potential for cartilage destruction and osteonecrosis with repeated injections, this therapy should be used judiciously.

SELECTING THE MOST APPROPRIATE AGENT

In selecting therapies for OA, the prescriber should consider patient variables such as age, childbearing status, progression of arthritis, and underlying illnesses. There is evidence that acetaminophen 4 g daily is as effective as an NSAID. Further, there is no evidence that one NSAID is more effective than another. The COX-2 inhibitors are typically reserved for

patients at increased risk of GI disorders such as peptic ulcer disease (patients over age 65, patients with a history of peptic ulcer disease or GI bleeding, patients taking oral anticoagulants and oral corticosteroids). The recommended treatment order appears in Table 38-2 and Figure 38-3.

First-Line Therapy

Acetaminophen, 1 g every 6 hours, has been shown to be effective in reducing the pain of OA within 4 weeks and lasting for up to 2 years. The addition of codeine to acetaminophen may further reduce the pain, but often patients discontinue this combination due to the side effects associated with codeine (constipation, drowsiness). For this reason, the addition of codeine is usually reserved for short-term use if acetaminophen or other options fail.

Table 38.2

Recommended Order of Treatment for Osteoarthritis

Order	Agents	Comments
First line	Acetaminophen	Useful as long as symptoms remain mild, intermittent, and do not affect the range of motion of affected joint(s)
	Tramadol	Centrally acting analgesic useful for moderate to moderately severe pain
Second line	Low-dose NSAIDs, such as celecoxib, ibuprofen, diclofenac, or the combination drug diclofenac and misoprostol	Begin NSAID therapy if inflammatory response has occurred as manifested by more constant and disabling pain.
Third line	Intra-articular corticosteroids	Therapeutic option that depends on size of joint involved and degree of inflammation
	Short-term narcotic analgesics, such as codeine or propoxyphene	A single joint should not receive an injection more than once every 6 mo.
		Used for a limited time because of potential for dependence and withdrawal

Second-Line Therapy

For patients without risk factors for GI disturbance, if acetaminophen therapy fails to provide relief, ibuprofen or a similar nonselective NSAID agent should be considered for second-line therapy. The choice of the specific NSAID should be based on the cost and convenience of therapy. Naproxen is typically given twice daily, ibuprofen three or four times daily. Further, prescription drugs may be much more expensive than over-the-counter agents. For patients with risk factors for GI hemorrhage, a COX-2 inhibitor may be a better second-line choice. Alternatively, the use of a traditional NSAID coupled with a proton-pump inhibitor may be sufficient to provide analgesia along with gastric protection.

Third-Line Therapy

Intra-articular steroids may be useful when an effusion is present and there are clear signs of local inflammation.

Special Populations

Geriatric

For elderly patients, the practitioner usually prescribes an NSAID with a shorter half-life in a smaller dosage than for a younger adult. Patients over age 65 should be considered at risk for GI hemorrhage and treated with either a COX-2 inhibitor or a combination of a COX-1 NSAID and a gastric protective agent such as misoprostol or a proton-pump inhibitor.

Women

Many of the NSAIDs are category C agents, which means that caution should be used in women of childbearing age and pregnant women.

MONITORING PATIENT RESPONSE

In addition to routine questions about the efficacy of the drug (eg, pain relief), baseline and ongoing monitoring for NSAID therapy should include a complete blood count (CBC), urinalysis, and serum creatinine, potassium, and aspartate aminotransferase measurements. These studies should be repeated at 1 to 3 months, then every 3 to 6 months thereafter for the duration of therapy. In patients at risk for GI hemorrhage, the clinician should consider evaluating the patient for stool occult blood, anemia, and other signs of bleeding.

PATIENT EDUCATION

Patients taking NSAIDs need to be aware of their potentially harsh effects on the GI system, ranging from mild GI discomfort to gastric bleeding. The practitioner may emphasize strategies for dealing with some of these adverse effects, including taking NSAIDs with food or milk or at meals.

Drug Information

Patients should be reminded that a specific NSAID should be used regularly for 2 to 3 weeks before switching to another NSAID. This period is needed to assess whether the medication is effective.

Practitioners should keep up with information regarding NSAIDs through the FDA's website (www.fda.gov). In 2004, rofecoxib (Vioxx), a COX-2 inhibitor, was voluntarily withdrawn from the market due to an increased risk of cardiovascular events associated with its use. This withdrawal has prompted increased scrutiny regarding the safety of the other COX-2 inhibitors, and investigations are ongoing.

Patients receiving a corticosteroid injection for joint pain need to be informed that a single joint should not be injected more frequently than every 6 months. Patients should be cautioned to limit activity of the injected joint for several days after the injection. Otherwise, the reduced pain perception of the joint may allow the patient to cause further joint damage, enhancing the progression of OA.

Patient-Oriented Information Sources

The National Institute of Arthritis and Musculoskeletal and Skin Diseases (NIAMS) is a government-sponsored group that provides information on OA and its treatment (http://www.niams.nih.gov/hi/topics/arthritis/oahandout.htm). This information is also available in Spanish. The Arthritis Foundation (http://www.arthritis.org/conditions/DiseaseCenter/oa.asp) provides information on the web and in print.

Nutrition/Lifestyle Changes

The practitioner should provide the patient with information about the continued use of physical therapy, exercise, and weight loss.

Complementary and Alternative Medications

Glucosamine, a form of an amino acid, is a naturally occurring substance in the body. It is believed to be involved in the development and repair of cartilage. Exogenous replacement of this substance is thought to help build on existing cartilage. Evidence-based reviews of this agent suggest that moderate improvements in pain relief and function can be achieved when administered at 1,500 mg/day. This effect is thought to be similar in magnitude to that of low-dose NSAIDs or acetaminophen.

Chondroitin, a large protein-like molecule that can impart elasticity to collagen, has shown similar, but slightly less, efficacy compared to glucosamine. The dosage of chondroitin used on most of the studies was 800 to 1,200 mg/day.

These agents may have GI side effects. Since they are considered food supplements, there is little FDA regulation and the preparations may vary in potency and effectiveness.

Capsaicin cream (Dolorac, others) may help relieve pain. The cream can be applied three or four times a day; patients must wash their hands after each use.

RHEUMATOID ARTHRITIS

RA is a chronic inflammatory disease characterized by symmetric polyarthritis and joint changes, including erythema, effusion, and tenderness. The course of RA is characterized by remissions and exacerbations. RA can affect several organs, but it usually involves synovial tissue changes in the freely movable joints (diarthroses). The most commonly affected joints include the wrists, PIP joints, and metacarpophalangeal joints. RA may also affect the elbows, neck, hips, knees, ankles, and feet.

RA affects approximately 1% of all adults and is three times more prevalent in men than women. New onset of RA is seen throughout the life span, including infancy, but most cases occur in the fifth or sixth decade. Almost 50% of people diagnosed with RA are disabled within 10 years of diagnosis.

CAUSES

The cause of RA continues to be the subject of research. Theories of causation include genetic factors, infectious agents, and an antigen–antibody response. It is unlikely that a single factor is responsible for all cases of RA.

PATHOPHYSIOLOGY

The major physiologic changes associated with RA include synovial membrane proliferation followed by erosion of the subarticular cartilage and subchondral bone. Although the precise etiology of RA is unknown, mounting evidence points to a series of immunologic events. It is unclear whether an infectious, viral, or genetic agent prompts these events.

Specific major histocompatibility complex (MHC) class II alleles and human leukocyte antigen (HLA) are seen more frequently in patients with RA. Some think that a predisposition to RA depends on a binding site for HLA. The presumed pathogenesis begins with antigenic stimulation of T lymphocytes that possess the appropriate MHC molecules. T- and B-cell proliferation ensues, stimulating the blood vessels in the synovial membrane. As the synovial membrane swells, polymorphonuclear leukocytes, lymphocytes, and macrophages are drawn toward the area, presumably to phagocytize the invading antigen. During this process, lysosomal enzymes are released, and this enzymatic process causes major destruction in the joint cartilage. The ensuing inflammatory process attracts additional lymphocytes and plasma cells to the area, and a chain of inflammatory events ensues.

The principal site of cellular involvement is the synovial membrane. The normal joint capsule is lined with synovial membrane approximately one or two cells thick. This membrane is highly vascularized compared with the largely avascular and acellular underlying stroma. The subsynovial tissue is made up of connective tissue, including areolar, fatty, and fibrous tissues.

Early Phase

In the early phase of RA, the synovial microvasculature undergoes significant changes. The capillaries become distended as plasma and other fluids accumulate. High endothelial venule formation enhances the movement of lymphocytes to the synovial lining, allowing formation of abnormal blood vessels. The result of these processes is damaged vascular endothelium (Moncur & Williams, 1995).

Concomitant with these microvascular changes are synovial proliferation and hypertrophy. The synovial tissue becomes edematous and exhibits frond-like villi. Synovial fluid becomes less viscous, while leukocytes proliferate. Most of these leukocytes are neutrophils.

Progression

As RA progresses to the chronic form, continued hyperplasia and hypertrophy of the synovial lining occur. The thickness of the synovial lining increases up to fivefold from the normal one or two cell layers. The proliferation of the synovium persists, with lymphocytic tissue and plasma cells forming around blood vessels. This proliferative tissue extends into the joint space, joint capsule, ligaments, and tendons (Firestein, 1998; Moncur & Williams, 1995).

Severe, Chronic Rheumatoid Arthritis

In severe RA, pannus forms as a result of the release of lysosomal enzymes. Pannus is granulation tissue composed of lymphocytes, plasma cells, fibroblasts, and macrophages. Growing much like a tumor, pannus can invade the cartilage, activate chondrocytes, and release enzymes that can degrade cartilage and bone. This destructive process begins at the synovium and extends to the unprotected area at the junction of the cartilage and subchondral bone. These inflammatory cells can erode surrounding tissue, tendons, and cartilage. When pannus invades the joint margins, decreased range of motion and ankylosis may ensue. Pannus is a specific feature of RA, differentiating it from other forms of arthritis.

DIAGNOSTIC CRITERIA

Although RA characteristically affects the joint structures, it is a systemic disease with potential extra-articular manifestations. The typical RA complaint of morning joint stiffness is usually preceded by fatigue; more severe cases may be preceded by constitutional symptoms such as fever and weight loss (Ross, 1997). Throughout the disease, the patient also may have generalized symptoms such as weakness, fatigue, mild fever, anorexia, and weight loss. End-organ involvement may occur in patients with high rheumatoid factor (RF) titers.

Diagnosis is based on the identification of key findings, as well as the results of certain diagnostic tests. Key symptoms include morning stiffness in involved joints that persists for at least 1 hour; symmetric joint involvement; and painful, swollen joints. The morning stiffness tends to abate as activity increases.

The most common extra-articular manifestation of RA is joint nodules. These occur in 15% to 20% of patients with RA and are most commonly seen in patients with erosive disease. These subcutaneous nodules may develop in any area of the body that is exposed to pressure. Some of these areas are the olecranon bursa, knuckles, ischial spines, Achilles tendon, extensor surfaces of the forearm, and the bridge of the nose (in patients who wear glasses). These nodules may also form internally on the heart, lungs, and intestinal tract. The nodules are firm and rubbery, occur in clusters, and may be either freely mobile or attached to underlying connective tissue. The treatment of the nodules is confined to the treatment of the underlying disease. These nodules may occur in other connective tissue diseases (eg, systemic lupus erythematosus), so alone they are not a criterion for diagnosing RA.

BOX 38–3. DIAGNOSTIC CRITERIA FOR RHEUMATOID ARTHRITIS

1. Morning stiffness exceeding 1 hour *and* involvement of at least three joint groups with soft tissue swelling (both must be present)
2. Swelling of at least one of the following groups: proximal, interphalangeal, metacarpophalangeal, or wrists
3. Symmetric joint swelling
4. Subcutaneous nodules
5. Positive rheumatoid factor
6. Radiologic changes associated with RA

An ocular manifestation of RA is sicca syndrome; patients have a sensation of grittiness in the eyes, accumulation of dried mucus, and decreased tear production. Scleritis and episcleritis are occasional sequelae of sicca syndrome. Additional extra-articular manifestations of RA include vasculitis, pulmonary fibrosis, and pericarditis.

In approximately 70% to 90% of patients with RA, the RF titer exceeds 1:80. An elevated RF titer alone is insufficient to diagnose RA; it must be coupled with associated clinical findings (Firestein, 1998).

Additional diagnostic tests may include an erythrocyte sedimentation rate (ESR), which is usually elevated in any inflammatory process. Also, antinuclear antibody levels are elevated in approximately 30% of patients. Radiography, although not necessary for diagnosis, may be useful in tracking the course of the disease. The American College of Rheumatology criteria for an RA diagnosis appear in Box 38-3.

INITIATING DRUG THERAPY

The inconsistent course of RA in each patient, with remissions and exacerbations, is a major determinant of the appropriate therapy.

Physical and occupational therapies are considered mainstays of nonpharmacologic therapy in patients with RA. These therapies help protect the joints and maintain strength, function, and mobility. Reduction of joint stress is an additional goal of therapy. Patients should engage in activity to their fullest possible extent, with adequate rest after activity, but they should avoid vigorous exercise and heavy labor during acute exacerbations of the disease. Hydrotherapy and hot and cold packs may be used to relax muscle spasms and facilitate joint movement. Warm showers and paraffin treatments may help relieve morning stiffness.

Surgery can help relieve symptoms, improve function, and correct deformities. The most common surgical procedures for RA include tendon transfers, osteotomy, synovectomy, arthroplasty, and total joint replacement. The most widely replaced joints are the hip and the knee.

In pharmacotherapy for RA, the "pyramid approach" to treatment was widely used until recently (Blackburn, 1996). The pyramid consisted of NSAIDs and rest, followed by the addition of corticosteroids and, finally, disease-modifying antirheumatic drugs (DMARDs). Because newer evidence has supported the earlier use of DMARDs, DMARDs are now used once NSAIDs or corticosteroids can no longer control symptoms. The drug classes discussed in the following sections are presented in order of their introduction to the RA treatment regimen.

Goals of Drug Therapy

The goals of drug therapy for RA include reducing pain, stiffness, and swelling; preserving mobility and joint function; and preventing further joint damage.

Nonsteroidal Anti-inflammatory Drugs

The NSAIDs, the most commonly used class of drugs in the world, form the cornerstone of RA treatment. The newer NSAIDs have replaced aspirin as the first-line agent in RA treatment for several reasons. First, the side effect profile, particularly related to GI bleeding, is greatly diminished with the NSAIDs. Second, compliance with the treatment regimen is enhanced because patients need to take fewer pills per day. Finally, the pharmacokinetic actions of the NSAIDs are better understood and anticipated. Despite the advantages of NSAIDs, however, aspirin is probably just as effective in reducing the inflammation associated with RA.

The NSAIDs are typically used to help relieve pain and improve symptoms during the diagnostic process. These agents are continued through the initiation of a DMARD to maintain reduced symptoms. This approach allows the NSAIDs to exert their anti-inflammatory action while the DMARD takes effect. See the discussion of NSAIDs in the Osteoarthritis section of this chapter for more information; also see Table 38-1.

Corticosteroids

Once reserved for second-line therapy, corticosteroids are being used much earlier in RA treatment. In addition to their anti-inflammatory properties (decreased joint swelling, pain, and morning stiffness), corticosteroids may slow the development of joint erosions in progressive disease. These agents are often used as bridge therapy until effective DMARD therapy is instituted.

Low-dose corticosteroids (prednisone 10 mg or equivalent) are beneficial in patients who are beginning DMARD therapy. Because the therapeutic effect of DMARDs may not be seen until several weeks to months after initiating therapy, corticosteroids may be used to provide almost immediate symptom relief. Corticosteroids are also indicated in elderly patients with recent onset of RA.

The difficulty in therapy with corticosteroids lies in the fine dosing line that divides therapeutic effects from long-term side effects. Low doses, such as prednisone (Deltasone, others) 5 to 7.5 mg every morning, may be beneficial. The lowest dose possible should be given by gradually decreasing the dose in 1-mg decrements.

Injectable corticosteroids can be used if symptoms are restricted to one or two joints that have not responded to first-line treatment. They may also be of limited benefit for acute flare-ups of RA.

Additional measures that enhance the effect of cortico-steroids include smoking cessation, limitation of alcohol intake, and weight-bearing exercises for 30 to 60 minutes each day.

The most common side effects of corticosteroid therapy include cataracts, glaucoma, mild glucose intolerance, and cutaneous atrophy. Less common adverse events include myopathy, hypothalamic–pituitary–adrenal axis dysfunction, and osteoporosis. Osteoporosis may be avoided by taking a calcium supplement (1,500 mg/day) along with vitamin D (800 mg/day). Hormone replacement therapy may be initiated or maintained in postmenopausal women taking corticosteroid therapy. Testosterone levels should be monitored in men; if levels drop, then replacement is needed.

Disease-Modifying Antirheumatic Drugs (DMARDs)

As stated previously, the early use of DMARDs is advocated because of the high degree of inflammation that is present early in the disease (Table 38-3). Radiographic evidence of joint damage usually is present in the first year of the disease, and functional deterioration due to this damage may be irreversible. Therefore, early initiation of DMARD therapy may be the best course of action to take in meeting the long-range goals of RA treatment. DMARD therapy should be initiated within 3 months after onset of symptoms.

Methotrexate

The most commonly prescribed DMARD is methotrexate (Rheumatrex). The patient best suited for treatment with methotrexate is one who has morning stiffness and synovitis.

Mechanism of Action

Methotrexate, a folic acid antagonist, is thought to affect leukocyte suppression, decreasing the inflammation that results from immunologic byproducts. When treatment stops, exacerbation of symptoms may occur as early as 2 weeks after cessation.

Dosage

Methotrexate is available for oral, subcutaneous, intramuscular, or intravenous use. For most patients, a starting dose of 7.5 mg orally once per week is recommended. If a significant decrease in symptoms is not noted by week 6 of therapy, the dosage is increased by 2.5 mg/week every 2 to 4 weeks until symptom control is attained. Most patients respond to 12.5 to 15 mg/week. The maximum weekly oral dose is 25 mg. Injectable methotrexate may be used if there is an inadequate response to oral therapy.

Time Frame for Response

Approximately 70% to 75% of patients respond favorably to methotrexate therapy, but it may take 3 to 8 weeks of therapy for improvement to be noted. More than 50% of patients stay on the treatment for more than 5 years. However, if patients have difficulty tolerating the side effects, methotrexate should be discontinued or the dosage lowered.

Contraindications

Methotrexate is contraindicated in pregnant patients and those with leukopenia or liver disease. Patients with an increased risk for toxicity include those with a history of alcoholism, obesity, diabetes, and renal and hepatic disease.

Adverse Events

The most commonly reported side effects of methotrexate are nausea and abdominal pain. These effects may be minimized by switching to parenteral therapy. Oral ulcers, leukopenia, anemia, and thrombocytopenia are also common. However, these adverse reactions may be minimized by administering 1 mg folic acid daily. Although methotrexate may inhibit folic acid metabolism, it does not seem to affect the efficacy of the therapy.

The most serious side effect of therapy is liver toxicity, which occurs more frequently in patients with diabetes, obesity, alcohol use, and existing liver disease. Women who wish to conceive should stop taking the drug for five ovulatory cycles before attempting to conceive. Women of childbearing age who are not sterilized should use a reliable form of contraception, because methotrexate has been implicated in spontaneous abortion and birth defects.

Pneumonitis is another potentially serious side effect of therapy. A baseline chest x-ray should be obtained, and patients should be instructed to report new onset of a dry cough, dyspnea, or fever. Methotrexate should be immediately discontinued if the patient has pulmonary problems, because immutable pulmonary damage may occur.

Baseline laboratory values should be obtained before initiation of therapy and should include a CBC and liver function, BUN, and serum creatinine tests. During therapy, these values should be monitored every 4 weeks; creatinine and albumin values should be monitored every 3 months. Decreasing albumin levels, even in the absence of creatinine changes, suggest liver dysfunction. A transient yet marked increase in serum aminotransferase levels may be seen, with stabilization occurring with continued treatment or dose reduction. If the AST or ALT persists at levels of two to three times the upper limit of normal, then methotrexate should be discontinued and a liver biopsy obtained.

Sulfasalazine

Like methotrexate, sulfasalazine (Azulfidine) is an effective DMARD that relieves symptoms relatively quickly. The best candidates for treatment are patients with significant synovitis. Before initiating sulfasalazine therapy, the practitioner needs to obtain baseline laboratory test values, including CBC and aminotransferases. The levels should be monitored every 2 weeks for 1 month after initiation of therapy, then monthly for 5 months. If laboratory values remain stable for the first 6 months of therapy, a CBC should be checked every 3 months.

Mechanism of Action

Sulfasalazine's mechanism of action is not clearly understood but is thought to be due to its conversion to sulfapyridine and 5-acetylsalicylic acid in the gut. Research has

Table 38.3

Overview of Selected Disease-Modifying Antirheumatic Drugs

Generic (Trade) Name and Dosage	Selected Adverse Events	Contraindications	Special Considerations
methotrexate (Rheumatrex) 7.5 mg/wk in single dose or 2.5 mg q12h, up to 22.5 mg/wk	GI effects, leukopenia, oral ulcers, thrombocytopenia, pulmonary toxicity, hepatotoxicity	Pregnancy and 5 mo before conception Caution in alcohol drinkers and liver disease	May take 3–6 wk to achieve clinical benefit Can induce spontaneous abortion and birth defects Monitoring includes CBC, serum creatinine, and liver function tests at 4- to 8-wk intervals.
sulfasalazine (Azulfidine) 500–1000 mg/d in divided doses; may increase up to maximum 2 g/d	GI effects, heartburn, dizziness, headache, rash, neutropenia, thrombocytopenia, orange-yellow color of skin	Contraindicated in intestinal or urinary obstruction Safety in pregnancy not established in RA treatment, although drug has proved safe in patients with inflammatory bowel disease in pregnancy	May take 3–6 wk to achieve clinical effect Causes reversible sterility in men; recommend that men cease therapy 90 d before starting a family Monitoring includes liver enzyme evaluation. CBC is necessary early in therapy but required less with prolonged use.
gold compounds *Injectable:* aurothioglucose (Solganal); gold sodium thiomalate (Myochrysine) 10 mg/wk IM, up to a total dose of 1 g; maintenance dose ~50 mg/mo *Oral:* auranofin (Ridaura) 3 mg bid	GI effects, rash, itching, stomatitis, vasomotor reactions, bone marrow suppression, nephritis, pneumonitis, exfoliative dermatitis, proteinuria	Uncontrolled diabetes Liver and renal disease, systemic lupus erythematosus, blood dyscrasias Lack of long-term studies in pregnant women, so not recommended during pregnancy or lactation	May take 6–8 wk for injectable form and 3–6 mo for oral form of drug to establish effectiveness Monitoring includes routine CBC with differential, platelet count; urinalysis to measure protein; renal and liver function tests.
hydroxychloroquine (Plaquenil) 400–600 mg/d in divided doses	GI effects, rash, CNS effects, ocular effects	Avoid in pregnancy and lactation.	Six months may be needed for clinical effect. Can trigger exacerbation of psoriasis Prolonged therapy may cause retinal damage. Monitoring should include periodic CBC and eye examination every 3–6 mo to monitor for retinal damage.
D-penicillamine (Depen, Cuprimine) 125 mg/d as single dose; may increase at monthly intervals to maximum daily dose of 1.5 g	GI effects, rash, itching, renal effects, autoimmune reactions, cytopenia	Not recommended in pregnancy or lactation—causes damage to fetal connective tissue	From 4 to 6 mo may be needed to establish clinical effect of therapy. Monitoring should include CBC with differential and platelets and urinalysis every 2–6 wk.
azathioprine (Imuran) 50–100 mg in single daily dose; can increase after 6–8 wk; 3.5 mg/kg is maximum daily dose	GI effects, bone marrow suppression, infection, hepatotoxicity, alopecia	Renal disease Avoid during pregnancy and lactation.	From 6 to 8 and up to 12 wk may be needed to establish clinical effect. Monitoring should include CBC with differential and platelets weekly for the first month, then biweekly for the second and third months, then monthly.
cyclophosphamide (Cytoxan, Neosar) 1 mg/kg/d increased to 2 mg/kg/d after 6 wk	Alopecia, hemorrhagic cystitis, sterility, GI effects, increased susceptibility to infection, thrombocytopenia	Contraindicated for RA during pregnancy and lactation	In renal impairment, decrease dose. Four months may be needed to establish clinical effect. Monitoring includes CBC with differential platelets, urinalysis for blood repeatedly, erythrocyte sedimentation rate, BUN, serum creatinine.
cyclosporin A (Sandimmune, Neoral) 5 mg/kg/d divided into 2 doses	Hypertension, tremor, nephrotoxicity, hepatotoxicity, increased susceptibility to infection, hyperkalemia	Contraindicated for RA during pregnancy and lactation	Approximately 8 wk may be needed to establish clinical effect. Decrease dose by 50% if hypertension or nephrotoxicity results. Monitoring includes CBC with differential, BUN, serum creatinine, serum bilirubin, liver enzymes repeatedly.

(continued)

Table 38.3

Overview of Selected Disease-Modifying Antirheumatic Drugs (*Continued*)

Generic (Trade) Name and Dosage	Selected Adverse Events	Contraindications	Special Considerations
etanercept (Enbrel) 25 mg SQ twice weekly	Upper respiratory tract infections, pain at the injection site, headache	Concurrent infections or hypersensitivity to etanercept	Use caution in patients predisposed to infection.
infliximab (Remicade) 3 mg/kg IV infusion at baseline, 2 wk, 6 wk, then every 8 wk thereafter	Urticaria, infusion reactions, dyspnea, hypotension	Concurrent infections or hypersensitivity to infliximab	Use caution in patients predisposed to infection.
adalimumab (Humira) 40 mg SQ every other week; 40 mg weekly as monotherapy	Redness, swelling, bruising, or pain at the site of injection, headache, upset stomach, diarrhea, infection, rash	Pregnancy; pre-existing infection	Comcomitant immunosuppressants can increase risk of serious infection.
anakinra (Kineret) 100 mg SQ daily	Redness, swelling, bruising, or pain at the site of injection, headache, upset stomach, diarrhea, infection, rash	Sensitivity to *Escherichia coli*-derived proteins; pre-existing infection	Routine monitoring of white blood cells is recommended; comcomitant immunosuppressants can increase risk of serious infection.
Leflunomide (Arava) 100 mg PO daily for 3 days; 20 mg daily thereafter	Diarrhea, hair loss, weight loss, rash, infection	Pregnancy	If 20 mg daily is not tolerated, then 10 mg daily may be used. Long half-life; cholestyramine will enhance elimination if agent is to be discontinued.

shown the anti-inflammatory features of this conversion, as well as its ability to decrease the production of inflammatory cytokines and the production of IgM RF.

Dosage

Sulfasalazine is available in oral form in 500-mg tablets. Dosing is started at 1,000 mg/day in two divided doses. The daily divided dose is gradually increased to 2,000 mg over 2 weeks. Therapeutic serum levels are usually attained in 4 to 5 days.

Time Frame for Response

Good response with a daily dose of 3,000 to 4,000 mg has been reported, but dosing should not be increased to this level until the patient has been taking 2,000 mg/day for at least 3 months and has some relief of symptoms. The potential for toxicity rises for patients taking these higher doses.

Adverse Events

The most common adverse reactions to sulfasalazine are dose dependent and include nausea and diarrhea. Other reported adverse events include dizziness, intestinal or urinary obstruction, oral ulcers, thrombocytopenia, orange-yellow pigmentation of the skin, headache, and depression. Any of these common side effects may become intolerable and cause discontinuation of the drug. Reversible sterility has been reported in men; therapy should be discontinued 3 months before attempting to father a child.

Agranulocytosis, the gravest adverse reaction to sulfasalazine, has been reported in fewer than 2% of patients, but it dictates immediate discontinuation of the drug.

Antimalarials

Historically, the antimalarials hydroxychloroquine (Plaquenil) and chloroquine have been used to treat arthritis. They are attractive because of their low side effect profile and high effectiveness. The drugs are discontinued in fewer than 9% of patients because of side effects. However, because these drugs cannot limit the progression of RA, they are currently used as an adjunct to methotrexate therapy or as single-agent therapy in early, mild RA without bone erosion.

Mechanism of Action

The antimalarials inhibit antigen processing by elevating cellular pH, which changes the degeneration of antigen. Thus, the presentation of the antigen to T cells is impaired. After absorption, these drugs concentrate in the retina, kidneys, bone marrow, and liver. The concentration of the drugs in specific organs dictates the regimen for baseline and ongoing monitoring of antimalarial therapy. Specifically, eye examinations should be performed every 6 to 12 months because of potential retinal accumulation of the drug. A CBC should be performed periodically.

Dosage

Hydroxychloroquine and chloroquine are available in oral form and are rapidly and completely absorbed. Dosing is calculated by patient weight, but the typical dosage for hydroxychloroquine is 200 mg twice daily or 400 mg daily.

Time Frame for Response

Therapeutic effects are usually noted within 2 to 6 months of treatment.

Contraindications

The antimalarials should not be used in pregnancy or during lactation. Patients with pre-existing retinal field changes should not use an antimalarial agent due to the ocular effects of long-term antimalarial therapy.

Adverse Effects

The most common adverse effects of the antimalarials are nausea, diarrhea, and abdominal discomfort. Less common side effects include photosensitivity and skin pigmentation. A maculopapular, pruritic rash encompassing the entire body may occur and cause extreme discomfort. Although neuromyopathy has been reported rarely, deep tendon reflexes should be monitored regularly for diminished activity.

Gold Compounds

Because of their high side effect profile, gold compounds are used much less frequently in treating RA, but they are an option for patients who have not responded to the previously mentioned drugs either alone or in combination.

Mechanism of Action

The mechanism of action of the gold compounds remains obscure, even though they have been used since the 1930s. It is thought that the gold compounds inhibit humoral immunity and decrease lysosomal enzyme release. The greatest effect seems to be reduction of lymphocyte, monocyte, and neutrophil activity (Gardner & Gilliland, 1998).

Dosage

Gold compounds are available in oral and injectable forms. Auranofin (Ridaura), the oral form of gold, is usually prescribed in a dosage of 3 mg twice daily; the maximum daily dose is 9 mg. The therapeutic response rate to gold compounds has been estimated at 30% to 50%.

Dosing of injectable gold sodium thiomalate (Myochrysine) should start at 10 mg. The dose is then increased to 25 mg 1 week later, and 50 mg in week 3. A weekly dose of 50 mg is continued for the next 20 weeks, bringing the total accumulated dose to 1,000 mg (1 g). At this point, the patient is evaluated for therapeutic response to the injectable form. If the patient reports symptom relief, treatment may continue with a dose of 50 mg every other week for an indefinite period. If substantial symptom relief has not occurred by 20 weeks, the drug should be discontinued.

Time Frame for Response

Oral gold therapy typically takes 4 to 6 months to produce a clear benefit. Injectable gold products may shorten this time, but only by 1 to 2 months. Almost 75% of patients discontinue therapy with gold compounds within 5 years because of inefficacy or toxicity.

Contraindications

Gold compounds should be used cautiously in patients with uncontrolled diabetes mellitus, liver or renal disease, systemic lupus erythematosus, and a history of blood dyscrasias. Gold compounds should not be prescribed for pregnant or lactating women because there is no scientific evidence that supports their safety during these periods (ACR, 1996b).

Adverse Events

The major systems that exhibit toxic effects are the hematologic, renal, and dermatologic systems. Oral gold compounds seem to be less toxic, but they are also less effective in symptom management. The rate of adverse reactions to gold therapy is approximately 35%.

Baseline and ongoing laboratory monitoring for patients on gold therapy is aimed at anticipating hematologic and renal reactions. Laboratory values should be measured at the time of the weekly gold injection and should include a CBC with differential and platelet count, alternating with a urinalysis. Liver function tests should also be performed periodically. With oral gold therapy, a monthly CBC and urinalysis is sufficient (ACR, 1996b; Moncur & Williams, 1995).

The most common adverse reactions to gold are transient and reversible and include itching, stomatitis, diarrhea, and skin reactions. More severe dermatitis should prompt the clinician to discontinue the therapy until the rash disappears, and then restart therapy at a lower dose.

Leukopenia, agranulocytosis, thrombocytopenia, and anemia are the most common hematologic side effects. Thrombocytopenia usually appears abruptly, whereas granulocytopenia may develop more gradually. Aplastic anemia associated with gold therapy is usually associated with a high mortality rate. The hematologic side effects are usually transient and require little more than treatment with glucocorticoids. Decrease in any cell count on the CBC should prompt the clinician to discontinue gold therapy (ACR, 1996b; Moncur & Williams, 1995).

Rare but potentially serious side effects include exfoliative dermatitis and nephrotic syndrome. Although transient proteinuria is common, an increase in urinary protein to more than 300 mg in 24 hours is cause for discontinuation of therapy; treatment can be prudently restarted once the urine clears.

Azathioprine

Azathioprine (Imuran) is an alternative agent that is usually reserved for patients who do not respond to methotrexate, sulfasalazine, and gold compounds. It is a purine agonist and is not indicated for initial DMARD treatment. Baseline and ongoing monitoring should include CBC with differential and platelet count and liver function tests weekly for the first month of therapy, then biweekly for the second and third months. If these profiles remain stable, monitoring can be decreased to monthly serum values (ACR, 1996b). Azathioprine interferes with the synthesis of adenine and guanine. It suppresses T-cell function, leading to the inhibition of leukocyte proliferation.

Dosage

Azathioprine is available in oral form. Dosing is based on patient weight and is initiated at 1 to 1.25 mg/kg/day (50 to 100 mg). The maximum daily dose is 2.5 mg/kg. Peak effect is usually attained in 6 to 12 weeks.

Adverse Events

The most common side effects include nausea, vomiting, oral ulcers, alopecia, and skin rash. The side effects may be diminished by reducing the dosage or by discontinuing the drug completely (ACR, 1996b).

The most serious side effect of azathioprine therapy is hematologic toxicity: leukopenia, thrombocytopenia, and anemia have been reported. If the white blood cell count drops to less than 3,000/mm³, azathioprine should be discontinued (ACR, 1996b).

A hypersensitivity reaction to azathioprine has been reported consisting of fever, arthralgias, hypertension, and hepatotoxicity. Again, azathioprine therapy should be stopped if this occurs.

Interactions

Caution should be exercised in prescribing azathioprine to patients taking allopurinol therapy. Because azathioprine metabolism is inhibited by allopurinol, these patients require a much smaller dose of azathioprine (approximately 25% of the usual dose). Azathioprine should be avoided during pregnancy and lactation, as well as in patients with known renal disease (ACR, 1996b).

Cyclosporine

Cyclosporine (Sandimmune, Neoral) is approved for RA treatment either as a single agent or in combination with methotrexate. Its immunosuppressant effect is derived from the inhibition of T-cell cytokines. Specifically, cyclosporine inhibits transcription of interleukin-2, a crucial activator of T-cell activity (Kellick et al., 1998).

Dosage

Cyclosporine is available in oral form. Dosing is based on patient weight and is started at 2.5 to 5 mg/kg/day in two divided doses. The dosage may be gradually increased to the upper threshold based on symptom resolution. Therapeutic effects are usually seen within 8 weeks of therapy.

Baseline and ongoing monitoring includes CBC with differential, blood pressure, and serum bilirubin, liver enzymes, and creatinine measurement. Blood pressure should be measured weekly during initial dosage adjustment and again after any dosage increase. Laboratory values are measured biweekly for the first 4 weeks, then monthly for 6 months and then every 3 months after dose stabilization. Cyclosporine is contraindicated during pregnancy and lactation.

Adverse Events

The most common side effects of cyclosporine include nausea, vomiting, diarrhea, abdominal pain, and headaches. Hypertrichosis, gingival hyperplasia, tremor, increased susceptibility to infection, and hyperkalemia have also been reported. These adverse reactions usually subside with dose reduction and a gradual return to therapeutic dosing levels.

The most serious side effects are nephrotoxicity and hypertension. Nephrotoxicity is dose related and occurs at dosages of more than 5 mg/day. A rise in the serum creatinine level is anticipated with cyclosporine therapy; the level may be as high as 25% above the normal range. Nephrotoxicity has been reported more frequently in patients concomitantly taking NSAIDs. It is not clear whether the nephrotoxic

effects are reversible. The daily dose should be decreased by 50% in patients who experience nephrotoxicity or hypertension. Patients experiencing hypertension on cyclosporine therapy may need to take antihypertensive medication.

Baseline and ongoing monitoring includes CBC with differential and platelet count and urinalysis; these tests are repeated every 2 weeks for the first 6 weeks, then monthly.

D-Penicillamine

D-Penicillamine (Depen, Cuprimine) can inhibit T-cell–mediated immunity by obstructing the conversion of monocytes to macrophages (Firestein, 1998; Kellick et al., 1998). D-Penicillamine is available in oral form. Dosing is started at 125 to 250 mg/day in a single dose for 3 months. The dose may then be increased to 500 mg/day for another 3 months. If no results are achieved at this dose, the drug should be discontinued because efficacy is probably not present. If partial efficacy is realized, the dose can be gradually increased by 125 mg every 2 to 3 months to a maximum daily dose of 1.5 g. Once therapeutic results are achieved at the higher dose, the dosage can be gradually decreased to 500 mg/day.

Because of its toxic side effect profile, D-penicillamine use has dramatically declined since approximately 1980. The most common adverse effects include rash, itching, and a change in taste sensation. Serious hematologic side effects include leukopenia, thrombocytopenia, and aplastic anemia. D-Penicillamine should be stopped if the patient has a white blood cell count of less than 3,000/mm³ or a platelet count of less than 100,000/mm³ (ACR, 1996b).

Proteinuria may herald the onset of glomerulonephritis or nephrotic syndrome. D-Penicillamine should be discontinued in patients with proteinuria in excess of 1 g/24 hours, measured via quantitative urinary protein levels. These levels should be obtained every 1 to 2 weeks as indicated by the patient's signs and symptoms. Any blood in the urine is also cause for discontinuing D-penicillamine.

Additional adverse events include various autoimmune syndromes, such as Goodpasture syndrome, myasthenia gravis, polymyositis, systemic lupus erythematosus, pemphigoid, and Sjögren syndrome. Adverse reactions usually present within the first 18 months of therapy. D-Penicillamine should not be used during pregnancy or lactation because it is known to damage fetal connective tissue (ACR, 1996b).

Cyclophosphamide

Cyclophosphamide (Cytoxan, Neosar) can relieve the inflammatory symptoms of RA as well as inhibiting the bony progression of the disease by reducing the development of new joint erosions. Cyclophosphamide is derived from nitrogen mustard and is cytotoxic. Its mechanism of action is based on its ability to decrease the levels of circulating T and B cells. Cyclophosphamide is indicated in patients who have not responded to the aforementioned drugs but who have severe disease (Kellik et al, 1998; Moncur & Williams, 1995).

Cyclophosphamide is available in oral form. Dosing is based on patient weight and is started at 1 mg/kg/day. After 6 weeks, the dose is doubled to 2 mg/kg/day. Peak effect is usually seen by 4 months of treatment. Baseline and ongoing monitoring of patients should include CBC with differential and platelet count, urinalysis, BUN, serum creatinine, and

ESR (ACR, 1996b). Cyclophosphamide is contraindicated in pregnancy and lactation (ACR, 1996b).

Adverse reactions usually involve the hematologic and renal systems. A major side effect of cyclophosphamide is hemorrhagic cystitis. Patients should take cyclophosphamide in the morning and should drink at least 3 L of fluid daily. Additional side effects include alopecia, sterility, nausea, thrombocytopenia, sterility, and increased susceptibility to infection.

Immunomodulators

The immune system has long been implicated in the development and progression of RA. Drugs that affect the major components of the system, the monocytes, B and T cells, and complement, can decrease the destructive processes of RA. These immunomodulating drugs decrease the activity of these cells directly or inhibit the cytokines that promote communication among these cells.

Leflunomide

A new immunomodulator recently approved for RA treatment, leflunomide (Arava) exerts both anti-inflammatory and antiproliferative actions, retarding erosions and joint space narrowing. It is a prodrug that undergoes rapid conversion to its active metabolite. The metabolite has a half-life of 15 to 18 days, with extensive enterohepatic recirculation.

Mechanism of Action

The drug is a competitive inhibitor of dihydrofolate reductase. This inhibition decreases the production of pyrimidines (amino acid building blocks), decreasing the proliferation of B and T lymphocytes. This action is similar to methotrexate, making this agent a reasonable alternative to patients who cannot tolerate or who have an inadequate response to methotrexate. Since leflunomide inhibits pyrimidine synthesis and methotrexate inhibits purine synthesis, these agents may be used in combination.

Dosage

Since the half-life of the drug is so long, therapy with leflunomide is usually initiated with a 100-mg loading dose for 3 days, and then the agent is continued at 20 mg/day if tolerated. If the side effects are too severe, the dose can be lowered to 10 mg/day.

Time Frame for Response

Benefit from leflunomide can be seen as early as 4 weeks but may take up to 3 months.

Contraindications

Like other disease-modifying agents, leflunomide is contraindicated in pregnancy. Since the half-life is so long, a typical washout period for women who wish to conceive is about 2 years. However, agents interrupting the enterohepatic recirculation (eg, activated charcoal or cholestyramine) can be used to reduce the half-life of the metabolite to about

1 day. The dosing of cholestyramine, as recommended by the manufacturer, is 8 g/day for 11 days.

Due to the hepatotoxicity, patients with a history of alcoholism or with pre-existing liver disease should not receive leflunomide.

Adverse Reactions

About 5% of patients receiving leflunomide monotherapy have elevated liver enzymes. While this number appears low, there are reports of more than 10 patients dying while on leflunomide therapy; the deaths are thought to be related to the hepatotoxicity of the agent.

The side effect profile also includes GI symptoms, weight loss, alopecia, and hypertension. Minor decreases in hemoglobin and hematocrit were also found.

Interactions

Leflunomide is an inhibitor of the CYP2C9 enzyme and therefore may increase the levels of agents metabolized through this pathway.

Tumor Necrosis Factor Antagonists

Etanercept, infliximab, and adalimumab are tumor necrosis factor alpha (TNF-alpha) inhibitors used in RA treatment. These agents are often used in combination with methotrexate to further reduce the signs and symptoms of RA.

Mechanism of Action

These agents act by binding the circulating TNF-alpha. TNF-alpha has been found in the joints of RA patients, and increased levels in the joints are associated with reduced function. By binding to TNF-alpha, these agents reduce the chemotactic effect of TNF-alpha by reducing interleukin-6 and C-reactive protein. This in turn reduces the infiltration of inflammatory cells into joints. Also, when these agents bind to surface TNF-alpha, cell lysis occurs.

Dosage

All three of these agents are injectables. Etanercept is self-administered at 25 mg twice weekly subcutaneously as monotherapy. Infliximab is administered intravenously at a dose of 3 to 5 mg every 4 weeks or 3 to 10 mg every 8 weeks. Infliximab is usually started at 3 mg at week 0, then another dose 2 weeks later, then another dose 4 weeks later, then every 4 to 8 weeks. Typically, infliximab is administered in conjunction with methotrexate because infliximab antibodies develop when administered as monotherapy. Adalimumab is given at 40 mg every other week as a subcutaneous injection. Adalimumab may be administered concomitantly with methotrexate, glucocorticoids, or NSAIDs. It may also be used as monotherapy; typically the dose for monotherapy is 40 mg weekly.

Time Frame for Response

All of the TNF inhibitors produce a rapid response, within days to weeks.

Contraindications

Patients should be assessed at baseline for infections or risk factors for infections. There have been reports of tuberculosis developing in patients taking infliximab; the theory is that the immunomodulation allows latent TB to flare. This usually occurs within the first 2 to 5 months of therapy. Other serious infections have also occurred with these agents, and careful consideration of the patient's history is important when prescribing them.

Adverse Events

Side effects include injection site reactions (etanercept and adalimumab) or infusion reactions (infliximab). Caution must be used when administering these agents to patients predisposed to infection. Sepsis and fatal infections have occurred in patients receiving TNF-alpha blocking agents. If a patient develops an infection while taking a TNF-alpha blocking agent, the agent should be discontinued until the infection resolves.

Anakinra

Anakinra (Kineret) is the recombinant form of human interleukin-1 receptor antagonist, except for the replacement of methionine at one of the N-terminals.

Mechanism of Action

The levels of naturally occurring interleukin-1 receptor antagonist are generally lower in RA patients. It is thought that this lower level of endogenous substance allows for interleukin-1 to promote inflammation. By exogenously providing this antagonist to RA patients, the joint inflammation process is interrupted.

Dosage

Anakinra is given as 100 mg subcutaneously daily. In patients with severe renal dysfunction (creatinine clearance below 30 mL/min), it should be administered every other day. Anakinra is supplied in prefilled syringes containing 0.67 mL (100 mg)

of drug. These syringes must be kept refrigerated and should not be frozen or shaken.

Time Frame for Response

In patients who responded to anakinra, the effect was seen within 12 weeks of initiation of therapy.

Contraindications

The primary contraindication to anakinra is sensitivity to *Escherichia coli*-derived proteins. Similar to the other immunomodulators, pre-existing infection or risk of infection may be a contraindication since there is an increased risk of bacterial infection in patients taking anakinra. Anakinra should not be administered in combination with etanercept due to the increased risk of infection.

Adverse Events

The most common adverse effect of anakinra is skin irritation at the injection site. This occurs in more than half the patients and usually resolves within a few weeks.

Patients also may experience a decrease in white blood cells. Routine monitoring of these is recommended at baseline and then monthly for the first 3 months, then quarterly for the first year.

Interactions

No known pharmacokinetic drug interactions exist. Pharmacodynamically, agents that suppress the immune system should be used with caution, if at all, due to the increased risk of serious infections.

Selecting the Most Appropriate Agent

In selecting a DMARD or combining DMARDs, the clinician needs to consider the toxicities of the medications, including the interactions with other prescribed drugs. Some patients may have difficulty adhering to the monitoring requirements for some of the more toxic drugs. Other patients may not be able to adhere to a strict dosing schedule. In addition, the time required to achieve benefit can be protracted with certain

---

Table 38.4

Recommended Order of Treatment for Rheumatoid Arthritis

Order	Agents	Comments
First line	DMARD (eg, methotrexate) along with NSAID	Continue NSAID alone as long as symptoms are limited to morning stiffness. Initiate with progression of disease; continue NSAID for anti-inflammatory effect.
Second line	Addition of corticosteroids (eg, prednisone)	May help slow the progression of joint erosions; can also be used for intermittent flare-ups. Consider estrogen replacement and calcium and vitamin D supplements in postmenopausal women.
	Combination therapy with DMARD	Add a second DMARD or immunomodulator.
Third line	Hydroxychloroquinine	Begin third-line therapy if second-line therapy is ineffective after 6 mo.
	Gold compound	Choice of drug depends on possible drug toxicities, time to expected benefit, and comorbid conditions.
	Sulfasalazine	Depends on size of joint(s) involved
	Intra-articular corticosteroids	Effects usually last an average of 3 mo. Repeated use may increase cartilage destruction.

DMARDs, which may be unacceptable to the patient. Finally, the cost of the various therapies varies widely. The DMARDs currently approved for treatment of RA are described in Table 38-4.

The selection of therapies depends on the stage of disease, comorbidities, and response to prior therapies. Early RA is usually treated with NSAIDs until the full diagnosis of RA is made. Once the diagnosis is established, a DMARD should be started. The clinician needs to adjust the DMARD dose or attempt combinations of drugs based on the patient's response, bone erosion, and toxicity. Flares of RA are best treated with both intra-articular and oral corticosteroids.

Appropriate drug choices for RA therapy proceed in accordance with the progression of disease. Like OA treatment, RA treatment begins with analgesics and NSAIDs and continues with NSAIDs and DMARDs and possibly corticosteroids, and, as needed, antimalarial agents, gold, sulfasalazine, corticosteroids, and immunomodulators may be tried. Table 38-4 and Figure 38-4 review the recommended order of treatment.

Special Populations

Geriatric

Caution should be used when starting elderly patients on NSAIDs due to the increased risk of GI hemorrhage. Further, many elderly patients have decreased renal function, and NSAIDs may contribute to a decline in this function. Several DMARDs and some immunomodulators are renally excreted, and doses should be adjusted in the elderly due to their decreased renal function.

Pediatric

In children, aspirin therapy is stopped if the child is exposed to varicella or influenza because of the risk for Reye's syndrome. Also, children receiving vaccinations may have a diminished response if they are taking immunomodulators such as anakinra.

Women

Women considering pregnancy should stop taking DMARDs and immunomodulating agents since many of these agents are teratogenic. At least five half-lives of the drug should pass before the woman attempts to conceive. For leflunomide, cholestyramine-assisted elimination should be used to shorten the half-life of the agent. Women should use effective contraception while taking these agents.

MONITORING PATIENT RESPONSE

Because the drugs used for treating arthritis have many adverse effects and because most are used for long-term treatment, monitoring should include baseline studies against which later results can be compared. CBC with differential, urinalysis, creatinine, serum bilirubin, liver enzymes, ESR, BUN, platelet studies, and eye examinations are among the tests performed periodically during therapy.

PATIENT EDUCATION

Patient education depends on the type of agent selected. The patient should know that routine blood work is important to detect adverse events before they become serious and life-threatening. Patients taking DMARDs and immunomodulators should report illness immediately, as the risk of serious infections is increased in these patients.

Patient-Oriented Information Sources

Support groups, education of family members, and assistive devices can help with activities of daily living. The American Rheumatism Association (800-282-7023) can provide information and assistance. The National Institutes of Health (NIH), in conjunction with the American Society of Health-System Pharmacists (ASHP) and the United States Pharmacopeia (USP), has a drug information website with information about thousands of medications (http://www.nlm.nih.gov/medlineplus/druginformation.html).

Nutrition/Lifestyle Changes

Weight loss programs and healthy habits such as adequate rest are key to the success of a treatment program. Patients should consider occupational therapy as needed to help with household chores. The patient should avoid repetitive joint motion and vibrations from electrical appliances or tools to reduce

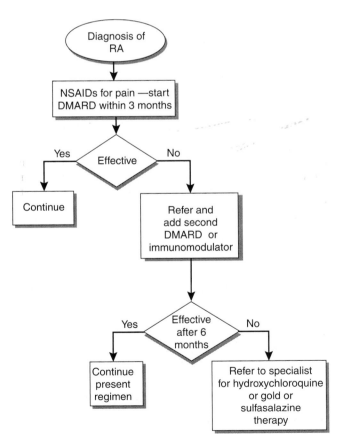

Key ⬭ Starting point for decision making; ▭ clinical actions (assessing, prescribing, monitoring); ◇ decision point.

Figure 38–4 Treatment algorithm for rheumatoid arthritis (RA).

exacerbations. Splinting the affected joint helps relieve pain and prevent deformity. Patients should remove the splint at least once daily and for any exercise activities. Patients should be instructed on strategies to avoid physical and emotional stress, which may precipitate an exacerbation.

Complementary and Alternative Medications

Folk remedies have been used for RA for many years. Although most of these remedies cause no harm, there is little scientific evidence supporting their efficacy. Some of the more commonly used approaches include shark cartilage, chondroitin, herbs, vitamins, acupuncture, magnet therapy, climate therapy, and a variety of diets. Clinicians should be aware of the therapies being considered or used by the patient; joint treatment goals should be established and monitored. Just as in traditional medicine, patients using complementary approaches either alone or as adjunctive therapy require ongoing monitoring for safety and efficacy of the selected approach.

Chiropractic treatment has helped many patients with RA, and more insurance carriers are reimbursing for chiropractic services. Chiropractic treatment as an adjunct to traditional measures should be viewed as mainstream therapy.

A recent review of the literature suggests that gamma-linolenic acid (GLA) may have a moderate effect on reducing pain and joint tenderness. This agent is found in borage seed oil (9% GLA), black currant oil (6% GLA), or evening primrose oil (2% GLA). The dose should be about 540 mg/day of GLA.

■ Case Study 1

J.W., a 46-year-old African-American woman, presents to your office with the chief complaint of bilateral stiffness of the shoulders, hands, and wrists in the morning. She reports she is otherwise healthy, takes no medications, and is employed as a systems analyst for a large bank. She recalls having some minor flu-like symptoms approximately 3 weeks before her visit. The stiffness makes it difficult for her to work for any extended period. She has also started wearing a wig because she cannot raise her arms in the morning to fix her hair. She has lost 10 pounds over the past 8 months but has not consciously dieted. She finds it increasingly difficult to drive, particularly when making turns and driving in reverse.

Diagnosis: Rheumatoid arthritis of the shoulders, hands, and wrists

1. List specific goals of treatment for J.W.
2. Which NSAID and which DMARD (assuming RA is confirmed) would you prescribe, and why?
3. How would you monitor J.W. in terms of efficacy and adverse effects? Specifically, what laboratory tests would you order?
4. List one or two adverse reactions for the selected agent that would cause you to change therapy.
5. If the above occurred, what would be the choice for second-line therapy, and why?
6. Discuss specific patient education based on your first-line therapy choices.
7. Describe one or two drug/drug or drug/food interactions for both the NSAID and the DMARD.
8. What dietary and lifestyle changes should be recommended for J.W.?
9. What over-the-counter and/or alternative medications would be appropriate for J.W.?

■ Case Study 2

G.P., a 66-year-old, right-handed white man, seeks treatment for swelling and decreased range of motion in the third finger of his right hand. He tells you he retired at age 65 after 40 years of assembly-line work. He reports that his physical activity has decreased and his weight has increased 20 pounds since retiring. His hobbies include woodworking and playing cards.

Although he describes several years of joint pain that gradually worsened, his activities were not limited until approximately 6 months ago, when he noted an insidious onset of swelling in the right third DIP joint. Over the years, he has sporadically taken acetaminophen, aspirin, and ibuprofen to control the pain. He reports that none of the drugs provided better relief than the others. He is concerned that he will continue to lose movement in the finger that is already affected, as well as in the fingers of his left hand. His medical history is remarkable for hypertension and three episodes of gout.

Diagnosis: Osteoarthritis

1. List specific goals of treatment for G.P.

2. What drug therapy would you prescribe, and why?

3. How would you monitor in terms of efficacy and adverse effects? Specifically, what laboratory tests would you order for G.P.?

4. List one or two adverse reactions for the selected agent that would cause you to change therapy.

5. If the above occurred, what would be the choice for the second-line therapy, and why?

6. Discuss specific patient education based on your first-line therapy choice.

7. Describe one or two drug/drug or drug/food interactions for your chosen drug therapy.

8. What dietary and lifestyle changes should be recommended for this patient?

9. What over-the-counter and/or alternative medications would be appropriate for G.P.?

Bibliography

Starred entries are cited in text.

*American College of Rheumatology Ad Hoc Committee on Clinical Guidelines. (1996b). Guidelines for monitoring drug therapy in rheumatoid arthritis. *Arthritis and Rheumatism, 39,* 723–731.

American College of Rheumatology (2000). Recommendations for the medical management of osteoarthritis of the hip and knee. *Arthritis and Rheumatism, 43*(9), 1905–1915.

American College of Rheumatology (2002). Guidelines for the management of rheumatoid arthritis. *Arthritis and Rheumatism, 46*(2), 328–346.

*Blackburn, W. D. (1996). Management of osteoarthritis and rheumatoid arthritis: prospects and possibilities. *American Journal of Medicine, 100*(Suppl.), 24S–30S.

Easton, B. T. (2001). Evaluation and treatment of the patient with osteoarthritis. *Journal of Family Practice, 50*(9), 791–797.

*Firestein, G. S. (1998). Rheumatoid arthritis. *Scientific American, 21,* 1–14.

*Gardner, G. C., & Gilliland, B. C. (1998). Rheumatoid disorders. In E. B. Larsen & P. G. Ramsey (Eds.), *Medical therapeutics* (3rd ed., pp. 790–794). Philadelphia: Lippincott-Raven.

*Hawkey, C. J., Karrasch, J. A., Szczepanski, L., Walker, D. G., Barkun, A, Swannell, A. J., & Yeomans, N. D. (1998). Omeprazole compared with misoprostol for ulcers associated with nonsteroidal antiinflammatory drugs. *New England Journal of Medicine, 338,* 727–734.

*Kellick, K. A., Martins-Richards, J., & Chow, C. (1998). Management of arthritis. *Primary Care Practice, 2*(1), 66–80.

*Marlowe, S. M. (1998). Evaluating rheumatic complaints. *Primary Care Practice, 2*(1), 3–19.

*Moncur, C., & Williams, H. J. (1995). Rheumatoid arthritis: status of drug therapies. *Physical Therapy, 75,* 511–525.

Oddis, C. V. (1996). New perspectives on osteoarthritis. *American Journal of Medicine, 100,* 10S–15S.

O'Dell, J. R. (1996). Rheumatoid arthritis: when more than one DMARD is needed. *Journal of Musculoskeletal Medicine, 13*(12), 21–28.

O'Dell, J. R. (2004). Drug therapy: therapeutic strategies for rheumatoid arthritis. *New England Journal of Medicine, 350*(25), 2591–2602.

Olsen, N. J., & Stein, C. M. (2004). Drug therapy: new drugs for rheumatoid arthritis. *New England Journal of Medicine, 350*(21), 2167–2179.

*Ross, C. (1997). A comparison of osteoarthritis and rheumatoid arthritis. *Nurse Practitioner, 22,* 20–39.

Soeken, K. K., Miller, S. A., & Ernst, E. (2003). Herbal medicines for the treatment of rheumatoid arthritis. *Rheumatology, 42*(5), 652–659.

*Yeomans, N. D., Tulassay, Z., Laszlo, J., Racz, I., Howard, J. M., van Rensburg, C. J., Swannell, A. J., & Hawkey, C. J. (1998). A comparison of omeprazole with ranitidine for ulcers associated with nonsteroidal anti-inflammatory drugs. *New England Journal of Medicine, 338,* 719–726.

Visit the Connection web site for the most up-to-date drug information.

OSTEOPOROSIS

■ VIRGINIA P. ARCANGELO

Osteoporosis is a progressive systemic disease characterized by a decrease in bone mass and microarchitectural deterioration of bone tissue, resulting in bone fragility and increased susceptibility to fractures. More than 44 million American women over 50 and 14 million men are at risk for osteoporosis, with an estimated 61 million by the year 2020. The estimated national direct expenditures (hospitals and nursing homes) for osteoporotic and associated fractures was $17 billion in 2001 ($47 million each day), and the cost is rising (National Osteoporosis Foundation, 2004).

Bone fracture is the major cause of mortality and morbidity in patients with osteoporosis. The most common fractures are vertebral compression fractures and fractures of the distal radius and proximal femur. One in two women and one in eight men older than 50 years of age will have an osteoporosis-related fracture in their lifetimes.

CAUSES

The three types of osteoporosis are postmenopausal, senile, and secondary (Box 39-1). Many risk factors are associated with osteoporosis (Box 39-2).

Skeletal growth and the majority of bone mass are achieved during the first two decades of life, with bone density peaking around age 30. Between the ages of 30 and menopause, bone mass remains relatively stable. At menopause women have a period of 5 or more years during which there is an accelerated rate of bone loss. Some women lose up to 5% of their bone mass per year during this time.

PATHOPHYSIOLOGY

Two types of bone are discerned at the macroscopic level: cortical bone and trabecular bone. Cortical bone has a dense structure, whereas trabecular bone has a spongy appearance. Long bones have a thick outer layer of cortical bone and a thin inner layer of trabecular bone, whereas short bones consist of mostly trabecular bone with a thin layer of cortical bone.

Bone is in a constant state of remodeling (re-forming). Osteoblasts are responsible for bone formation, osteoclasts for bone resorption. A balance is normally achieved between osteoblast and osteoclast activity. When bone resorption occurs at a faster rate than bone remodeling, osteoporosis is

the result because the bones then become brittle and prone to fracture. Bone loss is greater in trabecular bone than in cortical bone.

Maximal mineral content of cortical bone occurs between the second and fourth decades of life, followed by a slow decline. In general, women have less bone mass than men, so even a small loss is more significant in women. Cortical bone loss in women is approximately 3% per decade until menopause, when the rate of bone loss accelerates to 9% per decade. Women lose approximately 15% of trabecular bone during the first 5 to 7 years after menopause. The rate returns to normal approximately 20 years after menopause. Generalized bone loss in men occurs at a rate of approximately 4% per decade throughout life.

Diagnostic Criteria

Medical history and a drug history are essential in the diagnosis. Bone mineral density (BMD) is related to bone mass at maturity and subsequent bone loss. Dual-energy x-ray absorptiometry (DEXA scan) measures BMD and is used to diagnose osteoporosis. A BMD of –1 to –2.5 standard deviations (SD) signifies osteopenia. A BMD of –2.5 SD, or lower than the mean for a normal 30-to-35-year-old woman, is diagnostic of osteoporosis. Screening is recommended for all women older than 65 years and for younger postmenopausal women or men who have any risk factors. For every decrease in bone mass of 1 SD, the relative risk of fracture increases by 1.5 to 3.

INITIATING DRUG THERAPY

Prevention of osteoporosis should begin early in life with adequate intake of calcium and vitamin D. Children 9 to 18 years of age should consume 1,300 mg of calcium daily. Adults 19 to 50 years of age need 1,000 mg of calcium per day, and those 51 years of age and older require 1,200 mg each day. Because it is difficult to ingest that amount, supplements are usually needed. Weight-bearing exercise enhances bone mass and thereby helps prevent osteoporosis. Alcohol intake should be minimal, and those who smoke should stop.

Drugs used for the prevention and treatment of osteoporosis decrease bone resorption. They are called resorption-inhibiting

BOX 39–1. TYPES OF OSTEOPOROSIS

Type I: Postmenopausal Osteoporosis
Occurs in postmenopausal women between 51 and 75 years of age

Decreased estrogen causes an accelerated rate of bone loss, especially trabecular bone loss.

The most common fractures are of the vertebrae and distal femur. There is also tooth loss.

Type II: Senile Osteoporosis
Occurs in men and women older than 70 years of age

There is a proportional loss of cortical and trabecular bone.

The most common fractures are hip, pelvic, and vertebral.

Type III: Secondary Osteoporosis
Occurs in men and women at any age

Secondary to other conditions such as drug therapy and other diseases

Goals of Drug Therapy

The goals of drug therapy are minimizing bone loss, delaying the progression of osteoporosis, and preventing fractures and fracture-related morbidity and mortality. Once osteoporosis is diagnosed and drug therapy is started, it is continued for life. Table 39-1 provides an overview of the drugs used in treatment.

Calcium Supplements

Sufficient calcium is necessary for the prevention of osteoporosis. Postmenopausal women should take 1,200 to 1,500 mg of calcium a day. Calcium is absorbed most effectively when taken in small amounts throughout the day. Patients should not take calcium with meals that are high in fiber or with bulk-forming laxatives because such materials decrease absorption. The OTC antacid Tums is an excellent and inexpensive source of calcium.

Most brand-name calcium products are absorbed easily in the body. If the product information does not state that it is absorbable, how well a tablet dissolves can be determined by placing it in a small amount of warm water for 30 minutes, stirring occasionally. If it hasn't dissolved within this

drugs and include estrogens, bisphosphonates, calcitonin, and selective estrogen receptor modulators (SERMs). When these drugs are given, the rate of bone resorption decreases within weeks and bone formation increases within months. Remodeling spaces fill in and an increase of BMD of 5% to 10% occurs with treatment. This process takes 2 to 3 years.

The National Osteoporosis Risk Assessment (NORA) Program was initiated to gather information on women at risk for osteoporosis and fracture. More than 200,000 women were enrolled in a comprehensive osteoporosis education and risk-assessment program. Data on the women recorded the incidence of osteopenia, osteoporosis, and fractures and provided information on risk factors. It showed that health care providers are not adequately identifying women who have low bone mass and thus a higher risk of fractures. The study found that almost half of the postmenopausal women enrolled had low bone mass; 7% of the participants were found to have osteoporosis and nearly 40% had osteopenia. During the 1-year follow-up period, the rate of bone fracture was four times higher for women with osteoporosis and twice as high for women with low bone mass compared to women with normal bone density (Siris, Miller, Barret-Conner, et al., 2001). This study reinforced the need to initiate medical treatment for women who already have osteoporosis, but it is less clear what the recommendations should be for women who have osteopenia but who are not yet osteoporotic. If recommendations were made that all the patients in this group should begin treatment, many women who are at risk for fracture would be captured, but many women would also receive treatment unnecessarily, as the NORA data suggested that nearly half the total population of women have either osteoporosis or osteopenia. To treat everyone would be unnecessary and too costly.

BOX 39–2. RISK FACTORS FOR OSTEOPOROSIS

Female sex
Older age
Asian or white race
Family history
Petite stature
Low body weight
Amenorrhea
Menopause (either natural or surgical) without hormone replacement
Sedentary lifestyle
Low calcium intake
Excess alcohol intake
Smoking
Excess caffeine intake
Low testosterone level in men
Drugs
    Thyroid replacement drugs
    Lithium
    Glucocorticoids
    Anticonvulsants
    Chemotherapy
    Heparin
Disease states
    Anorexia/bulimia
    Cushing's syndrome
    Thyrotoxicosis
    Rheumatoid arthritis
    Type 1 diabetes mellitus
    Thalassemia

Table 39.1

Overview of Selected Agents Used to Prevent or Treat Osteoporosis

Generic (Trade) Name and Dosage	Selected Adverse Events	Contraindications	Special Considerations
Bisphosphonates			
alendronate (Fosamax) Prevention: 5 mg/d or 35 mg once a week Treatment: 10 mg/d or 70 mg once a week	GI upset, abdominal pain, gastroesophageal reflux disease, esophagitis, headache	Esophageal abnormalities, inability to be upright for 30 min, hypocalcemia, creatinine clearance <30	Swallow whole. Take with 8 oz. of water 30 min before eating or drinking. Sit or stand for 30 min after taking (do not lie down until after eating). Calcium supplements and aluminum- or magnesium-containing antacids may interfere with absorption, so should be given at a different time.
risedronate (Actonel) 5 mg/d or 35 mg once a week	Arthralgia, GI disturbances, headache, abdominal pain, rash, edema, chest pain, bone pain, dizziness, leg cramps, infection	Same as above	Same as above This drug is more tolerable for patients with GI problems than alendronate.
Selective Estrogen Receptor Modulators			
raloxifene (Evista) 60 mg qd	Hot flashes, leg cramps	Pregnancy, history of thromboembolic events	Medication is to be stopped 72 h before surgery or prolonged immobilization.
Other			
calcitonin (Miacalcin) 200 units (one spray) daily 100 units IM or SC daily	Rhinitis, GI upset, back pain, facial flushing (with injection)	Allergy to salmon or fish products, lactation Caution in renal deficiencies	Perform periodic nasal examinations to check for ulceration. Stop if nasal ulceration results. Switch nostrils each day. Injection recommended at bedtime because of possible facial flushing and nausea
Hormone Modifiers			
teriparatide (Forteo) 20 mcg daily SC	Hypercalcemia, dizziness, hyperuricemia, leg cramps, nausea, arthralgia	Paget's disease, previous bone radiation, skeletal malignancy, hypercalcemia, hyperparathyroidism; caution with kidney stones	Used in women with a high risk of fracture or who have failed other therapies

time it probably will not dissolve in the stomach. Chewable and liquid calcium supplements dissolve well because they are broken down before they enter the stomach. Calcium carbonate is absorbed best when taken with food. Calcium citrate can be taken any time. Calcium, whether from the diet or supplements, is absorbed best by the body when it is taken several times a day in amounts of 500 mg or less, but taking it all at once is better than not taking it at all.

While calcium supplements are a satisfactory option for many people, certain preparations may cause side effects, such as gas or constipation, in some individuals. If simple measures such as increased fluids and fiber intake do not solve the problem, another form of calcium should be tried. Also, it is important to increase supplement intake gradually; take 500 mg/day for a week, then add more calcium slowly.

Vitamin D is responsible for the maintenance of an adequate concentration of calcium and phosphorus in the extracellular fluid. It also works with parathyroid hormone to regulate calcium movement across the gastrointestinal (GI) tract. Supplemental vitamin D (400 to 800 units) should be taken daily when calcium supplements are taken.

Hormone Replacement Therapy

For many years, hormone therapy had been the sole FDA-approved pharmacologic therapy for the prevention and

treatment of osteoporosis. The recent report from the Women's Health Initiative (WHI) study on hormone therapy provides the first large-scale, randomized controlled trial for the use of estrogen in preventing osteoporosis. Results from the study showed that hormone therapy reduced the incidence of hip and vertebral fractures by 34%, with an overall reduction in fracture risk of 24% (Rossouw, Anderson, Prentice, et al., 2002). However, other findings from the study regarding the absence of benefits for cardiovascular events and the increased risk of breast cancer limit the indications for the use of hormone therapy. The evidence suggests that hormone therapy should be limited to menopausal or postmenopausal women who are at highest risk for osteoporosis and should not be considered as a form of treatment for osteoporosis.

Mechanism of Action

Estrogen prevents menopausal osteoporosis. Estrogen receptors are found on osteoclasts. When estrogen binds to these receptors, chemical mediators are secreted that decrease the activity of osteoclasts, causing decreased bone resorption. Estrogen slows bone loss significantly for at least as long as treatment continues. Practitioners should consider estrogen therapy for all estrogen-deficient women without contraindications. Hormone replacement therapy in women who have had a hysterectomy is estrogen alone, but in women with an intact uterus, practitioners must add progestin to prevent endometrial cancer. When treatment stops, bone mass decreases at a rate similar to that in post-menopausal women who are not taking hormone replacement therapy.

Transdermal hormone therapy is not effective for treating osteoporosis because it takes at least 12 months to be effective. Practitioners can, however, prescribe it for prevention.

Contraindications

Contraindications to estrogen include pregnancy, active or past history of thrombophlebitis or thrombolytic disorders, estrogen-dependent neoplasia, and undiagnosed genital bleeding. Chapter 59 discusses hormone replacement therapy in more detail.

Bisphosphonates

Alendronate (Fosamax) and risedronate (Actonel) are aminobisphosphonates used for preventing and treating osteoporosis. Others are being developed that can be taken once a month or several times a year.

Mechanism of Action

These drugs inhibit bone resorption and increase bone density. They are deposited in the bone at sites of mineralization and in resorption lacunae. The bone resorption and fracture rate declines, whereas bone density increases. In studies of alendronate, an increase in bone mass was shown in the spine and hip, with a 48% decrease in the rate of vertebral compression fractures. Bone turnover increases to previous levels after 6 to 9 months when the patient takes alendronate for 6 months and then stops. If the patient takes alendronate for 6 years, no decrease in bone mass is noted for 2 years after therapy stops. These drugs have been used successfully for prevention and treatment of decreased bone mass as a result of long-term use of glucocorticoids.

In large, randomized, controlled trials, alendronate showed consistent increases in BMD irrespective of the severity of the underlying bone density levels, and reduced the incidence of both vertebral and nonvertebral fractures (Cummings et al., 1998; Liberman et al., 1995). Among women with osteoporosis, the incidence of symptomatic vertebral fractures was decreased by 44% over 4 years and clinical fractures were reduced by 36% (Cummings et al., 1998). Risedronate similarly reduced the incidence of vertebral fractures by 41% over 3 years (Harris et al., 1999) and reduced hip fractures by 40% in elderly women who had low BMD but not in women who had risk factors alone (McClung, Geusens, Miller, et al., 2001).

Dosage

The dosage for alendronate is 5 mg/day for prevention and 10 mg/day for treatment. It has also been approved for use once a week at 35 mg for prevention and 70 mg for treatment. Intestinal absorption of the drug is poor, so patients should take it on awakening with 8 ounces of water and 30 minutes before consuming any food or other drink. The dosage for risedronate is 5 mg/day or 35 mg once a week for prevention and treatment.

Contraindications

Bisphosphonates are not prescribed to patients with a history of esophageal problems, gastritis, or peptic ulcer disease. Adverse events include GI disturbance, esophagitis, diarrhea, and abdominal pain. Absorption increases with intravenous administration of ranitidine. Bisphosphonates should be prescribed with caution when the patient also is using nonsteroidal anti-inflammatory drugs. Absorption decreases when these drugs are taken with food, calcium, or iron, so patients should take the medication at different times from these substances (ie, at least 30 minutes before or after taking food or liquid nourishment).

Adverse Events

Alendronate can cause esophagitis, usually within the first month of therapy. Ways to diminish esophagitis as well as to increase drug absorption include taking alendronate and risedronate with 8 ounces of water and remaining upright for 30 minutes after administration. Risedronate has fewer harsh effects on the GI system.

Calcitonin

Salmon calcitonin (Miacalcin) is another drug used in treating osteoporosis.

Mechanism of Action

Calcitonin works by inhibiting the action of osteoclasts. It is available in injectable form and as a nasal spray. It is not effective in preventing bone loss early in the post-menopausal period, but studies have shown that it increases bone mass in the spine and decreases the risk of vertebral compression fractures. Calcitonin also has an analgesic effect on pain associated with vertebral compression fractures.

In one study of postmenopausal women who used calcitonin daily, new vertebral fractures were decreased by 33% compared with placebo, though only a small increase was noted in BMD (Chestnut et al., 2000).

Dosage

The intranasal dosage of calcitonin is 200 U/day. The patient should alternate nostrils each day. The injectable dosage is 100 U subcutaneously or intramuscularly each day.

Adverse Events

An adverse event with the use of nasal calcitonin is rhinitis. The nasal mucosa should be inspected every 6 months for ulceration. Injection can cause local irritation. With both inhalation and injection, GI upset, flushing, rash, and back pain may occur. Recommendations are for patients to perform injections at bedtime because facial flushing and nausea may occur.

Selective Estrogen Receptor Modulators

The SERMs are indicated for treating and preventing osteoporosis. They reduce the risk of vertebral fractures but do not appear to have an effect on hip fractures.

Mechanism of Action

SERMs mimic the effects of estrogen on bones without replicating the stimulating effects of estrogen on the breasts and uterus. They decrease bone resorption and bone turnover. These agents also decrease total cholesterol and low-density lipoprotein cholesterol levels.

Dosage

Raloxifene (Evista) is the only available SERM. The dose is 60 mg once a day. Supplemental calcium and vitamin D are recommended.

Contraindications

Raloxifene is contraindicated in women who are lactating or who may become pregnant. It is also contraindicated in women who have a history of thromboembolic events. The patient must discontinue the drug 72 hours before prolonged immobilization, such as surgery requiring bed rest.

Adverse Events

Adverse events include hot flashes, GI distress, flu-like symptoms, leg cramps, deep vein thrombosis, and arthralgias. When taken with cholestyramine, absorption is disrupted.

Hormone Modifiers

Hormone modifiers contain recombinant human parathyroid hormone (PTH).

Mechanism of Action

PTH is the primary regulator of calcium and phosphate metabolism and regulates bone metabolism, renal tubular reabsorption of calcium and phosphates, and intestinal calcium absorption. It stimulates new bone formation in trabecular and cortical bone surface by preferential stimulation of osteoblastic activity over osteoclastic activity. This causes an increase in skeletal mass and an increase in markers of bone formation and resorption and bone strength.

A study showed women using teriparatide had an increased density of the spine of 10% to 14% and of the hip of 5%. In 18 months, vertebral fractures were reduced 60% to 70% and nonvertebral fractures 55% (Dempster, Cosman, & Kurland, 2001). It has been shown that teriparatide can prevent back pain in women with osteoporosis for up to 18 months beyond the end of treatment.

Dosage

Teriparatide (Forteo) is the only agent in this class currently. It is administered subcutaneously at a dosage of 20 micrograms daily. This is used in women at high risk for fracture or those who have failed to respond to or who are intolerant of other therapies.

Contraindications

Teriparatide is contraindicated in the following circumstances: Paget's disease, children, previous bone radiation therapy, history of skeletal malignancy, metabolic bone disease, hypercalcemia (which is usually transient), and hyperparathyroidism. It should be used cautiously in patients with a history of kidney stones.

Adverse Events

Teriparatide may increase calcium levels and increase the risk of digoxin toxicity if used together. Common adverse events include dizziness, nausea, leg cramps, arthralgia, and hyperuricemia.

Selecting the Most Appropriate Agent

The patient needs to take calcium and vitamin D in addition to any other drug selected. Results of the DEXA scan guide the provider's decision in selecting therapy for osteoporosis. If the T score is less than –1.0 SD from the norm, the patient is said to have no osteoporosis or osteopenia, but calcium intake and weight-bearing exercise are encouraged. A T score below –1.0 SD or less than –2.5 SD from the mean indicates osteopenia, and treatment with calcium and vitamin D should begin. Also, the practitioner should consider preventive resorption-inhibiting therapy. The risk of fracture almost doubles for each BMD decrease of 1 SD. The DEXA scan should be repeated in 2 years or sooner if the patient experiences menopause. The National Osteoporosis Foundation recommends pharmacologic treatment if the T score is below –2.0 SD from the mean, if the T score is –1.5 with other risk factors for osteoporosis or fracture, and if the woman is older than 70 with multiple risk factors, especially previous fractures (Fig. 39-1).

First-Line Therapy

Raloxifene, alendronate, or risedronate or hormone replacement therapy is used for prevention; raloxifene, alendronate, or risedronate is used for treatment (Table 39-2). Patients should also take calcium and vitamin D supplementation. Treatment decisions are based on patient history. For instance, if the patient has a history of esophagitis, alendronate is not the best choice; if the patient has a history of thromboembolic disease, raloxifene is not the appropriate therapy. In light of the findings of the WHI trial, hormone replacement therapy should not be chosen in patients with a history of cardiac disease, breast cancer, or thromboembolic disease. The risks and benefits of all therapies should be discussed with the patient before a decision is made.

Second-Line Therapy

Calcitonin or a hormone modifier is recommended for second-line therapy in women who have failed to respond to

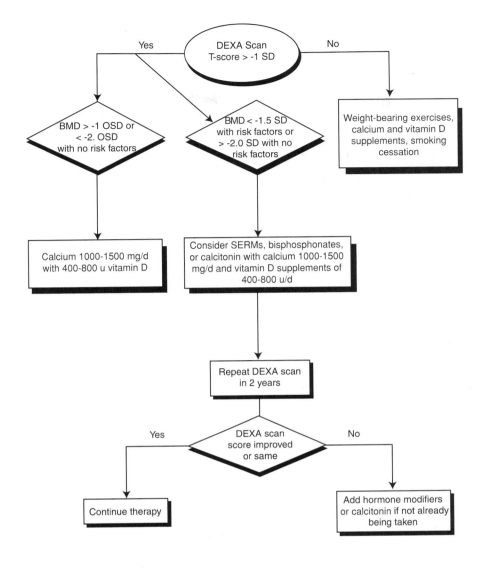

Key ⬭ Starting point for decision making; ▭ clinical actions (assessing, prescribing, monitoring); ◇ decision point.

Figure 39–1 Treatment algorithm for osteoporosis.

first-line therapy or who cannot tolerate hormone replacement therapy, bisphosphonates, or SERMs.

MONITORING PATIENT RESPONSE

The DEXA scan should be repeated every 2 years. Measurement of the density of the proximal femur is most helpful in predicting fractures, and measurement of the density of the lumbar spine is most effective in measuring the response to therapy. Within 2 years, resorption-inhibiting drugs increase the BMD of the lumbar spine by 5% to 10% in women with postmenopausal osteoporosis, causing the incidence of fractures to decrease by 50% (Cummings et al., 1993; Melton et al., 1993). Follow-up

Table 39.2

Recommended Order of Prevention and Treatment for Osteoporosis

Order	Agents	Comments
First line	Prevention: raloxifene, alendronate, or risedronate plus calcium and vitamin D	Treatment may be lifelong. These drugs are considered when estrogen therapy is contraindicated.
	Treatment: raloxifene, alendronate, risedronate, or calcitonin	
Second line	Addition of hormone modifiers or calcitonin if not being taken	

is recommended 1 to 2 months after the start of therapy, then every 3 to 6 months if the patient has osteoporosis. Follow-up is necessary every year if the therapy is prophylactic.

PATIENT EDUCATION

Drug Information

Bisphosphonates should be taken with 8 ounces of water, and the patient should remain upright for 30 minutes after administration. Information about osteoporosis can be obtained from the National Osteoporosis website (http://www.nof.org) or the National Institute of Health Osteoporosis and Related Bone Disease National Resource Center (http://www.osteo.org).

Lifestyle/Nutritional Changes

A well-balanced diet is important, as are weight-bearing exercises. Safety strategies are necessary, such as removing unstable rugs and keeping items that could cause a fall out of the way. Smoking cessation is essential. Excessive alcohol intake should be avoided.

Complementary and Alternative Therapy

Supplemental calcium and vitamin D are important adjuncts to therapy. Patients without osteopenia or osteoporosis should ingest 1,000 mg of calcium a day, and those with osteopenia or osteoporosis should ingest more—1,500 mg calcium daily and 400 to 800 U of vitamin D to facilitate the absorption of calcium.

■ Case Study

J.S., a 72-year-old woman of Asian descent, has just transferred to your practice. She had a hysterectomy 8 years ago and has not been on hormone replacement therapy. She is 5-foot-2 and weighs 102 lb. She has had a sedentary lifestyle (she was a secretary and retired 2 years ago). She drinks four glasses of wine a day. Her mother died at age 62 from complications of a hip fracture. J.S.'s sister was just diagnosed with metastatic breast cancer. You prescribe a DEXA scan, and the T score is −2.6 SD.

Diagnosis: Osteoporosis

1. List specific goals of therapy for J.S.
2. What drug therapy would you prescribe? Why?
3. What are the parameters for monitoring the success of the therapy?
4. Discuss specific patient education based on the prescribed therapy.
5. List one or two adverse reactions for the selected agent that would cause you to change therapy.
6. What OTC or alternative medicines might be appropriate for this patient?
7. What dietary and lifestyle changes might you recommend?
8. Describe one or two drug/drug or drug/food interactions for the selected agent.

Bibliography

Starred references are cited in the text.

Alendronate Once-Weekly Study Group (2002). Two-year results of once-weekly administration of alendronate 70 mg for the treatment of postmenopausal osteoporosis. *Journal of Bone Mineral Research 17*, 1988–1996.

Berg, A. O. (2002). *Postmenopausal hormone replacement therapy for primary prevention of chronic conditions: Recommendation and rationale, U.S. Preventive Task Force.* U.S. Preventive Task Force, Guidelines from Guide to Clinical Preventive Services, 2000–2003.

*Chesnut, C. H. III, Silverman, S., Andriano, K., et al. (2000). A randomized trial of nasal spray salmon calcitonin in postmenopausal women with established osteoporosis: The Prevent

Recurrence of Osteoporotic Fractures Study. PROOF Study Group. *American Journal of Medicine, 109*, 267–276.

*Cummings, S. R., Black, D. M., Thompson, D. E., et al. (1998). Effect of alendronate on risk of fracture in women with low bone density but without vertebral fractures: Results from the Fracture Intervention Trial. *JAMA, 280*, 2077–2082.

*Cummings, S. R., Black, D. M., Nevitt, M. C., et al. (1993). Bone density at various sites for prediction of hip fractures: The Study of Osteoporotic Fractures Research Group. *Lancet, 341*, 72–75.

Davidson, M. R. (2003). Pharmacotherapy for osteoporosis prevention and treatment. *Journal of Midwifery and Women's Health, 48*(1), 39–54.

*Dempster, D. W., Cosman, F., & Kurland, E. S. (2001). Effects of daily treatment with parathyroid hormone on bone microarchitecture and turnover in patients with osteoporosis: a paired

biopsy study. *Journal of Bone Mineral Research, 16,* 1846–1853.

Ettinger, B., Black, D, Pearson, J., et al. (1999). Reduction of vertebral risk factors in postmenopausal women with osteoporosis treated with raloxifene: Results from a 3-year randomized clinical trial. Multiple Outcomes of Raloxifene Evaluation (MORE) Investigators. *JAMA, 282,* 2077–2082.

Follin, S. L., & Hansen, L. B. (2003). Current approaches to the prevention and treatment of postmenopausal osteoporosis. *American Journal of Health System Pharmacy, 60*(9), 883–901.

Garnero, P., & Delmas, P. D. (1998). Osteoporosis. *Endocrinology and Metabolism Clinics, 26,* 913–933.

Gregg, E. W., Pereira, M. A., & Casperson, C. J. (2000). Physical activity, falls and fractures among older adults: A review of epidemiological evidence. *Journal of the American Geriatric Society, 48,* 883–893.

*Harris, S. T., Watts, N. B., Genant, H. K., et al. (1999). Effects of risedronate treatment on vertebral and nonvertebral fractures in women with postmenopausal osteoporosis: A randomized controlled trial. Vertebral Efficacy with Risedronate Therapy (VERT) Study Group. *JAMA, 282,* 1344–1352.

Heaney, R. P. (1998). Pathophysiology of osteoporosis. *Endocrinology and Metabolism Clinics, 27,* 255–265.

Kannus, P., Parkkari, J., Niemi, S., et al. (2000). Prevention of hip fracture in elderly people with the use of a hip protector. *New England Journal of Medicine, 343,* 1506–1513.

*Liberman, U. A., Weiss, S. R., Broll, J., et al. (1995). Effect of oral alendronate on bone mineral density and the incidence of fractures in postmenopausal osteoporosis. The Alendronate Phase III Osteoporosis Treatment Study Group. *New England Journal of Medicine, 333,* 1437–1443.

Marcus, R. (1996). The nature of osteoporosis. *Journal of Clinical Endocrinology and Metabolism, 81,* 1–5.

*Melton, L. J., Atkinson, E. J., O'Fallon, W. M., Wahner, H. W., et al. (1993). Long-term fracture prediction by bone mineral assesses at different skeletal sites. *Journal of Bone Mineral Research, 8,* 1227–1233.

*McClung, M. R., Geusens, P., Miller, P. D., et al. (2001). Effect of risedronate on the risk of hip fracture in elderly women. *New England Journal of Medicine, 344,* 333–340.

Miller, P. (2003). Analysis of vertebral fracture risk reduction data in treatments for osteoporosis. *Southern Medical Journal, 96*(5), 478–485.

*National Osteoporosis Foundation. (2003). Osteoporosis fast facts [on-line]. Available at http://www.nof.org.

Neer, R. M., Arnaud, C. D., Zanchetta, J. R., et al. (2001). Effect of parathyroid hormone on fractures and bone mineral density in postmenopausal women with osteoporosis. *New England Journal of Medicine, 344,* 1434–1441.

NIH Consensus Development on Osteoporosis Prevention, Diagnosis and Treatment (2001). *JAMA, 285,* 785–795.

*National Osteoporosis Foundation. America's bone health: The state of osteoporosis and low bone mass. Available at: http://www.nof.org/advocacy/prevalence/index.htm. Accessed July 30, 2004.

Nelson, H. D., Humphrey, L. L., LeBlanc, E., Miller, J., Takano, L., Chan, B. K., et al. (2002). *Postmenopausal hormone replacement therapy for the primary prevention of chronic conditions: A summary of the evidence for the U.S. Preventive Services Task Force.* Rockville, MD: Agency for Healthcare Research and Quality, 2002. Accessed December 2002. Available at: http://www.ahrq.gov/clinic/3rduspstf/hrt/hrtsum3.htm.

Orwell, E. S. (1998). Osteoporosis in men. *Endocrinology and Metabolism Clinics, 27,* 349–367.

Orwell, E. S., & Nelson, H. D. (1999). Does estrogen adequately protect postmenopausal women against osteoporosis? An iconoclastic perspective. *Journal of Clinical Endocrinology and Metabolism, 84,* 1872–1874.

Overgard, K., Hansen, M. A., Jensen, S. B., et al. (1992). Effect of salcatonin given intranasally on bone mass and fracture rates in established osteoporosis. *British Medical Journal, 305,* 556–561.

Reginster, J., Taquet, A. N., & Gosset, C. (1998). Therapy for osteoporosis. *Endocrinology and Metabolism Clinics, 27,* 453–463.

*Rossouw, J. E., Anderson, G. L., Prentice, R. L., et al. (2002). Risks and benefits of estrogen plus progestin in postmenopausal women: Principal results from the Women's Health Initiative randomized controlled trial. *JAMA, 288,* 321–333.

Reginster, J., Minne, H. W., Sorensen, O. H., et al. (2000). Randomized trial of the effects of risedronate on vertebral fractures in women with established postmenopausal osteoporosis. Vertebral Efficacy with Risedronate Therapy (VERT) Study Group. *Osteoporosis International, 11,* 83–91.

Singer, F. R. (2000). Osteoporosis. In R. Rakel (Ed.), *Conn's current therapy* (52nd ed., pp. 593–597). Philadelphia: W. B. Saunders.

*Siris, E. S., Miller, P. D., Barrett-Connor, E., et al. (2001). Identification and fracture outcomes of undiagnosed low bone mineral density in postmenopausal women: Results from the National Osteoporosis Risk Assessment. *JAMA, 286,* 2815–2822.

United States Preventive Services Task Force (USPSTF) (2003). Postmenopausal hormone replacement therapy for prevention of chronic conditions. *American Family Physician, 67*(2), 358–364.

*Women's Health Initiative (2002). Risks and benefits of estrogen and progestin in healthy postmenopausal women. *JAMA, 288,* 321–333.

Visit the Connection web site for the most up-to-date drug information.

FIBROMYALGIA

■ SUSAN SCHRAND AND ANDREW M. PETERSON

Fibromyalgia (FM) is a chronic condition of widespread musculoskeletal pain characterized by diffuse aches and stiffness, soft tissue tender points, fatigue, and nonrestorative sleep. It has been estimated that nearly 7 to 10 million Americans have FM, with women being 20 times more likely than men to acquire this condition. Most patients experience an onset of symptoms around the second or third decade of life, but FM has been identified as affecting people of all ages (Colorado Health Net, 1996).

Reiffenberger and Amundson (1996) reported that 5% to 6% of patients receiving care in family practice and general medicine offices are diagnosed with FM, and suggested that this condition may be present in up to 5% of the general population. Patients with FM are often seen by rheumatologists, and the number of office visits is only slightly less than for patients with rheumatoid arthritis. For family health care providers, Maurizio and Rogers (1997) stated that FM may be one of the most common conditions encountered. With a continued rise in prevalence of FM, Jones and Burckhardt (1997) estimated an annual financial toll of $15.9 billion in both direct and indirect health care costs, causing a significant public health concern.

CAUSES

There is no known cause or cure for FM, and its etiology has been long debated. Because of this lack of understanding and direction in disease management, people with FM may be among the more challenging patients for primary care providers. Patients often have a difficult time distinguishing specific events that precede their symptoms. Common factors precipitating FM include a flu-like viral illness, physical or emotional trauma, and withdrawal of corticosteroids. Symptoms that coincide with FM include migraine or tension-type headaches, irritable bowel, waking with stiffness and achiness, feeling underrested or unrefreshed after a full night of sleep, hypersensitivity to cold or heat, environmental sensitivities, abdominal pain, sensations of numbness and tingling in hands and feet, and anxiety and depression (Maurizio & Rogers, 1997).

PATHOPHYSIOLOGY

Three possible explanations for this syndrome that are being explored are deficiencies in pain mechanisms, changes in the central nervous system, and muscular abnormalities. Allodynia, or a reduction in pain threshold, is commonly associated with FM, but as Jones and Burckhardt (1997) noted, researchers are still trying to explain the origins of chronic pain symptoms. It has been discovered, for example, that peripheral pain nerves (nociceptors) in muscle tissue that has experienced repeated stretching or pressure can release neurotransmitters in the spinal cord. As these neurotransmitters enter the central nervous system, the result is allodynia, with its symptoms of increased response to and duration of pain after noxious stimuli. Research on this theory continues.

Because patients with FM commonly experience sleep disturbances and chronic pain, researchers are also focusing on neurohormones as a factor in the disease etiology. Neurohormones, including serotonin, endorphins, or substance P, can have effects on sleep patterns, mood, and pain response. With substance P being influenced by serotonin, any deficiency could lead to an exaggerated sensory perception of stimuli. Goldenberg (1998) cited one study that showed patients with FM having a threefold increase in substance P. The sleep disturbance may also disrupt the production of growth hormone, a substance essential for tissue repair, which is produced during non–rapid eye movement (REM) or stage 4 sleep.

More recently, Wassem and Stillion-Allen (2003) suggested that recent studies may classify FM into a disease of the immune and central nervous system activation. Some research has documented inconsistencies in the growth hormones somatomedin C and IGF-1, the sympathoadrenal systems, and the neuroendocrine axis.

Muscular changes have been identified through biopsy, but the results reveal only nonspecific changes. On microscopic examination, a "moth-eaten" appearance of muscle noted in patients with FM has been associated with nonpathologic conditions and disuse (Jones & Burckhardt, 1997). No evidence of an inflammatory process was found in either tendon or muscle tissue.

Psychological factors, especially depression, play a role in FM, but no universal pattern or striking psychological abnormalities have been documented (Rosenblum, Campbell, & Rosenbaum, 1996). Because the etiology is unknown and the objective findings are nonspecific, FM is frequently considered a psychosomatic disorder. Anxiety about illness stemming from chronic pain, along with the uncertainty of the diagnosis, is more likely to be a precipitating factor for psychological distress in patients with FM than a specific individual trait (Jones & Burckhardt, 1997).

DIAGNOSTIC CRITERIA

The term *fibromyalgia* has evolved from earlier terms, such as fibrositis, fibromyositis, muscular rheumatism, psychogenic rheumatism, and primary FM. To simplify matters, FM is now the only term used to describe this syndrome.

In 1990, the American College of Rheumatology (ACR) developed classification criteria to help clinicians better distinguish FM from other rheumatologic disorders, such as rheumatoid arthritis or neck or back pain syndromes, and to provide a better exclusion system for conducting research. To be diagnosed with FM, a patient usually meets the criteria listed in Box 40-1. Jones and Burckhardt (1997) warned that clinicians should use clinical judgment to best explain their patients' signs and symptoms rather than rule out FM if the patient does not meet the exact ACR criteria.

INITIATING DRUG THERAPY

The chronic nature and lack of visible outward signs of FM make it reasonable and helpful to involve family and friends of the patient in education about the disease. Understanding that FM is a disease process is a crucial factor in promoting health and improvement for patients with FM. In most cases, FM interferes with the patient's quality of life, either in personal relationships or the ability to work and be a productive member of society. The fact that others recognize the patient's physical and psychological suffering can be most beneficial (Carette, 1996). Patients and their families should be encouraged to understand that FM is not crippling. With supportive environments, both at home and in the health care system, the patient can learn to take an active, self-help approach to controlling the disorder. Practitioners need to emphasize wellness rather than illness (Simms, 1996).

Most current research about FM suggests that patient education should be a primary focus in managing patients with FM. Many patients express a sense of relief when their symptoms finally have a name (Jones & Burckhardt, 1997). Keeping patients up to date on information regarding new research findings and treatment modalities while encouraging them to participate in support groups can give them the tools needed to gain self-efficacy.

Several alternatives to traditional drug therapy have been tried at various times by various patients. Low-impact exercise is one of the few therapies studied that proves significantly beneficial in managing symptoms. Hence, encouraging a systematic, supervised exercise regimen is one of the most beneficial therapies that can be offered. However, patients with FM need to avoid any

---

BOX 40–1. AMERICAN COLLEGE OF RHEUMATOLOGY DIAGNOSTIC CRITERIA FOR FIBROMYALGIA

History of widespread pain (defined as pain in the left side of the body, in the right side of the body, above the waist and below the waist)

In addition to widespread pain, axial skeletal pain (cervical spine, anterior chest, or thoracic spine or low back). Shoulder and buttock pain is categorized with the side pains. Low back pain is categorized as lower segment pain.

Pain on digital palpation in at least 11 of 18 "tender points" (9 bilaterally). Tender points include:

- Occiput: bilateral, at the suboccipital muscle insertions
- Low cervical: bilateral, at the anterior aspects of the intertransverse spaces at C5–C7
- Trapezius: bilateral, at the midpoint of the upper border
- Supraspinatus: bilateral, at origins, above the scapular spine near the medial border
- Second rib: bilateral, at the second costochondral junctions, just lateral to the junctions on upper surfaces
- Lateral epicondyle: bilateral, 2 cm distal to the epicondyles
- Gluteal: bilateral, in upper outer quadrants of buttocks in anterior fold of muscle
- Greater trochanter: bilateral, posterior to the trochanteric prominence
- Knee: bilateral, at the medial fat pad proximal to the joint line

Adapted with permission from Wolfe, F., et al. (1990). The American College of Rheumatology 1990 criteria for the classification of fibromyalgia: Report of the Multicenter Criteria Committee. *Arthritis and Rheumatism, 33,* 160–172.

"impact-loading" exercises that involve jumping up and down, such as running sports. Walking, swimming, and bicycling are activities that can improve physical conditioning and minimize symptoms. Having the patient receiving adequate pharmacologic and psychological support prior to starting an exercise regimen will most likely promote adherence and increased tolerance to the recommended regimen (Wassem & Stillion-Allen, 2003). Even for the healthy person, commitment to a routine exercise program can be challenging, so encouraging and implementing an exercise regimen for people who live with chronic pain and an impaired quality of life may prove to be even more difficult for the practitioner.

Pacing is an important concept to relay to patients with FM. Learning to take life's activities more slowly—alternating days of rest and exercise and avoiding stressful situations—usually improves their sense of well-being (Bennett & McCain, 1995).

Goals of Drug Therapy

There is no generally applicable algorithm for the pharmacologic management of FM, so the goal is relief or control of symptoms. Most of the reviewed literature suggests beginning with low-dose tricyclic antidepressants (TCAs) but usually encourages practitioners to experiment with dosing and agents that are found to be most suitable for the individual patient and his or her current symptoms. There are some data suggesting that patients with a mixed FM and depression will do moderately well with TCA treatment. There appears to be a functional reduction in serotonergic activity in patients with FM, and antidepressants might enhance the activity of serotonin and norepinephrine neurotransmitters in the descending inhibitory pain pathways, leading to a reduction in pain.

Antidepressants

Tricyclic Antidepressants

Amitriptyline hydrochloride (Elavil) increases non-REM stage 4 sleep by inhibiting reuptake of serotonin rather than acting in an antidepressant manner (Maurizio & Rogers, 1997). Low doses of amitriptyline appear to cause REM suppression and prolong stages 3 and 4 of non-REM sleep.

Because the goal of FM therapy differs from that of depression therapy, drug dosages and onset of action differ significantly. Prescribing 10 mg of amitriptyline 2 to 3 hours before bedtime helps the patient gain more restful sleep and minimizes any "hangover" feeling the next day. Dosing may start as low as 5 mg/day for patients sensitive to anticholinergic side effects. (See Chapter 44 for details of anticholinergic side effects.) If the patient does not respond to the 10-mg daily dose after 1 week, the dosage is increased to 20 mg/day, and increments of 10 mg on a weekly basis are added. Doses that exceed 50 mg/day provide little additional benefit. Patients experiencing significant improvements should continue the dosage effective for them for approximately 3 months. After this time, a tapering regimen of 10 mg/month should begin until the minimum effective dosage is achieved. Patients may maintain their dosage regimen for years without complications, but abrupt discontinuation of a TCA may lead to rebound insomnia. Tapering of this medication is recommended (Simms, 1996).

Nortriptyline hydrochloride (Pamelor) is another drug in the TCA class that has provided symptomatic relief for patients with FM (Table 40-1). Similarly, doxepin may be used. The doses of these agents, like amitriptyline, are lower than those used for depression. These agents could be considered alternatives to amitriptyline, though there are no data suggesting that one is more effective than another for the treatment of FM.

Selective Serotonin Reuptake Inhibitors

Fluoxetine (Prozac), a selective serotonin reuptake inhibitor (SSRI), has been studied as a potential antidepressant agent for FM therapy, but it was found to contribute to sleep disturbances because of its stimulating characteristics (Simms, 1996). The full dosage of an SSRI would be recommended as therapy for patients with FM who have concomitant depression, but the decline in sleep quality may cause problems. Some clinicians manage this by prescribing an SSRI in the morning and a TCA at bedtime (Bennett & McCain, 1995). In a 12-week, flexible-dose, placebo-controlled trial, Arnold et al. (2002) found fluoxetine to be effective on most outcomes (ie, Fibromyalgia Impact Questionnaire total score and the McGill Pain Questionnaire), and it was well tolerated.

Skeletal Muscle Relaxants

Cyclobenzaprine hydrochloride (Flexeril, Cycloflex), a TCA structurally similar to amitriptyline, shows some short-term efficacy in FM. This drug, which has properties that reduce brain stem noradrenergic function and motor neuron efferent activity, is usually marketed as a muscle relaxant (Simms, 1996). Because of the lack of substantial drug trials, dosing recommendations vary in the literature. One study cited by Simms (1996) reported some benefits with dosing beginning at 10 mg/day for 1 week, 25 mg/day for weeks 2 through 12, and 50 mg/day for weeks 13 through 24. Dosing described by Goldenberg (1998) started at 10 to 40 mg/day in divided doses. Patients taking cyclobenzaprine in this regimen showed improvement in pain, fatigue, sleep, and tender point count. Bedtime dosing is highly recommended with this agent because of its potential to cause impairment and drowsiness.

Cyclobenzaprine, having similar properties to the TCAs, can cause anticholinergic side effects such as drowsiness, dizziness, lightheadedness, dry mouth, and muscle weakness and should usually be avoided when a patient is already taking TCAs.

Anti-inflammatory Agents

Nonsteroidal anti-inflammatory drugs (NSAIDs) are commonly used for analgesia, but because there does not seem to be any inflammatory process associated with FM, minimal relief is obtained with their use (Wassem & Stillion-Allen, 2003). In light of the associated symptoms of irritable bowel, NSAIDs are not the analgesics of first choice. Acetaminophen may be better tolerated for analgesia, especially in patients who have irritable bowel syndrome. Studies are underway to assess the combination of TCAs and NSAIDs for symptom relief, but at this time the combination cannot be suggested for therapy. See Chapter 38 for more information on NSAIDs.

Narcotic Analgesics

Because of the chronic nature of FM, narcotic analgesic drugs should be avoided for pain control because of their addiction potential. There may be some clinical situations that require management with narcotics, especially during disease flare-ups or during initiation of new therapies. Yunus and Arslan (2004) reserved use for patients who have failed to respond to other therapy attempts. Narcotics must be reserved for short-term use and with close collaboration with the prescriber. Yunus and Arslan reported that they had success using oxycodone, 10 to 30 mg/day in divided doses every 12 hours, with codeine, 30 mg, two to four times daily. They suggested avoiding this class of medication altogether in patients with known addiction potential. See Chapter 7 for more information regarding narcotic analgesics.

Table 40.1

Pharmacologic Therapy for Fibromyalgia

Generic (Trade) Name	Starting Dose and Range	Side Effects	Contraindications	Special Considerations
amitriptyline (Elavil)	Start at 5 mg per day. Increase by increments of 10 mg per week if no relief after one week of therapy. Continue effective dose for 3 months, then begin taper of 10 mg per month until minimum effective dose is achieved. Safe to maintain above dose for years	See Chapter 44, Table 44–4, for complete listing of side effects.	Hypersensitivity to any tricyclic drug Concomitant therapy with MAO inhibitors Recent MI Pregnancy Lactation	Abrupt discontinuation of drug may lead to rebound insomnia. Due to different dosing methods, there is no suggested plasma concentration to follow. Avoid alcohol. SSRI combination use may increase levels of TCAs.
cyclobenzaprine (Flexeril)	10–40 mg per day in divided doses	CNS: drowsiness, dizziness, fatigue GI: dry mouth, nausea, and constipation	Recovering MI Use caution in patients with urinary retention.	Avoid alcohol. Report any dizziness, blurred vision, or other CNS symptoms.
doxepin (Sinequan)	10–50 mg once daily	See Chapter 44, Table 44–4, for complete listing of side effects.	Hypersensitivity to any tricyclic drug Concomitant therapy with MAO inhibitors Recent MI Pregnancy Lactation	Abrupt discontinuation of drug may lead to rebound insomnia. Due to different dosing methods, there is no suggested plasma concentration to follow. Avoid alcohol.
fluoxetine (Prozac)	Start at 20 mg in a.m. May increase by weekly increments.	See Chapter 44, Table 44–4, for complete listing of side effects.	Hypersensitivity to any SSRI drug	
nortriptyline hydrochloride (Pamelor)	10–50 mg once daily	See Chapter 44, Table 44–4, for complete listing of side effects.	Same as for amitriptyline	Same as for amitriptyline

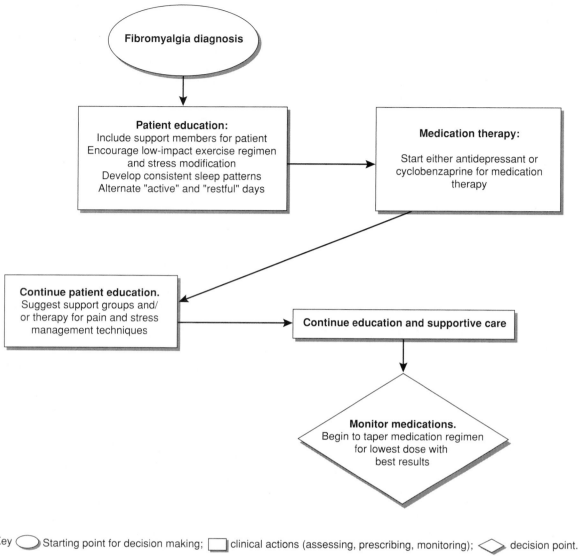

Key ◯ Starting point for decision making; ▢ clinical actions (assessing, prescribing, monitoring); ◇ decision point.

Figure 40–1 Treatment options for patients with fibromyalgia.

Selecting the Most Appropriate Agent

Figure 40-1 provides an algorithm for treating FM. Drug treatment is individualized to meet the patient's needs. First- and second-line therapies are summarized in Table 40-2.

First-Line Therapy

Amitriptyline is the first line of medication suggested for short-term treatment of FM, although nortriptyline or cyclobenzaprine may be tried as well. Once a minimum effective dosage is achieved, therapy may continue for years.

Table 40.2

Recommended Order of Treatment for Fibromyalgia

Order	Agents	Comments
First line	Tricyclic antidepressants (TCAs) initially for short term. Suggested agents include amitriptyline, nortriptyline, cyclobenzaprine.	Dosage schedules of these medications are adjusted to meet patient needs, and not in accord with recommended dosage for depression therapy. Patient should be monitored for side effects associated with TCAs and educated to recognize and report adverse events.
Second line	Additional therapy with a selective serotonin reuptake inhibitor such as fluoxetine (Prozac)	Dosage schedules of these medications are adjusted to meet patient needs, and not in accord with recommended dosage for depression therapy. Patients should be educated to recognize and manage possible side effects.

Discontinuation of therapy should be gradual (tapered) to avoid untoward effects.

Second-Line Therapy

Because a therapeutic regimen for FM remains largely undefined, second-line therapy may consist of tailoring and tapering first-line therapy and possibly adding an NSAID or an SSRI, such as fluoxetine, to the TCA regimen.

Third-Line Therapy

When first- or second-line therapy is unsuccessful, the practitioner may add or substitute one of the narcotic analgesics.

Special Population Considerations

Geriatric

Care must be taken when prescribing TCAs to patients over age 65. The anticholinergic effect can worsen existing glaucoma and benign prostatic hyperplasia in men. The sedative effects can affect a patient's ability to perform activities of daily living. Dosages above those recommended can cause confusion. Similarly, narcotic analgesia should be used with caution in the elderly due to the side effect profile.

Women

This disease primarily affects women. A recent review (Yunus, 2001) showed that the ratio of women to men is 9:1. He reported that women had more tender points than men, but in men with the disease, pain severity and physical functioning were not significantly different. He did not offer convincing evidence of the reason for the gender differences but postulated that there might be a complex interaction between physiology, psychology, and environmental factors.

The clinician must consider the dangers of prescribing teratogenic medications to women of childbearing age. Both amitriptyline and cyclobenzaprine are category D medications, and caution should be taken when prescribing to this age group (Lacy, Armstrong, Ingrim, & Lance, 1996–1997).

MONITORING PATIENT RESPONSE

Keeping in close contact with the patient to monitor pain relief, sleep quality, and general feelings of sickness and teaching the patient to recognize signs of anticholinergic effects are keys to careful monitoring. No radiologic studies are indicated for monitoring patients with FM, although annual liver function tests and baseline electrocardiograms are suggested for monitoring the use of TCAs.

PATIENT EDUCATION

FM is a disease commonly seen by the primary care provider. Helping patients understand its chronic nature and encouraging them to focus on their wellness is vital in managing the condition. Low-impact exercise, stress reduction, established sleep patterns, and strong support systems are essential factors for improving quality of life for people with this disease. The practitioner needs to be aware of pharmacologic and nonpharmacologic alternatives to assist patients with health promotion. As more research is done on FM, practitioners hope to gain a better understanding of how to manage care of patients with this disorder without becoming frustrated by its chronicity.

Drug Information

Since there is no specific treatment for FM, the practitioner should seek traditional sources of drug information such as the FDA, the *Physicians' Desk Reference*, *Drug Facts and Comparisons*, and the manufacturer of a specific agent. The practitioner can access information about ongoing clinical trials for FM at ClinicalTrials.gov (http://clinicaltrials.gov/ct/gui/action/FindCondition?ui=D005356&recruiting=true).

Patient-Oriented Information Sources

The National Fibromyalgia Association's website (http://fmaware.org/fminfo/brochure.htm) has information related to improving the quality of life of patients with FM. This site provides information about the disease and clinical trials involving FM treatment, along with products to support patients with the disease. The association has an online newsletter and offers support groups.

The National Library of Medicine (http://www.nlm.nih.gov/medlineplus/tutorials/fibromyalgia.html) has an online tutorial about the diagnosis and treatment of FM.

Complementary and Alternative Medications

Nearly 33% of Americans turn to complementary and alternative medicine to help manage their health (Eisenberg et al., 1993). Patients with complicated disease processes who feel that conventional medicine is failing to treat their symptoms effectively turn to alternative therapy to seek additional relief. Twenty FM patients involved in a pilot study reported improvement in pain, function, and mood with the use of a mind-body intervention combining patient education, meditation techniques, and movement therapy (Singh, Berman, Hadhazy, & Creamer, 1998).

Various methods of alternative medicine such as acupuncture, TENS, massage, biofeedback, and hypnotherapy produced some pain relief and have shown some efficacy in randomized controlled clinical trials (Ebell & Beck, 2001). Acupuncture has been examined in a meta-analysis and proved to be a useful adjunctive treatment for many patients with this disease. Millea and Holloway (2000) reported that although acupuncture is not curative, it can help to improve quality of life. A recent report from the Agency for Healthcare Quality and Research (2003) concluded that there was insufficient evidence to support the use of acupuncture in the treatment of FM.

One herbal remedy is being looked at as a topical anesthetic. Capsaicin (Zostrix) is a cream that comes in 0.025% or 0.075% strengths. The active ingredient comes from dried, ripe fruits of Capsicum and functions as a counter-irritant that depletes substance P from sensory nerve fibers. This cream is being investigated in various painful conditions, including diabetic neuropathy, postherpetic neuralgia, stump pain, and postmastectomy pain, to name a few. Markovits and Gilhar (1997) found capsaicin to be successful with pain relief and suggested that it might help to reduce the use of NSAIDs. They reported that the use of capsaicin 0.025% four times a day for 5 weeks led to relief of neck and shoulder pain in patients with FM, although no exact statistics were reported specific to FM pain relief. They mentioned that 74% of patients reported mild burning associated with capsaicin use. Evidence at this time remains inconclusive regarding its use in FM therapy, and it cannot be recommended.

■ Case Study

S.S., a 28-year-old white female, comes to you as a new patient with her chief complaint being chronic pain and poor sleep patterns. During your interview, you discover that she has been fighting global, diffuse body pain and feeling depressed for the past 2 years. She just recently received health insurance and would like to figure out why she is feeling so poorly. After a complete history and physical and a full panel of labs, you find all of her results to be within normal limits, with the exception of global tenderness.

Using the diagnostic criteria from the American College of Rheumatology, you note that she has 15 of the 18 tender points, widespread pain, and morning stiffness and fatigue. After diagnosing her with FM, you begin to form a plan of care.

1. List at least two specific goals for the treatment of this patient.

2. Which agent would you prescribe, and what were some considerations that led you to this choice?

3. How would you monitor the success of your treatment, and when would you do so?

4. List one or two adverse reactions for the selected agent that would cause you to change therapy.

5. Describe one or two drug/drug or drug/food interactions for the selected agent.

6. What would be the choice for second-line therapy should the adverse reactions you considered occurred?

7. Are there any OTC or alternative medications you would recommend she consider adding to your regimen?

8. How would you respond if this patient asked about the use of acupuncture to treat her disease?

Bibliography

*Starred references are cited in the text.

*Agency for Healthcare Quality and Research (2003). Technology assessment Report: Acupuncture for fibromyalgia. http://www.cms.hhs.gov/coverage/download/id83.pdf. Accessed July 7, 2004.

*Arnold, L. M., Hess, E. V., Hudson, J. I., Welge, J. A., Berno, S. E., & Keck, P. E. (2002). A randomized, placebo-controlled, double-blind, flexible-dose study of fluoxetine in the treatment of women with fibromyalgia. *American Journal of Medicine, 112*, 191–197.

*Bennett, R. M., & McCain, G. A. (1995). Coping successfully with fibromyalgia. *Patient Care, 15*, 29–45.

*Carette, S. (1996) Chronic pain syndromes. *Annals of Rheumatic Disease, 55*, 497–501.

*Colorado Health Net. (1996). Fibromyalgia definitions, facts and statistics. [On-line]. Available: http://www.coloradohealthnet.org/site/idx_fibro.html.

*Ebell, M., & Beck, E. (2001) How effective are complementary/alternative medicine (CAM) therapies for fibromyalgia? *Journal of Family Practice, 50*, 401.

*Eisenberg, D. M., Kessler, R. C., Foster, C., Norlock, F. E., Calkins, D. R., & Delbanco, T. L. (1993). Unconventional medicine in the United States: Prevalence, costs and patterns of use. *New England Journal of Medicine, 328*, 246–252.

*Goldenberg, D. L. (1998). Fibromyalgia and related syndromes. In: J. H. Klippel & P. A. Dieppe (Eds.), *Rheumatology* (2nd ed., pp. 1–12). Philadelphia: C.V. Mosby.

*Jones, K. D., & Burckhardt, C. S. (1997). A multidisciplinary approach to treating fibromyalgia syndrome. *Pain Management, 12*, 7–14.

*Lacy, C., Armstrong, L. L., Ingrim, N., & Lance, L. L. (1996–1997). *Drug information handbook: Pocket* (pp. 10, 59–61, 265–266) Cleveland: Lexi-Comp.

*Markovits, E., & Gilhar, A. (1997). Capsaicin: An effective topical treatment in pain. *International Journal of Dermatology, 36*, 401–404.

*Maurizio, S. J., & Rogers, J. L. (1997). Recognizing and treating fibromyalgia. *Nurse Practitioner, 22,* 18–31.

*Millea, P. J., & Holloway, R. L. (2000). Treating fibromyalgia. *American Family Physician, 62,* 1575–1580.

*Reiffenberger, D., & Amundson, L. (1996). Fibromyalgia syndrome: A review. *American Family Physician, 53,* 1698–1704.

*Rosenblum, R., Campbell, S., & Rosenbaum, J. (1996). *Clinical Neurology of Rheumatic Diseases* (pp. 12–13). Boston: Butterworth-Heinemann.

*Simms, R. W. (1996). Fibromyalgia syndrome: Current concepts in pathophysiology, clinical features, and management. *Arthritis Care and Research, 9,* 315–328.

*Singh, B. B., Berman, B. M., Hadhazy, V. A., & Creamer, P. (1998). A pilot study of cognitive behavioral therapy in fibromyalgia. *Alternative Therapies in Health and Medicine, 4*(2), 67–70.

*Wassem, R. A., & Stillion-Allen, K. A. (2003). Evidence-based management of the fibromyalgia patient. In search of optimal functioning. *Advance for Nurse Practitioners,* 34–41.

*Yunus, M. B. (April 2001). The role of gender in fibromyalgia syndrome. *Current Rheumatology Reports, 3*(2), 128–134.

*Yunus, M. B., & Arslan, S. (2004). Fibromyalgia syndrome: Can it be treated? *Consultant,* 289–302.

Visit the Connection web site for the most up-to-date drug information.

IX

Pharmacotherapy for Neurologic and Psychiatric Disorders

PARKINSON'S DISEASE

■ ROBERT W. BARAN AND ANGELA CAFIERO

Named for James Parkinson, an English physician who was first to document a case of the "shaking palsy" in 1817, Parkinson's disease (PD) affects more than 1.5 million Americans, with approximately 20 new cases per 100,000 people diagnosed yearly (National Parkinson's Foundation, 2004). PD is usually considered a disease that targets older adults, with a prevalence at 1 of every 100 persons over age 60, increasing to 2.5% in persons over 80 (National Parkinson's Foundation, 2004; Uitti, 1996). The prevalence of PD in one large nursing home population (N = 5,020) was estimated at 6.8% (Mitchell, Kiely, Kiel, et al., 1996). The mean age of onset is 54 to 63 years, and the prevalence in men and women is approximately equal (Lang & Lozano, 1988).

The mortality rate is projected to be two to five times greater in those with PD compared with age-matched control subjects. Total societal costs (direct plus indirect) of PD are difficult to ascertain, but the federal government spends more than $6 billion annually on PD-related treatment. Medication costs for the patient can exceed $5,000 per year, depending on the complexity of the regimen. The physical burden of progressive PD is compounded considerably by the financial burden that many patients must overcome.

CAUSES

The etiology of idiopathic PD is still in question (Stern, 1997). Hypotheses include aging, environmental toxins, genetic predisposition, and oxidative stress. Environmental factors such as ingesting well water or living on a farm (insecticides/herbicides) have been linked to idiopathic PD, but so have industrial toxins such as heavy metals (eg, manganese, iron). There appears to be an inverse relationship between the development of PD and the use of caffeine, coffee, or smoking.

Although PD has occasionally been labeled a "disease of the industrial age," ancient writers noted curiously similar afflictions (Lang & Lozano, 1988). Congruent with this possibly historical pathologic process, a genetic lineage has been identified that describes a mechanism of transmission between generations (Lazzarini, Myers, Zimmerman, et al., 1994). Some populations exhibit a pattern of autosomal dominance with low penetrance. The genetic link has been implicated in patients with younger-onset PD. After age 50, genetic factors do not play a role in the development of PD

(Olanow, Watts, & Koller, 2001). The oxidative stress hypothesis relates the generation of destructive free radicals to the endogenous metabolism of dopamine in the brain (Olanow, 1990). It is proposed that PD may result from a combination of these factors and predispositions, but that position can be viewed as a compromise until a definite etiology is confirmed.

In addition to the pathophysiologic process that results in classic PD symptoms, numerous drugs have been implicated as the cause of parkinsonian symptoms (Koller, 1997). The presentation associated with this pharmacologic etiology may be sufficiently different from idiopathic PD that such manifestations can be readily detected, but practitioners must first be alert to the possibility. For example, in the 1980s, injection of MPTP (1-methyl-4-phenyl-1,2,3,6-tetrahydropyridine), an illegal "designer drug," gained notoriety when errant synthesis of illegal drugs of abuse resulted in high levels of MPTP contamination. Injection of the preparation caused severe parkinsonism in several people (Tetrud & Langston, 1989). Since then, the action of MPTP has been used as a model for the PD pathologic process in primates. Box 41-1 identifies frequently prescribed pharmacologic agents commonly associated with the onset of drug-induced PD. The sudden onset of parkinsonian symptoms that are not unilateral (see section on Diagnostic Criteria) and that are temporally associated with the administration of the identified agents should be viewed with suspicion.

PATHOPHYSIOLOGY

Termed a *movement disorder*, which encompasses a broad variety of diseases, PD may be better termed an *extrapyramidal disease* because it originates in the basal ganglia.

The pyramidal tract is the primary, efferent, descending motor pathway in the central nervous system (CNS). It originates in the cerebral cortex and provides motor control to the periphery. The extrapyramidal tract parallels the pyramidal tract, but its output is largely directed to the cerebral cortex and the pyramidal tract, providing coordination and control. The extrapyramidal system filters excitatory impulses in the cortex through successive waves of neuronal inhibition and disinhibition. The extrapyramidal tract is located deep in the cerebral hemispheres and consists of the basal ganglia (including the caudate nucleus), the putamen, and

BOX 41–1. AGENTS ASSOCIATED WITH DRUG-INDUCED PARKINSONISM

Anticonvulsants (valproate, phenytoin)
Antipsychotics (phenothiazines, haloperidol)
Calcium channel blockers
Lithium
Methyldopa
Metolocpramide
Reserpine
Selective serotonin reuptake inhibitors
Vincristine
Cytosine arabinoside

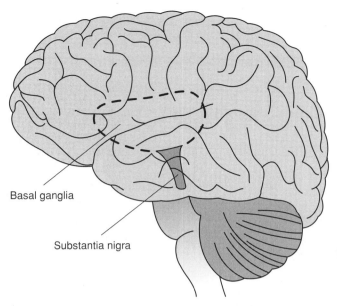

Figure 41–2 Location of substantia nigra in relation to basal ganglia.

the globus pallidus; the caudate nucleus and the putamen together make up the neostriatum or striatum (Fig. 41-1). The extrapyramidal system also encompasses structures in the brain stem, including the substantia nigra and the subthalamic nucleus.

PD is characterized by the pathologic loss of dopamine-producing neurons in the CNS. The substantia nigra of the extrapyramidal system is the region suspected to be most affected with nerve damage. Because neuronal projections originate in the substantia nigra and terminate in the striatum, there is a resulting depletion of dopaminergic transmission in the striatum. The anatomic position of the substantia nigra and its neuronal projections in relation to the basal ganglia (including the striatum) are shown in Figure 41-2.

Although the exact mechanisms are not well understood, the absence of an inhibitory dopaminergic influence in the extrapyramidal system contributes to the loss of motor coordination that defines parkinsonism. Augmentation and restoration of dopamine or inhibitory dopaminergic stimulus in the appropriate CNS regions is the primary goal of therapy. Notably, the first symptoms of disease are correlated with at

least a 60% to 80% loss of dopaminergic neuronal activity (Koller, 1997; Lang & Lozano, 1988), so a pathologic but presymptomatic phase is inferred during which neuronal death is ongoing.

Another neurotransmitter of importance in the extrapyramidal system is acetylcholine. With the deficiency of dopamine, the excitatory action of endogenous acetylcholine predominates, upsetting the balance of inhibitory and excitatory influences. The attenuation of cholinergic action is a secondary option in correcting the symptoms of PD. A simplified description of the relationship of dopamine and acetylcholine with respect to site of action is given in Figure 41-3.

Lewy bodies are a suspected pathologic feature of PD and other degenerative disorders. They were initially described as concentric, hyaline, cytoplasmic inclusions usually observed in selectively vulnerable neuronal populations (Lang & Lozano, 1988). In idiopathic PD, they are especially prevalent in nigral tissues. Unfortunately, Lewy bodies are not confined to PD, and their true significance can only be speculated on at this time. Nevertheless, they are frequently mentioned in the literature, and no discussion of PD would be complete without reference to them.

DIAGNOSTIC CRITERIA

Presenting symptoms may include any combination of motion-related symptoms, including abnormal involuntary movement, changes in skeletal muscle tone with an increase or decrease in resistance to passive motion, poverty of movement, or alteration of automatic-associated movement. The primary symptoms of PD are the hallmarks of the disease: limb muscle rigidity, resting tremor (abolished with movement), bradykinesia, and postural dysfunction or gait disturbance. At least two of the primary symptoms must be present for a diagnosis of PD. Although tremor, especially of the upper extremities, is often distinguished as the primary symptom of PD onset, this presentation may not be the case for every patient. Approximately 70% of patients manifest

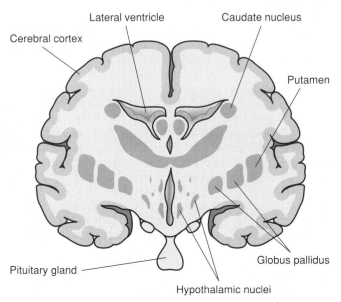

Figure 41–1 Frontal section basal ganglia.

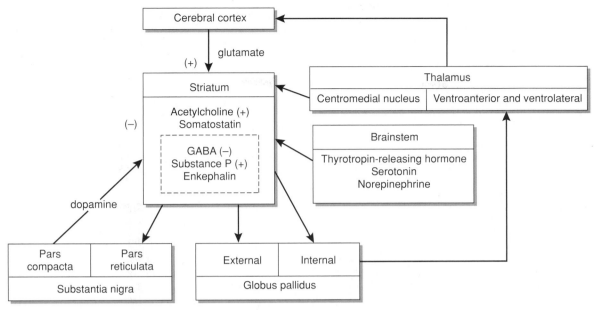

Figure 41–3 Excitatory and inhibitory effects of neuroregulators released by neurons along the basal ganglia pathways. GABA, substance P, and enkephalins are efferent neurons. Plus signs indicate an excitatory postsynaptic effect; minus signs indicate inhibitory effects.

this course (Koller, Silver, & Lieberman, 1994), but initial tremor in the lower extremities or the trunk is possible. Table 41-1 identifies the primary symptoms of PD and their features. The classic finding is initiation of symptoms unilaterally, with progression to bilateral symmetry. For the diagnosis of PD, all other disorders must be excluded.

The disability from the disease and its progression can be monitored using the easily implemented Hoehn and Yahr Scale of Disability in Parkinson's disease (Hoehn & Yahr, 1967; Box 41-2). One feature of the scale is its classification of early-stage disease by virtue of symptom asymmetry versus symmetry, indicative of the classic disease progression. Although other, more complex scales such as the United Parkinson's Disease Rating Scale (UPDRS) are available, the Hoehn and Yahr scale is distinguished by its elegance.

Both scales are validated and both are used in clinical practice and research.

In addition to the primary symptoms of PD, patients are subject to numerous secondary symptoms (Koller et al., 1994). Some of these are the end result or manifestation of the primary symptoms described earlier. Included in this category are constipation, difficulty voiding, dysphagia and drooling, shortness of breath, speech difficulties (microphonia), writing abnormalities (micrographia), blepharospasm (spasmodic twitching of the eyelids), blepharodiastasis (exaggerated separation of the eyelids, or inability to close the eyelids completely), dizziness, and masked facies (flat affect).

Table 41.1

Primary Signs and Symptoms of Parkinson's Disease

Signs and Symptoms	Features
Tremor	Occurs at rest in extremities. Initially unilateral, but often progressing to bilateral presentation. Distinguished in PD by a 4- to 6-Hz frequency (4 to 6 cycles per second).
Rigidity	Increased muscle tone at rest, exacerbated by movement. Constant resistance to range of motion, described as "cogwheel effect" due to the continual opposition of flexor and extensor muscles.
Bradykinesia	Delay in initiation of movement and poverty of all movements with halting and hesitation as a result.
Postural dysfunction and abnormal gait	Difficulties in balance and walking because of a combination of alterations in equilibrium and bradykinesia. Manifest as "freezing" episodes, poor compensation for positional changes, falls.

BOX 41–2. HOEHN AND YAHR SCALE OF DISABILITY IN PARKINSON'S DISEASE

Stage I
Unilateral involvement only; minimal functional impairment

Stage II
Bilateral involvement; no postural abnormalities

Stage III
Bilateral involvement with mild postural imbalance; patient leads independent life

Stage IV
Bilateral involvement with pronounced postural instability; patient requires substantial help with activities of daily living

Stage V
Severe, fully developed disease; patient restricted to bed or chair

These secondary symptoms can theoretically be linked to the effect of bradykinesia and rigidity.

Other secondary symptoms are psychological but are linked to the progression of parkinsonism as comorbidities, including depression, insomnia, nightmares, dementia, psychosis, and dizziness. Many of the secondary symptoms remit with appropriate PD treatment, and others can be treated with conventional modalities as appropriate. Psychosis is a more difficult problem for patients with PD because the classic neuroleptic medications used to treat psychotic symptoms (eg, hallucinations) exacerbate the motor symptoms of PD by antagonizing dopamine at its CNS receptor cites, thereby mimicking the disease process. Success in controlling psychosis has been reported with some of the newer, second-generation antipsychotic agents (Pfeiffer & Wagner, 1994). Low-dose clozapine (Clozaril), in particular, has been shown to control psychotic symptoms and has even permitted an increase in levodopa–carbidopa (Sinemet) dosing, with subsequent improved control of PD (Factor et al., 2003). However, due to its life-threatening adverse effect of agranulocytosis and frequent blood monitoring, the use of clozapine is limited. Quetiapine (Seroquel) has been shown to be effective for controlling psychosis while not compromising parkinsonian symptoms. Evidence for similar benefits with other agents of this class is lacking at this time. Clinically, quetiapine (Seroquel) has been used with some success in treating psychosis and replaces the use of clozapine.

When diagnosing a patient with PD, the practitioner needs to rule out other movement disorders such as chorea, athetosis, dystonia, hemiballismus, hepatolenticular degeneration, and a lengthy list of disorders that share a common appearance to the untrained eye. Most of these disorders are rare. Idiopathic PD, which is the most prevalent, is the focus of this chapter. Box 41-3 lists conditions to be ruled out when

BOX 41–3. DISTINGUISHING PARKINSON'S DISEASE FROM OTHER DISORDERS

Various disorders are characterized by signs and symptoms resembling those of Parkinson's disease. These conditions should therefore be ruled out when diagnosing and treating Parkinson's disease. Among them are the following:

- Alzheimer's disease
- Corticobasal ganglionic degeneration
- Drug-induced parkinsonism
- Essential tremor
- Multiple-system atrophies
- Neoplastic disease
- Olivopontocerebellar atrophy
- Postencephalitic parkinsonism
- Posthypoxic (head trauma) parkinsonism
- Progressive supranuclear palsy
- Shy-Drager syndrome
- Striatonigral degeneration
- Vascular (multi-infarct) parkinsonism

diagnosing parkinsonism. The clinical course and treatment of movement disorders may vary greatly depending on the specific clinical entity, so a diagnosis of idiopathic PD should be confirmed before considering the appropriateness of pharmacotherapeutic management.

INITIATING DRUG THERAPY

The management of PD is a unique challenge to the practitioner. The decision on when to initiate drug therapy is controversial, with no one modality being successful in all patients. Disease progress also differs from patient to patient, so implementation of therapy requires experimentation and individualization. Most providers initiate therapy when a patient begins to experience functional impairment.

As the understanding of the PD pathologic process grows, the promise of more effective therapies also grows. The future direction is for treatment focused on the presymptomatic stage of the disorder, thereby preventing disease progression. Selegiline (Eldepryl) is the only agent available that provides some approximation of this type of benefit. All other drug treatments simply focus on replacing neurotransmitter deficiencies and controlling symptoms.

Pharmacologic treatment is patient-specific; as any given agent loses its effect or becomes a source of intolerable side effects, a change in therapy should be tried. The alteration may include dose reduction, discontinuation of current agents, or addition of adjunctive agents. Patients typically take numerous combinations of agents over the course of their disease; a static, unchanging regimen is the exception rather than the rule.

Diet may play a role in stabilizing the response to drug therapy, particularly levodopa (Larodopa, Dopar) and levodopa–carbidopa (Sinemet). Because levodopa is an amino acid in chemical conformation, the ingestion of protein in the diet can compete with the transport of both exogenously provided levodopa and endogenously synthesized levodopa. This disruption of amine transport by food is thought to occur in the gastrointestinal tract and across the blood–brain barrier (Koller et al., 1994). Some patients respond favorably to limits on protein intake during the daytime hours, with the evening meal providing the bulk of daily protein intake (0.5 to 1 g/kg body weight daily); in this way, disruption of levodopa transport is avoided during the daytime hours, when control of parkinsonian symptoms is most desired.

Exercise is considered a valuable treatment modality for all patients with PD. Patients with PD may avoid activity and consequently enter a cycle of physical decompensation. A program of range-of-motion and aerobic exercise, tailored to the patient's ability, can help preserve muscle strength and coordination as the disease progresses. Although loss of strength is not necessarily part of the constellation of symptoms associated with PD, the maintenance of muscle tone promoted by a regular exercise routine can prolong physical function and maintain the ability to perform activities of daily living. The patient's sense of well-being and control is also served.

There has been increasing promise realized through surgical techniques to control parkinsonian symptoms. These techniques involve the ablation of various tissue sections in the extrapyramidal tract. The limitations to this type of surgery are obvious: unstable patients are poor candidates. In addition, the optimal extent and location of surgery are not yet well determined. Some techniques involve unilateral ablation, but more aggressive bilateral ablation has been given a trial. There is a risk of sensory and motor loss associated with these techniques. Other types of surgical procedures include deep brain stimulation and fetal transplantation. The best results are achieved in control of tremor, so that surgical correction of PD is most often reserved for younger patients whose predominant complaint is related to tremor.

Goals of Therapy

The overall goal of treatment is to cure the disease by slowing the degeneration of the nigrostriatal dopaminergic system, but unfortunately there is no therapy available currently to attain that goal. Our goal of treatment is to attain a satisfactory balance between symptom control and adverse drug effects. Establishing the goals of treatment, therefore, requires the involvement of patients and attention to their lifestyle preferences. Some patients may demand optimal muscle control because of the activities in which they prefer to participate (eg, sports, occupation). Other patients may forgo some symptomatic control of motor function and thereby avoid the detrimental CNS effects often caused by aggressive drug therapy; these patients may prefer to maximize cognitive function. In general, all the agents discussed in this chapter cause hallucinations, excitement, and insomnia when the dose is pushed past the desired response parameter. With extended use (months to years), all agents contribute to a loss of muscle control, CNS adverse effects, and "wearing off" effects. Because lifelong therapy is required, adjustment of the therapeutic combination rather than termination of therapy should be anticipated.

The following discussions identify the agents that are most efficacious in managing the symptoms of idiopathic PD (Table 41-2). All agents provide a rapid response (within hours to days) but may require cautious titration to achieve full therapeutic effect. In addition, patient tolerance has a significant impact on the dosing of any given agent or combination of agents.

Anticholinergics

The anticholinergic agents benztropine (Cogentin) and trihexyphenidyl (Artane) alter the relative balance of cholinergic and dopaminergic influences in the extrapyramidal system by inhibiting the cholinergic neurons. With the diminution of the influence of acetylcholine, nerve transmission may become more favorably controlled by dopamine. However, the anticholinergic agents are not very effective in controlling parkinsonian symptomatology. Resting tremor and sialorrhea are the symptoms that are responsive to the anticholinergic agents with any consistency. These agents have a minimal benefit in bradykinesia and rigidity. In addition, their use in patients with dementia or cognitive impairment and in geriatric populations is discouraged because anticholinergic side effects frequently manifest as confusion. Peripheral, bothersome adverse effects include dry mouth, blurred vision, constipation, urinary retention, and impaired sweating. Other difficult adverse effects include depression, irritability, insomnia, hallucinations, and tachyarrhythmia.

Abrupt discontinuation of anticholinergic agents can exacerbate PD symptoms. Anticholinergic agents are not as effective as levodopa and have a limited role in PD. These agents are typically used in younger patients with a resting tremor as the predominant symptom. Given that most patients find the adverse effects of anticholinergics intolerable and that the benefits offered are limited, further discussion of this drug category is obviated.

Dopaminergic Agents

Among the primary dopaminergic agents used in PD are levodopa and levodopa–carbidopa. Levodopa is a precursor to dopamine. Dopamine is easily degraded in the body and does not cross the blood–brain barrier. Supplementation with levodopa allows for absorption into the brain, and once in the CNS, it is converted into dopamine. The discovery of levodopa revolutionized the treatment of PD. The use of carbidopa inhibits the breakdown of levodopa in the periphery, thus allowing more levodopa to cross the blood–brain barrier. The combination of levodopa and carbidopa is the most effective treatment available for symptomatic PD. However, as the disease progresses, the duration of benefit from each dose of levodopa shortens (the "wearing off" effect) as the patient develops fluctuations in response.

Mechanism of Action

Levodopa is a precursor of dopamine that crosses the blood–brain barrier and is converted to dopamine in the brain by the enzyme dopa-decarboxylase. A cofactor of vitamin B_6 is necessary for this conversion, which occurs in the periphery as well as in the CNS. When levodopa is used alone, large doses are needed to achieve therapeutic levels in the brain because peripheral conversion of levodopa predominates.

Carbidopa prevents levodopa from being metabolized in the periphery. It inhibits the peripheral (but not the CNS) breakdown of levodopa by inhibiting its decarboxylation, thereby increasing available levodopa at the blood–brain barrier. As a result, when these agents are combined, less levodopa may be needed to achieve a therapeutic response and fewer peripheral side effects occur.

Levodopa is absorbed in the small bowel. It reaches peak plasma concentrations in 30 minutes to 2 hours for the immediate-release and controlled-release formulations, respectively. The extent of absorption depends on gastric contents. Protein-rich meals decrease and delay the absorption of levodopa from the intestines. Bioavailability of levodopa from the oral controlled-release formulation is approximately 70% to 75% compared with the immediate-release combination product. Onset of action ranges from 30 to 90 minutes with the immediate-release levodopa and 60 to 180 minutes with the controlled-release formulation (Olanow, Watts, & Koller, 2001). Levodopa undergoes extensive (85%) peripheral and hepatic metabolism. Pyridoxine (vitamin B_6) may reverse the therapeutic effects of levodopa by increasing the rate of aromatic amino acid decarboxylation in the periphery. When combined with carbidopa, the amount of levodopa required to achieve a therapeutic effect may be reduced by approximately 70%; concerns with pyridoxine are obviated. Carbidopa increases levodopa plasma levels and half-life from 1 hour to approximately 1.5 to 2 hours. Plasma levels of

Table 41.2

Overview of Selected Antiparkinsonian Agents

Generic (Trade) Name and Dosage	Selected Adverse Events	Contraindications	Special Considerations
Dopaminergics			
levodopa–carbidopa (Sinemet, Sinemet CR) Start: 100/10 tid Range: 200–2,000 mg levodopa component	Nausea, vomiting, dyskinesias	Hypersensitivity to levodopa	Withdraw monoamine oxidase inhibitors (MAOIs) at least 14 d before initiation of therapy.
levodopa (Larodopa, Dopar) 500–8,000 mg	Same as above	Same as above	Same as above
Dopaminergic Agonists			
pergolide (Permax) Start: 0.05 mg qd Range: 0.5–3 mg qd	Dyskinesias, nausea, constipation, postural hypotension, hallucinations	Hypersensitivity to pergolide or ergot derivatives	Start at 0.5 mg for 2 d, then increase by 0.1 mg every 3 d over next 12 d until therapeutic effect is achieved.
bromocriptine (Parlodel) Start: 1.25 mg PO bid Range: 2.5–100 mg bid	Dyskinesias, nausea, constipation, ataxia, insomnia, hallucinations	Hypersensitivity to pergolide or ergot derivatives Severe ischemic heart disease or peripheral vascular disease Pregnancy, lactation	
pramipexole (Mirapex) Start: 0.125 mg PO tid Range: 0.375–7.5 mg qd	Headache, dizziness, nausea, constipation, asthenia, hallucinations	Hypersensitivity to pramipexole	Gradually increase dose: 0.125 mg tid wk 1 0.25 mg tid wk 2 0.5 mg tid wk 3 0.75 mg tid wk 4 1 mg tid wk 5 1.25 mg tid wk 6 1.5 mg tid wk 7 If combined with levodopa, consider a dose reduction.
ropinirole (Requip) Start: 0.25 mg tid Range: 0.75 mg–24 mg qd	Dizziness, somnolence or insomnia, hypokinesia or hyperkinesia, nausea, constipation, postural hypotension, hallucinations	Hypersensitivity to pergolide or ergot derivatives Severe ischemic heart disease or peripheral vascular disease Pregnancy, lactation	Gradually increase dose by 0.75 mg/d for first several weeks.
Monoamine Oxidase-B Inhibitors			
selegiline (Eldepryl) Start: 2.5 mg bid Range: 5–10 mg qd	Insomnia	Hypersensitivity to selegiline and patients taking meperidine	Dose at breakfast and lunch. May require a dose reduction of levodopa–carbidopa of 10%–30% if excessive adverse reactions occur.
Catechol-O-Methyltransferase Inhibitors			
tolcapone (Tasmar) Start: 100 mg tid Range: 300–600 mg qd	Dyskinesia, nausea, sleep disorder, diarrhea	Hypersensitivity to tolcapone	Expensive
entacapone (Comtan) Start: 200 mg with each levodopa/carbidopa dose Range: 400–1,600 mg/d Max. 8 tablets (1,600 mg) per day	Orthostatic hypotension, diarrhea, hallucinations, dyskinesias	Nonselective MAOIs, hypersensitivity to entacapone	Administer with caution to patients with hepatic insufficiency.
Miscellaneous Agent			
amantadine (Symmetrel) Start: 100 mg bid Range: 100–400 mg qd	Dry mouth, blurred vision, constipation	Narrow-angle glaucoma, hypersensitivity to amantadine	Adjust dose for patients with renal dysfunction.

levodopa increase with the combination as a result of reduced peripheral degradation. The apparent half-life of levodopa is further prolonged by the controlled-release formulation (McEvoy, 1997; Olin, Hebel, & Herman, 1997).

Adverse Events

As a single agent, levodopa undergoes considerable peripheral degradation. Toxicities related to its peripheral conversion include nausea, vomiting, cardiac dysrhythmias, and postural hypotension. By combining levodopa with carbidopa, the amount of levodopa that is converted to dopamine in the periphery is decreased, reducing the adverse effects. For this reason, levodopa is no longer given alone but in combination with carbidopa. Levodopa-induced dyskinesias are involuntary, jerky movements of the head, neck, torso, limbs, and respiratory muscles. This can occur in response to levodopa administration. Dyskinesias are reversible and disappear with the reduction in levodopa dose. Long-term adverse CNS effects associated with levodopa use include akathisia, depression, delirium, agitation, paranoia, delusions, and hallucinations. In addition, there is a loss of efficacy over time—known as the "on–off" phenomenon—that may be related to fluctuating levels of levodopa in the serum and at postsynaptic dopamine receptors. Up to 50% of patients treated with levodopa develop motor fluctuations; the controlled-release combination product of levodopa–carbidopa may help to decrease the on–off phenomenon by providing a slower steady release of levodopa. Also, this formulation has a longer duration of action, which prevents fluctuations in levodopa levels.

Combination Therapy

Levodopa therapy is the cornerstone of PD treatment. Several studies have shown its efficacy (Diamond, Markham, Hoehn, et al., 1987; Markham & Diamond, 1981). Several formulations of levodopa–carbidopa are available. To block the peripheral conversion of levodopa to dopamine, 70 to 100 mg/day of carbidopa is needed. The maximum effective daily dose of carbidopa is 100 to 125 mg, beyond which there is little increase in the dopa-decarboxylase inhibitory effect. However, because of problems with peripheral degradation and side effects associated with levodopa, it is no longer given alone but in combination with carbidopa (Beizer, 1995). The current standard of care recommends a trial of levodopa as first-line therapy in patients who desire symptomatic control. The patient may be maintained on this monotherapy until levodopa component dosages exceeding 600 to 800 mg/day are required. Then, the addition of adjunctive agents to levodopa therapy or changing over to controlled-released formulations should be considered.

Levodopa–carbidopa is available in immediate- and sustained-release forms. Because of a delay in onset of action, a combination of immediate- and controlled-release preparations may be necessary. When adding a dopamine agonist, selegiline, or a catechol-O-methyltransferase (COMT) inhibitor to levodopa–carbidopa therapy, doses of the latter should be decreased. The controlled-release form of levodopa–carbidopa has been studied for the relief of dyskinesias or fluctuations in response associated with levodopa therapy, which can occur in up to 50% of patients. The dyskinesias are a result of an increase in the amount of levodopa at the dopamine 1 receptor, which can be resolved by decreasing the dose or converting to a controlled-release dosage form. These studies showed that the controlled-release formulation may decrease motor fluctuations without an increase in adverse effects (Hutton & Morris, 1992; Pahwa, Busenbark, Huber, et al., 1993; Poewe, Lees, & Stern, 1986). Studies have shown no efficacy advantage in decreasing motor fluctuations by initiating controlled-release levodopa–carbidopa over the immediate-release formulation (Koller et al., 1999). The controlled-release formulation reduces the number of doses needed; however, a higher dose of levodopa is necessary due to the decreased bioavailability of the controlled-release formulation.

Limitations with levodopa–carbidopa include the duration of effectiveness. Levodopa–carbidopa has been proven to be effective from 2 to 5 years. However, over time, it begins to "wear off," or an increase in fluctuations occurs in response to the medication. With the development of "wearing off," an increased dose of levodopa is necessary. Increasing the dose, changing to a sustained-release product, or adding an additional agent is considered.

Dosage

Levodopa therapy should be started at the lowest dosage, with the dosage increased gradually to minimize side effects. Levodopa–carbidopa may be initiated with either an immediate-release or controlled-release dosage form. The theoretic advantage of the controlled-release formulation has been discussed previously, but therapy usually is initiated with one tablet three times daily of the immediate-release formulation containing 100 mg levodopa and 25 mg carbidopa. This regimen provides the minimum amount of carbidopa to inhibit peripheral decarboxylation of levodopa to dopamine. The dose may be accelerated every few days until eight tablets (800 mg levodopa) are taken daily. At that time, transition to the formulation with 250 mg levodopa and 25 mg carbidopa may be made to allow an increasing daily levodopa dosage without exceeding 200 mg carbidopa per day.

If the controlled-release preparation is preferred for initial therapy, the usual dose is 200 mg levodopa combined with 50 mg carbidopa twice daily. Because the bioavailability of the controlled-release formulation is less than for the immediate-release formulation, patients switching to the controlled-release formulation may require 10% to 30% more levodopa than was provided in their previous immediate-release regimen. Levodopa–carbidopa may be prescribed up to a maximum of 2,000 mg levodopa and 200 mg carbidopa per day.

It is best to administer levodopa on an empty stomach or 1 hour before or after eating to facilitate absorption and minimize competition with dietary proteins. The patient should be maintained on the lowest dose that provides alleviation of symptoms. Slow titration of the dose can minimize adverse effects.

Dopamine Agonists

Dopamine agonists include pergolide (Permax), bromocriptine (Parlodel), pramipexole (Mirapex), ropinirole (Requip), and cabergoline (Cabsar). These agents directly stimulate postsynaptic dopamine receptors without affecting dopamine metabolism. Use of dopamine agonists causes less damage to the neurons since it does not involve dopamine metabolism. These agents are used as monotherapy or combination therapy. There is growing evidence in favor of using these agents as initial monotherapy to reduce the risk for development of the motor complications associated with levodopa therapy (Parkinson Study Group, 2000). These agents are less likely to cause dyskinesias. However, levodopa will eventually be necessary.

Both pergolide and bromocriptine are ergot derivatives that stimulate a wide array of neurotransmitters. Pergolide acts predominantly at the dopamine D_2 receptor but also is a weak agonist at the dopamine D_1 receptor. Bromocriptine is a potent D_2 receptor agonist and mildly antagonizes the D_1 receptor. In contrast, pramipexole, ropinirole, and cabergoline are synthetic non-ergot entities. In addition, pramipexole and ropinirole selectively bind only the D_2 and D_3 receptor families, although the significance of this selectivity is not established (Pharmacia and Upjohn Company, 1997; SmithKline Beecham, 1997; Tulloch, 1997; Watts, 1997).

The newer, non-ergot derived dopamine agonists have been shown to have fewer adverse effects than the older ergot-derived agents. Dopamine agonists and levodopa–carbidopa have been proven to be effective to alleviate symptoms; however, levodopa–carbidopa has been superior in sustaining long-term effects than the dopamine agonists, cabergoline, ropinirole and pramipexole (Parkinson Study Group, 2000). When used in combination with levodopa–carbidopa, the dose of the levodopa–carbidopa may need to be decreased. Typically, patients who are unresponsive to levodopa are considered poor candidates for dopamine agonist therapy (McEvoy, 1997). Dopamine agonists should be started at the lowest dosage and gradually titrated over several weeks to months to avoid adverse effects.

There are many advantages in using dopamine agonists as initial therapy. First, they do not require metabolic conversion to an active product to exert their pharmacologic effect and act independent of the dopamine neuron. Dopamine agonists directly stimulate subsets of dopamine receptors. They have a longer half-life then the levodopa–carbidopa formulations and thus require less frequent dosing. They do not undergo oxidative metabolism and do not generate free radicals, which could be linked to having neuroprotective effects (Albin & Frey, 2003).

Bromocriptine and Pergolide

The primary role of the ergot-derived dopamine agonists bromocriptine and pergolide in PD is as adjunctive treatment in patients in whom levodopa effectiveness is declining.

Bromocriptine is completely metabolized in the liver to inactive metabolites. Less than 5% of a dose is excreted in the urine. Most of the drug is excreted through the bile (McEvoy, 1997; *Physicians' Desk Reference*, 1997a). Bromocriptine is approximately 90% protein bound and has a half-life of 3 hours. Patients with reduced hepatic function may require adjustment of the bromocriptine dosage.

Although some studies have documented efficacy of bromocriptine as monotherapy in patients with newly diagnosed PD, efficacy for periods greater than 6 months is limited, and most patients require levodopa. Controlled, double-blind studies show that bromocriptine may provide additional control in patients maintained on optimal doses of levodopa and in patients who are beginning to acquire tolerance (the on–off phenomenon or "end-of-dose" failure of levodopa) (Koller et al., 1994). Bromocriptine has been shown to be as effective as levodopa in controlling parkinsonian symptoms when used as a substitute in patients whose symptoms are well controlled on levodopa. However, monotherapy is often limited by CNS disturbances (McEvoy, 1997). Bromocriptine and pergolide are considered to be equally effective in producing these beneficial effects.

There are limited data available on pergolide's pharmacokinetics. It is converted to at least 10 metabolites, 2 of which have dopamine agonist activity in animals. Radiolabeled pergolide was excreted by the kidneys (55%) and the lungs (5%), with 40% to 50% of the dose found in the feces over the next 7 days (Athena Neurosciences, 2000; Langtry &

Clissold, 1990). The half-life of pergolide is not known, but the mean body elimination half-life of total radioactivity was 27 hours (Langtry & Clissold, 1990). In patients with reduced hepatic function, pergolide dosage may require adjustment.

Pergolide may be useful in patients with a deteriorating response to bromocriptine. In addition, if the dose is taken at bedtime, the prolonged duration of pergolide's effect may make it particularly useful in patients with end-of-dose deterioration or early-morning akinesia and dystonia. Pergolide as initial monotherapy has been studied in a limited number of patients (Flahery, 1992; Langtry & Clissold, 1990).

Pergolide and bromocriptine are associated with a high incidence of adverse effects, including nausea, hallucinations, psychosis, confusion, and hypotension, particularly at the beginning of treatment (McEvoy, 1997). For this reason, these drugs are not routinely recommended as initial treatment for PD because they may be less well tolerated than levodopa. Orthostatic hypotension and other cardiovascular effects (palpitations, angina pectoris, and atrial premature contractions) may be more frequent with pergolide than with bromocriptine. Although pergolide may cause mild bradycardia or tachycardia, no significant arrhythmogenic properties are usually seen in patients without underlying cardiac problems. Pergolide should be administered cautiously in patients with cardiac arrhythmias or angina pectoris.

Ropinirole, Pramipexole, and Cabergoline

The newer, non–ergot-derived dopamine agonists are ropinirole, pramipexole, and cabergoline. These agents can be used as initial monotherapy to control symptoms and delay the use of levodopa or adjunctive therapy in conjunction with levodopa in patients who are experiencing "wearing off" phenomena.

Ropinirole has extensive first-pass metabolism, thus reducing its bioavailability to 55%. It is 40% bound to plasma proteins. Ropinirole is primarily metabolized by the liver to inactive metabolites. The elimination half-life is approximately 6 hours; clearance is reduced approximately 30% in patients older than age 65 years, but no effect on kinetics is observed in those with moderate renal impairment. Caution in patients with hepatic impairment is warranted (SmithKline Beecham, 1997).

Ropinirole has shown utility for de novo or adjunctive therapy of PD. In a placebo-controlled, double-blind, randomized 6-month study, ropinirole monotherapy was shown to benefit patients with early-stage (Hoehn and Yahr I to III) disease (Adler, Sethi, Hauser, et al., 1997). In other studies, significantly more patients taking ropinirole showed improvement, suggesting that ropinirole may be superior to bromocriptine as monotherapy. Moreover, ropinirole as adjuvant therapy significantly reduced the duration of "off" periods (Korczyn, 1996; Rascol, Lees, Senard, et al., 1996).

The bioavailability of pramipexole is greater than 90%. It can be administered with food, which does not alter the extent of absorption. Pramipexole is less than 20% bound to plasma proteins. Approximately 90% of a dose is recovered unchanged in the urine. No metabolites have been identified. The elimination half-life is 8 hours in healthy adults but increases to approximately 12 hours in elderly patients. Because it is eliminated primarily by the renal system, pramipexole should be used with caution in patients with renal insufficiency or failure. Dosage reduction based on creatinine clearance may be necessary in patients with impaired renal function (Nelson et al., 2002). The optimal dosage of pramipexole in geriatric patients may be less than it is in young adults (Pharmacia & Upjohn Company, 1997).

Like ropinirole, pramipexole can be used de novo or as an adjunct to levodopa–carbidopa. In two pivotal, placebo-controlled, double-blind, randomized studies (Parkinson's Study Group, 1997; Shannon, Bennett, & Friedman, 1997), pramipexole significantly improved the control of symptoms compared with placebo in patients with early-stage disease (Hoehn and Yahr I to III). Recent use of levodopa or other agonists was not permitted by study design. According to measures of motor response and activities of daily living, overall improvements of approximately 20% to 30% were noted in both studies. Study duration ranged from 10 weeks (Parkinson's Study Group, 1997) to 6 months (Shannon et al., 1997). Similar results were reported in a less rigorous investigation of early-stage patients (Hubble, Koller, Cutler, et al., 1995). Pramipexole as an adjunct to levodopa–carbidopa has also improved control in advanced disease with motor fluctuations characterized by the "wearing off" effect (Lieberman, Ranhosky, & Korts, 1997). All other PD medications were continued throughout this 32-week, randomized, placebo-controlled, double-blind trial. Significant improvements in UPDRS measures of motor function and activities of daily living, as well as a significant reduction in the duration of "off" time, were noted. Levodopa use was also significantly reduced. Another study of adjunctive pramipexole therapy in patients with advanced disease produced less impressive results, but included patients with the more severe on–off fluctuations (Molho, Factor, Weiner, et al., 1995).

Ropinirole and pramipexole may present the same dopaminergic or serotonergic adverse effect profile (Gottwald, Bainbridge, Dowling, et al., 1997). Postural hypotension, dyskinesias, somnolence, unsteadiness, hallucinations, and confusion have been reported with the use of both agents.

Ropinirole serum levels may be significantly increased by ciprofloxacin (Cipro) and estrogens. Given its renal route of elimination, pramipexole serum levels are greatly increased by cimetidine (Tagamet), an inhibitor of renal tubular secretion (Pharmacia & Upjohn Company, 1997). Cimetidine causes a 50% increase in the amount of pramipexole retained in the body and a 40% increase in half-life. As with all dopaminergic agonists, titration of dose to individual patient response is necessary to optimize treatment.

Cabergoline is a long-acting dopamine agonist. It not indicated for the treatment of PD in the United States, only for the treatment of hyperprolactinemia; however, it is indicated for PD in some European countries. Further discussion of this agent is not necessary.

Dopamine Metabolism Inhibitors: Selegiline

Selegiline (Eldepryl) is an irreversible monoamine oxidase type-B (MAO-B) inhibitor. It is selective for MAO-B at dosages lower than 20 mg/day. Primarily found in the brain, MAO-B is an enzyme responsible for the degradation of dopamine. By inhibiting this enzyme, selegiline increases nigrostriatal dopamine levels. Selegiline is approved for use as adjunctive therapy in patients who have developed tolerance to levodopa. The drug mildly improves clinical function, but when used in combination with levodopa, the levodopa dosage can be reduced by approximately 20% to 30% to avoid the development of dyskinesias. In addition, selegiline may have neuroprotective effects; however, this is still controversial (Beizer, 1995; Parkinson's Study Group, 1993; Tetrud & Langston, 1989). Selegiline may slow the rate of neuronal degeneration by blocking the formation of free radicals, which are formed with dopamine metabolism. This effect may account for its neuroprotective properties; however, selegiline does not halt disease progression. Early use of selegiline 5 mg twice a day may slow the progress of PD by approximately 9 months to 1 year. The mechanism for this protective effect involves inhibition of endogenous oxidative mechanisms that may contribute to premature nerve cell death (Olanow, 1997).

Selegiline is rapidly absorbed and achieves maximum plasma concentrations in 30 minutes to 2 hours. It is metabolized in the liver to three metabolites: *N*-desmethyldeprenyl (the major metabolite), amphetamine, and methamphetamine (Olin et al., 1997). Some of the symptom-relieving effects of selegiline may be attributed to these metabolites.

Dosage

Selegiline's use is limited to the amelioration of the end-of-dose fluctuations seen in patients who have become tolerant to levodopa. It is most effective when used with levodopa in these patients. A reduction of 10% to 30% in the total daily dose of levodopa may be permitted (or required by dyskinetic manifestations) when selegiline is added to existing therapy (Koller et al., 1994). It is given 5 mg two times a day, with the second dose being given in the early afternoon due to the amphetamine metabolite.

Controlled studies evaluating selegiline's effectiveness when used alone or in early PD have yielded conflicting results. Most evidence suggests that initial selegiline use may have a neuroprotective effect (Parkinson's Study Group, 1993), providing a greater time before levodopa therapy becomes necessary; other studies found no neuroprotective effects or clinical benefits compared with levodopa therapy alone (Fuller & Tolbert, 1991; Lees, 1995; Lieberman & Fazzini, 1991). The early use of selegiline as a component of therapy is recognized to offer a potential neuroprotective benefit with little risk to the patient (Koller et al., 1994). This therapeutic opportunity is particularly applicable to the younger patient with PD, in whom protection against disease progression offers the greatest potential benefit.

Adverse Events

Selegiline causes a high incidence of insomnia. To reduce the incidence of insomnia, it is best to give the second dose earlier in the day. Dosages greater than 20 mg/day are likely to produce pronounced stimulation. Selegiline use can also cause confusion, hallucinations, nausea, and orthostatic hypotension. These effects are usually mild and occur in fewer than 10% of patients. At dosages less than 10 mg/day, adverse effects associated with nonselective MAO inhibitors and tyramine-containing foods are rarely seen. Concomitant administration of selegiline and the selective serotonin reuptake inhibitors (eg, fluoxetine [Prozac], paroxetine [Paxil], sertraline [Zoloft]) should be avoided.

Dopamine Metabolism Inhibitors: Tolcapone, Entacapone

Tolcapone (Tasmar) and entacapone (Comtan) are selective and reversible inhibitors of the enzyme catechol-O-methyltransferase (COMT). COMT metabolizes levodopa to an undesirable toxic metabolite, 3-O-methyldopa, both centrally and peripherally (whereas dopa-decarboxylase converts levodopa to dopamine). When peripheral metabolism of levodopa by dopa-decarboxylase is inhibited by carbidopa, COMT becomes a primary route of peripheral levodopa degradation. The role of COMT inhibitors in PD is as an adjunctive therapy to levodopa in patients with advanced PD. These agents will decrease motor fluctuations, "off" time, and levodopa requirements. When used in combination with levodopa, the levodopa dosage may have to be decreased to minimize the risk of dyskinesias. Stalevo is a new fixed-dose combination product of entacapone and levodopa–carbidopa. Both COMT inhibitors must be used in conjunction with levodopa to produce an effect.

Mechanism of Action

Tolcapone prevents the peripheral (and, to a lesser degree, central) degradation of levodopa to 3-O-methyldopa by inhibiting COMT; entacapone inhibits only peripheral COMT. The result is that levodopa levels are increased approximately twofold in the CNS when a COMT inhibitor is administered with levodopa formulations (Jorga, Sedek, Fotteler, et al., 1997, Olanow, Watts, & Koller, 2001). The combination increases the amount of levodopa available for activity in the body (and the CNS), resulting in steady levodopa levels (Spencer & Benfield, 1996). More specifically, the initial levels of levodopa that are achieved with any given dose are relatively unchanged, but the subsequent degradation over time is slowed, thereby preserving levodopa levels and dopamine activity.

The bioavailability of tolcapone is approximately 65%, with a decrease of 10% to 20% when given with food. Plasma protein binding—largely to serum albumin—exceeds 99.9%. Tolcapone is virtually completely metabolized by COMT and by glucuronidation. A small amount is excreted unchanged in the urine (Roche Laboratories, 1997). The half-life of the parent compound is approximately 2 hours (Dingemanse, Jorga, Schmitt, et al., 1995), and no accumulation has been detected in otherwise healthy elderly patients (Jorga et al., 1997).

When entacapone is given in conjunction with levodopa–carbidopa, plasma levels of levodopa are greater and more sustained than after administration of levodopa–carbidopa alone. The onset of action is usually within 1 hour, and action is sustained for 6 to 8 hours. Since entacapone enhances the bioavailability of levodopa, it may also cause an increase in the occurrence of orthostatic hypotension. Diarrhea, hallucinations, and dyskinesias are other possible side effects. Entacapone may increase levels of other drugs metabolized by the COMT enzyme, such as epinephrine

and norepinephrine. Entacapone may interact with nonselective MAO inhibitors but can be given concomitantly with an MAO-B selective agent such as selegiline (Comtan, 2000).

Time Frame for Response

Adjunctive therapy with tolcapone provides beneficial effects for up to 12 months in patients with PD experiencing motor fluctuations on levodopa–carbidopa (Kurth, Adler, St. Hilaire, et al., 1997). In this placebo-controlled, double-blind, randomized trial, patients were limited to those with a predictable wearing-off response. In a second, similarly designed study (Rajput, Martin, St. Hilaire, et al., 1997), tolcapone significantly decreased the mean percentage of "off" time and total levodopa dose and significantly increased total "on" time compared with placebo. In a third study that included patients not experiencing motor fluctuations while taking levodopa–carbidopa, adjunctive therapy with tolcapone significantly improved measures of motor function and activities of daily living, as measured by the UPDRS (Waters, Kurth, Bailey, et al., 1997). Total levodopa dose was also significantly reduced compared with placebo. Improvements were maintained over a 12-month period.

Entacapone has been associated with an increase in "on" time, a decrease in "off" time, and improved motor function. In a placebo-controlled trial, entacapone increased the "on" time by 1.5 hours, and the mean duration of "on" response was increased by approximately 30 minutes with each dose. This allowed for a 16% decrease in the levodopa requirement (Rinne, Larsen, Siden, et al., 1998). Improvements were sustained over a period of 3 years.

Adverse Events

The adverse effect profile of the COMT inhibitors is largely related to an increased dopaminergic response; an increase in the incidence of dyskinesias has been noted when a COMT agent is added to levodopa therapy (Gottwald et al., 1997). Additional adverse effects include diarrhea, nausea, headache, mild somnolence, insomnia, urine discoloration, abdominal cramping, and orthostatic hypotension. These adverse reactions present within the first few days of therapy and can usually be controlled by reducing the dosage of levodopa by 15% to 30% (Olanow, Watts, & Koller, 2001). Severe hepatocellular injury has been reported with tolcapone. Because the incidence of hepatic failure may be increased 100-fold, tolcapone should be reserved for patients not responding adequately to other agents or those who are intolerant of alternative therapies. In addition, patients with hepatic dysfunction are not considered good candidates for tolcapone therapy, and the drug should be discontinued in any patient showing serum hepatic aminotransferase elevations or signs and symptoms of hepatic injury during treatment. Frequent monitoring (every 2 weeks) of liver function is required during tolcapone therapy, and the drug should be discontinued if no clinical benefit is realized within 3 weeks of initiation. Tolcapone has been taken off the market in Canada and several European countries, and a black-box warning limits the use of tolcapone in the United States. The severe hepatotoxicity that occurs with tolcapone has not been reported with entacapone.

Miscellaneous Agent: Amantadine

Amantadine (Symmetrel) is an antiviral agent with antiparkinsonian properties used to treat mild PD and drug-induced parkinsonism and as an adjunct in late PD. It is effective in the treatment of the resting tremor of PD when used alone or in combination with levodopa. This has been documented in several early studies (Fahn & Isgreen, 1975; Schwab et al., 1972; Timberlake & Vance, 1978). Its usefulness, however, in treating PD is limited because tachyphylaxis can develop within a few months of initiating therapy (Fahn & Isgreen, 1975; Koller et al., 1994). Long-term use is discouraged, and dose escalation is necessary in pursuit of continued efficacy. Sudden withdrawal of amantadine may cause exacerbation of parkinsonian symptoms.

When used to treat PD, amantadine is often classified as a dopaminergic agent, but its mechanism of action is not completely understood and it is inaccurate to place it in the same class as levodopa or the dopaminergic agonists. Amantadine's antiparkinsonian activity is believed to be due to its ability to block the reuptake of dopamine into presynaptic neurons, to stimulate dopamine release from the nerve storage sites, causing direct stimulation of postsynaptic receptors and possibly having anticholinergic effects (Beizer, 1995; Olin et al., 1997).

Amantadine is readily absorbed and is not metabolized. Blood levels peak in approximately 4 hours after oral administration in normal adults. It is excreted unchanged in the urine, with a mean elimination half-life of approximately 2 to 7 hours in patients with normal renal function and 24 to 29 hours in geriatric patients. Amantadine's clearance is reduced and its elimination half-life is significantly increased by two- to threefold in patients with renal insufficiency. A dosage reduction is recommended for patients age 65 years and older (Olin et al., 1997). Specific dosage adjustments are required for patients with renal impairment and are based on creatinine clearance values.

Amantadine is associated with a high incidence of insomnia. Because it is administered twice daily, it is best to take the second dose earlier in the day to reduce the incidence of insomnia. Amantadine has been reported to cause livedo reticularis, a rose-colored mottling of the skin usually involving the lower extremities. This can occur in up to 80% of patients and may be observed as early as 2 weeks after initiating therapy. This side effect is usually self-limiting and resolves after discontinuation of amantadine therapy. Other problematic side effects include urinary retention, orthostatic hypotension, peripheral edema, and congestive heart failure. Besides insomnia, other CNS side effects are common and include dizziness, confusion, disorientation, depression, nervousness, irritability, and hallucinations.

Selecting the Most Appropriate Agent

Since there is no therapy proven to slow the progression of disease, pharmacologic therapy is not considered until the patient's disability warrants it. The rationale for selecting any particular antiparkinsonian agent is the patient's age, stage of disease, therapeutic history, predominant symptoms, cost, and preferred level of symptomatic control (patient's activity level) (Fig. 41-4). The gold standard of care at nearly any Hoehn and Yahr stage remains levodopa–carbidopa in either the immediate- or controlled-release formulation. Pharmacotherapy is initiated upon bothersome symptoms and is tailored using the criteria mentioned above. It is important to monitor for signs and symptoms of adverse effects (eg, dyskinesias). Initiation of pharmacologic therapy should begin with a low dosage, with the dosage increased slowly to avoid adverse effects. The dosage of the first agent should be optimized before adding additional agents. Patients should be maintained on the lowest dosage of medication possible. Table 41-3 summarizes therapeutic choices.

First-Line Therapy

First-line therapy is often chosen by the stage of the disease, presenting symptoms, age of the patient, and other comorbidities. A younger patient usually has a long treatment span, and thus the use of levodopa–carbidopa should be reserved until other treatments have failed. Amantadine, anticholinergics, and dopamine agonists are acceptable starting options in these patients, and therapy should be tailored to symptoms. The use of levodopa–carbidopa may be supplemented and may eventually be necessary. Studies have shown that patients started on dopamine agonist therapy have a reduced risk for the development of motor complications compared to those started on levodopa (Parkinson Study Group, 2000). Patients with an older onset of disease have a shorter treatment time, and thus starting with levodopa–carbidopa is appropriate. Patients with cognitive impairment who may not tolerate a dopamine agonist may start with levodopa–carbidopa. Dosages are always dictated by the patient's tolerance of drug effects and the onset of side effects (eg, hallucinations, hypotension). Initiation of therapy with selegiline is often considered, even at the mildest stages of disease, in the hope of slowing disease progression by its possible neuroprotective effects.

Second-Line Therapy

The addition of adjunctive drugs is suggested once the threshold of levodopa–carbidopa therapy is reached to avoid accelerating the levodopa dose and increasing the risk of negative outcomes. Adjuncts may include the dopamine agonists or COMT inhibitors; amantadine or selegiline may be added if not previously instituted. The addition of dopamine agonists is often given a trial, but the advent of hallucinations or psychotic symptoms may be dose-limiting. Entacapone and selegiline increase existing levodopa serum (and CNS) levels, with the possibility of exacerbating the existing side effect profile. When using adjunctive therapy along with levodopa–carbidopa, a reduction in the levodopa–carbidopa dose may be necessary to avoid dyskinesias.

Third-Line Therapy

Third-line therapy consists of manipulating previously initiated drug doses or recombining agents. Patients at this stage are very likely to experience an erratic response to levodopa, but they also may experience severe hallucinations with the dopamine agonists. Augmentation with and adjustment of adjunctive medications may promote a longer duration of response; better, less variable control; and possibly a minimization of side effects. Lower doses with multiple agents may be successful.

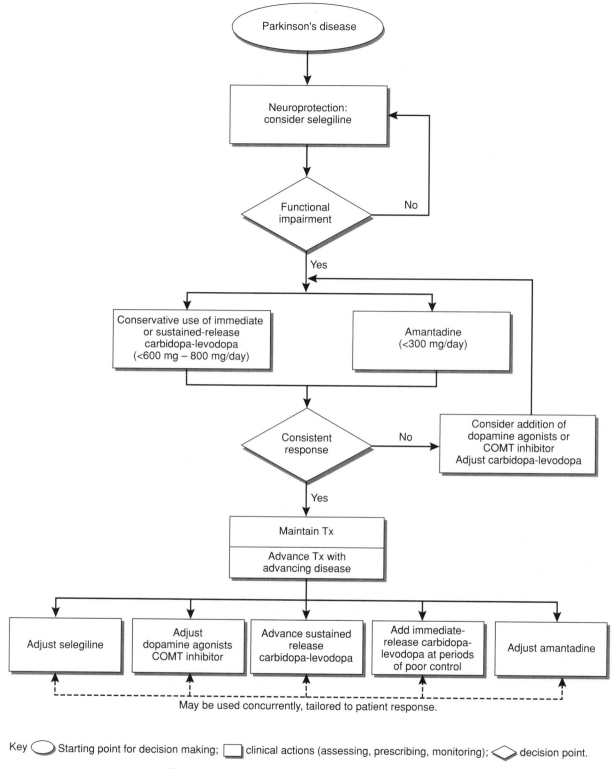

Figure 41–4   Treatment algorithm for Parkinson's disease.

MONITORING PATIENT RESPONSE

The greatest concern with the use of antiparkinsonian agents is their CNS effects, particularly in those who may exhibit preexisting intellectual deterioration, such as patients with dementia. All of these agents have CNS adverse effects that include hallucinations, agitation, delirium, insomnia, and confusion. Therefore, the patient's mental status should be assessed frequently. The Mini Mental Status Exam is an accessible instrument that can be quickly implemented for this purpose (Koller et al., 1994). Erratic motor responses associated with levodopa–carbidopa and the concern over its long-term efficacy require frequent monitoring of patient response. The

Table 41.3

Recommended Order of Treatment for Parkinson's Disease

Order	Agents	Comments
First line	Selegiline Amantadine Anticholinergics Dopamine agonist Levodopa–carbidopa	The early use of selegiline as a component of therapy is recognized to offer a potential neuroprotective benefit with little risk to the patient (Koller et al., 1994). Medications should be tailored to the symptoms, other comorbidities, and the patient's treatment span. In younger patients, amantadine, anticholinergics, or dopamine agonist is an appropriate starting agent. In older patients, levodopa–carbidopa should be initiated.
Second line	Levodopa–carbidopa (sustained release) COMT inhibitors Dopamine agonist	Once first-line therapy is optimized, use of an additional agent is necessary. Sustained-release levodopa–carbidopa is appropriate for motor fluctuations. When adding a dopamine agonist, selegiline, or a COMT inhibitor to levodopa–carbidopa therapy, doses of the latter should be decreased.
Third line	Multiple agents in combination	Tachyphylaxis can occur within a few months of initiating therapy.

dopaminergic agonists may be more likely to produce hallucinations, but combination levodopa–agonist therapy can mitigate adverse effects by permitting lower dosages of either agent. The use of other drug combinations may offer the same benefits. Geriatric patients may be disposed to CNS toxicities associated with antiparkinsonian drugs.

The individualization of therapy to patient response is the most prudent guide. Control of symptoms should meet the patient's functional needs. Goals of therapy should be set in conjunction with the patient's desires. The onset of drug-induced adverse effects may preclude full symptomatic control. Empiric manipulation of therapy (both dosage and drug combination) to achieve a satisfactory balance of symptom control and drug-induced adversities is to be expected. The Hoehn and Yahr scale is adequate for monitoring disease progress.

Disease progress is unique in any individual. Some patients may expect to be stable at an early stage of the disease for most of their lives. These patients may not require adjustments of therapy to maintain an adequate quality of life. Other patients exhibit progression to severe disease. Therefore, monitoring of patient response to drug therapy must account for individual patient presentations.

PATIENT EDUCATION

Education of the patient and the patient's family is essential so that the difficulties of progressing disease can be anticipated and management strategies planned. Decisions about drug therapy must involve the patient's preferences, so the patient must be fully aware of the consequences of both

disease and therapy. Patients should be aware that PD may progress to severe disability or may become relatively stable. In recognizing this, both the patient and the family can prepare emotionally and enlist the financial and social resources that eventually may be necessary.

Drug Information

There is no particular source for information. The website for the National Parkinson's Foundation (http://www.parkinson.org) has useful information for providers about current clinical trials. The journals *Neurology* and *Archives of Neurology* publish many articles on PD.

Patient-Oriented Information Sources

The National Parkinson's Foundation (http://www.parkinson.org) is a primary source of patient support. In addition, most health care systems, hospitals, and clinics offer regular programs in support of patients with PD. At these seminars, patients and families can share their experience and expertise, thereby empowering patients to maintain control of their lives.

Complementary and Alternative Medications

The use of vitamin E and coenzyme-Q10 remains controversial for PD therapy. These agents are reviewed in another chapter, but in general their beneficial mechanisms of action have been due to their antioxidant effects.

■ Case Study

D.H. is a 55-year-old white man who has been active as an office manager in the insurance industry for most of his career. He and his wife enjoy a full family life with two children, 25 and 30 years of age, who are independent but remain geographically and socially close. His activities include recreational golf and tennis with his children, and he expects to continue his chosen employment until retirement.

Lately, D.H. reports, he has experienced a tremor in his right hand that is not overly disruptive of work but has impaired his ability to participate in recreational activities. His wife has not noticed the tremor when D.H. is sleeping. None of his coworkers has noticed his physical symptoms, and he is confident that he can "hide" it indefinitely, but he has brought it to the attention of his children. They are not overly concerned but have encouraged D.H. to seek a medical opinion.

Diagnosis: Idiopathic Parkinson's disease

> 1. List one or two specific goals of treatment for D.H.
>
> 2. What drug therapy would you prescribe for D.H., and what is the rationale for the selection?
>
> 3. Describe how and when you would monitor for the success of the therapy.
>
> 4. Describe one or two adverse reactions to your treatment that would cause you to change therapy.
>
> 5. Describe one or two drug/drug or drug/food interactions for the selected agent.
>
> 6. What education would you provide to D.H. regarding the drug therapy? What would you tell the caregiver or spouse of the patient?
>
> 7. If the drug was not achieving the intended goal, what would be your second drug of choice?
>
> 8. What OTC and/or alternative medications, if any, would be appropriate for D.H.?
>
> 9. What dietary and lifestyle changes should be recommended for D.H.?

Bibliography

Starred references are cited in the text.

*Adler, C. H., Sethi, K. D., Hauser, R. A., et al. (1997). Ropinirole for the treatment of early Parkinson's disease. *Neurology, 49,* 393–399.

*Albin, R. L., & Frey, K. A. (2003). Initial agonist therapy of Parkinson disease. *Neurology, 60,* 390–394.

Anonymous. (1989). Pergolide and selegiline for Parkinson's disease. *Medical Letter on Drugs and Therapeutics, 31,* 81–83.

Athena Neurosciences. (2000). Permax (pergolide) package insert. San Francisco: Author.

*Beizer, J. L. (1995). Parkinson's disease. *American Pharmacy, 35*(1), 20–30.

Brannan, T., & Yahr, M. D. (1995). Comparative study of selegiline plus L-dopa versus L-dopa-carbidopa alone in the treatment for Parkinson's disease. *Annals of Neurology, 37,* 95–98.

Calne, D. B. (1993). Treatment of Parkinson's disease. *New England Journal of Medicine, 329,* 1021–1027.

Cedarbaum, J. M., Toy, L. H., & Green-Parsons, A. (1991). L-deprenyl (selegiline) added to Sinemet CR in the management of Parkinson's disease patients with motor response fluctuations. *Clinical Neuropharmacology, 14,* 228–234.

Chrisp, P., Mammen, G. J., & Sorkin, E. M. (1991). Selegiline: A review of its pharmacology, symptomatic benefits and protective potential in Parkinson's disease. *Drugs and Aging, 1,* 228–248.

*Diamond, S. G., Markham, C. H., Hoehn, M. M., et al. (1987). Multicenter study of Parkinson mortality with early versus late dopa treatment. *Annals of Neurology, 22,* 8–12.

*Dingemanse, J., Jorga, K. M., Schmitt, M., et al. (1995). Integrated pharmacokinetics and pharmacodynamics of the novel catechol-O-methyltransferase inhibitor tolcapone during first administration to humans. *Clinical Pharmacology and Therapeutics, 57,* 508–517.

Eden, R. J., Costall, B., Domeney, A. M., et al. (1991). Preclinical pharmacology of ropinirole, a novel dopamine D_2 agonist. *Pharmacology, Biochemistry, and Behavior, 38,* 147–154.

Elizan, T. S., Yahr, M. D., Moros, D. A., et al. (1989). Selegiline as an adjunct to conventional levodopa therapy in Parkinson's disease. *Archives of Neurology, 46,* 1280–1283.

*Factor, S. A., Feustel, P. J., Friedman, J. H., et al. (2003). Longitudinal outcome of Parkinson's disease patients with psychosis. *Neurology. 60,* 1756–1761.

*Fahn, S., & Isgreen, W. P. (1975). Long-term evaluation of amantadine and levodopa combination in parkinsonism by double-blind crossover analyses. *Neurology, 25,* 695.

*Flahery, J. F. (1992). Parkinson's disease. In M. A. Koda-Kimble & L. Y. Young (Eds.), *Applied therapeutics: The clinical use of drugs* (5th ed.). Vancouver: Applied Therapeutics.

*Fuller, M. A., & Tolbert, S. R. (1991). Selegiline: Initial or adjunctive therapy of Parkinson's disease? *DICP, 25*(1), 36–40.

Goetz, C. G., Tanner, C. M., Glantz, R. H., & Klawans, H. L. (1985). Chronic agonist therapy for Parkinson's disease: A 5-year study of bromocriptine and pergolide. *Neurology, 35,* 749–751.

*Gottwald, M. D., Bainbridge, J. L., Dowling, G. A., et al. (1997). New pharmacotherapy for Parkinson's disease. *Annals of Pharmacotherapy, 31,* 1205–1217.

*Hoehn, M. H., & Yahr, M. D. (1967). Parkinsonism: Onset, progression and mortality. *Neurology, 17,* 427–442.

*Hubble, J. P., Koller, W. C., Cutler, N. R., et al. (1995). Pramipexole in patients with early Parkinson's disease. *Clinical Neuropharmacology, 18,* 338–347.

*Hutton, J. T., & Morris, J. L. (1992). Long-acting carbidopa-levodopa in the management of moderate and advanced Parkinson's disease. *Neurology, 42,* 51–56.

*Jorga, K. M., Sedek, G., Fotteler, B., et al. (1997). Optimizing levodopa pharmacokinetics with multiple tolcapone doses in the elderly. *Clinical Pharmacology and Therapeutics, 62,* 300–310.

*Koller, W. C. (1992). Initiating treatment of Parkinson's disease. *Neurology, 42*(Suppl. 1), 33–38.

*Koller, W. C., Hutton, J. T., Tolorsa, E., et al. (1999). Immediate-release and controlled-release carbidopa/levodopa in PD: A 5-year randomized multicenter study. *Neurology, 53,* 1012–1019.

Koller, W. C., & Montgomery, E. B. (1997). Issues in the early diagnosis of Parkinson's disease. *Neurology, 49*(Suppl. 1), S10–S25.

*Koller, W. C., Silver, D. E., & Lieberman, A. (1994). An algorithm for the management of Parkinson's disease. *Neurology, 44*(Suppl. 10), S1–S2.

*Korczyn, A. (1996). A double-blind study comparing ropinirole and bromocriptine in patients with early Parkinson's disease (Abstract). *Neurology, 46*(Suppl.), A159.

*Kurth, M. C., Adler, C. H., St. Hilaire, M., et al. (1997). Tolcapone improves motor function and reduces levodopa requirement in patients with Parkinson's disease experiencing motor fluctuations. *Neurology, 48*, 81–87.

*Lang, A. E., & Lozano, A. M. (1988). Parkinson's disease: First of two parts. *New England Journal of Medicine, 339*, 1044–1053.

*Langtry, H. D., & Clissold, S. P. (1990). Pergolide: A review of its pharmacological properties and therapeutic potential in Parkinson's disease. *Drugs, 39*, 491–506.

*Lazzarini, A. M., Myers, R. H., Zimmerman, T. R., Jr., et al. (1994). A clinical genetic study of Parkinson's disease: Evidence for dominant transmission. *Neurology, 44*, 499–506.

*Lees, A. J. (1995). Comparison of therapeutic effects and mortality data of levodopa and levodopa combined with selegiline in patients with early, mild Parkinson's disease. *British Medical Journal, 211*, 1602–1607.

LeWitt, P. A., Ward, C. D., Larsen, T. A., et al. (1983). Comparison of pergolide and bromocriptine therapy in parkinsonism. *Neurology, 33*, 1009–1014.

*Lieberman, A., & Fazzini, E. (1991). Experience with selegiline and levodopa in advanced Parkinson's disease. *Acta Neurologica Scandinavica Supplementum, 136*, 66–69.

*Lieberman, A., Ranhosky, A., & Korts, D. (1997). Clinical evaluation of pramipexole in advanced Parkinson's disease: Results of a double-blind, placebo-controlled, parallel-group study. *Neurology, 49*, 162–168.

Lieberman, A.M., Neophytides, A., Liebowitz, M., et al. (1983). Comparative efficacy of pergolide and bromocriptine in patients with advanced Parkinson's disease. *Advances in Neurology, 37*, 95–108.

*Markham, C. H., & Diamond, S. G. (1981). Evidence to support early levodopa therapy in Parkinson's disease. *Neurology, 31*, 125–131.

McDowell, F., & Cedarbaumm, J. M. (1992). The extrapyramidal system and disorders of movement. In R. J. Joynt (Ed.), *Clinical neurology* (vol. 3). Philadelphia: J. B. Lippincott.

*McEvoy, G. K. (Ed.). (1997). Bromocriptine. In *AHFS drug information 97*. Bethesda, MD: American Society of Health-System Pharmacists.

McFarland, H. R. (1993). Treatment of Parkinson's disease. *Neurology, 43*, 1056–1057.

Miyasaki, J. M., Martin, W., Suchowersky, O., et al. (2002). Practice parameter: Initiation of treatment for Parkinson's disease: An evidence-based review. *Neurology, 58*, 11–17.

*Mitchell, S. L., Kiely, D. K., Kiel, D. P., et al. (1996). The epidemiology, clinical characteristics, and natural history of older nursing home residents with a diagnosis of Parkinson's disease. *Journal of the American Geriatrics Society, 44*, 394–399.

*Molho, E. S., Factor, S. A., Weiner, W. J., et al. (1995). The use of pramipexole, a novel dopamine agonist, in advanced Parkinson's disease. *Journal of Neural Transmission, 45*(Suppl.), 225–230.

*National Parkinson's Foundation. (2004). [On-line]. Available: http://www.parkinson.org.

Novartis Pharmaceuticals. (2000). Comtan (entacapone) package insert. East Hanover, NJ: Author.

*Nelson, M. V., Berchou, R. C., & LeWitt, P. A. (2002). Parkinson's disease. In J. T. DiPiro, R. L. Talbert, P. E. Hayes, G. C. Yee, G. R. Matzke, & L. M. Posey (Eds.), *Pharmacotherapy: A pathophysiologic approach* (5th ed.). New York: McGraw-Hill.

*Olanow, C. W. (1990). Oxidative reactions in Parkinson's disease. *Neurology, 40*(Suppl. 3), S32–S37.

*Olanow, C. W. (1997). Attempts to obtain neuroprotection in Parkinson's disease. *Neurology, 49*(Suppl. 1), S26–S33.

*Olanow, C. W., Watts, R. L., & Koller, W. C. (2001). An algorithm (decision tree) for the management of Parkinson's disease: Treatment guidelines. *Neurology, 56*, S1–S88.

*Olin, B. R., Hebel, S. K., Herman, R. C., eds. (1997). *Drug facts and comparisons*. St. Louis: Facts and Comparisons.

*Pahwa, R., Busenbark, K., Huber, S. J., et al. (1993). Clinical experience with controlled-release carbidopa/levodopa in Parkinson's disease. *Neurology, 43*, 677–681.

Parkes, J. D. (1981). Adverse effects of anti-Parkinsonian drugs. *Drugs, 21*, 341.

*Parkinson Study Group. (2000). Pramipexole vs. levodopa as initial treatment for Parkinson disease: A randomized controlled trial. *JAMA, 284*(15), 1931–1938.

*Parkinson's Study Group. (1993). Effects of tocopherol and deprenyl on the progression of disability in early Parkinson's disease. *New England Journal of Medicine, 328*, 176–183.

*Parkinson's Study Group. (1997). Safety and efficacy of pramipexole in early Parkinson disease. *JAMA, 278*, 125–130.

Pezzoli, G., Martignoni, E., Pacchetti, C., et al. (1994). Pergolide compared with bromocriptine in Parkinson's disease: A multicenter, crossover, controlled study. *Movement Disorders, 9*, 431–436.

*Pfeiffer, C., & Wagner, M. L. (1994). Clozapine therapy for Parkinson's disease and other movement disorders. *American Journal of Hospital Pharmacy, 51*, 3047–3053.

*Pharmacia & Upjohn Company. (1997). Mirapex (Pramipexole) package insert. Kalamazoo, MI: Author.

Physicians' Desk Reference. (1997a). Parlodel package insert.

Physicians' Desk Reference. (1997b). Permax package insert.

*Poewe, W. H., Lees, A. J., & Stern, G. M. (1986). Low-dose L-dopa therapy in Parkinson's disease: A 6-year follow-up study. *Neurology, 36*, 28–30.

Quinn, N. P. (1984). Anti-parkinsonian drugs today. *Drugs, 28*, 236.

*Rajput, A. H., Martin, W., Saint-Hilaire, M. H., et al. (1997). Tolcapone improves motor function in Parkinson patients with the "wearing-off" phenomenon: A double-blind, placebo-controlled, multicenter trial. *Neurology, 49*, 1066–1071.

*Rascol, O., Lees, A. J., Senard, J. M., et al. (1996). Ropinirole in the treatment of levodopa-induced motor fluctuation in patients with Parkinson's disease. *Clinical Neuropharmacology, 19*, 234–245.

*Rinne, U. K., Larsen, J. P., Siden, A., et al. (1998). Entacapone enhances the response to levodopa in parkinsonian patients with motor fluctuations. *Neurology, 51*, 1309–1314.

*Roche Laboratories. (1997). Tasmar (Tolcapone) package insert. Nutley, NJ: Author.

Ross, R. T. (1990). Drug-induced parkinsonism and other movement disorders. *Canadian Journal of Neurological Sciences, 17*, 155–162.

Sage, J. I., & Mark, M. H. (1994). Diagnosis and treatment of Parkinson's disease in the elderly. *Journal of General Internal Medicine, 9*, 583–589.

*Schwab, R. S., et al. (1972). Amantadine in Parkinson's disease. *JAMA, 222*, 792.

*Shannon, K. M., Bennett, J. P., Jr., & Friedman, J. H. (1997). Efficacy of pramipexole, a novel dopamine agonist, as monotherapy in mild to moderate Parkinson's disease. *Neurology, 49*, 724–728.

Shults, C. W. (2003). Treatments of Parkinson disease. *Archives of Neurology, 60*, 1680–1684.

Shults, C. W., Oakes, D., Kieburtz, K., et al, and the Parkinson Study Group. (2002). Effects of coenzyme Q$_{10}$ in early Parkinson disease: Evidence for slowing of the functional decline. *Archives of Neurology, 59*, 1541–1550.

*SmithKline Beecham. (1997). Requip (ropinirole) package insert. Pittsburgh: Author.

*Spencer, C. M., & Benfield, P. (1996). Tolcapone. *CNS Drugs, 5*, 475–481.

*Stern, M. B. (1997). Contemporary approaches to the pharmacotherapeutic management of Parkinson's disease: An overview. *Neurology, 49*(Suppl. 1), S2–S9.

*Tetrud, J. W., & Langston, J. W. (1989). The effect of deprenyl (selegiline) on the natural history of Parkinson's disease. *Science, 245*, 519–522.

*Timberlake, W. H., & Vance, M. A. (1978). Four-year treatment of patients with Parkinsonism using amantadine alone or with levodopa. *Annals of Neurology, 3*, 119.

*Tulloch, I. F. (1997). Pharmacological profile of ropinirole: A non-ergoline dopamine agonist. *Neurology, 49*(Suppl. 1), S58–S62.

*Uitti, R. J. (1996). Diagnosis and treatment of common movement disorders in nursing home residents. *Nursing Home Medicine, 4*, 149–160.

*Waters, C. H., Kurth, M., Bailey, P., et al. (1997). Tolcapone in stable Parkinson's disease: Efficacy and safety of long-term treatment. *Neurology, 49*, 665–671.

*Watts, R. L. (1997). The role of dopamine agonists in early Parkinson's disease. *Neurology, 49*(Suppl. 1), S34–S48.

Visit the Connection web site for the most up-to-date drug information.

HEADACHES

■ ELYSE L. DISHLER, GINA M. KARCSH, AND JOSHUA J. SPOONER

Headache is one of the most common complaints of patients coming to primary care offices. The pain of a headache can range from mild to severe. Headaches can be classified as primary or secondary. A primary headache is a headache with no underlying organic disease process; a secondary headache is one for which a recognized disease process exists. The practitioner must first rule out a secondary headache and then accurately diagnose the type of primary headache. The main types of primary headache, as classified by the International Headache Society, are tension-type headaches, migraine, cluster, and miscellaneous; benign cough headache, benign exertional headache, headache associated with sexual activity, idiopathic stabbing headache, and external compression headache. This chapter will focus on diagnosing and treating migraines and tension headaches.

Migraine is a neurologic syndrome causing not only throbbing head pain but also nausea, appetite change, photophobia, and phonophobia. The pain generally ranges from moderate to severe; it can be debilitating. In any given month, 8% of men and 14% of women with migraine miss at least part of a day of work or school. Migraines affect approximately 10% of the population; women are affected three times as often as men. The age of onset is from 15 to 35 years, but peak prevalence is from 35 to 45 years. Family histories of migraines, usually along the female line, are common in migraine patients.

Tension headaches have a dull quality, with pain that radiates bilaterally from the forehead to the occiput in a band-like fashion. The pain is mild to moderate and can last from 30 minutes to several days in severe cases. Tension headaches are common, with a lifetime prevalence of 78%. The pain of a tension headache is generally not as severe as that of a migraine.

Cluster headaches are far less common than migraine or tension headaches, occurring in 0.4% of the population. The pain is burning or boring and centered around one eye and is described by patients as being more severe than childbirth or passing a kidney stone. Attacks generally last 90 to 120 minutes and may occur one to eight times per day. Associated unilateral symptoms include lacrimation, nasal congestion, rhinorrhea, miosis, ptosis, eyelid edema, or conjunctival injection. A patient with symptoms suggestive of cluster headache should be referred to a neurologist or headache specialist.

CAUSES OF TENSION HEADACHES

There are multiple causes of these common headaches, many likely still undiscovered. It has been suggested that tension headaches result from underlying psychological issues, but this theory has not been proven true. In fact, anxiety and depression may be a result rather than a cause of recurring headache pain (Breslau et al., 2000). Inadequate sleep is a common precipitating factor, causing tension headache in 39% of healthy volunteers after sleep deprivation (Blau, 1990). Cigarette smoking has also been correlated with an increased number of days of headache per week (Payne et al., 1991). Underlying muscle tension in the cervical or pericranial muscles occurs more frequently in tension headache sufferers than in headache-free controls (Hatch, 1992).

A frequent cause of recurrent tension headaches is the overuse of over-the-counter and prescription analgesic medications, the so-called rebound phenomenon. The headache recurs as each dose of medication wears off, causing the patient to take another analgesic and thus continue the cycle of pain. Treating more than two headaches, either migraine or tension, per week can lead to chronic daily headache.

PATHOPHYSIOLOGY OF TENSION HEADACHES

The physiology of tension headaches is poorly understood and an active area of research. The most common theory is that the pain of these headaches is muscular and related to increased resting pericranial muscle tone. The flaw in this theory is that electromyographic (EMG) studies do not consistently detect elevated resting muscle tone in patients with chronic tension headaches.

One study showed increased muscle hardness in patients with chronic tension headaches that was present with or without the headache being present (Ashina et al., 1999a). What is unknown is whether this muscle hardness is the cause or the result of the pain. Further research implicates nitric oxide as a local mediator of tension headaches. Blocking nitric oxide production led to decreased pericranial muscle hardness and headache pain in patients with chronic tension headaches (Ashina et al., 1999b). It is hoped that continued research will allow for a better understanding of these headaches.

DIAGNOSTIC CRITERIA

The first step in determining the type of headache a patient has is to take a detailed headache history. The history should include the patient's age; the time of day when the attack occurs; the duration and frequency of attacks; precipitating or relieving factors; the quality, location, and intensity of the pain; and associated symptoms. The social history and family history are also important. The results of physical and neurologic examinations should be unremarkable in a patient with primary headache, other than revealing possible tenderness of pericranial muscles. Diagnostic alarms in the evaluation of a headache patient that require further testing include headache onset after age 50, sudden-onset headache, accelerating headache pattern, headache with fever and stiff neck, and abnormal results on the neurologic examination.

Tension headaches are not typically present upon awakening, but begin later in the day and progress with time. They last from 30 minutes to a few days and usually are mild to moderate in severity. The pain is bilateral and wraps from the forehead around to the occiput in a band-like, squeezing fashion. The pain often radiates down the neck and even into the trapezius muscles. The pain of tension headaches is rarely debilitating, but it can affect a person's ability to function, especially if prolonged or chronic. There are no associated symptoms of nausea, vomiting, photophobia, or phonophobia (Box 42-1).

INITIATING DRUG THERAPY FOR TENSION HEADACHES

Before initiating drug therapy, it is critical to determine the type and frequency of over-the-counter medication use. Patients with tension headaches and headaches in general frequently self-medicate and may present when experiencing rebound headaches from medication overuse. Treating more

than two headaches per week for more than a few consecutive weeks can lead to a chronic daily headache pattern where the patient gets a rebound headache as each medication wears off. Caffeine and butalbital products are notorious for causing rebound headaches. The initial treatment of rebound headaches consists of withholding all analgesics for 1 to 2 weeks.

It is also important to help identify any headache triggers and to encourage a healthy lifestyle. Often simple changes such as eating and sleeping in a consistent pattern, decreasing alcohol and tobacco use, and using good posture can decrease headache severity and frequency.

Adjuncts to pharmacologic therapy include relaxation therapy, biofeedback, self-hypnosis, and cognitive therapy. Some techniques of relaxation are progressive muscle relaxation and the use of autogenic phrases. With progressive muscle relaxation, patients learn to contract and then relax all of the major muscles from head to toe. Using autogenic phrases involves repeating statements about calmness, warmth, and heaviness, allowing the patient to relax deeply. Patients may also benefit from acupuncture or cervical physical therapy in the case of chronic tension headaches.

Goals of Drug Therapy for Tension Headaches

The primary goals of drug therapy should be to reduce the severity and frequency of headaches, thus improving the patient's quality of life and ability to function. The goals for patients with episodic tension headaches are to select appropriate analgesic agents that will have the fewest side effects. Prophylactic therapy should be considered in addition to abortive analgesic agents for patients with more than two significant headaches per week. In a patient with analgesic rebound headache, it is appropriate to start a prophylactic agent and abruptly stop analgesic medications (other than barbiturate drugs, which must be tapered) simultaneously. It is important to educate patients about analgesic rebound headache and to limit the use of analgesics to 2 days per week.

Acetaminophen and Aspirin

Acetaminophen at a dose of 1,000 mg can be very effective in treating mild to moderate tension headaches. The advantage of this drug is that it is well tolerated and has few drug/drug interactions and side effects. Acetaminophen should be avoided in patients with heavy alcohol consumption or chronic liver disease, as the drug is metabolized through the liver. Prolonged use of acetaminophen and aspirin or nonsteroidal anti-inflammatory agents (NSAIDs) should be avoided, as they can cause nephrotoxicity. The amount of acetaminophen should be limited to 2 g/day for patients taking coumadin, as the combination could increase the INR and the risk of bleeding.

Aspirin can also alleviate mild to moderate tension headaches. It inhibits prostaglandin synthesis, reducing the inflammatory response and platelet aggregation. Contraindications to aspirin use are a history of bleeding disorders, asthma, and hypersensitivity to salicylates or NSAIDs. Patients should avoid combining aspirin with other NSAIDs because decreased serum concentrations of NSAIDs result when the two are used together. The most common adverse

---

BOX 42–1. DIAGNOSTIC CRITERIA FOR EPISODIC TENSION HEADACHE

A. At least 10 previous headache episodes fulfilling criteria B through D with <180 per year or <15/month
B. Headaches lasting from 30 minutes to 7 days
C. At least 2 of the following pain characteristics:
   1. Pressing or tightening quality
   2. Mild or moderate intensity that may inhibit but not prevent activity
   3. Bilateral
   4. No aggravation by routine physical activity

D. None of the following:
   1. Photophobia or phonophobia
   2. Nausea or vomiting

Adapted from Headache Classification Committee of the International Headache Society. (1988). Classification and diognostic criteria for headache disorders, cranial neuralgia, and facial pain. *Cephalgia, 8*(Suppl. 4), 1–96.

effects associated with aspirin are gastrointestinal, such as nausea, vomiting, or heartburn.

NSAIDs

The NSAIDs work well for moderate tension headaches. They work by inhibiting the cyclooxygenase enzyme responsible for prostaglandin synthesis, thereby reducing inflammation. These drugs take effect in 30 to 60 minutes, similar to aspirin and acetaminophen. Commonly used NSAIDs are ibuprofen, naproxen, ketoprofen, and indomethacin.

Common side effects of NSAIDs are abdominal cramps, nausea, indigestion, and even headache. Occasionally these drugs cause peptic ulcers and gastrointestinal hemorrhage.

Any given NSAID should be tried in a patient twice before deciding whether it is successful or not. It is not uncommon for a patient to respond poorly to one NSAID and extremely well to another.

Antiemetic Agents

Although patients with tension headaches rarely suffer from nausea, antiemetic agents can augment the pain-relieving properties of analgesics. Commonly used antiemetics are promethazine and prochlorperazine. These medications can be sedating and have numerous other potential side effects, including rare but serious neurologic and bone marrow effects. Patients should be educated about these possible effects before starting on these medications and should be encouraged to use them sparingly.

Other Abortive Agents

For patients whose headaches do not respond to the above agents, certain combination agents can be considered. Some patients have a good response to over-the-counter agents containing acetaminophen, aspirin, and caffeine. However, these agents have a high rate of analgesic rebound headache when used regularly and probably should not be used more than 1 to 2 days per week.

Prescription combinations that can be used are butalbital/acetaminophen/caffeine (Fioricet, others) and butalbital/aspirin/caffeine (Fiorinal, others). The butalbital component is a barbiturate, which is both sedating and potentially habit-forming: these medications should not be used in patients with any history of substance abuse. Fiorinal and Fiorcet very commonly cause analgesic rebound headaches and should not be used for more than 3 days per month. If a patient is taking many butalbital-containing pills per day, they must be slowly tapered to avoid withdrawal symptoms. Patients taking these medications should be closely monitored. Table 42-1 gives an overview of selected drugs used to abort tension-type headaches.

Midrin (acetaminophen/isometheptene/dichloralphenazone) is another medication that may relieve tension headaches. It works by constricting dilated cranial and cerebral arterioles. It is contraindicated in patients with hypertension, glaucoma, hepatic disease, organic heart disease, and severe renal disease. It should not be used concurrently with NSAIDS, aspirin, or acetaminophen-containing products. Use of Midrin should be limited to 5 days per month.

Prophylaxis of Tension Headaches

If a patient has more than two tension headaches per week, prophylaxis should be considered. Medications proven to reduce the frequency of tension headaches in clinical studies are amitriptyline, paroxetine, fluoxetine, and venlafaxine (Adelman et al., 2000; Goebel et al., 1994; Langemark &

Table 42.1

Overview of Selected Drugs to Abort Tension Headaches

Generic Name and Dosage	Selected Adverse Events	Contraindications	Special Considerations
acetaminophen 650–1,000 mg q4–6h	Rare: hepatotoxicity, nephrotoxicity, agranulocytosis, rash	Chronic alcohol use, impaired liver or renal function	Avoid using with alcohol. Limit to 2 g/day if on Coumadin.
aspirin 650 mg q4h	Rare: GI bleed, angioedema Common: GI upset	Bleeding disorder, peptic ulcer disease, asthma	Avoid using with NSAIDs.
NSAIDs ibuprofen 200–600 mg q6h	Rare: anaphylaxis, GI bleed, hepatotoxicity, bone marrow suppression, bronchospasm Common: GI upset, fluid retension, rash, tinnitus, constipation	Recent GI bleed, 3rd trimester of pregnancy, renal disease	Use with caution if history of CHF, HTN, GI bleed. Lower doses in patients with renal of hepatic disease
naproxen 500 mg q 12h	Same as above	Same as above	Same as above
ketoprofen 50 mg q 6h	Same as above	Same as above	Same as above
isometheptene/dichloralphenozone/ acetaminophen (Midrin) 1–2 tabs q4h, not to exceed 8 tabs/day	Rare: severe HTN Common: dizziness, rash	Uncontrolled HTN, PVD, CAD MAOI use within 14 days	Lower doses in patients with renal or hepatic disease.
Barbiturates butalbital/caffeine/aspirin or acetaminophen (Fiorocet or Fiorinal) 1–2 tabs q 4h, not to exceed 6 tabs/day	Rare: anaphylaxis, GI bleed, bone marrow suppression Common: sedation, nausea, vomiting, abdominal pain, intoxicated feeling	Hepatic or renal dysfunction, paptic ulcer disease, history of substance abuse	May be habit-forming, avoid using with other sedating medications.

Table 42.2

Overview of Selected Drugs Used to Prevent Tension Headaches

Generic Name & Dosage	Selected Adverse Events	Contraindications	Special Consideration
Amitriptyline 10–75 mg PO at bedtime	Rare: seizures, MI, agranulocytosis Common: dry mouth, drowsiness, constipation, urinary retention, blurred vision	Recent MI; BPH; caution if history of seizures, CAD, glaucoma	Most widely used
Fluoxetine 20–40 mg PO daily	Common: insomnia, nausea, dry mouth, sexual symptoms	MAOI use within 14 days Same as above	
Paroxetine 20–40 mg PO daily	Same as above		

Olesen, 1994) (Table 42-2). Prophylactic medications should be started at low dosages and increased slowly. It can take 4 to 8 weeks before the full effect of these prophylactic agents is seen. Finding the appropriate prophylactic agent for a patient is a process of trial and error, as different medications work in different patients.

Amitriptyline, a tricyclic antidepressant, is the medication most commonly used to prevent tension headaches. It can be used in doses much lower than those used for treating depression, ranging from 10 to 75 mg. Common side effects include sedation, constipation, blurred vision, and dry mouth. Amitriptyline should be used with caution in patients with a history of coronary artery disease, urinary retention, glaucoma, and seizures. Usually only low doses of amitriptyline are needed, making discontinuation secondary to side effects uncommon.

Fluoxetine (Prozac) and paroxetine (Paxil) are used with some success in patients with chronic tension headaches. They are commonly used in doses of 20 to 40 mg, which may also concurrently treat depression and anxiety. Common side effects are nausea, somnolence, and insomnia, which often diminish after a few weeks. Patients may also experience sexual dysfunction, increased sweating, or nervousness; these side effects may or may not diminish with time. Fluoxetine and paroxetine can interact with many medications. These medications must be tapered down slowly and not abruptly stopped, as withdrawal symptoms may occur.

Venlafaxine (Effexor), a serotonin-norepinephrine reuptake inhibitor, may also prevent tension headaches in certain patients. The appropriate dosages are not currently known.

First-Line Therapy for Tension Headaches

Aspirin and acetaminophen are appropriate first-line agents. They should be used no more than 2 days per week, as with any other analgesic agents, to avoid rebound headaches. If used judiciously, these agents have few adverse effects and are very well tolerated. They work best for mild to moderate headaches.

Second-Line Therapy for Tension Headaches

NSAIDs are the next option for treatment of tension headaches. If one agent fails for two consecutive headaches, another agent in this class should be tried. NSAIDs seem to work well for more stubborn tension headaches. If they pro-

vide incomplete relief, an antiemetic agent may be added to augment their effect.

Another second-line agent to try is an over-the-counter caffeine-containing analgesic. These medications should be used infrequently and may be alternated with NSAIDs for different headaches.

Third-Line Therapy for Tension Headaches

If the above agents fail, then butalbital-containing compounds or Midrin may be used. These agents may also be reserved as backup if the above-mentioned agents fail to relieve a more severe tension headache. Again, butalbital-containing agents should never be used more than 3 days per month, as they easily trigger rebound headaches.

As mentioned earlier, any patient requiring treatment for two or more headaches per week or who has particularly severe tension headaches should be considered for a prophylactic agent (Table 42-3 and Fig. 42-1).

CAUSES OF MIGRAINE HEADACHE

Why some patients experience migraines while others do not is unknown, but it is clear that there is a genetic component to migraines and that migraines tend to cluster in families (Kallela et al., 2001). There are many possible migraine triggers, and each patient's triggers are unique. Triggers range from certain foods to too much or too little sleep to medications to hormonal factors and others. In some patients, no obvious triggers are found. Estrogen is thought to play a role in the development of migraines, which explains the female predominance of migraines. About 25% of migraine attacks

Table 42.3

Recommended Order for Treatment of Tension Headaches

Order	Agents	Comments
First line	Aspirin or acetaminophen	Not to be used more than 2 days a week
Second line	NSAIDs and/or caffeine-containing analgesics	Antiemetic may be added if needed
Third line	Midrin or butalbital-containing compounds	Not to be used more than 3 days a month

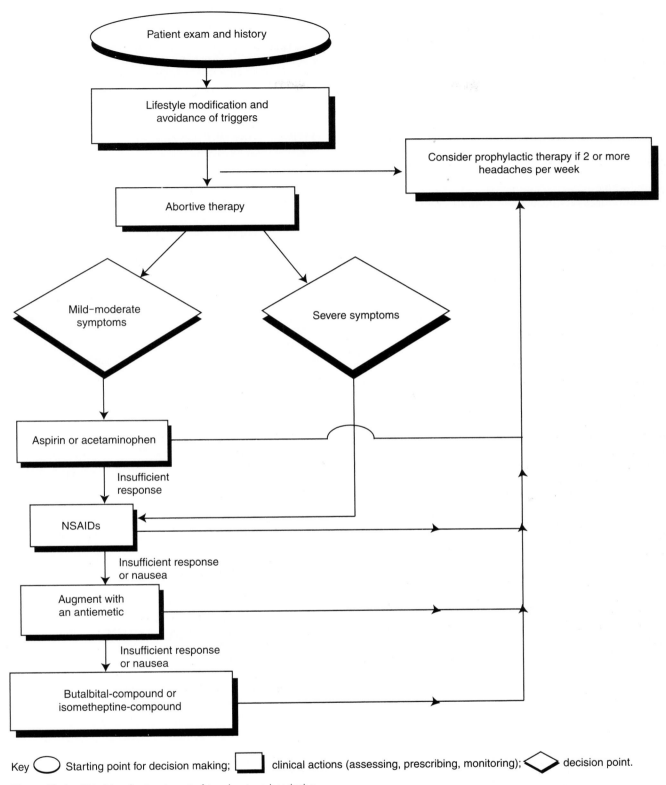

Key ⬭ Starting point for decision making; ▭ clinical actions (assessing, prescribing, monitoring); ◇ decision point.

Figure 42–1 Algorithm for treatment of tension-type headache.

occur within 4 days of a woman's menses, when estrogen has fallen to a low level (Fox & Davis, 1998). Box 42-2 lists migraine triggers. The best way to pinpoint triggers is to have the patient keep a diary of what he or she ate and did in the 12 hours before getting the headache to see if any patterns emerge.

PATHOPHYSIOLOGY OF MIGRAINE HEADACHES

The neuronal dysfunction theory is the currently accepted theory of migraine pathophysiology. According to this theory, migraine pain is thought to originate from the trigeminovascular system of the cerebrum. This system is a network of fibers that surrounds cranial blood vessels in close proximity, allowing for regulation of the environment of the vessel wall. The trigeminovascular system is an initiator and promoter of tissue inflammation, and when activated it releases neuropeptides that cause vasodilation and inflammation. Noradrenergic and, more significantly, serotonergic neurons regulate this activity. The trigeminovascular system may be activated by the cerebral cortex, thalamus, or hypothalamus in response to emotion or stress, circadian rhythm disruption, or environmental factors, including lights, strong odors, and loud noises (Lance, 1993).

Serotonin (5-hydroxytryptamine [5-HT]) is believed to play an important role in migraine development. There are seven classes of serotonin receptors, but only two have been associated with migraine pathophysiology. The 5-HT$_1$ receptors, located on presynaptic neurons, regulate the release of neurotransmitters. The 5-HT$_2$ receptors are excitatory receptors and can be found on postsynaptic neurons. Medications that are serotonin agonists specific to these receptors cause cranial artery vasoconstriction, thus often aborting migraine pain.

DIAGNOSTIC CRITERIA FOR MIGRAINE HEADACHE

The first step in making a precise diagnosis of migraine is to obtain a thorough headache history. Evaluation of the history should include age at onset; time of day when attacks occur; duration of attack; precipitating or relieving factors; nature, intensity, and location of headache pain; and any associated symptoms. The patient should also be questioned about any aura symptoms, such as visual symptoms (flashing lights, loss of peripheral vision, diplopia) or other sensory symptoms (vertigo, tinnitus, paresthesias, or hemiparesis). Because a family history is evident in many patients, asking if anyone in the family experiences migraines aids in the diagnosis. Specific diagnostic criteria for migraine with aura (classic migraine) and without aura (common migraine) are given in Box 42-3.

Patients most frequently experience migraines in the early morning, but a migraine attack can come at any time of day. Migraines are more often unilateral than bilateral, with the pain occurring around the eye or the temple. Migraine pain generally peaks 2 to 12 hours into the attack. Common symptoms accompanying migraine include nausea, anxiety, depression, irritability, fatigue, light and noise sensitivity, nausea, diarrhea or constipation, and hunger or anorexia. Patients may describe the pain of migraine as pounding, pulsating, or throbbing. A migraine sufferer often seeks refuge in a dark, quiet place.

INITIATING DRUG THERAPY FOR MIGRAINE HEADACHES

Practitioners must consider many factors when designing a treatment regimen for patients with migraine, such as the severity of the pain, duration of attack, concomitant disease states, current medication use, and any triggers. Migraine treatment needs to be highly individualized. Table 42-4 gives an overview of selected drugs used to treat migraine headaches.

The most effective treatment for migraines involves both nonpharmacologic and pharmacologic approaches. Nonpharmacologic approaches include various psychological techniques that aid in managing the migraine attack. Relaxation, stress management, and biofeedback are some techniques used to reduce migraine severity and frequency. Progressive muscle relaxation and use of autogenic phrases are examples of relaxation techniques (see the tension headache section above). It helps for patients to keep a diary detailing their headaches and the circumstances surrounding them to uncover any triggers or patterns.

BOX 42–3. DIAGNOSTIC CRITERIA FOR MIGRAINE

Migraine Without Aura
A. At least five attacks fulfilling B through D below
B. Headache attacks lasting 4 to 72 h (untreated or unsuccessfully treated)
C. Headache has at least two of the following characteristics:
   1. Unilateral location
   2. Pulsating quality
   3. Moderate or severe intensity (inhibits or prohibits daily activities)
   4. Aggravation by walking stairs or similar routine physical activity
D. During headache, at least one of the following:
   1. Nausea or vomiting
   2. Photophobia and phonophobia
E. At least one of the following:
   1. History, physical, and neurologic examinations do not suggest an organic disorder
   2. History or physical or neurologic examinations do suggest such disorder, but it is ruled out by appropriate investigations
   3. An organic disorder is present, but migraine attacks do not occur for the first time in close temporal relation to the disorder

Migraine With Aura
A. At least two attacks fulfilling B and C below
B. At least three of the following four characteristics:
   1. One or more fully reversible aura symptoms, including focal cerebral cortex or brain stem dysfunction
   2. At least one aura symptom develops gradually over more than 4 min, or two or more symptoms occur in succession
   3. No aura symptom lasts more than 60 min (if > 60 min, then diagnosis is migraine with prolonged aura). If more than one aura symptom is present, accepted duration is proportionally increased
   4. Headache follows aura with a free interval of less than 60 min (it may also begin before or simultaneously with the aura)
C. And at least one of the following:
   1. History, physical, and neurologic examinations do not suggest an organic disorder
   2. History or physical or neurologic examinations do suggest such disorder, but it is ruled out by appropriate investigations
   3. An organic disorder is present, but migraine attacks do not occur for the first time in close temporal relation to the disorder

Adapted from Headache classification committee of the International Headache Society. (1988). Classification and diagnostic criteria for headache disorders, cranial neuralgias, and facial pain. *Cephalgia, 8*(Suppl. 4), 1–96.

Goals of Drug Therapy

The main goal of pharmacologic therapy is relieve the migraine attack with minimal or no side effects. Short-term goals include decreasing the severity and duration of the headache and relieving nausea, if present. Long-term goals include diminishing the frequency and severity of attacks, improving the patient's quality of life, and allowing the patient to return to full functioning.

NSAIDs

The first-choice agents for mild to moderate migraines are NSAIDs and aspirin. These medications, like all migraine medication, work best when taken early in the attack. The most common side effects are gastrointestinal. The same doses as used for tension headaches are appropriate for migraines. Aspirin may be used in initial dosages of up to 900 mg. Aspirin alone is effective in up to 40% of migraine patients (Silberstein, 2002). As with tension headaches, a given NSAID should be used on more than one occasion before deciding whether it is efficacious.

Isometheptene and Caffeine Combinations

The isometheptene-containing drug Midrin can often abort mild to moderate migraines. The dosing is different than that used for tension headaches. Over-the-counter caffeine-containing compounds are also effective for milder migraines, but they can easily cause rebound headaches and should be used no more than 3 days per month.

5-HT₁ Receptor Agonists (Triptans)

Triptans are migraine-specific drugs that work as 5-HT_1 serotonin receptor agonists. These receptors are located on intracranial blood vessels, central nervous system neurons, and trigeminal terminals. Triptans cause cerebral vasoconstriction and can treat both the pain and nausea of migraine.

Triptans are indicated for moderate to severe migraines or for milder migraines that do not respond to NSAIDs, aspirin, or the above combination drugs. The triptans vary in their time to peak concentration and in their half-lives, which helps guide the selection of a triptan for a particular patient. If one triptan fails on two separate occasions, another triptan should be tried. Triptans work best when given early in the course of a migraine, but unlike many other agents, they may be effective even when given late in the course of a migraine.

Triptans should not be used more than 6 days per month and should not be used within 24 hours of any other vaso-constricting drugs, such as an ergotamine or Midrin. Triptans should be avoided in patients with basilar, hemiplegic, or retinal migraines; they must also be avoided in patients with coronary artery disease, cerebrovascular disease, or severe peripheral vascular disease.

The seven triptan drugs are sumatriptan, zolmitriptan, naratriptan, rizatriptan, almotriptan, frovatriptan, and eletriptan. Sumatriptan and zolmitriptan are available as a nasal spray, and sumatriptan has a subcutaneous form. These are useful for patients with severe nausea who cannot tolerate an oral medication. The injectable form of sumatriptan

Table 42.4

Overview of Selected Drugs Used to Treat Migraine Headaches

Generic Name and Dosage	Selected Adverse Events	Contraindications	Special Considerations
aspirin 650–1000 mg q4h	Rare: GI bleed, angioedema Common: GI upset	Bleeding disorder, peptic ulcer, asthma	Avoid use with NSAIDs.
NSAIDs—see Table 42.1 for dosing information isometheptene/dichloralphenazone/ acetaminophen (Midrin) 2 tabs at headache onset; 1 tab every hr to max of 5 tabs/day	Rare: severe HTN Common: dizziness, rash	Pregnancy, uncontrolled HTN, CAD, PUD	Use lower doses if hepatic or renal impairment.
Over-the-counter caffeine-containing compounds (Excedrin) 1–2 tabs q4h	Insomnia, agitation	Uncontrolled HTN	Avoid use with other vasoconstriction agents.
Triptans sumatriptan (Imitrex) 25, 50, 100 mg PO at headache onset; may repeat dose up to 100 mg in 2h 6 mg subcutaneous, may repeat dose in 2h 5 or 20 mg intranasal; may repeat dose in 2h	Rare: MI, severe HTN, arrhythmia, seizure Common: paresthesias, chest tightness, discomfort in lower mouth, mouth, abdomen, weakness, fatigue	Pregnancy, uncontrolled HTN, CAD, PVD, severe hepatic or renal disease, basilar or hemiplegic migraine	Interactions with oral contraceptives Propranolol SSRIs, verapami ketoconazole. Do not use with MAOI or within 24 h of another triptan or ergotamine drug; use at lowest possible doses.
naratriptan (Amerge) 2.5 mg q4h to max of 5 mg/day	Same as above Same as above	Same as above Same as above	Same as above and long half-life.
Rizatriptan (Maxalt, Maxalt-MLT) 5–10 mg PO q4h to max of 30 mg/day	Same as above	Same as above	Same as above and has form that melts in mouth.
zolmitriptan (Zomig) 2.5–5 mg q2h to max of 10 mg/day	Same as above	Same as above	Same as above
almotriptan (Axert) 0.25–12.5 mg q2h to max of 25 mg/day	Same as above	Same as above	Same as above
eletriptan (Relpax) 20–40 mg q2h to max of 80 mg/24 hrs	Same as above	Same as above	Same as above; rapid onset of action.
frovatriptan (Frova) 1.5 mg q2h to max of 7.5 mg/day	Same as above	Same as above	Same as above; slow onset, longest half-life
Ergotamine derivatives caffeine/ergotamine (Cafergot) 1–2 tabs q30min to max of 6 tabs/day supp PR q30min to max 2 supp/day	Rare: MI Common: Nausea, vomiting, irritability, palpitations, paresthesias, rebound headache	HTN, PVD, pregnancy, CAD	Do not use within 24 hrs of a triptan. Use no more than 3 days/month. Pregnancy category X.
dihydroergotamine	Usually managed by a neurologist		
Barbiturates—see Table 42.1 for dosing			
Opioids butorphanol (Stadol) Nasal Spray sp. in nostril, may repeat in 1h to max of 4 sp/day	Sedation, dizziness, nausea, vomiting	History of substance abuse	Use with caution if impaired renal, hepatic, pulmonary function. Use with caution in elderly
Tylenol with codeine 1 or 2 tabs q4h	Same as above	Same as above	May be used sparingly in pregnancy
Dexamethasone single dose of 4 mg or 4 mg BID × 2 days then 4 mg daily × 3 days	Rare and serious: steroid psychosis; PUD, CHF Common: nausea, GI upset, insomnia, mood swings	CHF, DM, HTN (uncontrolled)	Use as rescue medication only.

has the fastest onset of action of any of the triptans but has a short half-life, often giving limited headache relief. Frovatriptan has the longest half-life of the triptans, at 26 hours, making it useful for patients with long-lasting migraines.

Sumatriptan

Sumatriptan (Imitrex) increases the levels of serotonin in the brain, causing vasoconstriction, and reduces inflammation associated with migraines. Sumatriptan is available in tablets (25, 50, and 100 mg), a nasal spray, and a subcutaneous injection (see Table 42-4). Injectable sumatriptan offers the quickest onset of action (10 minutes), whereas the effects of the tablet take longer (30 to 90 minutes). If the headache recurs, the patient can take a second dose of medication, but only after a certain time and without exceeding the maximum dose. Patients with migraine with aura cannot take sumatriptan until the headache actually begins, because the drug has no effect on relieving aura symptoms. Two hours after oral administration of 100 mg sumatriptan, 58% of patients improved and 35% were pain free; after injection of 6 mg sumatriptan, 71% of patients improved within 1 hour, 79% improved within 2 hours, and 43% were pain free after 1 hour and 60% after 2 hours (Ferrari, 1998).

Patients with ischemic heart disease, Prinzmetal's angina, or uncontrolled hypertension should not use sumatriptan. When sumatriptan is administered intravenously, vasoconstriction is exerted on peripheral arteries, resulting in additional side effects and contraindications to its use. The vasoconstrictive potential of sumatriptan can lead to significant side effects such as dizziness, paresthesia, numbness, tightness in the chest, and a burning sensation. Sumatriptan should be avoided in patients with a history of cardiovascular disease. Drug interactions associated with sumatriptan primarily involve medications that increase the levels of serotonin, such as ergotamine derivatives, monoamine oxidase (MAO) inhibitors, and selective serotonin reuptake inhibitors (SSRIs).

Rizatriptan

Rizatriptan (Maxalt), an agonist for the 5-HT$_1$ receptor, causes cranial vessel vasoconstriction. Rizatriptan is available in a tablet and oral disintegrating formulation (Maxalt-MLT), offering an alternative way to treat a migraine. The usual dosage of both formulations is listed in Table 42-4. The effect of rizatriptan can be observed within 30 minutes and lasts from 14 to 16 hours. Contraindications to the use of rizatriptan can be found in Table 42-4. The most common adverse effects seen with rizatriptan include increases in blood pressure, dizziness, fatigue (dose-related), somnolence, and dry mouth. Patients must avoid use of another ergotamine derivative or 5-HT agonist, SSRIs, or MAO inhibitors because of excessive increases in serotonin levels. Patients taking propranolol (Inderal) should take only the 5-mg dose of rizatriptan because of a 70% increase in rizatriptan's area under the curve (a measure of bioavailability).

Naratriptan

Naratriptan (Amerge) is marketed as an alternative agent for patients who are taking repeated doses of other migraine therapies, specifically those who have recurrent headache or chest tightness when using oral sumatriptan. Naratriptan is available only in a tablet formulation (see Table 42-4) and reaches peak serum concentrations in 2 to 3 hours. Because of its long half-life of 6 hours, headache recurrences are not common. Contraindications and adverse effects are similar to those with the other 5-HT$_1$ agonists; however, patients with renal or hepatic impairment should avoid naratriptan because its clearance is significantly decreased. In contrast to the other agents, smoking increases the clearance of naratriptan, resulting in decreased serum concentrations. Naratriptan is metabolized through a different pathway, resulting in no significant drug interactions with MAO inhibitors.

Zolmitriptan

Zolmitriptan (Zomig) is indicated for treating migraine with or without aura. It comes in tablet form, nasal spray, and oral disintegrating form. The recommended initial dose of zolmitriptan is 2.5 mg (see Table 42-4). The onset of effect is attained within 45 minutes, resulting in a rapid therapeutic response but a relatively short duration of action. Contraindications and adverse effects are similar to the other triptans (see Table 42-4). If pain or tightness in the chest or throat occurs with the use of this agent or other 5-HT$_1$ agonists, the patient must discuss continued use of the medication with the health care provider. Cimetidine (Tagamet) or oral contraceptives can increase the toxicity profile of zolmitriptan, and patients should avoid concomitant use.

Eletriptan

Eletriptan (Relpax) is indicated for treating migraine with or without aura. It comes in 20- and 40-mg tablets. The recommended initial dose is 40 mg at the onset of a headache. Contraindications and adverse effects are similar to the other triptans (see Table 42-4). If pain or tightness in the chest or throat occurs with the use of this agent or other 5-HT$_1$ agonists, the patient must discuss continued use of the medication with the health care provider.

Frovatriptan

Frovatriptan (Frova) is indicated for treating migraines with or without aura. It comes in a 2.5-mg tablet, which is the recommended dose. Contraindications and adverse effects are similar to the other triptans (see Table 42-4). If pain or tightness in the chest or throat occurs with the use of this agent or other 5-HT$_1$ agonists, the patient must discuss continued use of the medication with the health care provider.

Ergotamine Derivatives

Before sumatriptan was approved for use, the most common agents used to abort migraines were ergotamine derivatives. These agents have fallen out of favor because of unpredictable patient responses. Ergotamines have partial agonist, antagonist, or both types of activity for serotonergic, dopaminergic, and alpha-adrenergic receptors, resulting in constriction of peripheral and cranial vessels.

Ergotamine tartrate (Ergostat) is available in tablet, sublingual, and suppository formulations. Its use should generally be avoided, as it commonly increases the incidence of migraines. Dihydroergotamine (Migranal) is available as an injection and nasal spray. This drug is mainly used to treat severe, refractory migraines and is usually managed by specialists. Cafergot, a combination of caffeine and ergotamine, is available in oral and suppository forms. Cafergot can also increase the incidence of migraines, and so it should be used infrequently.

Because ergotamines cause contraction of other arteries in the periphery, their use is absolutely contraindicated in patients with cardiovascular and cerebrovascular disease. Ergotamines also are contraindicated in patients with hepatic or renal disease, peripheral vascular disease, and sepsis. The ergotamines are pregnancy category X and should not be used in women of childbearing age who are not using birth control. Side effects can be severe; the most common include nausea and vomiting, tachycardia or bradycardia, arterial spasm, drowsiness, and tingling of the extremities.

Barbiturates

Butalbital-containing compounds such as Fiorinal and Fioricet should be used sparingly and only if the migraine-specific agents have repeatedly failed. If overused, these agents can lead to addiction, rebound headaches, and withdrawal symptoms. The most common side effects of butalbital-containing compounds are drowsiness and dizziness. Use should be limited to no more than six tablets per day and 3 days per month.

Opioids

Opioids are useful when used as rescue medications for severe migraines that do not respond to the above medications. They are also useful in patients who have infrequent migraines and have contraindications to other agents. They may be used sparingly for moderate to severe migraines during pregnancy. They have many potential side effects, namely lightheadedness and sedation, and may impair a patient's ability to function. If prescribed appropriately, they may prevent a migraine sufferer from visiting an emergency room.

Steroids

If a patient has a severe, persistent migraine that seems refractory to any abortive medications, a brief course of steroids may be used to break the attack. There have been no good studies about using steroids to treat status migrainosus (an intractable, prolonged migraine), but they are commonly used with good results. Dexamethasone may be used, unless contraindicated, for a 5-day course. Steroid use should be limited.

Antiemetic Agents

The antiemetic agents prochlorperazine and metoclopramide are affective adjunctive therapies for patients experiencing an acute migraine, whether or not nausea and vomiting accompany the migraine. Prochlorperazine comes in a suppository form, which is useful for patients unable to tolerate oral medications. These medications augment the effects of the above-mentioned abortive agents and may be taken before or together with these agents.

PROPHYLACTIC DRUG THERAPY FOR MIGRAINES

Prophylactic medications are used to reduce the frequency and severity of migraine attacks. Most prophylactic medications were discovered accidentally when being used for another purpose. Patients may or may not respond to a particular agent, and a therapeutic trial of a given agent should last for 2 to 3 months before the efficacy of the agent is assessed. The main classes of agents are the beta blockers, calcium channel blockers, tricyclic antidepressants, anticonvulsants, serotonin antagonists, and NSAIDs. The choice of prophylactic agent should be based on the patient's coexisting conditions and the medication's side effect profile. Figure 42-2 shows treatment for migraine prophylaxis. Table 42-5 gives an overview of selected drugs used to prevent migraines.

The current recommendations for starting prophylactic therapy are recurring migraines that affect the patient's function despite acute treatments: intolerance or failure of multiple acute treatments; overuse of acute medications; special circumstances such as hemiplegic migraines; and more than two headaches per week (Silberstein, 2002).

Medications should be started at low doses and titrated slowly until the desired effects occur. Dosages may need to be lowered if side effects occur. A full therapeutic trial takes at least 2 months. It may take months until an effective agent is found.

Beta Blockers

Beta blockers are often considered first-line agents for prophylactic treatment of migraines. Propranolol (Inderal), metoprolol (Lopressor), atenolol (Tenormin), and nadolol (Corgard) have been used, and all have similar efficacy. Only propanolol and timolol have been approved by the FDA for migraine prophylaxis. Beta blockers are contraindicated in patients with uncompensated congestive heart failure, bradycardia, second- or third-degree atrioventricular block, and asthma. Side effects include fatigue, vivid dreams, depression, impotence, bradycardia, and hypotension. Many pathways of the cytochrome P450 enzyme system metabolize beta blockers. Beta blockers have numerous drug interactions, and practitioners should consult a reference before administering beta blockers to avoid such interactions.

Tricyclic Antidepressants

Tricyclic antidepressants can also be used as first-line agents for migraine prophylaxis. The agents most commonly used include imipramine (Tofranil), nortriptyline (Pamelor), and amitriptyline (Elavil). Patients usually need only low doses for prophylaxis, lower than those generally used to treat depression. Patients should avoid use if they are currently taking an MAO inhibitor, have glaucoma, or are pregnant. Anticholinergic side effects commonly occur and include sedation, constipation, blurred vision, hypotension, and slowed conduction in the atrioventricular node. Tricyclic antidepressants also have many potential drug interactions; prescribers should consult a reference before administering them.

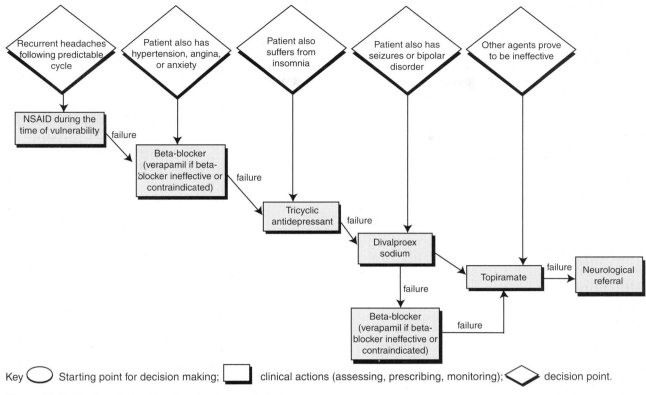

Figure 42–2 Treatment algorithm for migraine prophylaxis.

Table 42.5

Overview of Selected Drugs Used to Prevent Migraine Headaches

Generic Name and Dosage	Selected Adverse Events	Contraindications	Special Considerations

Beta blockers
propranolol
  (use long-acting)
  start 80 mg daily;
  goal 160–240 mg daily
	AV block, CHF,
	  agranulocytosis,
	  fatigue, dizziness,
	  constipation, depression
		Use with caution
		  in CHF, depression,
		  asthma, diabetes,
		  Raynaud's disease
			Useful if coexisting
			  HTN or CAD history

timolol
  start 5 mg bid;
  goal 10 mg bid
	Same as above	Same as above	Same as above

Tricyclic antidepressants
amitriptyline
  start 10 mg qhs;
  goal 10–75 mg qhs
	See Table 42-2		

Anticonvulsants
valproic acid
  (extended release)
  start: 500 mg qhs;
  goal: 1,000 mg qhs
	Hepatotoxicity,
	  bone marrow suppression,
	  nausea, vomiting,
	  somnolence, tremor,
	  alopecia
		Impaired renal or
		  hepatic function
			Check baseline
			  CBC and liver
			  function tests,
			  monitor levels and
			  liver function.
			Use with caution
			  in the elderly.

topiramate
  start 25 mg daily,
  goal 50–100 mg bid
	Metabolic acidosis,
	  kidney stones,
	  osteoporosis,
	  dizziness, somnolence,
	  memory difficulty, tremor,
	  mood disturbance
			Use with caution if liver
			  or renal impairment or
			  history of kidney stones.

Calcium Channel Blockers
verapamil
  80 mg tid
	Rare: CHF, AV block
	Common: constipation,
	  dizziness, hypotension,
	  edema
		AV block, CHF,
		  bradycardia,
		  atrial fibrillation
			Useful if coexisting HTN.

Anticonvulsants

Valproic acid (Depakene) and divalproex sodium (Depakote) can reduce the frequency, severity, and duration of migraines (Mathew, Saper, & Silberstein, 1995). Use of these drugs is contraindicated in patients with liver disease. Side effects such as tremor, weight gain, nausea, and hair loss limit their use as agents for prophylaxis. Numerous drug interactions can result when valproic acid or divalproex sodium is administered with other anticonvulsants. Increased effects or toxicity of valproic acid are seen with the administration of central nervous system depressants and aspirin. Valproic acid is contraindicated in pregnancy because it is toxic to the fetus.

Before starting valproic acid, a baseline complete blood count and liver function tests should be obtained. The dose should be increased very gradually, and follow-up liver function tests and valproate levels should be monitored. If tremor appears, the dose should be lowered.

Topiramate has been proven to prevent migraines in a recent double-blind study (Brandes et al., 2004). It is particularly effective for patients who have chronic daily headaches or who have failed to respond to many other prophylactic treatments. Topiramate has many potential side effects that limit its use, such as concentration and memory impairment, significant somnolence, mood disturbance, and tremor. It should be used with caution in patients with renal or hepatic impairment.

Calcium Channel Blockers

Verapamil (Calan) is the calcium channel blocker most commonly used to prevent migraines; however, it provides only a slight benefit in reducing the frequency of attacks. It is often considered a second- or third-line agent, for use when other agents are ineffective or contraindicated. The mechanism of action is believed to be the inhibition of serotonin release, which is not achieved until after up to 8 weeks of therapy. Its use is contraindicated in patients with bradycardia, heart block, ventricular tachycardia, or atrial fibrillation. Side effects include constipation, fluid retention, bradycardia, and hypotension. Numerous drug interactions are associated with calcium channel blockers; prescribers must consult a reference before administering.

NSAIDs

NSAIDs may be used for prophylaxis. Naproxen sodium is the most common agent used. NSAIDs can be used to prevent headaches that occur with a regular pattern (eg, menstrual migraine). Therapeutic effects are believed to result from inhibition of prostaglandin synthesis and inflammation that evolves from the trigeminovascular system. These agents may cause gastrointestinal and renal toxicity if used for a prolonged period. If the patient requires an NSAID on a chronic basis, renal function should be monitored.

Other Prophylactic Agents

Methylsergide and MAO inhibitors can also be used for migraine prophylaxis, but because they have multiple serious side effects, their use should be managed by a neurologist.

Gabapentin (Neurontin) has recently been established to be effective in the treatment of chronic daily headache at dosages of 1,800 to 2,400 mg/day. Angiotensin-converting enzyme inhibitors and angiotensin receptor blockers are also being studied as potential prophylactic agents.

SSRIs such as paroxetine and fluoxetine have been used with some success; they are particularly useful in patients also suffering from anxiety or depression.

Selecting the Most Appropriate Agent

It is important to initiate therapy at the first sign of a migraine (Fig. 42-3). The following section discusses the recommended therapy for migraines (Table 42-6).

First-Line Therapy

NSAIDs and aspirin are appropriate first-line treatments for mild to moderate migraines. They are inexpensive and generally well tolerated. The triptans are first-line therapy for moderate to severe migraines, with or without an antiemetic. The NSAIDs may be tried for more severe migraines, but they are often unsuccessful.

Second-Line Therapy

The over-the-counter caffeine-containing compounds and Midrin are appropriate treatment options for mild to moderate migraines that have not responded to the above agents. They can also be used as rescue medications if NSAIDs or aspirin fails to relieve a given attack. For more severe migraines, the ergotamine derivative along with an antiemetic can be used as second-line agents if multiple triptans have failed.

Third-Line Therapy

If the above agents are ineffective in treating mild to moderate migraines, then the triptans should be tired. For severe migraines that have not responded to triptans or ergotamine derivatives and antiemetics, butalbital compounds or opioids should be used.

CLUSTER HEADACHES

Patient suspected of having cluster headaches should be promptly referred to a neurologist. Some of the medications used to abort cluster headaches include inhaled oxygen, triptans, and ergotamine derivatives.

SPECIAL POPULATION CONSIDERATIONS
Pediatric

The most common headache type seen in children is migraine. Migraines may present differently in children than in adults. The pain is throbbing and pulsating but tends to be bifrontal or bitemporal. Children may have severe nausea and vomiting along with the pain. The headache usually persists for 1 to 3 hours but may last for longer than a day. Pediatric migraines are usually best managed by simple analgesics such

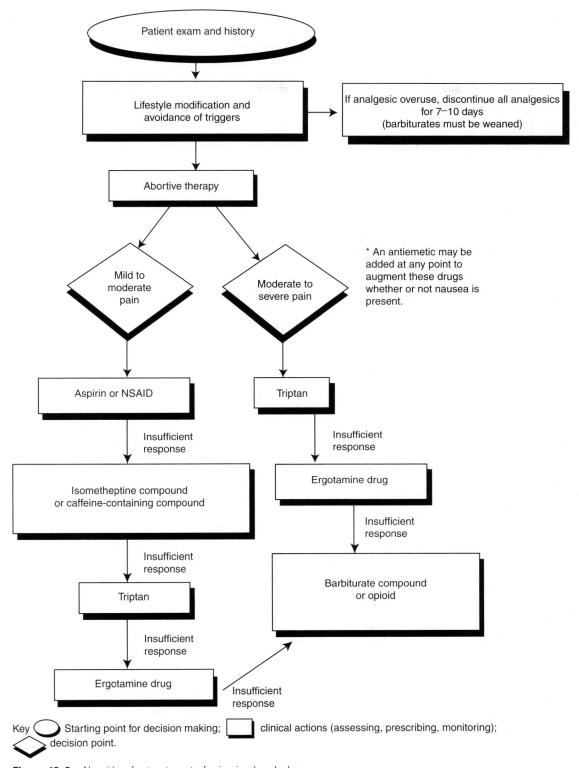

Figure 42-3 Algorithm for treatment of migraine headaches.

as acetaminophen and ibuprofen, with an antiemetic added if necessary. The triptan drugs are not recommended for use in children; if a stronger agent is required, an ergotamine derivative should be tried. Propanolol is the prophylactic drug used most commonly in children.

Tension headaches do occur in children. Recurrent tension headaches should prompt a search for any underlying stressors at home or at school, as well as a vision examination. Tension headaches are usually best managed by simple analgesics.

Geriatric

New-onset migraines do not often occur in the geriatric population. Changes in renal and hepatic function often occur

Table 42.6

Recommended Order for Treatment of Migraine Headaches

Order	Agents	Comments
First line	NSAIDs or aspirin Triptans for severe migraines	With moderate to severe migraines, can use antiemetic as needed
Second line	OTC caffeine-containing products or Midrin For severe migraine can use ergotamine derivative	
Third line	Triptans	Ergotamine derivatives and antiemetic can be used or butalbital compounds or opioids if triptans fail

with advancing age, so if a geriatric patient is experiencing migraines, adjustment of drug dosages is recommended.

A new headache pattern in an elderly patient should make the practitioner suspicious of organic disease or a medication side effect.

Women

As noted earlier, migraines occur more often in women than men, likely as a result of estrogen. Pregnancy is a primary concern if drug therapy is to be initiated, even though migraines can diminish during the second and third trimesters. Practitioners should consider drug therapy for pregnant women using the risk-versus-benefit approach. The agents selected should be those that are safe to use during pregnancy. The triptans and ergotamine derivatives are strongly contraindicated in pregnancy. Acetaminophen is the safest analgesic to use during pregnancy, but it is usually minimally effective. For more severe migraines, ibuprofen may be used in the first and second trimester only. Tylenol with codeine may be used sparingly throughout the pregnancy.

Menstrual migraines are a common problem that may be particularly responsive to Midrin and the triptans. Another difficult time for women is around menopause, when estrogen levels dramatically decline. In a recent cross-sectional analysis, women using hormone replacement therapy were found to be 40% more likely to have migraines than those who were not taking hormone replacement (Misakian, 2003). If a woman wishes to stay on hormone replacement therapy despite migraines, she can be given a reduced dose and can be switched to pure estradiol or synthetic ethinyl estradiol. Using continuous dosing instead of interrupted dosing may also reduce migraine frequency.

MONITORING PATIENT RESPONSE

Careful monitoring of therapy is important. The practitioner should document the frequency, intensity, and duration of migraines before starting any new therapy and should evaluate the patient periodically after implementing any drug or lifestyle change to assess its effectiveness. Prescribers should monitor how frequently patients are taking abortive therapies to ensure they are not using them excessively.

Patients should return to the office after a few attempts with a therapy to assess its effectiveness, and practitioners should switch to another agent if the therapy is unsuccessful. Practitioners also need to evaluate prophylactic therapies for patient compliance and effectiveness. They should note in the chart side effects to therapy and treatment failures to avoid repeating ineffective therapies.

PATIENT EDUCATION

Drug Information

Practitioners need to educate patients about their headaches and what they should realistically expect from treatment. The prescriber should attempt to identify any headache triggers (ie, diet, medication, or environmental factors) and should encourage the patient to avoid or minimize these triggers.

Practitioners also must educate patients about their drug therapy. They should tell patients how frequently they can take an abortive therapy, what the maximum daily dose is, and what side effects to expect from the medication. If the patient will be using a nasal spray or injectable medication, the prescriber should demonstrate proper administration technique. Also, prescribers need to encourage patients to take their prophylactic therapies as scheduled, emphasizing that taking prophylactic therapies on an as-needed basis will not improve the condition. If switching to a new therapy, the prescriber should remind the patient to stop using the old therapy and not to use the two therapies simultaneously (unless this is intended).

Nutrition

Foods that can trigger headaches include aspartame, caffeine, chocolate, monosodium glutamate, and red wine and other alcohol. The patient should be aware of any foods that trigger his or her headaches and should avoid them.

Complementary and Alternative Medicine

Some patients use feverfew to prevent migraines. One of the active ingredients in feverfew is sesquiterpene lactones, which has an anti-inflammatory effect that blocks the transcription of inflammatory proteins. A minimum of 0.2% is the recommended dosage. Side effects include nausea, flatulence, diarrhea, and indigestion. Withdrawal symptoms when stopping long-term use can include muscle stiffness, anxiety, and rebound migraines. It also has anticoagulant properties, so PT/INR levels should be checked periodically, and it should be stopped 2 weeks before surgical procedures.

Another nutritional supplement used for migraine prophylaxis is butterbur. This contains petasin and isopetasin, which have vasodilation properties and inhibit leukotriene synthesis, reducing inflammation. A dosage of 50 mg twice daily has been shown to reduce migraines (Grossman & Schmidramsl, 2001). There should be at least 7.5 mg petasin in the preparation. Side effects include abdominal pain, distended abdomen, and reduced urinary output.

Magnesium and riboflavin (vitamin B$_2$) have also been shown to reduce migraines.

■ Case Study

J.J., age 24, presents to your practice for the first time. She reports constant headaches. She smokes a pack of cigarettes a day but is in good health otherwise. She states that the headaches usually occur in the morning and last a few hours. The pain, localized to an area near her right temple, has a throbbing quality. The headache often results in nausea and vomiting and sensitivity to bright lights. She has tried to treat the headaches with acetaminophen, ibuprofen, and naproxen unsuccessfully. The headaches are causing her to miss work and she is afraid she will lose her job.

Diagnosis: Migraine headaches without aura

1. List specific goals of therapy for J.J.

2. What drug therapy would you prescribe? Why?

3. What are the parameters for monitoring success of the therapy?

4. Discuss specific patient education based on the prescribed therapy.

5. List one or two adverse reactions for the selected agent that would cause you to change therapy.

6. What would be the choice for the second-line therapy?

7. What over-the-counter and/or alternative medicines might be appropriate for this patient?

8. What dietary and lifestyle changes might you recommend?

9. Describe one or two drug/drug or drug/food interactions for the selected agent.

Bibliography

Starred references are cited in the text.

*Adelman, L. C., et al. (2000). Venlafaxine extended release for the prophylaxis of migraine and tension-type headache: a retrospective study in a clinical setting. *Headache, 40,* 572–580.

*Ashina, M., et al. (1999a). Muscle hardness in patients with chronic tension-type headaches: relation to actual headache state. *Pain, 75,* 201–205.

*Ashina, M, et al. (1999b). Effect of inhibition of nitric oxide synthetase on chronic tension-type headaches: a randomized crossover trial. *Lancet, 353,* 287–289.

Aukerman, M. D., Knutson, D., & Miser, W. F. (2002). Management of the acute migraine headache. *American Family Physician, 66,* 2123–2141.

*Becket, B. E., & Herndon, K. C. (1999). Headache disorders: migraine and cluster. In J. T. Dipiro et al. (Eds.), *Pharmacotherapy, a pathophysiologic approach* (4th ed., pp. 1027–1038). Stamford, CT: Appleton and Lange.

Blau, J. N. (1992). Migraine: theories of pathogenesis. *Lancet, 339,* 1202–1207.

*Blau, J.N. (1990). Sleep deprivation headache. *Cephalgia, 10,* 157–160.

*Brandes, J. L. et al. (2004). Topiramate for migraine prevention. *JAMA, 291*(8), 964–973.

*Breslau, N., et al. (2000). Headaches and major depression: is the association specific to migraine? *Neurology, 54,* 308–313.

Diener, H. C., Kaube, H., & Limmroth, V. (1998). A practical guide to the management and prevention of migraine. *Drugs, 56,* 811–824.

Feuerstein, M., Bortolussi, L., Houle, M., & Labbe, E. (1983). Stress, temporal artery activity, and pain in migraine headache: a prospective analysis. *Headache, 23,* 296–304.

*Fox, A. W., & Davis, R. L. (1998). Migraine chronobiology. *Headache, 38,* 436–441.

*Goebel, H., et al. (1994). Chronic tension-type headache: amitriptyline reduces clinical headache duration and experimental pain sensitivity but does not alter pericranial muscle activity readings. *Pain, 59,* 241–249.

*Grossman, W., & Schmidramsl, H. (2001). An extract of *Petasites hybridus* is effective in prophylaxis of migraines. *Alternative Medicine Review,* 6(3), 303–310.

*Hatch, J. P. (1992). The use of EMG and muscle palpation in the diagnosis of tension-type headache with and without pericranial muscle involvement. *Pain, 49,* 175–178.

*Kallela, M., et al. (2001). Familial migraine with and without aura: clinical characteristics and co-occurrence. *European Journal of Neurology, 8,* 441–449.

*Headache Classification Committee of the International Headache Society. (1988). Classification and diagnostic criteria for headache disorders, cranial neuralgias, and facial pain. *Cephalalgia,* 8(Suppl. 4), 1–96.

*Lance, J. W. (1993). Current concepts of migraine pathogenesis. *Neurology, 44*(Suppl. 3), 11–15.

*Langemark, M., & Olesen, J. (1994). Sulpiride and paroxetine in the treatment of chronic tension-type headache. An explanatory double blind trial. *Headache, 34,* 30–34.

Maizels, M. (1998). The clinician's approach to the management of headache. *Western Journal of Medicine, 168,* 203–212.

*Mathew, N. T., Saper, J. R., & Silberstein, S. D. (1995). Migraine prophylaxis with divalproex. *Archives of Neurology 52,* 281–286.

Millea, P. J., & Brodie, J. J. (2002). Tension-type headache. *American Family Physician, 66,* 797–806.

*Misakian, A. L. (2003). Postmenopausal hormone therapy and migraine headache. *Journal of Women's Health, 12*(10), 1027–1036.

Nelson, W.E., et al. (1996). *Nelson Textbook of Pediatrics* (15th ed.). Philadelphia: W. B. Saunders.

*Payne, T. J., et al. (1991). The impact of cigarette smoking on headache activity in headache patients. *Headache, 31,* 329–332.

Rios, J., & Passe, M. M. (2004). Evidence-based use of botanicals, minerals and vitamins in the prophylactic treatment of migraines, *Journal of the American Academy of Nurse Practitioners, 16*(6), 251–256.

Rasmussen, B. K., Jensen, R., & Olesen, J. (1991). A population-based analysis of the diagnostic criteria of the International Headache Society. *Cephalgia, 11,* 129–134.

Silberstein, S. D., Lipton, R. B., & Goadsby, P. J. (2002). *Headache in clinical practice* (2nd ed.). London: Martin Dunitz, Ltd.

*Silberstein, S. D. (2002). *Clinician's manual on migraine* (2nd ed.). Philadelphia: Current Medicine, Inc.

Snow, V., et al. (2002). Pharmacologic management of acute attacks of migraine and prevention of migraine headache. *Annals of Internal Medicine, 137,* 840–849.

Weitzel, K. W., Thomas, M. L., Small, R. E., & Goode, J. V. R. (1999). Migraine: a comprehensive review of new treatment options. *Pharmacotherapeutics, 19,* 957–973.

Visit the Connection web site for the most up-to-date drug information.

SEIZURE DISORDERS

■ ANDREW M. PETERSON AND KUNJAL PATEL

Epilepsy is a common neurologic condition that may be best defined as recurrent seizure activity. A single seizure does not constitute epilepsy unless a brain abnormality that would result in future seizure episodes can be identified. Such an abnormality may be detected on an imaging study (eg, magnetic resonance imaging or computed tomography scan), a physiologic study (eg, electroencephalography [EEG]), or a neurologic examination. Epilepsy affects approximately 1% of the population worldwide. It is estimated that 5% to 7% of all adults will experience one seizure in their lifetime.

Epilepsy is a variable condition with multiple facets, differing physical manifestations, differing prognoses and outcomes, and differing responses to treatment. If seizures occur frequently, neurons can be damaged, which may lead to changes in memory and other cognitive functions. This underscores the importance of controlling seizures. It is important for the practitioner to be aware of the various etiologies and to screen patients appropriately with accurate and reliable diagnostic testing.

Patients with epilepsy often harbor fears based on myths about their disorder as well as fears of significant lifestyle changes or long-term disability. Modern medicine has dispelled some of these fears, mostly because more than 90% of all people with epilepsy lead normal, healthy, and productive lives.

CAUSES

Epilepsy has a number of causes. By far the largest category of causes is idiopathic (unknown cause) epilepsy; approximately 65% of all cases of epilepsy are identified as idiopathic. Approximately 8% of cases are thought to be congenital, approximately 5% are thought to be due to trauma, and approximately 11% are thought to be vascular in origin. Seizures from degeneration, infection, and neoplasm are considerably less prevalent. Seizures can occur at any age, and although etiology varies by age, the idiopathic cause is still the most common at any age.

In newborns and infants, perinatal injuries, metabolic defects, and congenital malformations and infection are more likely causes of epilepsy. Some cases of epilepsy are hereditary or congenital (present at birth), and some are acquired (eg, serious head injury, a central nervous system [CNS]

infection, stroke, or dementia). Obviously, not all people with these disorders acquire epilepsy. This suggests that there is a certain threshold that may play a role in the development of epilepsy and may be based on individual biochemistry. Why a person may have a seizure at one time rather than another relates to cause. This further suggests that there may be immediate triggers that can provoke an attack in a predisposed person (eg, sudden seizure activity in people who are playing video games, working with a calculator, or listening to a particular piece of music). These sensory triggers are uncommon and are often referred to as *reflex epilepsy*.

Predisposing factors that may come into play more often are sleep deprivation, hyperventilation, fever from underlying illness, hormonal changes that can occur during menses, and drug or alcohol ingestion. All of these may lower the seizure threshold and provoke seizures in people who are predisposed.

A number of acute metabolic, infectious, medication-related, and other disorders (eg, alcohol or drug withdrawal, viral meningitis, or hypoglycemia from overdose of insulin in a patient with diabetes) are associated with seizures. However, on recovery from these disorders, a person is not necessarily predisposed to future seizures. These are known as *secondary* or *acute* seizures rather than epilepsy.

Pathophysiology

To understand the pathophysiologic process of an epileptic seizure, it is necessary to understand normal neuronal conduction. Normal cellular transmission from nerve cell to nerve cell depends on a normal distribution of positively or negatively charged ions between the inside and the outside of the cell. In normal human physiology, there is a resting membrane potential (270 microvolts) that leaves the inside of the cell negatively charged with respect to the outside of the cell. A stimulus is needed to produce a cellular discharge, and once stimulated, an action potential is generated in what is referred to as an *all-or-none phenomenon*. After the generation of the action potential, there is a brief period during which the nerve cell membrane is hyperpolarized, which makes it more difficult for a second action potential to be generated until the normal resting membrane ionic gradient is restored.

Communication between neurons occurs through highly specialized structures called *synapses*. There are hundreds of synapses on each neuron. In these synapses, neurotransmitters are released from vesicles in the neurons where they are stored and then diffuse across the synaptic region to contact specific receptors. Once stimulated, the receptors can open or close a specific ion channel. There are two types of ion channels—excitatory and inhibitory. The channels consist of a number of different protein substances. The main inhibitory one in the CNS is gamma-aminobutyric acid (GABA). There are several excitatory neurotransmitters as well, including glutamate and aspartate. These chemicals can activate several different receptors that, depending on their action, can excite or inhibit a group of nerve cells.

To produce an actual seizure, a large group of nerve cells (neurons) must fire abnormally and together. It is thought that this firing occurs within certain highly organized areas of the brain that tend to support seizure activity. This is known as an *epileptic focus*. When epileptic discharges (focus) occur, normal inhibitory circuits (GABA-ergic) begin to fire, which tends to limit the size of the focus. The implication is that a seizure may result from impairment of the inhibitory brain nerve cells or conditions in which there is abnormal excitation. The epileptic focus that is produced may lead to a focal seizure only in the involved area of the brain, or the discharge may travel through other pathways to become more generalized and involve the entire brain. Clinical manifestations of a seizure can be classified by type of seizure, but the manifestations depend on the balance between abnormal, excitatory, and inhibitory neuronal firing, the location of the epileptic focus, and the patterns and degree of spread of the epileptic focus.

Classification of Seizures

The International Classification of Epileptic Seizures (ICES) categorizes seizures in two major groups: partial seizures and generalized seizures. The terminology used by the ICES, however, is not always the same as that used by many clinicians. For instance, many practitioners call the ICES "absence" seizure a *petit mal*, and the designation "tonic-clonic" is often referred to as a *grand mal* seizure. A complex partial seizure is often referred to as a *psychomotor* or *temporal lobe* seizure, and a simple partial seizure has been called *focal* or *Jacksonian*.

Furthermore, classifying epileptic seizures by seizure type is difficult because seizures often appear within a cluster of other symptoms and signs. To help classify seizure type, physicians may look for precipitating factors, age of onset, severity, chronicity, diurnal or circadian cycling, anatomic location of seizure focus, and physical manifestations to help define the patient's treatment and prognosis.

Partial (Focal, Local) Seizures

Partial seizures begin in a localized area of the brain, although there may be generalization to involve both hemispheres. Simple partial (focal) seizures are seizures in which there is no alteration of consciousness and the first clinical and EEG change indicates an initial activation of nerve cells in a limited part of one cerebral hemisphere.

The patient's symptoms are determined by the anatomic location of the seizure focus. There may be motor, sensory, autonomic, or psychic symptoms. These may evolve into complex partial or secondary generalized tonic-clonic seizures. An EEG recorded during this time may show some low-voltage fast activity, rhythmic spikes, and slow-wave activity.

Complex partial seizures (psychomotor) are associated with impaired consciousness and with some form of automatic behavior (automatisms). This type of seizure can evolve from a simple partial seizure and can generate into a secondarily generalized tonic-clonic seizure. The EEG may show a unilateral or bilateral, low-voltage, fast activity with rhythmic spikes and slow waves. Complex partial seizures may be preceded by an aura.

Generalized (Convulsive or Nonconvulsive) Seizures

Generalized seizures involve both hemispheres of the brain from the onset, and early loss of consciousness is the rule. Generalized seizures may involve only loss of consciousness (similar to absence seizures), or they may result in generalized tonic-clonic, clonic, or myoclonic seizures.

Absence seizures (petit mal) usually have a sudden onset, are brief (often lasting less than 10 seconds), and interrupt ongoing activities. The patient exhibits a blank stare and is usually unresponsive when spoken to, although at times the patient may be able to relate what was said to him or her during the initial phase of the seizure. There may be some mild clonic or tonic jerking, but it is not prolonged. There is abrupt onset and abrupt discontinuation. There is no postictal confusion, which may be characteristic of other seizure types, and there are no other associated symptoms. The EEG shows a very rhythmic, 3 cycles/second spike-wave discharge during the event. There is often confusion as to the diagnosis of absence seizures versus complex partial seizures. Absence seizures are usually restricted to childhood and are provoked by hyperventilation.

A subtype of absence seizure is the *atypical absence seizure*, in which the alteration of consciousness may not be complete. A child experiencing this type of seizure may continue with some activities. There may be an associated loss of muscle tone of the face and neck muscles and there may be mild clonic twitching of the eyelids and mouth. The onset and discontinuation of this type of seizure is gradual.

Tonic-clonic seizures (grand mal) are associated with abrupt loss of consciousness. There may be some vague, ill-defined warning signs but no true aura. The patient experiences a sudden, sharp, bilaterally symmetric contraction of muscles and may cry, fall, or do both. The patient's head may be extended and appear cyanotic. There may be associated tongue biting and incontinence. Depressed consciousness that can be prolonged (several hours) characterizes the postictal period, during which the patient exhibits bilaterally symmetric clonic jerking of the extremities, increased salivation and frothing at the mouth, and deep respiration and relaxation of muscles. After the postictal period, the patient usually reports waking with muscle stiffness and headache. The EEG typically shows generalized high-voltage, spike-wave activity.

Clonic seizures consist of rapidly repetitive bilateral jerking of the extremities and facial muscles with loss of consciousness. The postictal phase is usually short.

Atonic seizures (drop attacks or astatic seizures) are characterized by a sudden loss of muscle tone, which may be only fragmentary. This type of seizure may be brief and not associated with loss of consciousness. It can occur in a repetitive, rhythmic, and successive manner and may be seen in patients with more diffuse neurologic insult and psychomotor retardation. Atonic seizures are frequently associated with Lennox-Gastaut syndrome.

Myoclonic seizures are sudden, brief, shock-like muscular contractions. They may be generalized or they may be confined to the face and trunk muscles, to one or more of the extremities, or to individual muscle groups. Myoclonic seizures can occur regularly in a repetitive manner, or they can be sporadic. These seizures may accompany other neurologic conditions, such as metabolic or toxic states, as well as epilepsy.

Tonic seizures consist of brief, generalized tonic contractions with associated head extension, possible stiffening of the back, and stiffening of all four extremities. These seizures can be associated with autonomic symptoms, a rapid heart rate, and cessation of breathing followed by cyanosis. This type of seizure is also seen in the Lennox-Gastaut syndrome and may be precipitated during slow-wave sleep.

Status Epilepticus

Status epilepticus is defined as seizure activity that persists for a long time or occurs so frequently that there is no recovery between attacks. Status epilepticus can be classified as either partial or primary generalized. Precipitating factors include drug noncompliance and sudden withdrawal from antiepileptic drugs (AEDs), fever, withdrawal from alcohol or sedative drugs, metabolic disorder, sleep deprivation, and, possibly, a new cerebral pathologic process.

Diagnostic Criteria

The accurate diagnosis of a seizure helps the health care provider decide whether to initiate or withhold drug treatment and which medications to prescribe. The diagnosis of epilepsy can often be made on the basis of history alone. A typical history, which includes a loss of consciousness associated with generalized tonic-clonic activity, tongue biting, incontinence, and prolonged postictal state, certainly would make the practitioner suspect a seizure. Unfortunately, many of the manifestations of epilepsy are subtle, making diagnosis and classification difficult.

One of the most useful and standard tests for assisting in the diagnosis of epilepsy is the EEG. The EEG is a brain-wave tracing showing voltage fluctuations versus time that is recorded from scalp electrodes placed in specific locations on the head (ie, montages). Neurologic imaging studies also help in the diagnosis of epilepsy. Computed tomography scanning of the brain is used to detect masses or lesions, bleeding, or stroke-like conditions. Cerebral arteriography may detect vascular malformation, aneurysms, and significant vascular disease. Magnetic resonance imaging, although helpful in diagnosing lesions, bleeding, and stroke-like states, also helps find more subtle brain abnormalities, including mesial temporal sclerosis. Positron emission tomography (PET) helps particularly in diagnosing partial epilepsy. PET scans measure regional cerebral blood flow and metabolism both during and between seizures. However, PET scanning is expensive, and some insurance carriers do not approve the test for reimbursement.

INITIATING DRUG THERAPY

The selection of the ideal AED depends on several factors, including seizure type and the age and sex of the patient. Treatment with AEDs starts after the diagnosis is confirmed and the patient has experienced two or more seizures. If a patient has one or more risk factors for recurrent seizures (EEG abnormalities, structural lesions, partial seizures, or a family history), then pharmacotherapy can be initiated.

Many epilepsy specialists advocate monotherapy as the first principle of management. If monotherapy fails, replacement by a second AED is recommended. Usually, when monotherapy with several drugs has failed, polytherapy may be tried. Whenever two or more drugs are used simultaneously, decisions regarding therapy become more complex and there is an increased risk of adverse events.

Monotherapy has several advantages. Management of toxicity is easier with monotherapy because adverse events often can be correlated with serum drug levels. Monotherapy also can promote patient compliance. The most frequent cause of failure to control seizure activity is the patient's lack of adherence to drug therapy. Monotherapy also makes it easier to monitor and control idiosyncratic side effects.

In contrast to monotherapy, polytherapy may increase the chance that chronic toxicity will develop in the patient. Some epilepsy specialists report that up to 75% of their patients have had complete seizure control on monotherapy.

The particular drug selected depends on the seizure type and toxicity. Table 43-1 and Figure 43-1 outline the recommended treatment order and algorithm of treatment.

Table 43.1

Recommended Order of Treatment for Epileptic Seizures

	Partial (Both Simple and Complex) Seizures	Generalized Tonic-Clonic Seizures	Absence Seizures	Atypical Absence, Myoclonic, and Atonic Seizures
First-line therapy	carbamazepine, phenytoin, fosphenytoin, valproic acid	carbamazepine, phenytoin, valproic acid, fosphenytoin	ethosuximide, valproic acid	valproic acid
Second-line therapy (alternative therapy)	felbamate, gabapentin, lamotrigine, phenobarbital, primidone, topiramate, tiagabine, vigabatrin, oxcarbazepine	felbamate, gabapentin, lamotrigine, phenobarbital, primidone, ethotoin, mephobarbital, mephenytoin, vigabatrin	clonazepam, paramethadione, trimethadione, methsuximide, phensuximide	clonazepam

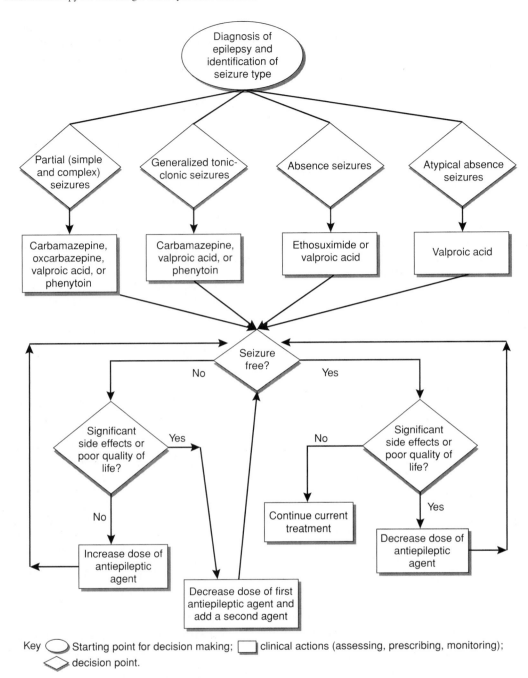

Figure 43–1 Treatment algorithm for epilepsy.

Surgical Treatment of Epilepsy

The surgical treatment of epilepsy has become an important therapeutic modality. Candidates for surgery are patients whose seizures are uncontrolled with medical therapy or who experience intolerable drug side effects. In general, patients with complicated epilepsy should be referred to a neurologist or epilepsy specialist for a decision regarding the need for surgical treatment.

Various surgical procedures can be performed, including anterior temporal lobectomy, amygdala-hippocampectomy, extratemporal focus removal, lesionectomy, corpus callosotomy, and hemispherectomy. Outcomes are good in general, and approximately 70% of patients are seizure free after a temporal lobectomy.

Goals of Drug Therapy

The drug treatment of patients with epilepsy is designed to reduce the number of seizures. A realistic goal for most patients is to control seizures completely (using monotherapy if possible). Linked with the seizure-control goal is the goal of returning to activities of daily living normally and without restriction (except driving; see Patient Education).

Hydantoins

One of the oldest and most effective AEDs is phenytoin (Dilantin). It is effective for a wide range of seizure types, including generalized tonic-clonic as well as simple or partial seizure activity. In either case, it can be used as a first-line drug for monotherapy. Phenytoin, an anticonvulsant, antiarrhythmic agent (class 1B), is currently the most commonly used anticonvulsant for generalized tonic-clonic (grand mal) seizure activity and for simple and complex partial seizures. It also is useful for preventing seizures after head trauma or neurosurgery.

Mechanism of Action

Phenytoin blocks post-tetanic potentiation by stabilizing neuronal membranes. It decreases seizure activity by increasing the efflux or decreasing the influx of sodium ions across cell membranes in the motor cortex during generation of nerve impulses. It also regulates neuronal excitability by blocking neuronal calcium conductance through altering calcium uptake in presynaptic terminals and preventing cyclic nucleotide buildup and cerebellar stimulation.

Phenytoin is a cytochrome P450 (CYP) 2C9 and 2C19 enzyme substrate and a CYP1A2, 2C9, 2D6, and 3A3/4 enzyme inducer. Drug interactions between phenytoin and other drugs occur frequently. It is metabolized in a nonlinear manner, exhibiting Michaelis-Menten enzyme kinetics. By definition, then, the enzymes that metabolize phenytoin are saturable. As the amount of drug approaches this saturation point, small incremental increases in a dose can result in disproportionately high serum levels. Further, as the saturation point is neared, the half-life of phenytoin increases. At typical concentrations in the general population the half-life of phenytoin ranges from 12 to 24 hours.

Dosage

The usual dosage is 300 to 400 mg/day in adults and 5 to 12 mg/kg/day in children. The therapeutic range is 10 to 20 mg/L. The therapeutic level of free, unbound phenytoin, in a person with a normal albumin level, is 1 to 2 mg/L. Contraindications to and special considerations with the administration of phenytoin are listed in Table 43-2.

Adverse Events

Patients receiving intravenous (IV) phenytoin are subject to adverse events such as hypotension, bradycardia, cardiac dysrhythmias, cardiovascular collapse (especially with rapid IV use), venous irritation, and thrombophlebitis. Phenytoin also has dose-related adverse events associated with elevated serum concentrations (Table 43-3). Other adverse events include gingival hyperplasia, hirsutism, coarsening of facial features, rash, hepatitis, megaloblastic anemia, thrombocytopenia, seizures (at elevated serum concentrations), mild sensory polyneuropathy, Stevens-Johnson syndrome, systemic lupus erythematosus (SLE), and folic acid deficiency. If seizures occur, they are usually controlled with diazepam (Valium) 5 to 10 mg (0.25 to 0.4 mg/kg in children).

In overdosages of phenytoin, the expected adverse event profile consists of unsteady gait, slurred speech, confusion, nausea, hypothermia, fever, hypotension, respiratory depression, and coma. The treatment for overdosage is supportive.

Interactions

Drug interactions between phenytoin, other AEDs, and other agents occur frequently (Table 43-4 and Box 43-1).

Fosphenytoin

Fosphenytoin (Cerebyx), the prodrug of phenytoin, is indicated for controlling generalized convulsive status epilepticus and preventing and treating seizures occurring during neurosurgery. It is indicated only for short-term parenteral administration when phenytoin is unavailable or inappropriate or deemed less advantageous. The safety and effectiveness of fosphenytoin in this use have not been systematically evaluated for more than 5 days. Its mechanism of action is the same as phenytoin's. After administration, plasma esterases convert fosphenytoin to phosphate, formaldehyde, and phenytoin (the active moiety).

Dosage

The dose, concentration in solutions, and infusion rates for fosphenytoin are expressed as phenytoin sodium equivalents. Fosphenytoin should always be prescribed in phenytoin sodium equivalents: 75 mg of fosphenytoin sodium = 50 mg of phenytoin sodium (see Table 43-2).

Contraindications to fosphenytoin include hypersensitivity to phenytoin or fosphenytoin or a rash that occurs during treatment (treatment should not be resumed if the rash is exfoliative, purpuric, or bullous). Caution must be used in patients with severe cardiovascular disease, hepatic disease, renal disease, diabetes mellitus, porphyria, fever, or hypothyroidism. It is not recommended for use in children younger than 4 years of age.

Adverse Events

The adverse event profile of fosphenytoin consists of nystagmus, somnolence, dizziness, ataxia, local intolerance to injection, paresthesia, nephrotic syndrome, and hypotension. The dose-related effects are the same as those with phenytoin, as are drug interactions. Adverse events of overdosage include unsteady gait, tremors, hyperglycemia, chorea, gingival hyperplasia, gynecomastia, slurred speech, mydriasis, confusion, agranulocytosis, granulocytopenia, hyperreflexia, coma, SLE, hypotension, and encephalopathy. The treatment is the same as for phenytoin toxicity. IV albumin (25 g every 6 hours) has been used to increase the bound fraction of the drug, and multiple doses of activated charcoal may be effective. In the case of fosphenytoin, an IV filter is not required during administration, whereas a filter is needed for IV phenytoin administration.

Carbamazepine

Carbamazepine (Tegretol) is an excellent anticonvulsant. Carbamazepine 10/11 epoxide, an active metabolite of

Table 43.2

Overview of Drugs Used to Treat Seizures

Generic (Trade) Name and Dosage	Selected Adverse Events	Contraindications	Special Considerations
phenytoin (Dilantin) Loading dose: 15–20 mg/kg in three divided doses q2–4h to decrease GI adverse events Maintenance dose: 300 mg/d or 5–6 mg/kg/d in three divided doses, or qd–bid using an extended-release form of the drug.	Nystagmus, ataxia, cognitive impairment, lethargy, gingival hyperplasia, increase in body hair, coarsening of facial features, acne, folate deficiency, skin rash	Hypersensitivity to phenytoin, other hydantoins, or to any of its components; heart block; sinus bradycardia Pregnancy category D	Avoid IM and SQ administration; it is painful, results in erratic absorption, and may cause local tissue damage. Maximum IV administration is 50 mg/min; in the elderly and in highly sensitive patients with pre-existing cardiovascular conditions, administration should be reduced to 20 mg/min. An in-line 0.22–5-μg filter is recommended for IVPB solutions because of the potential for precipitation. Normal saline solution should be injected through the same needle or IV catheter to prevent irritation. Therapeutic ranges: Neonates: 8–15 μg/mL total phenytoin, 1–2 μg/mL free phenytoin Children and adults: 10–20 μg/mL total phenytoin, 1–2.3 μg/mL free phenytoin Toxic: 30–40 μg/mL
fosphenytoin (Cerebyx) Nonemergent loading dose IV or IM Adults: phenytoin equivalent (PE) 10–20 mg PE/kg (maximum IV rate 150 mg PE/min) Initial daily maintenance dose: IV or, IM, 4–6 mg PE/kg/d	Nystagmus, dizziness, pruritus, ataxia, headache	Hypersensitivity to phenytoin or fosphenytoin or to any of its components; occurrence of any rash while on treatment (the drug should not be resumed if rash is bullous, purpuric, or exfoliative); not recommended for use in children <4 y Pregnancy category D	IV filter is not required; there is no precipitation problem with fosphenytoin. Therapeutic range: 10–20 μg/mL
carbamazepine (Tegretol) 6–12 y: 20–30 mg/kg/d in 2–4 divided doses per day; usual dose is 400–800 mg/d, maximum 1 g/d; 12 y–adult: usual dose 800–1200 mg/d in 3–4 divided doses; 6–12 μg/mL; 4–8 μg/mL if used in combination with other AEDs Toxic >15 μg/mL	May cause GI upset	Pregnancy category D	Oral suspension should not be administered simultaneously with other liquid medicinal agents or diluents. To avoid GI upset, take medication with food or water; splitting doses may also help reduce GI upset. The appearance of a rash does not automatically rule out using carbamazepine.
valproic acid (Depakote, Depakene) Children and adults: 30–60 mg/kg/d in 2–3 divided doses Children receiving more than 1 anticonvulsant: Rectal: 10–15 mg/kg/dose q8h Reduce dose in hepatic impairment	Lethargy, GI upset, weight gain, alopecia, hepatitis	Hypersensitivity to valproic acid, its derivatives or any component; hepatic dysfunction; hepatic failure resulting in death has occurred, and children <2 y are at considerable risk Pregnancy category D	Therapeutic range: 50–100 mg/mL; toxic >200 μg/mL Seizure control may improve at levels >100 μg/mL. Toxicity may occur at levels of 100–150 μg/mL. Take with food or milk, do not administer with carbonated drinks.
ethosuximide (Zarontin) Children 3–6 y: 15–40 mg/kg/d in 2 divided doses Children > 6 y and adults: 20–40 mg/kg/d in 2 divided doses	Nausea, GI upset, hiccups, headache	Hypersensitivity to ethosuximide or its components Pregnancy category C	Seldom-used drug for absence seizures in children
phenobarbital (Barbita, Solfoton) Infants: 5–8 mg/kg/d in 1–2 divided doses	Sedation, ataxia, cognitive impairment, hyperactivity, rash, problems with sleep,	Hypersensitivity to phenobarbital or any of its components Pre-existing CNS depression,	Avoid rapid IV administration (>50 mg/min). Do not add IV form to acidic solutions.

Table 43.2

Overview of Drugs Used to Treat Seizures (Continued)

Generic (Trade) Name and Dosage	Selected Adverse Events	Contraindications	Special Considerations
Children 1–5 y: 6–8 mg/kg/d in 1–2 divided doses Children 5–12 y: 4–6 mg/kg/d in 1–2 divided doses Children >12 y–adults: 1–3 mg/kg/d in 2–3 divided doses or 50–100 mg bid–tid	megaloblastic anemia (responds to folic acid)	severe uncontrolled pain, porphyria, severe respiratory disease with dyspnea or obstruction Use caution in patients with hypovolemic shock, CHF, hepatic impairment, respiratory dysfunction or depression, previous addiction to the sedative/hypnotic group, chronic or acute pain, renal dysfunction, and the elderly (because of its long half-life and addiction potential, phenobarbital is not recommended as a sedative in the elderly). Pregnancy category D	Avoid intra-arterial injection. CrCl <10 mL/min— administer q12–16 h. Tolerance, or psychological and physical dependence, may occur with prolonged use. Abrupt withdrawal in patients with epilepsy may precipitate status epilepticus. Therapeutic ranges: Infants and children: 15–30 μg/mL Adults: 20–40 μg/mL Toxic range: >40 μg/mL
primidone (Mysoline) Children <8 y: 10–25 mg/kg/d tid–qid Children ≥8 y–adults: Start at 100–125 mg qhs for 3 d; then increase to 100–125 mg bid for 3 d; then increase to up to 250 mg tid	Same as above	Hypersensitivity to primidone, phenobarbital, or to any of its components; porphyria Use caution in renal, hepatic impairment or pulmonary insufficiency Pregnancy category D	Abrupt withdrawal may precipitate status epilepticus. This drug is 20%–50% dialyzable; administer dose after dialysis or administer supplemental 30% dose. Folic acid as a supplement to avoid folic acid deficiency and megaloblastic anemia: Adults 5–12 μg/mL Children <5 y: 7–10 μg/mL Toxic level >15 μg/mL Be consistent with protein intake during primidone therapy (low-protein diets increase the duration of action). Avoid foods high in vitamin C because of displacement of drug from binding sites.
gabapentin (Neurontin) 900–1800 mg/d in 3 divided doses Children >12 y: 300 mg on day 1 at bedtime; 300 mg bid on day 2; 300 mg tid on day 3	Ataxia, fatigue, dizziness, somnolence, weight gain, GI upset	Hypersensitivity to gabapentin or its components Pregnancy category C	Dosage adjustments for patients with renal impairment: CrCl >60 mL/min: 1200 mg/d CrCl 30–60 mL/min: 600 mg/d CrCL 15–30 mL/min: 300 mg/d CrCl <15 mL/min: 150 mg/d
lamotrigine (Lamictal) Children 2–12 y with concomitant AEDs without valproic acid therapy: 5–15 mg/kg/d; max. 400 mg/d in 2 divided doses Children 2–12 y with concomitant valproic acid therapy: 1–5 mg/kg/d; max. 200 mg/d in 2 divided doses Adults: 100–400 mg/d in 1–2 doses/d Adults with concomitant valproic acid therapy: 50–200 mg/d in 2 divided doses	Dizziness, headache, rash, ataxia, tremor, GI upset, diplopia, Stevens-Johnson syndrome (rare)	Hypersensitivity to lamotrigine or any of its components Use with caution with lactation, hepatic or cardiac dysfunction, and in children. Pregnancy category C	Take without regard to meals; drug may cause GI upset. Immediately report development of a rash. Gradually decrease dosage (taper) over 2 wk when discontinuing drug therapy.
topiramate (Topamax) Adults: initial: 50 mg/d; titrate by 50 mg/d at 1-wk intervals to a target dose of 200 mg bid; CrCl <70 mL/min: administer 50% of dose and titrate more slowly	Cognitive difficulties, tremor, dizziness, ataxia, headache, fatigue, GI upset, renal calculi	Hypersensitivity to topiramate or any of its components Pregnancy category C	Maintain adequate fluid intake.

(continued)

Table 43.2

Overview of Drugs Used to Treat Seizures (*Continued*)

Generic (Trade) Name and Dosage	Selected Adverse Events	Contraindications	Special Considerations
tiagabine (Gabitril) Children 12–18 y: 4 mg qd for 1 wk; may increase to 8 mg daily in 2 divided doses for 1 wk; then may increase by 4–8 mg weekly to response or up to 32 mg in 2–4 divided doses/d. Adults: 4 mg qd for 1 wk; may increase by 4–8 mg wk to response or up to 56 mg in 2–4 divided doses/d	Dizziness, somnolence, asthenia, confusion, GI upset, anorexia, fatigue, impaired concentration, speech or language problems, confusion	Hypersensitivity to tiagabine or any of its components Pregnancy category C	Should be taken with food Use caution when taking with other CNS depressants.
oxcarbazepine (Trileptal) Initial dose: 300 mg bid; increased by 600 mg/d at weekly intervals Children 4–16 y: 8–10 mg/kg in 2 divided doses/d, not to exceed 600 mg/d	Dizziness, diplopia, ataxia, headache, weakness, rash, hyponatremia	Hypersensitivity to oxcarbazepine or any of its components	Very recent drug
levetiracetam (Keppra) 500 mg twice daily; max 1,500 mg daily	Somnolence, asthenia	Hypersensitivity to the agent; not indicated for children	No drug interactions, rapid titration; only as adjunct therapy
Zonisamide (Zonegran) 100 mg once daily, titrated up to 400–600 mg daily	Fatigue, dizziness, ataxia, anorexia	Hypersensitivity to sulfonamides; not indicated for children	Long half-life leads to long titration period of 100 mg every 2 weeks.

carbamazepine, plays a role in carbamazepine's anticonvulsant activity. It is a first-line drug choice for monotherapy in simple or complex partial seizures with secondary generalization.

Mechanism of Action

Carbamazepine is believed to alter synaptic transmission by limiting the influx of sodium ions across cell membrane channels. It may also work by other, unknown mechanisms. It has the advantage of being nonsedating within the therapeutic range and can be given twice daily with a sustained-release form that is now available.

Dosage

The usual starting dosage of carbamazepine is 200 mg twice daily, leading to a maintenance dose of 600 to 1,200 mg/day (divided into two or three doses). The therapeutic plasma concentration is 4 to 12 mg/L. Doses should be increased no more frequently than once a week in 200-mg increments.

Table 43.3

Relationship Between Total Serum Concentration of Phenytoin and Adverse Events

Serum Concentration	Adverse Events
>20 mg/L	Far lateral nystagmus
>30 mg/L	45 degrees lateral gaze nystagmus and ataxia
>40 mg/L	Decreased mentation and lethargy
>100 mg/L	Lethal

BOX 43–1. NON-ANTIEPILEPTIC DRUGS THAT INTERACT WITH PHENYTOIN

Non-AEDs Affecting Phenytoin Levels
Decreases Phenytoin Levels
Alcohol (long-term use)
Antacids, folic acid, rifampin, tube feedings

Increases Free-Phenytoin Levels
Aspirin, diazoxide, tolbutamide

Increases Total Phenytoin Levels
Alcohol (shortly after intake), amiodarone, chloramphenicol, chlordiazepoxide, chlorpheniramine, cimetidine, disulfiram, fluconazole, fluoxetine, imipramine, isoniazid, metronidazole, omeprazole, propoxyphene, sulfonamides, ticlodipine, trazadone

---

Adverse Events

Adverse events associated with carbamazepine include hematologic abnormalities, drowsiness, fatigue, ataxia, syndrome of inappropriate diuretic hormone secretion (SIADH), rash (Stevens-Johnson syndrome), gastrointestinal (GI) upset, confusion, and nystagmus (see Table 43-2). It can exacerbate seizures (particularly the myoclonic type). Carbamazepine also can induce its own microsomal enzymes, underscoring the need to monitor serum levels frequently during the first 6 months of therapy. It has few long-term dysmorphic tissue

Table 43.4

Summary of Interactions Between Select Antiepileptic Drugs

Added Drug	Effects of Added Drug on Other AED Levels								
	CBZ	GBP	LTG	PB	PHT	VPA	ESM	PRM	FBM
CBZ	Autoinduction	0	↓	↓, ↑	↓, ↑	↓	↓	↓ PRM ↑ PB	↓
GBP	0	—	0	0	0	0	?	?	?
LTG	0	0	—	0	0	↓	?	?	?
PB	↓ CBZ ↑ EPOX	0	↓	—	↓, ↑	↓	↓	X	↓
PHT	↓ CBZ ↑ EPOX	0	↓	↓, ↑	—	↓ Total, ↑ Free	↑	↓ PRM ↑ PB	↓
VPA	↑ EPOX	0	↑	↑	↓ Total, ↑ Free	—	Slightly ↑	↑ PB	↑
ESM	0	?	?	↑	Slightly ↑	0	—	0	?
PRM	↓ CBZ ↑ EPOX	?	?	X	↓, ↑	?	↓	—	?
FBM	↓ CBZ ↑ EPOX	?	?	?	↑	↑	?	?	—

AED, antiepileptic drug; CBZ, carbamazepine; EPOX, CBZ epoxide metabolite; ESM, ethosuximide; FBM, felbamate; GBP, gabapentin; LTG, lamotrigine; PB, phenobarbital; PHT, phenytoin; PRM, primidone; VPA, valproic acid; X, rarely used in combination; ↓, ↑, decreases and increases can occur; ↓, decreased level; ↑, increased level; ?, interaction not known; 0, no effect; PEMA = phenylethymalonamide metabolite of primidone.
Adapted from Brittan, J., & So, E. L. (1996) Symposium on epilepsy, part V: selection of antiepileptic drugs: a practical approach to antiepileptic drug therapy. *Mayo Clinic Proceedings*, 71, 778–789.

effects and may be safer in pregnancy than most other agents. It can be neurotoxic above a narrow therapeutic range, and there can be considerable toxicity during the initiation of therapy. Therefore, slow titration to the desired dose is necessary. Table 43-4 and Box 43-2 list drug interactions between carbamazepine, AEDs, and other drugs.

If toxicity occurs, expected adverse events include dizziness, ataxia, drowsiness, nausea, vomiting, tremors, agitation, nystagmus, urinary retention, dysrhythmias, coma, seizures, respiratory depression, and neuromuscular disturbances. Treatment consists of general supportive care, activated charcoal, and possibly induction of emesis or initiation of gastric lavage. Electrocardiogram, blood pressure, body temperature, pupillary reflexes, and bladder function should be monitored for several days after an overdose.

The suspension formulation is incompatible with chlorpromazine (Thorazine) solution and thioridazine (Mellaril) liquid. Carbamazepine suspension should be given at least 1 to 2 hours apart from that of other liquid medications.

Oxcarbazepine

Oxcarbazepine (Trileptal) is a newer AED. Its pharmacologic effect is exerted through the 10-monohydroxy metabolite (MHD) of oxcarbazepine. The exact mechanism by which oxcarbazepine and MHD work is unknown. However, studies indicate that the drug blocks sodium channels, resulting in stabilization of hyperexcited neural membranes and inhibition of repetitive neuronal firing. Increased potassium conductance and modulation of high-voltage activated calcium channels may contribute to the anticonvulsant effect.

Dosage

Oxcarbazepine is indicated for monotherapy or as adjunctive therapy in treating partial seizures in adults or in children 4 to 16 years of age. Oxcarbazepine is contraindicated in patients with a hypersensitivity to the drug or any of its components. Two other safety concerns with oxcarbazepine are in patients who have had a hypersensitivity reaction to carbamazepine (25% to 30% of whom will also experience a reaction to oxcarbazepine) and in patients at risk for hyponatremia (2.5% of patients).

The typical starting dosage is 300 mg twice daily, increasing by 600 mg per day at weekly intervals. The target maintenance dosage is 600 to 2,400 mg/day. There are no therapeutic levels established for this agent.

BOX 43–2. NON-ANTIEPILEPTIC DRUGS THAT INTERACT WITH CARBAMAZEPINE

Non-AEDs Affected by Carbamazepine
Decreased Levels due to Carbamazepine
Benzodiazepines, corticosteroids, cyclosporine, doxycycline, folic acid, haloperidol, oral contraceptives, theophylline, warfarin

Non-AEDs Affecting Carbamazepine Levels
Increases Carbamazepine Level
Cimetidine, danazol, diltiazem, erythromycin, fluoxetine, imipramine, isoniazid, propoxyphene, verapamil, nicotinamide

Decreases Carbamazepine Level
Alcohol (long-term use), folic acid

Adverse Events

Common adverse events include dizziness, somnolence, diplopia, fatigue, nausea, ataxia, vomiting, abnormal vision, abdominal pain, tremor, dyspepsia, and abnormal gait (see Table 43-2).

Oxcarbazepine is known to interact with valproic acid (Depakene), lamotrigine (Lamictal), carbamazepine, phenytoin, and phenobarbital (Barbita, Solfoton, Luminal). Oxcarbazepine inhibits CYP2C19 and induces the CYP3A4/5 enzyme system. It is a weak inducer of UDP glucuronyl transferase (which is responsible for the metabolism of some drugs, such as valproic acid and lamotrigine). Strong inducers of CYP enzymes (carbamazepine, phenytoin, and phenobarbital) have been shown to decrease plasma levels of the metabolite MHD (29% to 40%). Oxcarbazepine and MHD also cause lower plasma concentrations of dihydropyridine calcium antagonists and oral contraceptives.

Valproic Acid and Derivatives

Valproic acid is an extremely effective anticonvulsant that appears to enhance the action of GABA as well as increasing its availability. The drug also stabilizes neuronal membranes by blocking the sodium channel. This is an extremely efficacious drug for absence, generalized tonic-clonic, partial myoclonic, and atonic seizures. It also may be effective in infantile spasms and partial and mixed seizure types.

Dosage

The average daily dose is 1,000 mg in adults and 15 to 60 mg/kg in children (see Table 43-2). The appropriate therapeutic range is 50 to 140 mg/L.

Adverse Events

Principal adverse events include fatigue, tremor, GI upset, alopecia, behavioral changes, and weight gain. Other adverse events include a change in the menstrual cycle, anorexia, ataxia, headache, erythema multiforme, pancreatitis, thrombocytopenia, prolonged bleeding time, transient increased liver enzymes, liver failure, tremor, and nystagmus. Patients taking valproic acid should be monitored for malaise, weakness, facial edema, anorexia, jaundice, and vomiting. Thrombocytopenia, bleeding, and hepatotoxicity have been reported after 3 days to 6 months of therapy. Other adverse events include SIADH, drowsiness, impaired judgment, and fever. Severe hepatotoxicity has been reported, especially in children 2 years of age and younger who are also taking other anticonvulsants. Valproic acid is teratogenic and produces spina bifida in 1% to 2% of pregnancies.

Interactions

Drug interactions may occur with drugs that affect the CYP2C19, 2C9, 2D6, and 3A3/4 enzyme systems. Valproic acid may decrease total phenytoin levels, but may increase free phenytoin levels because of displacement resulting from protein binding. With carbamazepine, lamotrigine, and possibly clonazepam (Klonopin; increased absence seizures have been reported), the effects of valproic acid may be reduced (see Table 43-4). On the other hand, aspirin may increase valproic acid levels. Increased effects and possibly toxicity have been associated with the concomitant use of diazepam, CNS depressants, and alcohol.

Symptoms of toxicity include coma, deep sleep, motor restlessness, and visual hallucinations. Treatment is supportive and may include the use of naloxone (Narcan) to reverse the CNS depressant effects. The only drawback is that naloxone may block the action of other anticonvulsants.

Divalproex

Divalproex sodium (Depakote) is hepatically metabolized to valproic acid. As such, it is an excellent anticonvulsant for a wide range of seizure types. This drug can be used as a first-line choice for monotherapy in tonic-clonic, absence, myoclonic, and atonic generalized seizures. Although listed as an alternative monotherapeutic agent for partial, simple, or complex seizures with or without secondary generalization, divalproex is often used as a first-line drug for monotherapy in these seizure types as well. No hepatic enzyme induction is associated with divalproex, and there are rare idiosyncratic reactions. Occasionally, persistent GI upset necessitates discontinuation of therapy. Weight gain is common, and rarely severe hepatotoxicity occurs. This drug is teratogenic: spina bifida affects 1% to 2% of newborns whose mothers took divalproex. If this drug is used by women during the childbearing years, folic acid supplementation is needed.

Ethosuximide

Like valproic acid, ethosuximide (Zarontin) is one of the drugs of choice for absence seizures, although it is seldom used. It also is used for managing akinetic epilepsy and myoclonic seizures. The usual dosage is 20 to 40 mg/kg/day, with the therapeutic range between 40 and 100 mg/L (see Table 43-2). Common adverse events are GI upset and fatigue.

Barbiturates

Barbiturates such as phenobarbital are low-cost drugs that can be taken once daily. These drugs have a relatively broad spectrum and can be used as alternative monotherapy in generalized tonic-clonic seizures as well as in simple or complex partial seizures with or without secondary generalization. Unfortunately, barbiturates are usually sedating and have long-term cognitive, memory, and behavioral effects, and drug dependence may develop. Therefore, it is usually best to try to exhaust other alternatives before initiating therapy with barbiturates.

Phenobarbital

Phenobarbital is the most commonly used barbiturate-based anticonvulsant. In addition to the indications listed previously, phenobarbital is used for myoclonic epilepsies and for neonatal and febrile seizures in children.

Mechanism of Action

Its mechanism of action is believed to be interference with the transmission of impulses from the thalamus to the cerebral cortex, resulting in an imbalance in central inhibitory and facilitatory mechanisms.

Contraindications

The drug should be administered cautiously to patients with severe liver disease because of increased side effects. In addition, patients should avoid alcohol and other CNS depressants while taking phenobarbital. Phenobarbital may cause physical and psychological dependence.

Adverse Events

The principal adverse events, drowsiness and fatigue, make phenobarbital a difficult drug to use (see Table 43-2). It also may cause ataxia and blurred vision, nausea, vomiting, constipation, and, over a long period, cognitive impairment and behavioral disturbances. Other major adverse events include cardiac dysrhythmias, bradycardia, dizziness, lightheadedness, "hangover" effect, CNS excitation or depression, and gangrene with inadvertent intra-arterial injection. To a lesser extent, hypotension, hallucinations, hypothermia, Stevens-Johnson syndrome, rash, agranulocytosis, megaloblastic anemia, thrombocytopenia, laryngospasm, respiratory depression, and apnea (especially with rapid IV use) also may occur.

Phenobarbital dosage is 90 to 120 mg/day in adults and 2 to 5 mg/kg/day in children. If an overdosage or toxicity occurs, the expected signs and symptoms include unsteady gait, slurred speech, confusion, jaundice, hypothermia, hypotension, respiratory depression, and coma. Treatment is supportive but may also include an IV vasopressor (eg, dopamine or epinephrine) if the patient is unresponsive. Repeated doses of activated charcoal significantly reduce the half-life of phenobarbital; the usual dose is 0.1 to 1 g/kg every 4 to 6 hours for 3 to 4 days unless the patient has no bowel movement, causing the charcoal to remain in the GI tract. Urinary alkalinization with IV sodium bicarbonate helps promote elimination. Hemodialysis or hemoperfusion is of uncertain value. Patients in stage 4 coma due to high serum barbiturate levels may require charcoal hemoperfusion.

Interactions

Phenobarbital is a CYP1A2, 2D6, and 3A3/4 enzyme inducer that interacts with many of the AEDs (see Table 43-4). Other drug interactions include increased toxicity of propoxyphene (Darvon), benzodiazepines, CNS depressants, and methylphenidate (Ritalin; Box 43-3).

Primidone

Primidone (Mysoline) is related structurally to the barbiturates. It is metabolized to phenobarbital and to phenylethylmalonamide (PEMA). PEMA may enhance the activity of phenobarbital. Primidone is used in the management of grand mal, complex partial, and focal seizures. Its mechanism of action is thought to decrease neuronal excitability and raise the seizure threshold, similar to phenobarbital. The dosage of primidone is adjusted mainly with reference to the phenobarbital level if primidone concentrations are low (see Table 43-2).

Primidone has much the same adverse events as phenobarbital, with fatigue, cognitive impairment, and ataxia being dose related. Other adverse events include nausea,

---

BOX 43–3. NON-ANTIEPILEPTIC DRUGS THAT INTERACT WITH PHENOBARBITAL

Non-AEDs Affected by Phenobarbital
Decreases Phenobarbital Level
Beta blockers, chloramphenicol, chlorpromazine cimetidine, corticosteroids, cyclosporine, desipramine, doxycycline, folic acid, griseofulvin, haloperidol, meperidine, methadone, nortriptyline, oral contraceptives, quinidine, theophylline, warfarin

Non-AEDs Affecting Phenobarbital Levels
Increases Phenobarbital Levels
Chloramphenicol, propoxyphene, quinine

Decreases Phenobarbital Levels
Chlorpromazine, folic acid, prochlorperazine

Increased Toxicity
Benzodiazepines, central nervous system depressants, methylphenidate

---

vomiting, hematologic abnormalities, and an SLE-like syndrome. A skin rash may develop, and over time further cognitive impairment and behavioral changes may develop. Patients who have GI upset while taking primidone may take the medication with food.

Symptoms of toxicity include unsteady gait, slurred speech, confusion, jaundice, hypothermia, fever, hypotension, coma, and respiratory arrest. Treatment is supportive and includes urinary alkalinization with IV sodium bicarbonate to enhance elimination as well as repeated oral doses of activated charcoal, which significantly reduces the half-life of primidone. Hemodialysis and hemoperfusion may be initiated in patients who are in a stage 4 coma.

Drug interactions with primidone are similar to those with phenobarbital (see Table 43-4).

Gabapentin

Gabapentin (Neurontin) is a safe and well-tolerated anticonvulsant with uncomplicated pharmacokinetics. It reduces presynaptic GABA release and seems to be effective as an adjunct agent in the treatment of complex partial seizures and possibly generalized tonic-clonic seizures. There are insufficient data to support its use as monotherapy. It is structurally related to GABA, but the precise mechanism of action in epilepsy is unknown.

Dosage

Gabapentin is most effective as an adjunctive drug for refractory partial seizures. It is not metabolized. It may be given once or twice daily, and its half-life is 5 to 7 hours. The mean dosage in adults is approximately 1,800 mg/day, with a maximum of 3,600 mg/day. The therapeutic range is not well defined.

Adverse Events

Gabapentin is contraindicated in patients who are hypersensitive to the drug or to any of its components. Principal adverse effects are fatigue, dizziness, and blurred vision (see Table 43-2). Many of the CNS-like symptoms resolve in a few weeks. There have also been reports of modest weight gain.

Interactions

Gabapentin does not have any major drug interactions (antacids decrease its bioavailability), and serum level monitoring is not required.

Lamotrigine

Lamotrigine (Lamictal) seems to be efficacious for generalized tonic-clonic, absence (especially atypical), and complex partial seizures. It also may be effective in the Lennox-Gastaut syndrome (not approved for use in children younger than 2 years of age). Although its mechanism of action is not completely clear, it may act on excitatory amino acid release. It also is thought to inhibit voltage-sensitive sodium channels. Its half-life depends on concurrent medications. If lamotrigine is used as monotherapy or combined with valproic acid plus an enzyme inducer, its half-life is 24 hours. If combined with valproic acid alone, the half-life is 48 hours. If combined with an inducing agent such as carbamazepine or phenytoin, its half-life is 12 hours.

Dosage

The starting dosage for lamotrigine is 25 mg twice daily, with a slow titration of 50 mg/day every 2 weeks. The titration may even be slower, such as 25 mg every other day, in patients taking valproic acid. This slower titration should help lower the risk for rash.

Adverse Events

Overall, lamotrigine is well tolerated and does not appear to have any long-term cognitive side effects. The principal adverse events include fatigue, dizziness, diplopia, and ataxia (see Table 43-2). In approximately 5% to 10% of patients (most often in children), a rash may develop; this usually necessitates discontinuing the drug. Other adverse events include angioedema, nystagmus, and hematuria. Lamotrigine is contraindicated in patients with a hypersensitivity to lamotrigine or any of its components.

In case of an overdosage (signs include dizziness, headache, somnolence, and coma), treatment is supportive and may include multiple doses of activated charcoal or gastric lavage.

Interactions

The combined use of lamotrigine and carbamazepine may result in decreased lamotrigine serum concentrations and increased serum concentrations of carbamazepine and carbamazepine 10/11 epoxide. Valproic acid inhibits lamotrigine metabolism, whereas carbamazepine and phenytoin induce its metabolism. Phenobarbital and primidone tend to decrease lamotrigine levels by approximately 40% (see Table 43-4). Although acetaminophen (Tylenol) may decrease lamotrigine levels, caution must be used when giving lamotrigine concomitantly with a folate inhibitor because it is an inhibitor of dihydrofolate reductase.

Levetiracetam

Mechanism of Action

The mechanism of action of levetiracetam is not known. This agent has shown efficacy in the adjunctive treatment of adults with partial-onset seizures.

Dosage

Levetiracetam is started at a dosage of 500 mg twice daily and titrated up to 1,500 mg/day. Dosages of 2,000 to 4,000 mg/day have been used in clinical trials with good tolerability. The dose can be rapidly titrated at 100 mg/day weekly until the desired effect is seen.

Adverse Events

The primary adverse events associated with levetiracetam therapy include somnolence, asthenia, headache, and infection. Most of these occur within the first 4 weeks of therapy, with no dose-toxicity relationship seen. These adverse effects were seen twice as often in patients taking levetiracetam than in those taking placebo. There are no clinically relevant drug/drug interactions with this agent.

Tiagabine

Tiagabine (Gabitril) is used as adjunctive therapy in adults and children older than 12 years of age with partial seizures. Its mechanism of action is not known. However, in vitro experiments show that it enhances GABA activity. Tiagabine does not inhibit the uptake of dopamine, norepinephrine, serotonin, glutamate, or choline.

Dosage

The starting dosage of tiagabine is 4 mg two to four times daily, with an average maintenance dose of 48 mg/day (range 32 to 56 mg/day). Titration is slow, at 4 to 8 mg/day, increased weekly. There are no therapeutic levels established.

Adverse Events

Therapy should not stop abruptly because of the possibility of increasing seizure frequency. All adverse events are dose related and include dizziness, headache, somnolence, CNS depression, memory disturbance, ataxia, confusion, tremors, weakness, and myalgia (see Table 43-2). Tiagabine is a CYP2D6 and 3A3/4 enzyme substrate and is cleared more rapidly when given with other hepatic enzyme–inducing AEDs (ie, carbamazepine, phenytoin, primidone, and phenobarbital).

Topiramate

Topiramate (Topamax) is used as adjunctive therapy for partial-onset seizures in adults and as treatment for Lennox-Gastaut syndrome. It is thought to decrease seizure frequency by blocking sodium channels in neurons, by enhancing GABA activity, and by blocking glutamate activity.

Dosage

The dosage starts at 25 to 50 mg twice a day and is increased to 200 to 400 mg/day in weekly increases of 25 to 50 mg/day. There are no therapeutic levels established for this agent. The agent is not metabolized and about 70% of the drug is eliminated via the kidney. In patients with a creatinine clearance of below 40 mL/min, the dosage should be lowered by about 50%.

Adverse Events

Prominent adverse events are fatigue, dizziness, ataxia, somnolence, psychomotor slowing, nervousness, memory difficulties, speech problems, nausea, paresthesia, tremor, nystagmus, and upper respiratory infections (see Table 43-2). These may occur more frequently in patients taking more than 600 mg/day of topiramate, or when titration occurs too rapidly (3 to 4 weeks to maintenance dose). Other adverse events include chest pain, edema, confusion, depression, difficulty concentrating, hot flashes, dyspepsia, abdominal pain, anorexia, xerostomia, gingivitis, myalgia, back pain, leg pain, rigors, nephrolithiasis, and epistaxis.

Therapy should never be withdrawn abruptly. Proper hydration is essential to decrease the risk of kidney stones. If an overdosage occurs, hemodialysis can remove the drug, but in most cases drug removal is not required. Instead, overdosage is best treated with supportive measures.

Contraindications

Caution must be used in patients with hepatic or renal impairment, during pregnancy, and in breast-feeding mothers.

Interactions

Topiramate is a CYP2C19 enzyme substrate inhibitor; thus, concurrent administration with phenytoin can decrease topiramate levels by as much as 48%, administration with carbamazepine reduces them by 40%, and administration with valproic acid reduces them by 14%. Digoxin (Lanoxin) and norethindrone (Aygestin) blood levels are decreased when given with topiramate, and concomitant administration with other CNS depressants increases topiramate's sedative effects. If used with carbonic anhydrase inhibitors, the risk of nephrolithiasis increases.

Zonisamide

Zonisamide is a broad-spectrum, sulfonamide-derivative AED with activity in partial-onset seizures in adults. This agent is indicated only for use as adjunctive therapy. It appears to block sodium channels and select calcium channels. It has a half-life of 63 to 69 hours in healthy volunteers.

Dosage

The dosage of zonisamide is 100 mg once daily, giving it a distinct compliance advantage over other agents requiring more frequent dosing. The titration to the daily maintenance dose of 400 to 600 mg is slow, at a rate of 100 mg daily every 2 weeks. There are no guidelines for dose adjustment in patients with renal or hepatic impairment, though caution should be used in patients with decreased function in one or both of these systems.

Adverse Events

Since zonisamide is a sulfonamide derivative, patients with a history of hypersensitivity to this class of agents should not take it. Potentially fatal reactions such as Stevens-Johnson syndrome, toxic epidermal necrolysis, and agranulocytosis have been reported. Other important adverse events include fatigue, dizziness, ataxia, and anorexia. In children, there have been reports of high fever secondary to hyperhidrosis; zonisamide is not approved for use in children.

Benzodiazepines

The benzodiazepine antianxiety agents are discussed in depth in Chapter 45.

Clonazepam

Clonazepam (Klonopin) is effective as an adjunctive drug in some patients with myoclonic, atonic, and generalized tonic-clonic seizures. It also is used for prophylaxis of absence, petit mal, variant (Lennox-Gastaut), akinetic, and myoclonic seizures.

Mechanism of Action

Clonazepam is thought to act at the GABA receptor to enhance GABA action, thereby depressing nerve transmission in the motor cortex area. The drug has a half-life of 20 to 40 hours. Dosages are 2 to 6 mg/day in adults and 0.1 to 0.2 mg/kg/day in children. Tolerance to this drug is common.

Contraindications

Contraindications include hypersensitivity to clonazepam, any of its components, or other benzodiazepines; severe liver disease; and acute narrow-angle glaucoma. Caution must be used in patients with chronic respiratory disease or impaired renal function and in patients who are mentally challenged (may have more frequent drug-induced behavioral symptoms).

Adverse Events

Fatigue, sedation, and behavioral changes (eg, aggressiveness and confusion) are the principal adverse reactions. Tachycardia, chest pain, headache, constipation, nausea, and decreased salivation are other adverse reactions. Symptoms of overdose include somnolence, confusion, ataxia, or coma. Treatment is usually supportive. Flumazenil (Romazicon) has been shown to block selectively the binding of benzodiazepines to CNS receptors, resulting in a reversal of benzodiazepine-induced CNS depression but not respiratory depression.

Interactions

Clonazepam interacts with phenytoin, barbiturates (concurrent use may increase clonazepam clearance), and medications that interfere or react with the CYP3A3 and 3A4 enzyme substrates (phenytoin and barbiturates may increase clonazepam clearance). Concomitant use of CNS depressants may increase the risk of sedation.

Lorazepam

Lorazepam (Ativan) is used to treat status epilepticus. It has an unlabeled use for partial complex seizures.

Mechanism of Action

The drug is believed to depress all levels of the CNS, including the limbic system and reticular formation, probably through the increased action of GABA. Before IV use, the injection must be diluted with an equal volume of compatible diluent. If it is injected intra-arterially, arteriospasm and gangrene may occur. The injectable form contains benzyl alcohol 2%, polyethylene glycol, and propylene glycol, which may be toxic to newborns in high doses. Oral doses greater than 0.09 mg/kg produced increased ataxia without increased sedative benefit versus lower doses. Symptoms of overdose may include confusion, coma, hypoactive reflexes, dyspnea, and labored breathing. The treatment for overdose is supportive. Flumazenil may be used in the same fashion as clonazepam, but blood pressure and respiratory support may be required until drug effects subside.

Contraindications

Lorazepam is contraindicated in patients with a hypersensitivity to lorazepam or to any of its components. There is also a risk of cross-sensitivity with other benzodiazepines. It should not be used in comatose patients; patients with pre-existing CNS depression, narrow-angle glaucoma, severe, uncontrolled pain, and severe hypertension; and pregnant women. Caution must be used in patients with renal or hepatic impairment, organic brain syndrome, myasthenia gravis, or Parkinson's disease.

Adverse Events

Common adverse reactions include tachycardia, chest pain, drowsiness, confusion, ataxia, amnesia, slurred speech, paradoxical excitement, headache, and depression. Lightheadedness, rash, decreased libido, xerostomia, bradycardia, cardiovascular collapse, syncope, constipation, nausea, vomiting, decreased salivation, phlebitis, and blurred vision also may occur. Menstrual irregularities, increased salivation, blood dyscrasias, and physical and psychological dependence occur with prolonged use.

Interactions

Lorazepam has a decreased effect with oral contraceptives (combination products), cigarette smoking, and levodopa. Its effects are increased with morphine or other narcotic analgesics. An increased risk of toxicity occurs with the concomitant use of alcohol, CNS depressants, monoamine oxidase inhibitors, loxapine (Loxitane), and tricyclic antidepressants.

Diazepam

Diazepam is used to treat status epilepticus and as an adjunct in convulsive disorders. Its mechanism of action is the same as that of lorazepam.

Dosage

Dosage guidelines and further discussion appear in Chapter 45. In patients with cirrhosis, the dosage must be reduced by 50%. Symptoms of an overdose are the same as with lorazepam.

Diazepam should not be used by patients with severe or acute liver disease. Contraindications include hypersensitivity to diazepam or to any of its components. Other contraindications are similar to those for lorazepam. Caution should be used in patients taking other CNS depressants, patients with low albumin levels or hepatic dysfunction, and elderly patients and infants. Because of its long-acting metabolite and the risk for falls in the elderly population, diazepam is not considered a drug of choice.

Adverse drug effects resemble those of lorazepam. Diazepam is a CYP1A2 and 2C9 enzyme substrate. It is also a minor enzyme substrate for CYP3A3/4, and diazepam and desmethyl-diazepam are CYP2C19 enzyme substrates. Enzyme inducers may increase the metabolism of diazepam, resulting in decreased efficacy. Increased toxicity, sedation, and respiratory depression may result when diazepam is given with CNS depressants (eg, alcohol, barbiturates, and opioids). Cimetidine (Tagamet) may decrease the metabolism of diazepam. Valproic acid may displace diazepam from binding sites, which may result in an increase in sedative effects. Selective serotonin reuptake inhibitors (eg, fluoxetine [Prozac], sertraline [Zoloft], paroxetine [Paxil]) greatly increase diazepam levels by altering its clearance.

Selecting the Most Appropriate Agent

There are a number of excellent AEDs from which to choose for various seizure types. The goal of monotherapy is to promote patient compliance, minimize side effects and toxicity, and reduce cost. Table 43-1 provides the recommended order of treatment for various seizure types; see also Figure 43-1.

In general, first-line monotherapy drugs are tried before using second-line monotherapy drugs, and first-line drugs may be first combined before trying the various second-line, adjunctive agents. Whether the second-line, adjunctive agents will be effective in monotherapy is still to be determined. The choice of an AED is determined by ease of use (ie, dosing regimen), pharmacokinetics, interactions, need for monitoring, and toxicity (which could be dose related, idiosyncratic, chronic, or teratogenic). Ultimately, the optimal treatment for a given patient can be established by a process of trial and error and by knowledge of prior AEDs used.

First-Line Therapy

Selecting the appropriate therapy for each patient is difficult, but there is a science to choosing the best treatment:

- Select the appropriate drug and dose for the type and severity of the seizure being treated.
- Consider the patient's characteristics. For example, does the patient have renal insufficiency, liver disease, hypoalbuminemia, burns, pregnancy, or malnutrition? What concomitant medications does the patient take? How old is the patient? Does the patient comply with the medication regimen? What adverse events are associated with the medication?
- Assess the patient's concurrent diseases and condition.
- Determine the patient's socioeconomic status.

If the initial AED fails, the practitioner should taper this drug's dosage while starting another first-line AED, if available. Typical first-line drugs for partial seizures and generalized tonic-clonic seizures include carbamazepine, phenytoin, fosphenytoin, and valproic acid. First-line therapy for absence seizures includes valproic acid and ethosuximide. Valproic acid is the first-line drug for atypical, absence myoclonic, and atonic seizures.

Second-Line Therapy

Before switching to a second-line agent, the practitioner must optimize treatment with the selected first-line drug (unless the patient experiences intolerable adverse effects) and exhaust all possible first-line drug therapy choices. The practitioner at this point may, based on the patient's past medical history, initiate polytherapy (the addition of two or more medications).

Typical second-line drugs for partial seizures are felbamate (Felbatol), gabapentin, lamotrigine, phenobarbital, primidone, topiramate, tiagabine, and vigabatrin. Second-line drugs for generalized tonic-clonic seizures include felbamate, gabapentin, lamotrigine, phenobarbital, primidone, ethotoin (Peganone), mephobarbital (Mebaral), mephenytoin (Mesantoin), and vigabatrin (Sabril). Typical second-line drugs for absence seizures are clonazepam, paramethadione (Paradione), trimethadione (Tridione), methsuximide (Celontin), and phensuximide (Milontin). Clonazepam is the second-line drug used typically for atypical absence, myoclonic, and atonic seizures.

Third-Line Therapy

If all medications fail and the patient has intractable seizures, surgery may be a third-line treatment option. Before recommending surgery, the practitioner should make sure drug treatment errors have been ruled out (Box 43-4).

Special Population Considerations

Pediatric

The most common seizure syndrome in childhood is Lennox-Gastaut syndrome. This usually is associated with mental retardation. Characteristically, multiple seizure types can

---

BOX 43–4. COMMON DRUG TREATMENT ERRORS

- Incorrect or incomplete identification of seizure type(s), resulting in inappropriate choice of treatment (eg, the practitioner may be confused between brief complex partial seizures and absence seizures, or may fail to recognize juvenile myoclonic epilepsy)
- Drug selection that is appropriate for the patient's seizure type(s) but not for the patient (eg, phenytoin for an adolescent or valproate for a woman who is pregnant or likely to become pregnant in the near future)
- Correct diagnosis and drug choice, but incorrect dosage (eg, the patient is given too low a dose, only the starting dose is tried, or the patient receives too high a dose too quickly)
- Insufficient follow-up (eg, the patient is seen by a specialist and referred back to the general practitioner with an appropriate recommendation regarding treatment, but when this proves ineffective, further advice is not sought)

---

occur, including atypical absence, atonic (drop attacks), secondarily generalized tonic-clonic, and myoclonic and tonic seizures. EEGs show considerable slow-wave and spike-wave activity. Although patients respond to valproic acid, benzodiazepines, and lamotrigine, there is a poor prognosis for seizure control.

Simple febrile seizures are another important category of seizures that affect children between the ages of 6 months and 5 years. Febrile seizures occur in 4% of all children and are preceded by high fevers, underlying the importance of controlling high fevers in children. The seizure is generalized and usually lasts under 15 minutes. Approximately 33% of children experience a recurrence, although almost never within the first 24 hours. These patients usually have no preceding neurologic abnormality or family history of epilepsy. Long-term anticonvulsant therapy is not indicated for this seizure type.

Geriatric

Understanding the basic pharmacologic principles involved in the administration of AEDs is the key to the optimal use of these drugs in older patients. Drug clearance and metabolism are significant issues in this population. Many older patients have decreased renal and liver function, which may have a profound effect on drug metabolism and excretion. AED dosages may need to be adjusted.

AEDs are bound to different degrees by plasma proteins, particularly albumin. If a patient has a low albumin level (as elderly adults tend to have), and therefore low protein binding of the AED, therapeutic effect and toxicity may be experienced at dosages lower than the recommended ones.

In patients with liver disease, which is common in the geriatric population, the rates of hepatic biotransformation of drugs and of hepatic blood flow are decreased. Therefore, protein binding of AEDs may also be reduced by low protein and displacement by bilirubin or other substances that have the net effect of increasing both the total serum drug concentration and the percentage of free drug in the serum. In renal disease, there may be a decrease in the clearance of drugs eliminated entirely by the kidney. Renal failure also may complicate elimination of drugs principally cleared by the liver. Studies have shown that in the patients with uremia who are taking phenytoin, hepatic biotransformation processes continue or accelerate during the renal failure, but renal excretion of metabolites is decreased. Therefore, uremic patients tend to have lower total serum phenytoin concentrations but higher serum concentrations of the oxidized principal metabolite (hydroxyphenyl-phenylhydantoin).

Women

For woman taking anticonvulsant therapy, a major point for discussion is the risk during pregnancy. Several anticonvulsants are listed as pregnancy category C or D (ie, phenytoin, fosphenytoin, phenobarbital, primidone, valproic acid, ethosuximide, topiramate, and tiagabine), indicating a greater risk for fetal abnormalities. The practitioner must work closely with the woman who wishes to become, or is, pregnant to assess the risks involved and to choose the drug that is effective for the woman and safest for the fetus.

MONITORING PATIENT RESPONSE

For patients taking an AED, the health care practitioner should monitor:

- Frequency and severity of seizures
- Adverse events
- Plasma drug levels, if applicable

Therapy is considered to be a failure if the AED dosage is at the optimal level and seizures are still uncontrolled or adverse events become intolerable. Some patients have good clinical responses at serum drug concentrations below the therapeutic range; others can exhibit toxicity within the therapeutic range. Still others require serum concentrations above normal therapeutic values for seizure control, and these patients may tolerate very high levels without signs of toxicity.

Drugs should be added or subtracted as needed. Whenever a new AED is started or a dosage change is made, it takes five elimination half-lives (or the period over which a drug's plasma concentration falls to 50% of the peak level after a single dose) before the new steady-state serum concentration is achieved and before the full therapeutic impact of the new medication or dosage change can be assessed. Therefore, too much haste in changing an AED or discarding it as ineffective may have significant therapeutic implications.

When AEDs are administered in combination, it is important to note the types of drug interactions that may occur

(see Table 43-4). Even when monotherapy is used, some AEDs alter their own biotransformation when they are administered chronically (eg, carbamazepine and valproic acid). The existence of these interactions complicates the design of the therapeutic regimen when more than one AED is used, underscoring the desirability of using monotherapy whenever possible.

Phenytoin and Phenobarbital

For patients taking phenytoin, blood pressure, vital signs (with IV use), complete blood count (CBC), liver function tests, and plasma phenytoin levels should be monitored. Steady-state concentrations are reached in 5 to 10 days.

For patients taking phenobarbital, its concentration, mental status changes, CBC, liver function tests, seizure activity, and respiratory rate should be monitored. Prolonged use may result in vitamin D loss, and supplementation may be necessary.

Primidone and Valproic Acid

For patients taking primidone, serum primidone and phenobarbital concentrations, CBC (at 6-month intervals), neurologic status, excessive sedation, and CNS effects should be monitored. Monitoring for patients on valproic acid must include liver enzymes, CBC with platelets, and valproic acid levels. Patients should immediately report a sore throat, fever, fatigue, bleeding, or bruising that is severe or persists.

Lamotrigine and Tiagabine

During therapy with lamotrigine, the practitioner should monitor seizures (frequency and duration), serum levels of concurrent anticonvulsants, and signs of a rash. During therapy with tiagabine, periodic monitoring of the CBC, renal function tests, liver function tests, and routine blood chemistry are required.

PATIENT EDUCATION

More than 90% of patients with epilepsy lead normal lives. The patient should avoid sleep deprivation and excessive alcohol use, both of which can lower the seizure threshold and make recurrent seizure activity likely. The patient should avoid jobs that involve working at heights or near heavy machinery, flames, burners, or molten material, so there are some restrictions on careers (eg, firefighter, commercial driver, or airline pilot). Patients should never swim alone. Most sports are permitted, but those in which a sudden loss of consciousness could be deadly, such as skydiving, hang gliding, mountain climbing, and scuba diving, should probably be avoided.

Drug Information

The American Academy of Neurology's practice guideline center (http://www.aan.com/professionals/practice/guideline/index.cfm) provides information about epilepsy and medications for practitioners. Other sources of information on AEDs include the American Epilepsy Society (http://www.aesnet.org/Visitors/PatientsPractice/index.cfm) and the National Institute of Neurological Disorders and Stroke (http://www.ninds.nih.gov/).

Patient-Oriented Information Sources

Patients often have questions about epilepsy prognosis and treatment, first aid, educational needs, pregnancy, and driving and insurance. The American Epilepsy Foundation or the many epilepsy societies around the country can help answer those questions. These organizations provide both professional and lay support assistance, including counseling and psychotherapy, access to social workers, and financial assistance.

Nutrition/Lifestyle Changes

The ketogenic diet has been advocated as a means of treatment for patients with epilepsy. This diet, high in fat and low in carbohydrates, is usually used in children refractory to AEDs. However, there does not appear to be reliable evidence supporting the use of the ketogenic diet in people with epilepsy.

Driving is, of course, one of the most serious restrictions. Laws concerning driving vary from state to state, but in general driving is not advised for 6 months after the last seizure. Some exceptions are strictly nocturnal seizures or those related to the discontinuation of an anticonvulsant on a physician's advice. Individual state laws regarding the driving restriction need to be reviewed by the practitioner.

First aid for seizure activity consists primarily of protecting the patient's head and body from injury. It usually is not advisable to try to open the patient's mouth or to put objects in the patient's mouth. This can result in injury to the patient's mouth and airway as well as to the helpful bystander. However, removing dentures, excessive secretions, and foreign materials from the mouth after a tonic-clonic seizure phase is completed may be helpful. Turning the patient into a semiprone position in the postictal period helps to prevent aspiration.

■ Case Study

Accompanied by his girlfriend, B.C., age 23, visits your office. His girlfriend states, "He hasn't been himself in the last month. He has headaches and is completely confused and tired for no reason." B.C. denies using illicit drugs and any recent traumatic injuries. He thinks his problem started approximately a month ago when he and his girlfriend were at a club dancing. His friends told him that he became confused and began tugging at his clothes. Then he fell down and was unconscious for a few minutes. When he awoke, he felt extremely tired and did not know what was going on. He girlfriend recalls that he had been hit in the head with a softball during a game the day before they went dancing.

Past medical history discloses insulin use since early childhood (currently 10 U NPH in the morning and 10 U regular insulin before meals), Zantac at bedtime, and Advil (1 or 2 tablets twice a day) for headaches. The patient says he has no allergies.

Family history reveals healthy parents who died in a car crash when the patient was 10 years of age. Social history discloses a love of dancing, an active sex life, and occasional alcohol use at social events. B.C. does not smoke cigarettes or use recreational drugs.

On physical examination, B.C. is 5-foot-10 and 155 lb. His temperature is 37°C, pulse rate 78, blood pressure 118/76, and glucose level 90. Skin appears normal. Head and neck are normal, chest is clear for anterior and posterior sounds, cardiovascular rrr and (2) r/m/g, and laboratory values are within normal limits. EEG findings include sharp-wave discharges.

At a follow-up visit 2 months later, B.C. and his girlfriend report that things have gotten worse. The girlfriend states that as B.C. was eating dinner one night, he had a seizure. He was completely stiff for a short time and then his arms and legs began moving. She believes that he was unconscious for a few minutes. B.C. says he could not remember what had happened when he woke up.

Diagnosis: Generalized tonic-clonic seizure

→ 1. List specific goals of treatment for B.C.

→ 2. What AED would you prescribe? Why?

→ 3. What are the parameters for monitoring the success of this therapy?

→ 4. Describe one or two drug/drug or drug/food interactions for the selected AED.

→ 5. Discuss specific patient education based on the prescribed therapy.

(Continued)

■ Case Study (*Continued*)

➤ 6. List one of two adverse reactions to the selected AED that would cause you to change therapy.

➤ 7. If the above occurred, what would be your choice for the second-line therapy?

➤ 8. What over-the-counter and/or alternative medications would be appropriate for B.C.?

➤ 9. What dietary and lifestyle changes would you recommend for this patient?

Bibliography

Berg, A. T., Shinnar, S., Levy, S. R., & Testa, F. M. (1999). Status epilepticus in children with newly diagnosed epilepsy. *Annals of Neurology, 45*, 618–623.

Bourgeois, B. (1998). New antiepileptic drugs. *Archives of Neurology, 55*, 1181–1183.

Brittan, J., & So, E. L. (1996). Symposium on epilepsy. Part V: Selection of antiepileptic drugs: a practical approach to antiepileptic drug therapy. *Mayo Clinics Proceedings, 71*, 778–789.

Browne, T. R., & Holmes, G. L. (2001). Epilepsy. *New England Journal of Medicine, 344*(15), 1145–1151.

De Silva, M., McArdle, B., McGowan, M., Hughes, E., Stewart, J., Neville, B. G., et al. (1996). Randomized comparative monotherapy trial of phenobarbitone, phenytoin, carbamazepine or sodium valproate for newly diagnosed childhood epilepsy. *Lancet, 347*, 709–713.

Dichter, M. A., & Brodie, M. J. (1996). Drug therapy: new antiepileptic drugs. *New England Journal of Medicine, 334*, 1583–1590.

Freely, M. (1999). Drug treatment of epilepsy: fortnightly review. *British Medical Journal, 318*, 106–109.

French, J. A., Kanner, A. M., Bautista, J., Abou-Khalil, B., Browne, T., & Harden, C. L., et al. (2004a). Efficacy and tolerability of the new antiepileptic drugs, I: treatment of new-onset epilepsy: report of the therapeutics and technology assessment subcommittee and quality standards subcommittee of the American Academy of Neurology and the American Epilepsy Society. *Neurology, 62*(8), 1252–1260.

French, J. A., Kanner, A. M., Bautista, J., Abou-Khalil, B., Browne, T., & Harden, C. L., et al. (2004b). Efficacy and tolerability of the new antiepileptic drugs, II: treatment of refractory epilepsy: report of the therapeutics and technology assessment subcommittee and quality standards subcommittee of the American Academy of Neurology and the American Epilepsy Society. *Neurology, 62*(8), 1261–1273.

Greenwood, R., & Tennison, M. (1999). When to start and stop anticonvulsant therapy in children. *Archives of Neurology, 56*, 1073–1077.

Krumholz, A. (1999). Nonepileptic seizures: diagnosis and management. *Neurology, 53*(Suppl. 2), S76–S83.

Lacy, C., Armstrong, L., Goldman, M., & Lance, L. (1999–2000). *Drug interaction handbook* (7th ed.). Hudson, OH: Lexi-Comp, Inc.

LaRoche, S. M., & Helmers, S. L. (2004a). The new antiepileptic drugs: clinical applications. *JAMA, 291*(5), 615–620.

LaRoche, S. M., & Helmers, S. L. (2004b). The new antiepileptic drugs: scientific review. *JAMA, 291*(5), 605–614.

Mattson, R. H., Cramer, J. A., & Collins, J. F. (1992). A comparison of valproate with carbamazepine for the treatment of complex partial seizures and secondary generalized tonic-clonic seizures. *New England Journal of Medicine, 327*, 765–771.

Sillanpaa, M., et al. (1998). Long-term prognosis of seizures with onset in childhood. *New England Journal of Medicine, 338*, 1715–1722.

Sperling, M., et al. (1999). Seizure control and mortality in epilepsy. *Annals of Neurology, 46*, 45–50.

Visit the Connecion web site for the most up-to-date drug information.

44

DEPRESSIVE DISORDERS

■ ANDREW M. PETERSON AND FRANK NATALE

Depression is a mood disorder characterized by changes in cognition, behavior, and physical functioning. As an extreme and sustained emotion, depression alters a person's perception of the world and considerably affects his or her ability to function. It is estimated that one in five patients in this country are affected by a mood disorder at some point in their lifetime (Mulrow et al., 2000). The cardinal symptoms of depression include persistent feelings of sadness, anxiety, loss of interest or pleasure in usual activities, changes in appetite, insomnia or hypersomnia, fatigue, and restlessness or irritability.

In primary care settings, depression is the most common psychiatric problem, with a prevalence of 4.8% to 9.2%. Approximately 14 million people in the United States are currently experiencing symptoms of depression. It is estimated that the economic cost of this disorder rivals that of cardiac disease in the United States (Young, Campbell, & Harper, 2002). Today, although 80% to 90% of those affected can be treated effectively, only one third seek treatment. Approximately two thirds of depressed people experience suicidal ideation, and 10% to 15% actually commit suicide.

The incidence of depression increases with age, and women have a higher lifetime prevalence of depression, ranging from 5% to 26%, compared with men, whose prevalence ranges from 2% to 12%. Women between the ages of 25 to 44 have a risk of depression of 10% to 25% (Young, Campbell, & Harper, 2002).

CAUSES

In the past, depression was thought to result from a weakness in personality structure, and resolution of depression required the patient to make behavioral changes. Today, practitioners recognize that depression has various causes involving a complex interaction of social, genetic, environmental, and biochemical factors.

The risk for development of a major depressive illness is not attributable to a single factor, but to many. Family history of depression has been a known risk factor for major depression for years, but the genetic contribution is less defined than in other mental illnesses (eg, schizophrenia). First-degree relatives of depressed people have a greater prevalence of depression than the general population.

Although cultural propensity is not a risk factor, the display of symptoms may differ among cultures. This interaction of multiple risk factors is not fully understood and is the subject of ongoing research.

PATHOPHYSIOLOGY

Most current research focuses on neurochemical aspects of depression and has spurred several theories relating to the generation and maintenance of specific neurotransmitters in the central nervous system. The basis for these neurochemical theories is the hypothesis that abnormal neurotransmitter release or decreased postsynaptic receptor sensitivity is affected before and during a major depressive episode. At least four theories relate to this hypothesis (Box 44-1). Three of the four theories center on a functional or absolute deficiency in the neurotransmitters serotonin, norepinephrine, or both. A functional deficiency suggests that the body produces neurotransmitters but the postsynaptic receptors cannot fully transmit the neural impulse. This is in contrast to an absolute deficiency, in which the body produces no neurotransmitters or the postsynaptic receptors cannot transmit the signal at all.

Similar to the theories associated with the monoamine catecholamines norepinephrine and serotonin, some theories suggest that dopamine should be included as a contributor to depression. This is because some agents known to increase central dopamine levels have been associated with relief of depressive symptoms. Data supporting this component of the theory are preclinical, and additional clinical supporting studies need to be conducted.

The permissive hypothesis, a more contemporary theory, suggests that reduced serotonin activity sets the stage for a mood disorder, such as depression or mania, depending on the underlying norepinephrine level. A low serotonin level coupled with a low norepinephrine level suggests that depression results from an increased beta-adrenergic receptor sensitivity. This alteration in postsynaptic receptor sensitivity results in an imbalance between the effects of norepinephrine and serotonin and may create a functional deficiency in serotonin.

DIAGNOSTIC CRITERIA

Mildly depressed patients meet the minimum criteria for diagnosis, whereas moderately depressed patients display a greater degree of dysfunction. Severely depressed patients experience symptoms well in excess of the diagnostic criteria.

BOX 44–1. PATHOPHYSIOLOGIC HYPOTHESES OF DEPRESSION

Serotonin Hypothesis
A functional or an absolute deficiency in the neurotransmitter serotonin

Catecholamine Hypothesis
A functional or an absolute deficiency in the neurotransmitters norepinephrine, serotonin, or dopamine

Permissive Hypothesis
Diminished serotonin gives "permission" for a superimposed norepinephrine deficiency to manifest as depression

Beta-Adrenergic Receptor Hypothesis
Depression results from increased beta-adrenergic receptor sensitivity

BOX 44–2. DIAGNOSTIC AND STATISTICAL MANUAL OF MENTAL DISORDERS IV: CRITERIA FOR DIAGNOSING MAJOR DEPRESSIVE EPISODE

A. Five (or more) of the following symptoms have been present during the same 2-week period and represent a change from previous functioning. At least one of the symptoms must be #1 or #2.
   1. Depressed mood most of the day. In children or adolescents the mood can be irritable instead of depressed.
   2. Diminished interest or pleasure in all or almost all of usual activities
   3. Significant weight loss or weight gain, or decrease or increase in appetite
   4. Insomnia or hypersomnia
   5. Psychomotor agitation or retardation as observed by others
   6. Fatigue or loss of energy
   7. Feelings of worthlessness, or excessive or inappropriate guilt
   8. Diminished ability to think or concentrate, indecisiveness
   9. Recurrent thoughts of death, sucidal ideation, suicide attempt, or a specific plan for suicide
   10. The symptoms cause clinically significant distress or impairment in social, occupational, or other important areas of functioning.
B. The symptoms are not due to the direct physiologic effects of a substance or a medical condition.
C. Patient must not be purposefully altering diet to achieve weight loss or gain.

Their symptoms often greatly interfere with social and occupational functioning. Pharmacologic treatment is strongly recommended in patients with suicidal ideation. In addition, certain instances require aggressive treatment because without treatment patients may act out on their suicidal thoughts (Matthews & Fava, 2000).

The criteria for diagnosing a major depressive episode are listed in Box 44-2. A patient must exhibit at least five of these signs or symptoms in the same 2-week period along with symptoms of depressed mood or anhedonia, the inability to gain pleasure from normally pleasurable experiences (Snow, Lascher, & Mottur-Pilson, 2000). Changes in weight, sleep habits, and other target symptoms also can be identified when taking the patient's history.

Subtypes of major depressive disorder delineate the etiology and severity of the illness or episode. These subtypes include mild, moderate, and severe depression. The descriptors (known as *specifiers*) refer to the severity of dysfunction and delineate comorbid or distinguishing features, such as melancholy, catatonia, and psychosis.

Types of Depression

Postpartum Depression

The onset is usually within 6 weeks after childbirth, and symptoms last from 3 to 14 months. Prevalence of postpartum depression ranges from 3.5% to 33%. Women with a history of postpartum depression have a 50% risk for recurrence, and 30% of women with a history of depression not related to childbirth have postpartum depression (Evins, Theofrastous, & Galvin, 2000).

Seasonal Affective Disorder

Seasonal affective disorder (SAD) is a pattern of depressive or manic episodes that occurs with the onset of winter. As the days become shorter and the weather colder, there is an increase in depressive symptoms. SAD causes individuals to eat more, sleep more, experience chronic fatigue, and gain weight. In pronounced cases, significant social withdrawal may occur.

Dysthymia

Dysthymia is a chronic but less severe form of depression that is found in approximately 3% of the population (Snow, Lascher, & Mottur-Pilson, 2002). It is characterized by functional impairment and at least 2 years of depressive symptoms. Common symptoms include appetite disturbances, insomnia or hypersomnia, fatigue, difficulty making decisions, and low self-esteem.

INITIATING DRUG THERAPY

When prescribing drug therapy, the practitioner considers many indicators, among them the severity of symptoms (eg, mild, moderate, or severe), kind of depression (major, acute episode, postpartum, seasonal, dysthymia), the potential duration of therapy, the patient's age, sex, and concomitant conditions, and other factors.

Because the depth of depression plays a role in treatment planning, depression is categorized by the severity of symptoms. The severity is gauged by clinical interview or rating scales, or both, as well as by physical examination and diagnostic findings.

Adequate assessment and monitoring of depression have been the subjects of numerous trials and surveys. Various self-rating scales, such as the Hamilton Depression Scale (HAM-D) (Hamilton, 1967) and the Geriatric Depression Scale (Yesavage, 1988), have been developed. These short, easy-to-complete, self-rating scales are used frequently in general practice to determine the baseline level of depression and to monitor the patient's progress throughout treatment.

Other tools used in assessing the severity or source of depression include a typical health and medication history. Also useful is a physical examination with documentation of the patient's height, weight, and pertinent laboratory test findings, such as a complete blood count with differential, electrolytes, and kidney and liver function. Caution must be exercised in diagnosing a major depressive disorder because medications and illnesses can induce depression. These conditions must be ruled out before making the diagnosis (Box 44-3).

In addition, the practitioner investigates alternative reasons for depression, including vascular disease, neurologic dysfunction, thyroid dysfunction, vitamin B_{12} and folate deficiencies (particularly in the elderly), and even infection.

Nonpharmacologic therapy for depression includes several psychotherapeutic techniques such as cognitive therapy, behavioral therapy, and interpersonal therapy. Each has its advantages and disadvantages. The practitioner selects the specific therapy or combination of therapies based on the patient's needs. Psychotherapy is usually used for patients with concurrent psychosocial stressors. Although psychotherapy alone may be effective, patients meeting the criteria for major depression should be evaluated for medication therapy. Moderately depressed patients often need a combination of medication and psychotherapy. Severely depressed patients may be refractory to psychotherapy, and their risk for suicide should be assessed.

Goals of Drug Therapy

The goals of pharmacotherapy include treating the patient's depression and returning the patient to a normal level of functioning with a minimum of side effects. In general, all of the available antidepressants are equally effective, with response rates ranging from 60% to 70% in all depressed patients. A 4- to 6-week trial of continuous therapy with antidepressant medications is required to reach a maximum therapeutic effect. However, an accurate diagnosis remains the focal point of effective patient care (Breen & McCormac, 2002).

Antidepressant Drugs

Several drug classes are available for treating depression: the selective serotonin reuptake inhibitors (SSRIs), tricyclic antidepressants (TCAs), monoamine oxidase inhibitors (MAOIs), and atypical agents. They all appear to work by affecting one or more of the primary neurotransmitters theorized to be respon-

---

BOX 44–3. SELECTED CONDITIONS AND MEDICATIONS ASSOCIATED WITH DEPRESSION

Endocrine disorders
Addison's disease
Cushing's syndrome
Hypothyroidism

Gastrointestinal disease
Irritable bowel syndrome
Inflammatory bowel disease
Cirrhosis

Infections
AIDS
Influenza
Meningitis

Cardiovascular diseases
Congestive heart failure
Myocardial infarction

Neurologic disorders
Alzheimer's disease
Multiple sclerosis
Parkinson's disease
Stroke
Chronic headache

Cancer
Alcoholism
Drug use
Alcohol
Antihypertensives
reserpine
methyldopa
diuretics
propranolol
clonidine
Oral contraceptives
Steroids

Rheumatologic
Systemic lupus erythematosis
Chronic fatigue syndrome
Fibromyalgia
Rheumatoid arthritis

---

sible for depression. In theory, each of the antidepressants increases the amount of neurotransmitter available in the synapse, either by inhibiting its metabolic degradation or by decreasing the rate at which it is recycled (by the process called *reuptake*) back into the presynaptic neuron (Fig. 44-1). For example, SSRIs inhibit the reuptake of select isoforms of serotonin, thereby increasing the functional availability of serotonin in the synaptic cleft. TCAs are thought to work by inhibiting the reuptake of norepinephrine from the synaptic cleft, thereby increasing the amount available to stimulate the postsynaptic

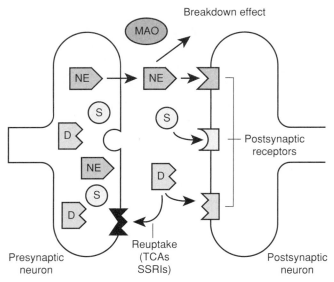

Figure 44–1 Schematic representation of the mechanism of action of antidepressant agents. Neurotransmitters (NE, S, D) are released from the presynaptic neuron into the synaptic space. They interact with the postsynaptic receptors and continue the neuronal transmission. After release from the postsynaptic neuron, these agents can be broken down by the enzyme monoamine oxidase (MAO) and the components recycled into the presynaptic neuron or they can be taken up again through the reuptake mechanism. Antidepressant agents can 1) block the MAO enzymes—MAO inhibitors; or 2) block the reuptake of the neurotransmitter. In effect, each mechanism increases the intrasynaptic concentration of the particular neurotransmitter.

neuron. Conversely, the MAOIs inhibit the metabolism of monoamines such as dopamine, serotonin, and norepinephrine. This nonselective inhibition also increases the relative amounts of each of these catecholamines available to stimulate the postsynaptic neurons. However, this nonselectivity may contribute to side effects.

Table 44-1 presents the antidepressants and the neurotransmitters primarily affected. Because all of these agents appear to have equal efficacy, the practitioner should select the most appropriate initial therapy based on side effect profiles, predicted patient compliance, and cost of therapy. The following discussion and accompanying tables and charts will help the practitioner in selecting the optimal initial agent for treating depression.

Selective Serotonin Reuptake Inhibitors

The SSRIs work primarily by binding to the serotonin transporter and inhibiting the reuptake of this neurotransmitter into the presynaptic neurons. Table 44-2 identifies starting dosages and expected dosage ranges of the SSRIs.

Time Frame for Response

The effects of these agents are apparent within 4 to 6 weeks of treatment. The length of therapy for first episodes of depression is 4 to 6 months after the initial response. Measures of efficacy include improved scores in the initial rating scales, self-reported improvement in the target symptoms originally described by the patient, and improved affect observed by the practitioner.

Just as effective as TCAs and older antidepressants, SSRIs are associated with fewer adverse reactions and a lower risk of dangerous overdose. Therefore, they have become first-line therapy for most patients with major depression.

Adverse Events

SSRIs are usually administered in the morning because of the potential to induce anxiety and insomnia. Insomnia is thought to be related to the suppression of rapid eye movement (REM) sleep and may be treated with a sedative–hypnotic drug such as the benzodiazepine temazepam (Restoril). Because long-term treatment of insomnia is not recommended, a gradual tapering of the sedative–hypnotic agent is advisable. If it appears necessary to continue a sedative–hypnotic, the practitioner should evaluate the reason for the sleep disturbance and treat accordingly. Some patients do, however, experience sedation with an SSRI, and these patients may be advised to take their medication at bedtime.

The SSRIs have virtually no potential for inducing orthostatic hypotension or cardiac conduction abnormalities, which makes them ideal for elderly patients or those with a history of dysrhythmias. They do have epileptogenic potential, so caution must be used in patients with a history of seizures.

A common side effect reported by patients taking SSRIs is sexual dysfunction. This is due to the increased serotonin activity at the 5-HT2 receptor site. Sexual dysfunction is

Table 44.1

Classification of Antidepressant Agents and Neurotransmitters Affected

Generic Name	Trade Name	NE	5-HT	D
Tricyclic Antidepressants				
amitriptyline	Elavil	+ + + +	+ + + +	0
desipramine	Norpramin	+	+ + +	0
doxepin	Sinequan	+	+ + +	0
imipramine	Tofranil	+ + +	+ +	0/+
nortriptyline	Pamelor	+ +	+ + +	0
protriptyline	Vivactil	+	+ + + +	0
trimipramine	Surmontil	+ +	+ +	0
Selective Serotonin Reuptake Inhibitors				
citalopram	Celexa	0	+ + + +	0
fluoxetine	Prozac	0	+ + + +	0
fluvoxamine	Luvox	0	+ + + +	
paroxetine	Paxil	0	+ + + +	0
sertraline	Zoloft	0	+ + + +	0
escitalopram	Lexapro	0	+ + + +	0
Monoamine Oxidase Inhibitors				
phenelzine	Nardil			
Atypicals				
amoxapine	Asendin	+ + +	+ + +	0
bupropion	Wellbutrin	+	0/+	+
maprotiline	Ludiomil	+ + + +	0	0
mirtazapine	Remeron	+	+ + + + +	0
nefazodone	Serzone	0/+	+ + +	0
trazodone	Desyrel	0	+ +	0
venlafaxine	Effexor	+ + + +	+ + + +	0/+

NE, norepinephrine; 5-HT, 5-hydroxytryptamine (serotonin); D, dopamine; + + + +, highly potent effect; +, minimally potent effect; 0, no effect.

Table 44.2

Overview of Antidepressant Agents

Generic (Trade) Name and Dosage	Selected Adverse Events	Contraindications	Special Considerations
Tricyclic Antidepressants			
amitriptyline (Elavil) Start: 25 mg tid Range: 50–300 mg	Sedation, dry mouth	History of cardiovascular disease	Therapeutic plasma concentration range: 60–200 ng/mL
amoxapine (Asendin) Start: 50 mg tid Range: 100–600 mg	Anticholinergic, sedation	History of epilepsy or cardiac dysfunction	Therapeutic plasma concentration range: 180–600 ng/mL
clomipramine (Anafranil) Start: 25 mg hs Range: 150–200 mg	Sedation, orthostatic hypotension	History of cardiovascular disease	Blood levels not used clinically
desipramine (Norpramin) Start: 25 mg tid Range: 50–300 mg	Sedation, dry mouth	Same as above	Therapeutic plasma concentration range: 125–250 ng/mL
doxepin (Sinequan) Start: 25 mg tid Range: 75–300 mg	Sedation, orthostatic hypotension	Same as above	Therapeutic plasma concentration range: 110–250 ng/mL
imipramine (Tofranil) Start: 25 mg tid Range: 50–300 mg	Sedation, orthostatic hypotension	Risk of falling, history of cardiovascular disease	Therapeutic plasma concentration: 180 ng/mL
maprotiline (Ludiomil) Start: 25 mg tid Range: 50–300 mg	Anticholinergic, sedation, seizures	History of epilepsy or cardiac dysfunction	Therapeutic plasma concentration range: 200–400 ng/mL
nortriptyline (Pamelor) Start: 25 mg tid Range: 50–200 mg	Sedation	History of cardiovascular disease	Therapeutic plasma concentration range: 50–150 ng/mL
protriptyline (Vivactil) Start: 5 mg tid Range: 15–60 mg	Sedation, orthostatic hypotension	Same as above	Therapeutic plasma concentration range: 100–200 ng/mL
trimipramine (Surmontil) Start: 25 mg tid Range: 15–90 mg	Sedation, cardiac conduction disturbances	Same as above	
Selective Serotonin Reuptake Inhibitors			
citolapram (Celexa) Start: 20 mg qd Range: 20–40 mg qd	Nausea, dry mouth, increased sweating, somnolence, insomnia	MAOI therapy	In trials, approximately 6% of men experienced difficulty with ejaculation, and 3% reported impotence.
fluoxetine (Prozac) Start: 10–20 mg each morning Range: 10–80 mg	Insomnia	Same as above	Take in morning to avoid insomnia.
fluvoxamine (Luvox) Start: 75 mg bid Range: 100–300 mg	Increases in blood pressure	Same as above	Monitor blood pressure.
paroxetine (Paxil) Start: 20 mg qd Range: 10–50 mg	Mild sedation	Same as above	May be useful in patients displaying insomnia as depressive symptom
sertraline (Zoloft) Start: 50 mg qd Range: 50–200 mg	Insomnia	Same as above	Take in morning to avoid insomnia. May be agitating.
escitalopram (Lexapro) Start: 10 mg qd Range: 10–20 mg qd	Nausea, diarrhea, increased sweating, somnolence, insomnia, fatigue	Same as above	Extensively metabolized in the liver. The dose for hepatic impairment is 10 mg qd.
Atypicals			
trazodone (Desyrel) Start: 50 mg tid Range: 50–600 mg	Orthostatic hypotension, priapism	Contraindicated in recovery phase of myocardial infarction	Therapeutic range: 800–1,600 ng/mL
venlafaxine (Effexor) Start: 25 mg tid or 37.5 mg bid Range: 75–375 mg	Increases in blood pressure	Do not use within 14 d of MAOI therapy	Monitor blood pressure closely. Tachycardia and hypotension above 200 mg/day may occur.

often a reason cited by patients for prematurely stopping their antidepressants (Breen, Rupert, & McCormac, 2002). The true incidence of sexual dysfunction remains undetermined and may vary from agent to agent. The manifestation is delayed or absent orgasm in both men and women, along with loss of libido. This side effect must be communicated to the patient prior to starting therapy. Treatment of this dysfunction is available, but lowering the dose, without compromising efficacy, may be the first strategy. If the symptoms persist, cyproheptadine (Periactin), amantadine (Symmetrel),

Table 44.3

Selected Antidepressant Drug Interactions Involving the Cytochrome P450 System

Agent-Drug Interaction Potential	Isozyme Inhibited	Drugs Affected
Addition of this agent . . .	will inhibit this isoenzyme . . .	resulting in increased levels of these drugs
fluoxetine—moderate mirtazapine—low nefazodone—high paroxetine—low sertraline—low venlafaxine—low	3A4	Type 1A antiarrhythmics Clozapine Benzodiazepines (alprazolam, triazolam, clonazepam) Calcium channel blockers Cannabinoids Carbamazepine Cyclosporine Estrogens Fentanyl HIV-1 protease inhibitors HMG-CoA reductase inhibitors Macrolide antibiotics Ondansetron Tricyclic antidepressants (amitriptyline, clomipramine, imipramine) R-warfarin Zolpidem
fluoxetine—high mirtazapine—low paroxetine—high sertraline—low venlafaxine—low	2D6	Narcotic analgesics Chlorpromazine Fluphenazine Haloperidol Perphenazine Risperidone Beta blockers (labetalol, metoprolol, pindolol, propranolol, timolol) Benztropine Cyclobenzaprine Dextromethorphan Donepezil Glimepiride Trazodone Tricyclic antidepressants
fluoxetine—low fluvoxamine—high mirtazapine—low nefazodone—low paroxetine—low sertraline—low venlafaxine—low	1A2	Clozapine Haloperidol Thioridazine Olanzapine Chlorpromazine Trifluoperazine Caffeine Diazepam Metoclopramide Ondansetron Propranolol Tacrine Theophylline Tricyclic antidepressants (amitryptyline, clomipramine, imipramine) Verapamil Warfarin Zolpidem

and yohimbine (Yohimex) may benefit some patients. In addition, sildenafil (Viagra), tadalafil (Cialis), or vardenafil (Levitra) may benefit some male patients who suffer from this sexual side effect.

Interactions

The selection of an SSRI for an individual patient is determined by the drug interaction profile. The SSRIs inhibit various components of the cytochrome P-450 system, thus causing elevations in other medications that are metabolized by this system (Breen & McCormac, 2002). Before prescribing an SSRI, the practitioner must take a thorough medication history and identify the potential for altering the pharmacokinetics or pharmacodynamics of medications that the patient will be taking concomitantly (Table 44-3 offers a guide to the major drug–drug interactions with the common SSRIs).

Of special note, SSRIs are contraindicated with MAOIs because the combination can lead to a sudden buildup of serotonin systemically. This results because the MAOIs inhibit the metabolism of serotonin (thereby increasing its circulating availability) and the SSRIs raise the level of serotonin at the synapse. The manifestation of excessive serotonin, which is potentially life-threatening, is termed *serotonin syndrome*. Signs and symptoms include heat stroke, vascular collapse, fever, and tachycardia.

Tricyclic Antidepressants

Prior to the emergence of the SSRIs, the TCAs were the mainstay of therapy for years. There are no proven significant

Table 44.4

Major Adverse Event Profile of Antidepressant Agents

Drug	Anticholinergic	Cardiac Conduction	Seizures	Orthostatic Hypotension	Sedation
Selective Serotonin Reuptake Inhibitors					
citalopram	0	0	+	0	0
fluoxetine	0	0	++	0	0
fluvoxamine	0	0	++	0	0
paroxetine	+	0	++	0	+
sertraline	0	0	++	0	0
escitalopram	0	0	++	0	0
Tricyclic Antidepressants					
amitriptyline	++++	+++	+++	+++	++++
desipramine	++	++	++	++	++
doxepin	+++	++	+++	++	+++
imipramine	+++	+++	+++	++++	+++
nortriptyline	++	++	++	+	++
protriptyline	++	+++	++	++	+
trimipramine	++++	+++	+++	+++	++++
Monoamine Oxidase Inhibitors					
phenelzine	++	+	++	++	++
tranylcypromine	++	+	++	++	++
Atypical Antidepressants					
amoxapine	+++	++	+++	++	+++
bupropion	+	+	++++	0	++++
maprotiline	+++	++	++++	+++	++++
mirtazapine	++	+	+	++++	+
nefazodone	0	+	++	+++	++
trazodone	0	+	++	++++	++
venlafaxine	+	+	++	+	++

++++ = highly potent effect; + = minimal effect; 0 = no effect.

differences in terms of efficacy between the TCAs and the SSRIs (Mulrow, Williams, & Chiquette, 2000). TCAs are potent inhibitors of the reuptake of norepinephrine and exert fewer effects on serotonin. Clomipramine (Anafranil) is a potent serotonin reuptake blocker, and its metabolite is a potent norepinephrine reuptake blocker (see Table 44-2). Amitriptyline (Elavil), for example, significantly increases the amount of norepinephrine and serotonin available to the postsynaptic neuron. In contrast, nortriptyline (Pamelor) has a relatively low effect on both norepinephrine and serotonin. These agents, therefore, attempt to restore the balance of neurotransmitters and work in accord with several of the aforementioned theories.

The TCAs are also active at acetylcholine and histamine receptors, which contributes to their side effect profile. This complex pharmacology, coupled with the cholinergic side effects, makes the TCAs a second-line choice for treating depression.

Adverse Events

The selection of a TCA for treating depression is based on the side effect profile (Table 44-4) along with successful treatment in patients who received TCAs in the past. In varying degrees, all TCAs can cause sedation, which is an important consideration, especially if the depression is characterized by insomnia. Administering a TCA at bedtime may help alleviate this symptom.

In addition, the hypotensive effect of each agent varies and should be considered when selecting a particular agent. For example, nortriptyline and desipramine (Norpramin) have less potential for inducing orthostatic hypotension, making them advantageous in elderly patients. Moreover, the epileptogenic potential and life-threatening cardiac conduction abnormalities associated with various agents must be considered when selecting a TCA for a given patient. Preexisting epilepsy and cardiac conduction abnormalities are often considered contraindications to the use of TCAs.

Therapeutic Ranges

Because the pharmacokinetic properties of the individual agents may vary according to the patient and few of the TCAs have established therapeutic ranges, routine monitoring of drug levels is not common. However, establishing the drug level at which a patient has improved is reasonable. In this way, the practitioner has documentation of an effective drug concentration for that patient. Later, if needed, changes in drug therapy may be determined based on this baseline information. Otherwise, drug levels should be evaluated only if the practitioner suspects that the patient is not adhering to therapy or if drug toxicity becomes a concern.

Interactions

Drug interactions with the TCAs tend to be pharmacodynamic, although some pharmacokinetic interactions do occur. Pharmacokinetically, TCA drug levels may increase in combination with certain SSRIs (see Table 44-3) and other cytochrome P450 enzyme inhibitors, such as cimetidine

BOX 44–4. FOODS WITH HIGH TYRAMINE CONTENT

- Aged cheese (Cheddar, blue, Gouda, Swiss)
- Yeast products
- Aged meats, processed meats, nonfresh meat
- Beef liver or chicken liver
- Sauerkraut
- Licorice
- Tap beer

(Tagamet), HIV protease inhibitors, and some antipsychotic agents. There are additive central nervous system effects with TCAs and anticholinergic drugs, such as diphenhydramine (Benadryl). In addition, TCA–MAOI interactions may significantly increase the level of circulating catecholamines and lead to a potentially fatal hypertensive crisis.

Monoamine Oxidase Inhibitors

The MAOIs were the first effective medications that were developed for the treatment of depression. They work by nonspecifically and irreversibly inhibiting type A and type B monoamine oxidases, leading to a decreased degradation of norepinephrine, serotonin, and dopamine in the synapse. However, the side effect profile and potential for life-threatening hypertensive crises have limited there use and relegated it a last-line treatment in clinical practice. Only skilled practitioners with extensive clinical expertise should prescribe MAOIs. See Table 44-2 for starting dosages and dosage ranges.

Adverse Events

Adverse reactions to the MAOIs are more common than any other class of antidepressant. Orthostatic hypotension occurring with high-dose therapy is probably the most common side effect. Attempts at preventing this reaction by applying support stockings, prescribing stimulants such as methylphenidate (Ritalin; 10 to 15 mg/d), or adding the mineralocorticoid fludrocortisone (Florinef; 0.025 to 0.05 mg/d) have met with reasonable success. However, caution must be used and the patient must be monitored carefully, especially when receiving the corticoid or the stimulant drug concomitantly. Hypertensive crisis can occur when MAOIs are taken with medications that stimulate excessive release of the neurotransmitters dopamine, epinephrine, and norepinephrine. In addition, patients taking MAOIs must be on a strict diet that eliminates tyramine-containing foods. Box 44-4 identifies certain foods that have an extremely high tyramine content and if ingested by patients taking MAOIs may cause a hypertensive crisis.

Concomitant use of TCAs and MAOIs can lead to a hyperpyretic crisis resulting in seizures and death. Similarly, using SSRIs and MAOIs together can lead to a serotonergic syndrome. Carefully monitored, these agents can be used together safely, but they should be prescribed and monitored only by experienced clinicians.

Atypical Antidepressants

The class of drugs labeled *atypical* represents agents used to treat depression that elude traditional classification. These agents are generally considered alternatives to the SSRIs or TCAs. The clinician decides which agent to use by assessing their side effect profile and specific effect on neurotransmitters. See Table 44-2 for starting dosages and dosage ranges.

Bupropion

The mechanism of action of bupropion (Wellbutrin) is poorly understood, but the drug is thought to affect norepinephrine reuptake primarily. Bupropion has mild dopaminergic effects and does not inhibit MAO. It is also used to treat sexual dysfunction and aid in smoking cessation.

Anticholinergic side effects, such as dry mouth, constipation, and visual disturbances, make this agent an alternative to SSRIs or TCAs. However, these side effects may be advantageous in select patients. There are several reports of seizure activity with bupropion, especially when daily doses exceed 450 mg or single doses exceed 150 mg. However, the incidence of seizures is lower with the new sustained-release preparation.

Trazodone

Trazodone (Desyrel) is a weak serotonin receptor antagonist that also blocks serotonin reuptake, though to a lesser degree. The agent is highly sedating in therapeutic doses, which limits its clinical use. Trazodone is used for treating insomnia associated with depression or drug use (eg, SSRIs), and it is known for its anxiolytic properties. Other side effects include orthostatic hypotension and priapism.

Nefazodone

Nefazodone (Serzone), structurally related to trazodone, acts similarly to trazodone but also inhibits the reuptake of norepinephrine and produces fewer side effects. Because it lacks significant anticholinergic and antihistamine effects, reports of blurred vision, urinary retention, and weight gain are relatively infrequent. Nefazodone interferes with the cytochrome P450 3A4 subsystem, and caution should be used in patients taking drugs metabolized by this enzyme system. In addition, nefazodone increases the levels of agents such as alprazolam (Xanax) and triazolam (Halcion); practitioners should avoid prescribing these agents concomitantly (see Table 44-3). Prior to initiating nefazodone, the washout period after discontinuing an SSRI should generally be 4 to 5 days for paroxetine (Paxil) and sertraline (Zoloft) and several weeks for fluoxetine (Prozac).

Venlafaxine

Venlafaxine (Effexor) and its active metabolite O-desmethylvenlafaxine blocks both norepinephrine and serotonin in clinically significant dosages, making this agent similar to the TCAs but without the anticholinergic side effects. Two dose-related side effects occur with venlafaxine: nausea and hypertension. Starting therapy with lower doses and gradually increasing the dose as tolerated minimizes the nausea. Patients need to be monitored for increases in diastolic blood pressure and should take multiple daily doses because of the medication's short half-life. The dosage should also be adjusted by 25% to 50% for patients with impaired renal or hepatic function.

Mirtazapine

Mirtazapine (Remeron) is a selective alpha$_2$-adrenergic receptor antagonist affecting both the norepinephrine and serotonergic systems. The role of mirtazapine in treating depression is similar to that of the TCAs. It has significant histamine-1 receptor blocking activity, thus causing sedation. In addition, because of its appetite stimulation, it may be a good choice for low-weight elderly or ill patients.

This agent may be useful in combination therapy because there have been no reports of drug interactions. However, there have been rare cases of reversible agranulocytosis.

Selecting the Most Appropriate Agent

A patient's past experience with antidepressant medications and current preferences should weigh heavily in the decision regarding the choice of initial drug. Past response tends to predict future response. Another consideration is the patient's perception about the efficacy and side effects she, he, or a family member has experienced. A negative perception of a drug may suggest potential for lack of adherence to drug therapy or an erosion of confidence in the therapy. If negative previous experience or intolerance to a medication is apparent, an alternative agent should be chosen.

First-Line Therapy

The SSRIs are accepted as the most common first-line agents. In selecting an SSRI, the practitioner must first understand the patient's target symptoms and the potentially interacting drugs he or she is taking. If insomnia is problematic in the patient, paroxetine (Paxil) may be the best choice. If the patient is taking drugs metabolized by the cytochrome P450 3A4 subsystem, then avoiding fluoxetine (Prozac) is wise. See Fig. 44-2 and Table 44-5 for an overview of treating a patient with depression.

The practitioner must also recognize the implications of the patient's economic and insurance status. Many managed care organizations have selected only one or two SSRIs as their formulary product. Occasionally, the prescriber must obtain prior authorization for a particular product if it is not on the formulary. In addition, if the product is not on the formulary, the patient often must pay a higher co-payment.

Second-Line Therapy

Patients failing to respond adequately to first-line treatments should be switched to an alternative antidepressant agent. Because most patients begin antidepressant therapy with an SSRI, an alternative agent should be considered. The options include an agent from the TCA or atypical class. The defini-

tive selection should include an assessment of the patient's underlying cardiac, neurologic, and comorbid conditions. For example, venlafaxine should be avoided in patients with uncontrolled hypertension because of its potential to increase blood pressure. Similarly, for an elderly man with a history of benign prostatic hyperplasia, TCAs and atypical agents with significant anticholinergic activity should be avoided because this action aggravates the condition.

Third-Line Therapy

If the first- and second-line agents fail, the clinician can try an agent from one of the remaining classes. Again, patient-specific indicators help the clinician decide on the next treatment regimen. For the most part, inexperienced general practitioners should not prescribe MAOIs. The side effects and the potential for dangerous drug and food interactions suggest that only clinicians well versed in managing this kind of therapy prescribe these agents.

Special Population Considerations

Children and Adolescents

The risk for underdiagnosis and undertreatment is extremely prevalent in this patient population. Children of parents who have been diagnosed with serious depression are at risk for developing anxiety and major depressive disorders in childhood (Ainsworth, 2000). Early childhood depression may manifest as acting out, changes in eating or sleeping patterns, or social withdrawal. These patients can seldom communicate a feeling of sadness because of the early language development level. From ages 5 through 8 years, low self-esteem, underachievement at school, and aggressive or antisocial behaviors (including stealing and lying) may indicate depression.

Approximately 4% of adolescents experience depression in a given year (Ainsworth, 2000). Depressed adolescents experience symptoms similar to depressed adults such as sleep disturbances, irritability, difficulty concentrating, and loss of energy.

Currently, fluoxetine (Prozac) is the only SSRI approved by the FDA for the treatment of depression in children 8 and up. Caution has been recommended in using other agents, such as paroxetine (Paxil) or venlafaxine (Effexor), with depressed children and adolescents. Compared to adults, adolescents are more likely to become agitated or to develop a mania while they are taking an SSRI. The FDA has issued a black-box warning due to increased risk of suicide in children and adolescents taking SSRIs.

Geriatrics

Geriatric patients often have significant changes in physiologic function, including reduced renal and hepatic function, decreased muscle mass, decreased serum albumin, and dietary alterations. These changes may affect the absorption, distribution, metabolism, and excretion of a variety of drugs, particularly antidepressants. Most practitioners agree that antidepressant therapy should be prescribed at one-third to one-half the usual starting adult dosage.

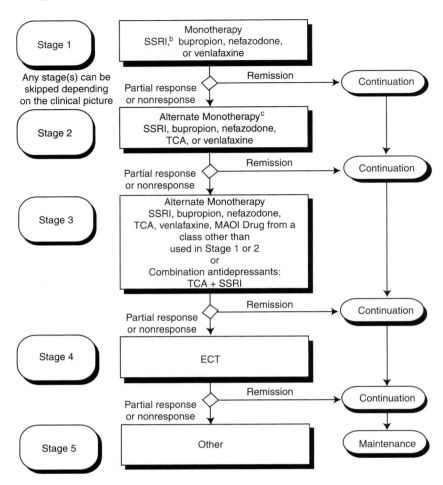

^aAdapted from Crismon et al. ⁹ The TMAP algorithms are in the public domain, and this figure may be reproduced without permission, but with the appropriate citation.
Abbreviations: EC = electroconvulsive therapy, MAOI = monoamine oxidase inhibitor, SSRI = selective serotonin reuptake inhibitor, TCA = tricyclic antidepressant.
^b SSRIs preferred.
^c Consider TCA or venlafaxine if not tried.

Figure 44–2 Texas Medication Algorithm Project (TMAP): Major depressive disorder without psychotic features.^a

Table 44.5

Recommended Order of Treatment in Antidepressant Therapy

Order	Agents	Comments
First line	SSRIs	Fluoxetine and sertraline may be good for patients with somnolence.
		Paroxetine may be good for patients with insomnia.
		Selection of agent should be based on patient's past experiences with medications and drug interactions.
		Cost may be a consideration.
Second line	TCA (desipramine or nortriptyline) or atypical antidepressant	These agents have the better side effect profile of the class and should be considered as agents of choice for the TCA class.
Third line	Atypical antidepressant or TCA	Depending on past response to other agents and side effect profile.

Late-onset depression commonly occurs in elderly patients, with nursing home residents nearly three times more likely to be depressed than the general population. These patients may also have an underlying neurologic or vascular disorder. Determining the root of the depression is essential to resolution.

Women

As noted earlier, younger women are more likely to experience depression than older women or men in general. Women of childbearing age are at the greatest risk. The decision to initiate antidepressant medication in a pregnant woman is a difficult one, and the risk of fetal exposure to the drug must be balanced against the risk of continued depression.

Postpartum depression is especially prevalent in women with a history of depression and a previous episode of postpartum depression. The risk is increased with concomitant marital problems, lack of social support, and medical issues with newborn children. The decision about which agent to use depends on the factors previously discussed as well as on the issue of breast-feeding and the risk of transmission of drugs through breast milk.

Ethnic

There are genetic variations in the metabolism of drugs in patients with varying ethnicity. The CYP450 2D6 enzyme system, responsible for the metabolism of many psychotherapeutic agents, is influenced by age, gender, and ethnicity. Up to 10% of Caucasians and nearly 19% of African Americans are consider "poor metabolizers" of drugs via the CYP450 2D6 system. Similarly, 33% of African Americans and 37% of Asians are poor metabolizers of drugs metabolized by the CYP450 2C19 system. The result of this poor metabolism can include quicker responses to drugs, greater than expected action of the agent, or even more pronounced side effects. As more data accrue on the effects of genetics on depression and cytochrome P450 metabolism, the effects of race and ethnicity on treating depression and selecting antidepressants will play a more prominent role.

MONITORING PATIENT RESPONSE

Drug therapy for depression can be divided into three phases: acute, continuation, and maintenance. Usually the patient needs additional contact with the practitioner or other health care provider (psychologist, social worker) during all phases of drug therapy. Assessments of efficacy, side effects, and adherence to the drug regimen should be made weekly, if possible.

Acute Treatment Phase

Drug therapy in the acute treatment phase relieves the depressive symptoms to the point of remission. The duration of this phase is 6 to 8 weeks, with apparent improvements occurring within the first 1 to 2 weeks. Patients should have frequent contact with their practitioner in the first stages of treatment, either by telephone or in person. If the full antidepressant effect does not occur for 4 to 6 weeks, earlier contact gives the patient validation that the practitioner cares about his or her well-being. In addition, earlier contact helps the practitioner identify side effects that may hamper a patient's adherence to the prescribed drug regimen.

Full assessment of the effects of the antidepressant should occur at the 4- to 6-week interval after drug therapy begins. At this point, the practitioner evaluates improvements in the target signs and symptoms, assesses adverse drug effects, and determines whether dosage increases or decreases are necessary. To assist the evaluation, several depression rating scales, such as the HAM-D, the Zung Self-Rating Scale for Depression, and the Beck Depression Inventory, may again be used as an objective measure of the change, or lack thereof, in a depressive state. The practitioner can use one or more of these scales routinely in diagnosing and treating depression, although this is not always feasible in the primary care setting.

Continuation Phase

The continuation phase represents the time after a treatment response is seen in the acute phase and usually lasts

> ## BOX 44–5. WARNING SIGNS OF SUICIDAL IDEATION
>
> - Pacing, agitated behavior, frequent mood changes, and chronic episodes of sleeplessness
> - Actions or threats of assault, physical harm, or violence
> - Delusions or hallucinations
> - Threats or talk of death (eg, "I don't care anymore," or "You won't have to worry about me much longer.")
> - Putting affairs in order, such as giving possessions away or writing a new will
> - Unusually risky behavior (eg, unsafe driving, abuse of alcohol or other drugs)

9 months to 1 year. The practitioner should continue antidepressant therapy for 4 to 6 months after symptoms have resolved. When therapy is to be discontinued, the practitioner advises the patient to taper the medication over 2 to 3 weeks to minimize the physical or psychological effects that occur with abrupt discontinuation of the medication. During this time, the patient should be monitored closely for resurgence of symptoms.

Maintenance Phase

For some patients, long-term therapy is indicated. Maintenance therapy should be considered in all patients with three or more prior episodes or any patient with two episodes within the past 5 years, a comorbid substance abuse or anxiety disorder, a family history of recurrent depression, or onset of depression earlier than 20 or later than 40 years of age. This phase of therapy uses the same effective antidepressant used during the acute and continuation phases for a minimum of 3 and up to 5 years or longer.

Elderly patients who had one episode of depression and those who had two or more previous episodes of depression have a risk of relapse of more than 80.5% (Breen, Rupert, & McCormac, 2002). These patients should receive antidepressant therapy indefinitely.

Emergencies

Suicide is the most feared consequence of inadequately treated (or unrecognized) depression. Up to two thirds of depressed patients have suicidal ideation, and 10% to 15% actually commit suicide (Box 44-5). The practitioner should be ever-vigilant for suicidal ideation and the potential for suicide. This is another reason for frequent contact between the practitioner and the patient. If the patient discloses thoughts of suicide, the practitioner and patient need to develop a plan for psychiatric referral or hospitalization. Contracting with the patient, such as by developing a written agreement to continue treatment without doing self-harm, may also be an effective means for minimizing the risk for suicide. All plans and actions should be documented in the patient's medical record.

PATIENT EDUCATION

Patients and caregivers should be instructed on the full range of issues surrounding depression and antidepressant therapy. Patients should be assured that depression is a biologic illness that occurs in a variety of people, and they should not feel ashamed of the disease. Moreover, the caregivers or significant others should also be counseled on the role they play in aiding in the patient's recovery. The more informed patients and significant others are of the illness, the more likely they will adhere to recommendations.

Expectations for a quick recovery can be detrimental to the healing process. Patients and caregivers should be informed that the antidepressant medication takes several (4 to 6) weeks to begin working and the patient might be required to continue taking the medication.

Teaching patients to recognize early signs and symptoms of behavior that may indicate a recurrence is crucial. Patients and family members should be instructed to contact the clinician if symptoms resume. A support group may also be a good resource for family and patients as a strategy for managing the illness.

Antidepressants and Suicide

Depression is a risk factor in patients with suicidal ideation, and up to 80% of depressed patients experience suicidal impulses. Since 1990, whether antidepressant drugs are linked to suicide has been an acrimonious debate. Some argue that depressed adolescents who are suicidal and treated with antidepressants may regain initiative and energy before improvement in cognition and mood, thereby becoming mobilized to attempt suicide (Matthews & Fava, 2000). Others argue that the medication prescribed to treat depression is responsible for causing adolescents to attempt suicide. In 2003, British drug regulators warned that the SSRIs, with the exception of fluoxetine, were unsuitable in minors experiencing depression. As a result, the FDA began public hearings in February 2004 to discuss this controversy. Currently, fluoxetine (Prozac) is the only FDA-approved antidepressant in patients 18 years and younger. However, other SSRIs such as sertraline (Zoloft), venlafaxine (Effexor), and paroxetine (Paxil) have been widely prescribed for adolescent depression. Until these hearings and more studies are concluded, the FDA has issued a warning to physicians to use extreme caution in prescribing SSRIs to patients less than 18 years of age.

Patient Information

The National Foundation for Depressive Illness, Inc. (NAFDI) (http://www.depression.org) was established in 1983 to educate the public and health care professionals about depression. This website contains useful information on the signs and symptoms of depression and provides public awareness on depression through a national "800" number.

The National Institute of Mental Health's website (http://www.nimh.nih.gov/publicat/depressionmenus.cfm),

also available in Spanish, is an excellent resource for depression. It describes the different types of depression along with the causes and treatments. This website also offers valuable information on how family and friends may contribute and assist in therapy.

The National Mental Health Association (NMHA) (http://www.nmha.org) is a nonprofit organization that provides beneficial information to the public and practitioners on mental illness. This website contains news releases along with an online bookstore. A calendar notes coming events relating to mental health. This website provides access to comprehensive mental health care and increases public awareness of mental health issues.

The Depression and Bipolar Support Alliance (DBSA) (http://www.dbsalliance.org) is a nonprofit organization that provides a wide range of information and support on depression and bipolar disorders. Their mission, as stated on the website, is to improve the lives of those affected by depression and bipolar disorder. The DBSA is a patient-directed national organization focusing on the most prevalent mental illnesses, with a network of approximately 1,000 support groups. This website is updated regularly to provide up-to-date, scientifically based information. The DBSA is guided by a scientific advisory board comprising researchers and clinicians in the field of mood disorders.

Complementary and Alternative Medications

The use of herbal products in the United States has dramatically increased in the past decade, resulting in consumer sales of $9 billion in 1999. Approximately $200 million was spent on the purchase of St. John's wort alone. The FDA does not classify herbal products as drugs, and as such they are not regulated under the same scrutiny as other medications.

St. John's wort (*Hypericum perforatum*) has been used for centuries for a variety of illnesses, but it is currently used almost exclusively as an herbal antidepressant. Most clinical trials have studied 900 mg/day of standardized extract (usually standardized to 0.3% hypericin content) divided in three daily doses. The clinical effect is usually seen within 2 to 3 weeks of initiating therapy (Ernst, 2002). The mechanism of action is unknown, although it is theorized that it inhibits MAO and the synaptosomal uptake of serotonin, dopamine, and noradrenaline (Butterweck, 2003).

St. John's wort appears to be well tolerated, with the most frequent side effects reported as nausea, fatigue, restlessness, rash, and photosensitivity. There have been reported cases of increase in heart rate, but no significant effect was seen on the PR interval (Gupta & Moller, 2003).

St. John's wort may activate hepatic cytochrome P450, so it has the potential to interact with medication that is metabolized by the P450 system. Therefore, it has been reported that St. John's wort decreases serum levels of theophylline, cyclosporine, warfarin, oral contraceptives, and indinavir. St. John's wort should not be taken in combination with any other antidepressant because of the risk of serotonin syndrome, especially in the elderly. Symptoms include changes in mental status, tremor, gastrointestinal disturbances, myalgia, restlessness, and headache.

■ Case Study

L.B. is a 55-year-old white female who presents to her family physician's office for a yearly routine physical. Her husband passed away 5 months ago after a 2-year battle with lung cancer. She has three children, two of whom are still in college. Her daughter accompanies her to the doctor's office and says she is concerned about her mother's recent behavior. She explains that her mother has been "sleeping all the time" and has lost 25 lb in the past 2 months without being on a diet. When the doctor examines L.B., she explains that she has become increasingly fatigued and "I have absolutely no energy." She no longer has any desire to participate in her lifelong hobbies of painting and photography because of frequent feelings of sadness. L.B.'s medical history is significant for hypothyroidism, hypercholesterolemia, and recently diagnosed hypertension. Her medications are levothyroxine (Synthroid) 0.075 mg daily, simvastatin (Zocor) 20 mg daily, hydrochlorothiazide (HydroDIURIL) 25 mg daily, lisinopril (Zestril) 10 mg daily, multivitamins 1 tab daily, and aspirin 81 mg daily.

Diagnosis: Major depression

1. What are reasonable treatment goals for L.B.? How would you incorporate her activities of daily living into these goals?

2. What medications and disease states may be contributing to L.B.'s depression?

3. What would be the first agent you would consider prescribing for L.B.? What considerations did you take into account when making this choice?

4. How would you monitor for improvement in L.B., and in what time frame would you expect to see these improvements?

5. What are some adverse reactions that may occur in L.B. based on your selection? Which of these would cause you or L.B. to stop the therapy?

6. If the initial drug therapy failed or L.B. chose to stop therapy, what would be your choice for second-line therapy?

7. L.B. asks you if she should take St. John's wort. How do you respond?

8. How would you monitor for suicidal tendencies in this patient?

9. Describe one or two drug/drug or drug/food interactions for the selected agent.

Bibliography

Starred items are cited in text.

*Ainsworth, P. (2000). *Understanding depression.* (Understanding Health and Sickness Series). Jackson, MS: University Press of Mississippi.

*Breen, R., & McCormac, R. J. (2002). A fresh look at management of depression. How to choose and use the newer antidepressant drugs. *Postgraduate Medicine, 112*(3), 28–40.

*Butterweck, V. (2003). Mechanism of action of St. John's Wort in depression. *CNS Drugs, 17*(8), 539–562.

*Ernst, E. (2002). The risk-benefit profile of commonly used herbal therapies: Gingko, St. John's wort, Ginseng, Echinacea, Saw Palmetto, and Kava. *Annals of Internal Medicine, 136*(1), 42–53.

*Evins, G. G., Theofrastous, J. P., & Galvin, S. L. (2000). Postpartum depression: A comparison of screening and routine clinical evaluation. *American Journal of Obstetrics & Gynecology, 182*(5), 1080–1082.

*Gupta, R. K., & Moller, H. J. (2003). St. John's wort. An option for the primary care treatment of depressive patients? *European Archives of Psychiatry & Clinical Neuroscience, 253*(3), 140–148.

*Hamilton, M. (1967). Development of a rating scale for primary depressive illness. *British Journal of Social and Clinical Psychology, 6,* 278–296.

Harris, P. A. (2004). The impact of age, gender, race and ethnicity on the diagnosis and treatment of depression. *Journal of Managed Care Pharmacy, 10*(2, Suppl S-a), S2–S7.

*Matthews, J. D., & Fava, M. (2000). Risk of suicidality in depression with serotonergic antidepressants. *Annals of Clinical Psychiatry, 12*(1), 43–50.

Miller, L. J. (2002). Postpartum depression. *JAMA, 287*(6), 762–765.

*Mulrow, C. D., Williams, J. W. Jr., Chiquette, E., Aguilar, C., Hitchcock-Noel, P., Lee, S., Cornell, J., & Stamm, K. (2000). Efficacy of newer medications for treating depression in primary care patients. *American Journal of Medicine, 108*(1), 54–64.

*Snow, V., Lascher, S., & Mottur-Pilson, C. (2000). Pharmacologic treatment of acute major depression and dysthymia. *Annals of Internal Medicine, 132*(9), 738–742.

*Yesavage, J. A. (1988). Geriatric depression scale. *Psychopharmacology Bulletin, 24,* 709–711.

*Young, S. A., Campbell, N., & Harper, A. (2002). Depression in women of reproductive age. Considerations in selecting safe, effective therapy. *Postgraduate Medicine, 112*(3), 45–50.

Visit the Connection web site for the most up-to-date drug information.

45

ANXIETY

■ ANNE DELLAIRA

Anxiety is defined as a vague, uneasy feeling with a source that often is nonspecific. People with anxiety frequently experience feelings of increased tension, apprehension, fear, restlessness, and worry along with physical symptoms such as increased heart rate, pupil dilation, trembling, and increased perspiration. With 14 different types, the anxiety disorders represent the largest group of psychiatric disorders (Table 45-1). The disorders discussed in this chapter are generalized anxiety disorder (GAD), panic disorder (PD), and obsessive-compulsive disorder (OCD). Anxiety often goes untreated in both children and adults, but millions of people seek help for what is broadly construed as anxiety or nervousness.

Approximately 25% of the U. S. population experiences pathologic anxiety during their lifetime. Epidemiologic studies report that 2% to 6% of adults have GAD. Approximately 1% of all patients have PD with resulting significant impairment, and 4% to 5% have agoraphobia. Approximately 12% of patients seen in anxiety disorder clinics present with GAD. OCD has a lifetime prevalence of 2.5%; it was once thought to be a rare disorder, but it is now known to be twice as common as schizophrenia or PD in the general population.

Anxiety disorders most commonly begin in early adulthood. They tend to be chronic, with interspersed periods of remissions and relapses of varying degrees, and they frequently continue into old age. Late onset of an anxiety disorder is rare. In the elderly, anxiety disorders as a whole are the most common psychiatric disorders. It is unknown whether they are a continuation of an illness with an onset from a younger age or whether they appear for the first time in old age.

There is considerable variation in the expression of anxiety across cultures, so it is important to consider the patient's cultural context. Patients from one culture may express anxiety vocally and physically, while patients from a different culture may express anxiety with silence and withdrawal. Sex differences also exist; approximately two thirds of patients with anxiety are female, but this ratio varies across the different types of anxiety.

CAUSES

Physiologic Factors

Most patients with an anxiety disorder first come to the attention of primary health care providers. Although the etiology of anxiety disorders is largely unknown, a wide range of medical illnesses, such as cardiovascular disease, pulmonary disease, hyperthyroidism, hypothyroidism, hyperadrenocorticism, pheochromocytoma, hypoglycemia, vitamin B_{12} deficiency, and neurologic conditions, may cause symptoms of anxiety. In addition, alcohol, amphetamines, cannabis, caffeine, cocaine, hallucinogens, sedatives, hypnotics, phencyclidine, and inhalants may cause substance-induced anxiety.

Genetic Factors

A positive family history is seen frequently in people with anxiety disorders. Twin studies suggest that heredity accounts for 30% of the cases of various anxiety disorders; environmental factors seem to be responsible for the remaining cases. More than 50% of people with PD have relatives with the disorder. A twin study reported that anxiety disorder with panic attacks occurs five times more frequently in monozygotic twins than in heterozygotic twins. Reports estimate that 20% of patients who have OCD have a first-degree relative with OCD.

PATHOPHYSIOLOGY

Anxiety is a phenomenon that all people experience. One type of anxiety, fear, is a normal fight-or-flight response to an observable threat. In contrast, pathologic anxiety is a fight-or-flight response to an internal or external threat that is real or imagined and causes the person to experience an unpleasant emotional state. Walter B. Cannon (1963) was the first to describe the fight-or-flight response, which is associated with anxiety. During this response, the person's autonomic nervous system, which consists of the sympathetic and parasympathetic nervous systems, prepares the person to deal with a threat (Box 45-1).

A pediatric autoimmune neuropsychiatric disorder associated with the streptococcal (group A beta-hemolytic streptococcal) infections is referred to as PANDA. In 1998, Swedo and her group first reported on children who developed neurologic abnormalities following a streptococcal infection known as St. Vitus' dance. It was thought to be a rare complication. Swedo's group was the first to make the connection that this is a form of OCD caused by an immune response. Before treating a child for OCD, PANDA must be ruled out.

Table 45.1

Summary of Anxiety Disorders

Anxiety Disorder	Definition
Panic Attack	A discrete period, in which there is a sudden onset of intense apprehension, fearfulness, or terror, often associated with feelings of impending doom. During these attacks, symptoms such as shortness of breath, palpitations, chest pain or discomfort, choking or smothering sensations, and fear of "going crazy" or losing control are present.
Agoraphobia	Anxiety about, or avoidance of, places or situations from which escape might be difficult (or embarrassing) or in which help may not be available in the event of having a panic attack or panic-like symptoms.
Panic Disorder Without Agoraphobia	Recurrent unexpected panic attacks about which there is persistent concern.
Panic Disorder With Agoraphobia	Recurrent unexpected panic attacks and agoraphobia.
Agoraphobia Without History of Panic Disorder	Agoraphobia and panic-like symptoms without a history of unexpected panic attacks.
Specific Phobia	Clinically significant anxiety provoked by exposure to a specific feared object or situation, often leading to avoidance.
Social Phobia	Clinically significant anxiety provoked by exposure to certain types of social or performance situations, often leading to avoidance behavior.
Obsessive-Compulsive Disorder	Characterized by obsessions (which cause marked anxiety or distress) and/or by compulsions (which serve to neutralize anxiety).
Posttraumatic Stress Disorder	Characterized by the reexperiencing of an extremely traumatic event accompanied by symptoms of increased arousal and by avoidance of stimuli associated with the trauma.
Acute Stress Disorder	Characterized by symptoms similar to those of posttraumatic stress disorder that occur immediately in the aftermath of an extremely traumatic event.
Generalized Anxiety Disorder	Characterized by at least 6 months of persistent and excessive anxiety and worry.
Anxiety Disorder Due to a General Medical Condition	Characterized by prominent symptoms of anxiety that are judged to be a direct physiological consequence of a general medical condition.
Substance-Induced Anxiety Disorder	Characterized by prominent symptoms of anxiety that are judged to be a direct physiological consequence of a drug abuse, a medication, or toxin exposure.
Anxiety Disorder Not Otherwise Specified	Used for coding disorders with prominent anxiety or phobic avoidance that do not meet the criteria for any of the specific Anxiety Disorders defined in this list (or anxiety symptoms about which there is inadequate or contradictory information).

Source: American Psychiatric Association. (2000). *Diagnostic and statistical manual of mental disorders,* (4th ed., text revision). Washington, DC: Author, with permission.

BOX 45–1. PHYSIOLOGIC REACTIONS TO THE FIGHT-OR-FLIGHT RESPONSE

The fight-or-flight response causes the following:

1. Epinephrine, norepinephrine, and cortisol are released into the blood.
2. The liver releases stored sugar into the blood to meet energy needs.
3. Digestion slows, allowing blood to be shifted to the brain and the muscles.
4. Breathing becomes rapid to allow for greater oxygen supply to the muscles.
5. The heart rate and blood pressure increase.
6. Perspiration increases to cool the body.
7. Muscles tense in preparation for action.
8. The pupils dilate.
9. All senses become more acute.
10. Blood flow to the extremities becomes constricted to protect the body from bleeding from injury.

This response is appropriate for extremely threatening situations, but the response would cause considerable damage to the body if people responded to all stressful situations in this manner.

Response to Stress

The fight-or-flight response is associated with significant stress. In 1980, Hans Selye, the "father of stress research," developed a stress framework by which he defined stress as the rate of wear and tear on the body. Stressors may be physical, chemical, psychological, or developmental. The demands and challenges of life are stressful and are handled through adaptation to changes to limit damage. Selye (1991) proposed that although stress cannot be perceived, it can be measured by the chemical and structural changes produced in the body. Selye referred to these changes as the general adaptation syndrome (GAS), reflecting the entire body's need to adjust to the changes.

The GAS has three stages. First, the alarm reaction occurs when the person mobilizes the various defense mechanisms of the body or mind to cope with a stressful physical or emotional situations. The second stage, resistance, represents the opposite of the alarm reaction: the person stops feeling tense and anxious and may state that he or she has become used to the situation. Exhaustion, the third stage, occurs when the stress continues over a prolonged period or the person is exposed to multiple stressors simultaneously, thus leaving him or her too exhausted to maintain normal functioning.

Neurotransmitters

Norepinephrine, serotonin, and gamma-aminobutyric acid (GABA) are the major neurotransmitters studied in relation to the pharmacologic treatment of anxiety. People with anxiety disorders, especially PD, are found to have malfunctioning noradrenergic systems with a low threshold for arousal. This, coupled with an unpredictable increase in activity, causes the anxiety symptoms.

The role of serotonin was identified by observing people with OCD who had favorable responses when treated with antidepressant medications such as the selective serotonin reuptake inhibitors (SSRIs). Drugs that release serotonin can precipitate anxiety in people with an anxiety disorder; selective reduction of serotonin levels restores normal functioning.

GABA and its associated receptors function as central nervous system (CNS) inhibitors. Although psychopharmacologic interventions support this role, the exact pharmacology of GABA receptors is still being examined.

DIAGNOSTIC CRITERIA

Anxiety disorders most commonly begin in early adulthood, tend to be chronic with interspersed periods of remission and relapse of varying degrees, and frequently continue into old age. In children, anxiety may develop, particularly in relation to school, and late onset of an anxiety disorder is rare but can occur. In the elderly, anxiety disorders are the most common psychiatric disorders seen.

Before a patient can be diagnosed with an anxiety disorder, he or she should undergo a thorough medical workup to rule out medical disease, neurologic problems, current medications that may cause anxiety symptoms, vitamin B_{12} deficiency, and drug or alcohol misuse. The history should focus on anxiety disorders in family members, environmental factors, family dynamics, cognitive functioning, work or school situations, or exposure to chemical substances.

If the patient's anxiety is not linked to any of these possibilities, the practitioner should consult the American Psychiatric Association's *Diagnostic and Statistical Manual of Mental Disorders, IV, Text Revision* (2000) to review the diagnostic criteria before diagnosing a particular anxiety disorder. Box 45-2 lists criteria for diagnosing GAD; Box 45-3 lists the criteria for diagnosing PD; and Box 45-4 lists the criteria for diagnosing OCD.

Comorbidity with major depression or personality disorders is common in patients with anxiety. These patients may self-medicate with alcohol or other substances to relieve their symptoms.

INITIATING DRUG THERAPY

Many people with anxiety disorders are terrified of beginning treatment and worried about possible addiction to, and side effects of, the drugs used to treat these conditions. These people also worry about the social stigma associated with having a psychiatric condition. Both pharmacotherapy and psychotherapy may be necessary for satisfactory treatment of these disorders. Frequently, a patient's health insurance policy does not cover the psychiatric treatment that he or she needs.

Nonpharmacologic therapy includes several psychotherapeutic techniques such as supportive counseling, behavioral therapy, cognitive therapy, and psychoanalytic therapy. In the past, before drug therapy was widely available and effective

---

BOX 45–2. APA CRITERIA FOR DIAGNOSING GENERALIZED ANXIETY DISORDER

A. Excessive anxiety and worry (apprehensive expectation), occurring more days than not for at least 6 months, about a number of events or activities (such as work or school performance).
B. The person finds it difficult to control the worry.
C. The anxiety and worry are associated with three (or more) of the following six symptoms (with at least some symptoms present for more days than not for the past 6 months).
   Note: Only one item is required in children.
   1. Restlessness or feeling keyed up or on edge
   2. Being easily fatigued
   3. Difficulty concentrating or mind going blank
   4. Irritability
   5. Muscle tension
   6. Sleep disturbance (difficulty falling or staying asleep, or restless, unsatisfying sleep)
D. The focus of the anxiety and worry is not confined to features of an Axis I disorder, for example, the anxiety or worry is not about having a panic attack (as in Panic Disorder), being embarrassed in public (as in Social Phobia), being contaminated (as in Obsessive-Compulsive Disorder), being away from home or close relatives (as in Separation Anxiety Disorder), gaining weight (as in Anorexia Nervosa), having multiple physical complaints (as in Somatization Disorder), or having a serious illness (as in Hypochondriasis) and the anxiety and worry do not occur exclusively during Posttraumatic Stress Disorder.
E. The anxiety, worry, or physical symptoms cause clinically significant distress or impairment in social, occupational, or other important areas of functioning.
F. The disturbance is not due to the direct physiologic effects of a substance (eg, a drug of abuse, a medication) or general medical condition (eg, hyperthyroidism) and does not occur exclusively during a Mood Disorder, a Psychotic Disorder, or a Pervasive Development Disorder.

From the American Psychiatric Association. (2000). *Diagnostic and statistical manual of mental disorders* (4th ed., text revision). Washington, DC: Author, with permission.

---

for anxiety disorders, therapy consisted of psychoanalysis or behavioral or cognitive therapy, or a combination of these modalities. Today, in many cases, these therapies can be helpful and useful in conjunction with drug therapy. Therapeutic modalities may vary among the historic psychotherapies.

In the past, proponents of Freudian theory recommended psychoanalysis because they thought that anxiety was the

Goals of Drug Therapy

The goal of therapy is to reduce the patient's anxiety and any depressive symptoms, return the patient to a normal level of functioning with a minimum of side effects, and improve the patient's quality of life.

The primary use of sedative-hypnotic and anxiolytic drugs is to produce calmness or sleep. Many CNS depressants have some ability to relieve anxiety, but only at doses that produce noticeable sedation. Most anxiolytic and sedative-hypnotic drugs produce a dose-dependent depression of the CNS.

The ideal anxiolytic drug should calm the patient without causing too much daytime sedation and drowsiness and without producing physical or psychological dependence. Pharmacologic agents used in the treatment of anxiety disorders can be classified into the following categories: antidepressants, benzodiazepines (BZDs), azapirones, other antianxiety agents, and beta-adrenergic blockers.

Benzodiazepines

The BZDs are important and widely prescribed sedative-hypnotics. Their pharmacologic properties include reduction of anxiety, sedation, muscle relaxation, and anticonvulsant and amnestic effects. Among the prominent BZDs are alprazolam (Xanax), clonazepam (Klonopin), lorazepam (Ativan), oxazepam (Serax), diazepam (Valium), and chlordiazepoxide (Librium). They are best prescribed for motivated patients with acute exogenous anxiety to a time-limited stress.

Mechanism of Action

The BZDs exert a therapeutic effect by binding to GABA-A receptors in the brain. They cause the GABA-A receptors to increase the opening of chloride channels along the cell membrane, leading to an inhibitory effect on cell firing. Other neurotransmitters, such as serotonin and norepinephrine, may play a role in the therapeutic effect of the BZDs. The exact mechanism of the BZDs' antianxiety effect is not yet fully understood. Most of the drugs in this class possess anxiolytic, sedative-hypnotic, and anticonvulsant properties.

The BZDs can be used for treating GAD and PD. Approximately 75% of patients with GAD respond moderately or better to BZDs. At this time, there is no evidence that one BZD is superior to another for this disorder. The high-potency BZDs, alprazolam, clonazepam, and lorazepam, have been effective in controlling panic attacks and anticipatory anxiety in panic attacks. The clinical indications for a specific BZD are not absolute, and considerable overlap in their use exists. Not only are they effective in pathologic anxiety, but also their calming effect is useful in nonpathologic anxiety states (temporary episodes of anxiety due to fear—such as of surgery or personal problems). BZDs have a wider therapeutic window than most other CNS depressants and are associated with fewer side effects.

The various BZDs differ little in their pharmacologic properties, but they differ significantly in their potency, their ability to cross the blood–brain barrier, and their half-lives. High-potency BZDs such as alprazolam, clonazepam,

---

BOX 45–3. APA CRITERIA FOR DIAGNOSING PANIC DISORDER WITHOUT AGORAPHOBIA

A. Both (1) and (2)
  1. Recurrent unexpected panic attacks
  2. At least one of the attacks has been followed by 1 month (or more) of one (or more) of the following:
     a. Persistent concern about having additional attacks
     b. Worry about the implications of the attack or its consequences (eg, losing control, having a heart attack, "going crazy")
     c. A significant change in behavior related to the attacks
B. Absence of Agoraphobia
C. The panic attacks are not due to the direct physiologic effects of a substance (eg, a drug of abuse, a medication) or a general medical condition (eg, hyperthyroidism).
D. The panic attacks are not better accounted for by another mental disorder, such as Social Phobia (eg, occurring on exposure to feared social situations), Specific Phobia (eg, on exposure to a specific phobic situation), Obsessive-Compulsive Disorder (eg, on exposure to dirt in someone with an obsession about contamination), Posttraumatic Stress Disorder (eg, in response to stimuli associated with a severe stressor), or Separation Anxiety Disorder (eg, in response to being away from home or close relatives).

From the American Psychiatric Association. (2000). *Diagnostic and statistical manual of mental disorders* (4th ed., text revision). Washington, DC: Author, with permission.

---

response of the ego to unconscious, unacceptable thoughts, feelings, and impulses that threatened to emerge into the conscious mind. To remain intact, the ego used defense mechanisms to protect the self from becoming overwhelmed by anxiety. Followers of the interpersonal theorists, such as Sullivan, May, and Peplau, thought that the anxiety disorders developed and were maintained as a result of dysfunctional family relationships.

Behavioral therapists treat anxiety as a learned behavior, arguing that anxiety is an internal conditioned response to a perceived threat or stimulus in the environment. They propose that people with anxiety learn to avoid the stimulus in order to reduce anxiety; therefore, behavior modification is the vehicle for changing behavior. Systematic desensitization is used to control external stimuli and internal sensations as well as anticipation of fear of a panic attack.

Cognitive therapists treat anxiety as a faulty thought pattern that evokes the physiologic symptoms of anxiety, feelings of loss of control, and fear of dying. Cognitive behavioral therapy (CBT) and drug therapy complement each other and tend to produce a greater therapeutic response.

BOX 45–4. APA CRITERIA FOR DIAGNOSING OBSESSIVE-COMPULSIVE DISORDER

A. Either obsessions or compulsions
   Obsessions as defined by (1), (2), (3), and (4)
   1. Recurrent and persistent thoughts, impulses, or images that are experienced, at some time during the disturbance, as intrusive and inappropriate and that cause marked anxiety or distress.
   2. The thoughts, impulses, or images are not simply excessive worries about real-life problems.
   3. The person attempts to ignore or suppress such thoughts, impulses, or images, or to neutralize them with some other thought or action.
   4. The person recognizes that the obsessional thoughts, impulses, or images are a product of his or her own mind (not imposed from without, as in thought insertion).

   Compulsions as defined by (1) and (2)
   1. Repetitive behaviors (eg, hand washing, ordering, checking) or mental acts (eg, praying, counting, repeating words silently) that the person feels driven to perform in response to an obsession, or according to rules that must be applied rigidly.
   2. The behaviors or mental acts are aimed at preventing or reducing distress or preventing some dreaded event or situation; however, these behaviors or mental acts either are not connected in a realistic way with what they are designed to neutralize or prevent or are clearly excessive.

B. At some point during the course of the disorder, the person has recognized that the obsessions or compulsions are excessive or unreasonable. **Note:** This does not apply to children.
C. The obsessions or compulsions cause marked distress, are time consuming (take more than 1 hour a day), or significantly interfere with the person's normal routine, occupational (or academic) functioning, or usual social activities or relationships.
D. If another Axis I disorder is present, the content of the obsessions or compulsions is not restricted to it (eg, preoccupation with food in the presence of an Eating Disorder; hair pulling in the presence of Trichotillomania; concern with appearance in the presence of Body Dysmorphic Disorder; preoccupation with having a serious illness in the presence of Hypochondriasis; preoccupation with sexual urges or fantasies in the presence of Paraphilia; or guilty ruminations in the presence of Major Depressive Disorder).
E. The disturbance is not due to the direct physiologic effects of a substance (eg, a drug of abuse, a medication) or a general medical condition.

Specify if:
With Poor Insight: if for most of the time during the current episode, the person does not recognize that the obsessions and compulsions are excessive or unreasonable

From the American Psychiatric Association. (2000). *Diagnostic and statistical manual of mental disorders* (4th ed., text revision). Washington, DC: Author, with permission.

---

and lorazepam have a great affinity for the BZD receptor. The onset and intensity of action of an oral dose of a BZD is determined by the rate of absorption from the gastrointestinal tract. Benzodiazepines are highly bound to plasma proteins (70% to 90%) and are highly lipid soluble. The duration of action is related to their lipid solubility as well as hepatic biotransformation to active metabolites. Oxazepam and lorazepam are metabolized to inactive compounds and therefore have shorter half-lives and durations of activity than other BZDs. This one-step inactivation to an inactive compound makes them the preferred drugs for the treatment of anxiety in elderly patients and patients with liver disease.

Accumulation of BZDs with a long half-life (long-acting BZDs) occurs from one dose to another. Long-acting BZDs take a longer time to reach steady-state levels, are removed more slowly, and cause more pronounced side effects (eg, sedation). However, use of these preparations reduces the likelihood and intensity of withdrawal symptoms when discontinued. Ultrashort-acting BZDs do not accumulate. High lipid solubility results in faster absorption, greater distribution in tissues, and faster entrance and exit from brain sites. Diazepam is a BZD with high lipid solubility used for anxiety (see Table 45-2 for more information).

On discontinuation of BZD therapy, relapse rates are high (see "Monitoring Patient Response"). Longer-acting agents, such as clonazepam, can minimize dose-rebound anxiety. Similarly, rapid-onset agents, such as diazepam or alprazolam, can provide acute anxiolysis, whereas short-acting agents such as lorazepam can minimize accumulation and oversedation. In the elderly, use of long-acting BZDs is discouraged because impaired liver and kidney function may precipitate severe and prolonged adverse effects.

Tolerance and Dependence Issues

Tolerance to the sedative (but not anxiolytic) effects of BZDs develops at moderate doses. BZDs can cause dependence if used continuously for more than several weeks. If the patient's anxiety is episodic, episodic use of BZDs may control symptoms. If anxiety is prolonged, BZDs may control anxiety, but this therapeutic benefit must be weighed against their capacity to cause dependence. Abuse potential does not appear to be a problem in people who do not abuse alcohol or other substances. See "Monitoring Patient Response" for information on tapering technique and withdrawal issues.

Table 45.2

Overview of Selected Drugs Used to Treat Anxiety

Generic (Trade) Name and Dosage	Selected Adverse Events	Contraindications	Special Considerations
Long-Acting Benzodiazepines *Note:* The use of long-acting benzodiazepines in the elderly is discouraged.			
clorazepate (Tranxene) Anxiety: 7.5–15 mg bid–qid. Adjust dose as needed within the range of 15–60 mg/d. Sustained-release forms may be given in a single dose of 11.25–22.5 mg hs in patients stabilized on 7.5 mg tid. Do not use to initiate therapy. Elderly or debilitated patients: initial dose 3.75–15 mg/d. May require adjustment of subsequent doses as needed. Children 9–12 y: 7.5 mg bid initially. May increase by 7.5 mg/wk but not to exceed 60 mg/d.	*CNS:* Drowsiness, dizziness, lethargy, mental depression, confusion, paradoxical excitement *EENT:* Blurred vision *Resp:* Respiratory depression *GI:* Constipation, diarrhea, nausea, vomiting *GU:* Urinary retention, incontinence *Derm:* Rashes *Misc:* Physical dependence, psychological dependence, tolerance	Hypersensitivity, cross-sensitivity with other benzodiazapines, preexisting CNS depression, severe, uncontrolled pain, narrow-angle glaucoma, pregnancy or lactation Use cautiously in preexisting hepatic disease, severe renal impairment, suicidal patients, past drug addiction, severe pulmonary disease, and geriatric or debilitated patients.	Half-life, including metabolites: 36–200 h Peak plasma level: 1–2 h Protein binding: 97%–98% Drowsiness may occur at initiation of treatment and with dosage increments. Avoid use of alcohol and other CNS depressants. Laboratory considerations: for patients on long-term therapy, check CBC and liver function studies periodically. May cause an increase in bilirubin, AST, and ALT. May cause decreased thyroid uptake of sodium iodide ^{123}I and ^{131}I.
chlordiazepoxide (Librium, Libritabs, Mitran, Reposans-10) Mild to moderate anxiety: 5–10 mg tid–qid Severe anxiety: 20–25 mg tid–qid Elderly or debilitated patients: 5 mg bid–qid Children: initial dose 5 mg bid–qid. A dose of 0.5 mg/kg/d q6–8h is also recommended for children >6 y. Not recommended for children <6 y.	*CNS:* drowsiness, dizziness, lethargy, mental depression, confusion, paradoxical excitement *EENT:* blurred vision *Resp:* respiratory depression *GI:* constipation, diarrhea, nausea, vomiting, dry mouth *GU:* urinary retention, incontinence *Derm:* rashes *Misc:* physical dependence, psychological dependence, tolerance	Hypersensitivity, cross-sensitivity with other benzodiazapines, preexisting CNS depression, severe, uncontrolled pain, narrow-angle glaucoma, pregnancy or lactation Some products contain tartrazine and should be avoided in patients who have intolerance. Use cautiously in preexisting hepatic disease, severe renal impairment, suicidal patients, past drug addiction, severe pulmonary disease, and geriatric or debilitated patients.	Half-life, including metabolites: 36–200 h Peak plasma level: 0.5–4 h Protein binding: 96% Avoid use of alcohol and other CNS depressants. Laboratory considerations: For patients on long-term therapy, check CBC and liver function studies periodically. May cause an increase in bilirubin, AST, and ALT. May cause decreased thyroid uptake of sodium iodide ^{123}I and ^{131}I. May alter 17-ketosteroids and 17-ketogenic steroids. May cause decreased response on metyrapone tests.
clonazepam (Klonopin) Panic disorder: 0.125 mg bid. Increase after 3 d toward a target dose of 1 mg/d. In some patients the dose may need to be increased to 4 mg/d.	*CNS:* Behavioral changes, drowsiness, slurred speech *EENT:* Abnormal eye movements, nystagmus, diplopia *Resp:* Respiratory distress, SOB, increased secretions, chest congestion *CV:* Palpitations *GI:* Constipation, diarrhea, hepatitis, changes in appetite *GU:* Dysuria, nocturia, urinary retention *Neuro:* Ataxia, hypotonia. *Hemat:* Anemia, eosinophilia, leukopenia, thrombocytopenia *Misc:* Fever, physical dependence, psychological dependence, tolerance	Hypersensitivity, cross-sensitivity with other benzodiazapine, and severe liver disease Use cautiously in chronic respiratory disease, narrow-angle glaucoma, pregnancy, lactation, children.	Rate of absorption: Intermediate Half-life, including metabolites: 18–50 h Peak plasma level PO: 1–2 h Protein binding: 97% Therapeutic serum levels: 20–80 ng/mL Do not discontinue abruptly. Abrupt withdrawal may precipitate status epilepticus. Withdrawal symptoms similar to those with barbiturates. Long-term use during pregnancy may result in withdrawal symptoms in the neonate. Take with food to minimize gastric irritation. Laboratory considerations: For patients on long-term therapy, check CBC and liver function studies periodically. May cause an increase in bilirubin, AST, and ALT. May cause decreased thyroid uptake of sodium iodide ^{123}I and ^{131}I.

(*continued*)

Table 45.2

Overview of Selected Drugs Used to Treat Anxiety (*Continued*)

Generic (Trade) Name and Dosage	Selected Adverse Events	Contraindications	Special Considerations
diazepam (Valium, Valrelease, Vazepam; IV: Valium, Zetran; Oral Solution: Intensol) Anxiety: 2–10 mg bid–qid. Increase dosage cautiously to avoid adverse effects. Sustained-release 15- or 30-mg tablets may be used when the optimal daily oral dose of diazepam is 5 or 10 mg tid. Elderly or debilitated patients: Initial dose 2–2.5 mg qd–bid. Increase gradually as needed and tolerated. May also use 15-mg sustained-release tablets if this is the optimal established dose. Children >6 mo: 1–2.5 mg PO tid–qid. Safety and efficacy have not been established in the neonate (≤30 d; injectable).	*CNS:* Drowsiness, dizziness, lethargy, mental depression, paradoxical excitement, slurred speech, transient amnesia, hallucinations *EENT:* Blurred vision *Resp:* Respiratory depression *CV:* Bradycardia, hypotension (IV only) *GI:* Constipation, diarrhea, nausea, vomiting *GU:* Urinary retention, incontinence *Derm:* Rashes *Misc:* Physical dependence, psychological dependence, tolerance	Hypersensitivity, cross-sensitivity with other benzodiazapines, preexisting CNS depression, severe, uncontrolled pain, narrow-angle glaucoma, and pregnancy or lactation Some products contain tartrazine, alcohol, or propylene glycol and should be avoided in patients who have known intolerance. Use cautiously in preexisting hepatic disease, severe renal impairment, suicidal patients, past drug addiction, children, and geriatric or debilitated patients.	Half-life, including metabolites: 20–100 h Peak plasma level PO: 0.5–2 h Protein binding: 98% Avoid use of alcohol and other CNS depressants. Laboratory considerations: For patients on long-term therapy, check CBC and liver function studies periodically.

Intermediate-Acting Benzodiazepines

alprazolam (Xanax) Initial dose: 0.25–0.5 mg tid. Titrate to maximal dose of 4 mg/d in divided doses. If side effects occur with starting dose, decrease dose. Elderly or debilitated patients: 0.25 mg bid–tid. Gradually increase as needed and tolerated. Panic disorder: Initial dose 0.5 mg tid. Depending on response, increase dose at intervals of 3–4 d in increments of 1 mg/d. Patients may require doses >4 mg/d. Do not exceed 10 mg/d. Children: Safety and efficacy for use in patients <18 y has not been established.	*CNS:* Drowsiness, dizziness, lethargy, mental depression, paradoxical excitement *EENT:* Blurred vision, nasal congestion *Resp:* Respiratory depression *GI:* Constipation, diarrhea, nausea, vomiting, dry mouth *Derm:* Rashes *Hemat:* Decreased hematocrit and neutropenia *Misc:* Physical dependence, psychological dependence, tolerance, weight gain, muscle rigidity	Hypersensitivity, cross-sensitivity with other benzodiazapines, preexisting CNS depression, severe, uncontrolled pain, narrow-angle glaucoma, and pregnancy or lactation Use cautiously in hepatic dysfunction, suicidal patients, past drug addiction, and geriatric or debilitated patients.	Half-life, including metabolites: 6–20 h Peak plasma level: 1–2 h Protein binding: 80% May be administered with food if GI upset occurs. Avoid driving or other activities that require alertness. Avoid use of alcohol and other CNS depressants. Patients on long-term or high-dosage therapy may experience withdrawal symptoms on abrupt cessation of therapy. Laboratory considerations: For patients on long-term therapy, check CBC and liver function studies periodically.
lorazepam (Ativan) Initial dose: 2–3 mg bid–tid (dose may vary from 1–10 mg/d). Elderly: initial dose: 1–2 mg/d in divided doses. Adjust dose based on need and tolerance. IM and IV routes are used for preoperative sedation. Children: Safety and efficacy for use in patients <12 y has not been established. Do not use injectable form in patients <18 y. May be used short term for insomnia due to anxiety, 2–4 mg/hs.	*CNS:* Drowsiness, dizziness, lethargy, mental depression, paradoxical excitement, amnesia, disorientation *EENT:* Blurred vision *Resp:* Respiratory depression *CV:* Bradycardia, hypotension: with rapid IV infusion, apnea, cardiac arrest *GI:* Constipation, diarrhea, nausea, vomiting, change in appetite *Derm:* Rashes *Misc:* Physical dependence, psychological dependence, tolerance	Hypersensitivity, cross-sensitivity with other benzodiazepines, preexisting CNS depression, severe, uncontrolled pain, narrow-angle glaucoma, and pregnancy or lactation Use cautiously in hepatic, renal, or respiratory dysfunction, suicidal patients, past drug addiction, and geriatric or debilitated patients.	Half-life, including metabolities: 10–20 h Peak plasma level PO: 2–4 h Protein binding: 85% Avoid use of alcohol and other CNS depressants. Laboratory considerations: For patients on long-term or high-dose therapy, check CBC and renal and hepatic function periodically.
oxazepam (Serax) Mild to moderate anxiety: 10–15 mg tid–qid Severe anxiety syndromes or anxiety associated with depression: 15–30 mg tid–qid	*CNS:* Drowsiness, dizziness, lethargy, mental depression, paradoxical excitement, impaired memory, slurred speech *EENT:* Blurred vision	Hypersensitivity, cross-sensitivity with other benzodiazepines, preexisting CNS depression, severe, uncontrolled pain, narrow-angle glaucoma, pregnancy or lactation	Half-life, including metabolites: 10–20 h Peak plasma level: 2–4 h Protein binding: 85% Avoid use of alcohol and other CNS depressants.

Table 45.2

Overview of Selected Drugs Used to Treat Anxiety (*Continued*)

Generic (Trade) Name and Dosage	Selected Adverse Events	Contraindications	Special Considerations
Older patients: initial dose 10 mg tid and if needed increase cautiously to 15 mg tid–qid Children: Dosage not established	*Resp:* Respiratory depression *CV:* Tachycardia *GI:* Drug-induced hepatitis, constipation, diarrhea, nausea, vomiting *Hemat:* Leukopenia (rare) *Derm:* Rashes *Misc:* Physical dependence, psychological dependence, tolerance, altered libido	Some products contain tartrazine and should be avoided in those patients who have intolerance. Use cautiously in preexisting hepatic disease, severe renal impairment, suicidal patients, past drug addiction, severe chronic pulmonary obstructive disease, and geriatric or debilitated patients.	Laboratory considerations: In long-term therapy, monitor CBC and hepatic function periodically. May cause decreased thyroid uptake of sodium iodide ^{123}I and ^{131}I.
buspirone (BuSpar) Initial dose: 5 mg tid. Increase dose 5 mg/d at intervals of 2–3 d as needed. Divided doses of 20–30 mg/d are common. Do not exceed 60 mg/d.	*CNS:* Drowsiness, dizziness, excitement, fatigue, headache, insomnia, nervousness, personality changes *EENT:* Nasal congestion, blurred vision, sore throat, tinnitus, and altered taste and smell *GI:* Nausea *CVP:* Chest pain, chest congestion, palpitations, tachycardia, hyperventilation and shortness of breath *Neuro:* Myalgia, incoordination, numbness, paresthesia *Derm:* Hair loss, facial edema, clamminess, sweating, rashes *Sexual dysfunction:* Irregular menses, decreased libido, delayed ejaculation, impotence *Other:* Weight gain or loss, fever, roaring sensation in head, malaise	Hypersensitivity, pregnancy, lactation, children, severe liver dysfunction and concurrent use of antianxiety agents or other psychoactive drugs	Half-life: 2–3 h Onset: 7–10 d Peak plasma level: 3–4 wk Optimal therapeutic results are usually after 3–4 wk. Some improvement will be seen in 7–10 d. Buspirone does not prevent withdrawal symptoms from other antianxiety agents, so gradual withdrawal from these medications is necessary. Patient must inform caregiver if any chronic abnormal movements occur, such as motor restlessness, or involuntary repetitive movements of facial or neck muscles. Alcohol and other CNS depressant use must be avoided while on this medication. Administration with food may decrease rate of GI absorption.
hydroxyzine HCl (Atarax) hydroxyzine pamoate (Vistaril) For mild to moderate anxiety: Begin with 25 mg tid. Optimum dose range is 75–150 mg/d in 3–4 divided doses. May increase to 300 mg/d. For very mild symptoms: Patients may be maintained on 25 to 50 mg/d. Drugs may be given IM or PO. Children: 50 mg/d in divided doses.	*CNS:* Drowsiness, dizziness, ataxia, headache, weakness *GI:* Dry mouth Hypersensitivity reactions Infection at IM injection site	Hypersensitivity, pregnancy, and lactation Use with caution in patients with hepatic dysfunction and geriatric patients.	Half-life: 3 h Peak plasma level PO: 2–4 h Additive CNS depression with other CNS depressants and alcohol. Give deep IM in large muscles. May cause false-negative skin tests using allergen extracts. Discontinue medication 72 h before skin test. Avoid driving or other activities that require alertness. Also used as an antipruritic and an antiemetic.
meprobamate (Equanil, Miltown) 1.2–1.6 g/d in 3–4 divided doses Sustained-release tabs: 400–800 mg AM and hs	CNS depression, nausea, vomiting, palpitations, tachycardia, dysrhythmias	Acute intermittent porphyria and allergy Use with caution in patients with epilepsy and in pregnancy.	Use for <4 mo. With prolonged use, wean the patient off the medication. Drug dependence may develop. This medication is rarely used now. It has been replaced by the benzodiazepines. Occasionally, elderly patients may have been on this medication for many years and continue to take the medication.

Adverse Events

The major adverse events of BZDs are drowsiness and ataxia. Mild, transitory cognitive and memory impairments are seen occasionally. This is of greater significance in elderly people and those with high sensitivity to these drugs. Reactions of rage, excitement, and hostility, although rare, have been reported after overdoses of chlordiazepoxide. Other reported side effects include increased depression, confusion, headache, gastrointestinal distur-

Table 45.3

Drug Interactions With the Benzodiazepines (BZDs)

Benzodiazepines	Interacting Drugs	Interaction
alprazolam (Xanax) chlordiazepoxide (Librium) clorazepate (Tranxene) diazepam (Valium) halazepam (Paxipam) lorazepam (Ativan) oxazepam (Serax)	cimetidine (Tagamet) ketoconazole (Nizoral) oral contraceptives metoprolol (Lopressor) disulfiram (Antabuse) propoxyphene (Darvon) fluoxetine (Prozac) propranolol (Inderal) isoniazid (Nydrazid)	Increased pharmacologic effect of the BZDs and excessive sedation and impaired psychomotor function may occur because of decreased hepatic metabolism.
	valproic acid (Depakene)	Clearance rate of BZDs may be increased.
	alcohol and other CNS depressants, such as barbiturates and narcotics	May cause increased CNS effects such as sedation and impaired psychomotor dysfunction
	antacids	May alter rate of GI absorption but not extent of GI absorption. Do not administer at same time.
	digoxin (Lanoxin)	Serum concentrations of digoxin may be increased. Monitor digoxin serum levels and signs and symptoms of digoxin toxicity (GI and neuropsychiatric symptoms and cardiac dysrhythmias).
	levodopa (Dopar)	Antiparkinson efficacy may be reduced with concurrent use of BZDs.
	neuromuscular blocking agents	Concurrent use of BZDs may potentiate, counteract, or have no effect on the actions of these drugs.
	phenytoin (Dilantin)	Data are conflicting, but phenytoin serum levels may be increased, resulting in toxicity; oxazepam levels may be increased as well.
	probenecid (Benemid)	May interfere with BZD conjugation in the liver, resulting in a more rapid onset or prolonged effect
	ranitidine (Zantac)	GI absorption of diazepam may be reduced.
	rifampin (Rifadin)	May decrease the pharmacologic effects of some BZDs because it may increase the oxidative metabolism of these agents
	scopolamine (Hyoscine HBr)	Concomitant use with parenteral lorazepam may increase the incidence of sedation, hallucinations, and irrational behavior.
	theophylline (Slo-Phyllin)	May antagonize the sedative effects of the BZDs

bances, menstrual irregularities, and changes in libido. Urticaria may occur in people with drug hypersensitivity, and drug interactions may occur with a variety of medications (Table 45-3).

Treatment of Benzodiazepine Overdose

Flumazenil (Mazicon) is a competitive BZD receptor antagonist that reverses the sedative effects of BZDs. Antagonism of BZD-induced respiratory depression is less predictable. Flumazenil is the only BZD receptor antagonist available for clinical use. It blocks many of the actions of BZDs but does not antagonize the CNS effects of other sedative-hypnotics such as ethanol, opioids, or general anesthetics. It is used for BZD overdose and after the use of drugs in anesthetic and diagnostic procedures. When given intravenously, it acts rapidly and has a short half-life (0.7 to 1.3 hours). Because all BZDs have a longer duration of action than flumazenil, sedation commonly recurs and repeated doses of flumazenil may be needed. Adverse effects of flumazenil include confusion, agitation, dizziness, and nausea.

Azapirones

An azapirone, buspirone (BuSpar) is an anxiolytic drug that inhibits the uptake of dopamine, serotonin, and norepinephrine. Buspirone is as effective in the treatment of GAD as BZDs and has minimal abuse potential. It is rapidly

absorbed from the intestinal tract but undergoes extensive first-pass metabolism. People with liver dysfunction have a decreased clearance of buspirone. Buspirone has no hypnotic, anticonvulsant, or muscle-relaxant properties. Patients taking buspirone do not acquire a cross-tolerance for alcohol or BZDs. It is generally well tolerated, with only a few patients experiencing adverse effects. When adverse effects do occur, they include nausea, dizziness, headache, and nervousness (see Table 45-2). Doses over 70 mg have caused jitteriness and dysphoria.

In contrast to BZDs, buspirone's therapeutic effect may take 1 to 2 weeks. Because of its delayed effects, this drug is not useful in patients who need immediate relief from anxiety, and patient education is needed to enhance compliance with the medication regimen.

Other Antianxiety Medications

Hydroxyzines are sometimes used to relief anxiety and tension associated with an anxiety state or as an adjunct in organic disease states with anxiety.

The use of hydroxyzines for long-term treatment of anxiety (more than 4 months) has not been assessed. Hydroxyzine HCl (Atarax) and hydroxyzine pamoate (Vistaril) are drugs more commonly used for sedating patients before and after surgery and for managing pruritus, chronic urticaria, and atopic contact dermatitis. See Table 45-2 for doses and adverse events.

Meprobamate (Equanil) has been used in anxiety disorders for short-term relief of symptoms. Long-term effectiveness (greater than 4 months) has not been assessed. Drug dependence and abuse can occur. This drug has been replaced by other antianxiety medications and is used infrequently today, but some elderly patients may have been on this drug for many years and have acquired drug dependence. See Table 45-2 for dosages and adverse events.

Antidepressants

Antidepressants are thought of as specific for treating depression, but they are effective in many anxiety disorders. There are three categories of antidepressants: tricyclic antidepressants (TCAs), nonselective serotonin reuptake inhibitors (NSRIs) and SSRIs, and monoamine oxidase inhibitors (MAO inhibitors; Table 45-4). Anxious patients often need long-term use of antidepressants to maintain benefit and prevent relapse. For further information on antidepressants, see Chapter 44.

Tricyclic Antidepressants

Tricyclics are effective in GAD and PA. Imipramine (Tofranil) is the prototypical TCA effective in controlling panic attacks in patients with PD and GAD. The TCAs have largely been supplanted by SSRIs as first-line interventions for the treatment of anxiety disorders.

Mechanism of Action

The TCAs block the reuptake of norepinephrine and serotonin into nerve endings, thus increasing the levels of norepinephrine and serotonin in the nerve cells. Imipramine does not have any direct effects on anticipatory anxiety or phobic avoidance behavior. The response is gradual, over a period of weeks. Other TCAs are equally effective in treating patients with PD.

When a TCA is given for PD, approximately 33% of patients feel overstimulated when treatment begins. To reduce this problem, the patient may need to start with a lower dose and gradually increase the dose until a therapeutic dose response occurs. BZDs can be used on a short-term basis to lessen these initial symptoms.

Adverse Events

Because PD is episodic, it is considered a chronic condition that requires long-term management with TCAs. However, approximately 33% of patients on TCAs discontinue their treatment because they cannot tolerate the side effects of the drugs.

The TCAs cause anticholinergic side effects such as dryness of the mouth and other mucosal surfaces, blurred vision, tachycardia, constipation, and urinary hesitancy. Other adverse effects are postural hypotension, carbohydrate craving, weight gain, excessive perspiration, and sexual dysfunction. They can also lower the seizure threshold and must be used cautiously in patients with seizure disorders. These drugs are contraindicated in patients with narrow-angle glaucoma, urinary hesitancy, and heart conduction abnormalities. TCAs enhance the CNS effects of alcohol. Plasma measurements of TCAs should be done in selected situations as needed. See Chapter 44 for more information.

Serotonin Reuptake Inhibitors

SSRIs have become the drugs of choice for treating most anxiety disorders. They have more benign side effects than TCAs, which makes them more acceptable to patients. They can be classified into NSRIs, such as clomipramine (Anafranil), which is structurally similar to cyclic antidepressants; and SSRIs, such as escitalopram (Lexapro), fluoxetine (Prozac, weekly Prozac), fluvoxamine (Luvox), paroxetine (Paxil), and sertraline (Zoloft). Nefazodone (Serzone) blocks 5-hydroxytryptamine (serotonin; 5-HT) receptors as well as inhibiting serotonin transport. Venlafaxine (Effexor XL) causes strong inhibition of serotonin and norepinephrine and weak inhibition of dopamine reuptake. See Table 45-4 and Chapter 44.

Medications indicated for treating OCD are the NSRI clomipramine (Anafranil) and the SSRIs fluoxetine (Prozac), fluvoxamine (Luvox), paroxetine (Paxil), sertraline (Zoloft), citalopram (Celexa), or escitalopram (Lexapro). More than 50% of patients treated with clomipramine have their symptoms controlled completely or controlled to subclinical levels; in other patients, the symptoms are reduced in intensity.

Dosage

The effective oral dosage of clomipramine for OCD is 150 to 250 mg/day. It takes approximately 4 to 6 weeks for the anti-obsessional effects to become evident, and it may take up to 12 weeks for patients to attain full benefits. SSRIs and clomipramine are palliative only and not a cure for OCD;

Table 45.4

Antidepressants Used in Treating Anxiety Disorders

Generic (Trade) Name	Initial Dose (mg)	Usual Dose (mg)
Tricyclic Antidepressants		
amitriptyline (Elavil)	10–50	150–300
amoxapine (Ascendin)	25–50	150–450
desipramine (Norpramin)	10–25	100–250
doxepin (Sinequan, Adapin)	10–25	150–300
imipramine (Tofranil)	10–50	150–300
maprotiline (Ludiomil)	25–50	150–200
nortriptyline (Pamelor)	25–50	150–200
protriptyline (Vivetil)	5–10	15–60
trimipramine (Surmontil)	25–50	150–300
Selective Serotonin Reuptake Inhibitors		
citalopram (Celexa)	20	20–40
escitalopram (Lexapro)	10	10–20
fluoxetine (Prozac)	10–20	10–80
fluoxetine (Prozac weekly)		
fluvoxamine (Luvox)	25–50	100–300
nefazodone (Serzone)	50–100	200–500
paroxetine (Paxil)	10–20	10–60
(Paxil CR)	12.5	12.5–75
sertraline (Zoloft)	25–50	75–200
veniafaxine (Effexor)	75 bid-tid	75–225
(Effexor XL)	37.5–75	75–225
Nonselective Serotonin Reuptake Inhibitors		
clomipramine (Anafranil)	20–50	150–450
Monoamine Oxidase Inhibitors		
phenelzine (Nardil)	15	45–90

once patients discontinue drug therapy, most of them relapse. SSRIs are very effective in patients with PD and GAD. An advantage of sustained-release venlafaxine (Effexor XL) is that it is taken once daily, starting with a dose of 37.5 mg that is increased weekly to a maximum dose of 225 mg (see Table 45-4 and Chapter 44).

Adverse Events

Common adverse events of SSRIs include nausea, headache, insomnia, drowsiness, nervous jitteriness, diarrhea, rash, urticaria, weight loss, and sexual dysfunction. Paroxetine (Paxil) and fluoxetine (Prozac) are associated with very significant inhibition of P450 IID6, which makes polypharmacy more difficult. Paroxetine (Paxil) may cause more weight gain and sexual inhibition than the other drugs. Approximately 15% of patients discontinue treatment because of side effects. The effects of an overdose of SSRIs are relatively benign, and death is rare. Caution should be used when SSRIs are given in combination with TCAs because SSRIs can inhibit one or more liver microsomal enzymes. The combination of SSRIs and MAO inhibitors has resulted in serious reactions such as hyperthermia, rigidity, and autonomic dysregulation that can be fatal. See Chapter 44 for more information.

Monoamine Oxidase Inhibitors

The MAO inhibitors are effective in controlling panic attacks in most patients with PD. Their effectiveness in GAD has not been explored because of the necessary dietary restrictions and dangerous drug interactions that make their use cumbersome.

Mechanism of Action

The MAO inhibitors inhibit the breakdown of 5-HT and norepinephrine in the synaptic cleft. The most commonly used MAO inhibitor is phenelzine (Nardil), which is given in a dose range of 45 to 90 mg/day.

Adverse Events

The MAO inhibitors have anticholinergic side effects such as blurred vision, dryness of the mouth and other mucosal surfaces, constipation, urinary hesitancy, and tachycardia. Weight gain, agitation, and sexual dysfunction frequently occur. Hypotension that is aggravated by postural changes may develop, but it usually diminishes in a few weeks. Palliative measures such as increased fluid intake, salt tablets, and low-dose fludrocortisone (Florinef) can be used to manage hypotension. The greatest danger with MAO inhibitors is hypertensive crisis, which can be caused by food or drug interaction and can result in cerebral hemorrhage and death. MAO inhibitors prevent the breakdown of monoamines, so the patient taking an MAO inhibitor must avoid sympathomimetic substances and foods that contain tyramine, such as cheese, liver, yogurt, yeast, soy sauce, red wine, and beer. For further information, see Chapter 44.

Beta-Adrenergic Blockers

Beta-adrenergic blockers neutralize the effects of epinephrine and norepinephrine on the beta-adrenergic receptors.

The anxiolytic effects of all beta blockers are peripheral rather than central. Their main effect is to slow the heart rate and reduce tremors that decrease the perception of physical distress in anxiety-producing situations. They do not directly affect psychic anxiety, vigilance, or hyperalertness. Beta blockers are useful in the treatment of patients with palpitations, irregular heartbeat, or muscular tremor caused by anxiety. It is advantageous to combine beta blockers with a BZD when physical distress and anxiety symptoms coexist.

Selecting the Most Appropriate Agent

General Anxiety Disorder

First-Line Therapy

SSRIs have quickly become the drug of choice for GAD. No evidence has shown any one SSRI to be superior to another; however, the SSRIs have significant differences in side effects and drug interactions. Patients may have to try several SSRIs until they find one that best relieves their symptoms. TCAs may be used, but the side effect profiles of TCAs have tended to limit their use as first-line therapy agents since SSRIs have come into use. Antidepressants all require weeks to become effective, so BZDs may be given along with an antidepressant until the antidepressant begins to work. Once this occurs, the patient is slowly tapered off the BZD.

Second-Line Therapy

Buspirone may be considered a first-line therapy in newly diagnosed patients or for patients with chronic anxiety, but it is usually used in second-line therapy. Buspirone may be more appropriate if sedation or psychomotor impairment would be dangerous. Buspirone differs from the SSRIs in its efficacy spectrum and side effect profile. Buspirone is available in immediate and sustained-release formulations. It has fewer side effects than the BZDs and minimal abuse potential. However, the therapeutic effect of the drug may take 1 to 4 weeks. Buspirone may be the most appropriate drug for patients with a history of substance abuse, personality disorder, or sleep apnea.

Third-Line Therapy

The BZDs are considered first-line therapy only for exogenous anxiety related to a time-limited stress. The BZDs used most frequently are alprazolam, clorazepate (Tranxene), and diazepam. There is no evidence that one BZD is superior to another in this disorder. When choosing the specific BZD for treatment, the practitioner must consider the drug's onset of action and its half-life and the patient's metabolism (Fig. 45-1 and Table 45-5).

The drug dosage should be increased gradually to reach therapeutic response levels without producing unacceptable adverse effects. Use of BZDs with a long duration of action can be a problem because they may cause daytime sedation and motor impairment.

Drugs such as lorazepam or oxazepam are preferred because rebound and hangover effects may be avoided. Use

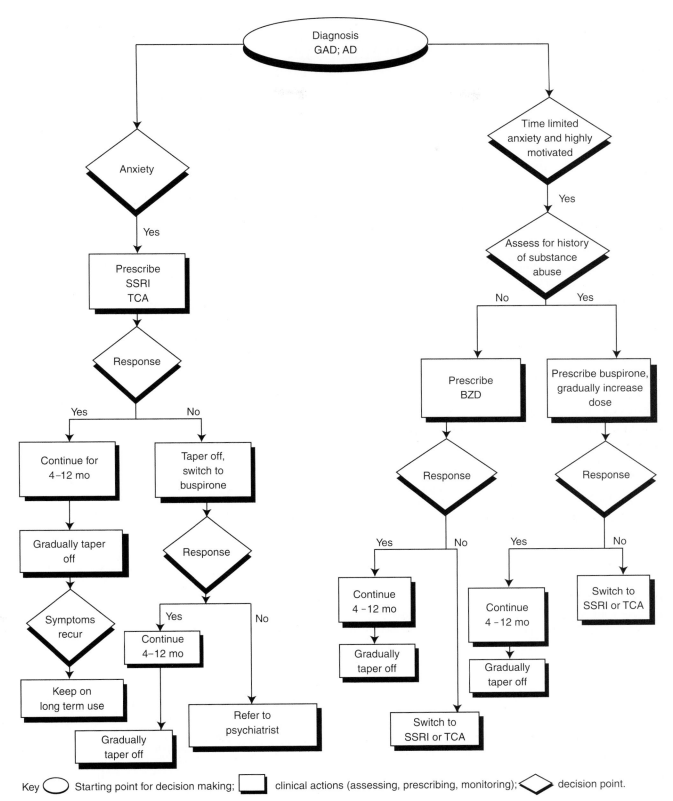

Key ◯ Starting point for decision making; ▭ clinical actions (assessing, prescribing, monitoring); ◇ decision point.

Figure 45–1 Treatment algorithm for generalized anxiety disorder (GAD).

of BZDs for more than 4 months may result in dependence, which can result in withdrawal symptoms and rebound effects. Concurrent psychotherapy may reduce the time needed for drug therapy as well as improving the patient's response rate (see Fig. 45-1).

Panic Disorder

First-Line Therapy

Panic disorder is episodic, and patients with PD frequently do well with SSRIs. Alprazolam (Xanax) is the only BZD

Table 45.5

Recommended Order of Treatment for Generalized Anxiety Disorder (GAD)

Order	Agents	Comments
First line	SSRI or TCA	Useful for anxiety disorder as well as a coexisting comorbidity
Second line	Buspirone	Takes 1–2 wk for effect
Third line		Select agent based on drug onset, half-life, and patient metabolism. Do not use if patient is alcohol or drug dependent. May be first-line drug in motivated patients with acute anxiety to a time-limited stress.

that is approved by the FDA for PD, but clonazepam (Klonopin) is also used. These drugs are used along with an SSRI if rapid relief from anxiety is needed. The practitioner needs to monitor symptoms, assess for side effects, and gradually increase the dosages of SSRIs and alprazolam or clonazepam if needed (Fig. 45-2).

Second-Line Therapy

Patients who do not respond to SSRIs may be changed to a TCA and monitored for effectiveness in decreasing panic attacks and controlling the severity of anxiety or panic symptoms while causing tolerable adverse events.

Third-Line Therapy

The MAO inhibitors can be very effective in controlling panic attacks. Before the patient begins therapy, however, the practitioner must assess his or her willingness to avoid the many tyramine-containing sympathomimetic drugs and foods, which can interact with MAO inhibitors to precipitate serious, life-threatening reactions. In addition, the patient should be referred to a psychiatrist for intensive therapy.

Obsessive-Compulsive Disorder

First-Line Therapy

Patients with OCD do well with clomipramine, an NSRI, as well as with SSRIs. The practitioner must monitor for a decrease in symptoms and assess for adverse events. If the patient has a good response to therapy without uncomfortable side effects, therapy may continue for up to 1 year (Fig. 45-3).

Second-Line Therapy

Buspirone (BuSpar) may be used for patients with OCD as a second-line drug. Response to drug therapy must be monitored and the patient referred for concurrent supportive therapy.

Third-Line Therapy

If the patient does not respond to drug therapy and psychotherapy and obsessions and compulsions interfere with activities of daily living, a psychiatric referral for intensive behavior therapy is indicated.

Table 45-6 summarizes drug therapy for anxiety disorders.

Special Population Considerations

Patients who have previously been treated for an anxiety disorder may have had drug treatment or psychotherapy that they found unsatisfactory. The practitioner should review with them what the treatments were, what adverse reactions they had, and the number of previous health care providers who treated them. Check with them for any history of drug withdrawal symptoms. If they report that a drug or treatment was unacceptable, plan a different but effective treatment. Assess for adverse effects to the new program. Also assess for drug-seeking behavior to rule out BZD dependence. Sometimes patients "shop around" for new health care providers when their previous provider has advised withdrawing from BZDs.

Patients with a history of prescription medication abuse and substance or alcohol abuse can become drug dependent. Buspirone, a nonaddicting drug, is a choice for their treatment regimen.

Pediatric

Four BZDs—clorazepate, chlordiazepoxide, diazepam, and alprazolam—have been approved by the FDA for use in children. Doses vary according to the child's age and weight. Clomipramine (Anafranil) remains the drug of choice in the treatment of OCD. Onset of action is in 2 to 4 weeks, with a final improvement over 8 to 10 weeks. The dosage of clomipramine is up to 200 mg/day or 3 mg/kg for children or adolescents. The SSRIs are effective in the treatment of OCD. Only sertraline (Zoloft) and fluvoxamine (Luvox) has been approved for the treatment of OCD in children.

Geriatric

Elderly patients may have decreased liver and renal function and metabolize and excrete drugs more slowly. They also may have neurologic disorders, cardiac disease, hypertension, hypotension, and glaucoma and may be taking drugs for these conditions. Elderly patients may be started on low doses of shorter-acting BZDs, TCAs, SSRIs, and buspirone, and the dosage may be gradually increased. Elderly patients may also experience paradoxical reactions to drugs (see Tables 45-2 and 45-3).

Women

Women are more likely than men to seek treatment for anxiety and depression. Women who are taking oral contraceptives drugs may have adverse drug interactions with BZDs

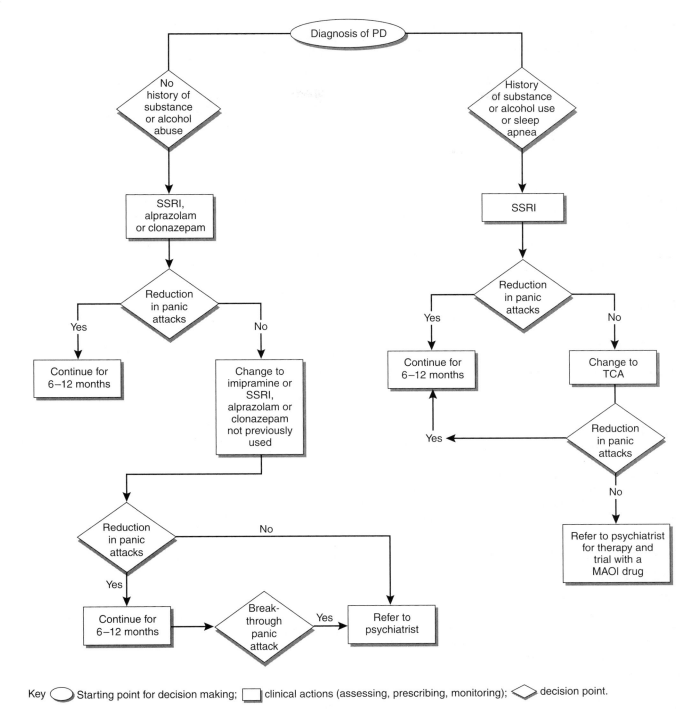

Key ◯ Starting point for decision making; ▢ clinical actions (assessing, prescribing, monitoring); ◇ decision point.

Figure 45–2 Treatment algorithm for panic disorder (PD).

(see Table 45-3). The practitioner needs to be alert for signs of anxiety disorders in men, because they are not as likely as women to report these symptoms. Rather, men are likely to report physical signs of anxiety and not identify the problem as emotional in origin.

Ethnic

Understanding a patient's cultural orientation or ethnic background is necessary for making a correct diagnosis and establishing an appropriate treatment plan. What we view as a problem such as anxiety or depression is not always perceived the same way by patients from other cultures. Complaints of anxiety or depression may not be reported by some patients because this is considered to be a mental disorder that is to be kept secret from people outside the family.

Research findings indicate that people from various racial or ethnic groups may metabolize some drugs differently because of their genetic makeup. An example of a drug that is metabolized differently is the antitubercular drug isoniazid (Laniazid). Researchers are beginning to examine other drug classifications for variations. Practitioners need to keep

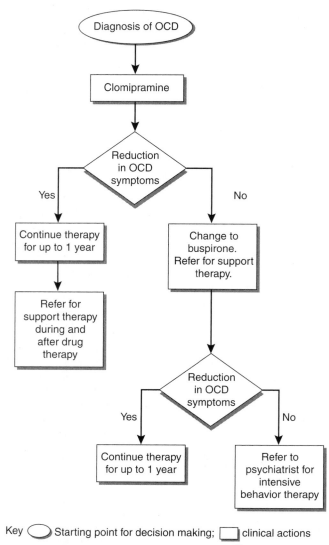

Key ⬭ Starting point for decision making; ▭ clinical actions
(assessing, prescribing, monitoring); ◇ decision point.

Figure 45–3 Treatment algorithm for obsessive-compulsive disorder (OCD).

current with research that examines genetic differences in the metabolism of drugs (see Chapters 2 and 3).

Monitoring Patient Response

Patients need to be monitored for self-reports of decreased anxiety symptoms. The practitioner should monitor patients closely for compliance with the medication regimen as well as side effects.

Most side effects from SSRIs are transient. Dose-related sexual effects, such as decreased libido or delayed ejaculation in men and anorgasmia in women, are common and typically do not resolve without intervention. Management of treatment-related sexual dysfunction includes reducing the SSRI dosage reduction and adding or switching to an antidepressant not associated with sexual dysfunction, such as bupropion (Wellbutrin, Wellbutrin SR), nefazodone (Serzone), or mirtazapine (Remeron). Another strategy includes the use of sildenafil (Viagra) or buspirone (BuSpar).

A non-life-threatening discontinuation syndrome of flu-like symptoms may occur after abrupt cessation of an SSRI. This syndrome can be minimized by gradually tapering the dose.

An overdose of TCAs can lead to anticholinergic delirium, ventricular arrhythmias, significant hypotension, seizures, and death. A TCA overdose is a medical emergency and requires close clinical and cardiac monitoring.

Many patients do not like buspirone because it takes 1 to 4 weeks to take effect. Frequently patients stop taking this medication because they think it is not helping their symptoms. Patient education and monitoring for compliance must be ongoing.

There have been no well-documented fatal overdoses of BZDs, but deaths have resulted from the ingestion of multiple drugs and overdoses of BZDs and other drugs. Prolonged use of BZDs can lead to dependence and withdrawal on discontinuation. Although the duration of therapy is not standardized, most clinicians prescribe the medication for 4 to 6 months and then try decreasing the dosage; however, the relapse rate of anxiety is approximately 60% to 80% within the first year that the patient is off the medication.

There are three components of a withdrawal syndrome: relapse is the return of the original symptoms of anxiety, rebound is a return of symptoms at greater severity than originally experienced, and withdrawal is the appearance of new symptoms.

When a BZD is discontinued, the severity of the withdrawal syndrome depends on how rapidly the drug is tapered, the half-life of the drug, and the duration of therapy. The withdrawal syndrome increases in severity with increased dosage and duration of use: for instance, more patients experience withdrawal symptoms after taking a BZD for 8 months than those taking it for less than 3 months. Withdrawal is relatively infrequent with short-term use, but it can occur with therapy as brief as 3 weeks. Abrupt discontinuation is frequently associated with withdrawal, usually of greater severity. Therefore, the rate of discontinuation should

Table 45.6						
Pharmacotherapy for Selected Anxiety Disorders						
	SSRIs	**TCAs**	**Buspirone**	**BZD**	**MAOIs**	**CBT**
GAD	+	+	+/−	+	+	+
PA	+	+	+	+	−	+
OCD	+	−	+/−	+/−	+	+

GAD, generalized anxiety disorder; PA, panic disorder; OCD, obsessive-compulsive disorder; SSRI, selective serotonin reuptake inhibitors; TCAs, tricyclic antidepressants; BZD, benzodiazepines; MAIOs, monoamine oxidase inhibitors; CBT, cognitive behavioral therapy.
(Adapted from Liebowitz, N. R. [2004]. Anxiety disorders. In R. Rakel & E. Bope [Eds.], *Conn's current therapy* [56th ed.]. Philadelphia: Elsevier.)

> ### BOX 45–5. SYMPTOMS OF BENZODIAZEPINE WITHDRAWAL
>
> **Frequent**
> Anxiety
> Insomnia
> Irritability
> Muscle problems
>
> **Common**
> Nausea
> Depression
> Ataxia
> Hyperreflexia
> Blurred vision
> Fatigue
>
> **Rare**
> Psychosis
> Seizures
> Delirium
> Confusion

be slowed to moderate the symptoms. Drugs with shorter half-lives are also more associated with withdrawal phenomena than those with longer half-lives. The tapering period should be at least 4 weeks, and the rate of tapering should be approximately a 10% dosage decrease every 3 to 4 days. Box 45-5 lists BZD withdrawal symptoms.

Patients on long-term (more than 4 months) BZD therapy need periodic blood counts and liver and thyroid function testing. BZDs can cause elevations in lactate dehydrogenase, alkaline phosphatase, alanine aminotransferase, and aspartate aminotransferase levels. Use of BZDs may cause leukopenia, blood dyscrasias, anemia, thrombocytopenia, eosinophilia, and decreased uptake of I-125 and I-131 sodium iodide (see Table 45-2; see also Chapter 44 for a discussion of monitoring concerns related to antidepressant medications).

PATIENT EDUCATION

Drug Information

The patient should know the name of the drug prescribed, dose, frequency of administration, expected outcome of therapy, drug interactions, adverse events, and the amount of time it will take for the drug to take effect. The patient should also know how to report adverse events to the primary caregiver. The patient should be taught to take the drug as ordered and not to increase the dose or stop the drug without first contacting the primary care provider.

The patient should know that the therapeutic effect of the drug needs to be monitored and that the dosage may need to be increased or another drug may be more helpful. If laboratory tests are needed, the patient should know the name of the laboratory test, what the test is, and the frequency of monitoring. The patient also needs to tell all health care providers what medications he or she is taking.

The National Institutes of Health's website (www.nih.gov/medlineplus/anxiety.html) provides useful patient information, as does the Anxiety Disorder Association of America's website (www.adaa.org).

Lifestyle Information

The patient should know that the physical symptoms of anxiety (eg, increased heart rate, palpitations, pupil dilatation, trembling, increased perspiration, muscle tension, and sleep disturbances) are not life threatening. The practitioner should instruct the patient about how combination treatment consisting of medications, psychotherapy, and relaxation therapy can control anxiety. Instruction on performing relaxation exercises is helpful. The practitioner should describe the various psychotherapeutic modalities so that the patient may select the one thought to be most appropriate. If the patient does not seek psychotherapy, the primary caregiver may need to provide emotional support. The patient who does not respond well to drug and relaxation therapy must be referred to a psychiatric specialist.

Providing written instructions is important because the patient may have trouble concentrating on or fully comprehending verbal instructions. After providing all instructions and materials, the practitioner should review the patient's comprehension of the instructions and willingness to comply with the medication regimen. This review should be part of each patient visit.

FUTURE DIRECTIONS IN ANXIOLYTIC PHARMACOLOGIC TREATMENT

Psychopharmacologists are developing new anxiolytic drugs that are fast-acting and free from the unwanted effects associated with BZDs. Drugs that are partial agonists at the BZD receptors have been studied in Europe, but no BZD partial agonists have been approved for anxiolytic use in the United States. Zolpidem, a structurally and pharmacologically similar agent, has been recently marketed as a hypnotic.

Neurosteroids are pharmacologic agents that target the BZD receptor. They now need to be tested in humans. Researchers are targeting various serotonin 5-HT receptor subtypes. Studies of neuropeptide receptor agonists and antagonists with anxiolytic properties have been conducted, but these agents need more clinical testing.

■ Case Study

L.P., age 23, is a white woman who graduated from college last year. She began working as an accountant 1 month after graduating. Approximately 2 months ago, she moved into a two-bedroom apartment with another woman who works at the same accounting firm. She states that her roommate recommended that she see a doctor to find out if she has anemia or "some sort of fatigue syndrome." She states that she has felt "restless" and "on edge" for most of the past

(Continued)

■ Case Study (*Continued*)

9 months. She becomes easily fatigued and irritable and has difficulty concentrating and falling asleep. She states that sometimes her mind "just goes blank," and she is worried that her work performance is no longer excellent. She reports that all her life she had good grades in school and was very successful in everything she attempted. Although she has been "a worrier from the day I was born," now she worries more than she ever has and feels nervous "all the time." L.P. reports that she has a good relationship with her boyfriend but they do not get to see each other very often because he is attending graduate school 100 miles away. She reports having a satisfying sexual relationship with him. She denies having any problems with relationships with her parents, roommate, or peers. She denies having any financial worries unless she is fired from her job for poor work performance. She reports that she has always been healthy and has taken good care of herself. The only medication she takes is birth control pills, which she has taken for the past 4 years without any adverse effects.

Diagnosis: Generalized anxiety disorder

1. List specific treatment goals for L.P.
2. What drug therapy would you prescribe? Why?
3. What are the parameters for monitoring the success of the therapy?
4. Describe specific patient monitoring based on the prescribed therapy.
5. List one or two adverse reactions for the selected agent that would cause you to change therapy.
6. What would be the choice for second-line therapy?
7. What dietary and lifestyle changes should be recommended for this patient?
8. Describe one or two drug/drug or drug/food interactions for the selected agent.

Bibliography

Starred references are cited in the text.

*American Psychiatric Association. (2000). *Diagnostic and statistical manual of mental disorders* (4th ed., text revision). Washington, DC: Author.

*Cannon, W. B. (1963). *Wisdom of the body.* New York: Norton.

Davis, R. D., & Winter, L. (2001). Antianxiety agents. In J. L. Jacobson, *Psychiatric secrets* (2nd ed.). New York: Hanley & Belfus.

DiPiro, J. T., Talbert, R. L., Yee, G. C., Matzke, G. R., Wells, B. G., & Posey, L. M. (Eds.). (1999). *Pharmacotherapy: a pathophysiologic approach* (4th ed.). Norwalk, CT: Appleton & Lange.

Ferri, F. (2004). *Practice guide to the care of the medical patient* (6th ed.). St. Louis: Mosby, Inc.

Goldstein, M. Z. (2002). Depression and anxiety in older women. *Primary Care Clinics in Office Practice, 29*(1).

Gutierez, K. (1999). *Pharmacotherapeutics: clinical decision making in nursing.* Philadelphia: W. B. Saunders.

Herbert, F. B. (2001). Obsessive-compulsive disorder in children and adolescents. In J. L. Jacobson (Ed.), *Psychiatric disorders* (2nd ed.). New York: Hanley & Belfus.

Kaplan, H., & Sadock, B. (1999). *Comprehensive textbook of psychiatry* (7th ed.). Baltimore: Williams & Wilkins.

Kercher, E. E. (2002). Anxiety disorders. In J. Marx, R. Hockenberger, & R. Walls (Eds.), *Rosen's emergency medicine: concepts in clinical practice* (5th ed.). St Louis: Mosby, Inc.

Lauderdale, S. A., & Shiekh, J. I. (2003). Anxiety disorders in older adults. *Clinics in Geriatric Medicine, 19*(4).

Liebowitz, N. R. (2004). Anxiety disorders. In R. Rakel & E. Bope (Eds.), *Conn's current therapy* (56th ed.). Philadelphia: Elsevier.

Moore, D. P., & Jefferson, J. W. (2004). Secondary anxiety disorder due to a general medical condition, DSM-IV-TR #293.89; substance-induced anxiety disorder, DSM-IV TR #292.80. *Handbook of Medical Psychiatry* (2nd ed.). St. Louis: Mosby, Inc.

*Selye, H. (1991). History and present status of the stress concept. In A. Monat & R. S. Lazarus (Eds.), *Stress and coping* (3rd ed.). New York: Columbia University Press.

Semia, T. P., Beizer, J. L., & Higbee, M. D. (2003). *Geriatric dosage handbook* (9th ed.). Hudson, OH: Lexi-Comp.

Shader, R. I., & Greenblatt (2000). Pharmacotherapy of acute anxiety: a mini update (Supported in part by a grant [MH-34223] from the Department of Health and Human Services) http://www.org/g4/GN401000128/CH126.html

Sood, A. B., Weller, E., & Weller, R. (2004). SSRIs in children and adolescents. *Current Psychiatry, 3*(3), 83–89.

Swede, S. E., Leonard, H. L., Garvey, M., et al. (1998). Pediatric autoimmune neuropsychiatric disorders associated with streptococcal infections: clinical descriptions of the first 50 cases. *American Journal of Psychiatry, 154*(1), 264–271.

Tancer, M. E., & Hussain, S. (2004). Panic disorder. In R. Rakel & E. Bope (Eds.), *Conn's current therapy* (56th ed.). Philadelphia: Elsevier.

Visit the Connection web site for the most up-to-date drug information.

INSOMNIA AND SLEEP DISORDERS

VERONICA WILBUR

Sleep, a naturally recurring state of restfulness for the body, is a necessary element of our daily life and occurs in a daily rhythmic pattern. Sleep disorders can affect the quality of sleep and therefore how individuals function on a daily basis. A problem with sleep is a symptom of another underlying problem. Sleep disorders include insomnia, snoring and sleep apnea, narcolepsy, and chronic sleep deprivation. Pharmacologic therapy is not appropriate for snoring and sleep apnea but has a role in the management of the other diagnoses. The key to an appropriate treatment plan is to recognize the type of sleep disorder.

INSOMNIA

Although most people occasionally have problems falling or staying asleep, insomnia can be defined as persistent trouble sleeping. Some experts argue, however, that problems sleeping at any time may be referred to as *insomnia*; they define the condition as loss of sleep for a short period. The loss of sleep may be due to physiologic causes such as restless leg syndrome, gastroesophageal reflux, or fibromyalgia, or sleep loss may simply be due to ignoring sleep cues. Sleep that is not refreshing also can be classified as insomnia. The World Health Organization and World Federation of Sleep Research Societies (1995) reported that the prevalence of sleep complaints is 36% in the United States. Of those 36%, approximately 10% of cases are classified as a serious or chronic health problem (Silva, Chase, Sartorius, & Roth, 1996). In primary care practice, 5% to 20% of all patients may report insomnia (Lustbader, Morgan, Pelayo, Vasquez, & Yuen, 1997). Complaints are more prevalent in women and increase with age, especially in those over age 65: up to 67% of elderly people have frequent sleep problems, but only one in eight is diagnosed and treated (Sleep America Poll, 2004).

In 1993, two Gallup surveys by *USA Today Magazine* from the National Commission of Sleep Disorders revealed that 95% of cases of insomnia remain undiagnosed. Insomnia can have social and economic consequences, as measured through direct and indirect costs.

The National Sleep Foundation (2004) estimated that the cost of sleep deprivation and sleep disorders equals $100 billion annually. This cost is seen in lost productivity, medical expenses, sick leave, and property and environmental damages. Up to 40% of people medicate themselves, commonly treating their insomnia with a host of over-the-counter drugs and other remedies before seeking the help of a health care provider. In the United States, more than $1 billion is spent yearly on sleep medications. According to a more recent Sleep America poll (2004), little has changed regarding these demographics since the early 1990s.

CAUSES

Insomnia can be of physiologic or psychological origin, and it is important to rule out the physiologic causes before labeling insomnia as psychological. Changes in a patient's biological clock can contribute to insomnia (eg, hyperarousal states, time zone and schedule changes), as can the sleep environment. The three main physiologic causes of insomnia are restless leg syndrome, gastroesophageal reflux, or fibromyalgia (Dement & Vaughan, 1999). Estimates are that up to half of all cases of insomnia are psychological in origin. In addition, 10% to 15% of cases result from drug or substance abuse. Medical causes are responsible for 10% of insomnia cases. Finally, primary or idiopathic sleep disorders account for 10% to 20% of all cases of insomnia (Box 46-1).

Insomnia can have both nocturnal symptoms and daytime consequences. This serious health care issue affects the quality of life, productivity, and safety of both the patient and society. Insomnia can be classified as *acute* or *transient*, lasting a few days; *short term*, lasting a few weeks; or *chronic* or *learned*, lasting months and years. It can also be classified as "difficulty falling asleep," "difficulty maintaining sleep," and "early morning awakening."

Acute insomnia is often related to environmental factors, such as sleeping in an unfamiliar place or excessive heat, noise, light, or movement of the bed partner. Transient insomnia often is related to stress or environmental changes. Usually, an acute emotional shock (either positive or negative) triggers this type of insomnia. Chronic, or learned,

BOX 46–1. CAUSES OF INSOMNIA

Medical
Endocrine problems (eg, hypothyroidism, hyperthyroidism, degenerative disease)
Neurologic and cardiovascular problems that cause difficulties with breathing
Pain
Renal problems (eg, urinary frequency)
Respiratory problems (eg, COPD, asthma)
Sleep apnea

Psychiatric
Anxiety
Excess stress
Major depression

Drug and Alcohol Abuse
Sedatives and stimulants

Primary Sleep Disorders
Excessive arousal and wakefulness
Poor sleep hygiene: related to lifestyle
Sleep state misperception: achievement of adequate sleep but not perceived by patient

---

PATHOPHYSIOLOGY

To understand how insomnia develops, it is first necessary to understand the physiologic process of sleep. The brain seeks to balance alertness and sleepiness on a continuum between sleep debt, biological alerting, and environmental stimulation. Sleepiness is a function of the brain fighting to get enough sleep to cover the debt. This system of sleep debt versus sleep arousal is intricately linked to circadian rhythms and exposure to light. Additionally, various internally regulated biologic systems govern the circadian pattern of the sleep–wake cycle. The interaction of these biologic systems includes changes in body temperature, cardiac and renal functions, and hormone secretion throughout the day. The term *circadian* means "approximately 1 day" and refers to the fact that endogenous rhythms last approximately 24 hours.

Normal sleep is divided into two phases: rapid eye movement sleep (REM) and non-REM (NREM). During the REM stage, which accounts for approximately 20% of the sleep cycle, the brain is active and most dreaming occurs. NREM, which constitutes approximately 80% of the sleep cycle, is a phase of deep rest in which pulse, respiration, and brain activity all slow. NREM sleep can be divided into four phases. Stages I and II are called light NREM sleep. Stage I is the lightest sleep, and fleeting dreams often occur during the transition between the awake state and stage I. Stage II, which accounts for 50% of NREM sleep, lasts approximately 15 to 20 minutes and is characterized by fragmented thoughts with distinctive EEG changes. Hypnotics commonly increase stage II. Stages III and IV are called delta or deep NREM sleep. This stage begins after approximately 30 to 45 minutes and lasts 40 to 70 minutes. During stages III and IV, blood pressure, cerebral glucose metabolism, and heart and respiratory rates are at the lowest in the circadian cycle. The total sleep pattern begins with light NREM, followed by deep NREM, and then by REM. This cycle lasts approximately 90 to 100 minutes and occurs four to six times per night. Box 46-2 summarizes the sleep stages.

insomnia has been defined as a condition lasting at least 3 weeks. Characteristics of chronic insomnia include somatized tension and acquired habits that prevent either the initiation or maintenance of sleep. Life stresses such as shift work, a family tragedy, or physical pain can exacerbate learned insomnia. As Regestein et al. reported in 1993, learned insomnia also may be associated with a hyperarousable state. This study, which examined daytime alertness in patients with primary insomnia, concluded that the measurement of hyperarousal, as measured by alpha waves on the electroencephalogram (EEG), may be useful to refine the description of insomnia populations. Insomnia can start with an initially stressful event, but the hyperarousable state of chronic insomniacs extends well beyond the heightened levels of stress.

Whether insomnia is labeled as transient or chronic, Dement and Vaughn (1999) argued that insomnia is significant for any length of time and needs thoughtful evaluation and possible treatment.

Many adolescents have an increased need for sleep, but they may have difficulty getting to sleep, difficulty awakening in the morning, or both. Adolescents who lead very busy lives may not get enough sleep.

Older adults may report early-morning awakening or general sleep disturbances. Central nervous system (CNS) changes are also thought to affect the sleep of the elderly. Frequent nighttime awakenings may result from secondary changes in circadian rhythms and loss of effective circadian regulation of sleep. Such changes can affect the quality of life. Many elderly patients exhibit daytime sleepiness, which shows that age does not diminish the need for sleep but reduces the ability to sleep.

BOX 46–2. STAGES OF SLEEP

Stage I
Light NREM: dreamlike state, lasts a few minutes

Stage II
Relatively light NREM: fragmented thoughts, lasts 15 to 20 min

Stage III–IV
Deep NREM: lowering of blood pressure, cerebral glucose metabolism, heart rate, and respiratory rate, starts 35 to 40 min after falling asleep and lasts 40 to 70 min

REM Sleep
Starts after 90 min of sleep, lengthens towards the end of the night
This cycle alternates throughout the night at intervals of 90 to 100 min, four to six times per night

Required amounts of sleep and of NREM sleep vary with age. Newborns sleep approximately 17 to 18 hours each day but have only two phases of sleep, NREM and REM. These two phases cycle every 60 minutes instead of every 90 minutes like adults. Children require 10 hours of sleep. In the early adult years, the total amount of sleep decreases to around 8 hours, which is normal for older adults as well as younger adults, with some variation among individuals. The total amount of REM sleep stays more constant at 15% to 20% throughout an adult's lifetime. Deep NREM sleep constitutes approximately 20% to 30% of total sleep in young children.

Insomnia is seen more often in people over age 65. The stages and architecture of sleep change, resulting in lighter stage II and decreases in stage III and IV sleep. This results in a decrease in deep NREM sleep. The circadian clock also becomes advanced, causing early-morning awakening in the elderly.

Light cues are important in the process of sleep. The absence of light cues tends to promote longer sleep–wake cycles. Two peaks in the daily need for sleep have been identified: the first at bedtime and the second in mid-afternoon. A study by Regestein et al. (1993) suggested that insomniacs have higher daytime alertness compared with normal subjects, which leads to higher hyperarousal states. Bonnet and Arand (1996) studied normal sleepers and found that sleep deprivation produces a primary hyperarousal state. They concluded insomniacs become more aware of small defects in the quality of sleep and daytime fatigue.

DIAGNOSTIC CRITERIA

Typical complaints of insomnia are malaise, fatigue, and too little sleep. These problems can lead to mild or moderate impairment in concentration and psychomotor abilities. The diagnosis is based on the patient's history, although a complete workup includes looking at all potential medical and psychological causes. The practitioner must determine the onset and duration of symptoms, along with the patient's regular sleeping schedule and general quality of sleep. The practitioner should interview other family members and significant others regarding any psychiatric or substance abuse problems of the patient. If the patient does not sleep alone, the practitioner also should elicit information from the bed partner. Questions about sleep also should be included in the review of systems; Box 46-3 lists suggested questions.

A complete physical examination is important to rule out medical causes of insomnia. Insomnia can be drug related (eg, stimulating medications or alcohol). Finally, the practitioner should investigate psychiatric causes of insomnia.

The use of sleep questionnaires or diaries and screening tools for depression and anxiety can add to the evaluation of insomnia. Sleep patterns may be measured by using a special wristwatch that measures wrist movements, a process called *actigraphy*. In humans, movement of the wrist throughout the night is much less frequent than during the day, which enables the practitioner to estimate the patient's sleep and wake times. This tool, however, is not very accurate in assessing total sleep time of insomniacs. Polysomnography (all-night monitoring of EEG, respiration, muscle activity, and other physiologic parameters) may reveal shallow sleep that is fragmented by multiple arousals. If the

---

BOX 46–3. SELECTED SLEEP HISTORY QUESTIONS

- What kind of work does the patient do? Is there shift work involved, and which shift?
- What time does the patient go to bed?
- What kind of bed partner does the patient have (restless, still, wakeful sleeper), if any?
- Does the patient regularly take any prescription or over-the-counter drugs?
- How many times during the night does the patient awaken?
- What does the patient do if he or she cannot go to sleep?
- Does the patient take daytime naps?

---

patient is depressed, the polysomnogram manifests changes in the REM latency stage. Polysomnograms are indicated when the primary suspected cause of insomnia is sleep apnea. The American Sleep Disorders Association, however, does not recommend the routine use of polysomnography, because a patient may not sleep normally at a sleep disorders center.

INITIATING DRUG THERAPY

In combination with behavioral management, the practitioner can consider using certain pharmacologic agents, but only with caution. In 1990, the NIH issued a consensus statement on the treatment of sleep disorders in older adults strongly recommending that hypnotic medications not become the mainstay of insomnia treatment because they are widely overused and have great potential to become habit-forming.

A wide range of therapies may be necessary to treat insomnia, because multiple causes of insomnia are the rule rather than the exception. Nonpharmacologic therapy includes evaluating for the key causes and treating with the appropriate intervention first: counseling, behavioral management, and lifestyle alterations for psychiatric problems. Patients with insomnia often have major depression, anxiety, obsessive disorders, or dysthymic disorders, and psychotherapy needs to focus on the specific psychiatric disorder.

In 1990, Everitt et al. conducted a comparison study of the clinical decision making of physicians and nurse practitioners when evaluating sleep. Overall, 60% of the nurse practitioners elicited a sleep history, but only 17% prescribed medications as first-line intervention. In contrast, 47% of physicians elicited a comprehensive sleep history and 46% prescribed pharmacologic treatment as the initial therapy. This suggests that a detailed sleep history is crucial to help the practitioner promote effective nonpharmacologic therapy, such as relaxation techniques, meditation, and exercise.

Reviewing proper sleep hygiene can enhance the patient's sleep pattern. A thorough examination of sleep hygiene issues can help identify important lifestyle changes that may enhance sleep, and its importance should not be underestimated. The practitioner should implement only one or two behavioral changes at a time. Follow-up and a strong patient–provider relationship are key. Additional measures, such as exposure to bright light, may help those with circadian rhythm disturbances. Light therapy can retrain the light pacemaker and may be effective for night-shift workers, travelers, and those with delayed or advanced sleep phase disorders.

Goals of Drug Therapy

The goal of pharmacotherapy is to promote the patient's ability to fall asleep, maintain sleep, or awaken refreshed. Another goal is to use the agent for as short a time as possible. Each drug has a different onset and duration of action. Selection of a pharmacologic agent depends on the origin of the insomnia (eg, pain, medical conditions), as previously discussed. If given in adequate doses, all hypnotics promote sleep; the key is to determine the *minimal* dose that will provide efficacy with few or no side effects.

Hypnotics, or sleeping pills, are the primary drugs used for insomnia, although other antidepressant agents also may be helpful (see Chapter 44). The practitioner should carefully consider selection of a hypnotic and prescribe use for as short a time as possible. Short-term use is defined as no more than 2 to 3 weeks combined with behavioral interventions; however, specific patients require occasional chronic hypnotic therapy. They may need to use a hypnotic agent two or three times a week over longer periods than 2 to 3 weeks. Careless use of sedative-hypnotics can be dangerous in patients with sleep apnea or a history of substance abuse.

The sedative-hypnotic drugs act by exerting a calming or anxiolytic effect, causing drowsiness and aiding in the sleep process. This group of drugs includes a variety of barbiturate, nonbarbiturate (eg, benzodiazepine agonists), and nonprescription drugs (eg, antihistamines).

Barbiturates

Barbiturates are structurally related to compounds that act throughout the CNS. They act at the level of the presynaptic and postsynaptic membranes and also have a cellular component to their action. It is unclear at which level the sedative-hypnotic effects occur. As a class, barbiturates usually are no longer recommended for the treatment of insomnia. This category of drugs includes amobarbital sodium (Amytal Sodium), butabarbital (secbutabarbital), mephobarbital (Mebaral), and secobarbital sodium (Seconal Sodium). The only barbiturates still indicated for use with insomnia are amobarbital sodium and butabarbital. Table 46-1 identifies starting doses and expected dosing ranges of the barbiturates still in use; however, with the advent of newer, safer agents, few reasons exist to use barbiturates to treat insomnia.

Adverse Events

The danger with barbiturates is that they can produce all levels of CNS depression, from mild sedation to coma to death. This is due to excessive sedation, short-term efficacy, and the potential for severe adverse reactions on withdrawal or overdose. Cardiac side effects include bradycardia, hypotension, and syncope. The respiratory system can experience hypoventilation, apnea, and respiratory depression. Barbiturate use rarely may cause Stevens-Johnson syndrome, which is sometimes fatal. Prolonged use of high doses in this class can lead to tolerance and physical or psychological dependence. Withdrawal syndrome can occur and is sometimes fatal.

Interactions

Serious side effects can result from drug/drug interactions with barbiturates. Alcohol may increase CNS depression. Barbiturates can decrease the effects of oral anticoagulants, corticosteroids, oral contraceptives and estrogens, beta-adrenergic blockers, theophylline (Slo-Phyllin), metronidazole (Flagyl), doxycycline (Vibramycin), griseofulvin (Grifulvin V), phenylbutazones, and quinidine (Cardioquin).

Benzodiazepines

Benzodiazepines are synthetically produced sedative-hypnotics. This group of structurally related chemicals selectively acts on polysynaptic neuronal pathways throughout the CNS. Benzodiazepines appear to enhance the effects of gamma-aminobutyric acid (GABA), an inhibitory neurotransmitter in the CNS. The subclass of benzodiazepines that is used to treat insomnia is believed to facilitate the effects of GABA in the ascending reticular activating system, which increases inhibition and blocks thalamic, hypothalamic, and limbic arousal.

When choosing a benzodiazepine, the practitioner should select an agent with an onset of action that matches the patient's problem, yet has a short duration of effect, lacks rebound insomnia, and causes few or no mental problems (eg, hangover, lack of motor coordination, or memory disturbance) (see Table 46-1). The prescriber also should consider the patient's metabolic requirements. Agents with a short half-life, such as alprazolam (Xanax), lorazepam (Ativan), or oxazepam (Serax), may be best for patients with depressed renal or hepatic function.

The benzodiazepines most commonly used for treating sleep disorders are divided into short-, intermediate-, and long-acting agents; flurazepam (Dalmane) and quazepam (Doral) are examples of the latter. Agents with short-term effects and short-term onset are best for patients who have difficulty falling asleep. The only agent in this category is triazolam (Halcion). Chloral hydrate also has a short-term effect but is intermediate in duration. Agents with intermediate onsets and usually longer half-lives are useful for patients with problems staying asleep. These include temazepam (Restoril) and estazolam (ProSom). Two agents with a rapid onset of action, flurazepam and quazepam, assist with falling asleep and also have a longer duration of action, which can assist in maintaining sleep.

Researchers are looking at the three GABA receptor subtypes in the hope of developing a benzodiazepine that can target the receptors with a agonist or partial agonist agent. This would ameliorate anxiety without causing corresponding sedation and motor impairment.

Adverse Events

Benzodiazepines have various actions, depending on their half-lives. Drugs of this class can produce drowsiness and

Table 46.1

Overview of Selected Drugs Used to Treat Insomnia

Generic (Trade) Name and Dosage	Selected Adverse Events	Contraindications	Special Considerations
Barbiturates			
amobarbital sodium (Amytal Sodium, Navamobarb) Start: 50–100 mg PO Range: 100–200 mg PO qhs	Somnolence, confusion, residual sedation nightmares, nausea and vomiting, constipation, diarrhea, hypoventilation *Potentially fatal side effects:* apnea, respiratory depression, Stevens-Johnson syndrome	Hypersensitivity to barbiturates, marked liver impairment, nephritis, respiratory disease, previous addiction to sedative-hypnotics, pregnancy	Use cautiously with acute or chronic pain, seizure disorder, lactation, fever, hyperthyroidism, diabetes mellitus, severe anemia, pulmonary or cardiac disease, asthma, impaired kidney function. For geriatric patients, reduce dosage and monitor carefully.
butabarbital (Secbutabarbital, Secbuto-arbiton) Start: 50 mg PO qhs Range: 50–100 mg PO qhs	Same as above plus circulatory collapse	Same as above	Same as above
Benzodiazepines			
alprazolam (Xanax) tablets 0.25, 0.5, 1, 2 mg Start: 0.25–0.5 mg PO tid; maximum 4 mg/d in divided doses Range: 0.25–2 mg tid–qd	*CNS:* transient mild drowsiness, sedation, depression, lethargy, apathy, fatigue, lightheadedness, disorientation, headache, mild paradoxical excitatory reaction in first 2 wk *GI:* constipation, diarrhea, dry mouth, nausea	Hypersensitivity to benzodiazepines, acute narrow-angle glaucoma, pregnancy, lactation	Use cautiously with impaired liver or kidney function, debilitation. Drug dependence and withdrawal result when abruptly discontinued, especially when used for longer than 4 mo. Use cautiously with elderly patients and gradually increase as tolerated.
estazolam (ProSom) tablets: 1, 2 mg Start: 0.5–1 mg qhs Range: 0.5–2 mg qhs	*CNS:* transient mild drowsiness, sedation lethargy, apathy, fatigue, lightheadedness, asthenia, mild paradoxical excitatory reaction in first 2 wk *GI:* constipation, diarrhea, dyspepsia *CV:* bradycardia, tachycardia *GU:* incontinence, urinary retention, changes in libido	Same as above	In addition to above: Drug–drug interactions: increased CNS depression with ethanol, omeprazole; increased effects of estazolam with cimetidine; increased sedative effects of estazolam with theophylline Drug dependence, withdrawal syndrome
flurazepam (Dalmane) 15–30 mg PO qhs Start: 15 mg PO qhs Range: 15–30 mg PO qhs	*CNS:* transient mild drowsiness, sedation lethargy, apathy, fatigue, lightheadedness, asthenia *GI:* constipation, diarrhea, dyspepsia *CV:* bradycardia, tachycardia *GU:* incontinence, urinary retention, changes in libido	Same as above	Same as above Has a long half-life
lorazepam (Ativan) 2–4 mg PO qhs	*CNS:* transient mild drowsiness, sedation, depression, lethargy, apathy, fatigue, lightheadedness, disorientation, headache, mild paradoxical excitatory reaction in first 2 wk *GI:* constipation, diarrhea, dry mouth, nausea	Same as above	Use cautiously with patients with impaired liver or kidney function. Debilitation, drug dependence and withdrawal result when abruptly discontinued, especially when used for more than 4 mo. Use cautiously with elderly patients and gradually increase as tolerated.
quazepam (Doral) 7.5–15 mg PO qhs	*CNS:* transient mild drowsiness, sedation, depression, lethargy, apathy, fatigue, lightheadedness, disorientation, restlessness, confusion *GI:* constipation, diarrhea *CV:* bradycardia, tachycardia *GU:* incontinence, urinary retention, changes in libido	Same as above	Drug–drug interactions: increased CNS depression with ethanol, quazepam; increased effects of cimetidine, disulfiram, oral contraceptives; increased sedative effects with theophylline
temazepam (Restoril) Start: 15 mg PO qhs Range: 15–30 mg PO qhs	Same as above	Same as above	Drug–drug interactions: increased CNS depression; increased sedative effects with theophylline

(continued)

Table 46.1

Overview of Selected Drugs Used to Treat Insomnia (*Continued*)

Generic (Trade) Name and Dosage	Selected Adverse Events	Contraindications	Special Considerations
triazolam (Halcion) Start: 0.125 mg PO qhs Range: 0.125–0.5 mg PO qhs *Elderly:* 0.125–0.25 mg PO qhs	Same as above	Hypersensitivity to benzo-diazepines, acute narrow-angle glaucoma, pregnancy, lactation	Same as above
Nonbenzodiazepines zolpidem (Ambien) Start: 10 mg PO qhs Range: 5–10 mg PO qhs	*CNS:* morning drowsiness, hangover, headache, dizziness, suppression of REM sleep *GI:* nausea	Hypersensitivity to zolpidem	Use cautiously in patients with acute intermittent porphyria, impaired hepatic or renal function, in addiction-prone patients, and in pregnancy and lactation.
zaleplon (Sonata) Start: 10 mg PO qhs Range: 5–20 mg PO qhs	*General:* back pain, chest pain *CV:* migraine *GI:* constipation, dry mouth *MS:* arthritis *CNS:* depression, hypertonia, nervousness *Derm:* rash, pruritus	Pregnancy, lactation	Pregnancy category B Pregnancy category C Patient must use just before bedtime because of quick onset.
modafinil (Provigil) 200 mg q am; maximum 400 mg daily	*Serious:* arrhythmias, syncope, visual changes, abuse/dependency *Common:* headache, nausea/vomiting, rhinitis, diarrhea	Sensitivity to class, caution with coronary artery disease, mitral valve prolapse, impaired liver failure	Start at 100 mg daily in elderly.

impaired motor function, which may be persistent. Other side effects can include short-term memory loss, confusion, and shakiness. Prolonged use of benzodiazepines can lead to physical dependency; abrupt discontinuance can trigger withdrawal symptoms. The newer agents in the class have fewer side effects, but for optimal therapy the drug selected should address the patient's specific sleep problem.

Interactions

Patients taking benzodiazepines must be cautious with the concomitant use of alcohol. Use of low-dose contraceptives may slightly decrease clearance of lorazepam and temazepam; the patient may need to alter the dosage or switch to oxazepam. Use of erythromycin (E-mycin) can decrease triazolam clearance by 50%; thus, prescribers must consider reducing the dosage of triazolam in patients taking both drugs concomitantly.

Benzodiazepine Receptor Agonists

This class of hypnotic has been developed to improve the safety profile of the barbiturate-type compounds. The benzodiazepine receptor agonists have one of the safest profiles in compounded medicines. They have a very short half-life with no development of tolerance after extended use. However, there is some question as to the potential for addiction to these drugs if used for longer than 4 weeks. All medications in this class have a half-life of 5 hours, therefore avoiding residual next-day effects. The drugs have greater receptor specificity of the GABAa BZ complex, which has been identified as being responsible for the sedative-hypnotic activity.

Zolpidem

A newer hypnotic agent that is a non-benzodiazepine is zolpidem (Ambien). Zolpidem also modulates the GABA receptors to suppress neurons, causing sedation and relaxation. Zolpidem has a strong hypnotic component and improves the overall quality of sleep while producing less daytime impairment than other hypnotics. Onset of action is rapid and it peaks quickly, which limits the hangover effects. Zolpidem has no carryover anxiolytic effects, which makes it less desirable for patients with concomitant anxiety.

Zaleplon

Another non-benzodiazepine is zaleplon (Sonata), which is chemically unrelated to benzodiazepines, barbiturates, and other drugs with hypnotic properties. Zaleplon is known to interact with the GABA-BZ omega 1 receptor, which causes sedation, muscle relaxation, and anticonvulsant activity. This interaction is also hypothesized to be responsible for the pharmacologic properties of benzodiazepines. Zaleplon works well for patients who have difficulty falling asleep. The onset of action is rapid, within 1 hour after oral administration, but the medication has a short half-life of 1 hour. Zaleplon can be taken as little as 5 hours before the scheduled wake-up time, with no lingering effects of daytime sedation. It may not be the agent of choice for patients who have difficulty maintaining sleep because of its short elimination half-life.

Antihistamines

Antihistamines are one of the most commonly used classes of over-the-counter sleep-inducing agents. The most commonly used agent is diphenhydramine (Benadryl). The main mechanism of diphenhydramine is unknown, but it chiefly acts as a CNS depressant. No scientific evidence exists in the literature supporting the use of diphenhydramine to relieve insomnia or prolong sleep.

Some side effects of diphenhydramine include excessive daytime drowsiness, impaired psychomotor function, and increasing tolerance to the drug. A better approach may be to use one of the sedating antidepressants before using a trial of diphenhydramine. If a patient taking diphenhydramine is stopped while driving under the influence of antihistamines, in many states he or she can be charged with driving under the influence (DUI).

Antidepressants

Sedating antidepressants also may be used in the treatment of insomnia, especially for patients with a subcomponent of depression. The most commonly used antidepressants in this category are imipramine (Tofranil), amitriptyline hydrochloride (Elavil), and nortriptyline (Pamelor). If the patient has a panic or anxiety subcomponent as well, some newer agents may assist with sleep. These include nefazodone hydrochloride (Serzone) and venlafaxine (Effexor), which also have some sedating as well as antianxiety effects (see Chapter 44).

Selecting the Most Appropriate Agent

As emphasized earlier, sedative-hypnotics should be used on a short-term basis only. For treatment of acute insomnia, the suggested duration of hypnotic use is 1 week, but some patients may need a longer course. Practitioners should schedule follow-up visits to monitor the effectiveness of therapy. The time between follow-up visits can vary, but in general they should fall between every 1 and 2 weeks. Starting the medication at the lowest possible dosage should minimize side effects. The practitioner should ask the patient about the effects the drug is having on sleep and daytime functioning. Changes may exist with dreaming, learning, memory, and adaptation to stress. Having the patient complete and bring in a sleep log for review can help pinpoint initial management needs and can continue to assist with evaluation for signs of improvement (Table 46-2 and Fig. 46-1). Pharmacologic therapy along with cognitive therapy should be initiated for at least 7 to 8 weeks (Cochran, 2003).

First-Line Therapy

As stated previously, the key to pharmacologic therapy is identifying the sleep defect. The practitioner should match the patient's need for an agent to both the classification of insomnia and the aspect of sleep that is altered. In cases of acute/transient and short-term insomnia, it is important to look for underlying physical and behavioral causes. Medications are indicated based on the subset of insomnia. When the problem is difficulty falling asleep, the agent should have a quick onset. Zaleplon is the best choice, given its quick onset and clean side effect profile. Patients with difficulty maintaining sleep require a drug with an extended duration, so the practitioner should base the choice of agent on the half-life to decrease side effects. Temazepam has a shorter half-life than other benzodiazepines.

Chronic insomnia often has underlying psychological components, and the best drug choice here usually is in the sedating-antidepressant class. Amitriptyline is the first choice, but it should be used cautiously.

Diphenhydramine is the only agent available to treat any sleep defect in pregnant women. The practitioner must assess the potential side effects and benefits for the both the fetus and mother before instituting therapy.

Second-Line Therapy

If the patient continues to have insomnia with first-line treatments, alternatives include switching to a benzodiazepine agent or using the other benzodiazepine receptor agonist, zolpidem. Again, the prescriber must consider the kind of sleep defect being treated and select a drug with the appropriate onset and half-life.

Third-Line Therapy

The practitioner should reassess the insomnia situation for patients who fail to respond to both first- and second-line therapies. Insomnia that has become chronic benefits most from continual evaluation and behavioral therapy along with the smallest dose possible of hypnotic medication. An antidepressant may play a key role at this level.

Special Population Considerations
Pediatric

Use of barbiturates in the pediatric population is usually limited to those who have seizure disorders. In general,

Table 46.2

Recommended Order of Treatment for Sleep Disorders

Order	Agents	Comments
First line	Nonbenzodiazepine hypnotics (zolpidem, zaleplon)	Cleanest side effect profiles
Second line	Benzodiazepine hypnotics	Consider short-acting agents, especially with patients who have renal or hepatic problems.
	Short half-lives: alprazolam, lorazepam, oxazepam	
	Rapid onset: triazolam, flurazepam, quazepam	
	Long half-lives: temazepam, estazolam	
Third line	Barbiturates, antidepressants	May have serious side effects
		Helpful when treating concomitant depression

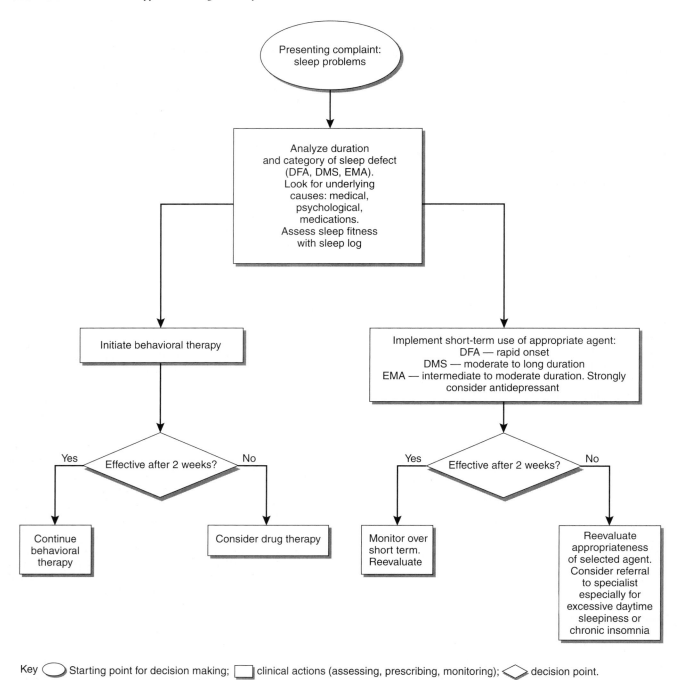

Figure 46–1 Treatment algorithm for insomnia (DFA: difficulty falling asleep, DMS: difficulty maintaining sleep, EMA: early morning awakening).

benzodiazepines are not indicated for children younger than 15 years of age. Caution is necessary when very young patients use antihistamines because of potential delirium or paradoxical excitation. Melatonin may be considered as treatment for a limited time (Ivanenko, Crabtree, Tauman, & Gozal, 2003).

Geriatric

It is important to evaluate the geriatric patient for underlying comorbidities that contribute to insomnia. Treating the underlying illnesses is important and may assist with re-establishing good sleeping patterns. Extreme caution is

essential when prescribing hypnotic medications to elderly patients because these drugs can increase the potential for delirium and subsequent falls. In 1996, Zisselman et al. analyzed hospital costs for the elderly when sedative-hypnotics were used to promote sleep. They found a statistically significant increase in cost resulting from increased length of hospital stay for patients who took sedative-hypnotics. In 1990, Shorr et al. analyzed the quantity of prescriptions given to elderly patients along with the number of refills. Their concern was the overuse of the agents and the risks at which they place elderly patients over time. They found that many different physician groups were overprescribing sedative-hypnotics.

Consistent monitoring of the elderly patient can be extremely important, especially when a long-acting hypnotic is prescribed. Antihistamines can cause delirium or paradoxical excitation.

Women

No sex differences exist in terms of the pharmacokinetics of the various agents used to treat sleep disorders. Caution is essential when prescribing all drugs to lactating women and women of childbearing age. Both antihistamines and zaleplon are pregnancy category C, whereas the barbiturates and benzodiazepines are pregnancy category D. Zolpidem, in category B, is in the lowest-risk pregnancy category.

MONITORING PATIENT RESPONSE

Sleep can be a reliable predictor of psychological and physical health. Differences in monitoring are related to whether the insomnia is an acute or chronic problem. Brief episodes of acute insomnia can warrant treatment, with the goal of preventing it from progressing and becoming chronic. A short course (up to 4 weeks) of sedative-hypnotic therapy is the current treatment of choice. Cognitive therapy can be included to improve the chance of an optimal response.

When insomnia becomes a chronic problem, consistent interaction between the patient and health care provider is important, as is the use of behavioral techniques. With chronic insomnia, issues of drug tolerance for the older benzodiazepines and rebound insomnia usually become paramount.

Current FDA guidelines allow only short-term prescription of hypnotic agents. Tolerance and rebound insomnia have been cited as problems associated with these agents, but few studies have borne this out. In practice, many people take low-dose hypnotic agents for long periods with few side effects. Caution is warranted, however, if a patient requires escalation of a previously stable dosage. Careful analysis of changes in the patient's sleep patterns is necessary in this event.

Patient Education

Patient education plays a key role in the treatment of insomnia. A key side effect of most hypnotic agents is excessive drowsiness or hangover from the medication. The clinician must alert the patient to this possibility and monitor the side effects of each agent prescribed (see Tables 46-1 and 46-2).

Patient-Oriented Information Sources

Major sleep centers across the country have web sites that are useful resources for patients and health care providers. These sites can provide information about diagnosis of sleep disorders and current research and therapies (Box 46-4).

Nutrition/Lifestyle Changes

Good sleep habits include setting a routine bedtime, getting regular exercise, using the bed for sleeping only, and getting in bed only when ready for sleep. Stimulants such as caffeine, alcohol, and excess fluids should be avoided before bedtime.

BOX 46–4. SLEEP WEB SITES

National Center on Sleep Disorders Research (NCSDR)
http://www.nhlbi.nih.gov/about/ncsdr

National Heart, Lung, and Blood Institute (NHLBI) Health Information Network
http://www.nhlbi.nih.gov

Restless Legs Syndrome Foundation
http://www.rls.org

Sleep Foundation
http://sleepfoundation.org

Complementary and Alternative Medications

Herbs and botanicals are often used as a "natural" way of promoting sleep. However, this is not without a certain danger, especially if these treatments are taken in conjunction with prescription drugs. Older patients are often likely to use herbal treatments: in 1997, it was reported that up to 3 million individuals over 65 use such therapy (Desai & Grossberg, 2003).

Melatonin, an endogenous hormone, is synthesized by the pineal gland from tryptophan. It is mainly secreted at night and its level peaks during normal sleep hours. In 1997, Lavie and Peretz discovered that endogenous melatonin opens the nocturnal sleep gate and increases nocturnal melatonin secretion. Melatonin does not induce sleep but acts as a gatekeeper in the cascade of events that enables the CNS to favor sleep over wakefulness. Most studies have examined the use of melatonin to treat sleep disorders resulting from jet lag; few have looked at the use of melatonin in primary insomnia. A 1996 study by Attenburrow and Dowling on melatonin and primary insomnia examined healthy volunteers compared with the elderly. Through analysis of urine concentrations of endogenous melatonin, the study found that the elderly volunteers had a lower concentration of the melatonin metabolite and a delayed onset to peak secretion. These findings supported the possibility that some patients, especially those with delayed sleep phase insomnia, may benefit from the administration of exogenous melatonin; however, further study is necessary.

Valerian is a traditional sleep remedy that is derived from the perennial herb *Valeriana officinalis*. The direct physiologic activity is mediated by the active sesquiterpene components of the volatile oil. This creates a synergistic effect with neurotransmitters such as GABA and produces a direct sedative effect. Effective dosage ranges from 300 to 600 mg of the valerian root; 2 to 3 g of the dried root is soaked in a cup of hot water for 10 to 15 minutes, and the patient then drinks the tea. Administration can occur 30 minutes to 2 hours before bedtime. Significant herb or drug interactions have not been reported by the German E Commission.

RESTLESS LEG SYNDROME AND PERIODIC LIMB MOVEMENT DISORDER

Restless leg syndrome (RLS) and periodic limb movement disorder (PLMD) are neurologic disorders. RLS is characterized by an intense need to move the legs, accompanied by paresthesias and dysesthesias that worsen usually in the evening. Sometimes the sensations can occur in other large muscle groups, but most often the legs are involved. Moving around relieves the feeling, but only for a short time, as the sensation soon returns. These sensations interfere with sleep. PLMD is characterized by episodes of highly repetitive and stereotyped limb movements only during sleep.

Both disorders interfere with sleep and contribute to sleep deprivation and decreased alertness and daytime function. Indications are that 2% to 15% of the population may experience RLS, but the diagnosis is made rarely in primary care.

CAUSES

As a primary CNS disorder, RLS can be found in patients with end-stage renal disease, anemia, and sometimes in pregnancy (Gigli et al., 2004). RLS can also be hereditary or drug induced. Allen (2004) argued that iron deficits may be a strong cause of RLS, altering the iron–dopamine linkage, but this hypothesis needs further study.

PATHOPHYSIOLOGY

RLS and PLMD are sensory-motor disorders that are not well understood. Primary RLS has a strong hereditary component, with 40% to 60% of patients having a familial association. Onset of familial RLS is before the age of 30 years, and studies have indicated the strong action of a single major gene (Zucconi & Ferini-Strambi, 2004). Secondary RLS can be associated with neuropathies from changes in axonal and small-fiber neural pathways. Patients with rheumatoid arthritis and diabetes also have shown a greater prevalence of RLS, again presumably from changes due to neuropathy. Parkinson's disease is frequently associated with RLS, pointing to a commonality in reduced dopaminergic functioning (Zucconi & Ferini-Strambi, 2004). A strong link has been established to the dopaminergic system by the positive response to the dopaminergic agonist classification of drugs (Allen, 2004).

DIAGNOSTIC CRITERIA

RLS is diagnosed primarily through the patient history. Clinical criteria have been established by the International Restless Legs Syndrome Study Group (Box 46-5).

PLMD is associated more with stereotyped repetitive movements of limbs (legs alone, or legs more than arms) that occur only during sleep. PLMD is generally diagnosed only through a sleep test.

BOX 46–5. DIAGNOSTIC CRITERIA FOR RESTLESS LEG SYNDROME

1. A compelling urge to move limbs associated with paresthesias/dysesthesias
2. Motor restlessness as evidenced by:
   - Floor pacing
   - Tossing and turning in bed
   - Rubbing legs
3. Symptoms worse or exclusively present at rest with variable and temporary relief by activity
4. Symptoms worse in the evening and at night

The physical examination for RLS and PLMD should include a full neurologic examination with emphasis on the spinal cord and peripheral nerve function. A vascular examination is also necessary to rule out vascular disorders. Secondary causes of RLS should be evaluated by a serum ferritin level and serum chemistry to rule out uremia and diabetes. Polysomnography is not routinely indicated for RLS but can be helpful to establish the diagnosis. Box 46-6 lists other possible diagnoses.

INITIATING DRUG THERAPY

Pharmacotherapy should be tailored for each patient. Patients with relatively mild symptoms may not need medications. Nonpharmacologic therapy should be instituted, including mental alerting activities and cessation of alcohol, nicotine, and caffeine. Any medications that may precipitate or worsen RLS symptoms, such as antidepressants and dopamine antagonists, should be avoided. Correction of underlying serum iron deficits may be helpful. Short-term studies have shown that drug therapy has significant benefits, but little is known about long-term treatment. A 3-year study of 70 patients by Clavadetscher et al. (2004) found that a good long-term response with

---

BOX 46–6. DIFFERENTIAL DIAGNOSES FOR RLS AND PLMD

1. Nocturnal Leg Cramps
   - Painful, palpable involuntary muscle contractions
   - Focal with sudden onset
   - Unilateral
2. Akathisia
   Excessive movement without accompanying sensory complaints
3. Peripheral Neuropathy
   - Usually tingling, numbness, or pain sensations
   - Not associated with motor restlessness
   - Not helped by movement
   - Evening or nighttime worsening

drug therapy can be achieved in 80% of patients. This study helped to establish the benefit of pharmacologic therapy in RLS.

Goals of Drug Therapy

The goal of drug therapy is to calm the restless legs or periodic limb movements. Some patients can be refractory to pharmacologic treatment but still achieve partial relief of their symptoms. Pharmacologic agents for RLS include dopaminergic agents, dopamine agonists, opioids, benzodiazepines, anticonvulsants, and iron (see Table 46-1). Other than dopamine agonists, many of these drugs are being used in an "off label" manner.

Dopaminergic Agents

These drugs are dopamine precursor combinations such as carbidopa–levodopa (Sinemet). These agents are useful for intermittent RLS because they have a quicker onset than dopamine agonists. This is useful for relief of sleep onset insomnia and RLS that occurs long car or airplane journeys. Dosage of these agents is lower than used for Parkinson's disease.

Adverse Events

The carbidopa–levodopa agents may actually worsen RLS symptoms in up to 80% of patients. The therapeutic effect may be reduced if taken with high-protein food. Insomnia, sleepiness, and gastrointestinal problems are other adverse events.

Dopamine Agonists

The initial dopamine agonists used for RLS were bromocriptine and pergolide, which were prone to side effects. The newer dopamine agonists are not ergot based; while they have fewer side effects, they can cause initial nausea and lightheadedness, nasal stuffiness, edema, and rarely daytime sleepiness. Increasing the dose slowly will help to mitigate these side effects. See Chapter 41 for further discussion.

Opioids

Opioids are reserved for the most severe cases of RLS or PLMD that are refractory to treatment with other pharmaco-

logic agents. This class of medications can be used on a daily or intermittent basis. Clinical experience by sleep experts suggests that only a few patients will require opioids (Silber, 2004).

Benzodiazepines

Benzodiazepines (see Table 46-1) are used concomitantly with a dopamine agonist when use of a sole agent has failed. Clinical experience is particularly crucial with clonazepam and temazepam. These drugs may be helpful for patients who cannot tolerate the other medications. Caution is necessary when using these agents with the elderly, and they can cause daytime sleepiness and cognitive impairment.

Anticonvulsants

Anticonvulsants are considered when dopamine agonists have failed and in patients who describe the RLS discomfort as pain. Gabapentin is helpful in patients with RLS and peripheral neuropathy. It is useful in treatment of daily RLS. As with the dopamine agonists, lower dosages of gabapentin (100 to 600 mg one to three times daily) can be successful. The side effect of hypersomnia often limits the dosage. Other side effects can include nausea, sedation, and dizziness. See Chapter 43 for further discussion.

Selecting the Most Appropriate Agent

For treatment purposes, RLS can be classified as *intermittent* (not often enough to require drug therapy), *daily* (troublesome enough to require drug therapy), and *refractory* (not adequately treated by a dopamine agonist). The ideal agent will minimize or abate the symptoms of RLS. No one pharmacologic agent appears to help all patients, and often a combination of medications is needed. The severity of RLS can vary, and pharmacologic treatment needs to be individualized. See Box 46-7 for considerations when selecting a pharmacologic agent (Fig. 46-2).

First-Line Therapy

Dopaminergic antagonists such as low-dose carbidopa–levodopa should be reserved for patients with intermittent RLS. The first choice of therapy for daily RLS is one of the dopamine agonists. The largest placebo-controlled trial has been conducted on ropinirole (Requip) (Trenkwalder, Gar-

---

BOX 46–7. CONSIDERATIONS IN PHARMACOLOGIC AGENT SELECTION IN RLS

Age of patient	Benzodiazepenes can cause cognitive impairment in elderly.
Severity of symptoms	Mild symptoms: no medication, or levodopa or dopamine agonist
	Severe symptoms: strong opioid
Frequency/regularity of symptoms	Patients with infrequent symptoms may benefit from prn medication.
Presence of pregnancy	No safety and efficacy clinical trials on treatment of RLS with medications in pregnancy
Renal failure	Need to decrease dosage if drugs are renally excreted

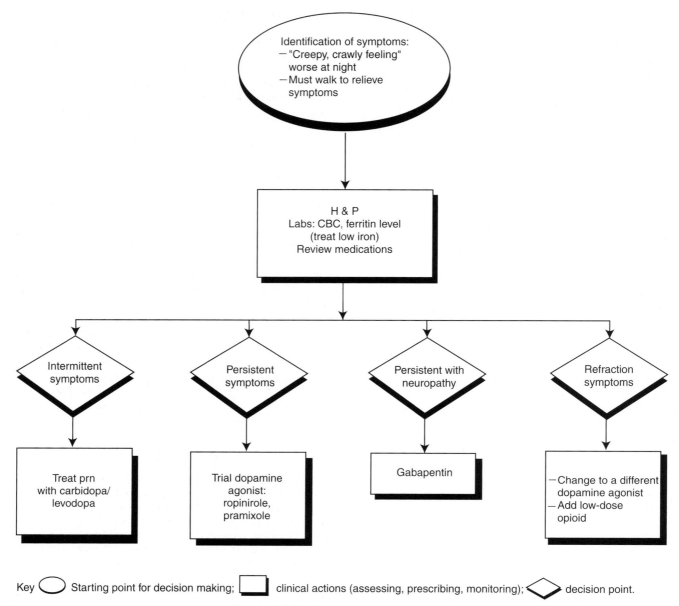

Figure 46–2 Algorithm for treatment of RLS.

cia-Borreguero, & Montagna, 2004). Other medications in this class include pramipexole (Mirapex) and pergolide (Permax). Nausea, dizziness, dyskinesia, and somnolence are potential side effects of both the dopaminergic antagonists and agonists.

Second-Line Therapy

Pharmacologic agents approved for neuropathic pain such as gabapentin (Neurontin) can be used alone or in conjunction with other agents. It is especially helpful for patients who describe RLS symptoms as painful. Other anticonvulsant agents such as carbamazepine (Tegretol) can be considered, but the older agents carry an increased risk of side effects such as dizziness, drowsiness, and lack of coordination. Patients also may experience nausea with these older agents. An opioid or opioid receptor agonist, tramadol (Ultram), may be added or used alone at low dose. If either

the anticonvulsant or opioid fails, a repeat trial of dopamine agonists should be attempted (Silber, 2004).

Third-Line Therapy

Patients who continue to have symptoms may be refractory to treatment. Therapeutic doses may not have been obtained, or the patients could not tolerate the side effects of the medications. Substitution of different medications in the dopamine agonist class or adding higher-potency opioids should be considered. Consultation with a sleep specialist should be considered.

Monitoring Patient Response

Most patients will have remittance of symptoms with the first therapeutic dose of medication. This supports the theory that dopaminergic abnormality is a cause of this disorder. Another indicator of improvement is a decrease in excessive daytime sleepiness from lack of REM sleep. Patients need to be monitored for side effects of the pharmacologic agents. The long-term efficacy of these pharmacologic agents is uncertain, and monitoring for relapse of symptoms is important. It is also important to monitor for dependence when benzodiazepines or opioids are used.

PATIENT EDUCATION

Many patients who have RLS use over-the-counter sleep medications, and poor sleep hygiene may contribute to the lack of sleep in RLS sufferers. Implementing cognitive sleep hygiene techniques may provide a modest improvement in short-term sleep symptoms (Edinger, 2003). Patients should inform all of their health care providers about their RLS diagnosis, and health care providers should be aware that the patient's inability to keep his or her limbs still is not due to lack of cooperation. Improper restraint of patients with this syndrome has resulted in mortality and morbidity.

Drug Information

A higher dosage of ropinirole (Requip) is needed compared to pramipexole (Mirapex) to achieve the same therapeutic effect. This may contribute to side effects and tolerability of the drug.

Patient-Oriented Information Sources

The Restless Legs Syndrome Foundation supports research and provides information for patients and health care providers. Extensive international research is also being conducted on this serious sleep problem (see Box 46-4).

NARCOLEPSY

Narcolepsy is a sleep disorder caused by malfunctions in the primary brain mechanism that induces sleep. Individuals with narcolepsy achieve REM sleep in less than a minute, bypassing the other sleep stages. The other features of narcolepsy include excessive daytime sleepiness, cataplexy (attacks of muscle weakness), sleep paralysis, and hypnagogic hallucinations. Narcolepsy is the second leading cause of excessive daytime sleepiness and has an overall incidence in the world of 0.2 to 1.6 per thousand individuals (Stanford Center for Narcolepsy, 2004). Narcolepsy can have a dramatic impact on virtually all areas of life.

CAUSES

Narcolepsy usually starts in the second or third decade of life, but it has been identified in children as young as 3 years old. Excessive daytime sleepiness or cataplexy may be the first symptoms, but most often cataplexy is delayed 2 to 3 years. Cataplexy attacks are often precipitated by highly specific situations or triggers of strong emotions. Hypnagogic hallucinations can be present but are rarely the first manifestation of narcolepsy.

PATHOPHYSIOLOGY

The pathophysiology of narcolepsy is not well understood. It appears to be a disease where daily periods of internal clock-dependent alerting appear to be missing. Narcolepsy is sporadic and without a familial predisposition. Some evidence has shown a genetic component with specific human leukocyte antigens. It is possible that hypocretin-producing cells express toxins that provoke an autoimmune cascade that triggers narcolepsy.

DIAGNOSTIC CRITERIA

The International Classification of Sleep Disorders states that individuals with narcolepsy have excessive sleepiness, cataplexy, sleep paralysis, and hypnagogic hallucinations (the "narcoleptic tetrad"). Many narcolepsy patients also have disrupted nighttime sleep and automatic behaviors. Not all patients with narcolepsy have all symptoms of the narcoleptic tetrad, but excessive sleepiness is present in virtually every patient.

Silber et al. (2002) researched whether including HLA typing provides a higher reliability of diagnosis. They used clinical and neurophysiologic data to evaluate 69 patients in four categories: definite narcolepsy, probable narcolepsy with two subgroups (confirmed by laboratory study), and probable narcolepsy (clinical). Seventy-four percent of patients had a positive HLA that helped to confirm the diagnosis of narcolepsy.

INITIATING DRUG THERAPY

There is no cure for narcolepsy, and pharmacologic therapy must be initiated to control the attacks. Evaluation for cataplexy, hypnagogic hallucinations, and sleep paralysis is important to identify the best agent for treatment. Most often antidepressants are used to block the REM paralysis of cataplexy. The mainstay of pharmacologic therapy until now has been amphetamines and amphetamine-like drugs such as methylphenidate (Ritalin). These are used to combat the abnormal sleepiness. A new pharmacologic agent that accomplishes the same effect as the amphetamines is modafinil (Provigil). This was approved in 1998 and is a non-amphetamine drug.

Goals of Drug Therapy

Pharmacologic therapy should be titrated to promote the optimal dose of stimulation. The health care provider needs to work with the patient to identify personal treatment goals such as staying awake in a classroom or social situation or while driving. The main goal is to achieve as normal a life as possible, staying awake in situations of normal daily living.

Psychostimulants

Modafinil (Provigil) is a psychostimulant that has unique properties to promote wakefulness. The potential for abuse of modafinil is much lower than with other stimulants, although it still needs to be monitored. The mechanism of action of modafinil is not well understood, but it appears to attenuate the central alpha-1 adrenergic system. The primary sites of action are the subregions of the hippocampus, the centrolateral nucleus of the thalamus, and the central nucleus of the amygdale. Modafinil can produce euphoria and psychoactive effects similar to other CNS stimulants. Absorption of the drug occurs rapidly, with peak plasma concentration in 2 to 4 hours and a half-life of 15 hours. Distribution of the drug is throughout the tissues, and it moderately bound to plasma proteins. The drug is metabolized in the liver and excreted in the urine. In a recent study of the long-term efficacy of modafinil conducted by the Narcolepsy Multicenter Study Group (Mitler, Harsh, Hirshkowitz, & Guilleminault, 2000), the most common adverse side effects of the drug were headache, nausea, nervousness, and anxiety. Most side effects are mild to moderate and transient (see Table 46-1).

SPECIAL POPULATIONS

Pediatrics

Modafinil has not been studied in children. The alternative drug of choice would be methylphenidate.

Geriatrics

Care must be taken when prescribing modafinil to the elderly population. The oral clearance of modafinil is reduced in the elderly by 20% to 50%. Renal failure does not influence the pharmacokinetics of the drug but does increase the inactive metabolite accumulation. Liver impairment can reduce the modafinil clearance and double serum concentrations.

MONITORING PATIENT RESPONSE

Narcolepsy is a life-long disease process, and patients must use the medications for their entire lives. Patient response is monitored by improvement in the disease's severity. Achieving the goals identified by the patient can help to improve compliance.

PATIENT EDUCATION

Patients and their families need to be aware of all available options to treat narcolepsy. Psychological distress is a consequence, not the cause, of the disease. Discussion of potential side effects of the drugs is important for compliance. Offering counseling and support groups when necessary is important.

Drug Information

Patients who are switched from amphetamine stimulants to modafinil may not experience the same euphoric effects, and this may make the switch undesirable to the patient. Amphetamines tend to produce a feeling of improved well-being and arousal, while modafinil increases arousal without a change in affect.

Patient-Oriented Sources

Health care providers and patients can find information about narcolepsy from a variety of sources. Online support groups exist (see Box 46-4).

■ Case Study 1

S.H., age 47, reports difficulty falling asleep and staying asleep. These problems have been ongoing for many years, but she has never mentioned them to her health care provider. She has generally "lived with it" and self-treated the problem with over-the-counter Tylenol PM. Currently she is also experiencing perimenopausal symptoms of night sweats and mood swings. Current medical problems include hypertension controlled with medications. Past medical history includes childhood illnesses of measles, chickenpox, and mumps. Family history is positive for diabetes on the maternal side and hypertension on the paternal side. Her only medication is an angiotensin-converting enzyme inhibitor and diuretic combination for hypertension control. She generally does not like taking medication and does not take any other over-the-counter products.

Diagnosis: Insomnia

→ 1. List specific goals of therapy for S.H.

→ 2. What drug therapy would you prescribe? Why?

→ 3. What are the parameters for monitoring the success of the therapy?

→ 4. Discuss specific patient education based on the prescribed therapy.

→ 5. List one or two adverse reactions for the selected agent that would cause you to change therapy.

6. What would be the choice for second-line therapy?

7. What over-the-counter and/or alternative medicines might be appropriate for this patient?

8. What dietary and lifestyle changes might you recommend?

9. Describe one or two drug/drug or drug/food interactions for the selected agent.

■ Case Study 2

J.F., age 73, reports a "funny sensation in my legs at night." To get rid of this sensation, she has to move. She can sleep only 2 or 3 hours at a time before the sensation wakes her up. This problem has been ongoing from her early twenties but has steadily worsened with age. She finds herself walking around a lot in the early evening. She has tried to self-treat the problem with over-the-counter Tylenol PM. Current medical problems include hypertension, hyperlipidemia, coronary artery disease, and depression. Family history is positive for coronary artery disease on the paternal side. Medications include Prinivil 10 mg qd, Zocor 40 mg qd, Lexapro 10 mg qd, and ASA 81 mg qd. She does not want to take any more medication but wants to help her legs stop moving at night.

Diagnosis: Restless leg syndrome

1. List specific goals of therapy for J.F.

2. What drug therapy would you prescribe? Why?

3. What are the parameters for monitoring the success of the therapy?

4. Discuss specific patient education based on the prescribed therapy.

5. List one or two adverse reactions for the selected agent that would cause you to change therapy.

6. What would be the choice for second-line therapy?

7. What over-the-counter and/or alternative medicines might be appropriate for this patient?

8. What dietary and lifestyle changes might you recommend?

9. Describe one or two drug/drug or drug/food interactions for the selected agent.

■ Case Study 3

D.W., age 35, mentions during a routine visit that he has been having horrible nightmares. He states that during the nightmares he is aware of his surroundings but just cannot seem to move. He also reports excessive daytime sleepiness, which he cannot understand since he is usually in bed by 10 PM and doesn't get up until 8 AM. This has been a problem for about the past 6 months. His family history is negative for any illnesses and sleep disorders. He does not take any medications or over-the-counter products routinely.

Diagnosis: Possible narcolepsy

(Continued)

■ Case Study 3 (*Continued*)

➤ 1. List specific goals of therapy for D.W.

➤ 2. What drug therapy would you prescribe? Why?

➤ 3. What are the parameters for monitoring the success of the therapy?

➤ 4. Discuss specific patient education based on the prescribed therapy.

➤ 5. List one or two adverse reactions for the selected agent that would cause you to change therapy.

➤ 6. What would be the choice for second-line therapy?

➤ 7. What over-the-counter and/or alternative medicines might be appropriate for this patient?

➤ 8. What dietary and lifestyle changes might you recommend?

➤ 9. Describe one or two drug/drug or drug/food interactions for the selected agent.

Bibliography

Starred references are cited in the text.

Ahmed, M. (2004). Circadian rhythm sleep disorders. [On-line] Available: http://sleepmed.bsd.chicago.edu/circadianrhythm.html.

*Allen, R. (2004). Dopamine and iron in the pathophysiology of restless legs syndrome (RLS). *Sleep Medicine, 5*, 385–391.

Anacoli-Israel, S. (1997). Sleeping problems in older adults: putting myths to bed. *Geriatrics, 52*(1), 20–28.

*Attenburrow, M., & Dowling, B. (1996). Case-control study of evening melatonin concentration in primary insomnia. *British Medical Journal, 312* [On-line], 1263. Available: http://gw5.epnet.com

Bateson, A. (2004). The benzodiazepine site of the $GABA_A$ receptor: an old target with new potential? *Sleep Medicine, 5*(Suppl. 1), S9–S15.

Belinger, J., Fins, A., Goeke, J., McMillan, D., Gersk, T., Krystal, A., & McCall, W. (1996). The empirical identification of insomnia subtypes: a cluster analytic approach. *Sleep, 19*, 398–411.

Boeve, B., Silber, M., & Ferman, T. (2003). Melatonin for treatment of REM sleep behavior disorders in neurologic disorders: results in 14 patients. *Sleep Medicine, 4*, 281–284.

*Bonnet, M., & Arand, D. (1996). The consequences of a week of insomnia. *Sleep, 19*, 453.

Brostrom, A., Stromberg, A., Dahlstrom, U. & Fridlund, B. (2004). Sleep difficulties, daytime sleepiness, and health-related quality of life in patients with chronic heart failure. *Journal of Cardiovascular Nursing, 19*(4), 234–242.

Brown, D. (1999). Managing sleep disorders: solutions in primary care. *Clinician Reviews, 9*(10), 51–69.

Bruck, D. (2001). The impact of narcolepsy on psychological health and role behaviours: negative effects and comparisons with other illness groups. *Sleep Medicine, 2*, 437–446.

Buyssee, D. (2004). Insomnia, depression, and aging: assessing sleep and mood interactions in older adults. *Geriatrics, 59*(2), 47–51.

*Clavadetscher, S., Gugger, M., & Bassetti, C. (2004). Restless legs syndrome: clinical experience with long-term treatment. *Sleep Medicine, 5*, 495–500.

Clinical Pharmacology (2004). *Melatonin.* [On-line]. http://www.gsm.com.

Clinical Pharmacology (2004). *Valerian, valeriana officinalis.* [On-line]. http://www.gsm.com.

*Cochran, H. (2003). Diagnose and treat primary insomnia. *Nurse Practitioner, 28*(9), 13–27.

Dato, C. (1999). Sleeping disorders. In J. Singleton, S. Sandowski, C. Green-Hernandez, et al. (Eds.), *Primary care* (pp. 686–691). Philadelphia: Lippincott Williams & Wilkins.

*Dement, W., & Vaughan, C. (1999). *The promise of sleep.* New York: Dell.

Desai, A. K., & Grossberg, G. T. (2003). Herbals and botanicals in geriatric psychiatry. *American Journal of Geriatric Psychology, 11*, 498–506.

Drake, C., Roehers, T., & Roth, T. (2003). Insomnia cause, consequences, and therapeutics: an overview. *Depression and Anxiety, 18*, 163–176.

Dunn, S. (1998). Insomnia. In *Primary care consultant* (pp. 320–321). St. Louis: Mosby.

*Edinger, J. (2003). Cognitive and behavioral anomalies among insomnia patients with mixed restless legs and periodic limb movement disorder. *Behavioral Sleep Medicine, 1*(1), 37–53.

*Everitt, D. E., Avorn, J., & Baker, M. W. (1990). Clinical decision-making in the evaluation and treatment of insomnia. *American Journal of Medicine, 89*, 357–362.

*Gigli, G., Adorati, M., Dolso, P., et al. (2004). Restless legs syndrome in end-stage renal disease. *Sleep Medicine, 5*, 309–315.

Gillian, J. C., & Byerley, W. (1990). The diagnosis and management of insomnia. *New England Journal of Medicine, 322*, 239–248.

Hauri, P. (1987). Specific effects of sedative/hypnotic drugs in the treatment of incapacitating chronic insomnia. *American Journal of Medicine, 83*, 925–926.

Hauri, P. (1998). Sleep disorders: insomnia. *Clinics in Chest Medicine, 19*, 157–168.

Hening, W., Walthers, A., Allen, R., et al. (2004). Impact, diagnosis and treatment of restless legs syndrome (RLS) in a primary care population: the REST (RLS Epidemiology, Symptoms, and Treatment) primary care study. *Sleep Medicine, 5*, 237–240.

*Ivanenko, A., Crabtree, V., Tauman, R., & Gozal, D. (Jan/Feb. 2003). Melatonin in children and adolescents with insomnia: a retrospective study. *Clinical Pediatrics*, 51–58.

Karch, A. (2000). *2001 Lippincott's nursing drug guide.* Philadelphia: Lippincott Williams & Wilkins.

Katz, D., & McHorney, C. (2002). The relationship between insomnia and health-related quality of life in patients with chronic illness. *Journal of Family Practice, 51*(3), 229. [On-line]. Available: http//www.jfponline.com/content/2002/03/jfp_0302_00229.asp.

Kryger, M., Monjan, A., Bliwise, D., & Ancoli-Israel, S. (2004). Sleep, health and aging: bridging the gap between science and clinical practice. *Geriatrics, 59*(1), 24–30.

Late-life insomnia: psychiatric and medical comorbidity common. (2004). *Geriatric Psychopharmacology Update, 8*(7), 1–7.

*Lavie, P. (1997). Melatonin: role in gating nocturnal rise in sleep propensity. *Journal of Biological Rhythms, 12*, 657–668.

Leger, D., Guilleminault, C., Biol, D., et al. (2002). Medical and socioprofessional impact of insomnia. *Sleep, 25*(6), 625–629.

Lindberg, E., & Gisiason, T. (2000). Epidemiology of sleep-related obstructive breathing. *Sleep Medicine Reviews, 4*(5), 411–433.

*Lustbader, A., Morgan, C., Pelayo, R. et al. (1997). Psychiatry: insomnia. In L. Rucker (Ed.), *Essentials of adult ambulatory care* (pp. 607–615). Baltimore: Williams & Wilkins.

Lyznicki, J., Doege, T., Davis, R., & Williams, M. (1998). Sleepiness, driving, and motor vehicle crashes. *Journal of the American Medical Association, 279*, 1908–1913.

Medical Letter of Drugs and Therapeutics. (1995). (Issue 962). Melatonin: therapeutic uses [On-line]. Available: http://gw5. epnet.com

Mendelson, W., Thompson, C., & Firanko, T. (1996). Adverse reactions to sedative/hypnotics: three years' experience. *Sleep, 19*, 702–706.

*Mitler, M., Harsh, J., Hirschowitz, M., & Guilleminault, C. (2000). Long-term efficacy and safety of modafinil (Provigil) for the treatment of excessive daytime sleepiness associated with narcolepsy. *Sleep Medicine, 1*, 231–243.

Morrish, E., King, M., Smith, I., & Shneerson, J. (2004). Factors associated with a delay in the diagnosis of narcolepsy. *Sleep Medicine, 5*, 37–41.

National Center on Sleep Disorders Research and Office of Prevention, Education, and Control. (1997). *Problem sleepiness in your patient.* U.S. Department of Health and Human Services. NIH Publication No. 97-4073.

National Center on Sleep Disorders Research and Office of Prevention, Education, and Control. (2000). *Restless legs syndrome: detection and management in primary care.* U.S. Department of Health and Human Services. NIH Publication No 00-3788.

National Center on Sleep Disorders Research and Office of Prevention, Education, and Control. (1997). *Working group report on problem sleepiness.* U.S. Department of Health and Human Services.

National Heart, Lung, and Blood Institute Working Group on Insomnia. (1999). Insomnia: assessment and management in primary care. *American Family Physician, 59*, 3029–3038.

National Institutes of Health Consensus Development Program. (1990). *The treatment of sleep disorders of older people.* NIH Consensus Statement. [On-line]. Available: http://home.mdconsult.com/das/article/body/jorg

National Sleep Foundation. (1999). *Is melatonin a treatment for insomnia and jet lag?* [On-line]. Available: http://www.sleepfoundation.org/publications/melatonin.html

National Sleep Foundation (2004). *Melatonin: The basic facts.* [On-line]. Available http://www.sleepfoundation.org/publications/melatoninthefact.cfm.

National Sleep Foundation. (2002). Sleep in America poll. [On-line]. Available: http://www.sleepfoundation.org.

Neubauer, D. (1999). Sleep problems in the elderly. *American Family Physician, 59*, 2551–2558.

Pagel, J., Zafralotifi, S., & Zammit, G. (1997). How to prescribe a good night's sleep. *Patient Care, 31*(4), 87–1002.

Quan, S., & Zee, P. (2004). A sleep review of systems: evaluating the effects of medical disorders on sleep in the older patient. *Geriatrics, 59*(3), 37–42.

*Regestein, Q., Dambrosia, J., Hallett, M., et al. (1993). Daytime alertness in patients with primary insomnia. *American Journal of Psychiatry, 150*, 1529–1534.

Requip improves symptoms of restless legs syndrome at 1 week, studies show. (July 5, 2004). *Health & Medicine Week,* 952.

Roth, T., & Drake, C. (2004). Evolution of insomnia: current status and future directions. *Sleep Medicine, 5*(Suppl. 1), S23–S30.

Schwartz, J., Feldman, N., Fry, J., & Harsh, J. (2003). Efficacy and of modafinil for improving daytime wakefulness in patients treated previously with psychostimulants. *Sleep Medicine, 4*, 43–49.

*Shorr, R., Bauwens, S., & Landefeld, C. S. (1990). Failure to limit quantities of benzodiazepine hypnotic drugs for outpatients: placing the elderly at risk. *American Journal of Medicine, 89*, 725–732.

*Silber, M. (2004). Calming restless legs. *Sleep, 27*(5), 839–841.

*Silber, M., Krahn, L., & Olson, E. (2002). Diagnosing narcolepsy: validity and reliability of a new diagnostic criteria. *Sleep Medicine, 3*, 109–113.

*Silva, J., Chase, M., Sartorius, N., & Roth, T. (1996). Special report from a symposium held by the World Health Organization and the World Federation of Sleep Research Societies: an overview of insomnias and related disorders—recognition, epidemiology, and rational management. *Sleep, 19*, 412–416.

*Sleep Facts and Stats (2004). 2004 Sleep in America Poll. [On-line]. Available: http://www.sleepfoundation.org/NSAW 1/pk_sleepfacts.cfm.

Smith, D., Simonson, W., & Zammit, G. (1999, March). *New ideas for the management of sleep disorders.* Symposium conducted at the meeting of the American Medical Directors Association Annual Symposium, Orlando, Florida.

Stanford Center for Narcolepsy. (2004). http://med.stanford.edu/school/Psychiatry/narcolepsy/symptoms.html.

Terzano, M., Rossi, M., Palomba, V., et al. (2003). New drugs for insomnia: comparative tolerability of zopiclone, zolpidem and zaleplon. *Drug Safety, 26*(4), 261–282.

Trenkwalder, C., Garcia-Borreguero, D., Montagna, P., et al. (2004). Therapy with ropinirole: efficacy and tolerability in RLS 1 Study Group. *Journal of Neurological and Neurosurgical Psychiatry, 75*(1), 92–97.

Trevena, L. (2004). Practice corner: sleepless in Sydney—is valerian an effective alternative to benzodiazepines in the treatment of insomnia? *ACP Journal Club, 141*(1), 14.

Vitiello, M., Larsen, L., & Moe, K. (2004). Age-related sleep change: gender and estrogen effects on the subjective-objective sleep quality relationships of healthy, noncomplaining older men and women. *Journal of Psychosomatic Research, 56*, 503–510.

Wallace, K., & Morbunas, A. (1997). Commonly abused prescription sedative-hypnotic drugs. *Topics in Emergency Medicine, 19*(4), 23–24.

Wagner, D. (1996). Sleep disorders I: disorders of the circadian sleep–wake cycle. *Neurologic Clinics, 14*, 651–670.

What are the risks when elderly patients combine herbal and prescription medications? (2004). *Geriatric Psychopharmacology Update, 8*(1), 1–6.

*Zisselman, M., Rovner, B., Yuen, E., & Louis, D. (1996). Sedative-hypnotic use and increased hospital stay and costs in older people. *Journal of the American Geriatric Society, 44*, 1371–1374.

*Zucconi, M., & Ferini-Strambi, L. (2004). Epidemiology and clinical findings of restless legs syndrome. *Sleep Medicine, 5*, 293–299.

Visit the Connection web site for the most up-to-date drug information.

47

ATTENTION-DEFICIT/ HYPERACTIVITY DISORDER

■ TARA WEIKEL CHAPMAN AND ANDREW M. PETERSON

Attention-deficit/hyperactivity disorder (ADHD) has become a commonly diagnosed condition among today's children. Hallmark symptoms include hyperactivity, impulsivity, and inattention. The American Psychiatric Association (APA) estimated in the *Diagnostic and Statistical Manual of Mental Disorders* (DSM-IV) that 3% to 5% of school-aged children had ADHD. The disorder is more common in boys than in girls, with a ratio ranging from 4:1 to 9:1 (APA, 2000; Spencer et al., 2002). Research is increasingly revealing that ADHD also affects adults, with estimates of prevalence ranging from 2% to 7% (Wender, 1995). This realization is changing perceptions of ADHD because it is becoming imperative to understand the disorder as diagnosed in adulthood.

Researchers have found that many of the core symptoms of ADHD are treatable. Treatment should be individualized to the patient's symptoms. The treatment plan usually is multimodal. Even when treatment begins early in childhood, the patient may still show symptoms in adolescence or adulthood. The outcome of the childhood disorder is uncertain, as is determining which children will have the disorder.

CAUSES

Many causes of ADHD have been suggested, but none has yet to be accepted. Evidence suggests that the disorder may have a genetic link (Farone & Biederman, 1994). Estimates are that children who have a sibling with ADHD have a two to three times greater chance of being diagnosed with ADHD (Dulcan et al., 1997). Although genetic factors appear to play a role, no genes have been isolated to allow diagnosis of the disorder before symptoms appear. ADHD has been associated with the dopamine transporter gene and the dopamine D_4 gene (Adler & Chua, 2002; Daley, 2004). Other theories involve dietary intake of certain chemicals and sugars, but data are lacking.

PATHOPHYSIOLOGY

Neurotransmitter dysfunction is a proposed mechanism for ADHD, and several different pathways for this dysfunction have been studied. These include a baseline norepinephrine

level that is too high, a central epinephrine level that is too high, a problem with the functioning of epinephrine in the peripheral system, or problems involving dopamine receptors or dopamine-mediated functions (Pliszka, McCracken, & Maas, 1996). All these mechanisms may work together to cause ADHD symptoms. The complete pathophysiologic process of these mechanisms is not completely understood, but there appears to be a connection between the D_4 receptor and activity of the major neurotransmitters, epinephrine, norepinephrine and dopamine (Adler and Chua, 2002; Daley, 2004).

Risk factors may be involved in the development of ADHD, although many are only associations and do not indicate that ADHD is present. The practitioner must ascertain the patient's drug history and examine for visual disturbances and hearing dysfunction as possible causes of the child's behavior (Dulcan et al., 1997). A rare genetic disorder, generalized resistance to thyroid hormone, has been associated with ADHD (Hauser et al., 1993). Fragile X syndrome, fetal alcohol syndrome, glucose-6-phosphate dehydrogenase deficiency, and phenylketonuria are also associated risks for development of ADHD (Dulcan et al., 1997). Limited numbers of cases have been associated with other risk factors, including such pregnancy variables as poor maternal health, young maternal age, maternal use of alcohol or cigarettes, toxemia or eclampsia, postmaturity, and extended labor (Dulcan et al., 1997; Markussen et al., 2003). Medical conditions and malnutrition in infancy may also play a role in ADHD, although this has not been proved (Dulcan et al., 1997).

DIAGNOSTIC CRITERIA

The diagnostic criteria for ADHD are listed in Box 47-1. Children are required to show symptoms by 7 years of age, and most children show symptoms for many years before the diagnosis is made (APA, 2000). For a definitive diagnosis, the child also must show symptoms in more than one setting, such as both at home and in school. The adult with ADHD may display symptoms both at home and work. Adult patients also have trouble maintaining relationships as a result of their inattentiveness. In both children and adults, the

BOX 47–1. CRITERIA FOR DIAGNOSING ATTENTION-DEFICIT/HYPERACTIVITY DISORDER

A. Either (1) or (2)
1. Six (or more) of the following symptoms of inattention have persisted for at least 6 months to a degree that is maladaptive and inconsistent with developmental level:

   Inattention
   a. often fails to give close attention to details or makes careless mistakes in schoolwork, work, or other activities
   b. often has difficulty sustaining attention in tasks or play activities
   c. often does not seem to listen when spoken to directly
   d. often does not follow through on instructions and fails to finish schoolwork, chores, or duties in the workplace (not due to oppositional behavior or failure to understand instructions)
   e. often has difficulty organizing tasks and activities
   f. often avoids, dislikes, or is reluctant to engage in tasks that require sustained mental effort (such as schoolwork or homework)
   g. often loses things necessary for tasks or activities (eg, toys, school assignments, pencils, books, or tools)
   h. is often easily distracted by extraneous stimuli
   i. is often forgetful in daily activities
2. Six (or more) of the following symptoms of hyperactivity-impulsivity have persisted for at least 6 months to a degree that is maladaptive and inconsistent with developmental level:

   Hyperactivity
   a. often fidgets with hands or feet or squirms in seat

   b. often leaves seat in classroom or in other situations in which remaining seated is expected
   c. often runs about or climbs excessively in situations in which it is inappropriate (in adolescents or adults, may be limited to subjective feelings of restlessness)
   d. often has difficulty playing or engaging in leisure activities quietly
   e. is often "on the go" or often acts as if "driven by a motor"
   f. often talks excessively

   Impulsivity
   g. often blurts out answers before questions have been completed
   h. often has difficulty awaiting turn
   i. often interrupts or intrudes on others (eg, butts into conversation or games)

B. Some hyperactive–impulsive or inattentive symptoms that caused impairment were present before age of 7 years.
C. Some impairment from the symptoms is present in two or more settings (eg, at school [or work] and at home).
D. There must be clear evidence of clinically significant impairment in social, academic, or occupational functioning.
E. The symptoms do not occur exclusively during the course of a Pervasive Developmental Disorder, Schizophrenia, or other Psychotic Disorder and are not better accounted for by another mental disorder (eg, Mood Disorder, Anxiety Disorder, Dissociative Disorder, or Personality Disorder).

From American Psychiatric Association. (2000). *Diagnostic and statistical manual of mental disorders* (4th ed., text revision). Washington, DC: Author, with permission.

---

symptoms must interfere with the person's ability to function. The criteria are further broken into subtypes, and based on the symptoms, the patient's disorder is coded (Box 47-2).

Diagnosing ADHD in a child may be difficult because children often behave differently in the health care setting, therefore making it impossible for the provider to observe symptoms. For this reason, the practitioner must use other methods to evaluate behavior. Such methods include rating scales, which usually are administered by parents and teachers. All scales are similar, but each has its own criteria and rating system. Some commonly used scales include the parent-completed Child Behavior Checklist (Achenbach, 1991; Biederman et al., 1993), the Teacher Report Form of the Child Behavior Checklist (Achenbach, 1991; Edelbrock, Costello, & Kessler, 1984), the Conners Parent and Teacher Rating Scale (Ullmann et al., 1985), the Barkley Home Situations Questionnaire and School Situations Questionnaire

(Barkley, 1990), and the Child Attention Problems Profile (Barkley, 1990; Barkley et al., 1989). These rating scales have been found to be accurate measures of ADHD behavior (Dulcan et al., 1997). Practitioners may use these rating scales to follow a child's behavior after the initial diagnosis of ADHD.

Making the initial diagnosis also requires detailed parent interviews that focus on a family history of ADHD or other psychiatric disorders, psychosocial adversity (eg, poverty, parental psychopathology or absence, family conflict), school behavior, learning, attendance and test reports, and medical evaluations (Dulcan et al., 1997).

A confounding factor in the diagnosis is the probability of comorbid disorders. Mood disorders, anxiety disorders, learning disorders, and communication disorders are more common in the child with ADHD (APA, 2000). Laboratory findings, physical examination, and evaluation of concurrent

BOX 47–2. DIAGNOSTIC AND STATISTICAL MANUAL OF MENTAL DISORDERS—IV: CODING BASED ON TYPE

314.01 Attention-Deficit/Hyperactivity Disorder, Combined Type: if both Criteria A1 and A2 are met for the past 6 months

314.00 Attention-Deficit/Hyperactivity Disorder, Predominantly Inattentive Type: if Criterion A1 is met but Criterion A2 is not met for the past 6 months

314.01 Attention-Deficit/Hyperactivity Disorder, Predominantly Hyperactive-Impulsive Type: if Criterion A2 is met but Criterion A1 is not met for the past 6 months

Coding note: For individuals (especially adolescents and adults) who currently have symptoms that no longer meet full criteria, "In Partial Remission" should be specified

From American Psychiatric Association. (2000). *Diagnostic and statistical manual of mental disorders* (4th ed., text revision, p. 93). Washington, DC: Author, with permission.

---

medical problems cannot be used to confirm the diagnosis. Minor physical anomalies such as hypertelorism, a highly arched palate, and low-set ears may be more common in this population (APA, 1994), but such characteristics do not mean that the child has ADHD. Many children diagnosed with ADHD can be expected to have some impaired social functioning in adult life.

The diagnosis of ADHD in the adolescent is less clear since as an ADHD child matures into adolescence, the symptoms change (Nahlik, 2004). Moodiness, laziness, boredom, or impatience may be common symptoms in the ADHD adolescent but may also be typical adolescent behavior or even another mood disorder.

Diagnosis in an adult consists of a complete psychiatric evaluation; childhood history; information from spouse or significant others, parents, or employers; and a review of school records. A medical history and physical examination can be used to rule out comorbid conditions. As with childhood diagnosis, rating scales and questionnaires may also be used (Weiss & Murray, 2003), such as the Conners Abbreviated Teacher's Rating Scale and the Wender Utah Rating Scale.

Practitioners cannot use a patient's response to stimulant therapy to determine ADHD status. A child not diagnosed with ADHD has the same response of reduced hyperactivity, impulsivity, and inattentiveness as a child diagnosed with ADHD (Goldman et al., 1998).

INITIATING DRUG THERAPY

Many practitioners today follow a multimodal treatment plan. Multimodal treatment plans seem logical because dif-ferent symptoms respond to different types of treatment. The Multimodal Treatment Study (MTA) showed that children receiving intensive behavioral management combined with medication fared better than those receiving intensive behavioral management alone (Anonymous, 1999). The core symptoms of the disorder (ie, inattention, hyperactivity, and impulsivity) respond to medication, with or without the behavioral intervention. Behavioral symptoms seem to respond to environmental modification, while skills in sports, academics, and social situations may not respond to medication or behavior modification. Relationship problems usually are can be treated through psychotherapy.

Nonpharmacologic aspects of a multimodal treatment plan consist of behavior modification, parent training, family therapy, social skills training, academic skills training, individual psychotherapy, cognitive behavior modification, and therapeutic recreation. These are discussed further in the Nutrition/Lifestyle section later in this chapter.

Goals of Drug Therapy

When a child is diagnosed with ADHD, questions arise regarding the outcome of this disorder. Parents want to know if there is a cure and, if so, what treatment will increase the chance for cure. However, the outcome of ADHD cannot be predicted, and the child will not always "grow out of it." Three outcomes have been identified. The first possible outcome is developmental delay, which occurs in approximately 30% of diagnosed children; this means that the child will outgrow the symptoms. The second possible outcome, which occurs in 40% of children, is continual display, which is marked by adult life with ADHD. Continual display may lead to social and emotional difficulties. The third possible outcome is developmental decay (30% of children with ADHD), which involves the continual display of core ADHD symptoms along with pathologic conditions such as substance abuse and antisocial personality disorder. Developmental decay is the most severe outcome (Sudak, 1998).

Medication therapy is usually one of the first options in treating patients newly diagnosed with ADHD. Pharmacotherapy offers several alternatives. The classes of medications used include stimulants, nonstimulant medications such as atomoxetine (Strattera), bupropion (Wellbutrin), tricyclic antidepressants (TCAs), selective serotonin reuptake inhibitors (SSRIs), monoamine oxidase (MAO) inhibitors, alpha-adrenergic agonists, and neuroleptics. Although it is not clear how these medications actually affect the primary symptoms of ADHD, it is known which neurotransmitters they affect (Table 47-1).

The long-term benefits of medication therapy have not been determined. It is clear that they work in the short term to improve symptoms, but there is a lack of long-term studies (Goldman et al., 1998). The following information addresses concerns for the pediatric population using these medications.

Stimulants

A stimulant is usually the first-choice medication, based on 60 years of research and clinical experience (Dulcan et al., 1997). Daley (2004) reported that nearly 70% of patients

Table 47.1

Neurotransmitters Affected by Pharmacotherapy

	NE	DA	5-HT	Comments
methylphenidate		I		Blocks reuptake
dextroamphetamine	I, ↑	I		Blocks reuptake of NE, DA
				Causes release of NE
atomoxetine	↑			Blocks reuptake of NE
pemoline		I		Unknown, thought to be DA
clonidine				Stimulates alpha$_2$ adrenoceptors
bupropion	I	I	I	Weak blocker of NE, 5-HT
nortriptyline	↑		↑	5-HT > NE
imipramine	↑		↑	5-HT > NE

NE, norepinephrine; DA, dopamine; 5-HT, serotonin; I, inhibits; ↑, increases concentrations in system.

will respond to stimulant therapy. The most commonly used stimulants are methylphenidate (Ritalin, Concerta), amphetamine salts (Adderall, Dexedrine), and pemoline (Cylert).

Dosage

Amphetamines should be started at the lowest dosage and titrated upward until the desired response is seen. Dosing is usually based on weight and titrated to a dosage that controls the symptoms of ADHD. Table 47-2 lists medications and their dosages.

For immediate-release methylphenidate, the typical starting dose for children under age 6 is 5 mg before breakfast and 5 mg at lunch. The dose may be increased by 5 to 10 mg weekly, with a maximum recommended dose of 60 mg. Long-acting preparations are available if the immediate-release formulation is impossible or inconvenient to give, or if rebound is a problem. The long-acting methylphenidate Ritalin LA should be started after the patient is taking 20 mg of the immediate-release preparation. For patients taking 10 to 20 mg of immediate-release methylphenidate daily, Concerta 18 mg or Metadate ER 10 or 20 mg may also be used.

Mechanism of Action

As mentioned previously, it is not clear how stimulants help to reduce the core symptoms of ADHD. In addition to increasing levels of epinephrine and norepinephrine, these agents also can bind to central dopamine receptors and increase the systemic levels of dopamine.

Adverse Events

The primary adverse events related to stimulant therapy include palpitations, tachycardia, elevated blood pressure, and potentially arrhythmias. Changes in appetite, nausea, vomiting, and other gastrointestinal disturbances may occur. The neurologic adverse events range from headache and insomnia to seizure activity, particularly in patients predisposed to seizures.

In general, adverse events are manageable, results are quick and predictable with the first dose, and the medications are easy to titrate (Buitelaar et al., 1995). The adverse events of the stimulants, such as headaches, dizziness, appetite suppression, tics, dyskinesias, sleep disturbances, abuse potential, and in

particular growth retardation (below height or weight on normal growth charts), may be of concern. One study found a significant difference in growth between patients who took stimulants and those who did not. Other studies have shown a decrease in height or weight in patients taking stimulants. The clinician must assess the growth progress, need for continued treatment, and overall functioning of the ADHD patient every 1 to 3 months (Daley, 2004).

Determining the long-term effect of stimulants on children is difficult. To minimize these effects, it is reasonable for the patient to take drug-free periods, usually over the summer. These periods also allow for reassessment of ADHD. Because children frequently seem to show symptoms in structured settings such as school, weekend "drug holidays" are also reasonable, permitting dosage adjustments and disease assessment. Rebound hyperactivity may be more prominent. No studies have been done to compare the effectiveness of weekend holidays versus summer holidays.

While there is concern about the potential for addiction and future substance abuse, a review by Kollins (2003) suggested that the abuse potential for methylphenidate is less than that of other stimulants, such as cocaine. Other data indicate that there is less likelihood of substance abuse later in life when ADHD children take stimulant medication (Daley, 2004).

The stimulants are contraindicated in children with certain comorbid disorders. Practitioners should not prescribe methylphenidate to patients with marked anxiety, tension, or agitation; glaucoma; or a history of tics or Tourette's syndrome. Pemoline should not be prescribed to patients with impaired hepatic dysfunction. Dextroamphetamine is contraindicated in patients with cardiovascular disease, hypertension, arteriosclerosis, hyperthyroidism, glaucoma, or substance abuse.

Nonstimulant Medications

Atomoxetine

One of the newest nonstimulant medications is atomoxetine (Strattera). This agent is the first nonstimulant with an FDA-approved indication for treating ADHD. It is currently the only agent approved for the treating adult ADHD. This agent also is not a controlled substance, and existing data suggest no real potential for abuse or diversion.

Table 47.2

Overview of Agents Used to Treat ADHD

Generic (Trade) Name and Dosage	Selected Adverse Events	Contraindications	Special Considerations
atomoxetine (Strattera) Children <12 y: 0.5 mg/kg/day for 3 days Increase up to 1.2 mg/kg/day Adolescents/adults >70 kg: 40 mg initially 80 mg target dose with a maximum of 100 mg/d	Increased heart rate and blood pressure, abdominal pain, decreased appetite Urinary retention in adults	Patients on monoamine oxidase inhibitors, narrow-angle glaucoma	Atomoxetine does not appear to promote the development of new tics and therefore may be a good choice for patients unable to take stimulant medications due to pre-existing tics.
bupropion (Wellbutrin) Children: Start: 50 mg qd Range: 3–6 mg/kg/d Adults: 100 mg, bid; then increase 100 mg, tid; max. 4.5 mg/d	Insomnia, anorexia, dizziness, anxiety, confusion, xerostomia, constipation, nausea, agitation, fever, headache, vomiting, seizures	Seizure disorders, bulimia, anorexia nervosa Within 14 d of MAOIs	Monitor weight.
clonidine (Catapres) Children: Start: 0.05 mg hs Range: 0.55 mg tid–qid Adults: 0.1 mg bid; max. 2–4 mg/d	Dizziness, drowsiness, anxiety, confusion, xerostomia, constipation, impotence, nausea, hypotension	Hypersensitivity to clonidine	Monitor blood pressure (standing and supine), respiratory rate and depth, and heart rate.
dextroamphetamine (Dexedrine) Children >6 y and adults: 5 mg once or twice a day Increase weekly by 5 mg to a maximum dose of 40 mg/d	Nervousness, insomnia, arrhythmias, dry mouth, anorexia	Cardiovascular disease, hypertension, arteriosclerosis, hyperthyroidism, glaucoma, alcohol or drug abuse	Monitor growth and CNS activity. High abuse potential Not recommended for children <3 y Avoid late evening dosing.
imipramine (Tofranil) Children: Start: 10–25 mg/d Range: 1–3 mg/kg/d Adults: 25 mg, tid–qid; max. 300/d	Dizziness, drowsiness, xerostomia, constipation, nausea, fever, headache, weight gain, skeletal weakness, increased appetite	Same as above	Monitor blood pressure, pulse, ECG, CBC, mental status. May cause allergic reaction in patients with sulfa allergy Increases photosensitivity Lowers seizure threshold
methylphenidate (Ritalin) Children >6 y: 0.5–1 mg/kg/d initially; 5 mg before breakfast and lunch. Increase weekly by 5–10 mg to a maximum of 60 mg/d Adults: 10–15 mg/d up to 40–60 mg/d in divided doses, bid–tid	Tachycardia, nervousness, insomnia, anorexia, dizziness, drowsiness	Marked anxiety, tension, or agitation Glaucoma History of tics or Tourette's syndrome in patient or family	Monitor blood pressure, weight, height, heart rate, tics, sleep habits May potentiate effects of anticoagulants and anticonvulsants Abuse potential Not recommended for children <6 y
methylphenidate extended release (Ritalin SR, Concerta) Ritalin SR: May be used when 8h dose of SR-titrated equals 8h dose of regular Concerta: Start 18 mg in AM; can increase to max. 54 mg in 18-mg increments weekly. If on immediate release already: 10 mg bid–tid (start with 36 mg qd) or 15 mg bid–tid (start with 54 mg qd).			
nortriptyline (Pamelor) Children: Start: 10–25 mg/d Range: 1–3 mg/kg/d Adults: 25 mg, tid–qid; max. 150 mg/d	Dizziness, drowsiness, xerostomia, constipation, nausea, fever, headache, weight gain, skeletal weakness, urinary retention	Acute post-myocardial infarction During or within 14 d of MAOIs	Monitor blood pressure, pulse, mental status, weight. Increases risk of arrhythmia in patients receiving thyroid replacement therapy
pemoline (Cylert) Children >6 y and adults: 37.5 mg/d initially Increase weekly by 18.75 mg to maximum of 112.5 mg/d	Insomnia, anorexia	Impaired hepatic dysfunction	Use caution with antiseizure medications. Monitor liver enzymes. Monitor weight.

Mechanism of Action

Unlike stimulant medications, atomoxetine inhibits the reuptake of norepinephrine by inhibiting the presynaptic norepinephrine transporter (Christman et al., 2004). The agent has a relatively short half-life in normal metabolizers (5 hours) and an extended half-life in poor metabolizers (21 hours). The primary route of hepatic metabolism is the CYP2D6 pathway, and about 7% of Caucasians and less than 1% of Asians are considered poor CYP2D6 metabolizers (Christman et al., 2004).

Dosage

In children, the starting dosage is 0.5 mg/kg/day; the dose is increased after a minimum of 3 days to a target dose of 1.2 mg/kg/day. For adolescents and adults over 70 kg, the starting dose is 40 mg; the dose is increased to an 80-mg target dose after a minimum of 3 days. The maximum recommended dose is 1.4 mg/kg/day for children and 100 mg for adolescents and adults; dosages should be adjusted only after 2 to 4 weeks of treatment at the lower dose. The capsules are supplied in 10, 18, 25, 40, and 60 mg. The agent can be given once a day or in divided doses.

Since this agent undergoes significant metabolism via the CYP 2D6 system, slow metabolizers or patients taking agents with strong CYP 2D6 effects (eg, paroxetine, fluoxetine), the starting dose should be maintained for up to 4 weeks before dose adjustments are made. Patients with significant hepatic impairment should be started on a dose 50% of the usual starting dose.

Time Frame for Response

Atomoxetine is rapidly absorbed from the gastrointestinal tract, leading to 63% bioavailability in extensive metabolizers and 94% bioavailability in poor metabolizers. The onset of action is quick, and dose adjustments are made in the first week. Despite the short half-life in extensive metabolizers, the duration of activity remains consistent throughout the day.

Contraindications

Atomoxetine should not be taken with MAO inhibitors because it increases synaptic norepinephrine concentrations. Further, due to the risk of angle closure, this agent should not be administered to patients with narrow-angle glaucoma.

Adverse Events

The increase in norepinephrine leads to an increase in blood pressure and heart rate, so this agent should be used cautiously in hypertensive patients or those with underlying cardiovascular disorders. In adults, there was a 3% rate of urinary retention or hesitation. Other common adverse effects include abdominal pain, vomiting, decreases in appetite, headache, irritability, and dermatitis. Atomoxetine dose not appear to promote the development of new tics and therefore may be a good choice for patients who cannot take stimulant medications due to pre-existing tics.

Interactions

This agent is a substrate of the CYP2D6 hepatic enzyme system, and levels of this agent can be increased when CYP2D6 inhibitors are administered.

Antidepressants

Efficacy of treatment with TCAs has been established, but not as substantially as with the stimulants (Spencer et al., 1996). TCAs are most often used as second-line agents in patients who experience depression or other significant side effects with the stimulants, who do not respond to the stimulants, or who have tics or Tourette's syndrome (Riddle et al., 1988; Spencer et al., 1993). They have a longer duration of action, so the patient does not need to take a dose during school hours. Also, no rebound effects are seen (Dulcan et al., 1997).

The TCAs also were effective in treating the core symptoms of ADHD. The sole controlled study that has been conducted using desipramine found that desipramine was significantly more effective for treating core symptoms than placebo (Wilens et al., 1995). The rest of the drugs, including bupropion, fluoxetine (Prozac), and venlafaxine (Effexor), have been studied only in open trials. Some clinicians have used them based on personal experience.

Dosage

Doses should be divided and the medication should be kept away from children because of the risk of overdose. Deaths have been reported in children taking desipramine (Norpramin); hence, imipramine (Tofranil) and nortriptyline (Pamelor) are the first-choice TCAs (Dulcan et al., 1997).

Contraindications

Adequate monitoring is necessary, and practitioners must measure baseline vital signs and electrocardiograms (Table 47-3). Cardiac disease, a history of sudden death in the family, unexplained fainting, cardiomyopathy, or early cardiac disease may contraindicate the use of TCAs (Dulcan et al., 1997).

Table 47.3

Recommended Order of Treatment for ADHD

Order	Agents	Comments
First line	Stimulants	Methylphenidate works quickly with first dose, is available in extended release, and is easy to titrate. If patient does not respond, dextroamphetamine or pemoline can be tried. Pemoline takes 3–4 wk to work.
Second line	Nonstimulants	Nortriptyline works in 1–3 wk. Imipramine works in 2–4 wk. Similar side effect profiles.
Third line	Bupropion	Takes 4 wk to show effects. May impair cognitive skills.

Adverse Events

Toxicity manifests as irritability, mania, agitation, anger, aggression, forgetfulness, or confusion. Blood tests are necessary to determine whether the patient is experiencing toxicity (Dulcan et al., 1997).

When discontinuing TCA therapy, the prescriber needs to taper the dose over 2 to 3 weeks to prevent anticholinergic withdrawal symptoms such as nausea, cramps, vomiting, headaches, and muscle pains. Of concern with the TCAs is the potential for cardiac side effects, overdose, sedation, anticholinergic effects, and decreasing efficacy with continued use (Dulcan et al., 1997).

Bupropion

Like the stimulants, bupropion (Wellbutrin) increases the reuptake of dopamine, but bupropion also is a weak blocker of serotonin and norepinephrine. Again, it is unknown how these effects reduce ADHD symptoms. Studies show that the overall efficacy of bupropion does not differ from that of methylphenidate (Barrickman et al., 1995). Adverse events are transient, which last only for the first 2 weeks of treatment (Barrickman et al., 1995), include drowsiness, fatigue, nausea, anorexia, dizziness, "spaciness," anxiety, headache, and tremor. Rash and urticaria were also seen (Conners et al., 1996). The most significant problem is a decrease in the seizure threshold, most often seen in patients with eating disorders (Dulcan et al., 1997). Bupropion also may exacerbate tics (Spencer et al., 1993). Data in children are limited.

Table 47-2 lists the appropriate dose for bupropion. The dosage should not exceed 150 mg/day because of the increased risk for seizures with higher doses. Because of this increased risk, bupropion is contraindicated in patients with a history of seizure disorders.

Clonidine

Clonidine (Catapres) has been found to help with mood, activity level, cooperation, and tolerance of frustration. It is not effective in treating inattention but may be used to treat behavioral symptoms in children with tics (Steingard et al., 1993) or in those who fail to respond to stimulants. In combination with stimulants, it may allow a lower dosage of stimulant medication.

Complications usually involve bradycardia, hypotension, and sedation. Sedation tends to decrease after several weeks and can be minimized with dose titration. The onset of action is slow, from 1 month to several months. When discontinuing clonidine, the prescriber needs to taper the dose to prevent withdrawal symptoms such as increased motor restlessness, headache, agitation, elevated blood pressure and pulse rate, and possible agitation of tics (Dulcan et al., 1997).

Other adverse events include dry mouth, nausea, photophobia, hypotension, dizziness, and allergic skin reactions when the patch is used. Before prescribing the patch, the practitioner must determine the equivalent dose in tablets (see Table 47-2).

Guanfacine hydrochloride (Tenex), a longer-acting alpha-adrenergic agonist with a better side effect profile, has been studied only in open trials (Chappell et al., 1995; Horrigan & Barnhill, 1995). Even though interest has been shown in

using SSRIs to treat ADHD, no trials have supported their use for the core symptoms (Dulcan et al., 1997). Because of their dietary restrictions and drug interaction profile, MAO inhibitors are not used to treat ADHD, even though efficacy has been shown (Dulcan et al., 1997). Thioridazine (Mellaril) has been suggested as an alternative treatment of ADHD, but because of its limited effectiveness, sedation, cognitive dulling, and risk of tardive dyskinesia or neuroleptic malignant syndrome, it should be used only in unusual circumstances (Green, 1995).

Special Population Considerations

Stimulants are also considered the best treatment option for adults. However, adults may have a difficult time because the frequency of dosing increases may lead to reduced compliance due to missed or forgotten doses. If ADHD is properly diagnosed, abuse of the drug usually is not a problem. In adults, tics and growth retardation are not a concern, but hypertension is. Methylphenidate is the stimulant most commonly used in adults because it is effective for nervousness, lack of concentration, anger, and fatigue (Wender et al., 1981, 1985).

Selecting the Most Appropriate Agent

Because of the number of therapeutic options available, this section suggests only a general outline to follow. Nonpharmacologic therapy differs for children and adults. Nonpharmacologic therapy should be individualized for each patient (see Table 47-3). Figure 47-1 outlines the therapeutic plan for a child, adolescent, and adult.

First-Line Therapy

The stimulants are the usual first-line therapy. Methylphenidate is usually the first stimulant the practitioner tries because of its immediate action and ease of titration.

Second-Line Therapy

Most practitioners try the TCAs after a patient fails to respond to stimulant therapy. Currently, either nortriptyline or imipramine is used. Prescribers must consider the time frame of action for these agents. The longer onset of action and more extensive side effect profile make these agents less desirable than the stimulants.

Third-Line Therapy

After the TCAs, bupropion is the next agent of choice. Again, prescribers must keep in mind the time it takes for the drug level to become therapeutic. This agent also may impair cognitive skills.

MONITORING PATIENT RESPONSE

To determine the efficacy of the drugs used to treat ADHD, practitioners must use the rating scales mentioned previously; no laboratory values or diagnostic tests can determine the patient's improvement.

Treatment is indicated for as long as the patient is showing core symptoms of ADHD. Practitioners can best determine

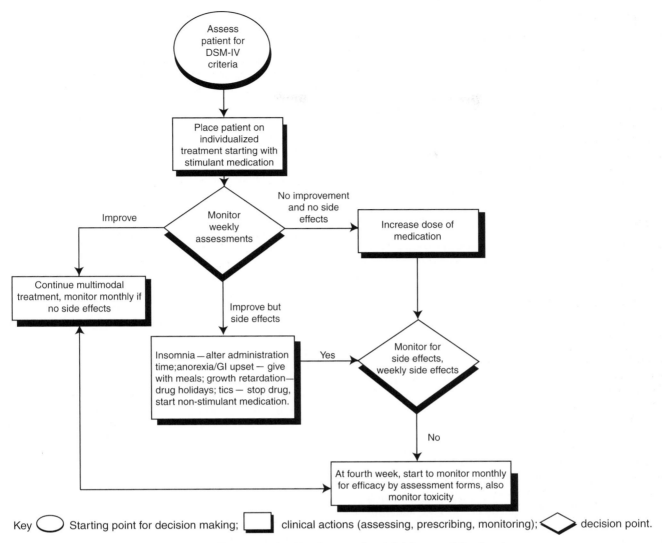

Figure 47–1 Treatment algorithm for attention-deficit/hyperactivity disorder.

the need to continue treatment by considering the patient's response during the "drug holidays." If symptoms are no longer present, treatment may not be needed. Continued assessment of the patient even when he or she is not using medication is essential. Monitoring parameters for the agents used to treat ADHD are summarized in Table 47-4. Medication should be given at the lowest effective dosage.

Studies show that stimulants' general side effects of insomnia, decreased appetite, dizziness, stomachache, and headache are usually mild and do not necessitate discontinuation of the drug (Ahmann, Waltonen, & Olson, 1993; Barkley et al., 1990; Efron, Jarman, & Barker, 1997). One study even suggested that these effects are more common in children with ADHD before treatment, although this has never been studied because of the difficulty of design (Efron et al., 1997). In narrower studies involving sleep disturbances, the data are conflicting on whether treatment causes the child to have less satisfactory sleep and to take longer to fall asleep (Kent et al., 1995; Tirosh et al., 1993). Sleep difficulties may actually be related to the ADHD, which causes symptoms that prevent the child from sleeping. Because sleep disturbances cannot be generalized, it is reasonable to assess the patient and determine whether

altered bedtimes or altered medication times are appropriate interventions.

In reviewing the complication of tics and dyskinesias, one study determined that transient tics develop in approximately 9% of children. The development of tics does not depend on prior personal or family history (Lipkin, Goldstein, & Adesman, 1994). Even though this study showed that tics or dyskinesias are not a contraindication, most health care professionals use stimulants cautiously in patients with prior histories.

Most of the other adverse events were discussed earlier. If any adverse event occurs that is disturbing to the patient, reasonable alternatives are to lower the dose or discontinue the medication. Table 47-5 summarizes the most common adverse events. If the patient is using a stimulant and the outcome is poor, substituting another stimulant is reasonable before trying another medication class.

PATIENT EDUCATION

Medications prescribed for ADHD must be taken exactly as prescribed to get the full benefit. If any adverse events occur that are disturbing, the patient should contact the health care

Table 47.4

Monitoring Parameters for Pharmacotherapy

Drug	Monitoring Parameters
atomoxetine	Blood pressure, pulse rate, mental status, weight periodically
bupropion	Weight monthly
clonidine	Blood pressure (standing and supine), respiratory rate and depth, heart rate monthly
dextroamphetamine	Growth, CNS activity monthly
imipramine	Blood pressure, pulse rate, ECG, CBC, mental status periodically
methylphenidate	Blood pressure, weight, height, heart rate, tics, sleep habits, drug use monthly
nortriptyline	Blood pressure, pulse rate, mental status, weight periodically
pemoline	Liver enzymes, weight periodically

provider immediately. Parents and adult patients should be aware of adverse events to watch for, as previously discussed. Patients need to be evaluated on a regular basis to determine their treatment needs.

Drug Information

The FDA's website (www.fda.gov) is a good source of initial prescribing information. Sources such as Facts and Comparisons can also provide information about the use of these agents.

Patient-Oriented Information Sources

The National Institute of Mental Health (NIMH) has an excellent website related to ADHD (http://www.nimh.nih.gov/healthinformation/adhdmenu.cfm). This site provides

Table 47.5

Summary of Adverse Events

	MTH	Dextro	Pem	Clon	Bupr	Imip	Nort
Tachycardia	X						
Nervousness	X	X					
Insomnia	X	X	X		X		
Anorexia	X		X		X		
Dizziness	X			X	X	X	X
Drowsiness	X				X	X	X
Arrhythmias		X					
Anxiety				X	X		
Confusion				X	X		
Bradycardia							
Xerostomia				X	X	X	X
Constipation				X	X	X	X
Nausea				X	X	X	X
Agitation					X		
Fever, headache					X	X	X
Vomiting					X		
Seizures					X		
Tremor							
Increased appetite						X	
Weight gain						X	X
Skeletal weakness						X	X
Urinary retention							X

MTH, methylphenidate; Dextro, dextroamphetamine; Pem, pemoline; Clon, clonidine; Bupr, bupropion; Imi, imipramine; Nort, nortriptyline.

access to booklets describing strategies for dealing with ADHD directed at parents of young children as well as adolescents. There are also links to local providers, clinical research trials, and other resources. CHADD (Children and Adults With Attention Deficit Disorder) at www.chadd.org is a great source of information and support for parents and patients with ADHD.

Nutrition/Lifestyle Changes

Dietary additives and supplements, such as dyes and preservatives, have long been implicated as a cause of ADHD symptoms. Daley reviewed literature suggesting that removal of these from the diet in certain children may help, but the impact of the removal was less than that seen with stimulant medications (Daley, 2004).

Parent training involves teaching parents to recognize situations in which their child could learn or improve social skills. Parents must actively participate in the child's social life, using punishment effectively by clear instruction, positively reinforcing good behavior, ignoring some behaviors, and using negative reinforcement, such as time out, to decrease the child's stimulation. This method has been shown useful for the short term and is an alternative for parents who do not want to proceed directly to medication therapy (Anastopoulos et al., 1993; Barkley, 1987, 1990).

As mentioned previously, the parents also may have ADHD (Dulcan et al., 1997). Family therapy can help teach all members how to negotiate and solve problems together as a unit. Because family therapy may be expensive, parent support groups can promote effective problem-solving techniques and unity (Dulcan et al., 1997).

Social skills training is based on the patient's deficits. Studies show that group training is more effective than individual training because self-observation usually is impossible for this patient population—both children and adults (Dulcan et al., 1997).

Academic skills training helps to refine a child's ability to organize, take notes, improve study habits, and prioritize activities. This methodology has not been tested, but in clinical practice it has been found useful if academic deficiencies are present (Dulcan et al., 1997).

Psychotherapy is not useful as treatment of ADHD but can help patients with moralization, self-esteem, and compliance problems. It may also be useful for patients with comorbid illnesses such as anxiety and depression. Psychotherapy may be needed only as difficulties arise (Dulcan et al., 1997). Psychotherapy also can help adolescents become responsible for their own medication regimen (Dulcan et al., 1997).

Cognitive behavior modification teaches stepwise problem solving and self-monitoring by using the reinforcement techniques of rewarding for good behavior and removing rewards for unwanted behavior. Although initially believed to be a good strategy, cognitive behavior modification was later found not to improve outcomes when added to medication therapy (Abikoff, 1985; Abikoff et al., 1988; Abikoff & Gittelman, 1985a,b). Some adolescents and children may benefit, but young children are very unlikely to benefit (Abikoff & Hectman, 1996). Practitioners of behavior modification try to determine how the child is responding to the environment and base interventions on the child's responses (Dulcan et al., 1997).

Therapeutic recreation is based on the idea that development of sports skills or other recreational abilities can have a positive effect on a child or adolescent with ADHD. This can be accomplished through existing programs, such as those offered by the YMCA or the Big Brothers Big Sisters organizations, or even by promoting a role model relationship with a college or high-school student to build self-esteem (Dulcan et al., 1997).

All these techniques offer different benefits, so individual assessment and reassessment are important to determine which techniques (if any) are making a difference for the patient. Some parents may want to try one or more of these methods before trying medication, and practitioners should permit the parents to try whatever methods they feel will be best for their child.

As with children, nonpharmacologic treatment also is beneficial for adults. "Coaching" involves daily encouragement to progress toward set goals. Educational programs help adults to identify their problem, understand it, and not blame themselves for it. Cognitive remediation also is used to teach attention enhancement, memory, problem solving, family relationships, time management, organization skills, and anger control (Kane et al., 1990). Medication should not be used as a substitute for treating behaviors with behavior modification. Each patient's therapeutic plan should be assessed and reassessed for success and usefulness.

Complementary and Alternative Medications

There are several herbal medications that may have an impact on a person with ADHD. *Gingko biloba*, a plant-derived medication, has shown some efficacy in improving memory and improving concentration. This may prove useful in ADHD patients with inattention problems. Similarly, glutamine, a naturally occurring amino acid, may also improve concentration, alertness and memory. However, neither of these agents has been proven in controlled clinical trials to improve these symptoms in patients with ADHD (Daley, 2004).

■ Case Study

Sam, age 8, is always interrupting his teacher, jumping out of his seat in class, fidgeting relentlessly, and butting into other children's games. At home, he runs around recklessly and is uncontrollable. His mother comes to you and wonders why he will not listen. She is concerned because his grades at school are dropping. After medical evaluation, you find nothing wrong with Sam physically, and he is taking no other medications. Through questioning, you determine that he has trouble concentrating on his homework, often forgets he has homework, loses pieces of games frequently, and hates to sit and read. His mother is unsure of the time frame over which these behaviors developed, but she thinks it has been since her second child was born 5 years ago. While in your office, Sam did not seem to be hyperactive or inattentive, but you notice he is easily distracted by people passing in the hallway because the door is slightly ajar.

Diagnosis: ADHD

1. List specific goals of treatment for Sam.

2. What would be the first-line drug therapy for Sam? Why?

3. What monitoring parameters would you institute for Sam's parents? For his teachers?

4. Discuss specific patient education you would provide to Sam's parents based on the prescribed therapy.

5. Describe one or two drug/drug or drug/food interactions that you would be wary of when prescribing this agent.

6. List one or two adverse reactions to the agent you selected that would cause you to change therapy.

7. If the adverse reactions you described above occurred, what would be your second-line therapy for Sam? Why?

8. What over-the-counter and/or alternative medications would be appropriate for Sam?

9. What dietary and lifestyle changes would you recommend to Sam's parents?

Bibliography

Starred references are cited in the text.

*Abikoff, H. (1985). Efficacy of cognitive training interventions in hyperactive children: a critical review. *Clinical Psychology Review, 5,* 479–512.

*Abikoff, H., Ganeles, D., Reiter, G., Blum, C., Foley, C., & Klein, R. G. (1988). Cognitive training in academically deficient ADDH boys receiving stimulant medication. *Journal of Abnormal Child Psychology, 16,* 411–432.

*Abikoff, H., & Gittelman, R. (1985a). Hyperactive children treated with stimulants: is cognitive training a useful adjunct? *Archives of General Psychiatry, 42,* 953–961.

*Abikoff, H., & Gittelman, R. (1985b). The normalizing effects of methylphenidate on the classroom behavior of ADDH children. *Journal of Child Psychology, 13,* 334.

*Abikoff, H., & Hechtman, L. (1996). Multimodal therapy and stimulants in the treatment of children with ADHD. In P. Jensen & E. D. Hibbs (Eds.), *Psychosocial treatment for child and adolescent disorders: empirically based approaches* (pp 501–546). Washington DC: American Psychological Association.

*Achenbach, T. M. (1991). *Manual for the Teacher's Report Form and 1991 Profile.* Burlington, VT: University of Vermont Department of Psychiatry.

*Adler, L. A., & Chua, H. C. (2002). Management of ADHD in Adults. *Journal of Clinical Psychiatry, 63*(Suppl. 12), 29–35.

*American Psychiatric Association. (2000). *Diagnostic and statistical manual of mental disorders* (4th ed., text revision). Washington, DC: Author.

*Ahmann, P. A., Waltonen, S. J., Olson, K. A., et al. (1993). Placebo-controlled evaluation of Ritalin side effects. *Pediatrics, 91,* 1101–1106.

*Anastopoulos, A. D., Shelton, T. L., DuPaul, G. J., & Guevremont, D. C. (1993). Parent training for attention-deficit hyperactivity disorder: its impact on parent functioning. *Journal of Abnormal Child Psychology, 21,* 581–596.

*Anonymous (1999). A 14-month randomized clinical trial of treatment strategies for attention-deficit/hyperactivity disorder. The MTA Cooperative Group. Multimodal Treatment Study of Children with ADHD. *Archives of General Psychiatry, 56*(12), 1073–1086.

*Barkley, R. A. (1987). *Defiant children: a clinician's manual for parent training.* New York: Guilford.

*Barkley, R. A. (1990). *Attention deficit hyperactivity disorder: a handbook for diagnosis and treatment.* New York: Guilford.

*Barkley, R. A., McMurray, M. B., Edelbrock, C. S., & Robbins, K. (1989). The response of aggressive and nonaggressive children to two doses of methylphenidate. *Journal of the American Academy of Child and Adolescent Psychiatry, 28,* 873–881.

*Barkley, R. A., McMurray, M. B., Edelbrock, C. S., & Robbins, K. (1990). Side effects of methylphenidate in children with attention deficit hyperactivity disorder: a systemic, placebo-controlled evaluation. *Pediatrics, 86,* 184–192.

*Barrickman, L. L., Perry, P. F., Allen, A. J., et al. (1995). Bupropion versus methylphenidate in the treatment of attention-deficit hyperactivity disorder. *Journal of the American Academy of Child and Adolescent Psychiatry, 34,* 649–657.

*Biederman, J., Faraone, S. V., Doyle, A., et al. (1993). Convergence of the Child Behavior Checklist with structured interview-based psychiatric diagnoses of ADHD children with and without comorbidity. *Journal of Child Psychology and Psychiatry, 34,* 1241–1251.

*Buitelaar, J. K., Van der Gaag, R. J., Swaab-Barneveld, H., & Kuiper, M. (1995). Prediction of clinical response to methylphenidate in children with attention-deficit hyperactivity disorder. *Journal of the American Academy of Child and Adolescent Psychiatry, 8,* 1025–1032.

*Chappell, P. B., Riddle, M. A., Scahill, L., et al. (1995). Guanfacine treatment of comorbid attention-deficit hyperactivity disorder and Tourette's syndrome: preliminary clinical experience. *Journal of the American Academy of Child and Adolescent Psychiatry, 34,* 1140–1146.

*Christman, A. K., Fermo, J. D., & Markowitz, J. S. (2004). Atomoxetine, a novel treatment for attention-deficit hyperactivity disorder. *Pharmacotherapy, 24*(8), 1020–1036.

*Conners, C. K. (1969). A teacher rating scale for use in drug studies with children. *American Journal of Psychiatry, 126,* 884–888.

*Conners, C. K., Casat, C. D., Gualtieri, C. T., et al. (1996). Bupropion hydrochloride in attention deficit disorder with hyperactivity. *Journal of the American Academy of Child and Adolescent Psychiatry, 35,* 1314–1321.

*Daley, K. C. (2004). Update on attention-deficit/hyperactivity disorder. *Current Opinion in Pediatrics, 16,* 217–226.

*Dulcan, M. K., Dunne, J. E., Ayres, W., et al. (1997). Practice parameters for the assessment and treatment of children, adolescents, and adults with attention-deficit/hyperactivity disorder: AACAP Official Action. *Journal of the American Academy of Child and Adolescent Psychiatry, 36,* 85S–121S.

*Edelbrock, C., Costello, A. J., & Kessler, M. K. (1984). Empirical corroboration of attention deficit disorder. *Journal of the American Academy of Child Psychiatry, 23,* 285–290.

*Efron, D. E., Jarman, F., & Barker, M. (1997). Side effects of methylphenidate and dextroamphetamine in children with attention deficit hyperactivity disorder: a double-blind, crossover trial. *Pediatrics, 100,* 662–666.

*Farone, S. V., & Biederman, J. (1994). Genetics of attention-deficit hyperactivity disorder. *Child and Adolescent Psychiatry Clinics of North America, 3,* 285–301.

Gittelman, R. L., Mattes, J. A., & Klein, D. F. (1988). Methylphenidate and growth in hyperactive children. *Archives of General Psychiatry, 45,* 1127–1130.

*Goldman, L. S., Genel, M., Benzman, R. J., et al. (1998). Diagnosis and treatment of attention-deficit/hyperactivity disorder in children and adolescents. *Journal of the American Medical Association, 279,* 1100–1107.

*Green, W. H. (1995). The treatment of attention-deficit hyperactivity disorder with nonstimulant medications. *Child and Adolescent Psychiatry Clinics of North America, 4,* 169–195.

*Hauser, P., Zametkin, A. J., Martinez, P., et al. (1993). Attention deficit-hyperactivity disorder in people with generalized resistance to thyroid hormone. *New England Journal of Medicine, 328,* 997–1001.

Hechtman, L. (1993). Aims and methodological problems in multimodal treatment studies. *Canadian Journal of Psychiatry, 38,* 458–464.

*Horrigan, J. P., & Barnhill, L. J. (1995). Guanfacine for treatment of attention-deficit hyperactivity disorder in boys. *Journal of Child and Adolescent Psychopharmacology, 5,* 215–223.

Jensen, P. S. (1993). Development and implementation of multimodal and combined treatment studies in children and adolescents: NIMH perspectives. *Psychopharmacology Bulletin, 29,* 19–25.

*Kane, R., Mikalac, C., Benjamin, S., & Barkley, R. A. (1990). Assessment and treatment of adults with ADHD. In R. A. Barkley (Ed.), *Attention deficit hyperactivity disorder: a handbook for diagnosis and treatment* (pp. 613–654). New York: Guilford.

*Kent, J. D., Blader, J. C., Koplewics, H. S., et al. (1995). Effects of late-afternoon methylphenidate administration on behavior and sleep in attention-deficit hyperactivity disorder. *Pediatrics, 96,* 320–325.

Klein, R. G., Landa, B., Mattes, J. A., & Klein, D. F. (1988). Methylphenidate and growth in hyperactive children. *Archives of General Psychiatry, 45,* 1127–1130.

Klein, R. G., & Mannuzza, S. (1988). Hyperactive boys almost grown up: methylphenidate effects on ultimate height. *Archives of General Psychiatry, 45,* 1131–1134.

*Kollins, S. H. (2003). Comparing the abuse potential of methylphenidate versus other stimulants: a review of available evidence and relevance to the ADHD patient. *Journal of Clinical Psychiatry, 64*(Suppl. 11), 14–18.

Levin, G. M. (1995). Attention-deficit/hyperactivity disorder: the pharmacist's role. *American Pharmacy, NS35,* 11–20.

*Lipkin, P. H., Goldstein, I. J., & Adesman, A. R. (1994). Tics and dyskinesias associated with stimulant treatment in attention-deficit hyperactivity disorder. *Archives of Pediatric and Adolescent Medicine, 148,* 859–861.

*Markussen, K., Dalsgaard, S., Obel, C., et al. (2003). Maternal lifestyle factors in pregnancy risk of attention deficit hyperactivity disorder and associated behaviors: review of the current evidence. *American Journal of Psychiatry, 160,* 1028–1040.

*Nahlik, J. (2004). Issues in diagnosis of attention-deficit/hyperactivity disorder in adolescents. *Clinical Pediatrics, 43,* 1–10.

*Pliszka, S. R., McCracken, J. T., & Maas, J. W. (1996). Catecholamines in attention-deficit hyperactivity disorder: current perspectives. *Journal of the American Academy of Child and Adolescent Psychiatry, 35,* 264–272.

*Richters, J. E., Arnold, L. E., Jensen, P. S., et al. (1995). NIMH collaborative multisite multimodal treatment study of children with ADHD: I. Background and rationale. *Journal of the American Academy of Child and Adolescent Psychiatry, 34,* 987–1000.

*Riddle, M. A., Hardin, M. T., Cho, S. C., Woolston, J. L., & Leckman, J. F. (1988). Desipramine treatment of boys with attention-deficit hyperactivity disorder and tics: preliminary clinical experience. *Journal of the American Academy of Child and Adolescent Psychiatry, 27,* 811–813.

Rowe, K. S., & Rowe, K. J. (1994). Synthetic food coloring and behavior: a dose response effect in a double-blind, placebo-controlled, repeated-measures study. *Journal of Pediatrics, 125,* 691–698.

*Spencer, T., Biederman, J., Steingard, R., & Wilens, T. (1993). Bupropion exacerbates tics in children with attention-deficit hyperactivity disorder and Tourette's syndrome. *Journal of the American Academy of Child and Adolescent Psychiatry, 32,* 354–360.

*Spencer, T. J., Biederman, J., Wilens, T. E., & Faraone, S. V. (2002). Overview and neurobiology of attention-deficit/hyperactivity disorder. *Journal of Clinical Psychiatry, 63*(Suppl. 12), 3–9.

*Spencer, T., Biederman, J., Wilens, T., Harding, M., O'Donnell, D., & Griffin, S. (1996). Pharmacotherapy of attention-deficit hyperactivity disorder across the life cycle. *Journal of the American Academy of Child and Adolescent Psychiatry, 35,* 409–432.

*Steingard, R., Biederman, J., Spencer, T., Wilens, T., & Gonzales, A. (1993). Comparison of clonidine response in the treatment of attention-deficit hyperactivity disorder with and without comorbid tic disorders. *Journal of the American Academy of Child and Adolescent Psychiatry, 32,* 250–253.

*Sudak, H. S. (1998). Attending to attention deficit disorder: diagnosis and treatment. *Notebook: Pennsylvania Hospital, 6*(1), 1–2.

*Tirosh, E., Saeh, A., Munvez, R., & Laurie, P. (1993). Effects of methylphenidate on sleep in children with attention-deficit hyperactivity disorder. *American Journal of Disorders in Children, 147,* 1313–1315.

*Ullmann, R. K., Sleator, E. K., & Sprague, R. L. (1985). Introduction to the use of ACTERS. *Psychopharmacology Bulletin, 21,* 915–919.

*Ward, M. F., Wender, P. H., & Reimherr, F. W. (1993). The Wender Utah Rating Scale: an aid in the retrospective diagnosis of childhood attention deficit disorder. *American Journal of Psychiatry, 150,* 885–890.

*Weiss, M., & Murray, C. (2003). Assessment and management of attention-deficit hyperactivity disorder in adults. *Canadian Medical Association Journal, 168,* 715–722.

*Wender, P. H. (1995). *Attention-deficit hyperactivity disorder in adults.* New York: Oxford University Press.

Wender, P. H., Reimherr, F. W., & Wood, D. R. (1981). Attention deficit disorder ("minimal brain dysfunction") in adults. *Archives of General Psychiatry, 38,* 449–456.

Wender, P. H., & Solanto, M. V. (1991). Effects of sugar on aggressive and inattentive behavior in children with attention deficit disorder with hyperactivity and normal children. *Pediatrics, 88,* 960–966.

*Wender, P. H., Wood, D. R., & Reimherr, F. W. (1985). Pharmacological treatment of attention deficit disorder, residual type (ADD, RT, "minimal brain dysfunction," "hyperactivity") in adults. *Psychopharmacology Bulletin, 212,* 222–231.

*Wilens, T. E., Biederman, J., Mick, E., & Spencer, T. J. (1995). A systematic assessment of tricyclic antidepressants in the treatment of adult attention-deficit hyperactivity disorder. *Journal of Nervous and Mental Disorders, 183,* 48–50.

Visit the Connection web site for the most up-to-date drug information.

48

ALZHEIMER'S DISEASE

■ ANGELA CAFIERO, KATHERINE WALTMAN, AND
TRACY OFFERDAHL-McGOWAN

Alzheimer's disease (AD), also known as *senile dementia of the Alzheimer's type*, is the most common cause of dementia accounting for approximately 60% of all dementias. AD is typified by a slow, progressive decline in cognition. Patients initially complain of short-term (recent) memory loss, forgetfulness, and a decreased ability to learn and retain new information.

Estimates suggest that approximately 4.5 million people have AD (Hebert et al., 2003). The number is expected to grow to 11.3 to 16 million by 2050 (Hebert et al., 2003). A majority of individuals with AD are residing in the community, which represents a huge emotional and financial burden on the patient, friends, and family members, as well as on society as a whole. The cost of care (including general, medical, and long-term care at a facility outside of the home) per patient is estimated at approximately $40,000 to $60,000 a year.

Patients may have sporadic or familial AD. Sporadic AD is the classic form of AD, occurring most often in patients 65 years of age or older (late onset). Familial AD is less common and affects patients with genetic mutations of amyloid precursor protein (APP), presenilin-1, and presenilin-2. Familial AD may be of early onset (age 65 years) or of late onset (Lendon et al., 1997). Genetic causes (eg, apolipoprotein E4 allele) have also been linked to sporadic or late-onset AD. Symptoms of AD can be divided between cognitive symptoms or noncognitive symptoms. Treatment is based on the particular domain of the symptoms. Cognitive symptoms, such as loss of short-term memory, usually present first in mild AD, whereas the noncognitive behavioral symptoms are seen in more moderate to severe AD. Currently, AD is incurable although pharmacologic agents have been used to slow the progression of the disease. The average life span for patients with AD is reduced by as much as 70% and generally ranges from 8 to 10 years after diagnosis (Brookmeyer, 2002; Small et al., 1997). Women are at a slightly higher risk for developing AD than men. Prevalence increases with age, with AD affecting approximately 50% of those older than 85 years of age. Patients commonly die from indirect causes of AD such as aspiration, infection, malnutrition, or pulmonary embolism (Morris, 1994).

CAUSES

Apolipoprotein E (ApoE), a protein involved in cholesterol transport, is linked to the development of AD. The E4 allele (homozygote E4/E4) is thought to increase the risk of AD, whereas the E2 allele may be protective, particularly for sporadic AD. Advanced age and family history are the most significant risk factors for AD. The risk factors and protective factors for AD are listed in Box 48-1.

PATHOPHYSIOLOGY

Pathologic changes in AD include formation of neurofibrillary tangles and senile plaques, cortical atrophy, and neuronal (cholinergic, glutamatergic) destruction and loss. In AD patients, acetylcholine levels are decreased and an excessive stimulation of glutamate causes neuronal toxicity. These changes affect several areas of the brain, including the hippocampus, amygdala, cerebral cortex, and ultimately the motor cortex. As a result of these changes, short- and long-term memory, learning, language, behavior, and eventually motor skills are impaired.

Neurofibrillary Tangles

Neurofibrillary tangles and senile (also known as *neuritic* or *β-amyloid*) plaques are the hallmark pathologic lesions in AD. Tau protein, the principal component of neurofibrillary tangles, becomes hyperphosphorylated in AD. The abnormal phosphorylation of tau protein leads to the formation of paired helical filaments and finally neurofibrillary tangles. As a result, microtubule assembly is inhibited and critical organelles may collapse, causing abnormal intracellular transport and neuronal cell death.

Senile Plaques

Senile plaques are brain lesions that contain a core of β-amyloid protein (BAP) and a shell of damaged neurites. APP is the parent protein of BAP. Proteases normally cleave APP through the BAP region, which prevents intact BAP from entering the extracellular fluid. When abnormal

BOX 48–1. RISK FACTORS AND PROTECTIVE FACTORS FOR ALZHEIMER'S DISEASE

Risk Factors
Advanced age
Family history (eg, genetic abnormalities)

Possible Risk Factors
Female sex
Low education level
Head injury

Possible Protective Factors
Estrogen replacement therapy
High education level
NSAID use

NSAID, nonsteroidal anti-inflammatory drug.
Adapted from Small, G. W., Rabins, P. V., Barry P. P., et al. (1997). Diagnosis and treatment of Alzheimer's disease and related disorders: Consensus statement of the American Association for Geriatric Psychiatry, the Alzheimer's Association, and the American Geriatrics Society. *Journal of the American Medical Association, 278,* 1363–1371.

proteolysis occurs, leaving BAP intact, increased extracellular BAP becomes involved in senile plaque formation and neuronal degeneration. Senile plaques are also composed of protease inhibitors, tau protein, ApoE, and glial cells, which may be involved in the pathologic process of AD and are areas of interest to researchers. Neurofibrillary tangles and senile plaque density correlate with increase severity of AD.

Neuronal Destruction

The neuronal cell damage and death seen in AD results in impaired neurotransmitter function. The cholinergic and glutamatergic systems are significantly involved. In particular, cholinergic neurons in the nucleus basalis of Meynert are damaged. Destruction of cholinergic neurons leads to decreased levels of acetylcholine, a neurotransmitter that aids in learning and memory. The symptomatic presentation of AD (memory loss and cognitive impairment) appears to be associated with acetylcholine deficiency. The cholinergic system has been the subject of a vast amount of research and pharmacologic development (eg, acetylcholinesterase inhibitors). Overstimulation or erratic stimulation of the glutamatergic system in the synapse causes neuronal toxicity leading to neuronal death. This disruption is thought to impair learning and memory.

The autoimmune system or inflammatory mediators may be linked to late-onset AD. Glial cells, complement cascade components, and cytokines are present in plaque areas. These cells and inflammatory mediators may contribute to neuronal cell damage and loss. Their role in AD is under investigation, as is the use of anti-inflammatory drugs and 3-hydroxy-3-methylglutaryl-coenzyme A (HMG Co-A) reductase inhibitors to prevent cell damage.

DIAGNOSTIC CRITERIA

The clinical diagnosis of AD can be made using the National Institute of Neurological and Communicative Disorders, and Stroke and the Alzheimer's Disease and Related Disorders Association (NINCDS-ADRDA) criteria (Box 48-2), or the *Diagnostic and Statistical Manual of Mental Disorders* (4th ed.), known as the DSM-IV. The diagnosis can be *confirmed* only by autopsy.

Patients and their caregivers should be intimately involved in the diagnostic process. A complete history and physical examination that includes a neurologic and mental status evaluation (Table 48-1) is essential. The Mini–Mental State Examination (MMSE) may be used to screen for cognitive impairment. The clock-drawing task (CDT) is another initial evaluation tool that is quick and can be performed by any health care professional (Fig. 48-1). Additional tools that are useful for monitoring changes in function, behavior, and cognition are the Functional Activities Questionnaire and the Revised Memory and Behavior Problems Checklist.

BOX 48–2. NINCDS-ADRDA* CRITERIA FOR ALZHEIMER'S DISEASE

Criteria for Clinical Diagnosis of Probable Alzheimer's Disease
- Dementia established by clinical examination, documented by the Mini–Mental State Examination or similar test, and confirmed by neuropsychological tests (eg, Mini–Mental State Examination) or other validated tests.
- Deficits occurring in two or more areas of cognition (eg, memory, calculation, judgment).
- Progressive worsening of memory and other cognitive functions.
- No disturbance of consciousness.
- Onset between ages 40 and 90 years.
- Absence of systemic disorders or other brain diseases that could account for progressive deficits.

Diagnosis Is Supported by the Following
- Progressive deterioration of specific cognitive functions.
- Impaired activities of daily living and altered patterns of behavior.
- Family history of similar disorder, particularly if confirmed neuropathologically.
- Normal lumbar puncture.
- Normal (age-related) nonspecific changes in EEG, such as increased slow-wave activity.
- Evidence of cerebral atrophy on CT, with progression documented by serial studies.

*National Institute of Neurological and Communicative Disorders, and Stroke–Alzheimer's Disease and Related Disorders Association.
From Wiser, T. H. (1994). Alzheimer's cognitive disturbances. *US Pharmacist, 19,* 58, with permission.

Table 48.1

Mini–Mental State Examination for Cognitive Function

Function	Test	Maximum Score
Orientation	What is the year? season? date? month? day?	5
	Where are we—what state? county? town or city? hospital floor?	5
Registration	Repeat after me: "apple," "table," "penny." (*Physician names objects and asks the patient to repeat until accurate.*)	3
Attention and calculation	Spell "world" backwards.	5
Recall	What were the three words you named before? (*Patient should answer "apple," "table," "penny."*)	3
Language	What is this? (*Physician points to two common objects, eg, a pencil and a watch.*)	2
	Repeat after me: "No ifs, ands, or buts."	1
	Take a piece of paper in your right hand, fold it in half, and put it on the floor.	3
	Close your eyes.	1
	Write a sentence.	1
	Copy this design:	1

Adapted from Folstein, M. F., Folstein, S. E., & McHugh, P. R. (1975). "Mini–Mental State": A practical method for grading the cognitive state of patients for the clinician. *Journal of Psychiatric Research, 12*, 796.

INITIATING DRUG THERAPY

A careful assessment of baseline diagnostic findings is essential before initiating drug therapy. The patient, family, and caregiver should be informed of the severity of cognitive and functional impairment. Baseline scores on the MMSE, CDT, and Functional Activities Questionnaire can help guide decisions related to drug therapy. Reversible causes of dementia must also be considered and eliminated because several medications and medical conditions may cause or aggravate dementia (Box 48-3).

Before starting drug therapy for the cognitive symptoms of AD, the patient or family should demonstrate a clear understanding of the efficacy and expected outcomes of treatment, as well as the potential adverse events, costs, and incurability of the disease. The choice not to initiate drug therapy is also a reasonable option.

Pharmacologic management of the noncognitive symptoms is tailored to the individual symptom. These medications are usually initiated when the patient progresses to the moderate to severe stages of AD. The use of both noncognitive and cognitive therapies may be necessary as the disease progresses.

Nonpharmacologic psychotherapies, such as behavior-oriented, emotion-oriented, cognition-oriented, and stimulation-oriented approaches, can be useful for some patients with AD. These treatments may have some initial benefit, but can be associated with an increase in patient frustration, agitation, and depression. The risks of these psychotherapies, especially cognition-oriented treatments, may outweigh the benefits.

Other nonpharmacologic interventions include using calendars, clocks, and written notes or instructions. The caregiver should attempt to maintain a predictable routine with the patient. Drastic changes in the environment, as well as confrontation and arguments, should be avoided. Recognition of precipitants of agitation, psychosis, and anxiety can assist the caregiver and health care provider to best develop a patient-specific treatment plan.

The patient's ability to drive should be evaluated and as AD progresses, the patient should be advised to stop driving because dementia may increase the risk of accidents. The patient's use of a stove should be evaluated because, if left on and unattended, it can be harmful. Families should be taught how to prevent falls and wandering. They should also be informed about the possibility of physical violence and suicide that is associated with more severe disease. Capable patients may want to discuss with their families advance directives, living wills, desires for nursing home placement, and powers of attorney.

Patient and family education are the most important nonpharmacologic interventions for AD. Depending on the stage of impairment, the patient requires some or full assistance with activities of daily living, such as dressing, toileting, and particularly, driving. Support for patients and families is vitally important at any stage of AD (Box 48-4), and anyone involved with a patient with AD should be educated on the availability of support groups to deal with the wide

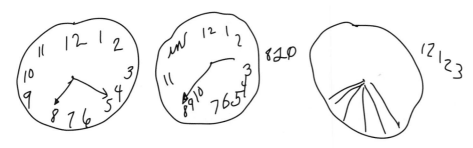

Figure 48–1 Clock drawing task completed by various elderly subjects. They were asked to draw a clock that represented 20 minutes after 8. The clock at left represents a normal result. The middle clock and the clock at right were drawn by elderly patients with dementia. (Adaptation based on a clock drawing test courtesy of Pfizer Inc., and Ensai Inc.)

BOX 48–3. POTENTIALLY REVERSIBLE CAUSES OF DEMENTIA

Medications
Anticholinergics (eg, benztropine, diphenhydramine)
Antidepressants (eg, amitriptyline, imipramine)
Antipsychotics (eg, thioridazine)
Anxiolytics (eg, diazepam, lorazepam)
Cardiovascular agents (eg, digoxin, propranolol)
Corticosteroids
Histamine (H_2) blockers (eg, cimetidine)
Metoclopramide

Metabolic Disorders
Dehydration
Hyperthyroidism and hypothyroidism
Hyponatremia
Hypercalcemia

Intracranial Infection or Disease
Meningitis
Neurosyphilis
Normal-pressure hydrocephalus
Subdural hematoma
Tumor
Toxoplasmosis

Miscellaneous
Toxins (eg, lead, mercury, alcohol)
Vitamin B_{12} deficiency
Depression
Psychoses

Adapted from Wiser, T. H. (1994). Alzheimer's disease. *US Pharmacist, 63,* with permission.

variety of issues associated with AD. Other resources for the caregiver include the use of respite care centers and day care centers.

Goals of Drug Therapy

The optimal goal of drug therapy is to maintain and maximize the patient's functional ability, quality of life, and independence for as long as possible while minimizing adverse events and cost (Small et al., 1997). A multidisciplinary approach to therapy, which includes the family, a physician, a psychiatric specialist, a nurse, a social worker, and a pharmacist, is the ideal. Drug therapy choices for the cognitive symptoms include the cholinesterase inhibitors, memantine (Namenda), and selegiline (Eldepryl).

Selected Agents for Cognitive Symptoms

Cholinesterase Inhibitors

Cholinesterase inhibitors, also known as the *acetylcholinesterase inhibitors,* play a key role in the pharmacologic treatment of AD. This drug class includes tacrine (Cognex), donepezil (Aricept), rivastigmine (Exelon), and galantamine (Reminyl), which are indicated for mild to moderate dementia of the AD type. These agents are used to slow the progression of the cognitive, functional, and behavioral domains of AD. Patients and families may report improvement—or lack of continued decline—within 3 to 6 weeks of beginning treatment.

If no effect is seen within 3 to 6 months of treatment or the patient is experiencing an adverse effect, another agent from this class may be tried. They are not curative and the improvements correlate with approximately a 6-month symptom decline in untreated patients. It is unknown how long treatment with these agents should be continued. However, once a patient progresses to severe AD, these agents are no longer solely recommended. Additional pharmacologic therapy may be necessary once the disease progresses into the severe stages. Thoughtful discussions with caregivers or families may guide the decision to discontinue therapy.

Cholinesterase inhibitors inhibit one or both types of the cholinesterase enzymes, butyrylcholinesterase or acetylcholinesterase. Butyrylcholinesterase is primarily found in the periphery and inhibition of this enzyme leads to many of the adverse effects of the cholinesterase agents. Acetylcholinesterase is found more centrally and thus is the primary focus of inhibition for the use in AD.

Tacrine was the first cholinesterase inhibitor approved by the U.S. Food and Drug Administration (FDA) for treating the cognitive symptoms of mild to moderate AD. This agent has fallen out of use due to the severe hepatotoxicity associated with it, 4 times a day dosing, and the approval of safer cholinesterase inhibitors. Donepezil is the second cholinesterase inhibitor approved for this indication. Both agents are thought to improve cognitive symptoms by reversing cholinesterase inhibition to increase the concentrations of acetylcholinesterase in the cerebral cortex. The effects of tacrine and donepezil, however, depend on functioning cholinergic neurons, and their efficacy likely decreases as AD progresses.

Rivastigmine is the third cholinesterase inhibitor with its potential advantage of being pseudo-irreversible. It inhibits the enzyme for about 10 hours, making this

BOX 48–4. ALZHEIMER'S DISEASE SUPPORT GROUPS AND RESOURCES

Alzheimer's Association
Phone: 1-800-272-3900
Web site: http://www.alz.org

Alzheimer's Disease Education and Referral (ADEAR) Center
Phone: 1-800-438-4380
Web site: http://www.alzheimers.org

Eldercare Locator Service (ELS)
Phone: 1-800-677-1116
Web site: http://www.eldercare.gov

an intermediate-acting agent. Galantamine is the fourth approved cholinesterase inhibitor on the market. Besides inhibiting the cholinesterase enzyme, it also allosterically modulates the nicotinic receptor.

The cholinesterase inhibitors have been shown to slow the progression of AD. These medications have also had positive effects on the noncognitive or behavioral symptoms of AD. They have been shown to reduce apathy, psychosis, anxiety, depression, and agitation. Although these medications appear to improve the cognitive function of patients with AD, there is no evidence that they alter the course of the disease.

Dosage

The cholinesterase inhibitors may modestly improve cognitive function or delay decline in cognitive function. The observed delay in cognitive decline correlates with approximately a 6-month decline in patients treated with placebos. Clinical studies of these agents versus placebo show that maximum efficacy by the maximum dose. Thus, it is necessary to titrate the cholinesterase inhibitor to the maximum tolerated dose.

Donepezil therapy is initiated at a 5-mg dose, taken at bedtime (to minimize gastrointestinal [GI] side effects). The dosage may be increased after 4 to 6 weeks to a maximum dose of 10 mg/d if tolerated. Donepezil 10 mg/d is slightly more effective than the 5-mg dose; therefore, increasing to 10 mg/d is appropriate for patients who do not respond within 6 weeks of treatment with the 5-mg dose. Rivastigmine doses should be started at 1.5 mg twice a day and increase to 3 mg twice a day after 2 weeks of treatment. Further dose increases should be based on clinical response and can be attempted on a biweekly basis. The maximum dose is 6 mg twice a day. Galantamine is usually started at a dose of 4 mg twice a day and titrated up every 4 weeks as tolerated to a maximum dose of 24 mg/d (12 mg twice daily).

Adverse Events

The major adverse effects of the cholinesterase inhibitors are cholinergic, most commonly nausea, vomiting, and diarrhea (5%-47%). Rivastigmine has been associated with the highest incidence of these GI disturbances (19%-47%). These effects are dose dependent and can be minimized by slowly titrating to higher doses (Table 48-2).

A major adverse effect of tacrine, but not the other cholinesterase inhibitors, is the development of reversible hepatocellular damage. This occurs in approximately 30% of patients taking tacrine. As a result, strict hepatic enzyme monitoring is required with the medication. Tacrine has a limited use due to this adverse effect.

Bradycardia can occur with the use of the cholinesterase inhibitors. Hyperacidity can occur with tacrine, donepezil, and rivastigmine. Although these effects are not common, they are of concern in patients who have cardiac conduction deficits, a history of peptic ulcer disease, or who currently take nonsteroidal anti-inflammatory drugs (NSAIDs). Although the manufacturer recommends administering donepezil at bedtime to minimize adverse effects, if insomnia or nightmares occur, dosing should be switched to the morning. Despite the GI effects associated with a rapid increase in dose, these agents appear to be well tolerated.

Interactions

Drug interactions with the cholinesterase inhibitors include synergy with other cholinergic agents (eg, succinylcholine [Quelicin]). Tacrine, donepezil, and galantamine are metabolized by the P450 enzyme system. Tacrine is a substrate for isoenzyme 1A2; donepezil and galantamine are substrates for 2D6 and 3A4. A potential advantage of rivastigmine is that it is metabolized by hydrolysis and thus is not susceptible to the drug interactions associated with the P450 enzyme

Table 48.2

Overview of Cholinesterase Inhibitors, Vitamin E, and Selegiline

Generic (Trade) Name and Dosage	Selected Adverse Events	Contraindications	Special Considerations
donepezil (Aricept) Start: 5 mg every evening Range: 5–10 mg/d	*GI:* nausea, vomiting *CV:* bradycardia, syncope	Hypersensitivity to agent or piperidine derivatives	Dose in the evening to avoid adverse GI events.
rivastigmine (Exelon) Start 1.5 mg bid for 2 wk, then increase by 1.5 mg bid; max. 6 mg bid Range: 3–6 mg bid	Nausea, vomiting, anorexia, dyspepsia, fatigue, headache malaise	Hypersensitivity to agent or carbamate derivatives	Initial response seen within 12 wk of therapy
galantamine (Reminyl) Start: 4 mg bid × 4 wk Range: 4–12 mg bid	Nausea, vomiting, diarrhea, anorexia, abdominal pain, dyspepsia, dizziness, sleep disturbances	Hypersensitivity to agent Severe hepatic, renal impairment	Moderate hepatic, renal impairment should not exceed a dose of 16 mg/d
tacrine (Cognex) Start: 10 mg qid Range: 10–40 mg qid	*GI:* nausea, vomiting *CV:* bradycardia, syncope Hepatic: elevated transaminases	Hypersensitivity to agent Prior history of jaundice with agent	Alanine aminotransferase monitoring required.
vitamin E Start: 1000 IU bid	Falls, syncope, bleeding	Hypersensitivity to agent	May increase INR and risk of bleeding in vitamin K–deficient patients or those taking warfarin.
selegiline (Eldepryl) Start: 5 mg in AM and at lunchtime	Orthostatic hypotension, insomnia	Hypersensitivity to agent	Monitor blood pressure. Dose in morning and at lunchtime to minimize insomnia.

INR, international normalized ratio

system. Inhibitors of these isoenzymes would cause an increase drug concentration of the cholinesterase inhibitor and thus more susceptible to cholinergic adverse effects.

Memantine (Namenda)

Memantine is a new drug to a new class of agents the N-methyl-D-aspartate (NMDA) receptor antagonists. This drug was approved in 2003 for the treatment of moderate to severe AD. It has a novel mechanism of action, which focuses on the glutamatergic system as compared to the cholinesterase inhibitors effect on the cholinergic system. Memantine blocks the activation of the NMDA receptor during an abundance of glutamate. Thus, this blocks overstimulation of the NMDA receptor and neuronal degeneration is inhibited. It dose not interfere with the pathologic activation of the NMDA receptor during learning and memory formation.

Clinical trials have shown that memantine used alone in patients with moderate to severe AD has produced reduced clinical deterioration over 28 weeks. When memantine was added to donepezil therapy, it resulted in significantly better cognition and activities of daily living compared to placebo over 24 weeks. Memantine should be started at 5 mg once daily and titrated every week, if tolerated, to a maximum dose of 10 mg twice daily. Food has no effect on the onset or absorption of memantine. In general, memantine was well tolerated compared to placebo. Memantine is minimally metabolized by the P450 enzyme system and thus not susceptible to P450 enzyme interactions. It is largely excreted renally via tubular secretion and, thus, there is the potential for decreased renal clearance with other drugs that undergo tubular secretion (eg, amantadine, ranitidine).

Overall, clinical trials have been positive regarding the use of memantine for moderate to severe AD. With a different mechanism of action and indication for moderate to severe AD, memantine has a unique role for treatment of AD. In the past, once a cholinesterase inhibitor failed, no other viable option for therapy was available. Now, the addition of memantine to a cholinesterase inhibitor may be an option.

Selegiline

Selegiline (Eldepryl), a selective monoamine oxidase (MAO) type B inhibitor, is a potential treatment option for patients with moderate AD. The drug is thought to have antioxidant or neuroprotective properties. The evidence for the use of selegiline is still limited.

Selegiline may be tried for patients who cannot tolerate cholinesterase inhibitors because some evidence indicates that it not only delays disease progression, but it may improve cognition—although improvement in cognition was not observed in the study by Sano and colleagues (1997). There does not appear to be a combined role for the use of selegiline and vitamin E because their effects together may be worse than with either agent used alone. Again, patients and families should be educated about the potential risks and benefits of the use of these agents.

Based on efficacy data, a dosage of 5 mg orally twice a day is recommended. Orthostatic hypotension, hallucinations, agitation, and insomnia are possible adverse events, although selegiline is in general well tolerated at doses of 10 mg/d or less. Nonselective inhibition of MAO can occur at daily doses exceeding 10 mg. Doses greater than 10 mg/d increase the risk of hypertensive crisis with tyramine-containing foods (eg, cheese, wine). For further discussion of tyramine and MAO inhibitors, refer to Chapter 44. Drug interactions with carbamazepine (Tegretol), selective serotonin reuptake inhibitors (SSRIs), tricyclic antidepressants, venlafaxine (Effexor), or meperidine (Demerol) can cause increased toxicity (agitation, delirium, seizures, and death) as well.

Atypical Agents

Ergoloid mesylates (eg, Hydergine) have been studied for treating cognitive impairment in dementia. Their use is not recommended because of lack of clear efficacy data.

Epidemiologic data also suggest that NSAIDs, cyclooxygenase inhibitors (COX-2), and estrogen replacement therapy (ERT) may protect patients against AD. The use of these agents, however, is not recommended because of the lack of well-designed efficacy trials, adverse effects, and the potential risks of therapy (American Psychiatric Association [APA], 1997). A discussion of the potential benefits versus the risks may be warranted in patients requiring arthritis treatment or in patients considering ERT. Long-term use of particular NSAIDs or COX-2 inhibitors has been associated with an increased risk of stroke and cardiovascular events.

The use of HMG Co-A reductase inhibitors (statins) has been gaining notoriety for the use of preserving cognitive function in patients with cognitive impairment. The exact mechanism for preserving cognitive function is still unknown; however, it is postulated that reducing the cholesterol content in the brain could decrease the formation of the plaques. There are not enough data to support using a statin in all patients with cognitive impairment.

In patients over the age of 60 using the statins, lovastatin and pravastatin, one observational study showed up to a 73% lower risk of developing AD compared to those not taking one of these agents. Because it is not a true cause-and-effect relationship, it is not routinely recommended for use as AD prevention.

Selected Agents for Noncognitive Symptoms

Antipsychotic Agents

The noncognitive symptoms of AD include agitation, psychosis, anxiety, depression, and sleep disorders. Approximately one half of patients with dementia experience agitation. Many patients with AD also experience psychotic symptoms, such as delusions, hallucinations, and paranoia. Agitation and psychosis, which may be particularly frightening for families and caregivers, should be treated if the patient is causing harm to self or others.

The choice of an antipsychotic agent is based on cost and adverse events. Choosing an agent with a low degree of anticholinergic activity seems warranted in patients with AD. High-potency agents, such as haloperidol (Haldol), are associated with fewer anticholinergic effects as compared to low-potency agents, such as chlorpromazine (Thorazine). The atypical antipsychotics are associated with less extrapyramidal symptoms than the typical agents; thus, these agents are preferred.

Recent developments have associated the atypical agents risperidone (Risperidal) and olanzapine (Zyprexa) with an increased risk of stroke in patients using these agents for behavioral disturbances associated with dementia. A warning on the package insert of these agents reports that they are not approved by the FDA for the treatment of behavioral disturbances associated with dementia. It is important for the practitioner to weigh the risks versus benefits of using these agents. Also, assessment of whether the patient has a history or risk factors for a stroke will provide insight into the use of these agents. The role of the other atypical antipsychotics has not been evaluated for this indication.

Cost may limit the use of atypical antipsychotics. The role of the newer atypical antipsychotic agents (eg, quetiapine [Seroquel], ziprasidone [Geodon]) remains to be determined. Regardless of the agent chosen, the lowest effective dose should be used. The practitioner should reassess the need for these medications periodically (every 3-6 months).

Benzodiazepines

Benzodiazepines have been prescribed to treat behavioral problems related to dementia. Because they do not appear to be as effective as the antipsychotics for treating behavioral problems, benzodiazepines are often reserved for treating symptoms of anxiety or for episodic agitation. These agents can be used as needed in situations that precipitate acute anxiety.

If a benzodiazepine is prescribed, lorazepam (Ativan) or oxazepam (Serax) are appropriate choices. They are inexpensive, have a short half-life, and hepatic metabolism is not significantly altered in the elderly. All benzodiazepines should be started at the lowest dose. The suggested starting dose for lorazepam is 0.5 to 1 mg orally every 4 to 6 hours, and the starting dose for oxazepam is 10 mg orally 3 times day. The advantage of lorazepam is that it is available parenterally.

Adverse effects of the benzodiazepines include falls, sedation, delirium, and loss of inhibition. Routine use is not recommended because of limited efficacy, adverse effects, and potential for worsening AD symptoms. The use of benzodiazepines for anxiety associated with dementia should be reevaluated periodically.

Data on using various other agents (trazodone [Desyrel], valproate [Depakene], carbamazepine [Tegretol], buspirone [BuSpar], SSRIs, and β blockers) for treating anxiety associated with AD are limited. These agents may have a role in treating agitation in patients who do not tolerate or respond to antipsychotic agents or benzodiazepines.

Antidepressants

Because there is a high incidence of depression associated with dementia, pharmacologic treatment is often necessary. Patients may not meet explicit criteria for a depressive syndrome, but it is recommended that these patients still be offered treatment. Treatment may improve cognition, mood, apathy, function, behavior, appetite, sleep, and overall quality of life. Because there is no evidence that one class of antidepressants is superior to another in treating depression, the prescriber may base the choice of an agent on the individual patient, cost, side effect profile, and potential drug interactions.

In many clinical practices, SSRIs, such as sertraline (Zoloft), paroxetine (Paxil), or citalopram (Celexa), have become a first-line therapy for depression in the elderly. The recommended starting dose of sertraline is 25 mg taken orally each morning. Patients who experience anxiety or insomnia with this agent can be given a trial of paroxetine, which is more sedating. Citalopram, in addition to its antidepressant effects, has proved beneficial in improving certain emotional symptoms of AD (panic, bluntness, depressed mood, confusion, irritability, anxiety, and restlessness) in patients with and without depression. SSRIs in general have fewer side effects (particularly anticholinergic) than the tricyclic antidepressants (TCAs) or MAO inhibitors, but they may be more costly to the patient.

The TCAs (eg, nortriptyline [Pamelor]) may also have a beneficial role. However, the TCAs have more anticholinergic side effects that have limited their use. Psychostimulants, such as methylphenidate (Ritalin), have been used for treating apathy, but they should be used with caution in patients with AD because they may worsen agitation and cause sleep disorders.

Selecting the Most Appropriate Agent for Cognitive Symptoms

First-Line Therapy

Once the decision has been made to initiate drug therapy, cholinesterase inhibitors may be tried in patients with mild to moderate AD (Fig. 48-2). Donepezil is considered the first choice because fewer adverse events are associated with its use and the once-daily dosing schedule. These medications, however, are expensive and only modestly benefit cognitive function. Patients with severe AD may be offered memantine in conjunction with a cholinesterase inhibitor (Table 48-3). The combination therapy is expensive and could only provide moderate benefit.

Second-Line Therapy

Second-line therapy is a trial of a different cholinesterase inhibitor. In conjunction, some providers may add vitamin E. Vitamin E has a benign side effect profile and minimal cost and may be added to acetylcholinesterase inhibitor regimens in patients with mild to moderate AD.

Third-Line Therapy

Another trial of a different cholinesterase inhibitor if the patient is mild to moderate AD. Selegiline may be considered for patients who experience adverse events (eg, bleeding) with vitamin E and who are unable to tolerate acetylcholinesterase inhibitor therapy.

Special Population Considerations

Estrogen replacement therapy (ERT) may have a potential benefit for postmenopausal women with AD. The exact

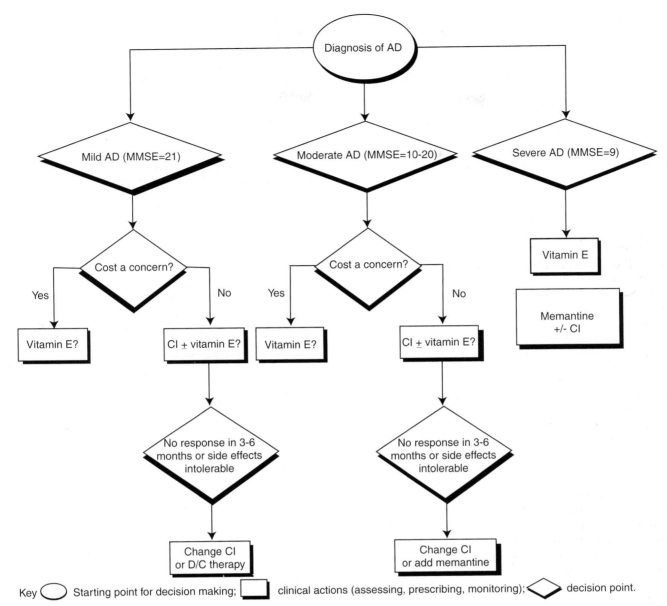

Figure 48–2 Treatment algorithm for the cognitive symptoms of Alzheimer's disease (AD). Initial treatment is determined by the severity of disease. A Mini-Mental State Exam (MMSE) score of 21 suggests mild AD whereas a score of 9 suggests severe disease.

role in AD is unknown but ERT has neurotrophic, antioxidant, and anti-inflammatory effects. Epidemiologic studies suggest that ERT may be protective and may benefit women with AD. Controlled clinical trials show no clinical benefit with the use of ERT and an increase in adverse drug effects. However, due to the risks associated with ERT, use of estrogen is not recommended or approved for the treatment of AD. See Chapter 59 for a more detailed discussion.

MONITORING PATIENT RESPONSE

Consensus guidelines suggest that the primary care provider should schedule appointments with patients with AD and families every 3 to 6 months to monitor cognitive and behavioral symptoms and to assess the patient's response to pharmacotherapy. If clinical improvement does not occur with a cholinesterase inhibitor after 3 to 6 months of treatment, the practitioner may consider switching to another cholinesterase inhibitor. Until all cholinesterase inhibitors have been tried should the provider assess whether the patient should stop the medication. The MMSE is a useful objective measure of cognitive response to therapy, but input from family and caregivers must also be recognized. Discontinuing the medication may be considered at any time during therapy if there is a perceived lack of efficacy. If a marked decline in cognitive function is noted within the first 3 to 6 weeks after discontinuing drug therapy, the practitioner may consider restarting the acetylcholinesterase inhibitor. When patients progress to severe

Table 48.3

Recommended Order of Treatment of the Cognitive Symptoms Associated with Alzheimer's Disease

Order	Agents	Comments
First line	Cholinesterase inhibitors (CIs)	Donepezil will be most likely the first-line CI for mild to moderate AD due to its convenient once-daily dosing and ability to achieve maximum dose rapidly.
	Memantine	Memantine is reserved for patients with moderate to severe AD; clinical trials show that it may be used in conjunction with a CI.
Second line	CIs	A trial of second CI is warranted.
	Vitamin E	Use of vitamin E may be added to the CI or used as monotherapy in patients who cannot afford CIs.
Third line	CI	Another trial of a different CI.
	Selegiline	Selegiline may be considered in a patient who cannot tolerate CIs or vitamin E.

impairment (ie, MMSE score <10), addition of memantine may be an option.

Ability to perform activities of daily living (ADLs), such as bathing, dressing, toileting, and feeding, and instrumental activities of daily living (IADLs), such as transferring, housekeeping, shopping, and paying bills, should be assessed to help determine the functional status of the patient and response to treatment. Assessment of the noncognitive symptoms of AD could be a sign of disease progression.

In patients receiving antipsychotic medications, response is usually seen within the first day of therapy. If patients continue to have delusions, hallucinations, or agitation, doses can be gradually increased at 4- to 7-day intervals.

In contrast, response to antidepressant medications is seen within 4 to 6 weeks. The psychostimulants (eg, methylphenidate) should be effective within 2 to 3 days of treatment and may be used while awaiting the onset of antidepressant effect with the SSRIs or TCAs. Evidence of suicidal ideation should be taken seriously and immediately addressed by the practitioner.

If patients with sleep disorders continue to require regular pharmacotherapy, psychiatric referral is necessary to assist in determining the source of the insomnia. Nonpharmacologic interventions, such as limiting daytime napping, moderate daytime exercise, and avoiding large meals or beverages at bedtime, should be reinforced with the patient and family. If the insomnia is not disruptive or problematic for the family or patient, no treatment may be a viable option.

Treatment with any of these agents may be continued until the risk of pharmacotherapy outweighs the benefit to the patient or family. Clear communication with the patient, family, and caregivers cannot be overemphasized because evaluation of pharmacotherapeutic efficacy and decisions to stop or continue treatment depend on this input.

PATIENT EDUCATION

Regardless of the agents chosen for AD treatment, patients, families, and caregivers must have realistic goals of drug therapy. Their goals should include increasing length of time of self-sufficiency, delaying the need for nursing home placement, and reducing the burden on the caregiver. It is important that the family and patients understand the available agents are expected to slow the disease progression.

They need to understand that no currently available agents are curative and only modest improvements can be expected.

Tacrine must be taken between meals for optimal absorption. Compliance with 4 times daily dosing and liver function monitoring with tacrine must be emphasized. Patients taking donepezil should be instructed to take it in the evening to avoid experiencing adverse GI events. If insomnia or nightmares occur, the drug may be given in the morning. Donepezil may be taken with or without food. Rivastigmine should be taken with food and have a slow dose titration to minimize the GI side effects. Galantamine can be taken without regard to food and should be slowly titrated to minimize adverse effects. Memantine appears to be well tolerated. Because vitamin E may predispose certain patients (eg, those with vitamin K deficiency) to bleeding, patients and families should be informed to report unusual bruising, blood in urine or stool, bleeding gums, and the like immediately to their health care provider. The practitioner should inform patients taking selegiline to take the first dose of the day in the morning and the second dose at lunchtime to minimize insomnia.

Patient-Oriented Information Sources

The various support resources available for patients and families of patients with AD are shown in Box 48-4.

Complementary and Alternative Medications

Vitamin E

Vitamin E, an antioxidant, has an emerging role in AD treatment. Due to its antioxidant effects, vitamin E can stabilize free radicals and the damage they produce. Patients with moderate AD started on vitamin E can expect approximately a 7-month delay in reaching a poor functional outcome or end point (ie, death, institutionalization, loss of the ability to perform basic ADLs, or severe dementia; Sano et al., 1997). This difference is seen within 2 years of initiating treatment. Indefinite treatment with vitamin E is a reasonable approach.

Vitamin E may be effective because of its antioxidant effects. A starting dose of 1000 IU given orally twice a day appears to be appropriate because this was the regimen used in the trial supporting its efficacy (Sano et al., 1997). Vitamin E, because of its benign side effect profile, minimal cost, and lack of significant drug interactions, has become a good choice for treating AD. It has been suggested that vitamin E may also have a role in the treatment of mild AD and can be used in combination with a cholinesterase inhibitor (APA, 1997).

Minimal adverse effects are associated with vitamin E. Because vitamin E may worsen coagulation problems (causing bleeding) in patients with vitamin K deficiency or taking warfarin (Coumadin), it is suggested that these patients receive lower doses (200-800 IU/d; APA, 1997). An increase in syncope and falls was also noted for vitamin E (and selegiline) in the study by Sano and colleagues (1997). Patients should be monitored for an increase in such events if they are receiving either of these agents.

Herbal Agents

Ginkgo biloba extract, thought to have antioxidant properties, has been studied in a well-designed, controlled trial of patients with mild to severe AD or multi-infarct dementia. Modest improvement of cognition was recorded in results of the Alzheimer's Disease Assessment Scale. Caregivers also recognized improvement in function (Le Bars et al., 1997).

Treatment was well tolerated, with some GI side effects reported. Additional well-designed studies should be conducted before routine use is recommended. Because this product is not regulated by the FDA as a medication, its safety remains unknown, and ginkgo biloba products may vary in extract concentrations and contents. Patients who choose to take this product should be cautioned that it may interact with warfarin or aspirin, increasing their risk of bleeding.

Huperzine A is another herbal product that reportedly benefits patients with AD. It appears to be a reversible cholinesterase inhibitor and may be more potent than either tacrine or donepezil. It has been used in China for treating dementia and appears to have fewer side effects and toxicities than tacrine or donepezil, as well as a longer half-life.

■ Case Study

M.W. is a 70-year-old white woman with a medical history of hypertension, osteoarthritis, irritable bowel syndrome, and total hysterectomy. She visits the primary care clinic with her daughter, who is concerned because M.W. has "bounced" a few checks and can no longer pay her bills without assistance. M.W. admits that she has been forgetful and appears anxious as she describes an incident in which she went shopping and could not remember where she parked her car. Her daughter states that her mother's memory has progressively worsened over the past year. M.W.'s medications include fosinopril (Monopril) 20 mg/d, raloxifene (Evista) 60 mg daily, calcium (Os-Cal 500) 3 times daily, and acetaminophen (Tylenol) 1000 mg every 6 hours. A careful evaluation and work-up was ordered.

Diagnosis: Mild AD with a MMSE score of 22.

1. List specific goals of treatment for M.W.

2. What over-the-counter or alternative medications would be appropriate for this patient?

3. What dietary and lifestyle changes should be recommended for this patient?

4. What drug therapy would you prescribe? Why?

5. How would you monitor for success with this therapy?

6. Discuss specific patient education based on the prescribed therapy.

7. Describe one or two drug–drug or drug–food interactions for the selected agent.

8. List one or two adverse reactions for the selected agent that would cause you to change therapy.

9. What would be the choice for the second-line therapy?

Bibliography

Starred references are cited in the text.

American Psychiatric Association. (1994). *Diagnostic and statistical manual of mental disorders* (4th ed.). Washington, DC: Author.

*American Psychiatric Association. (1997). Practice guideline for the treatment of patients with Alzheimer's disease and other dementias in late life. *American Journal of Psychiatry, 154*(Suppl. 5), 1–39.

*Brookmeyer, R., Corrada, M. M., Curriero, F. C., et al. (2002). Survival following a diagnosis of Alzheimer's disease. *Archives of Neurology, 59*, 1764–1767.

Carr, D. B., Goate, A., & Morris, J. C. (1997). Current concepts in the pathogenesis of Alzheimer's disease. *American Journal of Medicine, 103*(Suppl. 3A), 3S–10S.

*Folstein, M. F., Folstein, S. W., & McHugh, P. R. (1975). Mini-Mental State: A practical method for grading the cognitive state of patients for the clinician. *Journal of Psychiatric Research, 12,* 189–198.

*Hebert, L. E., Scherr, P. A, Bienias, J. L., et al. (2003). Alzheimer disease in the U.S. population: Prevalence estimates using the 2000 census. *Archives of Neurology, 60*(8), 1119–1122.

Henderson, V. W., Paganini-Hill, A., Miller, B. L., et al. (2000). Estrogen for Alzheimer's disease in women: Randomized, double-blind, placebo-controlled trial. *Neurology, 54,* 295–301.

In't Veld B. A., Ruitenberg A., Hofman A., et al. (2001). Nonsteroidal anti-inflammatory drugs and the risk of Alzheimer's disease. *New England Journal of Medicine, 345,* 1515–1521.

*Le Bars, P. L., Katz, M. M., Berman, N., et al. (1997). A placebo-controlled, double-blind, randomized trial of an extract of ginkgo biloba for dementia. *Journal of the American Medical Association, 278,* 1327–1332.

*Lendon, C. L., Ashall, F., & Goate, A. M. (1997). Exploring the etiology of Alzheimer's disease using molecular genetics. *Journal of the American Medical Association, 277,* 825–831.

McKhann, G., Drachman, D., Folstein, M., et al. (1984). Clinical diagnosis of Alzheimer's disease: Report of the NINCDS-ADRDA Work Group under the auspices of the Department of Health and Human Services Task Force on Alzheimer's Disease. *Neurology, 34,* 939–944.

*Morris, J. C. (1994). Differential diagnosis of Alzheimer's disease. *Clinics in Geriatric Medicine, 10,* 257–257.

Medical Economics Company. (2000). Aricept (donepezil). In L. Murray (Ed.), *Physician's desk reference* (54th ed.). Montvale, NJ: Author.

Mulnard, R. A., Cotman, C. W., Kawas, C., et al. (2000). Estrogen replacement therapy for treatment of mild to moderate Alzheimer's disease: A randomized controlled trial. Alzheimer's Disease Cooperative Study. *Journal of the American Medical Association, 283,* 1007–1015.

National Advisory Council on Aging [NACA]. (1995). *Report to Congress on the scientific opportunities for developing treatments for Alzheimer's disease.* Washington, DC: Author.

Nyth, A. L., & Gottfries, C. G. (1990). The clinical efficacy of citalopram in treatment of emotional disturbances in dementia disorders: A Nordic multicenter study. *British Journal of Psychiatry, 157,* 894–901.

Reisberg, B., Doody, R., Stoffler, A., et al. (2003). Memantine in moderate-to-severe Alzheimer's disease. *New England Journal of Medicine, 348,* 1333–1341.

*Sano, M., Ernesto, C., Thomas, R. G., et al. (1997). A controlled trial of selegiline, alpha-tocopherol, or both as treatment for Alzheimer's disease. *New England Journal of Medicine, 336,* 1216–1222.

*Small, G. W., Rabins, P. V., Barry, P. P., et al. (1997). Diagnosis and treatment of Alzheimer disease and related disorders: Consensus statement of the American Association for Geriatric Psychiatry, the Alzheimer's Association, and the American Geriatrics Society. *Journal of the American Medical Association, 278,* 1363–1371.

Skolnick, A. A. (1997). Old Chinese herbal medicine used for fever yields possible new Alzheimer disease therapy. *Journal of the American Medical Association, 277,* 776.

Talbot, C., Lendon, C., Craddock, N., et al. (1994). Protection against Alzheimer's disease with ApoE2. *Lancet, 343,* 1432–1433.

Tariot, P. N., Farlow, M. R., Grossberg, G. T., et al. (2004). Memantine treatment in patients with moderate to severe Alzheimer disease already receiving donepezil: A randomized controlled trial. *Journal of the American Medical Association, 291,* 317–324.

*Wiser, T. H. (1994). Alzheimer's cognitive disturbances: a case study. *US Pharmacist, 19,* 52–78.

Wolozin, B. K. W., Rousseau, P., Celesia, G. G., et al. (2000). Decreased prevalence of Alzheimer disease associated with 3-hydroxy-3-methyglutaryl coenzyme A reductase inhibitors. *Archives of Neurology, 57*(10), 1439–1443.

Yankner, B. A., & Mesulam, M. M. (1991). β-Amyloid and the pathogenesis of Alzheimer's disease. *New England Journal of Medicine, 325,* 1849–1857.

Visit the Connection web site for the most up-to-date drug information.

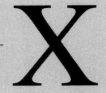

Pharmacotherapy
for Endocrine
Disorders

49

DIABETES MELLITUS

■ JANIS BONAT AND VIRGINIA P. ARCANGELO

Diabetes mellitus is the term used to represent a clinically and genetically heterogeneous group of disorders characterized by abnormally high blood glucose levels (hyperglycemia) as a result of either insulin deficiency or cellular resistance to the action of insulin. Four major classifications of diabetes have been defined: type 1 diabetes mellitus (formerly known as insulin-dependent diabetes mellitus), type 2 diabetes mellitus (formerly known as non–insulin-dependent diabetes mellitus), gestational diabetes mellitus, and diabetes secondary to other conditions (eg, hormonal abnormalities and pancreatic diseases).

According to the National Institute of Diabetes and Digestive and Kidney Diseases and the American Diabetes Association (ADA), diabetes was the sixth leading cause of death in the United States in 2000. Overall, the risk of death among people with diabetes is approximately twice that of people without diabetes. Direct annual medical costs for diabetes in the United States in 2002 were $92 billion, with indirect costs adding another $40 billion. Diabetes affects approximately 18.2 million people in the United States. Of this number, 90% to 95% have type 2 diabetes.

CAUSES

Type 1 diabetes is thought to be an autoimmune disease in which pancreatic beta cells are destroyed. The beta cells are responsible for secreting insulin, a major hormone that promotes cellular uptake and use of glucose and maintains metabolic functions throughout the body. If the beta cells are destroyed, the pancreas produces no insulin, causing glucose levels in the blood to skyrocket. Onset can occur at any time, but most patients are younger than 30 years of age.

Although type 1 diabetes is one of the most common chronic diseases in children, its etiology remains unclear. Suggested etiologies include genetic predisposition to the destruction of beta cells, infection, autoimmunity, and environmental factors. Viral agents are highly suspected in the pathogenesis of type 1 diabetes because mumps, rubella, varicella, measles, influenza, coxsackievirus, cytomegalovirus, and viral pneumonia have been reported to precede its onset. Furthermore, the incidence increases in the United States during the fall and winter, when viral infections are prevalent. Autoimmunity is evident because 80% of patients with type 1 diabetes test positive for specific human leukocyte antigen. It is likely that a combination of these factors contributes to the destruction of beta cells and the subsequent absence of insulin.

In type 2 diabetes, adipose and muscle cells become less sensitive to the actions of insulin or the pancreas produces less insulin than the body needs. In either situation, glucose levels in the blood escalate. Most patients with type 2 diabetes are older than 30 years of age. Box 49-1 lists risk factors for type 2 diabetes; the major risk factors are obesity and family history. Both beta cell defects and insulin resistance are found in patients with type 2 diabetes.

In gestational diabetes mellitus, pregnancy causes the woman to become intolerant to glucose. The causes are not fully clear, but they appear to be related to the anti-insulin effects created by progesterone, cortisol, and human placental lactogen. Usually, once the woman has delivered her infant, blood glucose levels return to normal; however, women who have had gestational diabetes have a 20% to 50% chance of developing diabetes in the next 5 to 10 years.

PATHOPHYSIOLOGY

In type 1 diabetes, the pancreatic beta cells are destroyed, causing a subsequent absence of insulin. In genetically susceptible people, an autoimmune attack occurs in which monocytes/macrophages and activated cytotoxic T cells infiltrate the islets. Multiple antibodies against beta cell antigens develop in the blood, and insulin reserve steadily decreases until the amount is insufficient to maintain a normal blood glucose level.

The pathogenesis of type 2 diabetes involves insulin resistance, impaired insulin secretion, elevated glucose production by the liver, or all these components. With insulin resistance, circulating insulin concentrations increase as compensation. Researchers have hypothesized that, in type 2 diabetes, the ability of insulin to inhibit hepatic glucose production and to stimulate its uptake and use by adipose and muscle cells is diminished. In lean patients with type 2 diabetes, the primary defect appears to occur in the beta cells. In overweight patients, who represent most patients with type 2 diabetes, the most likely primary defect is impairment of the target cells. Although abnormal hepatic glucose metabolism plays an important role in maintaining the diabetic state, it is probably not the earliest development and most likely follows impaired insulin sensitivity in the muscle.

BOX 49–1. MAJOR RISK FACTORS FOR TYPE 2 DIABETES MELLITUS

- Family history of diabetes (ie, parents or siblings with diabetes)
- Obesity (ie, 20% over desired body weight or body mass index >27)
- Race/ethnicity (eg, African Americans, Hispanic Americans, Native Americans, Asian Americans, Pacific Islanders have increased risk)
- Age older than 45 y
- Previously identified as having IFG (impaired fasting glucose)
- Hypertension
- High-density lipoprotein cholesterol level >35 mg/dL or triglyceride level >250 mg/dL
- History of gestational diabetes mellitus or delivery of babies weighing >9 lb
- Sedentary lifestyle
- Polycystic ovary syndrome

Insulin affects many body systems, and chronic hyperinsulinemia contributes to the pathogenesis and worsening of hypertension, dyslipidemia, and coronary heart disease. Hypertension, high plasma triglyceride levels, and low high-density lipoprotein (HDL) plasma levels correlate with hyperinsulinemia secondary to insulin resistance and a worsened cardiovascular risk profile. This collection of clinical markers or indicators associated with insulin resistance is referred to as the metabolic syndrome.

Epidemiologic and interventional studies consistently point to the relationship between good glycemic control and the prevention or slowing of the progression of long-term complications of diabetes. The Diabetes Control and Complications Trial (DCCT) presented definitive evidence to support the hypothesis that diabetic complications are related to the degree of hyperglycemia. In this landmark study, patients with type 1 diabetes were randomized to two groups and followed for an average of 6.5 years. One group received conventional therapy (one or two daily insulin injections, daily self-monitoring of glucose, and diabetes education) to normalize blood glucose levels; the other group received intensive therapy (three or more daily administrations of insulin and glucose monitoring 4 times daily). The incidence of microvascular complications was 60% lower in the group that

received intensive therapy than in the patients who received conventional therapy. Hence, intensive therapy delayed the onset of complications and slowed their progression. The United Kingdom Prospective Diabetes Study (UKPDS) Group answered the question as to whether the DCCT results could be extrapolated to include type 2 diabetics. In the UKPDS, patients with type 2 diabetes were randomized to intensive or conventional therapy and followed over a 10-year period. As in the DCCT, there was a significant (25%) risk reduction in microvascular end points with tight control.

DIAGNOSTIC CRITERIA

Patients with marked hyperglycemia present with the classic symptoms of polyuria (excessive urination), polydipsia (increased thirst), weight loss, polyphagia (increased hunger and caloric intake), and blurred vision. In type 1 diabetes, the onset of these symptoms usually is sudden and often preceded by ketoacidosis. In contrast, the course of development for type 2 diabetes is gradual, insidious, and frequently undiagnosed for years. The onset and sometimes the presence of symptoms often go unnoticed. Therefore, screening for diabetes as part of a routine medical examination is appropriate if a patient has one or more risk factors (see Box 49-1). The more risk factors that the individual has, the greater the chances are for him or her to develop or have diabetes. Because early detection and prompt treatment may reduce the impact of diabetes and its complications, screening is recommended for those at risk.

In general, the ADA strongly prefers the fasting plasma glucose (FPG) test instead of the oral glucose tolerance test (OGTT) for most screening and diagnostic purposes because the FPG test is more convenient for patients and less expensive. Fasting is defined as no intake of food or beverage other than water for at least 8 hours before testing. The OGTT is still the preferred test for pregnant women.

Normal glucose is defined as an FPG level less than 100 mg/dL and a 2-hour postload glucose (PG) value in the OGTT less than 140 mg/dL. An FPG level of 126 mg/dL or more or a 2-hour PG value in the OGTT of 200 mg/dL or more warrants repeat testing on a different day to confirm the diagnosis. Patients with an FPG of at least 100 mg/dL but less than 126 mg/dL have impaired fasting glucose (IFG). Patients with a 2-hour PG value of at least 140 mg/dL but less than 200 mg/dL in the OGTT are considered as having impaired glucose tolerance (IGT). Patients with IFG or impaired glucose tolerance are now referred to as having "pre-diabetes," indicating the relatively high risk for the development of diabetes. Diagnostic criteria are presented in Table 49-1.

Table 49.1

Criteria for the Diagnosis of Diabetes Mellitus

Normoglycemia	Impaired Glucose Metabolism	Diabetes Mellitus
FPG <100 mg/dL 2-h PG <140 mg/dL	FPG ≥100 and <126 mg/dL (IFG) 2-h PG ≥140 and <200 mg/dL (IGT)	FPG ≥126 mg/dL 2-h PG ≥200 mg/dL Random plasma glucose ≥200 mg/dL and symptoms of diabetes mellitus

FPG, fasting plasma glucose; IFG, impaired fasting glucose; IGT, impaired glucose tolerance; PG, plasma glucose.

Plasma glucose levels can be obtained from patients regardless of the time the patients last ate. Such levels are referred to as random plasma glucose levels. Any random plasma glucose level of 200 mg/dL or more is considered positive for diabetes and warrants additional testing, preferably by the FPG test on another day.

Certain drugs may cause hyperglycemia. These include glucocorticoids, furosemide, thiazide diuretics, products containing estrogen, beta blockers, and nicotinic acid.

INITIATING DRUG THERAPY

Effective treatment programs for diabetes mellitus require comprehensive training in self-management, ongoing support from the clinical care team, and, for many, intensive pharmacologic regimens. These programs must be individualized according to each patient's needs and should include the following features:

- Self-monitoring blood glucose (SMBG)
- Medical nutrition therapy
- Regular exercise
- Drug therapy individualized for each patient
- Oral glucose-lowering agents for some patients with type 2 diabetes
- Instruction in the prevention and treatment of acute and chronic complications, including hypoglycemia
- Continuing patient education and support
- Periodic assessment of treatment goals

Treatment of abnormal glucose levels consists of diet and exercise. The cornerstone of therapy for all patients with diabetes is diet, but the goals of therapy differ between types 1 and 2 diabetes. In general, patients with type 1 diabetes are usually thin and present at or below ideal body weight. Therefore, the goals of diet are directed toward regulation of caloric intake and proper spacing of meals and snacks. In the presence of exogenously administered insulin, these patients require proper timing of meals and routine activities to prevent episodes of hypoglycemia. Patients taking insulin should carry a source of simple sugar at all times in the event of hypoglycemia.

Because most patients with type 2 diabetes are overweight, the goal of treatment is directed toward weight reduction. Weight loss leads to improved glucose tolerance by enhancing the sensitivity of peripheral glucose receptors. Patients with type 2 diabetes can control the condition through diet and exercise alone. If these interventions fail to achieve desirable glycemic control, practitioners should initiate drug therapy.

Goals of Drug Therapy

The major goals of drug therapy in diabetes mellitus are as follows:

Glycemic control

- Hemoglobin A_{1c} (HbgA$_{1c}$) level $\leq 6.9\%$, preferably $\leq 6.5\%$

- Preprandial plasma glucose level 90–130 mg/dL
- Postprandial plasma glucose level <180 mg/dL

Blood pressure

- <130/80 mm Hg (125/75 for patients with proteinuria)

Lipids

- Low-density lipoprotein (LDL) level <100 mg/dL
- Triglyceride level <150 mg/dL
- HDL level >40 mg/dL

Microalbumin (random collection)

- <30 μg/mL creatinine

In type 1 diabetes, insulin is the mainstay of drug therapy. When diet and exercise alone do not achieve glycemic control of type 2 diabetes, drug therapy is indicated. In type 2 diabetes, oral agents with glucose-lowering effects are used. The ADA suggests that pharmacologic therapy be selected with consideration to the following factors:

- Degree of hyperglycemia and the presence or absence of symptoms
- Presence of comorbidity
- Patient motivation
- Patient preference

Table 49-2 provides an overview of the various oral agents.

Sulfonylureas

Sulfonylureas are a major group of oral hypoglycemic agents used to treat type 2 diabetes (see Table 49-2). They correct derangements of carbohydrate, lipid, and protein metabolism.

Mechanism of Action

Sulfonylureas bind to specific receptors on beta cells, causing adenosine triphosphate (ATP)-dependent potassium channels to close. The calcium channels subsequently open, leading to increased cytoplasmic calcium, which stimulates the release of insulin. Theorists have hypothesized that these drugs also have extrapancreatic effects involving the liver, muscle, and adipose cells, but because these agents are ineffective in patients with type 1 diabetes, it appears that their predominant hypoglycemic action is on the beta cells. When used alone, these agents have the most significant effect on blood sugar, especially in patients who are lean and insulinopenic.

The sulfonylureas are divided into first- and second-generation agents. The second-generation drugs are more potent and more widely used than are the first-generation agents. Comparison of these drugs by potency and other pharmacologic properties is presented in Table 49-3.

Approximately one third of patients with type 2 diabetes fail to respond adequately to sulfonylureas, most often because of markedly impaired beta cell function, not adhering to diet, or stressful events such as infection. After 10 years of

Table 49.2

Overview of Oral Antidiabetic Agents

Generic (Trade) Name and Dosage	Selected Adverse Events	Contraindications	Special Considerations
Sulfonylureas			
FIRST GENERATION			
tolbutamide (Orinase) 0.25–3 g in 1 or 2 divided doses	Hypoglycemia, increased risk of cardiovascular disease	Ketoacidosis, sulfa allergy	Onset occurs within 1 h, lasts 6–12 h. Give with morning meal. Effectiveness may decrease over time. Increased hypoglycemia may occur in elderly or debilitated patients. Signs and symptoms of hypoglycemia may be masked in patients taking beta blockers.
chlorpropamide (Diabinese) 100–750 mg qd Elderly start at 100 mg/d, and others at 250 mg/d	Hypoglycemia	Same as above	Onset is 1 h, lasts 72 h. Same as above
tolazamide (Tolinase) Initially 100–250 mg qd; increase weekly by 100–250 mg/d until desired blood glucose Maximum dose 1000 mg/d	Hypoglycemia, increased risk of cardiovascular mortality	Same as above	Onset occurs within 4–6 h, lasts 10–14 h. Same as above
SECOND GENERATION			
glyburide (DiaBeta, Micronase) Initially 2.5–5 mg qd; increase by 2.5 mg/wk until desired blood glucose Elderly patients start at 1.25 mg/d Maximum dose 20 mg/d	Hypoglycemia	Same as above	Onset occurs within 1.5 h, lasts 18–24 h. Same as above
glyburide, micronized (Glynase) Initially 1.5–3 mg qd; 0.75 mg in elderly Maximum dose 12 mg/d	Same as above	Same as above	Onset occurs within 1.5 h, lasts 18–24 h. Same as above
glipizide (Glucotrol) Initially 5 mg qd (2.5 mg in elderly); increase weekly to a maximum of 40 mg/d to desired blood glucose	Same as above	Same as above	Patients should take medication 30 min before a meal. Onset occurs within 1 h, lasts for 10–24 h. Same as above
glimepiride (Amaryl) Initially 1–2 mg with breakfast; increase by 2 mg/wk until desired blood glucose Maximum dose 8 mg/d	Same as above	Same as above	Onset occurs within 2–4 h, lasts 24 h. Same as above
BIGUANIDE			
metformin (Glucophage) Initially 500 mg bid; increase by 500 mg/wk until desired blood glucose Maximum dose 2550 mg/d in divided doses	GI distress: diarrhea, nausea, bloating, flatulence Rare lactic acidosis	Renal dysfunction, CHF, metabolic acidosis, ketoacidosis, impaired hepatic function, excess alcohol consumption, pregnancy	Patients should take with meals to minimize GI side effects. Medication must be temporarily held when patient is undergoing IV iodinated contrast study. Modest synergistic effect may occur when given with sulfonylurea. Medication should be held for patients undergoing surgery.
Thiazolidinediones			
rosiglitazone (Avandia) Initially 4 mg/d in single dose; if response is inadequate after 12 wk, increase to 8 mg/d in single dose	Anemia, edema, headache, reversible increase in ALT	Children, ketoacidosis	Monitor ALT at baseline, every 2 mo for the first 12 mo, and periodically thereafter. Discontinue medication if ALT is >3 times the upper limit of normal or if jaundice occurs. Medications may increase plasma volume; caution is necessary for patients with New York Heart Association class III and IV heart failure.

Table 49.2

Overview of Oral Antidiabetic Agents (*Continued*)

Generic (Trade) Name and Dosage	Selected Adverse Events	Contraindications	Special Considerations
pioglitazone (Actos) 15–30 mg/d Maximum 45 mg/d as monotherapy and 30 mg/d as combined therapy	Same as above	Same as above	Resumption of premenopausal ovulation may occur in anovulatory women. Unintended pregnancy may result. Same as above
α-Glucosidase Inhibitors acarbose (Precose) Initially 25 mg tid with the first bite of a meal; increase by 25 mg at 4- to 8-wk intervals to a maximum of 300 mg in three divided doses (150 mg if weight <60 kg)	Flatulence, diarrhea, abdominal pain/distention	Renal dysfunction, ketoacidosis, inflammatory bowel disease, colonic ulceration; predisposition to intestinal obstruction; disorders of digestion	Patients should take with first bite of each meal.
miglitol (Glyset) Same as above	Same as above	Same as above	Same as above
Meglitinide Analogs repaglinide (Prandin) Initially 0.5 mg with two to four meals daily if patient has never received any other treatment for diabetes; if previous treatment, 1–2 mg with two to four meals daily Double dose weekly to a maximum of 16 mg/d	Hyperglycemia, upper respiratory tract infection, headache, diarrhea, constipation, arthralgia, back or chest pain	Type 1 diabetes, ketoacidosis	As monotherapy or in conjunction with metformin, medication is to be taken within 30 min of a meal. Patient should skip a dose if he or she skips a meal and add a dose if he or she adds a meal.
nateglinide (Starlix) Initially 120 mg before each meal to a maximum dose of 360 mg/d	Same as above	Same as above	Same as above
Combination drugs SULFONYLUREA AND BIGUANIDE glyburide and metformin (Glucovance) 1.25 mg/250 mg; 2.5 mg/500 mg; 5 mg/500 mg Maximum dose 20 mg/2000 mg/d	Hypoglycemia, GI distress, diarrhea, flatulence Rare lactic acidosis	Same as above	Same as above
glipizide and metformin (Metaglip) 2.5 mg/200 mg 2.5 mg/50 mg 5 mg/500 mg	Same as above	Same as above	Same as above
THIAZOLIDINEDIONE AND BIGUANIDE rosiglitazone and metformin (Avandamet) 1 mg/500 mg 2 mg/500 mg 4 mg/ 500 mg 2 mg/1000 mg 4 mg/1000 mg	GI distress, diarrhea, flatulence Rare lactic acidosis, edema, headache Reversible increase in ALT	Same as above	Same as above

ALT, alanine aminotransfearse; CHF, Congestive heart failure; GI, gastrointestinal.

therapy, only 50% of initial responders have adequate glycemic control. For optimal response, careful patient selection should include the following criteria: duration of disease less than 5 years, no history of prior insulin therapy or good glycemic control on less than 40 U/d insulin, close to normal body weight, and FPG less than 180 mg/dL.

Adverse Events/Contraindications/Interactions

The most important complication of the use of sulfonylureas is hypoglycemia. In the elderly population, this risk is greatest secondary to comorbidity, polypharmacy, or poor social situations (eg, isolation, financial constraints). In younger

Table 49.3

Comparison of Oral Sulfonylureas

Drug	Equivalent Therapeutic Dose (mg)	Duration of Action (h)	Doses per Day	Adverse Events (%)	Hypoglycemic Reactions (%)
First Generation					
tolbutamide	1000	6–12	2–3	3	<1
tolazamide	250	12–24	1–2	2	1
acetohexamide	500	12–18	2	4	1
chlorpropamide	250	24–72	1	8	4–6
Second Generation					
long-acting glipizide	10	12–24	1–2	5	2–4
long-acting glipizide	5–10	24	1	5	<1
long-acting glyburide	5	16–24	1–2	7	4–6

patients, hypoglycemia may be associated with alcohol abuse or overexertion. Long-acting agents (eg, chlorpropamide [Diabinese]) place elderly patients with other underlying disorders at risk for prolonged and sometimes fatal hypoglycemic episodes. Drugs with active metabolites also may increase the risk of hypoglycemia in patients with impaired renal function. Hence, patient education must include recognition of symptoms as well as prevention and treatment plans for hypoglycemia. Sulfonylureas can cause weight gain of about 2 to 3 kg. They cannot be used in patients with sulfa allergies.

Biguanides

Biguanides are oral hypoglycemics used in conjunction with diet as first-line monotherapy or in combination with other classes of diabetic drugs, including insulin, to treat type 2 diabetes (see Table 49-2). Their mechanisms of action and side effect profiles differ from those of the sulfonylureas, offering notable advantages. Biguanides do not cause hypoglycemia (when used as monotherapy) and do not promote hyperinsulinemia or weight gain.

Mechanism of Action

This class inhibits hepatic glucose production and moderately improves peripheral sensitivity to insulin. Gluconeogenesis and glycogenolysis are inhibited in the liver. Glycemic control is achieved without stimulating insulin secretion, so hypoglycemia does not develop. Other advantages of biguanides over sulfonylureas include their tendency to induce weight loss and promote favorable effects on lipid profiles. In addition, in certain patients, biguanides can be combined effectively with sulfonylureas, thiazolidinediones, or insulin because their mechanisms of action differ. Biguanides are the agents of choice in patients who exhibit secondary failure to sulfonylureas. In view of their many beneficial effects, biguanides appear to be a more rational choice than sulfonylureas for first-line therapy in patients with newly diagnosed type 2 diabetes. Metformin (Glucophage) is the only available biguanide. There is now a combination of glyburide and metformin (Glucovance) and glipizide and metformin (Metaglip) available. Metformin is also now available in liquid form (Riomet).

Dosage

The dose is started low and increased weekly as needed to the maximum. Patients usually take the medication before meals in the morning and evening. The dose is carefully titrated in elderly patients. With metformin, the starting dose is 500 mg twice a day with increases every 1 to 2 weeks to a maximum of 2550 mg/d. Peak action is within 2 to 2.5 hours, and the effects last for 10 to 16 hours. Steady-state levels of the drug are achieved in 24 to 48 hours. Metformin also comes in an extended-release formula. It is started at 500 mg daily with the evening meal and increased to a maximum of 2000 mg daily.

Contraindications

Contraindications include renal dysfunction, serum creatinine level of 1.4 mg/dL or higher, heart failure, and pregnancy. This class also is contraindicated in children, alcoholics, binge drinkers, those over 80 years old, and those with dehydration. Patients must stop taking metformin when undergoing radiologic studies with iodinated contrast, when experiencing metabolic acidosis, and before surgery until they resume normal oral intake.

Adverse Events/Interactions

The most common side effect of metformin therapy is gastrointestinal (GI) upset, which includes diarrhea, nausea, vomiting, abdominal bloating, flatulence, anorexia, and a metallic taste in the mouth. Such problems occur in approximately 30% of patients during the initiation of therapy and usually resolve with continued treatment. To minimize these adverse effects, treatment is started with a low dose and increased slowly at no less than weekly intervals.

Because GI upset is rare late in therapy, any sudden onset of severe vomiting or diarrhea at that time should alert providers to the possibility of lactic acidosis, a rare but potentially fatal complication of metformin therapy. In such cases, patients should discontinue metformin immediately until they can be evaluated and stabilized. From data collected in Europe over 20 years, the reported worldwide incidence of metformin-induced lactic acidosis is 0.03 cases/1000 patient-years. Risk of lactic acidosis increases with advancing age and worsening renal function. Therefore, metformin is contraindicated in patients with renal disease or dysfunction and acute or chronic metabolic acidosis. In addition, metformin should be temporarily withheld in patients undergoing radiologic studies requiring the use of iodinated contrast media because of their effects on renal excretion. Renal impairment is suggested in men with serum creatinine levels of 1.5 mg/dL or more and in women with levels of 1.4 mg/dL or more. Renal dysfunction may be secondary to a variety of comorbid conditions such as cardiopulmonary insufficiency, liver disease, alcoholism, and infection. These conditions predispose patients to impaired perfusion of tissues and decreased elimination of lactate and are therefore contraindications to the use of metformin. In addition, patients should temporarily discontinue metformin during any situation in which an acute decline in renal function may occur (eg, aggressive diuresis, dehydration from gastroenteritis, surgery).

The concomitant use of metformin with cimetidine increases the risk of hypoglycemia. The concomitant use of metformin with glucocorticoids or alcohol increases the risk of lactic acidosis.

Thiazolidinediones

This class of antidiabetic agents (see Table 49-2) reduces insulin resistance at sites of insulin action.

Mechanism of Action

Thiazolidinediones (TZDs) bind to the nuclear steroid hormone receptor perixosome proliferator-activated receptor-gamma (PPARγ) and increase insulin sensitivity in skeletal muscle and fat. Clinically, they decrease peripheral insulin resistance and at higher doses may decrease hepatic glucose production. Like biguanides, they improve the action of insulin without directly stimulating insulin secretion from the pancreatic beta cells. There is an improvement of endothelial function, preservation of beta cell function, and a decrease in albumin excretion.

The patient's alanine aminotransferase (ALT) levels are monitored for possible hepatic toxicity every 2 months for the first year after the patient starts the drug and periodically thereafter. The patient must stop taking the medication if ALT levels are greater than 3 times the upper limit of normal. Hypoglycemia may develop in patients taking this class of drug with insulin or sulfonylureas because the TZDs are potent sensitizers of insulin. If this occurs, the drug should be discontinued or the dose of insulin or sulfonylurea should be reduced.

Pioglitazone (Actos) has been shown to increase HDL levels.

Adverse Events/Contraindications

Pioglitazone (Actos) may cause reduced concentrations of combined oral contraceptives; therefore, patients using oral contraceptives should consider alternative contraception methods. The administration of rosiglitazone (Avandia) 4 mg twice daily had no clinically significant effects on the pharmacokinetics of combined oral contraceptives.

In premenopausal anovulatory women with insulin resistance, ovulation may resume when drugs of this class are used. Thus, the patient may be at risk of unintended pregnancy, and contraception should be considered. Because of increased plasma volume from this class of drugs, TZDs are not recommended for patients with New York Heart Association class III or class IV heart failure. Another contraindication is active liver disease.

TZDs can stimulate weight gain from plasma volume expansion and generation and redistribution of fats into the subcutaneous compartments.

α-Glucosidase Inhibitors

Mechanism of Action

The enzyme α-glucosidase, found on the brush border of the intestine, is necessary for the absorption of starch and disaccharides. This class of drugs (see Table 49-2) acts by slowing the absorption of carbohydrates from the intestines, minimizing the postprandial rise in blood sugar. The result of this delay is decreased levels of postprandial glucose and HgbA$_{1c}$. The α-glucosidase inhibitors are most useful in patients with postprandial hyperglycemia and patients with very high HgbA$_{1c}$ levels and poor dietary adherence. They are useful in patients from ethnic groups with high-carbohydrate diets, such as Asians and Hispanics.

Dosage

Agents from this class can be prescribed alone or with a sulfonylurea. Patients should take each dose with the first bite of each meal. Dosages are increased gradually (at 4- to 8-wk intervals) to avoid GI side effects. The starting dose is 25 mg 3 times a day at the start of each meal. This regimen lasts for 4 to 8 weeks; then the dose may be increased to 50 mg 3 times a day. After 3 months at 50 mg, the dose can be increased to 100 mg 3 times a day. Peak concentration occurs in 2 to 3 hours.

Contraindications

Acarbose (Precose) is contraindicated in patients with diseases of the bowel (eg, inflammatory bowel disease, absorptive disorders, history of bowel obstruction) or cirrhosis. Patients with motility disorders of the upper GI tract should not be treated with acarbose.

Adverse Events/Interactions

The most common side effects involve the GI tract. Increased fermentation secondary to the delay in carbohydrate absorption increases intestinal gas, causing flatulence, diarrhea, and abdominal distention.

A 1-hour postprandial glucose measurement is useful to assess the therapeutic response during the dosage titration period. Additional monitoring should include serum aminotransferases every 3 months during the first year of therapy. Intestinal adsorbants such as charcoal antagonize this class of drugs. The α-glucosidase inhibitors may decrease the levels of propranolol and ranitidine.

Meglitinide Analogs

Meglitinide analogs are rapid-acting insulin secretagogues that stimulate the release of insulin from the pancreas in response to a meal (see Table 49-2). Binding at characterized sites closes the ATP-dependent potassium channels in the membranes of the beta cells. This causes a depolarization of the beta cells and an opening of calcium channels. The resulting increased influx of calcium causes insulin secretion.

Meglitinide analogs are effective in patients who become hypoglycemic while taking sulfonylureas and have acceptable FPG readings but high postprandial blood glucose levels. They also are effective for patients with irregular meal schedules because patients take them at meals. Repaglinide (Prandin) and nateglinide (Starlix) are the two drugs available in this class. They lower postprandial blood glucose concentrations without any significant effects on FPG level.

Meglitinide analogs can be used as monotherapy or in combination with other oral agents. The starting dose of repaglinide is 0.5 mg before meals if the HgbA$_{1c}$ level is less than 8.0. If the HgbA$_{1c}$ concentration is greater than 8.0, the starting dose is 1 to 2 mg before meals. Patients must add a dose if they add another meal or skip a dose if they skip a meal. The dose may be doubled to 4 mg before meals to a maximum of 16 mg a day. Nateglinide is similarly administered with a starting dose of 60 to 120 mg before meals.

The peak level is achieved in 1 hour. In 96 hours, the body excretes 90% of the medication. Meglitinide analogs are contraindicated in patients with diabetic ketoacidosis.

Adverse Events

Adverse events include hypoglycemia, GI disturbances, upper respiratory infections, headache, diarrhea, constipation, arthralgias, and back or chest pain. Concomitant use with beta blockers or alcohol increases the risk of hypoglycemia. Ketoconazole, miconazole, erythromycin, and other cytochrome P450 3A4 inhibitors may potentiate the drug, as may nonsteroidal anti-inflammatory drugs, aspirin, sulfonamides, and warfarin. Drugs such as rifampin, barbiturates, thiazides, phenothiazines, phenytoin, sympathomimetics, calcium channel blockers, and isoniazid may antagonize it.

Insulin

Insulin is the drug therapy of choice for all patients with type 1 diabetes and those patients with type 2 diabetes who cannot control their condition with diet and exercise alone or in whom oral therapy fails. Other clinical situations in which insulin therapy is appropriate include newly diagnosed cases of type 2 diabetes presenting with severe, symptomatic hyperglycemia, pregnancy, and surgery.

Just like the insulin that the pancreas normally produces, insulin as drug therapy regulates glucose metabolism in the muscle and other tissues (except the brain). It causes the rapid transport of glucose and amino acids intracellularly, promotes anabolism, and inhibits protein catabolism. In the liver, it promotes the uptake and storage of glucose in the form of glycogen, inhibits gluconeogenesis, and promotes the conversion of excess glucose into fat.

The major characteristics of insulin preparations are onset of action and duration of action (Table 49-4). Semisynthetic insulin, which is produced by recombinant DNA technology, has the identical amino acid composition as human endogenous insulin and is therefore referred to as "human" insulin. Human insulin preparations lower the risk of local reactions. An insulin analog, lispro insulin, is a two-amino

Table 49.4

Insulins

Preparation	Brand	Onset (h)	Peak (h)	Duration (h)
Very Rapid Acting				
Insulin analog	Humalog	<.5	0.5–3	3–5
Short Acting				
Insulin injection	Novolog	0.5	1–5	8
	Humulin R			
Regular (R)	Novolin R			
	Velosulin BR			
Intermediate Acting				
NPH	Humulin N	1–4	4–12	14–26
	Novolin N			
Lente	Humulin L	1–4	4–15	16–26
	Novolin L			
Long Acting				
Insulin extended zinc suspension (U)	Humulin U	4–6	8–20	24–36
Insulin glargine	Lantus	1–2	None	24
Combination				
NPH and Regular	70/30	0.5–3	Dual	12–14
	51/50			
Humalog mix	75% insulin lisproprotamine/ 25% insulin lispro	0.1–0.25	1–12	4–24

Table 49.5

Various Insulin Regimens

No. of Daily Injections	How Administered	Comments
2	Two thirds of insulin 15–30 min before breakfast and $^1/_3$ 15–30 min before the evening meal In AM, $^2/_3$ intermediate, $^1/_3$ short or rapid acting In PM, $^1/_2$ intermediate, $^1/_2$ rapid or short acting	This regimen is the most commonly prescribed. It is the most desirable to patients. There may be too little coverage at noon and too much insulin during the night. There is less dawn phenomenon and Somogyi effect.
3	40% intermediate and 15% short or rapid acting 15–30 min before breakfast 15% short or rapid acting before dinner 30% intermediate at bedtime	There is too little coverage at noon.
4	20%–25% of daily dose with rapid or short acting before each meal 25%–40% intermediate or long acting at bedtime	Use of insulin glargine provides most predictable basal control.

acid modification of regular human insulin. Aggregates do not form when lispro insulin is injected subcutaneously, allowing for a more rapid onset and shorter duration than regular insulin and minimizing the postprandial rise in blood sugar and the risk of late hypoglycemia. Another human insulin analog is insulin glargine.

Insulins are categorized as basal (NPH, lente, and glargine) or bolus (regular, lispro, and aspart). Initial insulin doses should be individualized in patients previously untreated with insulin. Preferably, a therapy with a basal insulin plus a bolus insulin 15 minutes before each meal is started. A minimum of two daily injections (split-dose regimen) should be considered to achieve regulation of blood glucose, especially in patients with type 1 diabetes.

The most common regimen is injection of a mixture of an intermediate-acting insulin (NPH) and rapid or short-acting insulin twice a day, 15 minutes before breakfast and 15 minutes before dinner. Usually, patients take a 2:1 ratio of NPH to rapid/short-acting insulin before breakfast and a 1:1 ratio before dinner. Patients take two thirds of the total daily dose in the morning and one third in the evening. Table 49-5 lists various insulin regimens. Most patients with type 1 diabetes, however, need three to four injections a day for optimal control. It is becoming more popular to use a bolus of rapid-acting insulin just before a meal and an injection of basal insulin at bedtime.

Dosage

To start insulin in patients with type 2 diabetes, an evening dose of 10 U basal insulin is started. Additional doses are added based on the FBG as follows:

- 2 U if FBG >120 mg/dL
- 4 U if FBG >140 mg/dL
- 6 U if FBG >180 mg/dL

Insulin doses should be individualized and closely monitored. In lieu of empiric estimations, however, the following guidelines can be used for total daily dosing:

- Children and adults: 0.5 to 0.6 U/kg/d
- Adults during illness or adolescents: 0.5 to 0.75 U/kg/d

- Adolescents during a growth spurt: 1.25 to 1.5 U/kg/d
- Pregnancy: 0.7 U/kg/d

If two doses are given a day, it is recommended that two thirds of the total daily dose be given in the morning with a 2:1 ratio of intermediate- to short-acting insulin and one third of the total daily dose be given before dinner with a 1:1 ratio of short-acting insulin and intermediate-acting insulin.

Doses should be adjusted based on the patient's clinical response, as evidenced by blood glucose levels. Adjustments are made in 1- to 2-U increments. Insulin must be decreased with hypoglycemia and increased with hyperglycemia. Table 49-6 provides some suggestions on when dosages need adjusting. For information on time frame for response, see Table 49-4. Use of insulin is contraindicated with hypoglycemia.

Insulin glargine is given at bedtime and cannot be mixed with other insulins.

The 1500 rule can be used to determine the change needed in the insulin dose. The insulin sensitivity factor (ISF) is determined by dividing a constant (1500) by the total daily dose (TDD) of insulin. This determines the change in blood glucose from 1 U of insulin. The formula is: ISF = 1500/TDD. For example, if the patient takes 50 U of insulin in 24 hours, the ISF is 1500/50 = 30.

Therefore each unit of insulin lowers the blood glucose level 30 mg/dL. If the SMBG at noon is 170, an addition of 2 U in the morning should lower the blood glucose level to 110 mg/dL.

Adverse Events

Hypoglycemia, hypokalemia, lipodystrophy, and local or systemic allergic reaction can occur with insulin. The dawn phenomenon, so-called for the worsening hyperglycemia that occurs in the early morning hours, is caused by the growth hormone surges that occur during sleep. The Somogyi effect, which also may be mistaken for inadequate control, is a rebound of hyperglycemia that occurs after an early morning episode of insulin-induced hypoglycemia. The hypoglycemia goes unnoticed because it happens while the patient is sleeping, at approximately 3:00 AM. Assessment clues include night sweats, nightmares, sleep disturbances,

Table 49.6

Adjusting Insulin Dosages Based on Clinical Response

Problem	Time Experienced	Possible Solutions
Hyperglycemia	Fasting	If the patient is receiving a single dose of an intermediate-acting insulin, split into two doses: $2/3$ of total dose before breakfast, $1/3$ of total dose before supper.
		If the patient is receiving split-dose insulin, increase presupper dose or move to later in the evening.
	Midmorning	Add Regular to morning dose to achieve a ratio of 2:1 (intermediate to Regular).
	Midafternoon	Increase morning NPH or Lente dose.
		Add Regular at lunch.
	Bedtime	Add or increase Regular with presupper dose.
	Early morning (2:00–3:00 AM)	Give the presupper dose later in the evening.
		Give Regular insulin at bedtime.
Hypoglycemia	Fasting	Decrease evening insulin dose.
	Midmorning	Decrease or omit prebreakfast dose of Regular insulin.
	Midafternoon	Decrease morning NPH or Lente.
	Bedtime	Add a bedtime snack.
		Decrease presupper dose of Regular insulin.
	Early morning (2:00–3:00 AM)	Consider Somogyi effect—decrease evening NPH.

Adapted from Francisco, G. E., & Brooks, P. J. (1999). Diabetes mellitus. In J. T. DiPiro, R. L. Talbert, G. C. Yee, et al. (Eds.), *Pharmacotherapy: A pathophysiologic approach* (4th ed., pp. 1219–1243). East Norwalk, CT: Appleton & Lange.

and early morning headaches. Monitoring of blood glucose when the hypoglycemia is thought to be occurring helps make the diagnosis.

Interactions

Salicylates, beta blockers, monoamine oxidase inhibitors, alcohol, and sulfa drugs potentiate insulin. Corticosteroids, isoniazid, niacin, estrogens, thyroid hormones, thiazides, phenothiazines, and sympathomimetics antagonize it.

Special Considerations

Pediatric/Adolescent

Until the mid-1990s, type 1 diabetes was the prevalent type of diabetes in children and adolescents. Recently, 40% of newly diagnosed cases of diabetes in children between 10 and 19 years of age have been type 2. The greatest risk factor is childhood obesity. Diabetes is often discovered with glucosuria on a random urinalysis. A red flag for type 2 diabetes in adolescents is acanthosis nigricans, dark pigmentation in skin creases and flexural area. This is a sign of insulin resistance and is present in 60% to 90% of adolescents with type 2 diabetes. Hypertension is present in 20% to 30% of adolescents with type 2 diabetes. In type 1 diabetes, children present with inappropriate polyuria, dehydration, poor weight gain, and ketonuria.

Treatment for type 1 diabetes in children is insulin therapy. Doses are

- 0.7 mg/kg before puberty
- 1.0 mg/kg mid puberty
- 1.2 mg/kg after puberty

These children should be treated by a specialist.

Treatment for type 2 diabetes is weight loss, medical nutritional therapy, exercise, and in many cases, medication. The only drugs approved for adolescents are insulin and metformin.

Geriatric

Diabetes in the elderly is often complicated by coexisting conditions. Complications develop at an accelerated rate probably because poor glycemic control has been long standing. Also the elderly usually have a decrease in renal function. Exercise programs for the elderly have to be started carefully with comorbid conditions in mind.

Pregnancy

There are two types of diabetes during pregnancy. One is pregestational diabetes, present before the pregnancy. This is treated by a specialist during pregnancy and is considered very high risk. The most common is gestational diabetes, which is glucose intolerance detected during pregnancy and associated with probable resolution after pregnancy.

During pregnancy, human placental lactogen plays a pivotal role in triggering glucose intolerance. It has an anti-insulin and lipolytic effect. Peripheral insulin sensitivity decreases to 50% of the first trimester during the third trimester. Basal hepatic glucose output increases by 30%.

Screening is recommended between weeks 24 and 48. The recommended test is the 50-g 1-hour glucose screening test, although some women require a 3-hour glucose tolerance test.

In the gestational diabetic, multiple daily SMBG are required and it can often be controlled by diet and medical nutritional therapy. If this does not control glucose levels, insulin is required.

Potential neonatal complications include shoulder dystonia, hypoglycemia, polycythemia, and respiratory distress.

Selecting the Most Appropriate Agent

Insulin is necessary in all cases of type 1 diabetes. In patients with type 2 diabetes, various oral agents as monotherapy or in combination therapy can be prescribed, because the oral agents act in different ways. Table 49-7 lists the potential decrease in $HgbA_{1c}$ with each agent. Table 49-8 shows first-,

Table 49.7

Capacity to Decrease HgbA$_{1c}$ by Agent

Agent	Decrease in HgbA$_{1c}$
insulin	>2%
sulfonylurea	1–2%
biguanide	1.5–2%
thiazolidinedione	0.5–1.8%
α-glucosidase inhibitor	0.5–1%
meglitinide	0.6–1.8%

second-, and third-line therapy for patients with type 1 diabetes. Table 49-9 shows first-, second-, and third-line therapy for patients with type 2 diabetes (Fig. 49-1).

First-Line Therapy

In type 1 diabetes, insulin is the first-line therapy. It usually is administered in a combination of intermediate- and short-acting insulin. The dosage is 0.5 to 0.6 U/kg/d. Several schedules can be used for administering insulin (see Table 49-5). The most common regimen is two injections a day, one in the morning and one in the evening. This promotes glycemic control both during the day and while the patient sleeps. The insulin dose required is divided into two thirds of the dose in the morning and one third of the dose in the evening. The morning dose is divided into two-thirds intermediate insulin and one-third short- or rapid-acting insulin. The evening dose is one-half intermediate insulin and one-half short- or rapid-acting insulin.

First-line therapy for type 2 diabetes is monotherapy with an oral agent. The agents used for first-line therapy are sulfonylureas, biguanides, thiazolidinediones, α-glucosidase inhibitors, and meglitinides. They act in different ways. The rule for initiating therapy with any of these agents is to start slowly and increase the dose every 1 to 2 weeks as needed. If intensification of treatment is required to meet goals (ie, HgbA$_{1c}$ <7.0%), the addition of another drug from a different class is recommended.

Sulfonylureas are the best choice if the patient has a blood glucose level over 250 mg/dL and is thin. Biguanides and the thiazolidinediones are the drugs of choice in patients with metabolic syndrome. The α-glucosidase inhibitors are most effective in patients with postprandial hyperglycemia but only mild fasting glucose elevations.

Second-Line Therapy

With failure to achieve optimal blood glucose levels in type 1 diabetes, practitioners must gradually increase the insulin dose, making adjustments 1 to 2 U at a time over 3 days. They must base adjustments on SMBG records. Table 49-10 lists how to determine adjustments.

Failure to achieve optimal blood glucose levels in type 2 diabetes necessitates the addition of another oral agent. Combinations of sulfonylureas and biguanides, thiazolidinediones, or α-glucosidase inhibitors are effective. Insulin may be added to oral medication regimens for effective control. Insulin is started at the lowest dose and increased every 1 to 2 weeks as needed.

Third-Line Therapy

In patients with type 1 diabetes, clinicians should add a thiazolidinedione or metformin to the regimen of insulin if control is still poor. They may add α-glucosidase inhibitors if postprandial blood glucose is high. Patients with type 1 diabetes may be appropriate candidates for an insulin pump.

In patients with type 2 diabetes, insulin is added if the addition of a second agent and third agent is unsuccessful. An intermediate or basal insulin at bedtime added to the daytime oral regimen can be very effective in treating those with type 2 diabetes to goal.

Combination Therapy

The following are suggestions for combination therapy for type 2 diabetes mellitus:

- **Sulfonylurea and biguanide** produced mealtime stimulation of endogenous insulin with the sulfonylurea and gluconeogenesis with the biguanide. This is recommended for a HgbA$_{1c}$ level above 8%.

Table 49.8

Recommended Order of Treatment for Type 1 Diabetes Mellitus

Order	Agents	Comments
First line	Insulin, usually a combined administration of intermediate and short acting; dose is 0.5–0.6 U/kg/d	Several schedules are used to administer insulin (see Table 49-5). The most commonly used regimen is two injections a day, in the morning and the evening. This promotes glycemic control both during the day and while sleeping. The insulin dose required is divided into $^2/_3$ of the dose in the morning and $^1/_3$ of the dose in the evening. The morning dose is divided into $^2/_3$ intermediate insulin and $^1/_3$ short- or rapid-acting insulin. The evening dose is $^1/_2$ intermediate insulin and $^1/_2$ short- or rapid-acting insulin.
Second line	Insulin dose is gradually increased.	Adjustments are made at 1 to 2 U at a time over 3 days. Adjustments are based on SMBG records.
Third line	Add a thiazolidinedione or metformin to regimen. α-glucosidase inhibitors can be added if postprandial blood glucose is high.	Insulin dose can be increased to 4 times daily using bolus/basal approach.

Table 49.9

Recommended Order of Treatment for Type 2 Diabetes Mellitus

Order	Agents	Comments
First line	Monotherapy with an oral agent: sulfonylureas *or* biguanides *or* thiazolidinediones *or* α-glucosidase inhibitors *or* meglitinides	The rule for initiating therapy with any of these agents is to start slowly and increase the dose every 1 to 2 wk as needed. The patient can be switched to another drug or class after 1 mo if the therapy is not effective in achieving glycemic control. Sulfonylureas are the best choice if the patient is thin, older than 40 y of age, has had diabetes for <5 y, and has a blood glucose >250 mg/dL. Glyburide is most effective in patients with fasting hypoglycemia, and glipizide is most effective in patients with postprandial hyperglycemia. Biguanides and the thiazolidinediones are the drugs of choice in the patient with metabolic syndrome X and when the blood glucose levels are <250 mg/dL. The α-glucosidase inhibitors are most effective in patients with postprandial hyperglycemia but only mild fasting glucose elevations.
Second line	Addition of another oral agent Combinations of sulfonylureas and biguanides, thiazolidinediones, or α-glucosidase inhibitors are effective. Also, metformin can be combined with a meglitinide or thiazolidinedione for effective control.	Again, the dose is started at the lowest level and increased every 1 to 2 wk as needed.
Third line	Triple oral therapy and/or addition of basal insulin	Oral medications at the same dose and a single asked time dose of 10 U of insulin with dose adjusted weekly (2 U if FPG > 120 mg/dL; 4 U if FPG > 140 mg/dL; 6 U if FPG > 180 mg/dL)

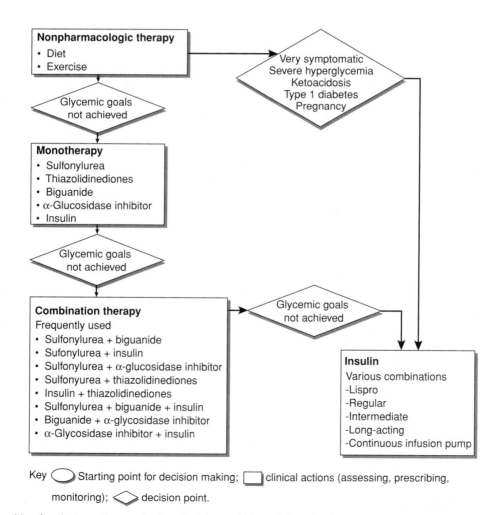

Figure 49–1   Algorithm for pharmacotherapy for Type 2 diabetes. (Adapted from the American Diabetes Association. [1995]. Algorithm for pharmacotherapy for NIDDM. *Diabetes Care, 18,* 1510–1518.)

Table 49.10

Measures of Control of Fasting Blood Glucose

Measure of Glucose	Goal	Levels When Adjustment to Regimen Is Indicated
Fasting glucose	90–130 mg/dL	<80 or >140 mg/dL
Bedtime glucose	110–150 mg/dL	<110 or >160 mg/dL
HgbA$_{1c}$	<7	≥7

- **Sulfonylurea and thiazolidinedione** improves insulin resistance and may enable a decrease in the dose of sulfonylurea.
- **Biguanide and thiazolidinedione** combination provides a synergistic effect on glycemic reduction. Liver and renal function must be monitored with this regimen.
- **α-Glucosidase inhibitor and another agent** is best used with an elevated postprandial blood glucose level.
- **Meglitinide and thiazolidinedione or biguanide** combination promotes a stimulation of insulin release and a decrease in peripheral insulin resistance and fasting hyperglycemia.

MONITORING PATIENT RESPONSE

Prolonged hyperglycemia of diabetes gives rise to long-term complications that involve lesions of the small (microvascular) and large (macrovascular) blood vessels. Microvascular complications include retinopathy, nephropathy, and neuropathy.

Control is measured using the patient's levels of blood glucose and HgbA$_{1c}$. Patients use SMBG to keep a daily record of blood glucose. HgbA$_{1c}$ measures blood glucose over 3 months. Table 49-10 lists the desired levels and levels that require changes in drug regimen.

PATIENT EDUCATION

Drug Information

Education is a hallmark of diabetes therapy. SMBG is essential for monitoring therapeutic response. Practitioners must educate patients about the signs and symptoms of hypoglycemia and instruct them to carry a source of glucose with them at all times. Possible sources are hard candy (not sugarless) or 4 ounces of orange juice. All patients with diabetes should have medical identification in the form of a Medic Alert bracelet or necklace.

In patients taking insulin, meals are to be eaten on a regular basis. If a rapid-acting insulin is used, it is taken immediately before eating. The α-glucosidase inhibitors are only taken if a meal is eaten.

Patient-oriented sources for information include:

www.diabetes.org is the site from the American Diabetes Association with information for managing the diabetic's life.

www.niddk.nih.gov/health/diabetes.htm is a site from National Institutes of Health that serves as an information clearinghouse.

www.diabetes.com provides information for the diabetic individual.

Nutritional and Lifestyle Changes

Diabetes management includes medical nutrition therapy (MNT), exercise, and, in most cases, drug therapy. Foods high in processed sugar and fat are to be avoided as is alcohol. Regular daily exercise helps to control blood sugar levels.

Patients with diabetes must follow "sick day guidelines" for the treatment of their condition when dealing with other illnesses. In general, practitioners should instruct people with diabetes not to stop their medication when they are ill. Infection, stress, and other variables increase plasma glucose levels, even though oral intake may be reduced. Practitioners should instruct patients to increase their fluid intake to approximately 8 ounces of water or sugar-free beverage every hour, especially if they have a fever. Patients should monitor blood glucose levels at home more frequently, as often as every 4 hours. Urine also requires testing for ketones. If the blood glucose concentration is greater than 300 mg/dL on two consecutive readings, fever is persistently high, and symptoms of severe dehydration and ketonuria develop, the patient requires formal evaluation. Sick day plans should be developed with patients before illness occurs.

Complementary and Alternative Medicine

In a recent study conducted at the U.S. Department of Agriculture, cinnamon reduced serum glucose levels and improved lipid profiles in patients with type 2 diabetes. Patients were randomized into 6 groups that received 1, 2, or 3 g cinnamon or placebo. All groups receiving cinnamon had a decrease of 18% to 30% in fasting serum glucose values and a reduction of 23% to 30% in triglycerides and 7% to 27% reduction in LDL levels. Total cholesterol level declined 12% to 26%.

A daily vitamin is recommended if the patient is on a weight reduction plan.

■ Case Study

R.S. is a 55-year-old moderately obese Hispanic woman (body mass index is 29). She was referred to you when her gynecologist noted glucose on a routine urinalysis. She subsequently has a FPG of 190 and 200 mg/dL on two separate occasions. She is thirstier than usual and has more frequent urination. She also complains of decreased energy over the last several months.

■ Case Study (*Continued*)

- Family history: sister, mother, and maternal grandmother have diabetes
- Social history: nonsmoker, drinks alcohol socially (1 drink about 3 times a month), and does not exercise.
- Review of systems: 20 lb weight gain over the past 2 years, has some blurred vision, has had 2 urinary tract infections in the past year and has frequent vaginal yeast infections
- Physical exam: unremarkable except blood pressure of 150/90
- Laboratory results: FPG 200 mg/dL, HgbA$_{1c}$ 10%, LDL 160 mg/dL, HDL 35 mg/dL, and triglycerides 266 mg/dL

Diagnosis: Type 2 diabetes mellitus

1. List specific goals for treatment for R.S.

2. What dietary and lifestyle changes would you recommend for A.S.?

3. What drug therapy would you prescribe? Why?

4. What is the goal for the FPG? Postprandial glucose? HgbA$_{1c}$?

5. Discuss specific education for R.S. based on the prescribed therapy.

6. List one or two adverse reactions for the therapy selected that would cause you to change the therapy.

7. If the HgbA$_{1c}$ after 3 months on the prescribed therapy is 8.8%, what would be the next line of therapy?

8. What over-the-counter or herbal medicines might be appropriate for R.S.?

9. Describe one or two drug–drug or drug–food interactions for the selected agent.

Bibliography

Adler, A. I., Stratton, I. M., Neil, H. A., et al. (2000). Association of systolic blood pressure with macrovascular and microvascular complications of type 2 diabetes (UKPDS 36): Prospective observational study. *British Medical Journal, 321,* 412–419.

ALLHAT Collaborative Research Group. (2000). Major cardiovascular events in hypertensive patients randomized to doxazosin vs chlorthalidone: The Antihypertensive and Lipid-Lowering Treatment to Prevent Heart Attack Trial (ALLHAT). *Journal of the American Medical Association, 283,* 1967–1975.

ALLHAT Study Group. (2002). Major outcomes in high-risk hypertensive patients randomized to angiotensin-converting enzyme inhibitor or calcium channel blocker vs diuretic: The Antihypertensive and Lipid-Lowering Treatment to Prevent Heart Attack Trial (ALLHAT). *Journal of the American Medical Association, 288,* 2981–2997.

*American Diabetes Association. (1995). Algorithm for pharmacotherapy for NIDDM. *Diabetes Care, 18,* 1510–1518.

American Diabetes Association. (2000). Type 2 diabetes in children and adolescents (Consensus Statement). *Diabetes Care, 23,* 381–389.

American Diabetes Association. (2004). Aspirin therapy in diabetes (Position Statement). *Diabetes Care, 27*(Suppl. 1), S72–S73.

American Diabetes Association. (2004): Gestational diabetes mellitus (Position Statement). *Diabetes Care, 27*(Suppl. 1), S88–S90.

American Diabetes Association. (2004). Hyperglycemic crises in diabetes (Position Statement). *Diabetes Care, 27*(Suppl. 1), S94–S102.

American Diabetes Association. (2004). Nephropathy in diabetes (Position Statement). *Diabetes Care, 27*(Suppl. 1), S79–S83.

American Diabetes Association. (2004). Postprandial blood glucose (Consensus Statement). *Diabetes Care, 24,* 775–778.

American Diabetes Association. (2004). Retinopathy in diabetes (Position Statement). *Diabetes Care, 27*(Suppl. 1), S84–S87.

Anderson, S., Tarnow, L., Rossing, P., et al. (2000). Renoprotective effects of angiotensin II receptor blockade in type 1 diabetic patients with diabetic nephropathy. *Kidney International, 57,* 601–606.

Arauz-Pacheco, C., Parrott, M. A., & Raskin, P. (2002). The treatment of hypertension in adult patients with diabetes mellitus [Technical Review]. *Diabetes Care, 25,* 134–147.

Bakris, G. L., Williams, M., Dworkin, L., et al. (2000). Preserving renal function in adults with hypertension and diabetes: A consensus approach: National Kidney Foundation Hypertension and Diabetes Executive Committees Working Group. *American Journal of Kidney Disease, 36,* 646–661.

Barteis, D. (2004). Adherence to oral therapy for type 2 diabetes: Opportunities for enhancing glycemic control. *Journal of the American Academy of Nurse Practitioners, 16*(1), 8–16.

Bartol, T. G. (2003). Treating type 2 diabetes to goal: The role of pharmacotherapy. *American Journal for Nurse Practitioners, 7*(11), 34–37.

Berl, T., Hunsicker, L. G., Lewis, J. B., et al. (2003). Cardiovascular outcomes in the Irbesartan Diabetic Nephropathy Trial of patients with type 2 diabetes and overt nephropathy. *Annals of Internal Medicine, 138,* 542–549.

Bode, B. W. (Ed.). (2004). *Medical management of type 1 diabetes,* 4th ed. Alexandria, VA: American Diabetes Association, 2004.

Brenner, B. M., Cooper, M. E., de Zeeuw, D., et al. (2001). Effects of losartan on renal and cardiovascular outcomes in patients with type 2 diabetes and nephropathy. *New England Journal of Medicine, 345,* 861–869.

Buchanan TA, Xiang AH, Peters RK, et al. (2002). Preservation of pancreatic [beta]-cell function and prevention of type 2 diabetes by pharmacological treatment of insulin resistance in high-risk Hispanic women. *Diabetes, 51,* 2796–2803.

Bullock, B. A., & Henze, R. L. (2000). *Focus on pathophysiology.* Philadelphia: Lippincott Williams & Wilkins.

Chiasson, J. L., Josse, R. G., Gomis, R., et al. (2002). Acarbose for prevention of type 2 diabetes mellitus: The STOP-NIDDM randomized trial. *Lancet, 359,* 2072–2077.

Chobanian, A. V., Bakris, G. L., Black, H. R., et al, the National Heart, Lung, and Blood Institute Joint National Committee on Prevention, Detection, Evaluation, and Treatment of High Blood Pressure, the National High Blood Pressure Education Program Coordinating Committee: The Seventh Report of the Joint National Committee on Prevention, Detection, Evaluation, and Treatment of High Blood Pressure. (2003). The JNC 7 report. *Journal of the American Medical Association, 289,* 2560–2572.

Ciulla, T. A., Amador, A. G., & Zinman, B. (2003). Diabetic retinopathy and diabetic macular edema: Pathophysiology, screening, and novel therapies. *Diabetes Care, 26,* 2653–2664.

*DCCT Research Group. (1995). Effect of intensive therapy on the development and progression of diabetic nephropathy in the Diabetes Control and Complications Trial (DCCT). *Kidney International, 47,* 1703–1720.

DCCT/EDIC Research Group. (2000). Retinopathy and nephropathy in patients with type 1 diabetes four years after a trial of intensive therapy. *New England Journal of Medicine, 342,* 381–389.

Diabetes Control and Complications Trial Research Group. (1993). The effect of intensive treatment of diabetes on the development and progression of long-term complications in insulin-dependent diabetes mellitus. *New England Journal of Medicine, 329,* 977–986.

Diabetes Prevention Program Research Group. (2002). Reduction in the incidence of type 2 diabetes with lifestyle intervention or metformin. *New England Journal of Medicine, 346,* 393–403.

Eknoyan, G., Hostetter, T., Bakris, G. L., et al. (2003). Proteinuria and other markers of chronic kidney disease: A position statement of the National Kidney Foundation (NKF) and the National Institute of Diabetes and Digestive and Kidney Diseases (NIDDK). *American Journal of Kidney Disease, 42,* 617–622.

Engelgau, M. E., Narayan, K. M. V., & Herman, W. H. (2000). Screening for type 2 diabetes [Technical Review]. *Diabetes Care, 23,* 1563–1580 [erratum appears in *Diabetes Care, 23,* 1868–1869, 2000].

Expert Committee on the Diagnosis and Classification of Diabetes Mellitus. (2003). Follow-up report on the diagnosis of diabetes mellitus. *Diabetes Care, 26,* 3160–3167.

Fagot-Campagna, A., Pettitt, D. J., Engelgau, M. M., et al. (2000). DM2 among North American children and adolescents: An epidemiologic review and a public health perspective. *Journal of Pediatrics, 136,* 664–672.

*Francisco, G. E., & Brooks, P. J. (1999). Diabetes mellitus. In J. T. DiPiro, R. L. Talbert, G. C. Yee, et al. (Eds.), *Pharmacotherapy: a pathophysiologic approach* (4th ed., pp. 1219–1243). East Norwalk, CT: Appleton & Lange.

Garg, J., & Bakris, G. L. (2002). Microalbuminuria: Marker of vascular dysfunction, risk factor for cardiovascular disease. *Journal of Vascular Medicine, 7,* 35–43.

Hayden, M., Pignone, M., & Phillips, C. (2002). Aspirin for the primary prevention of cardiovascular events: A summary of the evidence for the U.S. Preventive Services Task Force. *Annals of Internal Medicine, 136,* 161–171.

Heart Outcomes Prevention Evaluation (HOPE) Study Investigators. (2000). Effects of ramipril on cardiovascular and microvascular outcomes in people with diabetes mellitus: Results of the HOPE study and MICRO-HOPE study. *Lancet, 355:*253–259.

Heart Protection Study Collaborative Group. (2003). MRC/BHF Heart Protection Study of cholesterol-lowering with simvastatin in 5963 people with diabetes: A randomized placebo-controlled trial. *Lancet, 361,* 2005–2016.

Jovanovic, L. (Ed.). (2000). *Medical management of pregnancy complicated by diabetes* (3rd ed.). Alexandria, VA: American Diabetes Association.

Kilingensmith, G. (Ed.). (2003). *Intensive diabetes management* (3rd ed.). Alexandria, VA: American Diabetes Association.

Klein, R. (2003). Screening interval for retinopathy in type 2 diabetes. *Lancet, 361,* 190–191.

National Institute of Diabetes and Digestive and Kidney Diseases. (2003/2004). National Diabetes Statistics fact sheet: General information and national estimates on diabetes in the United States, 2003. Bethesda, MD: U.S. Department of Health and Human Services, National Institutes of Health. 2004 Rev. ed. Bethesda, MD: U.S. Department of Health and Human Services, National Institutes of Health.

Ohkubo, Y., Kishikawa, H., Araki, E., et al. (1995). Intensive insulin therapy prevents the progression of diabetic microvascular complications in Japanese patients with non-insulin-dependent diabetes mellitus: A randomized prospective 6-year study. *Diabetes Research and Clinical Practice, 28,* 103–117.

Rohlfing, C. L., Wiedmeyer, H. M., Little, R. R., et al. (2002). Defining the relationship between plasma glucose and HbA1c: Analysis of glucose profiles and HbA1c in the Diabetes Control and Complications Trial. *Diabetes Care, 25,* 275–278.

Rosenstock, J. (2001). Insulin therapy: Optimizing control in type 1 and type 2 diabetes. *Clinical Cornerstone, 4*(2), 50–64.

Sacks, D. B., Bruns, D. E., Goldstein, D. E., et al. (2002). Guidelines and recommendations for laboratory analysis in the diagnosis and management of diabetes mellitus. *Diabetes Care, 25,* 750–786.

Smeltzer, S. C., & Bare, B. G. (2000). *Brunner & Suddarth's textbook of medical-surgical nursing* (9th ed.). Philadelphia: Lippincott Williams & Wilkins.

The National Cholesterol Education Program (NCEP) Expert Panel on Detection, Evaluation and Treatment of High Blood Cholesterol in Adults (Adult Treatment Panel III). (2001). Executive summary of the third report of the National Cholesterol Education Program (NCEP) Expert Panel on Detection, Evaluation and Treatment of High Blood Cholesterol in Adults (Adult Treatment Panel III). *Journal of the American Medical Association, 285,* 2486–2497.

Tuomilehto, J., Lindstrom, J., Eriksson, J. G., et al. (2001). Prevention of type 2 diabetes mellitus by changes in lifestyle among subjects with impaired glucose tolerance. *New England Journal of Medicine, 344,* 1343–1350.

UK Prospective Diabetes Study Group. (1998). Effect of intensive blood-glucose control with metformin on complications in overweight patients with type 2 diabetes (UKPDS 34). *Lancet, 352,* 854–865.

UK Prospective Diabetes Study Group. (1998). Intensive blood-glucose control with sulphonylureas or insulin compared with conventional treatment and risk of complications in patients with type 2 diabetes (UKPDS 33). *Lancet, 352,* 837–853.

US Preventive Services Task Force. (2002). Aspirin for the primary prevention of cardiovascular events: Recommendation and rationale. *Annals of Internal Medicine, 136,* 157–160.

Vijan, S., Hofer, T. P., & Hayward, R. A. (2000). Cost-utility analysis of screening intervals for diabetic retinopathy in patients with type 2 diabetes mellitus. *Journal of the American Medical Association, 283,* 889–896.

Visit the Connection web site for the most up-to-date drug information.

THYROID DISORDERS

■ LOUIS R. PETRONE

Diseases of the thyroid gland are common clinical conditions, accounting for many office visits each year. Population-based studies have found that hypothyroidism exists to some degree in 4.6% to 9.5% of individuals, with higher rates occurring in the elderly (Canaris et al., 2000; Hollowell et al., 2002). These same studies found a 1.3% to 2.2% rate of hyperthyroidism. Both hypothyroidism and hyperthyroidism have been associated with adverse cardiovascular outcomes (Hak et al., 2000; Sawin et al., 1994). If these conditions are not treated properly, their morbidity can be high. Thyroid nodules are common, occurring clinically in approximately 5% of patients, but found using ultrasound studies in 22% of patients and in autopsy studies in 50% of patients. Although most thyroid nodules are nonmalignant and most thyroid cancers are not very aggressive, approximately 1200 deaths per year are attributed to thyroid malignancy. Therefore, clinicians should understand the therapeutic options for these conditions.

To diagnose and treat thyroid disease, a basic understanding of thyroid anatomy and physiology is necessary (Figs. 50-1 and 50-2). The gland is divided into two lobes that are separated by an isthmus. Histologically, the thyroid is composed of follicles that are made of cells that are cuboidal at rest but column shaped when activated by thyroid-stimulating hormone (TSH). These follicular cells encircle a mass of colloid that contains thyroglobulin, a glycoprotein that the follicular cells secrete. Iodine, which is consumed in the diet, is reduced to iodide in the gastrointestinal (GI) tract and readily absorbed. Iodide is then carried to the thyroid, where it is taken up by the follicular cells. In these cells, iodide is oxidized and incorporated into tyrosine residues of thyroglobulin to form monoiodothyronine (MIT). Two MITs are paired to make diiodothyronine (DIT), and combinations of MIT with DIT produce triiodothyronine (T_3) and thyroxine (T_4), respectively.

The pituitary gland secretes TSH, which controls the rate of release of T_3 and T_4. The hypothalamus secretes thyrotropin-releasing hormone (TRH), which modulates the release of TSH. All these hormones work in a negative-feedback system, in which low levels of thyroid hormones in the blood cause increased secretion of TSH and, subsequently, T_3 and T_4.

Once T_3 and T_4 are secreted into the bloodstream, proteins known as thyroid-binding globulins (TBGs) bind most of these hormones. Only a small amount of T_3 and T_4 is in the "free" or unbound state; the hormones in this state are the clinically significant ones. Free T_3 and free T_4 act at the cellular level to regulate metabolism by binding to nuclear receptors and affecting gene expression and protein synthesis. Any condition that can affect TBGs also can affect the level of free T_3 and free T_4. The thyroid produces only approximately 20% of circulating T_3, whereas monodeiodination of T_4 in the periphery produces the remainder.

Clinically, measurement of serum TSH and free T_4 are used most commonly to assess thyroid function. Given the availability of the free T_4 assay, total T_4 is used less frequently because actual thyroid function depends on the level of free T_4 rather than total T_4. Table 50-1 depicts relative levels of TSH and free T_4 in disorders of thyroid function.

HYPOTHYROIDISM

Hypothyroidism is a relatively common clinical entity, occurring in up to 5.9% of women and 0.2% of men. Patients may complain of symptoms of fatigue, constipation, weight gain, or change in menstrual periods, among others. Physical examination may reveal thyromegaly, bradycardia, or peripheral edema (Box 50-1). Total cholesterol and low-density lipoprotein (LDL) levels may be elevated in 90% to 95% of patients.

CAUSES

Hypothyroidism has several causes (Box 50-2). In the United States and other developed countries, hypothyroidism nearly always results from a problem with the production or release (or both) of thyroid hormones. Worldwide, iodine deficiency is most commonly the cause. Hashimoto (or autoimmune) thyroiditis is the most common precipitant of hypothyroidism in the United States. It results from the infiltration of the thyroid gland by lymphocytes, which results in progressive fibrosis and decreased function of the gland. Patients may present with goiter and be euthyroid or hypothyroid initially; antithyroid antibodies are positive in high titers.

Posttherapeutic hypothyroidism is another common cause, whereas other entities such as subacute thyroiditis or

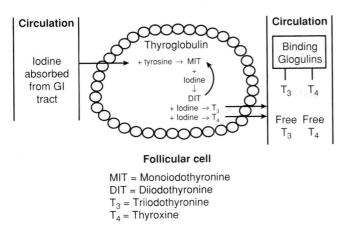

MIT = Monoiodothyronine
DIT = Diiodothyronine
T₃ = Triiodothyronine
T₄ = Thyroxine

Figure 50–1   Thyroid hormone synthesis.

postpartum thyroiditis can produce brief periods of hypothyroidism. Subacute and postpartum thyroiditis are discussed at the end of this chapter.

Many drugs may interfere with thyroid function and induce hypothyroidism (Box 50-3). These include amiodarone (Cordarone) and lithium (Eskalith). If patients discontinue these drugs, thyroid function should return to normal; however, many patients taking these drugs have serious coexisting conditions and cannot stop using them. Therefore, clinicians should monitor these patients regularly for hypothyroidism and treat them with thyroid replacement if appropriate.

PATHOPHYSIOLOGY

Hypothyroidism results from a relative deficit of thyroid hormones, usually T_4. The deficit may result from failure of the thyroid gland itself (primary hypothyroidism) or, less commonly, from failure of the pituitary gland or hypothalamus (secondary or tertiary hypothyroidism, respectively). Presenting symptoms of thyroid hormone deficiency are similar in all types of hypothyroidism.

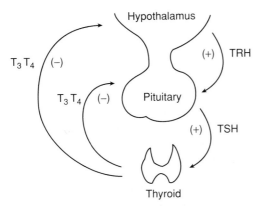

TRH = Thyroid Releasing Hormone
TSH = Thyroid Stimulating Hormone
T₃ = Triiodothyronine
T₄ = Thyroxine
(+) = positive effect
(−) = negative effect

Figure 50–2   Hypothalamic-pituitary-thyroid axis.

Table 50.1

Thyroid Function Testing in Common Thyroid Disorders

	TSH	Free T₄
Primary hypothyroidism	Increased	Decreased
Secondary or tertiary hypothyroidism	Decreased	Decreased
Mild thyroid failure	Increased	Normal
Hyperthyroidism	Decreased	Increased (or normal in T₃ thyrotoxicosis)
Subclinical hyperthyroidism	Decreased	Normal

DIAGNOSTIC CRITERIA

Primary hypothyroidism is confirmed, in the appropriate clinical setting, by the finding of an elevated TSH and a low free T_4 level. Secondary hypothyroidism, as a result of pituitary dysfunction, results in low free T_4 and low TSH levels. Tertiary hypothyroidism results from decreased production of TRH by the hypothalamus. Secondary hypothyroidism can be distinguished from tertiary hypothyroidism by imaging of the pituitary and hypothalamus. There is a TRH stimulation test in which exogenous TRH is administered and serum TSH response is measured, but this test is of limited value. Secondary hypothyroidism and tertiary hypothyroidism are not very common.

INITIATING DRUG THERAPY

The only course of treatment for hypothyroidism is replacement with thyroid hormone. Figure 50-3 shows an algorithm for the evaluation and treatment of hypothyroidism.

Goal of Drug Therapy

The goal of therapy is to return the patient to the euthyroid state with a TSH in the range of 0.5 to 4.0 mIU/mL. Clinicians should exercise caution not to overtreat hypothyroidism by suppressing the TSH to lower than normal levels because such overtreatment will put the patient at risk for

BOX 50–1. SYMPTOMS AND SIGNS OF HYPOTHYROIDISM

Fatigue	Bradycardia
Constipation	Delayed deep tendon
Menorrhagia	reflexes
Weight gain	Hyperlipidemia
Hair loss	Goiter
Cold intolerance	Hypothermia
Hoarseness	Periorbital swelling
Depression	Jaundice
Dry skin	Ataxia
Infertility	Edema
Difficulty with memory and concentration	Myalgias

BOX 50–2. CAUSES OF HYPOTHYROIDISM

Primary Hypothyroidism (Elevated TSH)
Autoimmune (Hashimoto, lymphocytic) thyroiditis
Treated Graves disease
Subacute thyroiditis
Silent thyroiditis
Iodine excess, including iodine-containing
    medication
Lithium therapy
Inadequate thyroid hormone replacement

Secondary Hypothyroidism (Low TSH)
Hypopituitarism

Tertiary Hypothyroidism (Low TRH, TSH)
Hypothalamic dysfunction

Other Causes of Elevated TSH
Nonthyroid illness
Adrenal insufficiency
Drugs (eg, metoclopramide and domperidone)
TSH-producing pituitary tumors
Thyroid hormone resistance syndromes

Modified from Mazzaferri, E. L. (1997). Evaluation and management of common thyroid disorders in women. *American Journal of Obstetrics and Gynecology, 176,* 507–514.

BOX 50–3. DRUG INTERACTIONS WITH T_4

Drugs That Decrease TSH Secretion
Dopamine
Glucocorticoids
Octreotide

Drugs That Alter Thyroid Hormone Secretion
Decreased Thyroid Hormone Secretion
Lithium
Iodide
Amiodarone
Aminoglutethimide

Increased Thyroid Hormone Secretion
Iodide
Amiodarone

Drugs That Decrease T_4 Absorption
Colestipol
Cholestyramine
Aluminum hydroxide
Ferrous sulfate
Sucralfate
Calcium carbonate

Drugs That Alter T_4 and T_3 Transport in Serum
Increased Serum TBG Concentration
Estrogens
Tamoxifen
Heroin
Methadone
Mitotane
Fluorouracil

Decreased Serum TBG Concentration
Androgens
Anabolic steroids (eg, danazol)
Slow-release nicotinic acid
Glucocorticoids

Displacement From Protein-Binding Sites
Furosemide
Fenclofenac
Mefenamic acid
Salicylates

Drugs That Alter T_4 and T_3 Metabolism
Increased Hepatic Metabolism
Phenobarbital
Rifampin
Phenytoin
Carbamazepine

Decreased T_4 5'-Deiodinase Activity
Propylthiouracil
Amiodarone
β blockers
Glucocorticoids

Modified from Surks, M. l., & Sievert, R. (1995). Drugs and thyroid function. *New England Journal of Medicine, 333,* 1688–1694.

hyperthyroidism and its attendant morbidities. Treatment of most cases of hypothyroidism usually is lifelong; exceptions include those cases that occur transiently in patients with postpartum or subacute thyroiditis (discussed later in this chapter).

Thyroid Hormone

Once they have made a diagnosis of hypothyroidism, practitioners should initiate treatment with thyroid hormone replacement in the form of levothyroxine (T_4). Table 50-2 lists the various preparations available. Natural thyroid extract derives from porcine thyroid glands and is a combination of T_3 and T_4. This preparation is not used much because of variability in the amount of T_3. T_3 replacement alone is available (liothyronine [Cytomel]), but also is not prescribed frequently because of its association with an increased risk of iatrogenic hyperthyroidism. It is sometimes given for short-term use before radioactive iodine scanning. A combination product of T_3 and T_4 (liotrix [Klotrix]) exists but offers no advantage over T_4 alone. Furthermore, this product increases serum T_3 above physiologic levels within several hours, leading to palpitations.

Several branded preparations of T_4 are available, any one of which may be used. Historically, authorities have recommended against the use of generic T_4. A controversial study of the bioavailability of generic preparations compared with brand name T_4, however, found no significant difference between generic and nongeneric T_4 and concluded that generic drugs may be used safely. The drug is readily

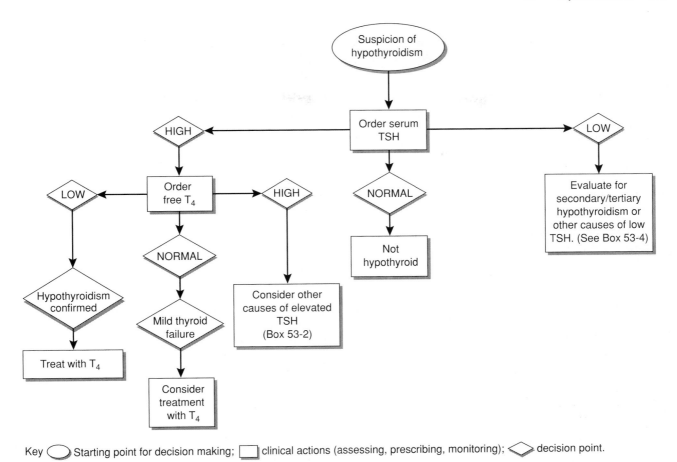

Key ⬭ Starting point for decision making; ▭ clinical actions (assessing, prescribing, monitoring); ◇ decision point.

Figure 50–3   Treatment algorithm for hypothyroidism.

absorbed from the GI tract. Serum T_4 levels peak at 2 to 4 hours, although the rise in serum T_3 levels is slower because of the time needed for conversion from T_4. Synthetic T_4 has a half-life of 1 week and requires approximately 6 to 8 weeks of therapy to reach steady state; therefore, patients may not notice improvement in symptoms for 1 week or more.

Dosage

When initiating therapy, clinicians must consider the patient's age, the duration of hypothyroidism, and any concomitant conditions. For adolescents and young adults, treatment can begin with the full replacement dose (100–125 mcg/d, or

Table 50.2

Overview of Drugs Used for Treatment of Hypothyroidism

Generic (Trade) Name and Dosage	Selected Adverse Events	Contraindications	Special Considerations
levothyroxin (Synthroid, others) Start: 12.5–100 mcg/d Maintenance: 75–150 mcg/d	Only with excessive dosing: dysrhythmias, palpitations, nervousness, tremor, weight loss	Untreated thyrotoxicosis, hypersensitivity to thyroid hormones, uncorrected adrenal cortical insufficiency	Goal TSH 0.5–4.0 mIU/mL (lower for treatment of thyroid cancer)
liothyronine (Cytomel) Start: 25 mcg/d Maintenance: 25–75 mcg/d	Only with excessive dosing	Same as above	Goal TSH 0.5–4.0 mIU/mL
liotrix (Thyrolar) (liothyronine and levothyroxine) Start: levothyroxine 50 mcg/d + liothyronine 12.5 mcg/d Maintenance: levothyroxine 100 mcg/d + liothyronine 25 mcg/d	Only with excessive dosing	Same as above	Goal TSH 0.5–4.0 mIU/mL
thyroid, dessicated (Armour) (liothyronine and levothyroxine) Start: 60 mg/d Maintenance: 60–120 mg/d	Only with excessive dosing	Same as above	Goal TSH 0.5–4.0 mIU/mL; not used much because of variability of T_3 content

1.6 ncg/kg/d, or approximately 0.75 mcg/lb/d). Children require approximately 4 to 10 mg/kg/d depending on age. In older adults or patients at risk for cardiac disease, thyroid hormone replacement should begin at 25 or even 12.5 mcg/d. Prescribers should increase the dosage incrementally (by 25 mcg/d every 4–6 weeks) until reaching the full replacement dose. Clinicians must monitor serum TSH levels and adjust the dose of T_4 accordingly. Many different dosage strengths (25–300 mcg) are available to allow titration to appropriate levels.

Interactions

Some drugs interfere with the absorption of thyroid hormone from the GI tract (see Box 50-3). These include cholestyramine (Questran), sucralfate (Carafate), aluminum-containing antacids, and calcium carbonate. Patients should not take T_4 several hours before or after ingesting these agents.

The concentration of total T_4 and T_3 depends on the concentration of serum TBGs. Any drug or condition that interferes with TBG levels can affect the interpretation of thyroid function tests. Furthermore, in patients who are taking T_4, the changing concentration of TBGs may necessitate adjustment of the dose. The most common causes of an increased serum TBG concentration are increased estrogen production (eg, as in pregnancy) and the administration of estrogen, either in the form of an oral contraceptive or as estrogen replacement therapy. Patients receiving these therapies will likely need higher doses of T_4 to maintain the euthyroid state because the estrogen increases the level of TBGs, and more thyroid hormone is in the bound, inactive state rather than in the free, active state. Androgens and niacin can decrease TBG concentrations and have opposite effects on thyroid function tests; patients taking these drugs will likely need lower doses of T_4.

Several drugs decrease the affinity of T_4 and T_3 to TBGs, causing displacement of hormones and resulting in a transient increase in free T_4 and T_3 levels. Salicylates and high doses of furosemide (Lasix) can exert this effect.

Another concern is for the patient taking oral anticoagulants. When hypothyroid patients become euthyroid, metabolism of vitamin K–dependent clotting factors increases. Thus, the patient's prothrombin time may increase, as does the risk of bleeding. The opposite occurs in patients treated for hyperthyroidism. Thus, clinicians need to monitor carefully coagulation studies in patients taking warfarin (Coumadin) who are being treated for thyroid disease.

Drugs like phenytoin (Dilantin) and carbamazepine (Tegretol) alter the metabolism of thyroid hormones. Patients who use these agents require more frequent monitoring of thyroid function.

Special Population Considerations

Pediatric

In children, developmental defects like thyroid aplasia or hypoplasia or inborn errors in thyroid hormonogenesis may result in thyroid deficiency. Routine screening of newborns allows early identification and treatment of this potentially devastating condition. Children with congenital hypothyro-idism require referral to a pediatric endocrinologist for treatment. Older children also may become hypothyroid as a result of lymphocytic (Hashimoto) thyroiditis or secondary to irradiation or surgery on the thyroid. Treatment is similar to that for adults, but children may require doses of up to 4.0 mcg/kg/d of T_4 due to rapid metabolism (National Academy of Clinical Biochemistry web site).

Geriatric

Clinicians need to maintain a high level of suspicion for thyroid disease in older adults because the presentation of illness may differ from that in younger patients. This difference is partly because of alterations in the rate of hormone secretion and clearance as well as increased nodularity and fibrosis of the thyroid gland. Furthermore, concomitant illnesses and medications can modify thyroid function in older adults. Symptoms of hypothyroidism may be subtle or nonexistent. Ataxia, paresthesias, and carpal tunnel syndrome may be the presenting symptoms of hypothyroidism in older adults. Psychiatric manifestations of thyroid disease (eg, depression or change in sensorium) also are more common in this age group. Older adults also are more susceptible to complications of therapy. Treatment should be initiated at a lower dose for elderly patients.

Pregnancy

Hypothyroidism in pregnancy deserves special mention. Because of the increased amount of thyroglobulin during pregnancy, more T_4 is bound in the circulation. Total T_4 and T_3 increase early in the first trimester, even in women without hypothyroidism. The free T_4 consequently declines to such a degree that symptoms of hypothyroidism may develop in many pregnant women with previously controlled hypothyroidism treated with T_4, necessitating a dose increase by approximately 50 mg until after delivery. Clinicians should evaluate thyroid function in pregnant women during every trimester by means of a TSH level. The serum total T_3 level returns to normal approximately 1 week after delivery, whereas the total T_4 level declines by 3 to 4 weeks if the patient is not using an oral contraceptive.

MONITORING PATIENT RESPONSE

Patients require clinical and laboratory evaluation with a serum TSH 6 to 8 weeks after initiating therapy or adjusting the dose of T_4. Because it takes this long for the TSH level to decline in response to T_4 replacement, a TSH test should not be ordered before this time. Clinicians should perform an interval history and physical examination, focusing on symptoms and signs of hyperthyroidism, which suggest overdosage, and residual symptoms of hypothyroidism to assess for underdosage.

Practitioners should check TSH levels 6 months after normalization to ensure stable metabolism of T_4, then annually unless new symptoms develop in the interim. Therapy is usually lifelong (although spontaneous recovery may occur in up to 20% of patients with hypothyroidism related to Hashimoto thyroiditis), so clinicians must encourage patients to comply with their medication regimens. The finding of a very high TSH but a normal free T_4 level suggests intermittent compliance with T_4 therapy.

PATIENT EDUCATION

Patients with primary hypothyroidism most likely will require lifelong replacement with thyroid hormone. Patients should not expect to see a difference in their symptoms until 2 to 4 weeks after beginning therapy. Follow-up laboratory testing is necessary relatively frequently until a therapeutic dosage that results in a stable TSH is reached; at that point, testing should be done annually.

Drug Information

Patients are advised against taking excessive thyroid hormone replacement because of the increased risk of drug-induced hyperthyroidism, osteoporosis, and dysrhythmias. Thyroid replacement should be taken on an empty stomach 30 minutes to 1 hour before ingestion of the first food of the day.

Patients on thyroid hormone replacement therapy should limit the use of adrenergic agents (eg, nonprescription decongestants). Patients should not take thyroid hormone at the same time as iron or calcium supplements, antacids, bile acid sequestrants, or simethicone; these preparations require administration at least 2 hours before or after administration of thyroid hormone. Finally, clinicians should reassure patients that although hypothyroidism is a chronic condition, treatment is usually safe and effective.

HYPERTHYROIDISM

Hyperthyroidism results from an excess amount of thyroid hormone. It occurs in up to 2.2% of the population (Hollowell et al., 2002), with a female-to-male ratio of 10:1 (Mulder, 1998).

CAUSES

Graves disease, an autoimmune disease that occurs most commonly in patients aged 20 to 50 years with a female-to-male ratio of 4 to 8:1, is the most common cause of overt hyperthyroidism (Box 50-4). It develops as a result of stimulation of the thyroid gland by TSH receptor autoantibodies on the follicular cell surface. The autoantibodies act like TSH in stimulating thyroid gland function. The gland is not susceptible to the usual negative-feedback mechanism of the thyroid hormones; thus, levels of thyroid hormone escalate.

Toxic nodular goiter (Plummer disease) is another frequent cause of hyperthyroidism, especially in older adults. In this condition, one or more thyroid nodules begins to "hyperfunction" and is not dependent on the feedback mechanisms of the pituitary–thyroid axis. As a result of the increased systemic T_4 produced by the nodule, TSH is suppressed, and the remainder of the gland begins to atrophy. Eye findings (ie, exophthalmos and lid lag sometimes found with Graves disease and thyrotoxicosis) are absent in this condition.

A less common cause of hyperthyroidism is thyrotoxicosis factitia, in which patients intentionally take T_4 in doses high enough to suppress their TSH. This finding is more common among those in the medical profession with access

---

BOX 50–4. CAUSES OF HYPERTHYROIDISM

Graves disease
Autonomously functioning nodule(s)
Lithium
Iodine excess, including iodine-containing
  medication
Thyrotoxicosis factitia
Excessive replacement of thyroid hormone
Subacute thyroiditis (transient)
Postpartum thyroiditis (transient)

TSH Suppression Unrelated to Hyperthyroidism
Nonthyroidal illness
Secondary or tertiary hypothyroidism
Recovery from hyperthyroidism
Drugs (eg, glucocorticoids, dopamine agonists)

Modified from Mazzaferri, E. L. (1997). Evaluation and management of common thyroid disorders in women. *American Journal of Obstetrics and Gynecology, 176*, 507–514.

---

to prescription medications. These patients may want to use T_4 to help with weight loss or to treat fatigue or depression.

Several forms of thyroiditis may result in hyperthyroidism with a characteristically low radioactive iodine uptake. These are discussed in a later section.

Amiodarone and other drugs that contain iodine, including radiographic contrast agents, may induce hyperthyroidism in patients with autonomously functioning nodules. Clinicians must monitor such patients closely to see if they need to receive these agents.

DIAGNOSTIC CRITERIA

The patient with hyperthyroidism classically exhibits symptoms of enhanced metabolic activity (ie, palpitations, sweating, heat intolerance, weight loss). Examination may reveal elevated blood pressure, tachycardia, a bruit over the thyroid gland, or exophthalmos in patients with Graves disease (Box 50-5). The diagnosis is confirmed by finding a low, or suppressed, TSH level with an elevated free T_4 level. A nuclear ^{123}I thyroid scan can confirm Graves disease, which causes a diffuse increase in uptake of radioactive iodine. Hyperthyroidism caused by a hyperfunctioning nodule appears as a localized area of increased radioiodine uptake (a "hot" nodule), with the remainder of the gland exhibiting generalized decreased uptake of the isotope.

INITIATING DRUG THERAPY

There are three main options to treat hyperthyroidism: (1) antithyroid drugs, (2) radioactive iodine ablation with ^{131}I, and (3) surgery (Table 50-3 and Fig. 50-4). In general, radioactive iodine is the treatment of choice for patients older than 40 years of age; it often is used in younger patients as well. Because of the high rate of permanent hypothyroidism after treatment and the eventual need for lifelong thyroid

BOX 50–5. SYMPTOMS AND SIGNS OF HYPERTHYROIDISM

Dyspnea	Goiter
Heat intolerance	Brisk reflexes
Palpitations	Tachycardia
Infertility	Tremor
Insomnia	Lid lag
Irritability	Exophthalmos
Nervousness	(with Graves disease)
Sweatiness	Weight loss
Frequent bowel	Amenorrhea or
movements	oligomenorrhea
Pretibial myxedema	
(with Graves disease)	

replacement, as well as concerns about subsequent cancers after exposure to radioiodine at a young age, many clinicians initially attempt to treat younger patients with antithyroid medications. Data on this issue have been conflicting, but many investigators are now beginning to use radioactive iodine as first-line therapy in young patients. Radioactive iodine is contraindicated in pregnancy; however, it may be used in women of childbearing age and in children. Women should postpone pregnancy until 6 months after radioiodine therapy. Lactating women should not receive radioiodine because it passes into breast milk.

Practitioners should follow patients treated with ^{131}I every 4 to 6 weeks for 3 months after radioiodine treatment, then less frequently. Because most patients with Graves disease become hypothyroid after treatment, clinicians must screen for symptoms and measure TSH and free T_4 levels intermittently. Conversely, when radioactive iodine is used to treat toxic nodules, the rate of posttherapeutic hypothyroidism is lower, likely related to the degree of suppression of the remainder of the gland by the nodule. If the free T_4 becomes low and the TSH elevated, patients should start T_4 supplementation with the goal of reaching the replacement dosage and maintaining euthyroidism. TSH levels should be done yearly or more frequently if the patient's clinical condition changes.

Surgery is reserved for patients with large goiters that compress vital structures or for those in whom there is a concern about a malignancy in the gland. It also may be used in pregnant women who are unable or unwilling to take antithyroid drugs. Before surgery, patients are often treated with antithyroid drugs until they are euthyroid, with inorganic iodide (discussed later) added 10 days after surgery.

Potential complications of surgery include hypoparathyroidism and injury to the recurrent laryngeal nerve, although in experienced hands these complications are rare. Hypothyroidism develops after thyroidectomy in up to 70% of cases depending on the extent of surgery, so postsurgical patients need regular follow-up and supplementation with T_4 as necessary.

Goals of Drug Therapy

The goals of therapy are to restore patients to the euthyroid state and eliminate the risks associated with chronic hyperthyroidism. Therapy usually is not lifelong. Patients usually stop taking antithyroid drugs after 1 to 2 years. If permanent hypothyroidism develops as a result of radioactive iodine treatment or surgery, however, then treatment of hypothyroidism (discussed previously) is lifelong.

Antithyroid Drugs

Antithyroid drugs commonly used are methimazole (Tapazole) and propylthiouracil (PTU [Propyl-Thyracil]; Table 50-4).

Mechanism of Action

These drugs act by inhibiting iodine organification. They also block the conversion of T_4 to T_3 in the periphery, although this mechanism has minimal clinical relevance. The drugs are rapidly absorbed and concentrated in the thyroid follicular cells. PTU has a short duration of action and thus requires multiple doses per day. Methimazole has a longer duration and may be dosed once a day, making it the drug of choice in most instances.

Dosage

The starting dose for PTU is 200 to 400 mg/d, whereas the initial dose of methimazole is 10 to 30 mg/d. Treatment usually continues for 12 to 24 months. Success rates for antithyroid drugs range from 10% to 75%, with remission rates inversely related to the duration of hyperthyroidism and the size of the goiter.

Table 50.3

Recommended Order of Treatment for Hyperthyroidism

Order	Agents	Comments
First line	Radioactive iodine	Usually recommended in patients older than age 40 y, but may be used for younger patients High incidence of hypothyroidism when used to treat Graves disease; less when used for toxic nodules
Second line	Antithyroid drugs	Often used in younger patients to induce remission of Graves disease; also used to prepare some patients for treatment with radioiodine or surgery
Third line	Surgery	Usually reserved for patients with large goiters or suspected malignancy

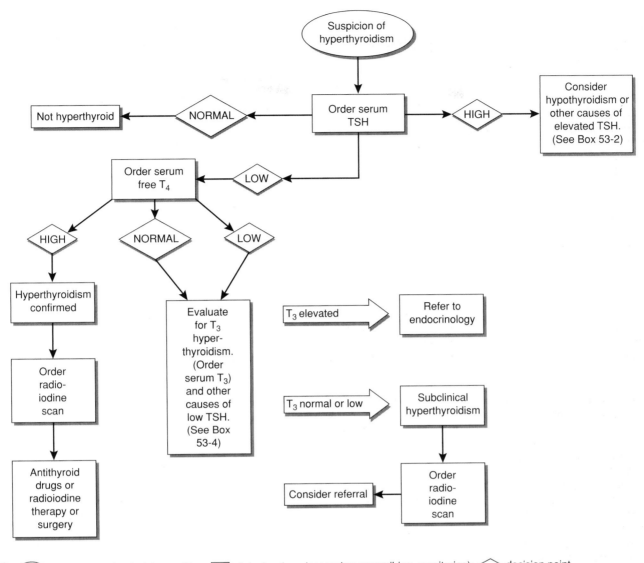

Key ⬭ Starting point for decision making; ▭ clinical actions (assessing, prescribing, monitoring); ◇ decision point.

Figure 50–4 Treatment algorithm for hyperthyroidism.

Antithyroid drugs also are used to prepare patients with severe hyperthyroidism for ablative therapy with either radioactive iodine or surgery, especially in those at risk for cardiac complications. The drugs usually are given for several weeks then stopped several days before definitive therapy, although patients sometimes may need to continue the drugs for several months after ^{131}I therapy to control persistent hyperthyroidism.

Adverse Events

Side effects are fairly minimal (Box 50-6), with the most common being rash, arthralgias, itching, and hepatic abnormalities. Patients who have difficulty with one medication may be given a trial of another, although cross-sensitivity among the antithyroid drugs may occur. Rarely (0.3% of patients), a potentially fatal agranulocytosis may result, which occurs somewhat more often with PTU than with methimazole. Clinicians should consider routine monitoring

of the complete blood count (CBC) during the first 3 months of therapy. They should warn patients who are taking these drugs to report symptoms of sore throat and fever immediately; they should obtain a CBC and stop the drug if the patient's white blood cell count is low.

Interactions

Because these drugs decrease iodine uptake and organification, they can interfere with subsequent radioactive iodine therapy. Higher doses of ^{131}I may be needed to increase success rates in these patients.

A study from Japan (Hashizume et al., 1991) demonstrated an increased remission rate in patients treated with high doses of antithyroid drugs combined with replacement doses of T_4 compared with those who received antithyroid drugs alone. The rationale was that by suppressing the TSH with T_4, there would be less stimulation of thyroid antigens. These results have not been confirmed in American and

Table 50.4

Overview of Drugs Used to Treat Hyperthyroidism

Generic (Trade) Name and Dosage	Adverse Effects	Contraindications	Special Considerations
Antithyroid Drugs			
propylthiouracil (PTU [Propyl-Thyracil]) Start: 100–600 mg/d Maintenance: 50–100 mg q8h	See Box 50–6	Hypersensitivity to drug	TSH 0.5–4.0 mIU/mL Monitor for fever, sore throat; check CBC.
methimazole (Tapazole) Start: 15–30 mg/d Maintenance: 5–15 mg/d		Same as above	Same as above
β Blockers			
propranolol (Inderal) Long acting: 80–160 mg/d	Fatigue, sexual dysfunction	Sinus bradycardia, heart block greater than first degree	For symptom control only Use with caution in asthma, diabetes, congestive heart failure, and depression.
atenolol (Tenormin) 50–200 mg/d	Same as above	Same as above	Same as above
Iodine-Containing Compounds			
SSKI (Lugol's solution) 0.1–0.3 mL tid sodium iodide (Iodopen) 0.5–1 g q12h	Rash, sialadenitis, vasculitis	Allergy to iodine	Administer after starting antithyroid drug.
Iodinated contrast agents: ipodate (Oragrafin) iopanoate (Telepaque) 0.5–2 g/d	Itching, skin rash, hives, diarrhea, nausea, vomiting; bruising/bleeding with iopanoate	Same as above	Reserved for severe thyrotoxicosis or thyroid storm Administer after starting antithyroid drug.
Other Agents			
lithium (Eskalith, others) Starting and maintenance: 900–1200 mg/d in divided doses	May have multisystem effects		Monitor lithium levels.
Glucocorticoids dosage depends on agent selected	May have multisystem effects		Adjunctive therapy for thyroid storm

BOX 50–6. COMPLICATIONS OF ANTITHYROID DRUGS

Serious and Rare Complications*
Agranulocytosis
Hepatitis (propylthiouracil)
Cholestatic jaundice (methimazole and propylthiouracil)
Aplastic anemia
Thrombocytopenia
Lupus-like vasculitis

Minor Complications
Fever
Pruritus
Urticaria
Arthralgia
GI distress
Hypoglycemia from insulin antibodies
Metallic taste

*These complications require immediate cessation of drug therapy. From Mazzaferri, E. L. (1997). Evaluation and management of common thyroid disorders in women. *American Journal of Obstetrics and Gynecology, 176,* 507–514.

European studies; thus, most authorities in the United States recommend against this therapy for Graves disease.

Adjunctive Agents Used to Manage Hyperthyroidism

β Blockers

The β blockers are used to treat the symptoms of hyperthyroidism. They do not affect thyroid hormone synthesis; rather, they act by decreasing the symptoms of adrenergic stimulation caused by the increased T_4 concentration. Practitioners should prescribe a nonselective β blocker like long-acting propranolol starting at a dose of 80 mg/d. Alternatively, atenolol may be used. These drugs can help prevent hyperthyroid-induced atrial fibrillation or control the ventricular rate in patients with established atrial fibrillation. Clinicians should consider anticoagulation to reduce the risk of stroke in patients with atrial fibrillation; treatment of these patients should be in consultation with a cardiologist. Prescribers should taper β blockers gradually and discontinue them as soon as the patient is euthyroid and asymptomatic. Patients in whom β blockers are not tolerated or are contraindicated (eg, those with asthma or congestive heart failure) may be treated with calcium channel blockers like diltiazem.

Iodine-Containing Compounds

Other agents used adjunctively in the treatment of hyperthyroidism are iodine-containing compounds like potassium iodide (in the form of saturated solution of potassium iodide [SSKI] 35 mg/drop or Lugol solution 7 mg/drop) and the iodinated contrast agents ipodate (Oragrafin) and iopanoate (Telepaque). These drugs are reserved for the treatment of severe thyrotoxicosis or thyroid storm. Such patients are usually treated in an intensive care unit under the care of an endocrinologist, intensivist, or both. Pharmacologic doses of iodine inhibit the release of thyroid hormones from the gland in the short term; however, because new hormone synthesis proceeds during treatment with iodine, iodine must be used in combination with antithyroid drugs, which are given 1 hour before the iodine compound.

Lithium

Lithium, which is chemically similar to iodine, is used rarely to block release of thyroid hormone from the gland in those patients who are intolerant of antithyroid drugs. The dose is 900 to 1200 mg/d, divided, and clinicians should monitor lithium levels.

Glucocorticoids

Glucocorticoids are occasionally used in thyroid storm. They reduce peripheral conversion of T_4 to T_3.

Treatment of Ophthalmopathy of Graves Disease

None of the aforementioned therapies for hyperthyroidism affects the ophthalmopathy of Graves disease. Anti-inflammatory drugs, immunosuppressive drugs (eg, prednisone and dexamethasone), and surgery are offered to patients as treatment for the ophthalmopathy. Sunglasses and artificial tears are used adjunctively for comfort.

Special Population Considerations

Geriatric

The term *apathetic hyperthyroidism* has been used to describe the atypical presentation of hyperthyroidism in some older patients. Rather than the usual symptoms of increased metabolic rate, these patients may present with weakness, dyspnea, anorexia, depression, or constipation. Physical examination may be unrevealing. Occasionally, new-onset atrial fibrillation or congestive heart failure is the initial presentation of hyperthyroidism in the older person.

Pregnancy

Radioactive iodine is contraindicated during pregnancy because it crosses the placenta and affects fetal thyroid development. PTU is the drug of choice for hyperthyroidism during both pregnancy and lactation because it crosses the placenta and enters the breast milk less than methimazole. Furthermore, use of methimazole during pregnancy increases the risk of a rare congenital abnormality, aplasia cutis congenita. During pregnancy, practitioners should prescribe the lowest dosages possible of antithyroid drugs that still maintain euthyroidism. The dosage usually decreases as pregnancy progresses and the severity of Graves disease lessens, then increases again after delivery. Clinicians should treat pregnant patients who have hyperthyroidism in consultation with an endocrinologist.

MONITORING PATIENT RESPONSE

Patients usually become euthyroid within 6 to 12 weeks of beginning antithyroid drugs; however, permanent hypothyroidism may develop many years after a course of therapy, so long-term follow-up is necessary. Patients taking antithyroid drugs should be evaluated every 1 to 3 months after starting treatment depending on the degree of hyperthyroidism and comorbid conditions. Once euthyroidism is achieved, practitioners can decrease the dose of antithyroid drugs and reevaluate the patient in 3 to 4 months. Clinicians should order free T_4 levels to monitor the patient because the TSH level remains suppressed for several months after the patient becomes euthyroid. They should continue to reduce and eventually discontinue the antithyroid drugs, after which they should see patients every 4 to 6 weeks for 3 to 4 months, and less frequently thereafter.

PATIENT EDUCATION

Patients with hyperthyroidism may have very troublesome symptoms that resemble those of anxiety disorders, such as panic attacks. Clinicians should advise them that these symptoms (which can be severe) will resolve with treatment of their thyroid disease.

Practitioners should review all treatment options with patients. They should tell patients that antithyroid drugs will put their disease into remission, but that the relapse rate is high. They should discuss the high likelihood of permanent hypothyroidism after radioactive iodine therapy. Patients will likely gain weight after therapy for hyperthyroidism, even if they do not become hypothyroid. Clinicians should emphasize the chronic nature of the condition and the importance of long-term follow-up regardless of the chosen treatment.

Drug Information

There can be increased effects of digitalis, metoprolol, and propanolol when the patient becomes euthyroid. The effects of anticoagulants can be altered. Drugs should be taken at equal intervals.

Complementary and Alternative Medicine

Bugleweed has been shown to treat a mildly overactive thyroid. It decreases thyroid hormone activity and increases the absorption and storage of thyroid hormone, causing a decreased metabolism. This is not used in patients with hypothyroidism.

Lemon balm is used in hyperthyroidism for its sedative effects.

Special Populations

Women of childbearing age with Graves disease may want to consider definitive treatment (radioiodine or surgery) before conception. Although it is acceptable to prescribe

PTU during pregnancy, clinicians must monitor thyroid function closely because of variations in the course of the disease in pregnancy.

THYROID NODULES

Thyroid nodules are encountered relatively often in clinical practice. The gland may have one or multiple nodules. Most are the result of adenomas, cysts, large collections of colloid, or focal areas of thyroiditis. Five percent of solitary nodules result from thyroid cancer, with higher rates in the very young and older age groups. Fine-needle aspiration biopsy (FNAB) is the initial diagnostic procedure to rule out carcinoma in a solitary nodule.

INITIATING DRUG THERAPY

Treatment of thyroid cancer is beyond the scope of this work; however, clinicians should be aware that high doses of T_4 are used in patients who have been treated for thyroid cancer in an effort to suppress the growth of any remaining cancer cells. Once a thyroid nodule is proved benign histologically, many clinicians attempt to reduce the size of the nodule medically (Fig. 50-5). T_4 is given in

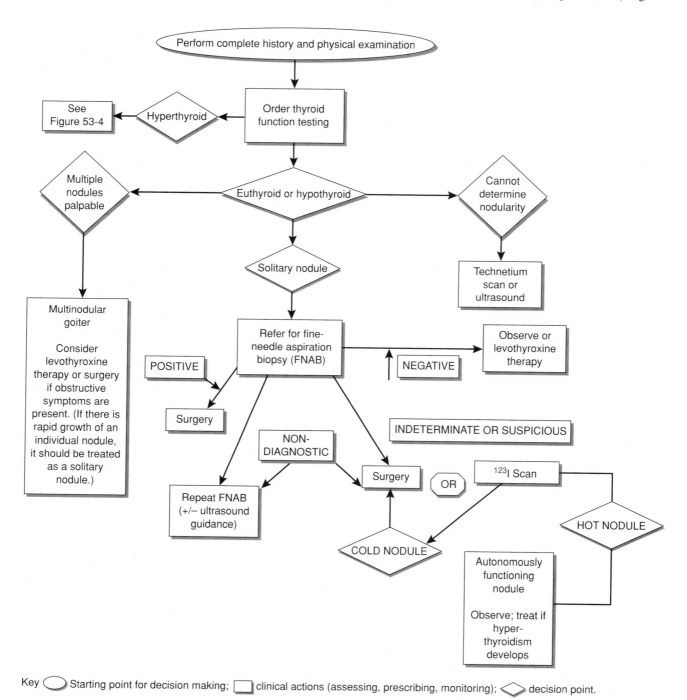

Figure 50–5   Evaluation and management of thyroid nodules.

higher than replacement doses (2.2 mcg/kg/d) in an attempt to turn off the secretion of TSH by the pituitary, with the presumption that growth of the nodule depends on TSH. With less circulating TSH, the nodule in theory will not increase in size and may decrease. The literature yields conflicting results in this regard, with some studies showing a significant effect on nodule size and others showing no effect.

Because of the likelihood of continued growth of a nodule and the possibility of development of further nodules, practitioners should consider suppressive therapy in patients with solitary and multiple nodules. The goal of therapy in these instances is to suppress the TSH to the low normal range, but not below, so as not to increase the patient's risk for hyperthyroidism. In fact, patients with autonomously functioning nodules should not receive T_4 because they often have relatively low or suppressed TSH levels already. Surgery is an alternative for patients with solitary nodules who do not respond sufficiently to T_4 therapy, whereas radioactive iodine and surgery are appropriate for such patients with multiple nodules.

MONITORING PATIENT RESPONSE

Patients require periodic evaluation to determine their responses to therapy. Clinicians should consider discontinuation of therapy if there is no response within the first 4 to 6 months. If the nodule grows while the patient is on T_4 suppression, or if there are other concerns about malignancy, practitioners should perform a repeat FNAB. Patients with hyperthyroidism as a result of toxic nodules respond to antithyroid drugs either in conjunction with or in lieu of ablative therapy.

PATIENT EDUCATION

Patients with thyroid nodules often are unaware of any problem. Therefore, practitioners need to emphasize the potential (although small) for malignancy and the need for further evaluation with FNAB.

If the nodule is found to be benign, clinicians must discuss treatment options. Attempting to shrink the nodule with T_4 is reasonable, but regular follow-up is necessary to ensure that patients are not being overtreated. If there is no difference in the size of the nodule after a reasonable trial, then T_4 may be discontinued; however, patients need to return for regular follow-up to be evaluated for increase in size of the nodule or development of new nodules.

SUBCLINICAL THYROID DISEASE

The entity of mild thyroid failure, previously known as *subclinical hypothyroidism*, presents a therapeutic challenge. This condition is defined as an elevated TSH level with a normal free T_4 concentration, usually in a patient with no symptoms. Many authorities believe that mild thyroid failure requires the same treatment as overt hypothyroidism because both entities have been associated with adverse cardiovascular outcomes.

Proponents of therapy for mild thyroid failure cite studies showing higher levels of LDL cholesterol and lower levels of high-density lipoprotein cholesterol in these patients, as well as increased systolic time intervals and decreased cognitive function. After treatment with T_4, some of these problems show improvement. Patients who have coexisting cardiovascular disease or dysrhythmias probably should not be treated for mild thyroid failure because the risks of therapy outweigh the potential benefits. If treatment is attempted, it should be with T_4 at doses to lower the TSH level to the normal range. The incidence of mild thyroid failure is higher in older adults, occurring in up to 20% of people older than 60 years of age.

A subclinical hyperthyroid entity has been defined by normal free T_4 and T_3 concentrations with a low TSH level in asymptomatic patients. This condition often results from overreplacement of T_4, autonomously functioning nodules, nonthyroid illness, or certain medications that decrease TSH (see Box 50-4). Risks of subclinical hyperthyroidism include increased bone turnover, which may predispose to osteoporosis and an increased risk of atrial fibrillation and other adverse cardiovascular outcomes. Antithyroid therapy similar to that of overt hyperthyroidism should be considered in consultation with an endocrinologist.

THYROIDITIS

After delivering a child up to 10% of women without previous thyroid disease have postpartum (also known as *painless* or *silent*) thyroiditis, a variant of Hashimoto thyroiditis. Patients present within 1 year after delivery with nonspecific symptoms of fatigue, palpitations, and depression. Tachycardia and goiter may be present on examination.

Patients often go through a hyperthyroid phase that resolves in a few months. Some have transient hypothyroidism that can last from 2 to 6 months. This condition is usually self-limited, so treatment is indicated only to relieve the symptoms of hyperthyroidism. The β blockers are the treatment of choice. Antithyroid drugs are not helpful because the hyperthyroidism that develops is a result of the gland's spilling of preformed thyroid hormone. Some patients require replacement doses of T_4 during the hypothyroid phase of their condition. Women with high titers of antithyroid peroxidase antibodies during or after the pregnancy are at increased risk for development of permanent hypothyroidism; these women should be followed closely.

Women with postpartum thyroiditis may experience symptoms similar to postpartum depression; therefore, practitioners should reassure these women that their symptoms will resolve once the condition subsides. Clinicians should encourage those women at higher risk for permanent hypothyroidism (those with a high titer of antithyroid peroxidase antibodies) to return for periodic follow-up.

Patients sometimes have subacute (DeQuervain) thyroiditis several weeks after an upper respiratory tract infection. They present with a painful, enlarged gland and symptoms and signs of hyperthyroidism, which is the result of leakage of thyroid hormones from the inflamed gland. If a radioiodine scan is performed, it shows diffusely decreased uptake of tracer (as opposed to the increased uptake seen in Graves disease).

This condition is self-limited and requires symptomatic treatment only. As in postpartum thyroiditis, β blockers are used to reduce tachycardia, tremor, and nervousness. Aspirin or other nonsteroidal anti-inflammatory drugs (NSAIDs) can reduce the pain in the gland. Rarely, steroids are needed to reduce swelling and pain. These patients may experience a brief period of hypothyroidism but do not usually become permanently hypothyroid, so that vigilant follow-up is not required.

Clinicians should reassure patients with subacute thyroiditis that their condition will resolve spontaneously, but may take weeks.

■ Case Study 1

M.E. is a 29-year-old woman with a 7-month history of heavy, irregular menses, a 5-pound weight gain, constipation, and decreased energy. Her past history is unremarkable. She takes no prescription medications but uses iron and calcium supplements. She has a family history of thyroid disease. On examination, her weight is 152 pounds, her heart rate is 64 bpm, and her blood pressure is 138/86. Her thyroid gland is mildly enlarged, without nodularity. She has trace edema in her lower extremities, and her reflexes are slow. Laboratory studies are as follows: TSH is 15.3 mIU/mL (elevated), free T_4 is 0.3 mIU/mL (decreased), total cholesterol is 276 mg/mL.

Diagnosis: primary hypothyroidism

1. List the specific goals of therapy for M.E.

2. What drug therapy would you prescribe and at what dose?

3. What are the parameters for monitoring the success of M.E.'s therapy?

4. Discuss specific patient education for therapy for hypothyroidism.

5. List one or two adverse reactions for the prescribed therapy that would cause you to change the drug or dose.

6. What would be the choice for second-line therapy?

7. What, if any, over-the-counter or complementary and alternative medicine would be appropriate for M.E.?

8. What dietary and lifestyle changes would be recommended for M.E.?

9. Describe one or two drug–drug or drug–food interactions for the selected treatment.

■ Case Study 2

J.C. is a 37-year-old woman who presents with "swollen glands" 2 weeks after an upper respiratory infection. She has no lingering respiratory symptoms but complains of neck pain and swelling. She denies palpitations, tremors and diarrhea, but has noted a weight loss of 4 pounds. Her blood pressure is 120/72, her pulse rate is 92, and her thyroid gland is tender to palpation and enlarged. Thyroid function testing reveals a TSH level less than 0.02 ngU/mL and a free T_4 of 3.0 ng/mL (elevated).

Diagnosis: subacute (DeQuervain) thyroiditis

1. List the specific goals of therapy for J.C.

2. What drug therapy would you prescribe and at what dose?

■ **Case Study** (*Continued*)

→ 3. What are the parameters for monitoring the success of J.C.'s therapy?

→ 4. Discuss specific patient education for therapy for hypothyroidism.

→ 5. List one or two adverse reactions for the prescribed therapy that would cause you to change the drug or dose.

→ 6. What would be the choice for second-line therapy?

→ 7. What, if any, over-the-counter or complementary and alternative medicine would be appropriate for J.C.?

→ 8. What dietary and lifestyle changes would be recommended for J.C.?

→ 9. Describe one or two drug–drug or drug–food interactions for the selected treatment.

Bibliography

Starred references are cited in the text.

Brander, A., Viikinkoski, P., Nickels, J., et al. (1991). Thyroid gland: US screening in a random adult population. *Radiology, 181*, 683–687.

Bullock, B. A., & Henze, R. L. (2000). *Focus on pathophysiology.* Philadelphia: Lippincott Williams & Wilkins.

*Canaris, G. J., Manowitz, N. R., Mayor, G., et al. (2000). The Colorado thyroid disease prevalence study. *Archives of Internal Medicine, 160*, 526–534.

Cooper, D. S. (2003). Hyperthyroidism. *Lancet, 362*, 459–468.

Garcia, M., Baskin, H. J., & Feld, S. (1995). *American Association of Clinical Endocrinologists (AACE) clinical practice guidelines for the management of hyperthyroidism and hypothyroidism.*

*Hak, A. E., Pols, H. A., Visser, T. J., et al. (2000). Subclinical hypothyroidism is an independent risk factor for atherosclerosis and myocardial infarction in elderly women: the Rotterdam Study. *Annals of Internal Medicine, 130*, 270–278.

*Hashizume, K., Ichikawa, K., Sakurai, A., et al. (1991). Administration of thyroxine in treated Graves' disease: Effects on the level of antibodies to thyroid stimulating hormone receptors and on the risk of recurrence of hyperthyroidism. *New England Journal of Medicine, 324*, 947–953.

*Hollowell, J. G., Staehling, N. W., Flanders, W. D., et al. (2002). Serum TSH, T_4, and thyroid antibodies in the United States Population (1988 to 1994): National Health and Nutrition Examination Survey (NHANES III). *Journal of Clinical Endocrinology and Metabolism, 87*, 489–499.

Kahaly, G. J. (2000) Cardiovascular and atherogenic aspects of subclinical hypothyroidism. *Thyroid, 10*, 665–679.

*Mandel, S. J., Brent, G. A., & Larsen, P. R. (1993). Levothyroxine therapy in patients with thyroid disease. *Annals of Internal Medicine, 119*, 492–502.

Mokshagundam, S., & Barzel, U. S. (1993). Thyroid disease in the elderly. *Journal of the American Geriatric Society, 41*, 1361–1368.

*Mulder, J. E. (1998). Thyroid disorders in women. *Medical Clinics of North America, 82*, 103–125.

*National Academy of Clinical Biochemistry Website: NACB laboratory medicine practice guidelines. Available at: http://www.nacb.org/lmpg/main.stm. Accessed February 18, 2004.

Parle, J. V., Maisonneuve, P., Sheppard, M. C., et al. (2001). Prediction of all-cause and cardiovascular mortality in elderly people from one low serum thyrotropin result: a 10-year cohort study. *Lancet, 358*, 861–865.

Pearce, E. N., Farwell, A. P., & Braverman, L. E. (2003). Current concepts: Thyroiditis. *New England Journal of Medicine, 348*, 2646–2655.

*Sawin, C. T., Geller, A., Wolf, P. A., et al. (1994). Low serum thyrotropin concentrations as a risk factor for atrial fibrillation in older persons. *New England Journal of Medicine, 331*, 1249–1252.

Smeltzer, S. C., & Bare, B. G. (2000). *Brunner & Suddarth's textbook of medical-surgical nursing* (9th ed.). Philadelphia: Lippincott Williams & Wilkins.

Surks, M. I., Ortiz, E. O., Daniels, G. H., et al. (2004). Subclinical thyroid disease: Scientific review and guidelines for diagnosis and management. *Journal of the American Medical Association, 291*, 228–238.

Uzzan, B., Campos, J., Cucherat, M., et al. (1996). Effects on bone mass of long term treatment with thyroid hormones: a meta-analysis. *Journal of Clinical Endocrinology and Metabolism, 81*, 4278–4289.

Visit the Connection web site for the most up-to-date drug information.

XI

Pharmacotherapy for Immune Disorders

51

ALLERGIES AND ALLERGIC REACTIONS

■ ANDREW M. PETERSON AND ANTHONY P. SORRENTINO

The term *allergy* is derived from the Greek words *allos* (differing from the normal or usual) and *ergon* (work or energy). To describe it in simple, nonclinical terms, allergy is an abnormal release of energy in the body. In clinical or physiologic terms, allergy is an exaggerated immune response resulting from an antibody–antigen reaction.

Antibodies are soluble protein molecules made by B lymphocytes in response to foreign substances. Antibodies, also referred to as *immunoglobulins*, are tailored specifically and uniquely to bind to each foreign substance and remove it from the circulation. Invasion or contact with a foreign substance results in the production and secretion of antibodies. Therefore, the foreign substance is an *anti*body *gen*erator—hence the term *antigen*. Antigens also are referred to as *allergens*; the terms are interchangeable.

All people come in contact with the same antigens, yet not all people display allergic symptoms. Allergy symptoms appear when the immune response is exaggerated or inappropriate, causing inflammation and tissue damage. This exaggerated response to an antigen is referred to as *hypersensitivity*. Hypersensitivity is a characteristic of an individual. It is manifested on the second or a subsequent contact with a particular antigen.

Allergens can be food-based, chemical, or environmental. Typical food allergens include milk or egg protein, peanut, shellfish, and wheat or soy. Parabens and lanolin, commonly found in make-up and sunscreens; thimerosal, a preservative found in contact lens solutions; and fragrance enhancers found in perfumes are common chemical allergens. Drugs, such as the local anesthetics lidocaine andbenzocaine, are also chemical allergens. Environmental allergens include mold, pollen and dust.

In contrast to allergy, *anergy* is the term used to describe the unexpected failure of the immune system to respond to the challenge of a foreign substance (antigen or allergen). Several skin test antigens may be applied to the skin (an anergy panel) to determine the status of the immune system. The antigens selected are those to which a majority of the population would be exhibit a reaction. Examples of these include *candida* species and histoplasmin. If the characteristic wheals do not appear in the prescribed period, the test can be interpreted as the patient not having prior exposure to the antigen or a potentially compromised immune system.

CLASSIFICATION OF ALLERGIC REACTIONS

The medical literature describes four types of hypersensitivity reactions (Coombs and Gell classification) that are listed and described in Box 51-1. There are four types of reactions under this classification system. Type I reactions involve the interaction between an antigen and a specific IgE antibody. These antibodies are bound to member receptors on mast cells and basophils. When an antigen binds to these antibodies, the cell releases histamine, leukotrienes, and prostaglandins. These vasoactive substances produce a vasodilation and increase capillary permeability, both of which allow for eosinophils and other inflammatory cells to infiltrate tissues, furthering the allergic response. The first contact results in the formation of the antibody. Subsequent contact with the same antigen results in the antibody–antigen reaction, resulting in this type I hypersensitivity reaction. The antibody–antigen reaction triggers the immune response that results in allergy symptoms (Fig. 51-1). Allergies can affect the airways, eyes, skin, or the entire body. Type I reactions are typically anaphylactic in nature and can be life-threatening.

Type II reactions, also known as cytotoxic reactions, occur when an antibody reacts with an antigenic component of a cell. This antibody–antigen reaction in turn activates killer T cells or macrophages to aid in the destruction of the antigenic cell. Complement activation is also involved in this process, furthering the cytotoxic process leading to tissue destruction. Transfusion reactions are typically type II allergic reactions.

Type III reactions result from immune complexes that activate the complement system. Activating this system promotes the migration and release of cells such as polymorphonuclear cells that can release proteolytic enzymes and factors that promote tissue permeability. Systemic lupus erythematosus (SLE) is a form of a type III allergic reaction.

Type IV reactions are also called delayed-hypersensitivity reactions. These cell-mediated reactions are the result of sensitized T lymphocytes coming into contact with a specific antigen. The delay typically takes 2 to 3 days or up to a week. Allergic dermatitis is an example of a type IV reaction.

Immunologic Versus Nonimmunologic Reactions

Some cutaneous reactions, such as contact dermatitis, may appear to be allergic reactions, but they do not involve the immune system. Irritant contact dermatitis is the most common cutaneous reaction and is often caused by skin irritants such as powders or chemicals found in gloves.

Contact dermatitis differs from allergic dermatitis in that there is direct tissue insult from the skin irritant. The cracked, dry skin occurring with contact dermatitis no longer can prevent allergens from entering the systemic cir-

culation. With latex allergies, for example, the powder already present in the glove can give rise to a contact dermatitis, thus allowing for the latex antigens to enter the circulation. This in turn increases the likelihood of an allergic reaction, resulting in allergic contact dermatitis. Because of this phenomenon, it is often difficult to distinguish allergic from nonallergic contact dermatitis. See Chapter 10 for more details on dermatitis.

General Treatment Overview of Allergic Reactions

The first step in treating an allergic reaction is to remove the allergen if possible. Remove the person from the environment causing the allergy, stop the offending drug, or wash off the offending chemical. Most allergic reactions clear up within a few days of removing the cause. Symptomatic cutaneous reactions such as pruritic rash, urticaria, or morbilliform eruptions, as well as reactions involving multiple organs are treated.

Cutaneous Reactions

Cutaneous reactions such as urticaria, pruritus, and hives are often secondary to the release of histamine, making antihistamine therapy the mainstay of treatment. There are two types of antihistamines used in the general treatment of allergic reactions: first generation and second generation. The first-generation antihistamines include diphenhydramine, hydroxyzine, and chlorpheniramine, among others. These agents are typically very effective, but they may also be very sedating. The second-generation agents, such as loratadine and fexofenadine, are nonsedating antihistamines (NSAs) that work fairly well at controlling mild to moderate symptoms of cutaneous reactions. However, if the symptoms persist for more than a few days, or are not well controlled, a first-generation antihistamine may be substituted, or added to, the NSA. Close communication with the patient regarding resolution of the symptoms is necessary, along with balancing the quality of life issues such as sedation, dry mouth, and urinary retention. If necessary, agents possessing more H_1- and H_2-antihistamine activity such as doxepin may be used instead. However, dose-limiting side effects such as dry mouth limit their utility. If the reaction is moderate to severe, or if there is no relief from antihistamine therapy, systemic glucocorticoids may be used. Short courses of treatment with oral prednisone or methylprednisolone are usually used. See Chapter 10 for more information on the use of oral steroids for treating cutaneous reactions.

Anaphylaxis and Anaphylactoid Reactions

Anaphylaxis is a type I hypersensitivity reaction involving IgE-mediated release of histamine, leukotrienes, and other mediators from already sensitized mast cells and basophils. The release of these mediators initiates a systemic chain of events that includes symptoms such as agitation, flushing, pruritus, urticaria, and wheezing. The onset of the reaction is quick, 1 to 30 minutes. The histamine release causes a smooth muscle contraction and vasodilation. The wheezing decreases oxygenation, whereas the vasodilation results in a

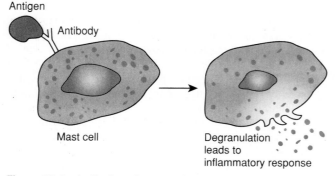

Figure 51–1 Antibody-antigen reaction.

release of fluids into the tissues, thus causing a lower effective plasma volume leading to shock. Prolonged vasodilation, coupled with decreased oxygenation, can lead to arrhythmias, convulsions, and death.

Anaphylactoid reactions are similar in appearance to anaphylaxis, but may occur after the *first* injection of certain drugs and contrast media. They are non-IgE mediated and the agent causes a direct release of histamine and other inflammatory toxics. They have a dose-related, toxic–idiosyncratic mechanism rather than an immunologically mediated one.

Treatment

Immediate treatment with epinephrine is imperative. Epinephrine effectively increases the blood pressure and is antagonist to the effects of histamine smooth muscle and other tissues.

For mild reactions such as generalized pruritus, urticaria, angioedema, or mild wheezing, 0.01 mL/kg aqueous epinephrine 1:1000 subcutaneously (usual dose 0.3–0.5 mL in adults; 0.3 mL maximum for children) should be given. If the reaction is caused by an injected antigen (eg, a drug), then a tourniquet may be applied above the injection site and half the above dose of epinephrine also injected into the site to reduce systemic absorption of the antigen. If the reaction is more severe, but does not have cardiovascular involvement (eg, collapse), then an injectable antihistamine such as diphenhydramine may be given to prevent further complications from histamine release such as laryngeal edema.

If the reaction does involve the cardiovascular system, then intravenous fluids should be rapidly infused to maintain volume. Hypovolemia is usually the major cause of the hypotension. Colloid plasma expanders such as dextran are rarely necessary. If fluid replacement is ineffective at restoring blood pressure, then dopamine or norepinephrine may be *cautiously* introduced. Alternatively, if the patient is in bradycardia, atropine may be used to increase heart rate. Patients with severe reactions should be observed in the hospital for 24 hours after recovery in case of relapse.

Systemic corticosteroids are indicated for all patients experiencing moderate to severe anaphylaxis. Typically, methylprednisolone, 1 to 2 mg/kg as an intravenous bolus, for children or adults, followed by 1 to 2 mg/kg every 6 to 8 hours for adults and 1 to 2 mg/kg/d 2 to 3 times a day for children is needed to prevent the onset of late-phase reactions.

Prophylaxis

The primary means of preventing an allergic reaction is avoidance. However, when this is not feasible or practical, immunotherapy is an effective means of preventing reactions, particularly anaphylactic reactions from insect bites. This form of "desensitization" is only effective when a specific allergen can be identified. Some ragweed and pollen allergies respond well to immunotherapy, though it may take several months before immunity is conferred.

Desensitization may be rapidly achieved in patients requiring drug therapy to which they have an established allergy. For example, patients with anaphylactic reactions to penicillin may be desensitized by using increasing concentrations of penicillin every 15 minutes. To ensure patient safety, desensitization is best done under constant supervision and in consultation with an experienced allergist. There are numerous protocols for penicillin desensitization and an increasing number for patients who are allergic to sulfa drugs.

ALLERGIC RHINITIS (HAY FEVER OR POLLEN ALLERGY)

Allergic rhinitis is an *airway allergy*. (Asthma, also an airway allergy, is discussed in Chap. 24.) Many people have hay fever. The National Institute of Allergy and Infectious Diseases states that pollen allergy affects nearly 9.3% of all people in the United States, not including those with asthma.

CAUSES

Common inhaled allergens that cause allergic rhinitis in sensitized people include pollen (grass, trees, weeds), dust mites, mold spores, enzymes (in detergents), and insect body parts. The two most common types of allergic rhinitis are seasonal and perennial (Table 51-1). The incidence of seasonal rhinitis is approximately 10 times greater than that of perennial rhinitis.

In seasonal allergic rhinitis, symptoms correspond with seasonal peaks in tree, grass, and weed pollens. During the spring, tree pollens such as alder, birch, and oak cause problems for many people. In the summer, grass pollens, such as timothy grass, can cause allergies. Weeds, such as mugwort and ragweed, pollinate in late summer and autumn. Pollens usually are windborne, and patients with seasonal allergic rhinitis often are said to have "hay fever." The most common cause of seasonal allergic rhinitis is ragweed pollen.

Patients with perennial allergic rhinitis have symptoms throughout the year, instead of only during certain months. They usually require chronic treatment. The most common causes of perennial rhinitis are animal dander and dust mites. In many cases, causative agents are difficult for patients to avoid because many such agents are indoor allergens. Perennial rhinitis may worsen when patients are exposed to nonnatural irritants such as paint, cleaners, or tobacco smoke.

Genetic predisposition plays a major role in the development of allergic rhinitis. The genetically determined tendency to produce increased quantities of IgE expresses itself

---

Table 51.1

Seasonal Versus Perennial Allergies

Causes of Seasonal Allergies	Causes of Perennial Allergies
Tree pollen (spring)	Mold (indoor)
Grass pollen (spring through fall)	Dust (dust mites)
Weeds (late summer)	Animal dander (skin flakes)
Leaf mold (early spring and late summer)	Animal fur
	Foods (nuts, shellfish, milk, eggs)

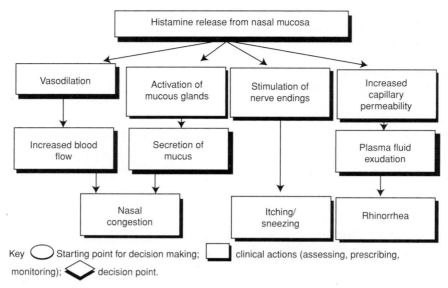

Figure 51–2   Results of histamine release in the nasal mucosa.

after prolonged exposure to an allergen. Consequently, allergic rhinitis is uncommon before 3 years of age. Those in later childhood or young adulthood are at greatest risk for development of new symptoms. In general, neither sex exhibits more of a predilection for allergic rhinitis; however, some sources indicate that the perennial form is more common in women.

Patients with a family history of asthma or eczema are more likely to have an allergic basis for rhinitis. The incidence of allergic rhinitis increases by approximately 30% when one parent has a history and is even higher when both parents have allergic disorders. Studies of pediatric populations have uncovered certain factors that may increase the expression of allergy: maternal smoking during pregnancy, month of birth (eg, being born during allergy season), and development of a viral infection in the upper respiratory tract.

PATHOPHYSIOLOGY

Initial exposure to the antigen/allergen stimulates the B lymphocytes (plasma cells) to produce an antigen-specific antibody (IgE) that binds to mast cell membranes (tissue-fixed antibody). The person is now sensitized to that specific antigen and susceptible to allergic reactions when re-exposed to it. On subsequent exposure, the antigen binds to the tissue-fixed IgE antibody and triggers breakdown of the mast cells (degranulation) and release of mediators (histamine, prostaglandins, leukotrienes, kinins, thromboxanes, and serotonin). Histamine, which is stored primarily in mast cells and basophils, is believed to be the mediator most responsible for the clinical signs and symptoms of allergic rhinitis.

Common symptoms in patients with allergic rhinitis are ocular pruritus (itching of the eyes) and conjunctival inflammation (inflammation of the membrane lining the eyelids).

Other symptoms of allergic rhinitis are irritability, lethargy, fatigue, and loss of appetite. Once released into the nasal mucosa, the mediators cause vasodilatation, increased capillary permeability, increased mucous production, and stimulation of nerve endings. The resulting symptoms are rhinorrhea (profuse, watery nasal discharge), nasal congestion (obstruction by mucus), and nasal pruritus. The most severe symptoms include violent episodes of sneezing (often a dozen or more times in a row) and total obstruction of nasal airflow resulting from copious amounts of mucus (Fig. 51-2).

The specific IgE antibody made in response to the allergen also may attach to eosinophils. Antigen-provoked degranulation of eosinophils also causes allergic symptoms. The symptoms associated with eosinophils are related to a late-phase allergic response, occurring hours to days after the initial reaction.

DIAGNOSTIC CRITERIA

The diagnosis of allergic rhinitis begins with a thorough history determining the presence of classic signs and symptoms and the time, place, and circumstances under which they occur. A family history is also important because it may establish the familial predisposition to allergy.

Physical examination of the patient with suspected allergic rhinitis begins with assessment of facial appearance, which often includes teary eyes and a red, swollen nose with scaling and crusting from frequent blowing and rubbing with facial tissues. There also may be dark circles under the eyes (allergic shiners), pinched nostrils, and a gaping mouth (from mouth breathing). The nasal mucous membranes are typically pale, swollen, and coated with a clear, watery secretion. Some erythema and bleeding may be noted. Swelling, streaks of erythema, and mucus may be present in the posterior pharynx. Other positive physical findings include swelling around and watery discharge from the eyes.

Table 51.2

Symptoms of Seasonal Allergies Versus Respiratory Infections

Symptoms	Seasonal Allergy (Hay Fever)	Upper Respiratory Infection
Head congestion/runny nose	Yes	Yes
Sneezing	Yes	Sometimes
Itchy, watery eyes	Yes	No
Cough	Usually dry	Dry or productive
Predictable seasonal patterns	Yes	Uncommon
Fever	No	Yes
Short duration (3–7 d)	No	Yes
Long duration (weeks)	Yes	No
Productive cough	Uncommon (except in asthma)	Yes

Nasal Smears

Practitioners may use the Wright stain for nasal secretions to detect eosinophils. Although eosinophilia suggests an allergic etiology for rhinitis symptoms (in infectious rhinitis, neutrophils predominate), it is not diagnostic. Conversely, no eosinophilia does not rule out allergy. Eosinophilia may be absent in patients who have superimposed infections or have not had a recent exposure to allergens.

Skin Testing

Skin testing with extracts of suspected allergens usually provides the most effective means of identifying specific sensitivities in patients with allergic rhinitis. In this test, a superficial scratch or prick is made in the skin and a diluted extract of antigen is applied. If the patient has allergen-specific IgE antibodies bound to tissue mast cells, a classic wheal-and-flare reaction appears over the next 15 to 30 minutes. To avoid false-negative results, patients should discontinue the use of antihistamines before they undergo skin testing. Clinicians should individualize this time frame based on the specific antihistamine that the patient is taking. In most cases, it is adequate to stop taking antihistamines 48 to 72 hours before testing. If patients do not stop taking antihistamines before skin testing, practitioners may mistakenly exclude a diagnosis of allergic rhinitis and subject patients to unnecessary further evaluations.

If the results of the scratch test are negative or unclear, practitioners may administer a more dilute extract of antigen intradermally. Clinicians should not use the intradermal test in patients with a positive response to scratch testing because of the risk of significant allergic reaction, including anaphylaxis.

Radioallergosorbent Testing

Radioallergosorbent testing (RAST) permits in vitro detection of serum IgE antibodies to allergens. Because only 1% of IgE molecules circulate in the blood (the remainder are bound to tissue), RAST results may not reflect the biologic situation. Although RAST is more specific, skin testing is less costly, more sensitive, and simpler to perform. Despite these shortcomings, RAST is helpful when the results of skin testing are unclear. The test is likewise useful when patients are unable to undergo skin testing because of dermatologic conditions or a history of anaphylactic reaction to the suspected allergen. RAST is also indicated for evaluation of children younger than 2 years, as well as for patients unable to discontinue using antihistamines, as required before skin testing.

Differential Diagnosis

Symptoms similar to those of allergic rhinitis may result from *mechanical nasal obstruction* (foreign body or anatomic factors); as a *side effect of medications* (oral contraceptives, hormone replacement therapy, tricyclic antidepressants, propranolol [Inderal], reserpine [Serpasil], methyldopa [Aldomet], and aspirin-containing compounds); or from *medical conditions associated with increased vasodilatation* (eg, hypothyroidism, cystic fibrosis, tumors, alcoholism, or pregnancy). Table 51-2 compares the symptoms of seasonal rhinitis with common cold symptoms to illustrate the similarities and differences between these conditions.

Although seasonal rhinitis usually is relatively easy to diagnose, identification of perennial rhinitis may be more elusive. Other nonallergic conditions could cause similar symptoms. *Vasomotor rhinitis* (congestion of the nasal mucosa without infection or allergy) could be difficult to differentiate from perennial rhinitis. In vasomotor rhinitis, however, irritants (eg, fumes, cold air, high humidity, alcoholic beverages, or emotional stress) rather than allergens usually trigger symptoms. Moreover, vasomotor rhinitis is associated with an absence of nasal, palatal, or conjunctival pruritus. In *nonallergic rhinitis with eosinophilia*, testing likewise fails to indicate a specific allergen.

INITIATING DRUG THERAPY

Allergic rhinitis may be treated through avoidance of the allergen, pharmacologic agents, and immunotherapy. The basic approach to pharmacologic management of allergic rhinitis is the use of antihistamines, nasal decongestants, and intranasal corticosteroids (Fig. 51-3).

The ideal treatment for allergic rhinitis is avoidance of the offending allergen. Complete avoidance often is not feasible, but most patients usually can reduce exposure. Basic strategies include the use of air conditioners in homes and automobiles to lessen exposure to pollen by keeping windows closed and use of dehumidifiers to discourage the growth of molds and mites. If possible, humidity

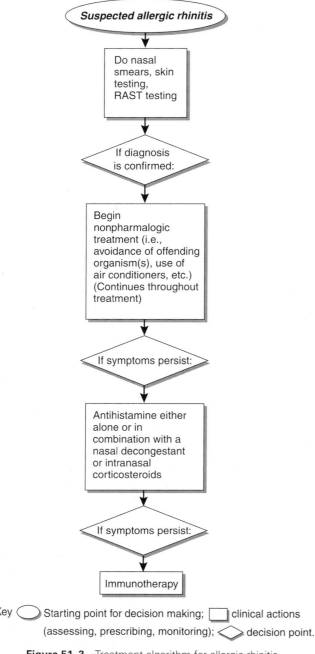

Key ⬭ Starting point for decision making; ▢ clinical actions
(assessing, prescribing, monitoring); ◇ decision point.

Figure 51–3   Treatment algorithm for allergic rhinitis.

should be maintained at 30% to 40% throughout the year. Patients can lessen exposure to mites by encasing mattresses in plastic, washing all bedding in very hot water each week, and removing carpeting and upholstered furniture. They can use high-efficiency particulate aerosol air cleaners to help filter out dust molds and pollen. Ideally, pets should be removed from the home; however, many patients and their families find doing so unacceptable. At a minimum, families should keep pets out of the allergic person's bedroom, as well as away from heating and cooling systems.

Immunotherapy, also known as *desensitization, hyposensitization,* or *allergy shots,* has been used for decades for the treatment of allergic rhinitis and asthma. It consists of repeated subcutaneous injections of gradually increasing concentrations of the allergens considered to be specifically responsible for the patient's allergy symptoms. The injections are purified extracts of the "trigger" substances, such as ragweed, grass, dust mite, and animal dander. Clinical benefits are related to the administration of high doses of allergens weekly or every other week. The duration of treatment is typically 3 to 5 years. Treatment is discontinued based on minimal symptoms over two consecutive seasons of exposure. The benefit is derived from a reduction in the percentage of histamine released after immunotherapy compared with before treatment. The result is milder or no symptoms of allergy. Immunotherapy is not first-line treatment. It is usually initiated when avoidance of the triggers and drug therapy fail to control the symptoms of hay fever and other allergies.

Goals of Drug Therapy

The goal of drug therapy for patients with allergies is to alleviate the symptoms with a little to no adverse effects from medications. This is accomplished primarily through decreasing the release or inhibiting the effect of histamine release and other mediators of inflammation from mast cells. Mast cells are distributed throughout the body; however, the greatest concentration of histamine occurs in the skin, respiratory system, and gastrointestinal (GI) mucosa. Relief of symptoms with minimal drug side effects should lead to an improved quality of life.

Histamine released in the GI tract does not cause allergy symptoms. It may result in hyperacidity by stimulating histamine type 2 (H_2) receptors and lead to peptic ulcer disease or gastroesophageal reflux disease. Treatment of these conditions is with H_2 blockers. It is the histamine released in the skin and respiratory tract (H_1 receptors) that causes classic allergy symptoms. The medications used to treat these symptoms are antihistamines (H_1 blockers), nasal decongestants, intranasal corticosteroids, and intranasal cromolyn. Suggestions for their selection are outlined in the following sections. The patient needs drug treatment of allergy symptoms as long as exposure to the triggers continues or until the patient becomes desensitized to the trigger, either naturally ("outgrowing the allergy") or through immunotherapy (described earlier).

Antihistamines

Antihistamines are classified according to their sedative effects or as first generation (older) and second generation (newer) depending on when they were marketed. The older antihistamines cross the blood–brain barrier, causing the greatest degree of sedation as well as central nervous system (CNS) effects. These agents can be subclassified on the basis of chemical structure. The main groupings include the ethanolamines, ethylenediamines, alkylamines, phenothiazines, and piperidines.

First-Generation Antihistamines

The first-generation antihistamines, such as diphenhydramine, chlorpheniramine, and brompheniramine, are the older antihistamines. As noted earlier, these tend to be more sedating than newer, second-generation agents such as loratadine or cetirizine.

Mechanism of Action

Antihistamines are drugs that exert their effect in the body primarily by blocking the actions of histamine at receptor sites. They are classified as pharmacologic antagonists of histamine. They do not prevent histamine release, but act by competitive inhibition. Most antihistamines can be classified as either H_1-receptor blockers, which block the smooth muscle response, or H_2-receptor blockers, which block the histaminic stimulation of gastric acid. If the concentration of antihistamine drug at the receptor site exceeds the concentration of histamine, then the effects of histamine are blocked. Antihistamines usually ameliorate itching, sneezing, ocular symptoms, and nasal discharge but do not always reduce nasal congestion.

Dosage

The dosage varies depending on the age and weight of the patients. Further, the frequency of dosing is typically every 4 to 6 hours as needed, but can be upwards of every 12 hours depending on the half-life of the drug as well as the formulation. For example, diphenhydramine (Benadryl) is given every 4 to 6 hours but carbinoxamine is dosed every 12 hours. These are often over-the-counter agents and are supplied as tablets, capsules, elixirs, or suspensions. Further, these formulations come in a variety of flavors, and some are even free of dye.

Time Frame for Response

The onset of action of these agents typically ranges from 15 to 30 minutes and lasts nearly as long as the dosing interval. Those agents with a longer half-life will take longer to get to steady state, but the initial effect is often seen fairly rapidly.

Some regular users of antihistamines find that tolerance, or drug failure, develops after several weeks or months. One reason for this decreased effectiveness is that some antihistamines are capable of hepatic enzyme induction, resulting in increased metabolism in the liver.

Essentially, the antihistamine drug hastens its own destruction and removal from circulation. The various antihistamine classes differ in their capacity to induce hepatic enzymes. Some practitioners have found that if tolerance develops, patients may benefit by switching to another antihistamine in a different chemical category. The effectiveness of this technique has not been evaluated by controlled studies.

Contraindications

Antihistamine therapy is contraindicated in lactating mothers. Additionally, the anticholinergic side effects of the first-generation antihistamines put patients with narrow-angle glaucoma at risk for an increase in intraocular pressure. Similarly, men with benign prostatic hyperplasia (BPH) should avoid these agents due the drug's ability to decrease urine flow. The sedating effects of these agents should also be considered when patients are required to perform hazardous tasks or drive.

Adverse Events

Knowledge of the chemical category to which an antihistamine belongs can help determine the relative degree of sedation and anticholinergic effects associated with the particular agent. In general, the ethanolamine derivatives, such as diphenhydramine (Benadryl), and the phenothiazine derivatives, such as promethazine (Phenergan), cause the greatest degree of sedation and anticholinergic effects. The most problematic anticholinergic effects are dry mouth, blurred vision, urinary hesitancy, constipation, confusion, and mental cloudiness.

The sedative effects of the older antihistamines vary among patients and may not cause problems for some. Tolerance to the sedative effect develops, and many patients find that sedation either disappears or becomes less bothersome after several days of continued use. Nonetheless, sedation may affect the patient's acceptance of the older antihistamine drugs.

Less Sedating Antihistamines

More recently, antihistamines have been developed that do not cross the blood–brain barrier to the extent exhibited by the older agents. These newer antihistamines, commonly referred to as *nonsedating antihistamines (NSAs)*, are considered to act peripherally and do not produce sedation or cause clinically important changes in mental status. In general, the anticholinergic effects of these agents are also minimal. The NSAs are listed and compared in Table 51-3.

Dosage

Loratadine (Claritin) is dosed as 10 mg once daily for adults and children 6 years and older. For children aged 2 to 5 years, the dose is 5 mg once daily. Cetirizine (Zyrtec) is given 5 to 10 mg once daily for children older than 6 years and adults. The lower dosage can be used for younger children or for patients with less severe symptoms. Children 2 to 5 years of age should be started on 2.5 mg once daily. Fexofenadine (Allegra) doses are for adults and children 12 and older, the starting dose is 60 mg twice daily or 180 mg once daily for the extended-release formulation. Children 6 to 11 years old should start at 30 mg twice a day.

Time Frame for Response

This class of agents has a rapid onset of action, with a time to maximum effect ranging from 1 to 2.5 hours. The half-life of these drugs is 8 to 28 hours, leading to a 1- to 3-day delay in reaching a steady state. Food can delay the absorption of cetirizine and loratadine, but not fexofenadine.

Contraindications

The contraindications to these agents are similar to the first-generation agents, but the lower propensity for anticholinergic

Table 51.3

Overview of Selected Antihistamines and Decongestants

Generic (Trade) Name and Dosage	Selected Adverse Events	Contraindications	Special Considerations
Nonsedating Antihistamines			
certirizine (Zyrtec) 5–10 mg PO qd Children 6–11 y: 5–10 mg qd	Somnolence, dry mouth, pharyngitis, dizziness	Known hypersensitivity to certirizine or hydroxyzine	Renal or hepatic impairment: Adults—5 mg qd; Children—not recommended Pregnancy category B
fexofenadine (Allegra) 60 mg PO bid 180 mg tablet PO qd	Viral infection (cold, influenza), nausea, dysmenorrhea, drowsiness, dyspepsia, fatigue	Known hypersensitivity to any of its ingredients	Not recommended in children <12 y Erythromycin and ketoconazole may increase plasma levels of fexofenadine. Pregnancy category C
loratadine (Claritin) 10 mg PO qd Children 6–11 y: 5 mg qd	Headache, somnolence, fatigue, dry mouth	Known hypersensitivity to any of its ingredients	Pregnancy category B
loratadine, 5 mg, pseudoephedrine, 120 mg (Claritin-D 12 Hour) One tablet PO bid, q12h	Headache, insomnia, dry mouth, somnolence, nervousness, dizziness, fatigue, dyspepsia, nausea, pharyngitis, anorexia, thirst		Not recommended in children <12 y Pregnancy category B
loratadine 10 mg, pseudoephedrine, 240 mg (Claritin-D 24 Hour) One tablet PO qd	Same as above		Same as above
Intranasal Antihistamines			
azelastine (Astelin Nasal Spray) Two sprays in each nostril bid; 100 doses per bottle, 2 bottles per package	Bitter taste, headache, somnolence, nasal burning, pharyngitis, dry mouth, paroxysmal sneezing, nausea, rhinitis, fatigue, dizziness	Known hypersensitivity	Amount of drug per actuation (spray): 137 mcg Supplied as two bottles of drug and one separate metered-dose spray pump per package. Not recommended in children 6–12 y
Oral Nasal Decongestants			
pseudoephedrine 60 mg q6h (240 mg); extended release, 120 mg q12h Children 6–12 y: 30 mg q6h (120 mg) Children 2–6 y: 15 mg q6h (60 mg)	Headache, insomnia, dry mouth, somnolence, nervousness, dizziness, fatigue, dyspepsia, nausea, pharyngitis, anorexia, thirst	Same as Claritin-D	
Topical Nasal Decongestants			
Systemic effects are unlikely from topical use, but use with caution in the conditions listed for oral agents. Adverse events are more likely with excessive use, in older adults, and in children.			
Intranasal Cromolyn			
cromolyn (Nasalcrom Nasal Solution) Patients >6 y: one spray in each nostril 3–6 times a day until symptom relief, then every 8–12 h	Common: burning, stinging, or irritation inside nose, increase in sneezing Rare: cough, headache, unpleasant taste, bloody nose		Comes in 13-mL bottle and 26-mL bottle—13-mL bottle = 100 sprays, 26-mL bottle = 200 sprays Not recommended in children <6 y

effects allows for wider use in the elderly, patients with glaucoma, and men with BPH.

Adverse Events

Common adverse events for this class of agents include headache, dyspepsia, nausea, and fatigue. Pharyngitis and dry mouth can also occur. More disturbing side effects include dizziness, myalgia, somnolence, and dysmenorrhea.

Interactions

To date, the nonsedating antihistamine loratadine (Claritin) and the miscellaneous antihistamine cetirizine (Zyrtec) do not carry the drug interaction warnings relating to erythromycin, ketoconazole, and itraconazole. Cetirizine, a metabolite of the antipruritic hydroxyzine (Atarax), has not been generally accepted as an NSA because it is reported to have a higher incidence of sedation than the other newer antihistamines. Nonetheless, it is an effective antihistamine approved by the U.S. Food and Drug Administration (FDA) for both seasonal and perennial rhinitis.

Antacids and grapefruit juice administered with Allegra may decrease absorption of Allegra. Zyrtec administered with sedating drugs may increase sedation.

Intranasal Antihistamines

Azelastine (Astelin), an intranasal antihistamine, is also available to treat allergic rhinitis. In placebo-controlled trials, it significantly improved the symptoms of rhinorrhea, sneezing, and nasal pruritus. The adverse events that occurred more frequently than in the patients treated with placebos were bitter taste (19.7% versus 0.6% for placebo) and somnolence (11.5% versus 5.4%). Prescribing information is noted in Table 51-3.

Nasal Decongestants

Mechanism of Action

Nasal decongestants are sympathomimetic amines chemically related to norepinephrine, a major neurotransmitter of the sympathetic nervous system. These drugs are vasoconstrictors. They offer relief from nasal congestion by constricting the blood vessels of the nasal mucosa that have been dilated by histamine. The results are a shrinking of swollen nasal passages and more air movement to make breathing easier. But, just as norepinephrine is a CNS stimulant, so are the synthetic oral and topical (nasal) decongestants.

Dosage

Fixed combination products containing antihistamines and sympathomimetic amines are convenient, but the effective dose of oral decongestants varies among patients. If use of a fixed combination causes side effects or does not relieve symptoms, then clinicians should titrate with single agents to achieve the required dosage.

Time Frame for Response

The onset of action for these agents, in immediate release form, is typically 15 to 30 minutes with a peak response within 30 to 60 minutes. The half-life of pseudoephedrine is 9 to 16 hours, but the effect of the decongestant activity wears off within 4 to 6 hours after administration.

Contraindications

Caution should be used when recommending over-the-counter oral decongestants. Patients with high blood pressure, heart disease, hyperthyroidism, narrow-angle glaucoma, and BPH may see exacerbation of their disease. In addition, use of oral decongestants is contraindicated in patients taking monoamine oxidase inhibitors (MAOIs). Pseudoephedrine causes the release of norepinephrine into the synapse and MAOIs inhibit the enzymatic degradation of norepinephrine. As such, the concomitant use of these agents increases the sympathetic activity of the nervous system and can lead to hypertensive crisis.

Adverse Events

Oral decongestants constrict blood vessels throughout the body and also act as CNS stimulants, thus increasing blood pressure and heart rate and causing palpitations. Stimulation of the CNS can lead to insomnia, irritability, restlessness, and headache. Many patients find that they can use oral decongestants only during the daytime because the stimulatory effects of these drugs can cause nervousness, agitation, and insomnia.

Products that contain the full and appropriate FDA-recommended dosage should be prescribed. For example, Dristan Advanced Formula contains the following in each tablet: phenylephrine 5 mg, chlorpheniramine 2 mg, acetaminophen 325 mg, and caffeine 16.2 mg. One tablet every 4 hours probably is not an adequate dose for an adult because the amounts of phenylephrine and chlorpheniramine are only one half the recommended adult dose.

Topical (Intranasal) Decongestants

Intranasal application (sprays or drops) of sympathomimetic amines provides a prompt and dramatic decrease of nasal congestion. A rebound phenomenon (rhinitis medicamentosa), however, often follows topical application of these drugs. In this scenario, the nasal mucous membrane becomes even more congested and edematous as the drug's vasoconstrictor effect wears off. This secondary congestion is believed to result from ischemia caused by the drug's intensive local vasoconstriction and local irritation of the agent itself. If the use of a topical decongestant is limited to 3 or 4 days, rebound congestion is minimal. With chronic use or overuse of these drugs, rebound nasal stuffiness may become quite pronounced. This phenomenon may begin a vicious cycle, leading to more frequent use of the drug that causes the problem. Should this occur, patients should discontinue topical decongestant therapy. They may use an oral decongestant, isotonic saline drops or spray, or both instead (Table 51-4). Side effects from topically administered agents include local irritation and rebound congestion.

Intranasal Corticosteroids

Nasal-inhaled corticosteroids are effective forms of therapy for allergic rhinitis. They help to relieve congestion and rhinorrhea by limiting the late-phase response and reducing inflammation. Corticosteroids have a wide range of inhibitory activities against multiple cell types (eg, mast cells, eosinophils, neutrophils, macrophages, and lymphocytes) and mediators of inflammation (eg, histamine, eicosanoids, leukotrienes, and cytokines).

Mechanism of Action

Corticosteroids exert their anti-inflammatory effect by disabling the cells that present antigen to antibody. Interfering with the antigen–antibody reaction reduces the stimulus for mast cell degranulation. With reduced mast cell degranulation, secretion of cytokines is diminished. The result is a weaker inflammatory reaction with milder or no symptoms of runny nose, nasal congestion, itching, and sneezing.

Table 51.4

Topical Nasal Decongestants

Generic	Trade	Concentration (%)	Patient Age			
			>6 mo	2–6 y	6–12 y	>12 y
phenylephrine	Neo-Synephrine	0.125	Yes	Yes	Yes	Yes
	Neo-Synephrine	0.25	No	No	Yes	Yes
	Neo-Synephrine	0.5	No	No	No	Yes
naphazoline	Privine	0.05	No	No	No	Yes
oxymetazoline	Afrin	0.025	No	Yes	Yes	Yes
	Children's Afrin	0.05	No	Yes	Yes	Yes
tetrahydrozoline	Tyzine Pediatric	0.05	No	Yes	Yes	Yes
	Tyzine	0.1	No	No	Yes	Yes
xylometazoline	Otrivin Pediatric	0.05	No	Yes	Yes	Yes
	Otrivin	0.1	No	No	Yes	Yes

Dosage

The dosage of the individual intranasal steroids is listed in Table 51-5. There are published differences in potency among the available agents. In general, mometasone furoate, fluticasone propionate, and budesonide have been rated as most potent, in vitro. However, the impact of this difference in potency has not been clinically established.

Time Frame for Response

The therapeutic effects of intranasal corticosteroids are not immediate. Clinicians must counsel patients that they may not experience maximal effects for 1 to 2 weeks. If nasal blockage is severe, patients should use a topical nasal decongestant for the first 2 to 3 days to reduce the swelling and increase the delivery of corticosteroid to the nasal mucosa. Use of nasal corticosteroids should not continue beyond 3 weeks in the absence of significant symptomatic improvement, according to the manufacturers' professional product information.

Contraindications

All intranasal corticosteroids are designated as pregnancy category C. This means that either animal reproduction studies have shown adverse effects on the fetus and there are no controlled studies in women, or there are no studies in women or animals. The drug should be given only if potential benefit justifies potential risk.

Adverse Events

The first intranasal corticosteroid, dexamethasone (Dexacort), was introduced in 1968. This drug is effective in treating

Table 51.5

Intranasal Corticosteroid Prescribing Information

Drug	Generic Name (Manufacturer)	Amount of Drug per Spray/Doses per Bottle or Canister	How Supplied	Suggested Dose	
				Adult	Pediatric (6–12 y)
Vancenase AQ	beclomethasone (Schering)	84 μg/120	19-g bottle with nasal spray pump	One or 2 inhalations per nostril qd	Same as adult
Vancenase Pockethaler	beclomethasone (Schering)	42 μg/200	7-g aerosol canister	One or 2 inhalations per nostril bid–qid	One inhalation in each nostril tid
Beconase AQ	beclomethasone (Glaxo SmithKline)	42 μg/200	25-g amber glass bottle with nasal spray pump	One or 2 inhalations in each nostril bid	Same as adult
Beconase Inhaler	beclomethasone (Glaxo SmithKline)	42 μg/200 aerosol canister	6.7-g and 16.8-g nostril bid–qid	One inhalation per each nostril tid	One inhalation in
Rhinocort Nasal Inhaler	budesonide (Astra)	32 μg/200	7-g aerosol canister	Four sprays in each nostril qd	Same as adult
Flonase Nasal Spray	fluticasone (Glaxo SmithKline)	50 μg/120	16-g bottle with spray pump	Two sprays in each nostril qd	Not recommended
Nasacort Nasal Inhaler	triamcinolone (Aventis)	55 μg/100	10-g aerosol canister	One spray up to 4 sprays in each nostril qd	One spray up to 2 sprays in each nostril qd
Nasarel or Nasalide Nasal Solution	flunisolide (Dura)	25 μg/200	25-mL bottle with spray pump	Two sprays in each nostril bid	Same as adult

Table 51.6

Common Adverse Events With Beclomethasone Intranasal Corticosteroid Products Based on Delivery System

Beclomethasone AQ Nasal Spray*		Beclomethasone Nasal Inhaler†	
Incidence above placebo		*Percentage of patients*	
Pharyngitis	6%	Irritation/burning	11%
Pain	3%	Sneezing	10%
Headache	2%	Rhinorrhea	1%
Nasal burning	2%	Epistaxis	2%
Tinnitus	2%		
Conjunctivitis	1%		
Coughing	1%		
Epistaxis	1%		
Myalgia	1%		

*Vancenase AQ, Beconase AQ.
†Vancenase Nasal Inhaler, Beconase Nasal Inhaler.

allergic rhinitis, but significant systemic absorption limits its use in long-term therapy. For that reason, it has not been included among the available intranasal corticosteroid preparations listed in Table 51-5. These preparations differ primarily with regard to their delivery systems. Triamcinolone (Nasacort) and budesonide (Rhinocort) are metered-dose aerosols manufactured with chlorofluorocarbons (CFCs), which is the propellant under pressure. The remaining products do not contain propellants under pressure. They are supplied as aqueous solutions in manually activated metered-dose nasal spray pumps, with separate patient instructions for use with every package. Although all the intranasal corticosteroids have some adverse effects, patients usually prefer the aqueous solutions because they cause less nasal irritation. Some of these formulations have a flowery odor that some patients may find annoying.

Probably the most disconcerting adverse effect of intranasal steroids is their potential for decreasing the rate of growth. The impact of this on final adult height is not known, but some short-term and long-term studies indicate that the impact on growth rate occurs primarily in the first year of use and may only have an overall reduction of about 1 cm.

Table 51-6 compares beclomethasone aqueous solution (Beconase AQ) with beclomethasone pressurized canister (Beconase Inhaler) for adverse effects to illustrate the differences between each system. All aqueous preparations contain preservatives. Benzalkonium chloride is the preservative in the beclomethasone, flunisolide, fluticasone, mometasone, and triamcinolone products, whereas budesonide contains potassium sorbate as the preservative.

Interactions

Other considerations in selecting an intranasal corticosteroid are that products under pressure can burst if punctured or exposed to temperatures above 120°F, and the U.S. Environmental Protection Agency requires warnings on these packages that CFCs harm the environment by destroying ozone in the upper atmosphere. Intranasal corticosteroid drug products that are offered in manual spray pumps must be primed before initial use. Clinicians should counsel patients to squeeze the pump a number of times until a fine spray appears. If patients do not use the pump for more than 1 week, they should reprime it.

Intranasal Cromolyn

Cromolyn is classified as a mast cell stabilizer. It prevents antigen-induced degranulation, thereby inhibiting the release of histamine and other cytokines that mediate inflammatory cell function. Cromolyn is of no value in treating acute allergic rhinitis. It is helpful only in preventing (prophylaxis) the nasal symptoms of allergic rhinitis. Treatment is more effective if it begins 2 to 4 weeks before exposure and continues throughout the exposure period. Intranasal cromolyn is available to patients as Nasalcrom 4% Nasal Solution. It does not require a prescription. Patient use information is noted in Table 51-3.

Selecting the Most Appropriate Agent

Nasal symptoms of allergic rhinitis include watery rhinorrhea (runny nose), paroxysmal sneezing (sudden fits of sneezing), nasal congestion (stuffy nose, sinus headache, or both), and postnasal drip that may cause coughing. Allergic rhinitis also may involve the conjunctiva (allergic conjunctivitis). The resulting symptoms are ocular pruritus (itching eyes), lacrimation (watery eyes), conjunctival hyperemia (bloodshot eyes), and chemosis (swollen eyelids). Drug treatment must be tailored to address the most bothersome

---

BOX 51–2. A STEPWISE APPROACH IS USED TO MANAGE THE SYMPTOMS OF ALLERGIC RHINITIS

1. Identify the offending allergens by history with confirmation of the allergy by skin test.
2. Teach the patient to avoid the offending allergens.
3. For mild symptoms, prophylactic treatment with cromolyn nasal spray (Nasalcrom) or treatment with an antihistamine/decongestant combination may be necessary. If unacceptable drowsiness occurs, switch to a nonsedating antihistamine.
4. For prominent symptoms, add topical corticosteroid nasal spray.
5. For treatment failures despite avoidance and pharmacotherapy, progress to immunotherapy.

Table 51.7

Recommended Order of Treatment for Allergies

Order	Agents	Comments
First line	Intranasal corticosteroids	Intranasal corticosteroids are the most potent agents available for relief of established seasonal or perennial rhinitis.
Second line	Antihistamines/Nasal decongestants	Either first- or second-generation agent can be used. Product selection is based on dosing frequency, potential for adverse effects, and cost. Second-generation antihistamines may be given only once or twice a day, and they are relatively nonsedating. First-generation antihistamines are given 3–4 times a day.
Third line	Intranasal cromolyn	Must be used prophylactically. Pseudoephedrine and phenylpropanolamine are the most popular oral nasal decongestants.

symptoms. See Box 51-2 and Figure 51-3 for a stepwise approach to treating allergic rhinitis. Table 51-7 lists the recommended treatment order for allergies.

First-Line Therapy

Intranasal corticosteroids are the most potent agents available for relief of *established* seasonal or perennial rhinitis. They provide efficacy with substantially reduced side effects compared with oral corticosteroids. Selection of the best agent depends on the patient's insurance formulary as well as the dosage form. Typically, aqueous formulations are better tolerated than nonaqueous formulations.

However, due to the long time frame for response, these agents are often given in combination with antihistamines. First-generation antihistamines were considered first-line agents for the prevention and treatment of allergic symptoms. However, the sedative side effects of the traditional antihistamines limit their usefulness in patients who must remain awake and alert. Fortunately, the NSAs, also known as newer or second-generation antihistamines, cause minimal sedation because they do not cross the blood–brain barrier into the CNS.

The various first- and second-generation antihistamines are equally effective in treating symptoms of allergic rhinitis. Product selection is based on dosing frequency (ie, duration of action), potential for adverse effects, and cost. Second-generation antihistamines may be given only once or twice a day, and they are relatively nonsedating. First-generation antihistamines are given 3 to 4 times a day. Some products are available in long-acting dosage forms that may be given only twice a day. Whether short acting or long acting, the first-generation antihistamines are more sedating than the second-generation drugs. First-generation antihistamines are also significantly less expensive than the second-generation drugs. These agents have the best results when patients take them before exposure to a known allergen. During seasonal attack, patients may need to take antihistamines around-the-clock for maximal effectiveness.

Second-Line Therapy

Because antihistamines do not reduce nasal congestion, they are often used in combination with nasal decongestants. Pseudoephedrine and phenylpropanolamine are the most popular oral nasal decongestants. Nasal decongestants are α-adrenergic receptor agonists. As such, they stimulate α-adrenergic receptors, causing vasoconstriction in the nasal mucosa, decreasing congestion, and opening nasal passages.

Side effects include CNS and cardiovascular stimulation. Elevation in blood pressure may also occur. Many prescription and nonprescription drugs contain a combined antihistamine and nasal decongestant. Some examples are given in Table 51-3.

Topical (intranasal) decongestants avoid systemic adverse effects. Prolonged use leads to rebound nasal congestion, however, so they are impractical for seasonal or perennial allergies. Their use should be limited to short periods (a few days).

Third-Line Therapy

Cromolyn, in the form of a metered-dose nasal spray, could be considered a first-line treatment for allergic rhinitis, but it is a prophylactic measure only. It is classified as a mast cell stabilizer in that it prevents or attenuates the allergen activation of nasal mast cells. To be efficacious, cromolyn must be administered continuously (usually 4 times a day) during seasonal allergen exposure or immediately before an anticipated exposure such as animal dander.

Intranasal cromolyn is an alternative to antihistamines and nasal decongestants for allergic rhinitis. It generally is considered less effective than intranasal corticosteroids, but it is virtually free of side effects.

Special Population Considerations
Pediatric

If one parent has allergies, the child has a 50% chance of having allergies. Allergies may also be more common in children who were formula fed, of low birth weight, or exposed to dogs, cats, or tobacco smoke early in life. In childhood, more boys have allergic rhinitis than do girls, but this difference begins to disappear after adolescence. No sex differences are found in adults.

To determine the dose of allergy medication for a child, practitioners should use weight if possible. Otherwise, they may base according to age. The official product literature usually provides child dosage recommendations by age and weight. For example, Children's Tylenol ALLERGY-D Liquid provides the following information in the *Physicians' Desk Reference* (PDR; Medical Economics Company, 2004):

If possible, use weight to dose; otherwise use age.
All doses may be repeated every 4 to 6 hours, if needed:
    4 to 11 months (12–17 pounds): 1/2 teaspoonful
    12 to 23 months (18–23 pounds): 3/4 teaspoonful
    2 to 3 years (24–35 pounds): 1 teaspoonful
    4 to 5 years (36–47 pounds): 1 1/2 teaspoonfuls

6 to 8 years (48–59 pounds): 2 teaspoonfuls
9 to 10 years (60–71 pounds): 2 1/2 teaspoonfuls
11 years (72–95 pounds): 3 teaspoonfuls

In determining the dose of medication for a child, practitioners must recognize that infants and small children are not merely "scaled-down" adults. Organs such as the GI tract, liver, and kidneys are not developed enough in children for them to handle medications. Estimating a child's dose based on the adult dose is not always safe. Most pharmaceutical manufacturers do not provide such comprehensive pediatric dosing guidelines. Usually, an age range for children's doses is stated in the official package insert or on the commercial package. If not, prescribers should contact the manufacturer or consult with a specialist who is experienced with the treatment. The PDR contains a Manufacturers' Index of addresses and telephone numbers.

As noted earlier, a major consideration in prescribing intranasal steroids in children is the impact on growth. The FDA has approved the use of mometasone for children older than 2 years of age and fluticasone for children older than 4 years. The other agents are approved for use in children older than 6 years of age.

Geriatric

Although few factors provoke rhinitis in older adults, treatments need to be more tailored because of slower metabolism and the potential for side effects. Also, this population is more likely to be taking multiple medications, and therefore runs a greater risk of drug interactions than most other patients.

Women

In women, allergic rhinitis symptoms may worsen during pregnancy. The antihistamines diphenhydramine, loratadine, and cetirizine are pregnancy category B agents, whereas desloratadine and fexofenadine are category C agents. All intranasal steroids are category C agents.

MONITORING PATIENT RESPONSE

Assessing the efficacy of treatment requires monitoring the patient's adherence to the drug therapy plan, quality of life, and degree of satisfaction with the care provided. Box 51-3 could be a useful office tool for this purpose.

BOX 51–3. QUESTIONS TO ASK THE ALLERGY PATIENT AT EVERY OFFICE VISIT

Monitoring Signs, Symptoms, and Functional Status
- Has your allergy been better or worse since your last visit?
  In the past 2 weeks, how many days have you had:
  (*Ask the patient to tell you how symptoms developed, what they were like, and how long they lasted.*)
    A runny, stuffy or itchy nose?
    Any wheezing or coughing?
    Any hives or swelling?
    Eczema or other skin rashes?
    Reactions to foods?
    Reactions to insects?
- Since your last visit, how many days has your allergy caused you to:
    Miss work or school?
    Reduce your activities?
    (For caregivers) change your activity because of your child's allergies?
- Since your last visit, have you had any unscheduled or emergency department visits or hospital stays?
- Since your last visit, have you had any times when your allergy symptoms were a lot worse than usual?
    If yes, what do you think caused the symptoms to get worse?
    If yes, what did you do to control the symptoms?
- Have there been any changes in your home, school, or work environment (eg, new smokers or pets)? Any new hobbies or recreational activities?

- Has there been difficulty sleeping at night due to symptoms of allergy?

Monitoring Pharmacotherapy
- What medications are you taking?
- How often do you take each medication? How much do you take each time?
- Have you had any unusual reactions to your medications?
- Have you missed or stopped taking any regular doses of your medications for any reason?
- Have you had trouble filling your prescriptions (eg, for financial reasons, not on formulary)?
- Have you tried any other medications?
- Has your allergy medicine caused you any problems (eg, sleepiness, bad taste, sore throat)?
- Have you had any night time awakenings?

Monitoring Patient–Provider Communication and Patient Satisfaction
- What questions do you have about your allergy management?
- What problems have you had in following your allergy management plan, such as taking your medications or reducing your exposure to allergens?
- Has anything prevented you from getting the treatment you need for your allergies?
- Have the costs of your allergy treatment interfered with your ability to get appropriate care?
- How can we improve your allergy care?

This information is provided by the Asthma and Allergy Foundation of America (AAFA) as part of its educational outreach to patients and their caregivers. The information was adapted from the 1997 National Asthma Education and Prevention Program's Guidelines for the Diagnosis and Treatment of Asthma published by the National Heart, Lung, and Blood Institute.

PATIENT EDUCATION

Patient education is extremely important in the prevention and management of allergy symptoms. Teaching each patient about the causes of allergic reactions, how triggers evoke symptoms, the various medications available and their use, when to self-treat and when to seek medical help, and how to assess whether treatment is working is highly desirable and appropriate during an office visit. But comprehensive teaching may not be practical because of time constraints. It may be more efficient to determine what the patient *does not* understand and fill in the gaps at that time. For example, at the end of the visit, practitioners could ask the patient three very basic questions about treatment:

- What is the name of the medication you are taking for allergy symptoms?
- What beneficial effects do you expect, and what side effects may occur?
- How do you take the medication (ie, dose, time of day, with meals, and what to avoid taking with it)?

If the patient can articulate the correct answers to these questions, little more needs to be discussed about treatment. Practitioners could provide verbally or in writing those things that the patient does not know or understand. Also, they should encourage patients to accept written materials that pharmacists provide when they fill prescriptions and to question any ambiguous or contradictory information.

Drug Information

A variety of sources provide information regarding the treatment of allergic rhinitis. The American Association of Allergies, Asthma, and Immunology provides practice parameters for the treatment of allergic rhinitis (www.aaaai.org). Further, the FDA provides drug information specific to the product, particularly in relation to children or pregnant women.

Patient-Oriented Information Sources

The American Association of Allergies, Asthma, and Immunology provides patient-directed information (http://www.aaaai.org/patients/resources/fastfacts/rhinitis.stm). Similarly, the FDA has information regarding medications in an easy to use format for patients.

Complementary and Alternative Medications

There is some suggestion that acupuncture and biofeedback may be effective means of treating allergic rhinitis. However, controlled studies evaluating the effectiveness of these treatment modalities are lacking. Further, although few studies have examined the effectiveness of specific homeopathic therapies, ephedra (now banned by the FDA) as well as *nux vomica* have been used to help in the treatment of nasal congestion and discharge.

ALLERGIC CONJUNCTIVITIS

The signs and symptoms of allergic conjunctivitis result from the same allergens that cause allergic rhinitis. Mast cells are abundant in the eyelid and conjunctiva, but are infrequently found in the eye. This limits allergic ocular inflammation to the lining of the eyelid and the ocular surface (the conjunctiva).

Histamine and arachidonic acid derivatives are the mediators that probably cause most ocular signs and symptoms. Mast cell activation, however, also leads to recruitment of eosinophils, which can be found in the conjunctiva 3 to 5 hours after mast cell degranulation.

Many patients experience ocular symptoms only when allergens directly contact the eyes. For example, patients with sensitivity to cat dander may not have reactions in a room with cats but experience symptoms if they bring their hands to their face. Patients who have symptoms even without direct contact need to be particularly rigorous in their

Table 51.8

Selected Ophthalmic Drugs for Allergic Conjunctivitis by Drug Class

Class	Generic (Trade) Name	Strength (Potency)	How Supplied	Dose
Corticosteroid	prednisolone (Pred-Mild)	$1/8$% (0.12%)	5- and 10-mL ophthalmic suspension	One drop in each affected eye tid–qid
Antihistamine	levocabastine (Livostin)	0.05%	2.5-, 5-, and 10-mL ophthalmic suspension	One drop in each affected eye qid
Antihistamine	emedastine (Emadine)	0.05%	5-mL ophthalmic solution	One drop in each affected eye qid
Antihistamine	olopatadine (Patanol)	0.1%	5-mL ophthalmic solution	One to 2 drops in each affected eye bid at 6- to 8-h intervals
Mast cell stabilizer	lodoxamide (Alomide)	0.1%	10-mL ophthalmic solution	One to 2 drops in each affected eye qid up to 3 mo
Mast cell stabilizer	cromolyn (Crolom)	4%	10-mL ophthalmic solution	One to 2 drops in each affected eye 4–6 times a day at regular intervals
NSAID	ketorolac (Acular)	0.5%	3-, 5-, 10-mL ophthalmic solution	One drop in each affected eye qid

efforts to eliminate or avoid allergens in their homes, workplaces, or school. Eye rubbing not only introduces allergens into the eye but may degranulate mast cells mechanically.

Practitioners should encourage patients to apply cool compresses to their eyelids rather than rubbing their eyes to alleviate symptoms. Artificial tears also may reduce symptoms and wash away allergens and inflammatory mediators from the conjunctiva. Often, however, these approaches are inadequate. In such cases, patients require pharmacologic intervention. The types of eye drop medications used to treat allergic conjunctivitis are corticosteroids, antihistamines, vasoconstrictor/antihistamine combinations, mast cell stabilizers, and nonsteroidal anti-inflammatory drugs (NSAIDs).

Topical corticosteroids are effective, but the use of these drugs is limited because they can induce cataracts and glaucoma. If topical corticosteroids are required, a lower-potency agent is preferred. Primary care practitioners should refer any patient who requires topical corticosteroids for more than 2 weeks to an ophthalmologist.

Oral antihistamines, which can help reduce ocular itching, may cause more problems by decreasing tear production. The NSAIDs provide temporary relief of ocular itching due to seasonal allergic conjunctivitis. They work by inhibiting biosynthesis of prostaglandin, a mediator of pain and inflammation. Prescribing information for the ophthalmic drops used to treat allergic conjunctivitis is noted in Table 51-8.

■ Case Study

G.B., an 18-year-old African American female college student, lives on campus with three other students. Her home is approximately 100 miles away. She has been at college since the beginning of the fall semester, approximately 2 weeks. She presents today with a chief complaint of fits of sneezing (sometimes 10 in a row); a runny, itchy, stuffy nose; and red, tearing eyes. Her temperature is 99°F; blood pressure is 118/78. She denies cough and headache. Her chest is clear. Her past medical history is unremarkable, except for "hay fever" when she was younger, which she "outgrew" during high school. These symptoms are the same. She is having difficulty studying because of the sneezing and itching nose, and she is embarrassed to be in class with these symptoms. She was nervous about meeting the challenges of college and making new friends. Her local physician prescribed lorazepam (Ativan) 1.0 mg as needed for stress, anxiety, or both. So far, she has taken two doses of a prescription for 30 tablets.

Diagnosis: allergic rhinitis/conjunctivitis

→ 1. List two specific goals of treatment of G.B.

→ 2. What would be your first class of agents to prescribe? Why? Within that class, which agent would you choose?

→ 3. What over-the-counter and/or alternative medications would be appropriate for G.B.?

→ 4. How would you monitor for the success of your selected treatment?

→ 5. What adverse events would you monitor for and what would you do if they occurred?

→ 6. Describe one or two drug–drug or drug–food interactions for the selected agent.

→ 7. What aspects of the drug would you emphasize in your patient education discussion with G.B.?

→ 8. What would you do if your first-line therapy was ineffective?

→ 9. What dietary and lifestyle changes should be recommended for G.B.?

→ 10. What would be the choice for the second-line therapy?

Bibliography

Starred references are cited in the text.

Conner S. J. (2002). Evaluation and treatment of the patient with allergic rhinitis. *Journal of Family Practice, 51*, 883–890.

Dykewicz, M. S., Fineman S., Nicklas R., et al. (1998). Joint Task Force Algorithm and Annotations for Diagnosis and Management of Rhinitis. *Annals of Allergy, Asthma & Immunology, 81*, 469–473.

Gendo K., & Larson E. B., (2004). Evidence-based diagnostic strategies for evaluating suspected allergic rhinitis. *Annals of Internal Medicine, 140*, 278–289.

Lichtenstein, L., & Fauci, A. (1996). *Current therapy in allergy, immunology, and rheumatology* (5th ed.). St. Louis: Mosby-Year Book.

*Medical Economics Company. (2004). *Physicians desk reference* (54th ed., p. 1675). Montvale, NJ: Author.

Middleton, E., Reed, C., Ellis, E., et al. (Eds.). (1998). *Allergy: Principles and practice* (5th ed., Vols. I and II). St. Louis: Mosby-Year Book.

National Institute of Allergy and Infectious Disease. (1997). *Disease state management sourcebook.* New York: Faulkner and Gray.

Patterson, R., Grammar, L., & Greenberg, P. (1997). *Allergic diseases: Diagnosis and management* (5th ed.). Philadelphia: Lippincott-Raven.

Wingard, L., Brody, T., Larner, J., et al. (1991). *Human pharmacology: Molecular to clinical.* St. Louis: Mosby-Year Book.

Yanez A., Rodrigo G. J., (2002) Intranasal corticosteroids versus topical H_1 receptor antagonists for the treatment of allergic rhinitis: a systematic review with meta-analysis. *Annals of Allergy, Asthma & Immunology, 89,* 479–484.

Visit the Connection web site for the most up-to-date drug information.

52

HUMAN IMMUNODEFICIENCY VIRUS

■ LINDA M. SPOONER

The first known case of human immunodeficiency virus (HIV) infection was documented in 1959 in a man from Kinshasha, Congo. How he became infected with the virus is unknown. Furthermore, how the disease grew to epidemic proportions also is unclear. In the United States, HIV infection was first recognized in 1981 after it was discovered that young homosexual men were contracting unusual cases of pneumonia and rare cancers that typically were not seen in immunocompetent patients.

HIV is the virus that causes acquired immunodeficiency syndrome (AIDS). A diagnosis of AIDS is based on the presence of an AIDS-defining condition (Box 52-1) or a $CD4^+$ T-cell count of less than 200/mm^3 (Centers for Disease Control and Prevention [CDC], 1992). Although rates of progression from HIV infection to AIDS vary greatly among individuals, the median is approximately 10 years in patients not receiving antiretroviral medications.

The two types of HIV that have been identified are HIV-1 and HIV-2. HIV-1 accounts for the majority of cases worldwide, whereas HIV-2 is primarily found in West Africa. HIV-2 is less efficiently transmitted and results in a slower disease progression than HIV-1. According to the CDC, there have been fewer than 100 cases of HIV-2 diagnosed in the United States, with the majority of cases originating from West Africa (CDC, 1995). Unfortunately, there are few data concerning the efficacy of antiretroviral medications for treatment of HIV-2 infection, although it is assumed that antiretroviral medications should be effective for either type of HIV.

Over the past two decades, HIV infection has reached epidemic proportions. The World Health Organization (WHO) estimates that 42 million people worldwide are infected with HIV, with over half the cases occurring in sub-Saharan Africa (WHO, 2004). Of these, 3.2 million children under the age of 15 are infected. In 2002, 5 million people were newly infected with HIV, and there were 3.1 million deaths attributed to HIV throughout the world. Explanations for these overwhelming numbers include limited access to health care and antiretroviral medications as well as lack of education about prevention and transmission of HIV.

AIDS is the fifth leading cause of death in people between the ages of 25 and 44 years in the United States. However, mortality rates have decreased by almost 70% from 1995 to 2002 (CDC National Center for Health Statistics, 2004). This phenomenon is a result of the availability of aggressive treatment with highly active antiretroviral therapy (HAART), which involves the use of various combinations of drugs to suppress the replication of the virus.

The management of patients infected with HIV is challenging for a number of reasons. First, HAART regimens can be complex, requiring a large pill burden as well as specific food and timing requirements. Second, adverse effects of the medications may affect a patient's ability to tolerate and comply with therapy. Third, nonadherence to HAART results in treatment failure as well as the development of resistance due to suboptimal serum concentrations of the antiretroviral drugs. The health care practitioner should collaborate with the individual patient to select a regimen that the patient can take successfully and still manage the potential adverse effects.

CAUSES

HIV is transmitted through four types of contact: sexual intercourse, bloodborne contact, perinatal transmission, and breast-feeding. *Prevention is the key to avoiding transmission* (Box 52-2). The most common route of transmission worldwide is through sexual contact with an infected person's genital fluids. The virus is also transmitted via intravenous transfer of infected blood through transfusions, intravenous drug use and needle sharing, or occupational exposure. An infected mother may transmit the virus to her baby prior to or during birth as well as during breast-feeding. It is important to note that HIV is *not* transmitted through casual contact (eg, contact with tears, saliva, toilet facilities).

PATHOPHYSIOLOGY

Unlike most viruses, HIV is a retrovirus. Each viral particle contains two single-stranded molecules of RNA, not DNA. Following infection of host cells, the viral enzyme reverse transcriptase allows synthesis of a DNA molecule that is then inserted into the DNA of the host cell, allowing the virus to replicate. In the case of HIV, the host cells are $CD4^+$ T lymphocytes, a white blood cell involved in cell-mediated

BOX 52–1. AIDS-DEFINING CONDITIONS

Candidiasis, pulmonary or esophageal
Cervical cancer
Coccidioidomycosis
Cryptococcosis
Cryptosporidiosis
Cytomegalovirus
Herpes simplex virus
Histoplasmosis (microscopy [histology or cytology],
    culture, or detection of antigen in a specimen
    obtained directly from the tissues affected or a
    fluid from those tissues)
HIV-associated dementia
HIV-associated wasting
Isosporiasis
Kaposi sarcoma
Lymphoma
Mycobacterium avium infection
Pneumocystis carinii pneumonia
Other pneumonias, recurrent (more than one episode
    in a 1-y period)
Progressive multifocal leukoencephalopathy
Salmonella septicemia
Toxoplasmosis
Tuberculosis

Adapted from Centers for Disease Control and Prevention. (1992).
1993 revised classification system for HIV infection and expanded
surveillance case definition for AIDS among adolescents and
adults. *Morbidity and Mortality Weekly Report, 41* (RR-17), 1–19.

BOX 52–2. PREVENTING HIV TRANSMISSION

Preventing Sexual Transmission

Abstinence, safe sexual practices, use of latex
condoms, risk factor modification, notification of
sexual partners, and education (especially to
adolescents) may be used to prevent sexual
transmission of HIV.

Preventing Blood Exposure Transmission

Since 1985, all donated blood is tested for the
presence of HIV. Implementation of universal
precautions training programs has decreased
transmission among health care workers. Needle
exchange and drug treatment programs are available
throughout the United States.

Preventing Perinatal Transmission

In 1994, Connor and colleagues conducted a study
evaluating the rates of perinatal HIV transmission in
women who received zidovudine during pregnancy.
Results indicated that taking zidovudine during
pregnancy reduces the risk of perinatal transmission
by 66% (Connor et al., 1994). Other ways to prevent
perinatal transmission include aggressive family
planning services (eg, HIV testing, counseling),
monitoring women closely during delivery, and no
longer recommending breast-feeding for infected
women.

immunity. As the virus replicates, it destroys the CD4$^+$ T
lymphocytes, thereby leading to immune deficiency.

HIV incorporates itself into the host cell through a number
of steps. A viral envelope surrounds HIV RNA. On the outer
surface of the envelope is an external glycoprotein (gp120).
This protein allows the virus to attach itself to the cell by
reacting specifically with the CD4$^+$ receptor on the T lymphocyte (CD4$^+$ T cell). Once this step is complete, a transmembrane glycoprotein (gp41) facilitates the fusion of the
viral envelope to the host cell and allows the HIV RNA to
enter the host cell. Next, reverse transcriptase catalyzes the
formation of a single-stranded DNA intermediate from the
viral RNA. This step is followed by duplication of the single-
stranded DNA to form a double-stranded DNA. Catalyzed by
the enzyme integrase, viral DNA is integrated into the host
cell's nucleus. After the DNA is transcribed and translated
back to RNA, the virus then makes long chains of polyproteins that are split by the enzyme protease to form new
copies of HIV RNA. To protect the viral RNA, a protective
core protein (p24) called a *capsid* surrounds the genetic
material. This process is rapidly repeated, producing an estimated 10 billion new particles each day. The average half-
life of a viral particle is 6 hours. The largest concentration of
viral particles can be found in lymph node tissue and genital
secretions.

DIAGNOSTIC CRITERIA

The signs and symptoms of HIV disease vary among patients.
The acute retroviral syndrome occurs 2 to 3 weeks following
exposure to the virus. During this time, the number of CD4$^+$
T lymphocytes (CD4$^+$ count) declines dramatically and the
number of HIV RNA particles in the plasma (viral load)
increases greatly. Clinically, the patient may experience fever,
swollen lymph nodes, sore throat, skin rash, muscle soreness,
headache, nausea, vomiting, and diarrhea (Schacker et al.,
1996). The specific symptoms and their duration vary among
patients, and their presence alone does not constitute a diagnosis. Diagnosis of HIV is based on the presence of virus in
the plasma as well as the absolute CD4$^+$ T-lymphocyte count.

The currently used method for diagnosing HIV-1 infection is the enzyme-linked immunosorbent assay (ELISA),
which detects circulating antibodies to the virus. This assay
is highly sensitive and specific (99% sensitivity and specificity), but false-positive results may occur in patients who
recently received influenza vaccine, have acute viral infections, or have autoantibody formation. False-negative results
may occur in newly infected patients whose antibody titer
has not risen to detectable levels. Antibodies develop within
6 months after infection in 95% of patients, and the median
time for antibody development is 2 months. If the ELISA

test is positive, a Western blot test is used to confirm diagnosis. Other confirmatory tests include an indirect immunofluorescence assay and a radioimmunoprecipitation assay.

Laboratory Parameters

Once the diagnosis of HIV has been confirmed using the above tests, determination of appropriate therapy should be guided by the patient's clinical status as well as two main laboratory parameters, the CD4$^+$ T-cell count and the plasma HIV RNA (viral load). Determination of these results allows the clinician to understand the patient's risk for opportunistic infections and risk for disease progression and to monitor response to drug therapy.

CD4$^+$ T-Cell Count

The CD4$^+$ T-cell count indicates the extent to which HIV has damaged the immune system. Normally, the CD4$^+$ T-cell count ranges between 500 and 1600/mm^3. As the viral infection progresses, the CD4$^+$ count declines, correlating with increasing immunosuppression. CD4$^+$ T-cell counts of less than 200/mm^3 are associated with an increased risk of AIDS malignancies, such as Kaposi sarcoma, and opportunistic infections, such as *Pneumocystis carinii* pneumonia, toxoplasmosis, and cytomegalovirus infection (see Chapter 53).

Plasma HIV RNA (Viral Load)

Quantification of HIV replication is determined by measuring the viral load in number of copies per milliliter of plasma. The primary assay used is the HIV-1 reverse transcriptase-polymerase chain reaction assay (RT-PCR), which has a lower limit of detection of 50 copies/mL. Clinical trials demonstrate that viral loads that are undetectable (eg, <50 copies/mL) are associated with longer duration of suppression of viral replication as compared with detectable levels. The viral load is a useful tool to monitor a patient's virologic status, disease progression, and HAART regimen.

HIV Drug Resistance Testing

Because of the significant association between the presence of drug-resistant HIV and failure of antiretroviral treatment regimens, HIV resistance assays have become useful mechanisms for guiding the selection of appropriate therapy. When used in combination with medication histories and patient counseling, these assays have assisted in attainment of more efficient and sustained viral suppression.

The two methods used to assess resistance include genotypic and phenotypic assays. Genotypic assays detect genetic mutations that may confer viral resistance. Interpretation of these genotypes requires an understanding of the mutations and their correlation with resistance to specific classes of antiretroviral medications. Phenotypic assays calculate the concentrations of antiretroviral drugs required to inhibit HIV replication by 50% and 90%. These values are known as the *inhibitory concentrations* and are abbreviated as the IC$_{50}$ or IC$_{90}$. The virus is reported as "susceptible," "resistant," or "resistance possible" for a variety of antiretroviral medications. Results of phenotypic assays are available within 2 to 3 weeks due to automation techniques, but they are more expensive to perform than genotypic assays.

Several limitations exist with HIV drug resistance testing. First, there is no standardized method for quality assurance for the available genotypic and phenotypic assays. Second, they are expensive to perform. Lastly, if drug-resistant virus comprises less than 10% to 20% of a patient's total virus population, the assays will not detect the resistant virus. Overall, these assays provide a method for making decisions on changing HAART in patients experiencing virologic failure, and their optimal role in patient management will be elucidated in future clinical trials.

INITIATING DRUG THERAPY

When discussing treatment of patients with HIV infection, it is helpful to classify them into two clinical categories: those with symptomatic disease (including AIDS) and those with asymptomatic disease (Panel on Clinical Practices, 2004). All patients in the first category as well as asymptomatic patients with CD4$^+$ T-cell counts less than 200/mm^3 should be offered treatment with HAART. The ideal time to initiate HAART for asymptomatic patients with CD4$^+$ T-cell counts greater than 200/mm^3 is unknown. Several factors must be considered prior to beginning therapy in this group of patients, including risk of disease progression, potential risks and benefits of early versus delayed therapy, and commitment of the patient to long-term therapy. Disease progression can be estimated based on data from observational cohorts that used CD4$^+$ T-cell counts and viral loads. Potential benefits of early therapy include early viral replication suppression, immune function restoration, disease-free survival prolongation, and possible decrease in HIV transmission risk. Risks of early therapy include adverse effects and toxicities of drug therapy, potential nonadherence to therapy (leading to drug resistance), and unknown duration of drug efficacy. Potential benefits of delayed therapy include avoidance of adverse effects as well as delay of the development of drug resistance. Risks of delayed therapy include possible irreversible damage to the immune system, increased risk of transmission of HIV to others, and more difficult viral replication suppression in the future. Although opinions vary, Table 52-1 provides a general guide for when to initiate therapy.

If treatment is deferred in the asymptomatic patient, CD4$^+$ T-cell count and viral load should be monitored closely. Depending on the values of these tests, discussion regarding initiation of therapy should be revisited. Before therapy is started for any patient, a thorough history and physical examination should be performed, in addition to a complete blood count, chemistry profile, liver function tests, lipid profile, CD4$^+$ T-cell count, viral load, and additional evaluation of various serologies (eg, toxoplasma immunoglobulin G, hepatitis B and C, etc).

Goals of Therapy

Because currently available antiretroviral regimens cannot achieve eradication of HIV, goals of therapy primarily focus on sustained suppression of viral replication to undetectable levels. There are four main goals of antiretroviral therapy (Panel on Clinical Practices, 2004). These include maximal and sustained suppression of viral load, restoration and preservation of immune system function, enhancement of

Table 52.1

Initiation of Antiretroviral Therapy

Clinical Category	CD4⁺ T-Cell Count	Plasma HIV RNA	Recommendations
Symptomatic	Any value	Any value	Therapy recommended
Asymptomatic, AIDS	<200/mm³	Any value	Therapy recommended
Asymptomatic	200–350/mm³	Any value	Therapy should be offered, but controversial
Asymptomatic	>350/mm³	>55,000 copies/mL	Some experts would treat, others would delay treatment and increase monitoring frequency
Asymptomatic	>350/mm³	<55,000 copies/mL	Most experts would defer treatment and monitor closely

Adapted from: Panel on Clinical Practices for Treatment of HIV Infection. (2004). *Guidelines for the use of antiretroviral agents in HIV-1-infected adults and adolescents.* (On-line) Available at http://AIDSinfo.nih.gov.

quality of life, and reduction in morbidity and mortality from HIV-related complications. Patients' responses to HAART are variable, although successful regimens can increase the CD4⁺ T-cell count by 100 to 200 cells/mm³/y. A higher CD4⁺ T-cell count is a good prognostic indicator of sustained viral suppression and improved quality and duration of life.

To maximize the benefits of HAART, it is important to select drug regimens carefully, because the first regimen selected is often the one that will be the most effective for the patient. There are three HAART regimens that may be used as initial therapy for HIV infection. These include nonnucleoside reverse transcriptase inhibitor-based regimens, protease inhibitor-based regimens, and triple nucleoside reverse transcriptase inhibitor-based regimens. Table 52-2 lists characteristics of all of the currently available antiretroviral medications.

Reverse Transcriptase Inhibitors

There are two subclasses of reverse transcriptase inhibitors (RTIs), the nucleoside reverse transcriptase inhibitors (NRTIs) and the nonnucleoside reverse transcriptase inhibitors (NNRTIs).

Nucleoside Reverse Transcriptase Inhibitors

There are seven NRTIs marketed in the United States. These include abacavir (Ziagen), didanosine (Videx), emtricitabine (Emtriva), lamivudine (Epivir), stavudine (Zerit), zalcitabine (Hivid), and zidovudine (Retrovir). There is one nucleotide RTI, tenofovir (Viread), which is similar in mechanism of action but is slightly different in structure than the nucleoside analogs. In addition, two combination products are available for dosing convenience: Combivir (zidovudine plus lamivudine) and Trizivir (zidovudine plus lamivudine plus abacavir).

The NRTIs must be phosphorylated in the target cells before becoming active. This intracellular phosphorylation results in an active triphosphorylated form that interferes with the transcription of viral RNA to DNA. This interference can occur through two mechanisms: chain termination and competitive inhibition.

The *chain termination* process results in the reverse transcriptase enzyme adding the NRTI to the growing chain of HIV viral DNA instead of the needed DNA nucleoside. The NRTI acts as a nucleoside analog in the DNA production, and its addition is relatively simple. Once this is accomplished, no more DNA nucleosides can be added to the chain, thus terminating its growth and halting the production of viral DNA.

Competitive inhibition occurs when the active (phosphorylated) NRTI competes with the cell's own nucleoside building block. By competing for the cell's building block, these agents also halt the production of viral DNA.

With the exception of abacavir, all NRTIs require elimination by the kidneys and therefore must be dose-adjusted for patients with renal insufficiency. This is an important concept because it helps to minimize the incidence of adverse effects.

The first NRTI that received Food and Drug Administration (FDA) approval in the United States was zidovudine. It has been studied extensively as a component of HAART and has proven to be effective in delaying progression of the disease, reducing the incidence of opportunistic infections, and prolonging survival. An important adverse effect of zidovudine is bone marrow suppression, which can lead to clinically significant anemia and neutropenia. Periodic monitoring of complete blood counts is essential to identifying this adverse event early so treatment can be instituted with hematopoietic growth factors, including erythropoietin and granulocyte colony-stimulating factors. The combination of zidovudine and stavudine should be avoided due to antagonistic effects observed in vitro and in vivo.

Lamivudine is one of the better-tolerated NRTIs. It recently received FDA approval for a 300-mg once-daily dosing regimen. Because it is effective for treatment of chronic hepatitis B, it should be added as a component of HAART in patients coinfected with HIV and hepatitis B.

Many of the NRTIs have been available for several years, including didanosine, stavudine, and zalcitabine. The bioavailability of didanosine is decreased in the presence of gastric acidity. Therefore it is formulated either with an antacid buffer or as an enteric-coated capsule to allow for improved absorption. Dosing of stavudine should be based on weight (see Table 52-2), and an extended-release preparation is currently being evaluated for FDA approval in the United States. Zalcitabine has fallen out of favor due to its propensity to cause severe peripheral neuropathy as well as its inconvenient dosing schedule. All three of these NRTIs have similar toxicities, including pancreatitis, peripheral neuropathy, and gastrointestinal (GI) disturbances.

Abacavir is an effective component of HAART. Patients who initiate treatment with this agent must be cautioned about the hypersensitivity reaction that occurs in 2.3% to 9% of patients. Symptoms of the hypersensitivity reaction include fever, rash, GI disturbances, lethargy, and malaise. These can occur at any time after initiating therapy (median, 11 days). Symptoms resolve after discontinuation of the drug but may recur and result in death if abacavir is restarted.

Tenofovir and emtricitabine are the two newest NRTIs available for use as a part of a HAART regimen. Both are well tolerated, dosed once daily, and can be taken without regard to meals.

Many NRTIs are used in combination as part of HAART. However, triple-NRTI regimens are less effective than protease inhibitor- or NNRTI-based regimens. Therefore, triple

Table 52.2

Overview of Drugs Used to Treat HIV Infection

Generic (Trade) Name and Adult Dosage	Selected Adverse Effects	Contraindications	Special Considerations
Nucleoside Reverse Transcriptase Inhibitors			
abacavir (Ziagen) 300 mg PO bid	Nausea, vomiting, diarrhea, headache, lactic acidosis, hepatic steatosis, hypersensitivity reaction (malaise, fatigue, nausea, vomiting, respiratory symptoms)	Hypersensitivity to any component Moderate to severe hepatic impairment	Take without regard to meals. Hypersensitivity reaction can be fatal (black box warning). Discontinue immediately. Do not rechallenge. Available in combination with zidovudine and lamivudine (Trizivir)
didanosine (Videx) >60 kg: 400 mg PO qd (enteric-coated capsule or buffered tablet) or 200 mg PO bid (buffered tablet) <60 kg: 250 mg PO qd (enteric-coated capsule or buffered tablet) or 125 mg PO bid (buffered tablet)	Nausea, vomiting, diarrhea, headache, pancreatitis, peripheral neuropathy, lactic acidosis, hepatic steatosis	Hypersensitivity to any component Pre-existing pancreatitis or painful peripheral neuropathy	Take 30 min before or 2 h after a meal. Dose adjustment required for renal insufficiency.
emtricitabine (Emtriva) 200 mg PO qd	Nausea, diarrhea, headache, skin hyperpigmentation, lactic acidosis, hepatic steatosis	Hypersensitivity to any component	Take without regard to meals. Dose adjustment required for renal insufficiency.
lamivudine (Epivir) 150 mg PO bid or 300 mg PO qd	Headache, fatigue, peripheral neuropathy, pancreatitis (in children), lactic acidosis, hepatic steatosis	Hypersensitivity to any component	Take without regard to meals. Dose adjustment required for renal insufficiency. Available in combination with zidovudine (Combivir) and in combination with zidovudine and abacavir (Trizivir)
stavudine (Zerit) >60 kg: 40 mg PO bid <60 kg: 30 mg PO bid	Nausea, vomiting, diarrhea, peripheral neuropathy, pancreatitis, lactic acidosis, hepatic steatosis	Hypersensitivity to any component Pre-existing pancreatitis Do not use with zidovudine	Take without regard to meals. Dose adjustment required for renal insufficiency.
tenofovir (Viread) 300 mg PO qd	Nausea, vomiting, diarrhea, headache, asthenia, lactic acidosis, hepatic steatosis (not yet reported)	Hypersensitivity to any component	Take without regard to meals. Dose adjustment required for renal insufficiency.
zalcitabine (Hivid) 0.75 mg PO tid	Severe peripheral neuropathy, oral ulcers, rash, pancreatitis (rare), amylasemia, lactic acidosis, hepatic steatosis	Hypersensitivity to any component Pre-existing pancreatitis or painful peripheral neuropathy Do not use with didanosine.	Take without regard to meals. Dose adjustment required for renal insufficiency.
zidovudine (Retrovir) 200 mg PO tid or 300 mg PO bid	Nausea, headache, malaise, bone marrow suppression, myopathy, lactic acidosis, hepatic steatosis	Hypersensitivity to any component Do not use with ribavirin	Take without regard to meals. Dose adjustment required for renal insufficiency.
Nonnucleoside Reverse Transcriptase Inhibitors			
delavirdine (Rescriptor) 400 mg PO tid	Nausea, vomiting, headache, rash, pruritus, increased bilirubin and transaminases	Hypersensitivity to any component Do not use with simvastatin, lovastatin, rifampin, cisapride, alprazolam, midazolam, ergotamine, St. John's wort	Take without regard to meals. Antacids decrease absorption; separate dosing by at least 1 h.
efavirenz (Sustiva) 600 mg PO hs	Rash (first 2 wk of therapy), hallucinations, nightmares, dizziness, impaired concentration, euphoria, confusion	Hypersensitivity to any component Avoid in pregnancy. Do not use with cisapride, midazolam, ergotamine, St. John's wort.	Take on empty stomach.
nevirapine (Viramune) 200 mg PO qd × 2 wk, increase to 200 mg PO bid	Nausea, headache, rash, hepatitis	Hypersensitivity to any component Severe hepatic impairment Do not use with St. John's wort.	Take without regard to meals. Dose titration may lessen incidence of rash. Severe, life-threatening hepatotoxicity reported; monitor transaminases closely during first 12–16 wk of therapy (black box warning)
Protease Inhibitors			
amprenavir (Agenerase) 1200 mg PO bid	Rash, nausea, diarrhea, headache, perioral paresthesia, increased transaminases, fat maldistribution, lipid abnormalities, hyperglycemia	Hypersensitivity to any component Oral solution contains propylene glycol; avoid use in pregnant women, children <4 y, hepatic or renal failure patients.	Avoid high-fat meals.

(continued)

Table 52.2

Overview of Drugs Used to Treat HIV Infection (*Continued*)

Generic (Trade) Name and Adult Dosage	Selected Adverse Effects	Contraindications	Special Considerations
atazanavir (Reyataz) 400 mg PO qd	Diarrhea, headache, prolonged PR interval, hyperbilirubinemia, fat maldistribution lipid abnormalities, hyperglycemia	Do not use with cisapride, dihydroergotamine, ergotamine, midazolam, triazolam, St. John's wort. Hypersensitivity to any component Avoid concomitant use with proton pump inhibitors.	Take with food.
fosamprenavir (Lexiva) HAART-naive patients: 1400 mg PO bid **or** 1400 mg PO qd plus ritonavir 200 mg PO qd **or** 700 mg PO bid plus ritonavir 100 mg PO bid HAART-experienced patients: 700 mg PO bid plus ritonavir 100 mg PO bid	Nausea, vomiting, diarrhea, headache, rash, increased transaminases, fat maldistribution lipid abnormalities, hyperglycemia	Do not use with cisapride, dihydroergotamine, ergotamine, midazolam, triazolam, St. John's wort. Hypersensitivity to any component Do not use with cisapride, dihydroergotamine, ergotamine, midazolam, triazolam, St. John's wort.	Take without regard to meals.
indinavir (Crixivan) 800 mg po q8h	Nephrolithiasis, nausea, hyperbilirubinemia, fat maldistribution lipid abnormalities, hyperglycemia	Same as above	Should be taken 1 h before or 2 h after meals. Drink 1.5 L fluid daily to avoid renal stones.
lopinavir/ritonavir (Kaletra) 400/100 mg PO bid	Nausea, vomiting, diarrhea, increased transaminases, fat maldistribution lipid abnormalities, hyperglycemia	Same as above	Take with food.
nelfinavir (Viracept) 1250 mg PO bid or 750 mg PO tid	Diarrhea, rash, increased transaminases, fat maldistribution lipid abnormalities, hyperglycemia	Same as above	Take with food.
ritonavir (Norvir) 600 mg PO bid	Circumoral and peripheral paresthesias, nausea, vomiting, diarrhea, increased transaminases, fat maldistribution lipid abnormalities, hyperglycemia	Same as above	Take with food. Separate dosing of buffered didanosine by 2 h. Check for drug interactions. Escalate dose over 2 wk.
saquinavir (Invirase): not recommended as sole protease inhibitor (Fortovase): 1200 mg PO tid	Nausea, diarrhea, abdominal pain, headache, fat maldistribution lipid abnormalities, hyperglycemia	Same as above	Take with large meal.
Fusion inhibitor enfuvirtide (Fuzeon) 90 mg SC bid	Local injection site reactions, nausea, vomiting, fever, rash, hypersensitivity reaction (<1%)	Hypersensitivity to any component	Store reconstituted solution in refrigerator and use within 24 h.

NRTI regimens should be reserved for patients who cannot tolerate protease inhibitors or NNRTIs due to adverse effects or drug interactions. NRTI combinations that should be avoided in all patients due to poor efficacy include tenofovir plus didanosine plus lamivudine, didanosine plus stavudine, stavudine plus zidovudine, zalcitabine plus stavudine, zalcitabine plus didanosine, and lamivudine plus emtricitabine. Many of these combinations demonstrate antagonism as well as an additive incidence of adverse drug reactions.

A class adverse effect observed with all NRTIs includes lactic acidosis and hepatic steatosis. Although this adverse effect is rare, it results in a high risk of death. This may be due to mitochondrial dysfunction that occurs on administration of NRTIs. The clinical presentation of lactic acidosis varies greatly among patients but often includes nonspecific GI symptoms (nausea, vomiting, abdominal pain) as well as generalized weakness, myalgias, and paresthesias. Hepatic steatosis may manifest as an enlarged fatty liver on computed tomography (CT) scan as well as increased liver transaminases.

Risk factors for development of this syndrome include pregnancy and postpartum state, obesity, female sex, and prolonged use of NRTIs. If this syndrome develops, the NRTIs should be discontinued immediately, and supportive care should be initiated. Because other clinical interventions such as administration of thiamine, riboflavin, and levocarnitine have not been adequately assessed in clinical trials, their efficacy cannot be determined at this time. Patients taking NRTIs should be cautioned about the signs and symptoms of lactic acidosis, and if these are observed, the patient should notify the practitioner immediately.

Non-nucleoside Reverse Transcriptase Inhibitors

By binding to reverse transcriptase, NNRTIs also interfere with the conversion of RNA to DNA. The three available NNRTIs are delavirdine (Rescriptor), efavirenz (Sustiva), and nevirapine (Viramune). Delavirdine is the least potent NNRTI and therefore is not recommended as part of initial HAART. Trials have shown that efavirenz-based regimens are more effective in suppressing viral replication than protease inhibitor-based regimens. Two studies that compared an efavirenz-based regimen with a nevirapine-based regimen found no significant difference in efficacy but a significant difference in toxicity (higher incidence of rash and hepatotoxicity with nevirapine). Based on the results of this trial, the Panel on Clinical Practices (2004) recommends efavirenz as the preferred NNRTI for NNRTI-based regimens.

The most frequently reported adverse effects of NNRTIs include GI disturbances, rash, and reversible elevations in hepatic transaminases and bilirubin. Efavirenz commonly causes central nervous system adverse effects, including dizziness, impaired concentration, abnormal dreams, and hallucinations. These events occur within the first few days of initiating therapy but resolve over 2 to 4 weeks with continued treatment. Nevirapine has been associated with life-threatening skin reactions such as Stevens-Johnson syndrome. To minimize the risk for developing the rash, patients should initiate nevirapine once daily for 14 days, then increase to twice daily. If rash occurs during the initial dosing regimen, the frequency of administration should not be increased until the rash has resolved.

Nevirapine has also been associated with severe, life-threatening hepatotoxicity, including hepatic necrosis and hepatic failure. Two thirds of cases occur within the first 12 weeks of treatment. This may also occur along with a hypersensitivity reaction that includes rash and fever. A black box warning in the nevirapine labeling notes that women with CD4$^+$ T-cell counts greater than 250 cells/mm^3 and men with CD4$^+$ T-cell counts greater than 400 cells/mm^3 have a considerably higher risk of hepatotoxicity. Therefore, all patients who initiate therapy with nevirapine should receive close monitoring of liver function tests and clinical symptoms throughout the treatment course. If hepatotoxicity occurs, nevirapine should be discontinued permanently.

All of the NNRTIs are metabolized by the cytochrome P450 (CYP450) 3A4 isoenzyme system in the liver. Each NNRTI also has variable effects on inhibiting or inducing this enzyme system. Therefore, caution should be used when administering NNRTIs with drugs dependent on CYP450 3A4 for metabolism, including protease inhibitors, phenytoin, phenobarbital, and clarithromycin. Concomitant use of rifampin with delavirdine is contraindicated because of increased metabolism of delavirdine that results in reduced serum concentrations and reduced efficacy. Rifampin may be used with caution with nevirapine. Rifampin must be used with an increased dose of efavirenz (800 mg daily). Concomitant use of St. John's wort is contraindicated with all NNRTIs due to risk of virologic failure secondary to the resulting suboptimal NNRTI concentrations.

Protease Inhibitors

The protease inhibitor (PI) class of drugs has revolutionized the treatment of HIV infection. Introduced in the mid-1990s, these agents have demonstrated efficacy in reducing viral load and elevating CD4$^+$ T-cell counts. They act near the final stage of HIV viral replication through inhibiting the protease-mediated cleavage of the polyproteins. These polyproteins are responsible for creating new HIV RNA copies. Inhibiting this final stage by use of PIs decreases the production of HIV RNA copies.

Eight PIs are available: amprenavir (Agenerase), atazanavir (Reyataz), fosamprenavir (Lexiva), indinavir (Crixivan), lopinavir/ritonavir (Kaletra), nelfinavir (Viracept), ritonavir (Norvir), and saquinavir (Invirase and Fortovase). These agents are active against both HIV-1 and HIV-2.

PI-based regimens provide excellent efficacy in virologic suppression. They frequently have been studied in combination with NRTIs. Regimens containing full-dose ritonavir are not recommended due to the high incidence of adverse effects (see Table 52-2). However, ritonavir can be used to increase the concentrations of other PIs, allowing greater exposure of the virus to the PI. These ritonavir "boosted" regimens demonstrate potent virologic suppression while reducing pill burden and adverse effects. One product, lopinavir/ritonavir, contains low-dose ritonavir to boost the concentration of lopinavir. This combination product is a first-line agent used in PI-based HAART regimens.

The pharmacokinetic characteristics of the PIs vary greatly across the class. Food affects the bioavailability of many of the PIs (see Table 52-2). For example, administration of atazanavir with food increases its bioavailability substantially and therefore should be administered with a meal. In contrast, concentrations of indinavir decrease by 77% with food, resulting in the requirement that this drug be taken on an empty stomach or with a small, low-fat snack (eg, pretzels).

The adverse effects of all PIs include GI disturbances, such as nausea, vomiting, and diarrhea. Diarrhea is especially problematic with nelfinavir, and it can be managed with over-the-counter antidiarrheals such as loperamide. All PIs can cause increases in levels of hepatic transaminases. Severe hepatotoxicity is more common in patients receiving regimens containing full-dose ritonavir or the ritonavir-saquinavir combination regimen. Risk factors for hepatotoxicity with PIs include hepatitis B or C coinfection, alcohol abuse, and concomitant use of hepatotoxic agents. This should be monitored carefully.

A class effect of the PIs includes fat maldistribution, also known as lipodystrophy. This results in accumulation of fat in the abdomen, breasts, and dorsocervical fat pad ("buffalo hump") as well as fat atrophy of the face and extremities. This occurs in 25% to 75% of patients receiving HAART. Fat maldistribution may be accompanied by metabolic abnormalities such as hyperlipidemia and hyperglycemia. There is no effective treatment for fat maldistribution. Unfortunately, changing to non–PI-based regimens does not result in substantial benefit, although data are conflicting in this regard.

PI therapy has been associated with hyperlipidemia, including increased levels of triglycerides, total serum cholesterol, and low-density lipoproteins. These lipid abnormalities may be associated with accelerated coronary artery disease in HIV patients. Atazanavir appears to have less effect on the lipid profile than other PIs. Management includes dietary modifications, exercise, blood pressure control, and smoking cessation, as well as addition of 3-hydroxy-3-methyl-glutaryl-coenzyme A (HMG-CoA) reductase inhibitors (statins). However, it is important to note that most statins cause drug interactions with the PIs. Therefore, pravastatin is the preferred agent because it does not have these interaction concerns.

Another class effect of PIs includes hyperglycemia. This may lead to new-onset diabetes mellitus as a result of insulin resistance and insulin deficiency. Patients should be cautioned about warning signs of hyperglycemia, including polydipsia, polyphagia, and polyuria. Data are inconclusive regarding efforts to change to non–PI-based regimens to reverse this adverse effect.

A unique adverse effect of indinavir includes nephrolithiasis. Patients receiving indinavir therapy must consume at least 1500 mL water daily to decrease the risk of this adverse effect. If stone formation occurs, indinavir should be discontinued temporarily, then resumed with increased fluid consumption once the situation has resolved.

All PIs are metabolized by the CYP450 3A4 isoenzyme system in the liver. Each of the PIs has a different effect on inducing or inhibiting the efficiency of this isoenzyme system. Therefore, caution must be used when combining PIs with any medications that are metabolized by CYP450 3A4 or that induce or inhibit this system. Concurrent use of PIs with ergot alkaloids, simvastatin, lovastatin, rifampin, and St. John's wort is contraindicated.

Fusion Inhibitor

Enfuvirtide (Fuzeon) is the only available agent in this class of antiretroviral drugs. It inhibits fusion of the virus to the cell membrane of the CD4$^+$ T cell, thereby preventing HIV from entering the cell. Because its mechanism of action is distinct from the intracellular agents previously discussed, it may be useful for patients with virus that is resistant to other currently available antiretroviral agents.

Enfuvirtide has been studied in treatment-experienced patients who demonstrated inadequate virologic suppression despite ongoing HAART. This agent has not been studied as initial therapy for treatment naïve patients. Its optimal role in the treatment of HIV has not yet been determined.

Enfuvirtide must be injected subcutaneously twice daily. Adverse effects include local injection site reactions, such as erythema, induration, and pain. Less than 1% of patients experience hypersensitivity reactions, including rash and fever. There are no known drug interactions with enfuvirtide.

Selecting the Most Appropriate Regimen

Although guidelines exist for the combinations of agents to be used in antiretroviral therapy, each patient must have a highly individualized regimen. Although current regimens are effective at keeping the viral load to undetectable levels, eradication of the virus is not yet attainable. This is due to the early development of latent CD4$^+$ T cells with a long half-life that, even with prolonged therapy, persist.

Previously Untreated Patients

One of the most important therapeutic interventions in the care of the patient with HIV infection is the initial treatment regimen (Tables 52-1 and 52-3). It is essential to select the most potent and appropriate therapy possible, keeping in

Table 52.3

Recommended Regimens for Treatment of HIV Infection in Previously Untreated Patients

NNRTI-Based Regimens	
Preferred regimen	efavirenz + lamivudine + (zidovudine or tenofovir or stavudine)*
Alternative regimens	efavirenz + (lamivudine or emtricitabine) + (didanosine or abacavir)*
	efavirenz + emtricitabine + (zidovudine or tenofovir or stavudine)*
	nevirapine + (lamivudine or emtricitabine) + (zidovudine or stavudine or didanosine)
PI-Based Regimens	
Preferred regimen	lopinavir/ritonavir + lamivudine + (zidovudine or stavudine)
Alternative regimens	atazanavir + (lamivudine or emtricitabine) + (zidovudine or stavudine or abacavir)
	fosamprenavir + (lamivudine or emtricitabine) + (zidovudine or stavudine or abacavir)
	fosamprenavir/ritonavir + (lamivudine or emtricitabine) + (zidovudine or stavudine or abacavir)
	lopinavir/ritonavir + emtricitabine + (zidovudine or stavudine or abacavir)
	nelfinavir + (lamivudine or emtricitabine) + (zidovudine or stavudine or abacavir)
	saquinavir (either formulation)/ritonavir + (lamivudine or emtricitabine) + (zidovudine or stavudine or abacavir)
Triple NRTI-Based Regimen	
Used only if one of the above regimens cannot be used	abacavir + lamivudine + (zidovudine or stavudine)
Preferred regimen	

*Cannot be used in pregnant patients or those not using effective contraception who may become pregnant.
Adapted from Panel on Clinical Practices for Treatment of HIV Infection. (2004). *Guidelines for use of antiretroviral agents in adults and adolescents.* [On-line]. Available: http://AIDSinfo.nih.gov.

mind adverse effects and adherence issues. Discontinuing preferred therapy due to nonadherence increases the risk of drug resistance and failure with alternate regimens.

Preferred regimens have been selected by the Panel on Clinical Practices based on optimal efficacy and durability demonstrated in clinical trials as well as tolerability and convenience of use. Alternative regimens demonstrate efficacy but have disadvantages in terms of virologic activity, durability of effect, tolerance, and pill burden. An alternative regimen may actually be preferred in some patients, depending on the individual situation.

There are three main regimens recommended for treatment-naïve patients: NNRTI-based, PI-based, and triple NRTI regimens. NNRTI-based regimens include one NNRTI plus two NRTIs. Efavirenz-based regimens are potent and convenient with a low pill burden, but cannot be used in pregnant patients due to concerns of teratogenicity. Nevirapine can be used as an alternative for pregnant patients or in women who wish to conceive. These regimens demonstrate far less fat maldistribution and dyslipidemia than PI-based regimens, and they allow the PIs to be spared for future use in the event of resistance development.

PI-based regimens contain a PI (with or without a "booster" dose of ritonavir) in combination with two NRTIs. These combinations have proven to be effective in numerous clinical trials The coformulation of lopinavir/ritonavir is part of the preferred PI-based regimen due to its virologic potency, tolerability profile, and low pill burden. All of the PI-based regimens are associated with metabolic complications, including fat maldistribution, hyperlipidemia, and hyperglycemia.

Triple NRTI regimens should be considered only for patients who cannot tolerate a NNRTI- or PI-based regimen due to toxicities, regimen complexity, or drug interactions. Although these regimens are very convenient due to their low pill burden, clinical trials have proven that they are less effective at suppressing viral replication than NNRTI- or PI-based regimens.

Treatment-Experienced Patients

When a treatment failure occurs, it is necessary to assess why this occurred to determine the appropriate therapy change (Table 52-4). Treatment regimen failure is a term that encompasses all potential reasons for failure that must be assessed, including nonadherence, drug toxicity, pharmacokinetic issues, resistance, and so forth (Panel on Clinical Practices, 2004). Treatment regimen failure often results in virologic, immunologic, and/or clinical failure. *Virologic failure* is defined as the failure to achieve nondetectable HIV RNA plasma levels within 24 to 48 weeks of initiating therapy or a rebound in viral load after prior virologic suppression. *Immunologic failure* results when $CD4^+$ T-cell counts decline while on therapy or if there is a failure to increase by 25 to 50 cells/mm^3 above baseline. *Clinical failure* results if an opportunistic infection occurs or recurs after receiving at least 3 months of HAART.

After the practitioner considers the causes and types of treatment failure, the drug regimen should be changed accordingly. The patient's previous treatment experience and drug resistance pattern must be considered because there may be cross-resistance between agents within the same therapeutic class. In addition, if an adverse effect or unacceptable toxicity caused a cessation of therapy, the practitioner should avoid alternative agents likely to cause that adverse effect. Furthermore, agents with complicated dosing schedules and strict diet and fluid requirements should be avoided if that is what caused the first treatment failure. Selecting agents that are free of side effects and strict dosing, diet, and fluid requirements is not easy, but each patient must be given the regimen to which he or she will most likely adhere.

When changing therapy, one or more of the agents in the regimen may need to be replaced. This will vary depending on the individual patient's situation. Expert advice from an HIV clinician is crucial to selecting the most appropriate option.

Special Population Considerations

Pediatric

Guidelines exist for treating HIV infection in the pediatric patient (Working Group on Antiretroviral Therapy and Medical Management of HIV-Infected Children, 2004). Although the principles remain the same, unique considerations in subsets of the pediatric population need brief discussion. These include diagnosis of disease, differences in $CD4^+$ T-cell counts, changes in pharmacokinetic parameters, and adherence issues.

Diagnostic testing on suspected HIV-infected infants can be performed as early as 2 days of age, and by 6 months in almost all infants. Testing in suspected infants should occur by 48 hours of life because in nearly 40% of infected infants the diagnosis can be made within this time frame. If the initial test is negative, repeat testing should be performed at 1 to 2 months and 3 to 6 months of age. HIV DNA polymerase chain reaction is the preferred virologic method for diagnosing HIV in infants. Antibody testing is not accurate due to the transfer of maternal HIV antibodies to the infant.

The $CD4^+$ T-cell counts in children younger than 6 years of age are typically higher than adult counts. Therefore, monitoring absolute $CD4^+$ T-cell counts may not be as reliable as measuring the percentage change in $CD4^+$ T-cell counts as disease progresses. Pediatric patients with a positive virologic test should have $CD4^+$ T-cell counts monitored every 3 months. Similarly, because of immunologic differences, particularly in those patients acquiring the disease perinatally, viral load (HIV RNA levels) may be difficult to interpret during the first year of life.

Pharmacokinetic variables, particularly volume of distribution and clearance, change as a person ages. These changes should be considered when designing drug therapy regimens for children. Similarly, the issue of medication adherence in this population is crucial. Some of the solution formulations for these agents may be unpalatable, depending

---

Table 52.4

Assessment of Treatment Regimen Failure

Reason for Failure	Assessment	Treatment Modification
Nonadherence	Identify reasons	Based on reason for nonadherence: reduce pill burden, decrease dosing frequency, improve access to medications
Tolerability	Adverse effects Persistence of adverse effects	Supportive care (eg, loperamide for diarrhea) Change the problematic drug in the regimen to another agent within the same class or in a different class
Pharmacokinetic issues	Review food requirements Review concomitant drugs for interactions	Counsel and educate about food requirements Substitute interacting medications with ones that do not interact Change the problematic drug in the regimen to another agent within the same class or in a different class
Resistance	Perform resistance testing	Based on results of resistance testing, change HAART regimen

on the child's preferences. Also, absorption of drugs can be affected by food, and timing of drug administration around food schedules can be extremely difficult. Mixing medications in bottles with formula may increase palatability but may create compatibility issues.

Women/Pregnancy

Several clinical studies have discovered gender-based differences in plasma HIV RNA levels, with women having significantly lower viral loads than men. It appears that this primarily occurs in the setting of very high viral loads. It has not been determined if a lower viral load threshold for initiating therapy should be considered for women at this point in time. Ongoing studies are also assessing variations in viral loads according to ovulatory cycles.

When considering the use of HAART in pregnant women with HIV infection, practitioners must consider two main issues: antiretroviral therapy of HIV in the mother and prophylaxis to reduce the risk of perinatal HIV infection (Public Health Service Task Force, 2003). The benefits and risks of using antiretroviral therapy must be assessed prior to initiating therapy in a pregnant patient. Current options for the individual patient can be found in the recommendations provided by the Public Health Service Task Force (2003), including special considerations for counseling the pregnant patient.

The acquisition of disease through exposure in utero is a major source of HIV infection in infants. Therefore, early identification of HIV-infected women is crucial before or during pregnancy. HIV counseling and testing for all pregnant women have been advocated by the American Academy of Pediatrics, the American College of Obstetricians and Gynecologists, and the U.S. Public Health Service.

One of the more remarkable aspects of zidovudine therapy was the discovery that this agent reduced the maternal–fetal transmission of HIV. The pivotal study by Connor and colleagues showed a maternal–fetal transmission rate of 8.3% with zidovudine versus 25.5% with placebo in expectant mothers between 14 and 34 weeks of gestation (Connor et al., 1994). Therefore, zidovudine chemoprophylaxis is recommended for all pregnant women in an effort to reduce perinatal transmission.

Health Care Workers/Occupational Exposure

As of December 2001, a total of 57 documented cases of HIV/AIDS seroconversion associated with occupational exposure were reported to the CDC (CDC, 2002). The primary means of transmission in this population is through an accidental needle stick. However, transmission can occur through exposure of HIV-infected blood to a health care worker's open wound or mucous membranes. The risk of HIV transmission after a percutaneous exposure to infected blood is approximately 0.3%; the risk decreases to approximately 0.09% for a mucous membrane exposure.

In theory, initiation of antiretroviral postexposure prophylaxis (PEP) soon after exposure may prevent or inhibit systemic infection by limiting the replication of virus in the lymphocytes and lymph nodes. As such, the CDC has published recommendations regarding the initiation and continuation of PEP in health care workers (CDC, 2001). The primary role of PEP is to prevent HIV infection after an accidental occupational exposure.

The data are scant regarding efficacy of PEP antiretroviral therapy in humans. However, the limited data suggest that zidovudine is the drug of choice for this therapy. No data exist that suggest combination therapy is superior to zidovudine monotherapy in PEP, but clinical data in non-PEP trials suggest that combination therapy could offer an advantage.

Current guidelines suggest a two- or three-drug approach to PEP. The basic two-drug approach consists of two NRTIs including zidovudine plus lamivudine, lamivudine plus stavudine, or didanosine plus stavudine. These basic regimens are used for "standard" occupational exposures, and the specific choice is based on resistance patterns in the particular geographic region. An expanded, three-drug regimen is used for increased risk of transmission or suspected resistance. These regimens include the two drugs used in the basic regimen plus either indinavir, nelfinavir, efavirenz, abacavir, or lopinavir/ritonavir. PEP therapy should be initiated within 24 to 36 hours after exposure and a regimen should be started while awaiting results of resistance, source identification, or both. Therapy should be continued for at least 4 weeks, and HIV antibody testing should be performed at baseline, 6 weeks, 12 weeks, and 6 months. Tables 52-5 and 52-6 outline the current recommendations for PEP (CDC, 2001).

Table 52.5

Recommended HIV PEP for Percutaneous Injuries

Exposure Type	HIV-Positive Class 1*	HIV-Positive Class 2†	Unknown HIV Status‡	Unknown Source	HIV-Negative
Less severe (solid needle and superficial injury)	Recommend basic 2-drug PEP	Recommend expanded 3-drug PEP	No PEP warranted; may consider basic 2-drug PEP for source with HIV risk factors	No PEP warranted; may consider basic 2-drug PEP in settings with likely exposure to HIV-infected patients	No PEP warranted
More severe (hollow needle, deep puncture, visible blood on needle)	Recommend expanded 3-drug PEP	Recommend expanded 3-drug PEP	No PEP warranted; may consider basic 2-drug PEP for source with HIV risk factors	No PEP warranted; may consider basic 2-drug PEP in settings with likely exposure to HIV-infected patients	No PEP warranted

*HIV-positive class 1: asymptomatic HIV or viral load <1500 copies/mL
†HIV-positive class 2: symptomatic HIV, AIDS, acute seroconversion, or viral load >1500 copies/mL
‡Unknown source: eg, a discarded needle from a sharps disposal container
Adapted from Centers for Disease Control and Prevention (2001). Updated U.S. public health service guidelines for the management of occupational exposures to HBV, HCV, and HIV and recommendations for postexposure prophylaxis. *Morbidity and Mortality Weekly Report, 50* (RR-11), 24–25.

Table 52.6

Recommended HIV PEP for Mucous Membrane Exposures and Nonintact Skin Exposures

Exposure Type	HIV-Positive Class 1*	HIV-Positive Class 2†	Unknown HIV Status‡	Unknown Source	HIV-Negative
Small volume (few drops)	Consider basic 2-drug PEP	Recommend basic 2-drug PEP	No PEP warranted; may consider basic 2-drug PEP for source with HIV risk factors	No PEP warranted; may consider basic 2-drug PEP in settings with likely exposure to HIV-infected patients	No PEP warranted
Large volume (splash)	Recommend basic 2-drug PEP	Recommend expanded 3-drug PEP	No PEP warranted; may consider basic 2-drug PEP for source with HIV risk factors	No PEP warranted; may consider basic 2-drug PEP in settings with likely exposure to HIV-infected patients	No PEP warranted

*HIV-positive class 1: asymptomatic HIV or viral load <1500 copies/mL
†HIV-positive class 2: symptomatic HIV, AIDS, acute seroconversion, or viral load >1500 copies/mL
‡Unknown source: eg, a discarded needle from a sharps disposal container
Adapted from Centers for Disease Control and Prevention (2001). Updated U.S. public health service guidelines for the management of occupational exposures to HBV, HCV, and HIV and recommendations for postexposure prophylaxis. *Morbidity and Mortality Weekly Report, 50* (RR-11), 24–25.

MONITORING PATIENT RESPONSE

Viral load should be measured at baseline for all patients. A repeat measurement should be obtained to ensure accuracy if HAART is being considered. If the patient has not begun treatment, viral load should be measured every 3 to 4 months.

Once therapy has been initiated or changed, viral load should be assessed immediately at that time and again 2 to 8 weeks later. Adherence to a potent HAART regimen should result in a significant decrease (~1 log$_{10}$) in viral load by 2 to 8 weeks. Subsequent testing should reveal an undetectable viral load by 16 to 24 weeks. At this point, the viral load testing should be repeated every 3 to 4 months to determine continuing effectiveness of the regimen. If the viral load is detectable after 16 to 24 weeks of therapy, the viral load should be confirmed with a repeat test, and a regimen change should be considered. Because variability exists between viral load assays, it is recommended that the same assay is always used to monitor viral load in an individual patient.

The CD4$^+$ T-cell counts are important not only because they indicate the risk for development of opportunistic infections, but also because they help the health care provider initiate therapy or evaluate the effectiveness of current therapy. If CD4$^+$ T-cell counts decline, a change in therapy may be warranted. Therefore, it is important to measure CD4$^+$ T-cell counts at diagnosis and recheck them every 3 to 6 months. More frequent measurements may be needed if a patient has a change in therapy, contracts an opportunistic infection, or has an increase in viral load. If any of these situations arise, CD4$^+$ T-cell counts should be monitored every 4 weeks. Laboratory values may vary throughout the day (there can be an increase by as much as 60 cells/mm^3 in the evening) and from laboratory to laboratory. Therefore, it is important for a patient to be tested at the same time of day and at the same laboratory, if possible.

Drug resistance testing is recommended for patients who experience virologic failure or suboptimal virologic suppression during therapy with antiretroviral agents. This allows optimization of the regimen and documentation of which drugs still retain activity. It is also useful for patients presenting with acute infection because resistant strains of virus can be identified immediately. Drug resistance testing is not rec-

ommended after discontinuation of therapy because the resistant mutants may become the minor species and would not be detected with currently available assays. Resistance testing is also not recommended for patients with viral loads of fewer than 1000 copies/mL because the assays cannot consistently determine resistance patterns with such low level viremia. Recommendations for resistance testing in pregnant patients are the same as for those who are not pregnant.

PATIENT EDUCATION

To minimize the likelihood of treatment regimen failure and development of drug resistance, the health care professional must be aware of who is at high risk for adherence issues as well as the most common reasons for inadequate adherence. Risk factors for inadequate adherence to antiretroviral regimens include alcohol and drug abuse, active mental illness, lack of disease and medication education, and lack of trust between the patient and clinician. Several treatment factors affect adherence, such as pill burden, frequency of dosing, food requirements, adverse effects, and cost.

Strategies the practitioner can use to minimize the risk of failure due to nonadherence include encouraging the patient to develop a strong relationship with the health care team, taking an active role in his or her therapy, and involving the patient's family and friends in the therapy. In addition, counseling on HIV and the consequences of inadequate adherence may encourage an otherwise indifferent patient to adhere to a regimen.

Another strategy the practitioner should use to promote drug adherence is preparing the patient for adverse events. The patient needs to know which adverse events are likely to occur, how to minimize the risk of experiencing adverse events, and which adverse events demand discontinuation of therapy. The patient also needs to understand the importance of following the strict dosing schedule in addition to the diet and fluid requirements for each agent (Panel on Clinical Practices, 2004). Table 52-2 provides information on dosing, diet, and fluid requirements of each agent.

Developing a plan for scheduling medications and carefully explaining to the patient how each medication should be taken is imperative. This plan should focus on daily pill taking as well as future events in a patient's life that threaten to interrupt the established schedule (eg, holidays or vacations). This plan must consider lifestyle factors such as work schedule and privacy issues (eg, taking medication at work or storage of medication at work). Regardless of how much or little assistance the patient needs in developing strategies for ensuring adherence, success is often determined by the patient's outlook. If the patient perceives that therapy will lead to an improved quality of life or increased length of life, chances for adherence are greater (Reynolds, 1998). Therefore, before attacking the logistics of a medication schedule, the health care provider must convince the patient of the benefits of continuing therapy.

Once the daily plan is developed, it should evolve into a long-term plan that allows the patient to adhere to therapy and allows the health care provider to monitor adherence. Aids for adherence include pill boxes that separate doses per day, beepers to wake patients for nighttime doses, or something as simple as a calendar that lists dosing schedules. Whatever method is used, the patient must remain adherent and be checked for adherence. The simplest way to check for adherence is to ask the patient. However, a patient may not confess to missed doses or may not be aware of missed doses. Pill counting is another option, but patients may remove missed doses to appear adherent. Blood or urine drug levels can be monitored, but laboratory costs and lack of data concerning interpretation make this method somewhat prohibitive. Testing the viral load may reveal adherence information, but if levels increase because of resistance, not nonadherence, the results will be misleading.

■ Case Study

A.P. is a 36-year-old man who was diagnosed with HIV infection 2 years ago. He has been feeling well for the past 2 years. His viral load has always been undetectable, and he maintains a healthy, active lifestyle by exercising three to four times a week and eating a balanced diet. His medications include a multiple vitamin and occasional omeprazole for heartburn. He has never received antiretroviral therapy. He comes to your office for a routine physical exam and blood work. The physical examination is unremarkable, and the laboratory results are as follows:

Electrolytes, serum creatinine, liver function tests: within normal limits

Complete blood count with differential: within normal limits

CD4+ T-cell count: 210 cells/mm^3

Viral load: 10,000 copies/mL

Diagnosis: asymptomatic HIV infection

1. List specific goals for treatment for this patient.

2. What drug therapy would you prescribe? Why?

3. What are the parameters for monitoring success of the therapy?

4. Discuss specific patient education based on the prescribed therapy.

5. List one or two adverse reactions for the selected agents that would cause you to change therapy.

6. What would be the choice for the second-line therapy?

7. What dietary and lifestyle changes should be recommended for this patient?

8. Describe one or two drug–drug or drug–food interactions for the selected agents.

Bibliography

Starred references are cited in the text.

Abramowitz, M. (2004). Drugs for HIV infection. *Treatment Guidelines from the Medical Letter, 2*(17), 1–8.

Ammassari, A., Trotta, M. P., Murri, R., et al. (2002). Correlates and predictors of adherence to highly active antiretroviral therapy: Overview of published literature. *Journal of Acquired Immunodeficiency Syndrome, 31*(3), S123–S127.

Bartlett, J. G. (2003). Antiretroviral therapy. In J. G. Bartlett & J. E. Gallant (Eds.), *Medical management of HIV infection* (pp. 82–89, 344, 345). Baltimore: Johns Hopkins University.

*Centers for Disease Control and Prevention. (1992). 1993 revised classification system for HIV infection and expanded surveillance case definition for AIDS among adolescents and adults. *Morbidity and Mortality Weekly Report, 41*(RR-17), 1–19.

*Centers for Disease Control and Prevention. (1995). Update: HIV-2 infection among blood and plasma donors—United States, June

1992–June 1995. *Morbidity and Mortality Weekly Report, 44* (32), 603–606.

*Centers for Disease Control and Prevention. (2002). Updated U.S. public health service guidelines for the management of occupational exposures to HBV, HCV, and HIV and recommendations for postexposure prophylaxis. *Morbidity and Mortality Weekly Report, 50*(RR-11), 1–52.

Centers for Disease Control and Prevention. (2002). *HIV/AIDS Surveillance Report, 14,* 1–40.

*Centers for Disease Control and Prevention National Center for Health Statistics (2004). *U.S. life expectancy at all-time high, but infant mortality increases.* [On-line]. Available: http://www.cdc.gov/nchs/releases/04news/infantmort.htm.

Cervia, J. S., & Smith, M. A. (2003). Enfuvirtide (T-20): A novel human immunodeficiency virus type 1 fusion inhibitor. *Clinical Infectious Diseases, 37,* 1102–1106.

*Connor, E. M., Sperling, R. S., Gelber, R., et al. (1994). Reduction of maternal-infant transmission of human immunodeficiency virus type 1 with zidovudine treatment. Pediatric AIDS Clinical Trials Group Protocol 076 Study Group. *New England Journal of Medicine, 331,* 1173–1180.

Lacy, C. F., Armstrong, L. L., Goldman, M. P., et al. (2004). *Drug information handbook* (12th ed.). Hudson, OH: Lexi-Comp.

*Panel on Clinical Practices for Treatment of HIV Infection. (2004). *Guidelines for use of antiretroviral agents in adults and adolescents.* [On-line]. Available: http://AIDSinfo.nih.gov.

*Public Health Service Task Force. (2003). Recommendations for use of antiretroviral drugs in pregnant HIV-1 infected women for maternal health and interventions to reduce perinatal HIV-1 transmission in the United States. [On-line]. Available: http://AIDSinfo.nih.gov.

*Reynolds, N. R. (1998). Initiatives to get HIV-infected patients to adhere to their treatment regimens. *Drug Benefit, 10* (11), 23–25, 29–30, 32.

*Schacker, T., Collier, A. C., Hughes, J., et al. (1996). Clinical and epidemiologic features of primary HIV infection. *Annals of Internal Medicine, 125,* 257–264.

Sperling, R. S., Shapiro, D. E., Coombs, R. W., et al. (1996). Maternal viral load, zidovudine treatment, and the risk of transmission of human immunodeficiency virus type 1 from mother to infant. *New England Journal of Medicine, 335,* 1621–1629.

*World Health Organization (WHO). (2004). *Global Summary of the HIV/AIDS epidemic, December 2002.* [On-line]. Available: http:// who.int/hiv/pub/epidemiology/epi2002/en/.

*Working Group on Antiretroviral Therapy and Medical Management of HIV-Infected Children. (2004). *Guidelines for the use of antiretroviral agents in pediatric HIV infection.* [On-line]. Available: http://AIDSinfo.nih.gov.

Visit the Connection web site for the most up-to-date drug information.

53

OPPORTUNISTIC INFECTIONS IN IMMUNOCOMPROMISED PATIENTS

■ EDINA ADVIC AND AMY S. MORGAN

People with impaired immune function, such as those infected with human immunodeficiency virus (HIV), are at risk for development of infections from microorganisms that rarely cause disease in immunocompetent hosts. These infections are called *opportunistic infections*. Bacteria, fungi, viruses, and protozoa cause opportunistic infections. Examples of opportunistic infectious agents include *Mycobacterium avium-intracellulare* complex (MAC), *Pneumocystis carinii*, cytomegalovirus (CMV), and *Toxoplasma gondii*. In the early years of the acquired immunodeficiency syndrome (AIDS) epidemic, opportunistic infections were a significant cause of morbidity and mortality. Since then, the quality of life for those infected with HIV has improved dramatically, and their life spans have lengthened considerably because of early detection and treatment of opportunistic infections, prevention of opportunistic infections through prophylactic regimens, and the use of highly active antiretroviral therapy (HAART). HAART has had a major impact on the incidence of opportunistic infections and is considered to be the most effective method for preventing them (Centers for Disease Control and Prevention [CDC], 2002). However, not all patients receive HAART. Therefore, effective prevention, detection, and treatment of opportunistic infections are still important.

CAUSES

Several microorganisms cause opportunistic infections in HIV-infected patients (Table 53-1), but three factors determine the likelihood of a microorganism causing disease. First and most important is the patient's immune status. HIV causes a decrease in the number of CD4$^+$ T lymphocytes, also known as T-helper lymphocytes. The risk for development of an opportunistic infection is inversely related to the CD4$^+$ T-lymphocyte count. A normal CD4$^+$ T-lymphocyte count is between 500 and 1400 cells/mm^3. The CD4$^+$ T-lymphocyte count at which a particular opportunistic infection occurs varies, depending on the microorganism (see Table 53-1).

Second, exposure to the microorganism is necessary for development of disease. Most opportunistic infections result from reactivation of latent infections. Latent infections occur when a person is exposed to an organism but does not develop active disease because the immune system can control the organism. However, when immune function declines, the organism is no longer controlled and active disease results. *P. carinii* pneumonia (PCP) and CMV infections are examples of reactivation diseases. Opportunistic infections also can result from recent exposures to microorganisms. Infections caused by MAC and *Cryptococcus neoformans* typically occur after recent exposure.

Third, the risk of development of a specific opportunistic infection depends on whether primary and secondary chemoprophylactic regimens targeted at specific microorganisms were used. Primary prophylactic drug regimens prevent first episodes of infection in patients with risk factors for that specific opportunistic infection. Secondary prophylactic drug regimens prevent the recurrence of infection after a patient has been treated for active infection. Patients receiving appropriate prophylactic regimens are less likely to acquire opportunistic infections.

PATHOPHYSIOLOGY

Opportunistic pathogens target several different anatomic sites. Because of decreased immune function, pathogens are able to replicate freely. The types of infections most commonly caused by opportunistic pathogens are outlined in Table 53-1. This chapter focuses on four opportunistic infections for which many patients receive prophylactic and therapeutic drug regimens in the ambulatory care setting—PCP, disseminated infection with MAC, CMV disease, and candidiasis.

PNEUMOCYSTIS CARINII PNEUMONIA

Although originally classified as a protozoan, *P. carinii* appears to be related more closely to the fungi. The incidence

Table 53.1

Causative Organisms of Opportunistic Infections

Organism	Most Common Types of Infection
Infections Occurring at a CD4$^+$ T-lymphocyte Count <500 Cells/mm^3	
Candida albicans	Oropharyngeal and esophageal
Mycobacterium tuberculosis (reactivation disease)	Pulmonary in early HIV
	Pulmonary and extrapulmonary in late HIV
Herpes zoster	Skin, with a dermatomal distribution
Infections Occurring at a CD4$^+$ T-lymphocyte Count <200 Cells/mm^3	
Cryptococcus neoformans	Meningitis
Herpes simplex	Orolabial, genital, and anorectal
Pneumocystis carinii	Pneumonia
Infections Occurring at a CD4$^+$ T-lymphocyte Count <100 Cells/mm^3	
M. tuberculosis (primary disease)	Pulmonary and extrapulmonary
Toxoplasma gondii	Encephalitis
Infections Occurring at a CD4$^+$ T-lymphocyte Count <50 Cells/mm^3	
Cytomegalovirus disease	Retinitis
	Encephalitis and polyradiculopathy
	Colitis
Mycobacterium avium complex	Disseminated disease

of PCP has declined since the beginning of the AIDS epidemic. However, it continues to be a concern because the mortality rate is 10% to 20% (Chaisson, 1999). Transmission appears to occur through inhalation of airborne pathogens.

DIAGNOSTIC CRITERIA

Usually, *P. carinii* affects the lungs. Extrapulmonary infection is uncommon. Early in the disease, patients may complain of unexplained fever and fatigue. As PCP progresses, patients experience persistent fever, shortness of breath, and a nonproductive cough that may be gradual or acute in onset. Physical examination reveals fever, tachypnea, tachycardia, and bibasilar rales.

Chest radiography findings may be normal during the early stages of disease, but as the disease progresses, diffuse bilateral interstitial infiltrates appear on the radiographs. Because *P. carinii* cannot be grown on culture media, laboratory diagnosis is usually made by examination of the sputum with special stains. Sputum is most commonly obtained through induction or bronchoalveolar lavage.

INITIATING DRUG THERAPY

Pharmacotherapy is used for both prevention and treatment of PCP. The CDC recommends chemoprophylaxis against PCP in patients with a CD4$^+$ T-lymphocyte count of fewer than 200 cells/mm^3, those with a history of oropharyngeal candidiasis (primary prophylaxis), or those who have experienced a prior episode of PCP (secondary prophylaxis).

Prompt initiation of therapy is important with active PCP because outcome is related to the severity of illness at the time drug therapy is initiated.

Goals of Drug Therapy

The goal of chemoprophylactic therapy is to prevent the occurrence or recurrence of PCP. Depending on the regimen, chemoprophylaxis has been effective in 90% of patients (Masur, 2003). Primary or secondary prophylaxis should be discontinued in patients receiving HAART with a CD4$^+$ T-lymphocyte count greater than 200 cells/mm^3 for 3 months or longer.

The goal of therapy for active disease is eradication of infection and reduction of clinical signs and symptoms of disease. Clinical response is usually seen in 4 to 8 days after treatment begins.

Trimethoprim–Sulfamethoxazole

Trimethoprim–sulfamethoxazole (Bactrim [TMP-SMZ]) is the gold standard therapy for both prevention and treatment of PCP. In addition, TMP-SMZ also provides prophylactic coverage against *T. gondii* and bacterial respiratory pathogens. Several different dosage regimens are used (Table 53-2). Dosage adjustment is required for renal dysfunction.

Adverse Events

Adverse effects of TMP-SMZ are common in HIV-infected patients and lead to drug discontinuation in 25% of patients (Masur, 2000). The most common adverse events are rash, pruritus, nausea, vomiting, fever, neutropenia, and thrombocytopenia. Mild to moderate skin reactions usually can be managed with antipyretics or antihistamines. Severe skin reactions and hematologic toxicity may require discontinuation of drug therapy. A complete blood count (CBC), electrolyte evaluations, liver function tests, and serum creatinine analyses should be monitored 2 to 3 times weekly after initiating TMP-SMZ for treating PCP; less frequent monitoring is required when the drug is used as prophylaxis. Because of its superior efficacy, TMP-SMZ therapy should be continued in patients with a non–life-threatening intolerance to the drug. If therapy is discontinued secondary to a non–life-threatening intolerance, it may be reinitiated through dose escalation.

Table 53.2

Overview of Selected Drugs Used to Prevent and Treat PCP

Generic (Trade) Name and Dosage	Selected Adverse Events	Contraindications	Special Considerations
trimethoprim–sulfamethoxazole (Bactrim, Septra) *Prevention* 1 SS or DS tab PO qd *or* 1 DS tab 3×/wk* *Treatment* (outpatient) 15 mg/kg/d of TMP component divided q6-8h	Rash, pruritus, fever, nausea, vomiting, diarrhea, anemia, leukopenia, elevated liver function tests	Prior life-threatening hypersensitivity reaction	Daily prophylaxis may be preferred to 3×/wk because protective against *T. gondii*. Use with caution in G6PD-deficient patients. Dosage adjustment required for renal dysfunction
dapsone *Prevention* 50 mg bid or 100 mg qd *or* 50 mg qd† *or* 200 mg† qwk *Treatment* 100 mg qd + TMP 15 mg/ kg divided q6-8h	Hemolytic anemia, methemoglobinemia, neutropenia	G6PD deficiency Life-threatening hypersensitivity reaction to TMP-SMZ or other sulfa-containing drugs	
aerosolized pentamidine (NebuPent) *Prevention* 300 mg/mo	Cough, metallic taste, bronchospasm		Must be administered with the Respigard II nebulizer. Pulmonary tuberculosis should be ruled out before use.
atovaquone (Mepron) *Prevention* 1500 mg qd *Treatment* 750 mg bid	Rash (transient)		Must be administered with food (preferably with high fat content)
clindamycin (Cleocin) + primaquine *Treatment* clindamycin 300–450 mg q6h + primaquine 15–30 mg qd	Rash, diarrhea, fever, hemolytic anemia	G6PD deficiency	

*SS tab = single-strength tablet (80 mg/400 mg TMP-SMZ); DS tab = double-strength tablet (180 mg/800 mg TMP-SMZ).
†Pyrimethamine 50–75 mg/wk should be added for prophylaxis against *T. gondii;* leucovorin 25 mg/wk should be added for protection against hematologic toxicity.

Interactions

TMP-SMZ increases the therapeutic effect of warfarin (Coumadin). Concomitant use may result in significant bleeding episodes. The international normalized ratio should be monitored with concomitant use, and the warfarin dosage should be adjusted as required.

Dapsone

Dapsone is used for preventing and treating PCP. In many situations, dapsone may be combined with pyrimethamine (Daraprim) when used for chemoprophylaxis to provide protection against both PCP and *T. gondii*. Dapsone must be combined with trimethoprim (Proloprim) to provide adequate efficacy for the treatment of active PCP. Dosage regimens for prophylaxis and treatment are listed in Table 53-2.

Adverse Events

Hematologic adverse events, which occur in 5% to 10% of patients receiving dapsone, include hemolytic anemia, methemoglobinemia, neutropenia, and thrombocytopenia (Warren et al., 1997). Hemolytic anemia usually occurs at doses exceeding 200 mg/d. Patients with significant glucose-6-phosphate dehydrogenase (G6PD) deficiency are at partic-ular risk for hemolytic anemia. Those with a high probability of G6PD deficiency, such as people of Mediterranean descent, should probably be screened for this deficiency before dapsone therapy is initiated. Other adverse events include rash and fever.

Interactions

Concomitant use of dapsone and didanosine (Videx) decreases serum concentrations of dapsone and may result in therapeutic failure. Therefore, administration of these drugs should be separated by 2 hours.

Pentamidine

Pentamidine (NebuPent, Pentam 300) is a second-line agent used for preventing and treating PCP. Pentamidine is administered by inhalation for prophylaxis and intravenously for treatment. The intravenous preparation requires dosage adjustment for renal dysfunction. The prophylactic regimen is outlined in Table 53-2.

Aerosolized pentamidine is well tolerated and results in drug discontinuation in only 2% to 4% of cases (Chaisson, 1999). A few patients may experience bronchospasm, cough, and a metallic taste with drug administration. Intravenous pentamidine can cause life-threatening adverse events, including nephrotoxicity, hypoglycemia, pancreatitis, and cardiac dysrhythmias.

Atovaquone

Atovaquone (Mepron) was initially used only for treating mild to moderate PCP. However, studies have demonstrated efficacious prophylactic use of the drug. Atovaquone blood levels increase significantly when the drug is administered with food, especially foods with a high fat content. In fact, therapeutic failure may result if atovaquone is not administered with meals. Table 53-2 outlines atovaquone dosage regimens.

Atovaquone is one of the best-tolerated PCP treatment drugs. The most common adverse event is a transient rash that usually does not require discontinuation of the drug. Some patients may find the liquid preparation unpalatable. Rifampin and rifabutin may decrease atovaquone serum concentrations. Concomitant use should be avoided.

Clindamycin and Primaquine

Clindamycin (Cleocin) and primaquine are used in combination for treating mild PCP when TMP-SMZ cannot be tolerated. Because the regimen involves two drugs and several doses a day, administration may be difficult for some patients (see Table 53-2).

Adverse effects also make this regimen problematic. Rash, diarrhea, and hepatic dysfunction occur in HIV-infected patients receiving clindamycin. Pseudomembranous colitis can result from clindamycin use and should be considered in patients experiencing diarrhea. Adverse effects of primaquine are usually mild and include fever and rash. Persons should be screened for G6PD deficiency because hemolytic anemia may occur with primaquine use.

Trimetrexate

Trimetrexate (Neutrexin) is a third-line agent used for treating PCP. It is available for intravenous administration only. Dosage adjustment is required for renal dysfunction.

The primary adverse event associated with trimetrexate is neutropenia. Leucovorin (Wellcovorin) is administered with trimetrexate to prevent neutropenia. Neutropenia can be alleviated by increasing doses of leucovorin or by decreasing the dose of trimetrexate.

Selecting the Most Appropriate Agent

Initial drug selection for both preventing and treating PCP is based on efficacy. The choice between oral or parenteral agents depends on the severity of disease. In general, patients with a partial pressure of oxygen (PaO_2) above 80 mm Hg are considered to have mild to moderate disease and can usually be treated with oral agents. Patients with a PaO_2 below 80 mm Hg and should be hospitalized and may require intravenous therapy. A survival benefit has been demonstrated in patients with severe disease who receive corticosteroids in addition to antimicrobial therapy. Table 53-3 provides PCP chemoprophylaxis and treatment, and Figure 53-1 outlines PCP treatment.

First-Line Therapy

TMP-SMZ is the drug of choice for preventing and treating PCP because of its superior efficacy. Every attempt should be made to reinstitute TMP-SMZ in patients with previous drug intolerance unless the adverse events were life-threatening.

Second-Line Therapy

For chemoprophylaxis, dapsone is used in patients who cannot tolerate TMP-SMZ; more than 60% of patients in this group tolerate dapsone. Dapsone has demonstrated protective efficacy against PCP and, unlike aerosolized pentamidine, achieves systemic drug levels and protects patients against extrapulmonary disease. Pyrimethamine may be added to dapsone to provide protection against toxoplasmosis.

For treatment, several second-line agents with efficacy similar to that of TMP-SMZ are available. The choice of drug depends on severity of disease, adverse effect profile, and drug adherence issues.

Dapsone/TMP and atovaquone are available in oral dosage forms only. Pentamidine is available for parenteral administration. The combination of dapsone and TMP is well tolerated and used commonly to treat mild to moderate PCP. Multiple daily doses of TMP may become an adherence issue in some patients. Atovaquone should be used only in patients with mild to moderate, stable disease. Patients must have a functional gastrointestinal (GI) tract because absorption of atovaquone is variable. Intravenous pentamidine is used in patients with severe disease. Adverse effects limit pentamidine use, and all attempts should be made to use TMP-SMZ first.

Table 53.3

Recommended Order of Prophylaxis Against PCP

Order	Agents	Comments
First line	Trimethoprim–sulfamethoxazole	Always the drug of choice because of superior efficacy, tolerance, and cost Provides protection against *T. gondii* and other bacterial pathogens
Second line	Dapsone ± pyrimethamine	Less expensive than third-line agents Pyrimethamine should be added to some regimens (see Table 53-2)

Third line	Aerosolized pentamidine (AP) *or* atovaquone	Choice depends on clinician and patient choice:
		  AP is administered monthly.
		  AP does not provide systemic protection against *P. carinii*.
		  Atovaquone may be unpalatable to some patients and must be administered
		    with food.

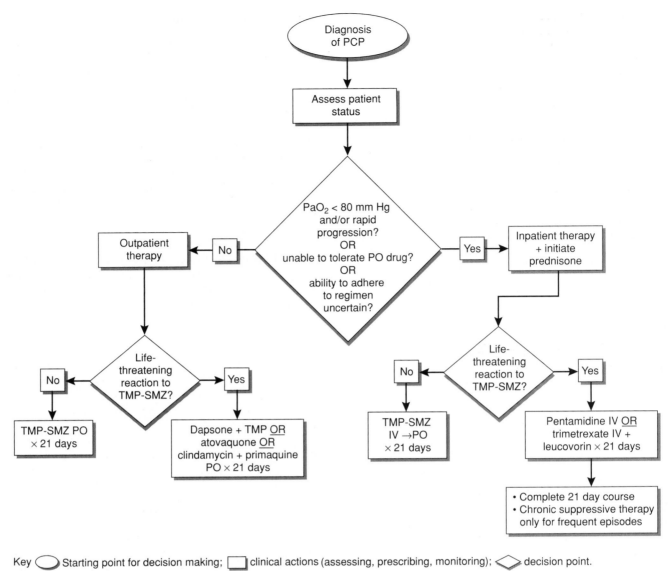

Key ◯ Starting point for decision making; ▭ clinical actions (assessing, prescribing, monitoring); ◇ decision point.

Figure 53–1   Treatment algorithm for *Pneumocystis carinii* pneumonia.

Third-Line Therapy

For chemoprophylaxis, aerosolized pentamidine is considered a third-line agent because it does not provide systemic drug levels like oral regimens, nor does it protect against extrapulmonary infections. In addition, it does not provide protection against other pathologic processes, such as toxoplasmosis. A once-daily dose of atovaquone appears to be effective for preventing PCP. However, it is more expensive than other oral regimens and may be unpalatable to some patients.

For treatment, the combination of clindamycin and primaquine is an option for patients with mild to moderate disease who cannot tolerate TMP-SMZ or dapsone. The number of daily doses required and the adverse effects associated with this regimen may make it impractical for some patients. Trimetrexate is usually reserved for patients with severe disease who have failed or who are intolerant to TMP-SMZ and pentamidine because it is less efficacious and drug administration is difficult.

Special Population Considerations

Pediatric

P. carinii pneumonia was the most common opportunistic infection in children before the use of prophylactic regimens. All newborns of HIV-infected mothers should receive PCP prophylaxis beginning at 4 to 6 weeks of age until HIV infection has been excluded in the infant, or for 1 year. After 1 year, the need for prophylaxis is based on age and the $CD4^+$ T-lymphocyte count as outlined by the CDC. Children with a prior episode of PCP should receive lifelong chemoprophylaxis. TMP-SMZ is the drug of choice for both prevention and treatment of PCP in children.

Women

Pregnant women should receive prophylaxis for PCP. The drug of choice is TMP-SMZ, followed by dapsone. Because of possible teratogenicity associated with drug use in the first trimester of pregnancy, some practitioners may withhold prophylaxis during this time. Others choose to administer aerosolized pentamidine because minimal systemic absorption occurs. Treatment of PCP in pregnancy should be individualized. Therapy should be chosen in consultation with an HIV specialist.

MONITORING PATIENT RESPONSE

Because the prognosis of PCP depends on the severity of disease when therapy is initiated, patients taking the drug as chemoprophylaxis should be taught to recognize symptoms of PCP and instructed to seek medical attention even for mild symptoms. Signs and symptoms of disease should be evaluated 2 to 3 times a week while the patient is receiving treatment for active PCP. Arterial blood gases and chest radiography are not necessary unless the patient's clinical status deteriorates. Chest radiographs obtained after therapy is completed may be useful for future comparison.

MYCOBACTERIUM AVIUM-INTRACELLULARE COMPLEX INFECTION

Mycobacterium avium-intracellulare complex is composed of two species of bacteria–*Mycobacterium avium* and *Mycobacterium intracellulare*. These bacterial organisms are ubiquitous in the environment, and transmission of MAC is thought to occur from the environment to the patient.

DIAGNOSTIC CRITERIA

Disseminated disease is the most common presentation of MAC in patients with AIDS. Patients experience persistent fever, night sweats, fatigue, weight loss, diarrhea, and abdominal pain.

Abnormal laboratory findings may include neutropenia and thrombocytopenia in patients with bone marrow involvement. Isolation of MAC from sputum and stool cultures is usually not helpful in diagnosing disease because MAC colonization is common.

Diagnosis is usually made when symptoms are present and MAC is isolated from blood, bone marrow, or other sterile sites. Drug susceptibility testing on MAC isolates is usually not warranted unless drug resistance is likely, patients fail to respond to initial therapy, or if relapse occurs.

INITIATING DRUG THERAPY

Pharmacotherapy is used for both preventing and treating disseminated MAC disease. Disseminated MAC infection develops in up to 40% of HIV-infected patients within 2 years of the diagnosis of AIDS without effective chemoprophylaxis (Karakousis et al., 2004). Therefore, primary prophylaxis is recommended in patients with a CD4$^+$ T-lymphocyte count of fewer than 50 cells/mm^3. Before initiating chemoprophylaxis, an appropriate evaluation is completed to ensure the patient does not have active MAC infection. Treatment is initiated with clinical and laboratory evidence of disseminated MAC disease.

Goals of Drug Therapy

The goal of chemoprophylaxis is to prevent the development of disseminated MAC infection. Depending on the regimen, chemoprophylaxis decreases the incidence of MAC disease by up to 69%. Some clinicians may choose to discontinue primary prophylaxis in patients receiving HAART with a CD4$^+$ T-lymphocyte count of greater than 100 cells/mm^3 for longer than 3 months (CDC, 2002).

The goal of pharmacotherapy for active disease is to eliminate symptoms and eradicate the infection. Symptomatic and bacteriologic improvement should occur within 2 to 4 weeks. The time to response may be longer with extensive disease. Chronic maintenance therapy (secondary prophylaxis) with full doses of drugs effective against MAC is required to prevent recurrence of disease. In the absence of signs and symptoms of MAC, secondary prophylaxis can be discontinued if patients have completed 12 months of MAC therapy and have a sustained increase in CD4$^+$ T-lymphocyte count greater than 100 cells/mm^3 in response to HAART.

Macrolides

Azithromycin (Zithromax) and clarithromycin (Biaxin) are used for prevention and treatment of disseminated MAC disease. Dosage regimens for each agent differ and are listed in Table 53-4. Clarithromycin dosage adjustment is required for renal dysfunction.

The most common adverse effects of the macrolides are GI problems and include nausea, vomiting, diarrhea, and abdominal pain. In addition, some patients may complain of altered taste while receiving clarithromycin. GI disturbances may resolve when medication is administered with food unless the medication is azithromycin, in which case capsules must be administered on an empty stomach (see Table 53-4).

Clarithromycin is an inhibitor of the hepatic cytochrome P450 enzyme system. Therefore, several important drug interactions may occur. Azithromycin is less likely to interact with concomitant drugs because it is has less effect on the cytochrome P450 enzyme system compared with clarithromycin. However, caution should be used with concomitant use of drugs metabolized by the same pathway. Table 53-5 outlines important drug interactions that occur with the macrolides.

Ethambutol

Ethambutol (Myambutol) is used in combination with other agents for treating disseminated MAC disease. Table 53-4 lists the ethambutol dosage regimen. Dosage adjustment is required in patients with severe renal dysfunction.

Ethambutol is well tolerated by most patients. The most important adverse effect is a dose-related optic neuritis, which is characterized by blurred vision, "floaters" in the visual field, and red/green color blindness. Optic neuritis is unusual with doses less than 20 mg/kg/d. Visual acuity should be assessed at baseline and at each visit, and patients should be interviewed at each visit to assess new visual complaints. Aluminum- and magaldrate-containing antacids decrease the absorption of ethambutol. Therefore, ethambutol should be administered 2 hours before or after these agents.

Overview of Selected Drugs Used to Prevent and Treat Disseminated MAC Disease

Generic (Trade) Name and Dosage	Selected Adverse Events	Contraindications	Special Considerations
azithromycin (Zithromax) *Prevention* 1200 mg/wk *Treatment* 500 mg qd	Diarrhea, nausea, abdominal pain	Concomitant use with pimozide, cisapride	Capsules must be administered 1 h before or 2 h after food. Tablets may be administered with or without food.
clarithromycin (Biaxin) *Prevention/treatment* 500 mg bid	Diarrhea, nausea, abdominal pain, abnormal taste	Same as above	Drug interactions Dosage adjustment required for renal dysfunction.
ethambutol (Myambutol) *Treatment* 15 mg/kg/d	Optic neuritis		Administer 2 h apart from antacids.
rifabutin (Mycobutin) *Prevention/treatment* 300 mg qd	Nausea, vomiting, uveitis, neutropenia	Concomitant use with ritonavir, delavirdine, and saquinavir (hard gel capsule).	Red-orange discoloration of body fluids
ciprofloxacin (Cipro) *Treatment* 750 mg bid	Nausea, vomiting, headache, insomnia		Administer 2 h apart from antacids. Dosage adjustment required with renal dysfunction.
levofloxacin (Levaquin) *Treatment* 500 mg qd	Nausea, vomiting headache, insomnia		Administer 2 h apart from antacids Dosage adjustment required with renal dysfunction
amikacin (Amikin) *Treatment* 10–15 mg/kg IM/IV qd	Nephrotoxicity, ototoxicity	Previous nephrotoxicity or ototoxicity to an amino glycoside	Dosage adjustment required with renal dysfunction and should be based on serum concentrations.

Rifabutin

Rifabutin (Mycobutin) is used for preventing and treating disseminated MAC infections. Table 53-4 lists the dosage regimens for rifabutin.

Rifabutin is usually well tolerated by most patients. Common GI complaints include nausea and vomiting, but taking the drug with food may decrease the nausea. Uveitis is an unusual adverse event that usually occurs at doses of 450 mg/d, or when used concomitantly with drugs that increase rifabutin serum concentrations. Patients complain of eye pain, redness, and blurred vision. Uveitis is treated with topical steroids and cycloplegic and mydriatic eye drops. Drug discontinuation usually is not required unless uveitis does not respond to treatment. Rifabutin may also cause neutropenia. An important counseling point for patients is that rifabutin causes discoloration of body fluid such as urine, sweat, and tears, which may in turn stain contact lenses.

Several important drug interactions occur with rifabutin. It induces the hepatic cytochrome P450 enzyme system and increases the clearance of drugs metabolized through this pathway. In addition, drugs that inhibit this pathway may increase rifabutin serum concentrations. Table 53-5 outlines important rifabutin drug interactions.

Fluoroquinolones

Ciprofloxacin (Cipro) and levofloxacin (Levaquin) are fluoroquinolone antimicrobials. They are used in combination with other drugs for treating disseminated MAC disease. The dosage regimens are outlined in Table 53-4. Dosage adjustment is required for renal dysfunction.

Ciprofloxacin is usually well tolerated. Nausea, vomiting, and diarrhea are the most common adverse events. Rash, headache, and central nervous system effects such as insomnia occur less commonly. Concomitant administration with divalent and trivalent cations, such as those contained in antacids, decreases the absorption of the fluoroquinolones. In fact, serum concentrations may be decreased by 50%, resulting in therapeutic failure. Therefore, both drugs should be administered 2 hours before or after these drugs. Other important drug interactions are outlined in Table 53-5.

Amikacin

Amikacin (Amikin) is an aminoglycoside antimicrobial used in the treatment of disseminated MAC disease. Amikacin is available only for parenteral administration and is usually administered intramuscularly for MAC infection. The dosage regimen is outlined in Table 53-4.

Like other aminoglycosides, the most common adverse events associated with amikacin are nephrotoxicity and ototoxicity. Risk factors for toxicity include increasing age, elevated amikacin serum concentrations, preexisting renal dysfunction, ototoxicity, and concomitant use of nephrotoxins or ototoxins. Baseline serum creatinine and blood urea nitrogen levels should be obtained, followed by periodic monitoring, especially in patients at risk for nephrotoxicity. Periodic serum amikacin levels also should be monitored, and baseline audiometry should be completed. Patients should be interviewed during each visit about hearing loss and vestibular dysfunction (eg, dizziness and vertigo), and audiometry should be repeated as needed.

Selecting the Most Appropriate Agent

Initial drug selection for prevention and treatment of MAC is based on efficacy. Patient tolerance and drug interactions

Table 53.5

Selected Clinically Significant Drug Interactions of MAC Therapy*

MAC Drug	Interacting Drugs	Effect	Recommendation
azithromycin/ clarithromycin	pimozide, cisapride	↑ pimozide and cisapride concentrations; may result in potentially fatal dysrhythmias	Do not use concomitantly.
	HMG-CoA reductase inhibitors (eg, lovastatin)	↑ serum concentrations of antilipid drugs; may result in myopathy	Monitor for myopathy (muscle pain, tenderness, weakness).
	warfarin	↑ anticoagulant effect may occur; bleeding may result	Monitor INR; adjust warfarin dose as required.
ciprofloxacin/levofloxacin	Divalent and trivalent cations: antacids, didanosine, sucralfate, multivitamins, iron and calcium products	↓ absorption of the fluoroquinolones may result in therapeutic failure	Administer these agents 2 h before or after fluoroquinolone
ciprofloxacin	theophylline	↑ theophylline concentration; possible toxicity	Monitor for signs of theophylline toxicity and serum concentrations, adjust doses as needed.
	warfarin	↑ anticoagulant effect may occur; bleeding may result	Monitor international normalized ratio (INR), adjust warfarin dose as required.
clarithromycin	atazanavir	↑ clarithromycin concentration	↓ clarithromycin dose by 50%
	carbamazepine	↑ carbamazepine concentrations; potential toxicity	Avoid combination if possible, monitor carbamazepine concentrations.
	fluoxetine	↑ fluoxetine concentrations	Monitor for adverse effects.
	Protease inhibitors[†]	↑ clarithromycin concentrations	Clarithromycin dosage adjustment required only with preexisting renal impairment.
	rifabutin	↑ rifabutin concentrations; ↑ risk uveitis	Monitor for uveitis (eye redness, blurred vision).
	rifampin/rifabutin	↓ clarithromycin concentrations	Clinical significance unknown.
	theophylline	↑ theophylline concentration; possible toxicity	Monitor for signs of theophylline toxicity and serum concentrations, adjust doses as needed.
rifabutin	clarithromycin	See above	See above
	delavirdine	↑ rifabutin concentrations; ↑ risk uveitis ↑ delavirdine concentrations	Do not use concomitantly.
	Oral contraceptives	May ↑ metabolism of estrogen and ↓ efficacy	Use alternative birth control methods.
	efavirenz	↓ rifabutin concentrations	Consider increasing rifabutin dose to 450–600 mg qd.
	fluconazole, ketoconazole, itraconazole	↑ rifabutin concentrations, ↑ risk uveitis	Monitor for uveitis (eye redness, blurred vision).
	variconazole	↑ rifabutin concentrations ↓ variconizole concentrations	Concomitant use contraindicated
	Protease inhibitors[†]	↓ Protease inhibitor concentrations	Do not use rifabutin concomitantly with saquinavir (hard gel capsule)
		↑ rifabutin concentration	Lower rifabutin dose is required when used with regimens containing amprenavir, indinavir, nelfinavir, or ritonavir.

*Note: This list is not all-inclusive. A drug interaction review should be performed each time a drug is added to a regimen containing these drugs.
[†]Protease inhibitors: amprenavir, indinavir, nelfinavir, saquinavir, ritonavir.
↑ = increased; ↓ = decreased.

are secondary considerations. The approach to prophylaxis and treatment is outlined in Figure 53-2 and Table 53-6.

First-Line Therapy

Based on efficacy, clarithromycin and azithromycin are the agents of choice for chemoprophylaxis. An additional benefit of these agents is the protection provided against bacterial pathogens as well as MAC. The choice between clarithromycin and azithromycin is usually based on drug tolerance, convenience, drug interactions, and cost. For example, some patients may prefer azithromycin because it is administered once weekly rather than twice a day, as with clarithromycin.

Treatment of active disease should always consist of at least two drugs because antimicrobial resistance occurs rapidly with monotherapy. Current recommendations for treating disseminated MAC disease are a combination of a macrolide and ethambutol with or without rifabutin. The decision about which macrolide to use is based on the same

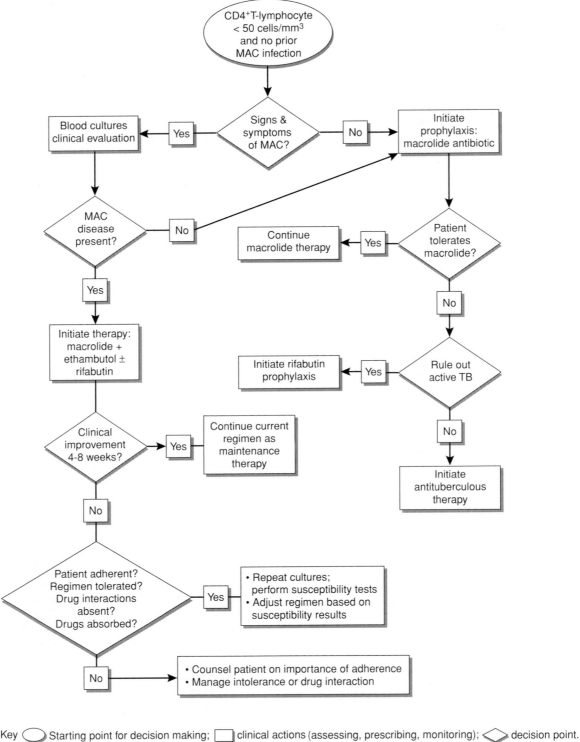

Figure 53–2 Prophylaxis and treatment algorithm for *Mycobacterium avium* complex infection.

considerations as chemoprophylaxis. Clinical trials show conflicting data regarding whether adding rifabutin to the drug combination is beneficial.

Second-Line Therapy

Rifabutin is recommended for chemoprophylaxis only if a macrolide cannot be tolerated because it is less effective.

Because rifabutin is in a class of drugs used to treat tuberculosis and use of it alone may cause *Mycobacterium tuberculosis* to become resistant to these drugs, active tuberculosis should be ruled out before initiating rifabutin chemoprophylaxis.

The second-line drugs for treating MAC disease are ciprofloxacin and amikacin. These drugs usually are added to the existing regimen if clinical response does not occur

Table 53.6

Recommended Order of Prophylaxis Against Disseminated MAC Disease

Order	Agents	Comments
First line	azithromycin or clarithromycin	Azithromycin can be administered weekly, clarithromycin must be administered bid. Similar tolerance
Second line	rifabutin	Less efficacious than macrolides

within 2 to 4 weeks or if relapse occurs on first-line therapy. Two drugs, rather than one, always should be added to a failing regimen to avoid the emergence of resistance. If rifabutin was not included in the initial regimen, it should be added to a failing regimen in addition to ciprofloxacin or amikacin. No treatment guidelines or formal studies address therapy for the clarithromycin-resistant MAC disease. Some experts suggest a fluoroquinolone plus ethambutol plus rifabutin with or without amikacin.

Some experts recommend that severe cases of MAC bacteremia should be treated with a macrolide and ethambutol plus an additional drug, such as ciprofloxacin, levofloxacin, rifabutin, or amikacin.

Special Population Considerations

Pediatric

Disseminated MAC infection occurs in children with advanced HIV disease. The CDC has developed recommendations for initiation of prophylaxis based on age and CD4$^+$ T-lymphocyte count. Macrolides are the preferred agents for prophylaxis. A drug regimen with three to five agents is used for treating active infection. The drugs used in children include macrolides, rifabutin, amikacin, ethambutol, and ciprofloxacin. Children with a history of disseminated MAC should have lifelong prophylaxis to prevent recurrence. The safety of discontinuing MAC prophylaxis among children whose CD4$^+$ T-lymphocyte counts have increased in response to HAART has not been studied (CDC, 2002).

Women

Recommendations for MAC prophylaxis in pregnant women are the same as those provided in the section on Selecting the Most Appropriate Agent. However, some practitioners may choose to avoid prophylaxis during the first trimester because drug administration during this period has been associated with teratogenicity. Azithromycin is the drug of choice for prophylaxis. Animal studies with clarithromycin have shown teratogenicity. Therefore, it should be used cautiously. Azithromycin and ethambutol is the drug regimen of choice for chronic maintenance therapy.

MONITORING PATIENT RESPONSE

The practitioner should monitor patients for clinical response, such as decreased fever, night sweats, and increased weight within 2 to 4 weeks of initiating therapy. The practitioner should question patients about recurrence of symptoms at each visit.

CYTOMEGALOVIRUS DISEASE

CMV is a herpes virus. CMV disease presents as retinitis in 75% to 85% of patients with AIDS and CMV infection (Martin et al., 1999). Between 75% and 100% percent of HIV-infected patients have serologic evidence of prior CMV infection (latent infection). Most disease is the result of reactivation of latent infection.

DIAGNOSTIC CRITERIA

Patients with CMV retinitis may experience blurring or loss of vision in the central part of their visual field, scotomata (blind spots), floaters, and photophobia. Ophthalmologic examination reveals whitening of the retina with or without hemorrhage. The diagnosis of CMV retinitis is usually made based on clinical findings because of the risks associated with invasive ocular procedures.

INITIATING DRUG THERAPY

Pharmacotherapy is used for prevention and treatment of CMV disease. Primary prophylaxis should be considered in patients who are seropositive for CMV and have a CD4$^+$ T-lymphocyte count under 50 cells/mm^3. However, the evidence to support the use of prophylaxis for CMV is not as convincing as with other opportunistic infections. Therefore, not all clinicians choose to initiate prophylaxis. Because the incidence of CMV has substantially declined with the use of HAART, this is considered one of the best interventions to prevent disease.

Early recognition of signs and symptoms of CMV and prompt initiation of therapy are important for preventing severe CMV retinitis. Patients should be taught to recognize early symptoms of retinitis and seek medical attention immediately. Depending on the regimen, therapy for active disease has two components. Induction therapy is used the first 3 weeks of therapy, followed by maintenance therapy (secondary prophylaxis). Maintenance therapy traditionally has been continued indefinitely. However, the use of HAART has changed this somewhat (discussed later).

Goals of Drug Therapy

The goal of primary prophylaxis is to prevent CMV disease. The goal of induction therapy is to halt the progression of CMV disease and relieve acute inflammation within 4 weeks. Symptoms caused by inflammation usually resolve in 2 to 3 weeks. Vision loss, however, may be irreversible. The goal of maintenance therapy (secondary prophylaxis) is to delay the progression of CMV disease. CMV retinitis usually recurs after several months of maintenance therapy. As noted earlier, the use of HAART has decreased the number of recurrences. Because of this, some practitioners may consider discontinuing maintenance therapy (secondary prophylaxis) in patients receiving HAART with an increase in

Table 53.7

Overview of Selected Drugs Used to Prevent and Treat CMV Retinitis

Generic (Trade) Name and Dosage	Selected Adverse Events	Contraindications	Special Considerations
valganciclovir (Valcyte) Induction 900 mg bid × 14–21 d Maintenance 900 mg qd	Neutropenia, anemia, nausea, vomiting, headache	Same as ganciclovir	Must be administered with food.
ganciclovir, oral (Cytovene) *Prevention/treatment* 1000 mg tid	Neutropenia, thrombocytopenia, diarrhea, vomiting	Sight-threatening CMV disease, platelet count <25,000/mm³, ANC <500/mm³ Hg B < m/dL Dosage adjustment required with renal dysfunction.	Must be administered with food (high-fat preferred).
ganciclovir, intravenous (Cytovene) *Induction* 5 mg/kg q12h × 14–21 d *Maintenance* 5–10 mg/kg/d	Neutropenia, thrombocytopenia	Platelet count <25,000/mm³, ANC <500/mm³	Dosage adjustment required with renal dysfunction.
ganciclovir, intraocular implant (Vitracert) 4.5-mg implant, 1 μg/h release	Blurred vision, retinal detachment, hemorrhage		Concomitant oral ganciclovir or valgenciclovir recommended.
foscarnet (Foscavir) *Induction* 90 mg/kg IV q12h × 14–21 d *Maintenance* 90–120 mg/kg/d IV	Nephrotoxicity, electrolyte imbalances, nausea		Dosage adjustment required with renal dysfunction. Controlled-rate infusion required.
cidofovir (Vistide) *Induction* 5 mg/kg IV each week × 2 weeks *Maintenance* 5 mg/kg IV q2 wk	Nephrotoxicity, uveitis, neutropenia probenicid: rash, fever, nausea, headache	SCr >1.5 mg/dL, CrCl <55 mL/min, 2+ proteinuria	Must be administered with probenicid and normal saline infusions to prevent nephrotoxicity.
fomivirsen (Viravene) 330 μg intravitreally on days 1 and 15, then each month	Intraocular inflammation, ↑ intraocular pressure		

ANC = absolute neutrophil count; HgB = hemoglobin.

CD4$^+$ T-lymphocyte counts exceeding 100 to 150 cells/mm³ for more than 6 months.

Ganciclovir

Ganciclovir/Valganciclovir

Ganciclovir (Cytovene) is used for prevention and treatment of CMV disease. It is available in oral, parenteral, and intraocular forms. All three dosage forms may be used to treat active disease. Oral ganciclovir also is used for prophylaxis. Oral ganciclovir is poorly absorbed and must be administered with food for maximum absorption. Valganciclovir (Valcyte) is available in an oral dosage form and is indicated for the treatment of CMV disease. It is a prodrug that is converted to ganciclovir in the intestine. Valganciclovir achieves serum concentrations similar to intravenous ganciclovir. For this reason and because it has better absorption than oral ganciclovir, valganciclovir has largely replaced parenteral and oral ganciclovir for the treatment of CMV disease. Valganciclovir should be administered with food for optimal absorption. Ganciclovir capsules and valganciclovir tablets are not interchangeable. Table 53-7 lists common dosage regimens for ganciclovir and valganciclovir. Dosage adjustment is required for renal dysfunction for both drugs.

Neutropenia (absolute neutrophil count [ANC] 500 cells/mm³) occurs in 15% to 40% of patients receiving intravenous ganciclovir and is the dose-limiting adverse effect

for both oral and parenteral preparations. Thrombocytopenia and anemia occur in 5% to 10% of patients receiving intravenous ganciclovir (Martin, 2003). Because valganciclovir is a prodrug of ganciclovir, adverse effects are similar. CBCs should be performed twice weekly during induction and every 1 to 2 weeks during maintenance therapy. Neutropenia is managed by coadministration of granulocyte colony-stimulating factor 300 mg/d titrated to 2 to 3 times a week dosing to maintain an ANC greater than 1000 cells/mm³. Ganciclovir should be discontinued for a platelet count of less than 25,000 cells/mm³. Other adverse effects include nausea and vomiting. Diarrhea is more common in patients receiving valganciclovir than ganciclovir. The ganciclovir intraocular implant may result in transient blurred vision, retinal detachment, and hemorrhage.

Foscarnet

Foscarnet (Foscavir) is used for treating CMV disease. Foscarnet is available for intravenous administration only. Induction and maintenance doses are listed in Table 53-7. Dosage adjustment is required for renal dysfunction.

Nephrotoxicity occurs in 10% to 20% of patients and is the major dose-limiting adverse event of foscarnet (Jacobson, 1997). Hydrating the patient with a normal saline infusion before drug administration may decrease the risk for development of nephrotoxicity. Foscarnet also may cause serious metabolic and electrolyte disturbances that include hypocalcemia, hypomagnesia, hypokalemia, and either hypophosphatemia or hyperphosphatemia. Foscarnet should be infused at less than 1.0 mg/kg/min to avoid these adverse effects. Nausea also occurs in 25% to 40% of patients receiving foscarnet (Martin, 2003). Adverse neurologic events include headache, agitation, perioral numbness, tremors, weakness, finger paresthesias, and seizures. Anemia may occur but is less common than with ganciclovir. Foscarnet may cause painful genital ulceration that resolves within 2 weeks of drug discontinuation.

Patients receiving foscarnet should have renal function, electrolyte, magnesium, calcium, and phosphate values monitored weekly. The CBC should be monitored weekly during induction, then every other week during maintenance therapy. Dosage adjustment and mineral and electrolyte replacement should occur as necessary. Drugs that cause nephrotoxicity, such as aminoglycosides and amphotericin B (Fungizone), should be avoided in patients receiving foscarnet.

Cidofovir

Cidofovir (Vistide) is used in treating CMV retinitis. Because it has a prolonged antiviral effect, cidofovir can be dosed intermittently. Induction and maintenance doses are listed in Table 53-7. Dosage adjustment is required with renal dysfunction. The use of cidofovir is contraindicated in patients with a serum creatinine level greater than 1.5 mg/dL, a creatinine clearance of less than 55 mL/min, or 2+ proteinuria on urinalysis.

Nephrotoxicity is the major dose-limiting adverse event of cidofovir and includes significant proteinuria and renal failure. Pretreatment with normal saline and probenecid (Benemid) is required to minimize nephrotoxicity. Probenecid causes rash, fever, nausea, and headache in over 50% of patients. Neutropenia occurs in 15% of patients and can be managed as outlined for ganciclovir. In addition, cidofovir use may result in uveitis and ocular hypotony.

Serum creatinine and electrolyte levels should be measured and a urinalysis should be obtained before each dose of cidofovir. Cidofovir should be discontinued if proteinuria is 2+ or greater or if the serum creatinine level increases by at least 0.5 mg/dL or is greater than 2.0 mg/dL. Ophthalmologic examinations, including measurement of intraocular pressure, should be performed each month. Patients should be questioned regarding the development of red eyes, photophobia, and blurred vision. The drug should be discontinued if the intraocular pressure is 50% below baseline. Cidofovir should not be used concomitantly with nephrotoxins such as aminoglycosides and amphotericin B.

Fomivirsen

Fomivirsen is administered intravitreally for treating CMV retinitis. The dosage regimen is listed in Table 53-7. Fomivirsen administration is associated with intraocular inflammation and elevation in intraocular pressure.

Selecting the Most Appropriate Agent

Oral ganciclovir is the only agent used for prophylaxis of CMV disease. Selection of an antiviral regimen for treating active disease depends on the likelihood of immune reconstitution with HAART, the phase of antiviral therapy (induction versus maintenance), severity of CMV retinitis, antiviral efficacy, patient characteristics in relation to the drug's adverse effects profile, and convenience. Figure 53-3 and Table 53-8 outline the initial treatment of CMV retinitis.

First-Line Therapy

Oral ganciclovir is the only available agent that has been studied for primary prophylaxis of CMV disease. However, many clinicians choose not to use oral ganciclovir for prophylaxis because most patients do not benefit from it. Moreover, there is a potential for development of antiviral resistance because of poor drug absorption and suboptimal serum levels. In addition, the drug is expensive. The efficacy of using prophylactic therapy in the era of HAART is not clear.

First-line agents used for the treatment of CMV retinitis are valganciclovir or intraocular ganciclovir implant plus oral valganciclovir. The main treatment decision is whether to use systemic or local therapy. When considering the use of a local therapy, the risk of a surgical procedure must be weighed against the benefit of having high intraocular drug levels. Many practitioners consider the implant the therapy of choice in patients with immediately sight-threatening disease and in patients who are unlikely to have immune reconstitution with HAART. A systemic therapy such as oral valganciclovir should be combined with the intraocular insert due to increased risk of CMV involvement in the contralateral eye or extraocular CMV disease. When considering systemic therapy, valganciclovir is usually preferred because it can be administered orally rather than the intravenous administration required for other agents (refer to second-line therapy). In patients with a small, peripheral area of retinitis oral valganciclovir in conjunction with the initiation of HAART is the preferred therapy.

Second-Line Therapy

Intravenous therapy is usually considered second-line therapy because it requires placement of a central venous catheter for chronic use for most of the regimens and oral therapy is available and equally effective. The efficacy of intravenous ganciclovir, foscarnet, and cidofovir for treatment of CMV is similar. The decision about which agent to use depends on the adverse events profile of the agent and patient preferences. For instance, a ganciclovir-based regimen is preferred in a patient with renal dysfunction because a common adverse effect of foscarnet and cidofovir is nephrotoxicity. However, foscarnet may be preferred in a person with a low neutrophil or platelet count because ganciclovir may cause neutropenia and thrombocytopenia. Cidofovir may be preferred if convenience is of paramount importance to the patient because it can be administered much less frequently than the other agents and an indwelling catheter is not required.

Third-Line Therapy

Intravitreal fomivirsen with valganciclovir is reserved for patients who have contraindications or intolerance or who have not responded to other therapies.

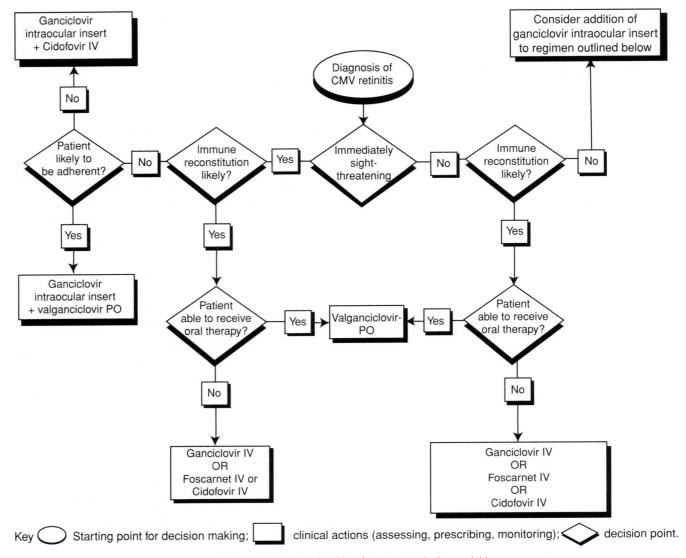

Figure 53–3 Treatment algorithm for cytomegalovirus retinitis.

Table 53.8

Recommended Order for CMV Retinitis

Order	Agents	Comments
First line	Valganciclovir *or* intraocular ganciclovir implant + valganciclovir	Valganciclovir is usually preferred because it can be administered orally. The intraocular insert combination may be preferred in patients with sight-threatening disease or those who are unlikely to have immune reconstitution with HAART.
Second line	Ganciclovir IV *or* foscarnet *or* cidofovir	Ganciclovir is preferred in patients with renal dysfunction. Foscarnet is preferred in patients with bone marrow suppression. Cidofovir is a good choice for patients who desire convenience.
Third line	Intravitreal fomivirsen + valganciclovir	Used only in patients who are intolerant or unresponsive to other therapies.

Special Population Considerations

Pediatric

CMV disease occurs frequently in children with advanced HIV disease. Primary prophylaxis with oral ganciclovir should be considered in children with a $CD4^+$ T-lymphocyte count of less than 50 cells/mm^3. Ganciclovir and foscarnet are the agents used most frequently for treating CMV retinitis in children.

Women

Pregnant women should not receive oral ganciclovir for primary prophylaxis, and this drug should be discontinued if pregnancy occurs because of the limited data available on the effects of this agent during pregnancy. However, because of the risks associated with recurrent CMV disease, chronic maintenance therapy should be continued during pregnancy. The drug regimen should be individualized and made in consultation with an HIV expert (CDC, 2002).

MONITORING PATIENT RESPONSE

The practitioner should teach the patient to monitor for symptoms of disease progression, such as blurred vision, new floaters, or loss of visual field. Dilated funduscopic examinations should be performed once a month.

CANDIDIASIS

Candidiasis is an infection caused by fungi of the *Candida* genus. *Candida albicans* is the most common causative species. *Candida* species commonly colonize the GI tract of humans. Colonization may be transient or progress to disease, depending on immune function and organism virulence. Infection usually occurs on a mucosal surface. The three types of mucocutaneous candidiasis that occur in HIV-infected patients are oropharyngeal, esophageal, and vulvovaginal. Vulvovaginal candidiasis is discussed in Chapter 37.

Oropharyngeal is the most common type of candidiasis; it occurs in up to 90% of patients with HIV infection (Vazquez, 1999). It often is the key event leading to the diagnosis of HIV infection. Although oropharyngeal candidiasis causes little mortality, it can significantly interfere with a patient's quality of life by decreasing the ability to eat, drink, and take medications.

Candidiasis that is refractory or resistant to therapy occurs in approximately 5% to 7% of patients (Powderly, 1999). Risk factors for drug resistance are a $CD4^+$ T-lymphocyte count of less than 50 cells/mm^3 and exposure to chronic antifungal therapy.

DIAGNOSTIC CRITERIA

Patients with oropharyngeal candidiasis may be asymptomatic or may experience a burning pain in the mouth, altered taste, or both. Clinical signs include white plaques on the gums, buccal mucosa, and tongue (often called *thrush*). Patients with esophageal candidiasis complain of difficult and painful swallowing, and oropharyngeal candidiasis usu-

ally is present. Diagnosis of oropharyngeal and esophageal candidiasis is usually made on a clinical basis. The infected site is rarely cultured unless therapeutic failure occurs.

INITIATING DRUG THERAPY

Pharmacotherapy is used primarily for treating acute episodes of oropharyngeal and esophageal candidiasis. The CDC does not recommend primary prophylaxis because treatment of acute disease is highly effective, mucosal disease does not cause death, there are concerns about drug interactions and development of fungal resistance, and because the drug regimens are expensive (CDC, 2002). Many practitioners do not recommend chronic suppressive therapy (secondary prophylaxis) for oropharyngeal candidiasis for the same reasons. However, chronic suppressive therapy should be considered when the patient has a history of frequent or severe episodes of esophageal candidiasis (CDC, 2002).

Goals of Drug Therapy

The goal of pharmacotherapy is resolution of signs and symptoms of candidiasis, as well as resolution or prevention of complications such as decreased oral intake. Between 90% and 100% of patients with oropharyngeal candidiasis show clinical response within 7 days of initiating therapy (Powderly, 1999).

Polyene Antifungals

The polyene antifungals consist of nystatin (Mycostatin) and amphotericin B (Fungizone), and are grouped together based on their mechanism of action. Nystatin is available as a pastille and an oral suspension for topical use. Amphotericin B is available as a parenteral formulation for intravenous administration. Amphotericin B oral solution may be compounded extemporaneously. Table 53-9 outlines dosage and administration guidelines.

Adverse Events

The adverse effects of these drugs vary. Nystatin is bitter tasting and can cause GI upset. Amphotericin B oral suspension may cause nausea and vomiting but does not have a bitter taste. Intravenous amphotericin B is associated with many adverse events. Infusion-related reactions such as fever, rigors, and hypotension may occur within 90 minutes of infusion. Management includes pretreatment with acetaminophen (Tylenol), diphenhydramine (Benadryl), or hydrocortisone. Meperidine (Demerol) is used to treat rigors. Tolerance to infusion-related effects usually occurs. Nephrotoxicity is the most worrisome adverse effect and occurs in up to 80% of patients receiving intravenous amphotericin B. It may be minimized by prehydration with normal saline and by limiting the use of other nephrotoxins, such as aminoglycosides. Nephrotoxicity may cause electrolyte imbalances. Nephrotoxicity usually resolves after drug discontinuation. Phlebitis also may occur with intravenous administration and can be avoided by ensuring that the concentration of amphotericin B does not exceed

Table 53.9

Overview of Selected Drugs Used to Prevent and Treat Candidiasis

Generic (Trade) Name and Dosage	Selected Adverse Events	Contraindications	Special Considerations
Topical Agents			
clotrimazole (Mycelex) 10 mg (1 troche) 5×/d	Nausea, vomiting, taste alteration		Troche should be dissolved slowly in mouth.
nystatin 100,000 U/mL (Mycostatin, Nilstat, Nystex) 5-mL, "swish and swallow" qid	Nausea, vomiting, bitter taste		Suspension should be swished to coat mouth thoroughly, then held for several minutes before swallowing. Administer between meals to promote prolonged contact with oral mucosa.
Systemic Therapy			
fluconazole (Diflucan) 100 mg qd (may be raised to a maximum of 800 mg qd for refractory disease)	Nausea, vomiting, rash, headache, hepatitis (rare)		Dosage adjustment required with renal dysfunction. Drug interactions: refer to Table 53-10. May decrease the effect of oral contraceptives.
itraconazole (Sporanox) *Capsules* 100 mg bid *Solution* 200 mg qd (may be raised to 100–200 mg bid for refractory disease)	Nausea, vomiting, diarrhea, hepatitis (rare)		Capsules and solution are not interchangeable. The solution must be administered 1 h before or 2 h after food. The capsules must be administered with food. Gastric acidity required for absorption. Solution should be swished in mouth for several minutes before swallowing.
caspofungin (Cancidas) 50 mg qd	Headache, nausea, vomiting		Dosage adjustment required with renal dysfunction.
ketoconazole (Nizoral) 200–400 mg bid	Nausea, vomiting, anorexia, rash, impotence and gynecomastia in men, hepatitis	Presence of achlorhydria or concomitant use of H$_2$ blockers or proton pump inhibitors	Gastric acidity required for absorption.
amphotericin B for IV infusion (Fungizone, Amphocin) 0.5–1 mg/kg/d	Nephrotoxicity, infusion-related reactions, phlebitis		Infusion-related reactions may be prevented by pretreatment with acetaminophen, diphenhydramine ± hydrocortisone. Rigors may be treated with mepeidine.
voriconazole (V fend) 100–200 mg bid	Visual disturbances, nausea, vomiting, diarrhea, rash, hepatitis		Tablets must be administred 1h before or after food.

0.1 mg/mL. Some clinicians also add heparin to the intravenous solution to prevent phlebitis.

Interactions

Important drug interactions occur with intravenous amphotericin B. Concomitant use of other nephrotoxins, such as aminoglycosides, increase the risk of amphotericin B–induced nephrotoxicity.

Imidazole Antifungals

Clotrimazole (Mycelex) and ketoconazole (Nizoral) are azole antifungals in the imidazole class. Clotrimazole is available as an oral troche for topical therapy. Ketoconazole is available as a tablet for systemic administration. Drug

absorption of ketoconazole does not occur unless the gastric contents of the stomach are at an acidic pH. Absorption of ketoconazole may be decreased in patients with advanced AIDS because this group tends to have decreased gastric acid secretion. Dosage guidelines are listed in Table 53-9.

The adverse effects of clotrimazole are alteration of taste and GI upset. Ketoconazole decreases serum testosterone concentrations, which may result in gynecomastia and breast tenderness in some men. Resolution occurs in some patients with continued therapy; in other patients, the effect persists until the drug is discontinued. Ketoconazole use is associated with transient increases in liver function test results and, rarely, fatal hepatotoxicity.

Ketoconazole-induced hepatotoxicity usually occurs within the first few months of therapy. Patients should be instructed to report symptoms of hepatotoxicity such as

Table 53.10

Selected Drug Interactions with Azole Antifungal Agents*

Interacting Drug(s)	Azole†	Effect	Management
Antacids Antiulcer agents (eg, cimetidine, ranitidine, omeprazole, etc)	I (capsules) K	↓ absorption of K, I, may result in therapeutic failure	Administer K, I 2 h before or after antacids Concomitant use with antiulcer agents should be avoided.
Anticonvulsants (carbamazepine, phenytoin, phenobarbital)	I, K, V	↓ I, K, and V concentrations, may result in therapeutic failure	Monitor clinical efficacy, ↑ dose of I, K as needed ↑ dose V required with concomitant phenytoin use Concomitant use of V with carbamazepine and phenobarbital contraindicated
Benzodiazepines (BZ) (alprazolam, triazolam)	F, I, K, V	↑ BZ concentration; toxicity may result	Concomitant use contraindicated with I, K Monitor for ↑ sedation, etc with F, V and adjust BZ dose as required
cisapride	F, I, K, V	↑ cisapride concentrations, fatal arrhythmias may result	Concomitant use contraindicated
Didanosine (ddI)	I, K	ddI buffer results in ↓ absorption of I, K	Administer drugs 2 h apart
HMG-CoA reductase inhibitors (eg, lovastatin)	F, I, K, V	↑ concentrations of antilipid drugs; may result in myopathy	Concomitant use with I contraindicated Monitor for myopathy (muscle pain, tenderness, weakness) with F, K, V
Indinavir (IND)	F, K	↑ concentrations of IND	↓ IND dose to 600 mg q8h with concomitant K; dosage adjustment not required for F
Oral contraceptives (OC)	F, K, I	↓ efficacy of OC	Use alternative birth control methods while patient receiving azole
Pimozide	K, I, V	↑ pimozide concentrations, fatal arrhythmias may result	Concomitant use contraindicated
Rifabutin	F, K, I, V	↑ rifabutin concentrations, ↑ risk uveitis ↓ V levels	Monitor for uveitis (eye redness, blurred vision) with F, K, I Concomitant use contraindicated with V
Rifampin	F, K, I, V	↓ azole concentrations, may result in therapeutic failure	Monitor clinical efficacy for F, K, I Concomitant use contraindicated with V
Saquinavir	F, K	↑ saquinavir concentration	No dosage adjustment required
Warfarin	F, K, I, V	↓ warfarin metabolism, ↑ therapeutic effect, may result in bleeding	Monitor international normalized ratio (INR), adjust warfarin dose as required
Zolpidem	K	↑ zolpidem concentrations, toxicity may result	Monitor for excess sedation, etc and adjust dose as required

*Note: This list is not all-inclusive. A drug interaction review should be performed each time a drug is added to a regimen containing these drugs.
†F = fluconazole; I = itraconazole; K = ketoconazole; V = voriconazole

fatigue, persistent nausea and vomiting, abdominal pain, dark urine, and jaundice. Liver function test results should be monitored at baseline, twice weekly during the first 2 months of therapy, and monthly thereafter in patients receiving ketoconazole.

No significant drug interactions have been reported with clotrimazole. Ketoconazole inhibits the hepatic cytochrome P450 enzyme system. Therefore, inhibition of metabolism of drugs administered concomitantly with ketoconazole may result in increased serum levels and toxic effects. In addition, drugs that reduce gastric acidity decrease ketoconazole absorption. Clinically important drug interactions are outlined in Table 53-10.

Triazole Antifungals

Fluconazole (Diflucan), itraconazole (Sporanox) and voriconazole (Vfend) are azole antifungals in the triazole class. Fluconazole is available as a solution for topical use and as a tablet and intravenous formulation for systemic administration. Itraconazole is available as a solution for topical use and as a capsule for systemic administration. Gastric acidity is required for itraconazole absorption. Itraconazole capsules must be administered with food; itraconazole solution must be administered on an empty stomach for maximum absorption. Voriconazole is available as a tablet and intravenous formulation for systemic administra-

Table 53.11

Recommended Order of Treatment for Oropharyngeal Candidiasis

Order	Agents	Comments
First line	Topical therapy (clotrimazole, nystatin) *or* systemic azole (fluconazole, itraconazole, ketoconazole)	Topical therapy may be used first to avoid early exposure to systemic azole therapy. Patient tolerance may be an issue with nystatin. Systemic azoles may be selected for patient convenience.
Second line	Itraconazole oral solution *or* amphotericin B oral suspension	Itraconazole solution is used in patients in whom fluconazole therapy fails. Amphotericin B oral suspension is sometimes effective in patients who do not respond to itraconazole therapy. Amphotericin B oral suspension must be prepared extemporaneously.
Third line	Amphotericin B IV *or* caspofungin	Caspofungin is safe and effective in refractory disease, but it is more expensive than amphotericin B. IV amphotericin B is used last because of difficulty of administration and toxicity.

tion. The intravenous formulation should not be used in patients with a creatinine clearance of less than 55 mL/min because the diluent used in the formulation can accumulate. Dosage adjustment is required for voriconazole in patients with hepatic dysfunction. Table 53-9 outlines dosage and administration guidelines for the triazole agents.

The triazole antifungal agents usually are well tolerated. The most common adverse effects reported with the oral agents are rash, mild to moderate nausea with or without vomiting, and diarrhea. GI disturbances usually resolve when the drug is administered with food. An exception is itraconazole solution, which should not be administered with food. Hepatotoxicity has been reported with the triazole drugs. Fluconazole, itraconazole, and voriconazole can cause transient increases in levels of serum aminotransferases, alkaline phosphatase, and γ-glutamyl transferase, which usually resolve with continued therapy. Occasionally, elevations in liver function test values result in drug discontinuation. Rare cases of clinically significant hepatitis have been reported. As with ketoconazole, patients should be instructed to report symptoms of hepatotoxicity. Voriconazole can cause mild, reversible vision disturbances that include blurred vision, enhanced or altered visual perception, change in color vision, and photophobia.

Like ketoconazole, the triazole drugs inhibit the hepatic cytochrome P450 enzyme system, fluconazole to a lesser extent than itraconazole and voriconazole. The clinically important drug interactions are outlined in Table 53-10.

Echinocandin Antifungals

Caspofungin (Cancidas) is the first echinocandin antifungal available in the United States. It is available for intravenous administration only. Dosage guidelines are listed in Table 53-9. Dosage adjustment is required in patients with hepatic dysfunction.

Caspofungin is well tolerated. The most common adverse effects are headache, nausea, vomiting, and infusion-related reactions. Concomitant administration of caspofungin with efavirenz, nelfinavir, nevirapine, phenytoin, rifampin, dexamethasone, or carbamazepine may result in decreased caspofungin concentrations. An increased caspofungin dose may be required.

Selecting the Most Appropriate Agent

Either topical or systemic therapy may be used for initial treatment of oropharyngeal candidiasis. Efficacy is similar between topical and systemic regimens. However, relapse occurs less frequently with systemic therapy.

Systemic therapy must be used for treating esophageal candidiasis; topical therapy is ineffective. Table 53-11 provides treatment strategies for oropharyngeal candidiasis and Figure 53-4 outlines treatment strategies for esophageal candidiasis.

First-Line Therapy

The first-line agents used to treat oropharyngeal candidiasis are topical clotrimazole or nystatin, or systemic therapy with an azole (fluconazole, itraconazole, or ketoconazole). Itraconazole solution should be selected over capsules due to better absorption. Factors that may be considered when deciding which agent to use include convenience, drug interactions, concern for development of azole resistance, and cost. Recurrent episodes in advanced AIDS may require systemic azole therapy for efficacy. Fluconazole and itraconazole solution are the preferred agents in this situation. Ketoconazole is rarely used due to variable absorption.

The first-line therapy for esophageal candidiasis is a systemic azole. Oral fluconazole and itraconazole solution are preferred because they are more efficacious than ketoconazole, and are easier to administer.

Second-Line Therapy

Itraconazole solution and an oral suspension of amphotericin B and are second-line agents for treating oropharyngeal candidiasis. Itraconazole solution may be used in patients in whom fluconazole therapy fails. Amphotericin B oral suspension may be effective in patients who do not respond to itraconazole therapy. Many clinicians will prescribe these agents before using intravenous therapy due to ease if administration.

Fluconazole refractory esophageal candidiasis may be treated with itraconazole solution. Caspofungin and voriconazole may also be used. The choice between voriconazole and caspofungin is usually based on drug tolerance, convenience

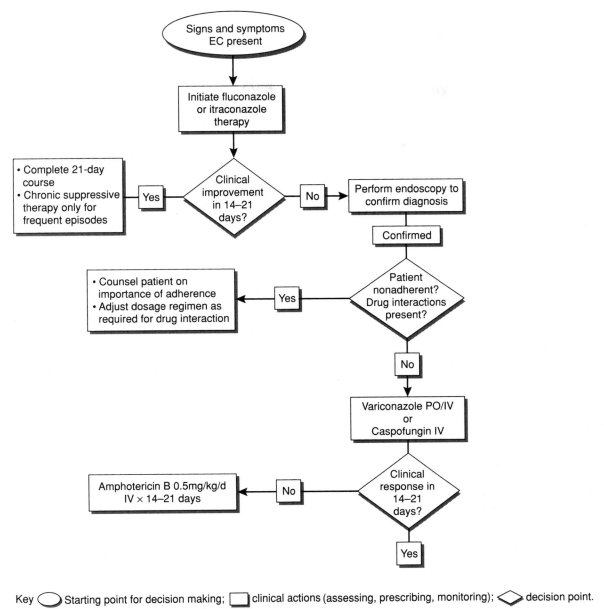

Figure 53–4   Treatment algorithm for esophageal candidiasis (EC).

(oral versus intravenous administration), drug interactions, and cost.

Third-Line Therapy

The third-line agents for treating oropharyngeal candidiasis are used for disease that is refractory to fluconazole or itraconazole therapy. Intravenous caspofungin or amphotericin B can be effectively used in patients with refractory disease (Infectious Disease Society of America [IDSA], 2003). Intravenous amphotericin B is typically used last because of difficulty of administration and toxicity associated with use; however, it is less expensive than caspofungin.

Esophageal candidiasis that is refractory to other systemic therapies may be treated with intravenous amphotericin B. However, immune reconstitution with HAART is often the most effective method for treating refractory oropharyngeal and esophageal candidiasis.

Special Population Considerations

Pediatric

Recurrent candidiasis (especially oropharyngeal candidiasis) is common in HIV-infected children. As with adults, primary prophylaxis is not recommended. Topical agents are preferred for initial therapy for oropharyngeal candidiasis. Oral azole antifungals are used for oropharyngeal disease refractory to topical agents and for esophageal candidiasis. Chronic maintenance (suppressive) therapy should be considered only in children who have severe recurrent oropharyngeal or esophageal candidiasis.

Women

Because of evidence of teratogenicity with the azole antifungal agents, pregnant women should not be treated with these agents. Women who are receiving triazole agents should be counseled to use effective birth control methods while being treated for candidiasis.

MONITORING PATIENT RESPONSE

The practitioner should monitor patients for resolution of signs and symptoms of candidiasis. If resolution does not occur within 14 to 21 days, patient adherence and potential drug interactions that might decrease antifungal levels should be considered. After all other causes of drug failure have been ruled out, cultures should be obtained and antifungal susceptibilities performed. Drug therapy should be adjusted when culture and susceptibility results are available.

PATIENT EDUCATION

The practitioner should teach patients about medication adherence, appropriate medication administration, adverse effects, drug interactions, and signs and symptoms of the target opportunistic infection. A nonthreatening assessment of the patient's medication adherence should occur at each clinic visit. This assessment helps to reinforce the importance adherence to the medication regimen and reveals potential problems with the drug administration, such as adverse events.

The practitioner should ask patients how they administer the medications, which may identify misunderstandings such as administration of an incorrect number of pills or inappropriate administration regarding meals.

The practitioner should teach patients about potential drug interactions and should instruct them to contact their health care provider before beginning any new medications. Patients also should be aware of the signs and symptoms of the opportunistic infections for which they are receiving prophylactic or treatment drug regimens. Successful management of opportunistic infections involves early recognition and treatment.

■ Case Study

T.T. is a 34-year-old man whose dentist discovered thrush during a routine dental visit. On questioning, he stated that he noticed small white patches on his gums approximately 1 month ago. He did not seek medical attention because it has not bothered him. He is a former intravenous drug user and has been in relatively good health since he quit using drugs 4 years ago. He is currently receiving omeprazole (Prilosec) to treat gastroesophageal reflux. He has no known drug allergies. His dentist referred him to the Infectious Diseases Clinic for evaluation for HIV.

T.T. is diagnosed with HIV infection. His CD4$^+$ T-lymphocyte count is 180 cells/mm^3 and his viral load is 200,000 copies/mL. T.T. is begun on a HAART regimen consisting of zidovudine (Retrovir), didanosine, and nelfinavir (Viracept).

Diagnosis: AIDS
Manifestations: oropharyngeal candidiasis
Required assessments: need for prophylaxis for opportunistic infections

1. List specific goals of chemoprophylaxis and treatment for T.T.

2. What over-the-counter and/or alternative medications would be appropriate for T.T.?

3. What dietary and lifestyle changes should be recommended for T.T.?

4. What drug therapy would you prescribe? Why?

5. What are the parameters for monitoring success of the chemoprophylaxis and therapy?

6. Discuss specific patient education based on the prescribed therapy.

7. Describe one or two drug–drug or drug–food interactions for the selected agent.

8. List one or two adverse reactions for the selected agent that would cause you to change therapy.

9. What would be the choice for the second-line therapy?

Bibliography

*Starred references are cited in the text.

American Thoracic Society. (1997). Diagnosis and treatment of disease caused by nontuberculous mycobacteria. *American Journal of Respiratory and Critical Care Medicine, 156*, S1–S25.

Benson, C. A. (2003). *Mycobacterium avium* complex and other atypical mycobacterial infections. In R. Dolin, H. Masur, & M. S. Saag (Eds.), *AIDS therapy* (2nd ed., pp. 475–490). Philadelphia: Churchill Livingstone.

*Centers for Disease Control and Prevention. (2002). USPHS/IDSA guidelines for the prevention of opportunistic infections in persons infected with human immunodeficiency virus. *Morbidity and Mortality Weekly Report, 51*(RR-8), 1–52.

Centers for Disease Control and Prevention. (2004). Updated guidelines for the use of rifamycins for the treatment of tuberculosis among HIV-infected patients taking protease inhibitors or nonnucleoside reverse transcriptase inhibitors. [On-line]. Retrieved November 12, 2004. Available: http://www.cdc.gov/nchstp/tb/tb_hiv_drugs/toc.htm.

*Chaisson, R. E. (1999). The management of *Pneumocystis carinii*, toxoplasmosis and herpes simplex virus infections in patients with HIV disease. [On-line]. Retrieved October 9, 1999. Available: http://www.medscape.com/viewprogram/663_pnt

Chaisson, R. E., & Bishai, W. R. (1999). MAC and TB infection: Management in HIV disease. [On-line]. Retrieved July 19, 1999. Available: http://www.medscape.com/viewprogram/664_pnt.

Dunn, J. P. (2003). Cytomegalovirus retinitis in 2003. The Hopkins HIV Report. [On-line] Retrieved September 14, 2004. Available: http://www.hopkins-aids.edu/publications/report/may03_4.html.

Fichtenbaum, C. J. (2003). Candidiasis. In R. Dolin, H. Masur, & M. S. Saag (Eds.), *AIDS therapy* (2nd ed., pp. 531–543). Philadelphia: Churchill Livingstone.

Haddad, N. E., & Powderly, W. G. (2001). The changing face of mycoses in patients with HIV/AIDS. [On-line] Retrieved October 7, 2004. Available: http://www.medscape.com/viewarticle/410402?src=search.

Hughes, W. T. (1998). Use of dapsone in the prevention and treatment of *Pneumocystis carinii* pneumonia: A review. *Clinical Infectious Diseases, 27*, 191–204.

*Infectious Disease Society of America. (2003). Guidelines for treatment of candidiasis. *Clinical Infectious Disease, 38*, 161–189.

*Karakousis, P. C., Moore, R. D., & Chaisson, R. E. (2004). Mycobacterium avium complex in patients with HIV infection in the era of highly active antiretroviral therapy. *Lancet Infectious Diseases, 4*(9), 557–565.

*Jacobson, M. A. (1997). Treatment of cytomegalovirus retinitis in patients with the acquired immunodeficiency syndrome. *New England Journal of Medicine, 337*, 105–114.

*Martin, D. F. (2003). Treatment of cytomegalovirus (CMV) retinitis in the era of highly active antiretroviral therapy. [On-line]. Retrieved October 8, 2004. Available: http://www.medscape.com/viewprogram/663_pnt.

*Martin, D. F., Dunn, J. P., Davis, J. L., et al. (1999). Use of the ganciclovir implant for the treatment of cytomegalovirus retinitis in the era of potent antiretroviral therapy: Recommendations of the International AIDS Society-USA Panel. *American Journal of Ophthalmology, 127*, 329–339.

*Masur, H. (2000). Management of opportunistic infections associated with HIV infection. In G. L. Mandell, J. E. Bennett, & R. Dolin (Eds.), *Principles and practice of infectious diseases* (5th ed., pp. 1500–1519). New York: Churchill Livingstone.

*Masur, H. (2003). Pneumocystosis. In R. Dolin, H. Masur, & M. S. Saag (Eds.), *AIDS therapy* (2nd ed., pp. 403–418). Philadelphia: Churchill Livingstone.

Michalets, E. L. (1998). Update: clinically significant cytochrome P-450 drug interactions. *Pharmacotherapy, 18*, 84–112.

Nichols, C. W. (1996). *Mycobacterium avium* complex infection, rifabutin, and uveitis: Is there a connection? *Clinical Infectious Diseases, 22* (Suppl. 1), S43–S47.

Nielsen, K. (1999). Pediatric HIV infection. [On-line]. Retrieved October 22, 1999. Available: http://www.medscape.com/viewprogram/663_pnt.

*Powderly, W. (1999). Fungal infections: Diagnosis and management in patients with HIV disease. [On-line]. Retrieved October 24, 1999. Available: http://www.medscape.com/Medscape/HIV/ClinicalMgmt/CM.v06/pnt-CM.v06.html.

Terrell, C. L. (1999). Antifungal agents: Part II. The azoles. *Mayo Clinic Proceedings, 74*, 78–100.

*Vazquez, J. A. (1999). Options for the management of mucosal candidiasis in patients with AIDS and HIV infection. *Pharmacotherapy 19*, 76–87.

*Warren, E., George, S., You, J., et al. (1997). Advances in the treatment and prophylaxis of *Pneumocystis carinii* pneumonia. *Pharmacotherapy, 17*, 900–916.

Whitley, R. J., Jacobson, M. A., Frieberg, D., et al. (1998). Guidelines for the treatment of cytomegalovirus diseases in patients with AIDS in the era of potent antiretroviral therapy. *Archives of Internal Medicine, 158*, 957–969.

Wright, J. (1998). Current strategies for the prevention and treatment of disseminated *Mycobacterium avium* complex infections in patients with AIDS. *Pharmacotherapy, 18*, 738–747.

Visit the Connection web site for the most up-to-date drug information.

XII

Pharmacotherapy for Hematologic and Oncologic Disorders

54

COAGULATION DISTURBANCES

■ ELLEN BOXER GOLDFARB AND ANGELA ALLERMAN

VENOUS THROMBOEMBOLIC DISEASE STATES AND ANTITHROMBOTIC THERAPY

Thromboembolic disease and risk factors for thromboemboli are frequently encountered in the ambulatory population, and an understanding of the pathogenesis of these conditions, along with the clotting cascade, is essential for determining appropriate treatment. Venous thromboembolism (VTE), atrial fibrillation, ischemic stroke, valvular heart disease, prosthetic cardiac valves, coronary and peripheral vascular disease, and hypercoagulable states are disorders warranting anticoagulant therapy. Prophylaxis of clotting events is also necessary in other situations, such as for patients undergoing orthopedic as well as other surgeries and those with prolonged immobility. Drugs used to manage these conditions include anticoagulants, which prevent clot extension and formation; antiplatelet agents, which interfere with platelet activity; and thrombolytic agents, which dissolve existing thrombi. Anticoagulants and antiplatelets are discussed in this chapter, whereas thrombolytics and anticoagulants, whose use is confined to the inpatient setting, are not. Coronary and peripheral arterial disease also will not be discussed in this chapter because they are related to atherosclerosis, which is reviewed in the chapters discussing hyperlipidemia and angina.

DISORDERS REQUIRING ANTICOAGULATION AND THEIR CAUSES

Venous Thromboembolism

Three components, known as *Virchow's triad*, contribute to venous thrombus formation, commonly called deep vein thrombosis (DVT): venous stasis, vascular endothelial wall injury, and hypercoagulability.

The most common causes and risk factors for DVT and VTE can be categorized according to the components of Virchow's triad. Venous stasis, resulting in pooling of blood, most frequently in the veins of the lower extremities, can be attributed to conditions such as obesity, pregnancy, prolonged immobility, heart disease, shock, stroke with paralysis, and vessel disease such as varicose veins. Vascular intimal injury may be related to recent surgery, especially abdominal and orthopedic surgery, recent trauma to the pelvis or lower extremities, childbirth, and previous venous thrombosis. Imbalances between the coagulation cascade and inhibitory systems in favor of clotting can result in hypercoagulable conditions. Hypercoagulability may be present secondary to inherited abnormalities of coagulation, malignancy, oral contraceptive use, and estrogen therapy. In addition, indwelling venous catheters and age older than 40 years also increases risk for venous thromboembolic disease (Morris et al., 2002). Risk factors for VTE should be identified and corrected, if possible (Salzman & Hirsh, 1994). Box 54-1 provides more information.

One complication of DVT is venous incompetence, which can develop into the postphlebitic syndrome and lead to chronic lower extremity edema, venous stasis ulcer formation, and chronic pain (Alpert & Dalen, 1994; Salzman & Hirsh, 1994). Another possible complication of and risk factor for DVT, which is related to venous incompetence, is the presence of varicose veins. It has been postulated that varicose veins may be an independent risk factor for the development of VTE. This is very controversial and few studies looking at this possibility have been done. There are various surgical as well as laser and radiofrequency procedures that may be done for the treatment of varicose veins, some of which also increase may risk for VTE (Anderson & Spencer, 2003). An initial, conservative, and frequently effective treatment for the manifestations of venous incompetence is compression stockings. Compression stockings decrease swelling and discomfort caused by postphlebitic syndrome and varicose veins. Graduated compression stockings, which are fitted to the individual and apply a prescribed amount of pressure, should be used. The stockings work by compressing the leg surfaces (with the most pressure at the ankle, decreasing pressure up the length of the leg) and forcing blood to flow from small superficial vessels to the larger deep veins and finally back to the heart. The stockings also help prevent backflow of blood by supporting leaky valves (Ball, 2003). In the setting of an acute DVT, compression stockings should be instituted only after therapeutic anticoagulation is achieved.

BOX 54–1. RISK FACTORS FOR DEEP VENOUS THROMBOSIS AND PULMONARY EMBOLISM

Reversible
Trauma, surgery,* pregnancy, estrogen therapy, prolonged or transient immobility, fractures, indwelling venous catheters

Acquired
Advancing age >40 y, malignancy,[†] previous venous thrombosis, hematologic disease, varicose veins, heart failure, stroke, inflammatory bowel disease, nephrotic syndrome

Inherited Disorders
Antiphospholipid antibodies, lupus anticoagulant, activated protein C resistance, antithrombin III deficiency, protein C deficiency, protein S deficiency, anticardiolipin antibodies,[‡] factor V Leiden, prothrombin gene mutation

---

*Especially orthopedic, gynecologic, neurosurgical, or urologic procedures.
[†]Especially of the lung, breast or viscera
[‡]May also be acquired

Patients with symptomatic calf vein thrombosis are more likely to have clot extension proximally compared with asymptomatic patients. DVTs that remain confined to the calf vein are at low risk for embolization (Hyers et al., 1998). However, 20% of calf vein thrombi may extend into the proximal veins (ie, femoral, popliteal, and iliac veins), where their large size can cause serious complications. Approximately 50% of proximal DVTs migrate to the pulmonary circulation. Embolization to the pulmonary circulation is considered a life-threatening emergency, with a mortality rate as high as 30% (Spandorfer et al., 2001). Lower extremity DVTs are the source of 90% of pulmonary emboli (Gorski, 2001).

Atrial Fibrillation

Atrial fibrillation is a cardiac arrhythmia characterized by loss of coordination of electrical and mechanical atrial activity. This causes impaired ventricular filling and pooling of blood, which leads to the formation of left atrial appendage thrombi (Spandorfer et al., 2001). Embolism of such atrial thrombi leads to cardioembolic stroke. Atrial fibrillation is a strong, independent risk factor for ischemic stroke and is weakly associated with transient ischemic attack (TIA; Hart et al., 2004).

Atrial fibrillation is the most common dysrhythmia, and its incidence increases with advancing age and is highest in those older than 65 years or younger than 65 years with hypertension or chronic heart disease. Several underlying cardiovascular conditions may cause atrial fibrillation. The most common causes are hypertension, ischemic heart disease, congestive heart failure (CHF), and rheumatic valvular disease. Additional cardiac causes include atrial enlargement,

atrial septal defect, and coronary artery bypass graft surgery. Noncardiac etiologies include thyrotoxicosis, hypothermia, fever, stroke, chronic pulmonary disease, electrolyte disorders, pulmonary embolism (PE), alcohol intoxication, and genetic predisposition (Spandorfer et al., 2001).

Several recent trials comparing treatment of atrial fibrillation and stroke prevention in patients with atrial fibrillation have concluded that the use of anticoagulation in these patients is mandatory in addition to ventricular rate or rhythm control medication or electrical cardioversion (Kellen, 2004).

Ischemic Stroke

An ischemic stroke, or cerebral infarction, results from obstructed cerebral blood supply due to underlying vascular disease or an embolic event. A TIA is an episode of brief ischemia resulting in temporary neurologic deficits that resolve within 24 hours and usually last less than 6 minutes. TIAs are most often caused by an embolus (Noble, 2001). A neurologic deficit that lasts longer than 24 hours is classified as a stroke.

Of the two general stroke categories, ischemic strokes occur in 85% of patients; hemorrhagic strokes account for the remaining 15%. Ischemic strokes are further classified by their etiology; 50% are due to atherothrombotic disease, 25% are attributable to cerebral small-vessel disease (lacunar infarcts), and 20% occur from cardioembolic sources (O'Rourke et al., 2004). Cardioembolic sources include atrial fibrillation (most common cardioembolic cause), mitral stenosis, prosthetic mechanical valves, recent myocardial infarction with left ventricular thrombosis, aortic atheroma, patent foramen ovale, atrial myxoma, infective endocarditis, and dilated cardiomyopathies. The remaining ischemic strokes are due to unusual etiologies, including hypercoagulable conditions, drug abuse, or unknown causes (Adams et al., 1994).

It was once thought that the most frequent cause of ischemic stroke was thrombosis of a cerebral artery. More recently, it has been recognized that emboli from other conditions such as thrombotic lesions in the carotid arteries and cardiac disorders resulting in thrombosis are the most common causes (Noble, 2001). Therefore, the focus of pharmacologic care must be prophylaxis of thromboemboli in the presence of risk factors.

Native and Prosthetic Valvular Heart Disease

The great risk of thromboembolism from valvular heart disease warrants consideration of anticoagulant therapy for all affected patients. Initiation of thrombosis in these patients is thought to be due to two mechanisms—one is the disruption of the vascular endothelial surface and the introduction of prothrombotic materials into the circulation and the second is the triggering of thrombosis in areas of stasis (Becker et al., 2002).

The risk of thromboembolism in native valvular heart disease is influenced by the position of the valve, for example, mitral versus aortic, heart chamber dimension, ventricular performance, and concomitant risk factors such as prior thromboembolism and atrial fibrillation. Mitral and aortic valve disease presents thromboembolic risk by different mechanisms. In the mitral position shear stress is low, blood flow is slow, and stasis occurs, allowing coagulation factor contact. In the aortic position, blood flow is rapid and shear stress is high, which causes red blood cell hemolysis and platelet and coagulation factor activation (Becker et al., 2002).

The incidence of embolism is highest in individuals with rheumatic mitral valve disease who have a 1 in 5 chance of having a clinically detectable embolus during the course of the disease. The incidence increases significantly in combination with atrial fibrillation. Mitral annular calcification, possibly with mitral stenosis or regurgitation, presents a risk of thromboembolism twice that of those without the condition according to the Framingham Heart study. Although because the true incidence of emboli in these patients is not known, anticoagulant therapy is usually reserved for those with concomitant risk such as atrial fibrillation. Thromboembolism in aortic valve disease has been noted but is uncommon. Without the coexistence of mitral valve disease or atrial fibrillation, anticoagulation is not indicated in these patients (Salem et al., 2001).

Prosthetic heart valves in either the mitral or aortic positions present a high risk for thromboembolism. The risk is great because of the artificial surface of the valve, which is thrombogenic. Anticoagulant therapy for thromboprophylaxis is recommended in all patients having prosthetic valve replacement. Bioprosthetic, tissue valves present a much lower risk of thromboembolism, averaging 1%/y. The risk is only of concern in the first 3 months postoperatively during which antithrombotic agents are used (Becker et al., 2002).

PATHOPHYSIOLOGY

The body's sophisticated system of checks and balances not only maintains normal hemostasis but promotes blood clotting in response to vascular endothelial injury. There are three major components of the coagulation system that work to preserve hemostasis with clot formation in response to vascular injury while maintaining blood fluidity. These components are composed of endothelial cells, platelets, and coagulation proteins (Spandorfer et al., 2001).

The endothelial cell lining of the vessel wall expresses anticoagulant and profibrinolytic properties. It produces inhibitors of platelet function and heparin-like substances that regulate activity of coagulation enzymes. In response to vascular injury, the endothelium preserves vascular integrity by triggering adhesion and aggregation of platelets and activates the coagulation factors of the clotting cascade to form a fibrin clot (Spandorfer et al., 2001).

Role of Clotting Cascade

In response to tissue injury, a series of complex enzymatic reactions (the clotting cascade) is initiated that leads to the formation of a stable fibrin clot. Circulating inactive coagulation factors are sequentially converted into activated coagulation factor complexes. The final step in the cascade is formation of thrombin (factor II), which leads to the conversion of fibrinogen to fibrin and the formation of a fibrin clot (Colman et al., 1994).

Platelets also participate in repairing tissue injury by adhering to the site of injured blood vessels, attracting other platelets to the site, and forming large platelet aggregates that help stabilize the platelet–fibrin clot. When platelets are activated, receptors for clotting factors are exposed. This also provides a stable environment for initiation of the clotting cascade (Colman et al., 1994).

The coagulation system is traditionally divided into the intrinsic and extrinsic pathways. Activity through the extrinsic pathway is initiated by components from both the blood and vasculature, with factor VII as the major initiating factor. Activation occurs when procoagulant components migrate to sites of vascular damage or when the blood is exposed to substances released as a result of vascular wall damage. In contrast, activity through the intrinsic coagulation pathway is initiated by activation of factor XII when blood comes in contact with a foreign surface (such as a prosthetic device) or damaged endothelial blood vessels. The pathways interact and eventually merge to form a final common pathway for clot formation (Fig. 54-1).

Several inhibitory processes limit the clotting process. One of the main regulatory proteins of the clotting cascade is antithrombin III, which inhibits factors IX, X, XI, XII and II (thrombin) (Colman et al., 1994; Hirsh et al., 1994). Two other regulatory proteins, proteins C and S, must be present in sufficient amounts because they prevent excessive clot formation by inhibiting factors V and VII. Deficiency in any of these proteins creates a predisposition to pathologic thrombosis (Spandorfer et al., 2001).

Thrombotic Process

Thrombi can form in any part of the cardiovascular system—the veins and arteries (including those of the brain), as well as the heart. Thrombi can cause local complications by obstructing vessels or by breaking off and traveling to a distant site. Arterial thrombi often form in the setting of pre-existing atherosclerosis or other vascular disease, especially at the sites of ruptured atherosclerotic plaques. In the heart, thrombi can develop on damaged cardiac valves, in a dilated or dyskinetic heart chamber, or on prosthetic valves. Although most intracardiac thrombi cause no symptoms, serious consequences can arise if the thrombi migrate to the systemic circulation, especially the brain. In the venous system, thrombi usually occur in the lower extremities as DVTs or in the pulmonary circulation as PEs. Venous thrombi form in areas of sluggish blood flow (venous stasis) and contain primarily red cells with only small amounts of platelets. In contrast, arterial thrombi form in areas of high blood flow and are composed primarily of platelet aggregates bound with fibrin strands (Hirsh et al., 1994).

Hypercoagulable States

Hypercoagulability may be inherited or acquired. The presence of a hypercoagulable state does not equal the presence of pathologic thrombosis, but increases the risk of thrombosis in those affected.

Hereditary risk factors for pathologic clotting can be distinguished by the mechanism by which they cause thrombosis. Functional deficiencies of coagulation factor regulatory proteins are those of antithrombin III, protein C, and protein S. These function as natural anticoagulant systems that allow balance between thrombin production and inhibition. When one is deficient, that balance is lost, inhibition of

COAGULATION PATHWAY

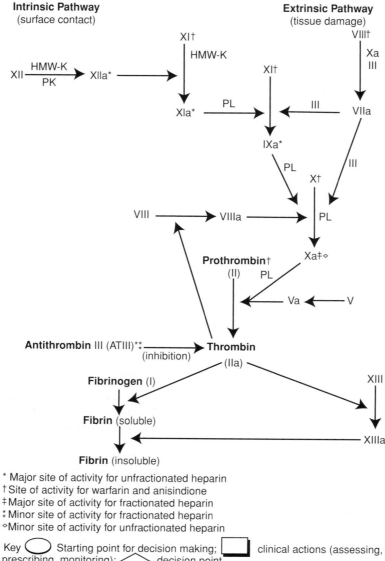

Figure 54–1 The coagulation system.

thrombin decreased, and increased clot formation occurs. Antithrombin III is created in the liver and irreversibly neutralizes clotting factors, including thrombin. Activity of antithrombin III is increased in the presence of heparin. Deficiency of antithrombin III is inherited as an autosomal, dominant trait, but can be acquired in liver disease, disseminated intravascular coagulation (DIC), and oral contraceptive use. Protein C and S are dependent on vitamin K and are made in the liver. Thrombin converts protein C to an activated form that then acts with protein S to prevent further generation of thrombin by inhibition of coagulation factors V and VIII. In the absence of these proteins thrombin remains uninhibited and promotes its own formation (Spandorfer et al., 2001).

In addition to a deficiency of protein C and S, these proteins can be ineffective in the presence of another inherited thrombosis risk factor, factor V Leiden. Factor V Leiden is a genetic mutation that causes coagulation factor V to be resistant to inhibition by activated protein C.

Another genetic mutation that causes increased risk for thrombosis is prothrombin gene mutation. This mutation causes increased levels of prothrombin, a coagulation protein, which, in the coagulation cascade, is activated and converted into thrombin and leads to the creation of a fibrin clot (Spandorfer et al., 2001).

Finally, hyperhomocysteinemia is another risk factor for pathologic thrombosis. Elevation is thought to be due to an abnormality in the enzymes that regulate homocysteine. Hyperhomocysteinemia may be inherited as a genetic mutation that causes one of the enzymes, 5,10-methylene tetrahydrofolate reductase (MTHFR) to be inactive. Homocysteine control and thrombosis prevention may be achieved with increased folate intake (Spandorfer et al., 2001).

A wide spectrum of acquired hypercoagulable states exist, such as antiphospholipid antibody (APA) syndrome, malignancy, hematologic disorders, vasculitis, and nephrotic syndrome. For the purposes of this chapter, only APA syndrome will be discussed. APAs are autoantibodies that often occur in systemic lupus erythematosus, but are frequently found in those who do not meet the disease criteria. There are two types of these antibodies, lupus anticoagulants and anticardiolipin antibodies (ACAs). Thrombosis, venous or arterial, is the main complication of APA syndrome, but thrombocytopenia and recurrent spontaneous abortion in affected women may also occur. APAs can persist for years or a lifetime, but what causes the sudden thrombotic event in these patients is unknown. The mechanism by which APAs cause thrombosis is not clear and is the subject of much debate. It is thought that the antibodies are directed against phospholipid-binding proteins and cause these proteins to be antigenic and initiate thrombosis (Khamashta et al., 1995).

Evaluation for the presence of hypercoagulable states should be done for select patients. Testing is recommended in those who are younger than 45 years of age at the time of first thrombosis and those with a thrombotic event of unknown etiology. Testing is only useful to help determine if family members should be evaluated and to decide the duration of anticoagulation therapy in those who have had a pathologic thrombosis. Empiric treatment for those found to possess an inherited or acquired hypercoagulable state in the absence of a thrombotic event is not recommended (Spandorfer et al., 2001).

DIAGNOSTIC CRITERIA
Venous Thromboembolism

Erythema, pain, swelling, venous distention and warmth in the leg are common presenting symptoms of a DVT. Objective confirmation is needed because the symptoms of DVT are nonspecific; many patients with clinical symptoms of DVT do not have DVT. Other conditions such as muscle strain, cellulitis, and postphlebitic syndrome may mimic symptoms of DVT. Approximately 50% of patients with a DVT have no symptoms (Gorski, 2001).

The methods used most often for detecting DVT are contrast-enhanced venography, ultrasonography, and magnetic resonance imaging (MRI). Contrast-enhanced venography is the gold standard for diagnosing DVT because of nearly 100% sensitivity and specificity; its disadvantages, however, include its high cost, invasiveness, and risk of allergic reactions due to radiopaque contrast agent. In venography, contrast agent is injected into the bloodstream, after which a series of x-rays is taken that allows visualization of the veins of both the upper and lower leg. Ultrasonography is the diagnostic method of choice because it is noninvasive, can be conducted at the bedside, and is relatively easy to perform. In ultrasonography, a DVT is diagnosed when there is lack of vein compressibility with pressure. Disadvantages of ultrasonography include insufficient sensitivity to the presence of calf vein thrombi, operator variability, and limitations caused by obesity, casts, and immobilization devices. MRI is said to be a sensitive and specific method to confirm suspected DVT. It is especially useful for examination of pelvic veins, which are not amenable to compression ultrasonography. Cost, the need for an experienced radiologist, and limitations related to the presence of metallic devices in the patient mean that MRI is seldom used as a diagnostic modality for DVT (Spandorfer et al., 2001).

PE is the most serious complication of DVT. The PE mortality rate is related to the size of the thrombus. A massive PE obstructs 50% of the pulmonary vasculature. The term *submassive* is used when less than 50% of the pulmonary circulation is affected. Death occurs from acute right-sided heart failure in untreated patients (Salzman & Hirsh, 1994). The diagnosis of PE is difficult when based on symptoms because presenting symptoms are not specific. Suspicion of PE is based on symptoms along with risk factors such as immobility, recent trauma or surgery, underlying malignancy, and oral contraceptive use. Sudden onset of dyspnea and pleuritic chest pain are the most common presenting symptoms. A presentation of pleuritic chest pain, tachypnea, and tachycardia, progressing to syncope, hypotension, and hypoxemia signal a massive PE. Diagnostic tests should be pursued whenever clinical information does not allow exclusion of PE (Spandorfer et al., 2001). Baseline tests for evaluating PE include a chest x-ray, with cardiomegaly being the most common abnormality seen in PE, electrocardiogram (ECG; to differentiate between PE and myocardial infarction), and arterial blood gas evaluations (to assess the severity of hypoxemia).

In ventilation/perfusion lung scanning (V̇/Q̇ scan), results are reported as high, intermediate, or low probability, or normal. A normal scan excludes clinically important PE and is sufficient evidence to withhold anticoagulant therapy. An abnormal scan, although suggestive of PE, can result from other disease states. Combining the level of clinical suspicion (high, moderate, or low) with the results of the V̇/Q̇ scan allows for a highly sensitive diagnostic assessment. Pulmonary angiography is the gold standard for confirmation of PE, but it is invasive, expensive, uses contrast dye, and is not always readily available (Spandorfer et al., 2001).

Alternatives to V̇/Q̇ scan and pulmonary angiography are spiral-helical computed tomography (CT) and magnetic resonance angiography (MRA). CT provides a view of the entire thorax, but does require contrast dye and exposure to large amounts of radiation. MRA uses gadolinium, a contrast material with no known adverse effects, but it is expensive and may not be appropriate for patients with metallic devices, claustrophobia, and obesity (Morris et al., 2002).

The D-dimer assay is a fairly new but useful screening test for PE. Several studies have shown levels less than 500 µg/L will rule out PE in 98% to 100% of cases. However, the test is nonspecific because any process that activates the coagulation cascade and fibrinolytic system, such as surgery, sepsis, and DIC, can cause D-dimer levels to rise (Morris et al., 2002). A study by Rathbun and colleagues (2004) evaluated D-dimer testing in patients with suspected PE and nondiagnostic lung scans or negative helical CT scans. It was thought that D-dimer could possibly be used as an exclusion test if the results were negative. However, the results showed D-dimer to be of limited clinical utility because D-dimers were negative in only 10% of inpatients and 31.8% of outpatients tested, all of whom had negative radiologic tests (Rathbun et al., 2004). Although study results are conflicting, some institutions do use D-dimer to rule out PE without using any radiologic testing.

Atrial Fibrillation

Symptoms associated with atrial fibrillation include palpitations, chest discomfort, and shortness of breath, weakness, hypotension, dizziness, and syncope. Clinical signs of atrial fibrillation include pulmonary edema, dyspnea, and possibly hemodynamic instability. The ECG is used to confirm the diagnosis. The hallmark of atrial fibrillation on ECG is an irregularly irregular ventricular rhythm. Other ECG characteristics of atrial fibrillation include absence of P waves and ventricular response rates of 100 to 180 bpm. A thorough history and physical examination is needed to rule out underlying causes of atrial fibrillation. An echocardiogram assesses left ventricular dysfunction, valvular heart disease, and atrial enlargement, and detects a left atrial thrombus. Transesophageal echocardiograghy may be used to identify atrial thrombi in preparation for treatment such as electrical cardioversion (Spandorfer et al., 2001).

Ischemic Strokes

Ischemic strokes are characterized by a sudden or progressive onset of a focal neurologic signs. The resulting neurologic deficits are dependent on the location of cerebral infarction. Most often the deficits are confined to one side of the body, right or left. The most common presenting stroke symptom is tingling, numbness, and weakness or paralysis on one side of the body. Incoordination, aphasia, dysarthria, and visual disturbances also can occur (Noble, 2001). Neurologic signs or symptoms may progress in approximately 25% of patients in the first 24 to 48 hours. Approximately 50% of patients are left with a permanent disability (Adams et al., 1994).

CT scan and MRI are used to detect the presence, extent, and progression of a cerebral infarction. Several tests can help detect the source of a presumed thromboembolic ischemic stroke. Noninvasive ultrasound determines if the extracranial arteries, such as the carotid arteries, are occluded or stenotic. An ECG differentiates between atrial fibrillation and myocardial infarction. Transthoracic and transesophageal echocardiograms visualize cardiac function and the presence of an atrial thrombus. Carotid-cerebral angiography can be performed to examine the arteries and veins of the brain and neck. This provides the most accurate visualization to detect abnormalities such as stenosis or occlusion that may have caused the ischemic event (Noble, 2001).

Native and Prosthetic Valvular Heart Disease

Signs and symptoms of valvular heart disease depend on the valve that is affected. In aortic stenosis the cardinal symptoms are dyspnea, angina, and exertional syncope. Aortic regurgitation is most often asymptomatic. Dyspnea is the hallmark symptom of mitral stenosis, although this usually is present with exertion and has a gradual onset over approximately 20 years. Mitral regurgitation also progresses slowly and may be asymptomatic for many years. The initial symptoms may be fatigue, exertional dyspnea, and palpitations that, in severe cases, may lead to pulmonary edema. Each valvular disorder is associated with a characteristic murmur (Noble, 2001).

Suspicion of valvular disease may begin with practitioner auscultation of heart sounds that include a murmur. ECGs may also be used to determine the possible cardiac effects of valve incompetence or stenosis, such as left ventricular hypertrophy in mitral and aortic regurgitation. Confirmation of the diagnosis of valvular disease is best accomplished by an echocardiogram and Doppler study. This can also help determine etiology and severity (Beare & Myers, 1994).

When physical symptoms of valvular disease lead to limitations in daily activities or cardiac decompensation occurs despite medical treatment, surgical intervention, frequently with prosthetic valve replacements are recommended. In the presence of a prosthetic heart valve, the condition of the heart and prosthetic valve is followed by physical assessment with cardiac auscultation, ECGs, and echocardiography. Patients are also assessed for signs and symptoms of stroke secondary to the risk presented by the presence of a prosthetic valve (Beare & Myers, 1994).

INITIATING DRUG THERAPY

Anticoagulants

Before starting anticoagulant therapy, several factors warrant consideration. Currently, warfarin (Coumadin) is the most widely used oral anticoagulant in the United States. Warfarin has a very narrow therapeutic index. Patients taking warfarin must be monitored regularly and must be able to accurately follow dosing instructions. Absolute contraindications to anticoagulation therapy with warfarin include, but are not limited to, recent hemorrhagic stroke, risk for or active major bleeding, recent trauma or traumatic surgery, the immediate postoperative period after central nervous system (CNS) or ocular surgery, or presence of spinal catheters and aneurysms or CNS tumors with high bleeding risk (*Drug Facts and Comparisons*, 2002). Cognitive impairment, severe psychiatric disease, chronic alcoholism, and severe hepatic or renal disease are relative contraindications to warfarin. Patients at risk for falls or trauma also are questionable candidates for warfarin therapy.

Baseline laboratory values including the prothrombin time (PT), international normalized ratio (INR), activated partial thromboplastin time (aPTT), urinalysis, complete blood count (CBC), and a liver profile are recommended before initiating warfarin therapy (Box 54-2 and Table 54-1). In women of childbearing age, pregnancy should be ruled out with a blood test to detect β-human chorionic gonadotropin. Obtaining the patient's telephone number and an alternative contact, such as a responsible family member or neighbor (obtain consent to contact others per HIPPA guidelines), is also advised. A detailed medical, surgical, and medication history is needed to assess the patient's risk for bleeding events. The indication for anticoagulation should be documented so that the target INR goal can be defined. Likewise, the duration of therapy should be determined. When all these issues are addressed, an initial warfarin dosing regimen is selected.

When using unfractionated heparin (UFH), a baseline aPTT, PT/INR, and a CBC should be performed before starting therapy. In addition, active major bleeding from the CNS or gastrointestinal (GI) tract must be ruled out. A digital rectal examination or guaiac test to detect blood in the stool is recommended. As with warfarin therapy, a detailed medical, surgical, and medication history is needed to assess the patient's risk for bleeding. Contraindications to heparin

BOX 54–2. INTERNATIONAL NORMALIZED RATIO: SENSITIVE TEST FOR CLOTTING TIME

The international normalized ratio (INR) is the universally accepted laboratory test for monitoring anticoagulation therapy. The INR has replaced the previously used prothrombin time (PT) ratio.

The PT is the time in seconds for a blood sample to clot after the addition of necessary laboratory reagents, including specific tissue thromboplastins. The PT measures the depression of three of the four vitamin K–dependent clotting factors (II, VII, and X) of the extrinsic coagulation cascade. The PT ratio is simply the patient's individual PT divided by a laboratory's control PT. In the 1960s, most commercial laboratories in the United States switched from a human brain tissue thromboplastin to a rabbit brain product. The rabbit-derived preparations were not as sensitive as the previous reagents. Thus, the sensitivity of the PT test was reduced, resulting in lower PT values. As a result, higher PT ratio goals were set, which increased the risk of hemorrhagic complications. The international sensitivity index (ISI) was developed by the World Health Organization (WHO) as a reference standard to correct this problem.

Mathematically, the INR is the PT ratio raised to the power of the ISI, or $INR = PT\ ratio^{ISI}$. The ISIs for commercially available tissue thromboplastins vary from lot to lot and from manufacturer to manufacturer. The WHO reference standard was assigned an ISI of 1.0, although most commercial laboratories use tissue thromboplastins with ISIs ranging from 1.0 to 2.88. The ISI for a particular reagent is identified in the package insert.

A greater potential for error in calculating the INR occurs when using thromboplastins with high ISIs because they are less sensitive than reagents with ISIs lower than 2.0. The INR can be determined using a calculator, if needed. Most laboratories commonly report both the PT and INR. However, only the INR should be used for dosing changes. Relying on the INR also minimizes variability in reported results if different laboratories, with different thromboplastin preparations, are used. The INR represents the best method for standardizing results from different thromboplastin reagents. The American College of Chest Physicians has standardized the desired target INR goal for anticoagulation therapy for each clinical indication. Current guidelines recommend an INR range of 2 to 3 for most indications of anticoagulation. INRs of 2.5 to 3.5 are reserved for patients with prosthetic heart valves or hypercoagulable conditions.

Table 54.1

Relationship Between the Prothrombin Time Ratio and the International Normalized Ratio for Thromboplastins With Varying International Sensitivity Index Values

Hospital	ISI	Control PT (s)	PT (s)	PT ratio	INR
A	1.3	14.8	33.9	2.3	2.9
B	2.3	11.4	18.2	1.6	2.9

PT, prothrombin time; PT ratio, observed PT divided by control PT;
ISI, international sensitivity index; INR, international normalized ratio
($INR = PT\ ratio^{ISI}$).
The INR takes into account the differences in thromboplastin sensitivity, thus giving a more accurate reflection of the level of anticoagulation.

use are hypersensitivity to heparin products, active bleeding, and severe thrombocytopenia. Before initiating heparin therapy, the target PTT should be defined, frequency of PTT monitoring established, and duration of therapy determined.

Low-molecular-weight heparin (LMWH) may be used in place of UFH. Baseline and periodic CBC and stool occult blood tests should be performed. Anti–factor Xa levels may be used to monitor patients with renal impairment, those experiencing bleeding or with abnormal coagulation parameters, pregnant patients, obese or low-weight patients, and children because dosing is based on weight. Contraindications to LMWH use are active major bleeding, hypersensitivity to LMWH or pork products when using enoxaparin (Lovenox), and history of thrombocytopenia associated with LMWH (Micromedex, 2004). When used in the outpatient setting, ability of the patient or caregiver to perform a subcutaneous (SC) injection must be established and SC injection teaching must be performed.

Antiplatelet Agents

A detailed medication history is needed before initiating therapy with antiplatelet agents. The data help reduce the risk of increased bleeding if concomitant medications are used, such as the nonsteroidal anti-inflammatory drugs (NSAIDs). Patients receiving aspirin should be questioned carefully regarding any medication allergies because antiplatelet agents are contraindicated in patients with a history of aspirin allergy or hypersensitivity to NSAIDs or salicylates. Patients with severe anemia or a history of coagulation defects also should not receive aspirin.

Before initiating therapy with clopidogrel (Plavix) or ticlopidine (Ticlid), a baseline CBC with differential and liver function tests should be performed. Patients also need to be assessed for any active major bleeding. Antiplatelet agents are contraindicated in patients with known hypersensitivity, impaired renal or liver function, thrombocytopenia, and active bleeding (Micromedex, 2004).

Goals of Drug Therapy

The goals of anticoagulation therapy in atrial fibrillation, native and prosthetic heart valvular disease, and in patients with a history of ischemic, cardioembolic stroke are to prevent development of future strokes. Anticoagulation treatment in patients with existing DVT/PE is initiated to prevent extension of the thrombus, thromboembolic complications, and production of a new thrombus. Anticoagulation prophylaxis after orthopedic surgery is initiated to decrease the risk of DVT or PE. The goals of antiplatelet therapy are to prevent and treat ischemic strokes from noncardioembolic sources.

Warfarin

Warfarin (Coumadin) is the most widely used oral anticoagulant in North America because of its good absorption (bioavailability), relatively predictable onset of action, and long duration of action (Hirsh et al., 1998) (Table 54-2).

Mechanism of Action

Oral anticoagulants exert their clinical effects through the extrinsic pathway of the clotting cascade. In contrast, heparin, an intravenous anticoagulant, influences the intrinsic coagulation cascade. In venous stasis or tissue injury, a series of stepwise enzymatic protein reactions is initiated that culminates in clot formation. Warfarin inhibits activation of the clotting factors that depend on vitamin K for synthesis—factors II, VII, IX, and X and the coagulation inhibitor proteins C and S. Oral anticoagulants disrupt the interconversion of vitamin K from the inactive epoxide form back into active vitamin K. The result is that the inactive epoxide accumulates, vitamin K is depleted, and the rate of clotting factor formation is decreased. Although the clotting factors are still synthesized in the liver, their physiologic activity is reduced, and clot formation is inhibited. Warfarin does not affect existing clotting factors.

The half-lives of clotting factors range from 6 hours (factor VII) to 60 hours (factor II) as indicated in Table 54-3. The average half-life of warfarin is 36 to 42 hours. The onset of anticoagulant effect depends on both the half-life of warfarin and the time required to deplete the vitamin K–dependent clotting factors. The anticoagulant effect of warfarin is monitored with the PT and INR, with the INR being the gold standard for warfarin titration. Initial prolongation of the PT/INR is seen in 8 to 12 hours secondary to the rapid depletion of factor VII, but peak antithrombotic effect of warfarin is delayed for 3 to 5 days as other factors with longer half-lives are depleted (*Drug Facts and Comparisons*, 2002). Clotting factors need to be decreased by 20% for effective anticoagulation. Therapeutic doses of warfarin decrease the amount of each vitamin K–dependent factor by 30% to 50% (Becker et al., 2002). In a hypercoagulable patient with thrombosis, warfarin should not be started alone, without overlap with a rapidly acting anticoagulant, because warfarin quickly depletes protein C and factor II, and will create a hypercoagulable state until a therapeutic dose is achieved. Box 54-3 presents additional information.

Dosage

Because of its long half-life, warfarin is administered once daily. Warfarin is completely absorbed after oral administration and is metabolized to inactive metabolites by the liver. Warfarin has a narrow therapeutic window. Therefore, the dose needed to exert clinical efficacy is similar to the dose that causes adverse effects (Benet & Goyan, 1995).

Individual patients vary widely in their ability to absorb and eliminate warfarin (pharmacokinetic variations) and in their rate of clinical response and dosage requirements (pharmacodynamic variations). Patient variability is not related to weight or sex but is dependent on diet, age, disease states, concomitant medications, and one's genetically predetermined rate of metabolism. Warfarin binds extensively to plasma proteins and is metabolized by the cytochrome P450 (CYP450) system of the liver. In a study evaluating the influences of vitamin K intake on warfarin dosing, it was discovered that individual sensitivity to warfarin is determined by CYP2C9 genotype and age and that the CYP2C9 genotype influenced warfarin dose requirements (Khan et al., 2004). Patients with genetic polymorphisms of the CYP2C9 enzyme may have impaired metabolism of warfarin and require lower doses than their counterparts (Spandorfer et al., 2001). A rare phenomenon of warfarin resistance, which may be acquired or inherited as an autosomal dominant trait, has only been documented in case studies. Resistance is thought to be due to altered pharmacokinetics of the drug or decreased pharmacodynamic effect. As of 1994, only four families had been described with the hereditary form of warfarin resistance. In these patients pharmacokinetics appeared normal and plasma levels of warfarin were high, ruling out noncompliance, decreased absorption, or increased elimination as a cause of the resistance. Due to the fact that high doses of warfarin were able to overcome the resistance, it was thought that the defect was tissue resistance possibly due to the presence of an enzyme or receptor site with decreased affinity to warfarin or an increased affinity to vitamin K (Diab & Feffer, 1994). Those with warfarin resistance require extremely high doses of warfarin, in the range of 5 to 20 times higher than usual, possibly 40 to 50 mg/d, to reach a therapeutic INR (Spandorfer et al., 2001).

Responsiveness to warfarin dosage also depends on the liver's ability to produce clotting factors and vitamin K reductase receptor affinity. Pharmacodynamic factors that may potentiate warfarin response include hypermetabolic states, such as hyperthyroidism and febrile states. These states are thought to increase the catabolic rate of vitamin K–dependent clotting factors in the liver. Hepatic disease, vitamin K deficiency states, and short-term alcohol bingeing can also increase sensitivity to warfarin by depressing the production of vitamin K–dependent clotting factors. Decreased dietary vitamin K absorption from fat malabsorption states, because vitamin K is fat soluble, and acute bouts of diarrhea can lead to a potentiated warfarin response. The elderly also seem to be more sensitive to warfarin, possibly because of alteration of pharmacodynamic parameters.

Note: If the patient receives a prescription for warfarin, the prescriber needs to choose among nine dosage strengths and colors (eg, a 1-mg tablet is pink, whereas a 5-mg tablet is peach). For safety's sake and to avoid confusing the patient, only one warfarin tablet strength should be prescribed (eg, 2.5- or 5-mg tablets, but not both). Patients also need to be taught to remember the tablet color, shape, and tablet strength with each new prescription and refill. In addition, there are several different manufacturers of warfarin and bioequivalence between products has been problematic. Therefore, brand interchange is not recommended (*Drug Facts and Comparisons*, 2002).

Table 54.2

Overview of Drugs Used to Treat Coagulation Disorders

Generic (Trade) Name and Dosage	Selected Adverse Events	Contraindications	Special Considerations
Anticoagulants			
warfarin (Coumadin) Start: 2.5–5 mg qd PO Range: 1–15 mg qd PO—must individualize dose	Bleeding	Contraindicated in pregnancy; for other contraindications, see text.	Used for prophylaxis and treatment of DVT, PE, and prophylaxis and treatment of atrial fibrillation. Monitored with the PT/INR. See text for drug interactions and dietary restrictions.
heparin SC: 8000–10,000 units q8h SC: 15,000–20,000 units q12h IV: 20,000–40,000 units/d—continuous infusion	Bleeding, thrombocytopenia	Contraindicated in active major bleeding (GI or intracranial), or in patients with thrombocytopenia	Used for prophylaxis and treatment of DVT, PE, atrial fibrillation with embolization, peripheral artery embolism, and surgical procedures. Monitored with the aPTT. Monitor CBC with platelets periodically for thrombocytopenia.
tinzaparin (Innohep) 175 anti-ka IU/kg SC qd	Bleeding, local irritation at injection site	Hypersensitivity to sulfites, LMWH Hypersensitivity to sulfites	Tinzaparin is used for treatment of DVT with and without PE; may affect PT/INR—check PT/INR just prior to a dose when using with warfarin.
dalteparin (Fragmin) 120 IU/kg Low risk: 2500 IU/d SC High risk: 5000 IU/d SC (ie, malignancy)	Bleeding, local irritation at the injection site	Active major bleeding (GI or intracranial); thrombocytopenia in association with positive in vitro testing for anti-platelet antibodies	A LMWH used for prophylaxis of DVT in patients undergoing abdominal surgery. Evaluate CBC periodically for bleeding effects.
enoxaparin (Lovenox) Orthopedic surgery: 30 mg SC bid Abdominal surgery: 40 mg SC qd DVT treatment: 1 mg/kg or 1.5 mg/kg qd DVT prophylaxis 40 mg SC qd	Bleeding, local irritation at the injection site, transient elevated liver function test values	Active major bleeding (GI or intracranial); thrombocytopenia in association with positive in vitro testing for anti-platelet antibodies. Hypersensitivity to heparin, LMWH, or patients with severe renal insufficiency	Low–molecular-weight heparin used for prophylaxis of DVT/PE after total hip replacement, total knee replacement, and abdominal surgeries in medical patients where immobility DVT/PE treatment. Evaluate CBC periodically for bleeding effects.
fondaparinux (Arixtra)	Bleeding, injection site bleeding and LFT elevation, thrombocytopenia and irritation	Active major bleeding, body wt <50 kg thrombocytopenia, severe hepatic impairment	Pentasaccharide used for DVT prophylaxis in patients following hip fracture and hip and knee replacement surgery.
Antiplatelet Agents			
aspirin (Bayer) 30–1500 mg/d PO	Bleeding, gastric ulceration, allergic reactions	Active stroke or stroke in progress; active GI bleeding, or aspirin allergy or hypersensitivity	Decreases the risk of death/nonfatal MI in patients with previous MI or unstable angina. Decreases the risk of recurrent ischemic stroke. Text discusses controversies with dosing
clopidogrel (Plavix) 75 mg qd PO	Bleeding, GI effects, rash (rare)	Active major bleeding (peptic ulcer or intracranial hemorrhage)	Reduces risk of MI, stroke, or vascular death in patients with atherosclerosis documented by recent stroke, MI, or established peripheral artery disease. Decreased risk of neutropenia compared with risk of neutropenia from ticlopidine
ticlopidine (Ticlid) 250 mg bid PO	Neutropenia, thrombocytopenia, rash, GI effects, hepatic impairment	Neutropenia or thrombocytopenia; active bleeding (GI or intracranial hemorrhage); severe hepatic impairment	Decreases the risk of thrombotic stroke in patients with a history of stroke or transient ischemic attack. Must monitor CBC and platelets every 2 wk for the first 3 mo of therapy because of neutropenia. Discontinue if the absolute neutrophil count drops below 1200, or if the platelet count falls below 80,000

(continued)

Table 54.2

Overview of Drugs Used to Treat Coagulation Disorders (*Continued*)

Generic (Trade) Name and Dosage	Selected Adverse Events	Contraindications	Special Considerations
			Reserved for patients allergic to or intolerant to aspirin because of neutropenia
Direct Thrombin Inhibiters			
lepirudin (Refludan) 0.4 mg/kg via slow IV bolus 0.15 mg/kg IV infusion	Bleeding, anemia, abnormal LFTs, allergic reactions	Hypersensitivity to hirudins	Direct thrombin inhibitor for prophylaxis and treatment for thrombosis in HIT.
argatroban 2 mg/kg/min as IV infusion	Bleeding, allergies, dyspnea, hypotension	Overt bleeding, hypersensitivity	

Initial Dose

It is difficult to predict an individual's warfarin requirement needed to reach the INR range that is considered therapeutic for the disease state. The common practice of administering a warfarin "loading" dose of 10 mg for 3 days is no longer recommended because the target INR is often exceeded in 20% to 50% of patients, which increases the risk for adverse events such as warfarin skin necrosis. Exceeding the target INR increases the risk of bleeding, prompts an interruption in therapy, and delays achievement of a stable dose. Large warfarin loading doses do not attain a therapeutic INR faster than starting a usual maintenance dose (Harrison et al., 1997).

Current recommendations are to start warfarin at an average maintenance dose of 5 mg daily and adjust the dose based on daily INR values. Table 54-4 presents a suggested dosing method (Spandorfer et al., 2001). Certain patient populations, such as the elderly, patients with congestive heart failure, those with underlying malignancy, or those with severely impaired renal or hepatic function or inadequate nutrition, are at high risk for bleeding, and should receive a lower initial dose of 2 to 4 mg daily. Larger starting doses such as 7.5 to 10 mg may be used if rapid effect is urgently needed but is unnecessary for most patients (Hyers et al., 2001). During the initial titration phase, daily dosage increases or decreases are commonly made in 2.5-mg increments based on INR values. If rapid anticoagulation is not necessary and the patient's risks for thrombosis and bleeding are not high, warfarin can be started on an outpatient basis with INR evaluations every 2 to 3 days (Spandorfer et al., 2001). Administering warfarin at the same time daily is recommended to reduce variability in effect.

Table 54.3

Normal Half-Lives of the Vitamin K–Dependent Clotting Factors and Proteins C and S

Activity	Vitamin K–Dependent Protein	Half-Life (hs)
Anticoagulant	Protein C	9
Anticoagulant	Protein S	60
Coagulant	Factor II	72
Coagulant	Factor VII	4–6
Coagulant	Factor IX	18–24
Coagulant	Factor X	48

From Spandorfer, J., Konkle, B. A., & Merli, G. J. (2001). *Management and prevention of thrombosis in primary care* (p. 106). London: Arnold.

Maintenance Dose

There is no linear relationship between the warfarin dosage and INR. Therefore, minor changes in dose can result in greater than expected changes in the INR. The maintenance warfarin dose varies widely among individuals. No accepted patient characteristics can predict the necessary maintenance dose. Calculating the total weekly warfarin dose, and then increasing or decreasing the weekly regimen by only 10% to 20% spread over the course of the week, can cause measurable changes in the INR. Some clinicians advocate

---

BOX 54–3. OVERLAPPING HEPARIN WITH WARFARIN

Acute thrombotic events; including DVT and PE, are initially treated with heparin in the inpatient setting. Warfarin should be started within the first 24 to 48 hours of heparin therapy, to avoid delaying hospital discharge. Overlapping therapy with both agents for at least 5 to 7 days is recommended until the INR is therapeutic.

The rationale for overlapping warfarin and heparin is to prevent a potential hypercoagulable condition. This may occur because when warfarin is started the initial increase in the INR is due to a fast drop in factor VII, which has the shortest half-life (6 hours) of the clotting factors. However, the full protective effects are not realized until factor II, which has a half-life of 60 hours, is depleted. Although changes in the INR may occur within 24 hours, it takes several days for the full anticoagulant effect to occur. Protein C, a vitamin K–dependent protein that has endogenous inhibitive effects on coagulation, also has a short half-life (4–6 hours) and is depleted quickly when warfarin is initiated. Thus, unless warfarin and heparin therapy are overlapped initially, there is a paradoxical risk of inducing a temporary hypercoagulable state. This hypercoagulable state would be due to the drop in protein C until factor II is depleted, which must occur before the full antithrombotic activity of warfarin can be reached.

Table 54.4

Anticoagulation Treatment—Oral Anticoagulation

Warfarin dosing requirements are highly variable and should be individualized based upon patient specific information. The following table represents a suggested dosing method to achieve a target INR of 2.5

INR	Day 1*	Day 2	Day 3	Day 4	Day 5
<1.5	5 mg	5 mg	7.5 mg	10 mg	10 mg
1.5–1.99	2.5 mg	2.5 mg	5 mg	7.5 mg	7.5 mg
2.0–2.49		1 mg	2.5 mg	5 mg	5 mg
2.5–2.99		0 mg	1 mg	2.5 mg	2.5 mg
3.0–3.5		0 mg	0 mg	1 mg	1 mg
>3.5		0 mg	0 mg	0 mg	0 mg

*Therapeutic aPTT obtained (eg, begin warfarin on day 1 of heparin therapy).
From Spandorfer, J., Konkle, B. A., & Merli, G. J. (2001). *Management and prevention of thrombosis in primary care*. London: Arnold.

administering the same dosage daily, whereas others agree that giving varying doses on alternate days is rational (Ansell, 1993). Patients with low education levels, cognitive impairments, or those receiving several other medications may benefit from a simple dosing schedule. If an alternating-day regimen is chosen, defining the actual dosage for each day of the week is recommended (eg, 5 mg administered on Tuesdays, Thursdays, Saturdays, Sundays, and 7.5 mg on Mondays, Wednesday, Fridays, rather than 5 mg alternating with 7.5 mg every other day). This helps to reduce patient confusion and avoid fluctuations in the INR. Sensitive patients with reduced requirements should receive warfarin daily, rather than alternating between drug and drug-free days, for example, 1.5 mg given every day, rather than 2 mg alternating with 0 mg every other day (Ansell, 1993; Benet & Goyan, 1995). Once a patient has reached a therapeutic INR with a consistent warfarin dose, INR monitoring should continue every 4 to 6 weeks.

Adverse Events

Bleeding is the most worrisome adverse event associated with oral anticoagulation therapy. As the intensity of anticoagulation increases, so does the bleeding risk. Refer to the section on monitoring warfarin therapy for a discussion of the INR. The highest risk of bleeding occurs when the INR exceeds a 4.0 to 5.0 range. In contrast, patients maintained at INRs of 2 to 3 have very low bleeding rates of approximately 1% (Hirsh et al., 1998). Other issues, such as individual patient characteristics, concurrent use of other antithrombotic medications such as aspirin or clopidogrel, and duration of therapy, also contribute to the propensity for hemorrhagic complications. The frequency of fatal bleeding, major bleeding, and minor bleeding is estimated at 0.6%, 3%, and 9.6%, respectively (Fihn et al., 1993).

Minor bleeding occurring from the oral or nasal mucosa, urine, stool, or soft tissues is the most common adverse effect of anticoagulation therapy. Bleeding complications in order of frequency are epitasis, purpura, hematuria, GI bleeding, and hemoptysis (Fihn et al., 1993; Landefeld & Byeth, 1993). Minor bleeding is usually managed by temporarily discontinuing warfarin therapy for 1 to 2 days, and then restarting at a reduced dosage, or reducing the target INR range.

Major bleeding is commonly defined as any bleeding resulting in hospitalization, necessitating transfusion, occurring in the intracranial or retroperitoneal areas, or causing death. Risk factors for major bleeding episodes include age older than 65 years; previous history of GI bleeding; and history of stroke, hypertension, severe cardiac disease, recent MI, severe anemia, or renal insufficiency (Hirsh, Dalen et al., 2001). Although controversial, most studies show that elderly patients have a higher frequency of bleeding. The greatest risk of bleeding occurs within the first 3 months of warfarin therapy (Levine et al., 1998). The rates of intracranial bleeding from several well-conducted trials have ranged from 0.3% to 1.4%. Although intracranial bleeding is a rare complication, it is the most frequent cause of fatal events (Levine et al., 1998). Management of major bleeding focuses on reversal of the anticoagulation effects of warfarin (Box 54-4). Any bleeding event should be adequately investigated because an underlying comorbidity, such as malignancy, may be the cause.

Other adverse reactions to warfarin therapy, which occur infrequently, include nausea, diarrhea, hypersensitivity/allergic reactions, hepatitis, elevated liver enzymes, jaundice, edema, fever, rash, dermatitis, urticaria, abdominal pain, flatulence/bloating, fatigue, lethargy, malaise, headache, dizziness, taste perversion, pruritus, alopecia, cold intolerance, and paresthesia including feeling cold and chills. Serious, but rare adverse effects of warfarin include skin necrosis, which usually appears within a few days of starting therapy and is thought to be associated with local thrombus, and purple toe syndrome, which occurs later in therapy and is thought to be due to cholesterol emboli and is not considered to be related to drug dose. These effects may require debridement or amputation of the effected area. Immediate cessation of warfarin therapy is warranted if these adverse reactions occur (Coumadin tablets package insert, 2001).

Interactions

An extensive list of medications either potentiate or inhibit the anticoagulant effect of warfarin. The potential mechanisms of drug interactions with warfarin include alterations in absorption, enhanced or decreased hepatic clearance, alteration in protein binding of warfarin, or enhanced or inhibited vitamin K metabolism and therefore enhanced or inhibited synthesis of vitamin K clotting factors. Interactions may also occur secondary to potentiation of anticoagulant effects by direct pharmacologic effect of concomitant medications on the PT or inhibition of platelet function. Medications that commonly effect warfarin include, but are not limited to, amiodarone; antibiotics such as erythromycin, metronidazole, and trimethoprim–sulfamethoxazole (TMP-SMZ); antifungals; salicylates; NSAIDS; H_2 antagonists; sucralfate; lipid-lowering medications; thyroid hormones; anticonvulsants; steroids; influenza vaccine; and vitamin E (Spandorfer et al., 2001). Drug interactions with warfarin and their level of evidence are displayed in Table 54-5. There is much patient variability when interacting drugs are added to or discontinued from warfarin therapy. Close laboratory monitoring and warfarin dosage adjustment is needed to prevent either supratherapeutic or subtherapeutic INRs, resulting in hemorrhagic effects or thromboembolic complications.

BOX 54–4. REVERSING THE ANTICOAGULANT EFFECTS OF WARFARIN

Managing patients with elevated international normalized ratios (INRs) is essential for safe and effective anticoagulation therapy.

Moderately Elevated INRs

For patients with INRs above therapeutic range but <5, simply decreasing the warfarin dose is a rational approach. The dose may be held for 24 hours, and then therapy restarted in a reduced regimen, which can bring the INR to within the target range (Bridgen et al., 1998). The INR may further increase for 1 day after warfarin is discontinued before declining. Holding the warfarin dose decreases the INR approximately 1 to 1.5 INR units per day exponentially. Patients who are maintained on warfarin and whose INR ranges between 2.0 and 3.0 require approximately 1 to 4 days for the INR to fall below 1.5 when therapy is discontinued. There is wide patient variation in the rate of decrease.

Highly Elevated INRs

Patients with highly elevated INRs or patients with active bleeding may need vitamin K in addition to temporary discontinuance of warfarin therapy. An initial drop in the INR occurs within 6 hours after vitamin K administration. However, the full effect does not occur for 24 hours. Doses of vitamin K larger than 1 mg may induce a state of warfarin resistance that can last for up to 2 weeks until the vitamin K–dependent clotting factors are depleted. The goals of vitamin K therapy are to reduce the INR to within the therapeutic range, without dropping below the target INR, and to prevent inducing a state of temporary warfarin resistance (Harrel & Kline, 1995). Therefore, much lower vitamin K doses than the formerly used dose of 10 mg are now advocated for reversing anticoagulation. Two recent studies reported that 1 or 2.5 mg oral vitamin K reduced the INR to the therapeutic range, without inducing a state of warfarin resistance (Crowther et al., 1998).

Parenteral Versus Oral Vitamin K

Previously, subcutaneous vitamin K was recommended to reverse warfarin's effect. However, new information suggests that oral vitamin K has advantages over the parenteral form. Intravenous vitamin K is often not practical in the ambulatory setting because of the risk of anaphylactic and hypersensitivity reactions. In addition, concerns have been raised about possibly erratic absorption of subcutaneous vitamin K. Advantages of oral vitamin K include a decreased risk of allergic reactions, convenience, and low cost (Harrell & Kline, 1995), although oral vitamin K is not useful for severe bleeding or malabsorption. In these situations parenteral vitamin K is recommended.

Oral vitamin K (Mephyton) is available in 5-mg tablets (Merck and Co., 1997). Parenteral vitamin K (Aquamephyton) is available in concentrations of 2 mg/mL in 0.5-mL ampules, and 10 mg/mL in 1-mL ampules, or 2.5- and 5-mL vials. Oral vitamin K tablets in 100-μg strengths can be purchased at health food stores without a prescription, or the parenteral preparation can be taken orally.

From Hirsh, J., Dalen, J. E. et al. (2001). Oral anticoagulants: Mechanism of action, clinical effectiveness, and optimal therapeutic range. *Chest, 119*(Suppl. 1), 8S–21S.

In addition, several herbal preparations can potentially interfere with the anticoagulant effect of warfarin. Although stringently performed clinical trials are lacking, bilberry, feverfew, garlic, ginger, and ginkgo biloba have limited data that show an increased anticoagulant effect when used with warfarin. Garlic has platelet-inhibitory effects that can increase the bleeding risk, and there are anecdotal reports of increases in the PT/INR in patients receiving warfarin (Tyler, 1996). Herbal products that can decrease the effect of warfarin include ginseng and green tea (Janetsky & Morreale, 1997; Taylor & Wilt, 1999). A web site for published scientific literature on herbal supplements can be accessed at www.nal.usda.gov/fnic/IBIDS. Patients must be educated to tell prescribing practitioners all medications and herbals that they are currently taking and alert them to addition, cessation, or change in dosage of any medications and herbals.

Excessive dietary vitamin K also interacts with warfarin by antagonizing its clinical effect. Therefore, the practitioner should discuss diet when prescribing this drug (see Patient Education section).

Unfractionated Heparin

Unfractionated heparin (UFH) augments the inhibitory effects of antithrombin III, thus disrupting the clotting cascade. It is indicated for the prevention of VTE and the treatment of DVT and PE, which will be the focus of heparin use described in this chapter. UFH may also be used in early treatment of unstable angina and acute myocardial infarction and for those undergoing cardiac bypass, catheterization, and stenting.

Mechanism of Action

UFH inhibits reactions that lead to clotting, but it does not alter the concentration of the normal clotting factors of the

Table 54.5

Drug and Food Interactions With Warfarin and Direction of Interaction

Type of Study	Potentiation	Inhibition	No Effect
Randomized controlled trials	Alcohol (if concomitant liver disease), amiodarone, anabolic steroids, cimetidine,[†] clofibrate, cotrimoxazole, erythromycin, fluconazole, isoniazid (600 mg/d), metronidazole, miconazole, omeprazole, phenylbutazone,* piroxicam, propafenone, propranolol, sulfinpyrazone (biphasic with later inhibition)*	Barbiturates, carbamazepine, chlordiazepoxide, cholestyramine, griseofulvin,* nafcillin, rifampin, sucralfate, high vitamin K content foods/ enteral feeds, large amounts of avocado	Alcohol, antacids, atenolol, bumetadine, enoxacin, famotidine, fluoxetine, ketorolac, metoprolol, naproxen, nizatidine, psyllium, ranitidine[‡]
Randomized controlled trials	Acetaminophen, chloral hydrate, ciprofloxacin, dextropropoxyphene, disulfiram, itraconazole, quinidine, phenytoin (biphasic with later inhibition), tamoxifen, tetracycline, flu vaccine	Dicloxacillin	Ibuprofen, ketoconazole
Observational studies	Acetylsalicylic acid, disopyramide, fluorouracil, ifosfamide, ketoprofen, lovastatin, metozalone, moricizine, nalidixic acid, norfloxacin, ofloxacin, propoxyphene, sulindac, tolmetin, topical salicylates	Azathioprine, cyclosporine, etretinate, trazodone	
Observational studies	Cefamandole, cefazolin, gemfibrozil, heparin, indomethacin, sulfisoxazole		Diltiazem, tobacco, vancomycin

*Has supporting level 1 evidence from both patients and volunteers.
[†]In a small number of volunteer subjects, an inhibitory drug interaction occurred.
[‡]Randomized, controlled trial evidence of potentiation in patients.
From Hirsh, J., Dalen, J. E., et al. (2001). Oral anticoagulants: mechanism of action, clinical effectiveness, and optimal therapeutic range. *Chest, 119*(Suppl. 1), 8S–21S.

blood. By binding with antithrombin III, UFH induces a structural conformation change that increases the inactivation rate of the intrinsic clotting cascade pathway, including factors XII, XI, X, IX, and thrombin (factor II). The heparin–antithrombin III complex has a high affinity for activated factor X (Xa) and thrombin. Small amounts of UFH combined with antithrombin III inhibit thrombosis by inactivating factor Xa and inhibiting the conversion of prothrombin to thrombin. Larger amounts can work, after active thrombosis has developed, to inhibit further coagulation by inactivating thrombin and preventing the conversion of fibrinogen to fibrin. UFH also prevents the formation of a stable clot by inhibiting activation of factor XIII, the fibrin stabilizing factor (*Drug Facts and Comparisons*, 2002). UFH is a very large molecule (ie, it has an average molecular weight of 15,000 Da with chains of 18–50 saccharide units), but only a small portion of the entire structure is necessary for binding with antithrombin III. Because the structure is so large, UFH can bind to both factor Xa and thrombin. Heparin derivatives with smaller structures cannot bind to thrombin, but can bind to and inhibit factor Xa (Hirsh, Warkentin et al., 2001).

Heparin is not absorbed from the GI tract. UFH has an immediate onset of action and is administered by intravenous infusion when rapid anticoagulation is needed, as in acute DVT, PE, or unstable angina. UFH may also be administered subcutaneously with peak levels occurring 2 to 4 hours after administration, depending on dose. Subcutaneous dosing must be at a sufficient dose to overcome the lower bioavailability, approximately 30%, associated with this route of administration. The duration of action and half-life are dependent on dose. The average half-life is 30 to 180 minutes, which may be significantly prolonged at high doses. UFH is metabolized by liver heparinase and the reticuloendothelial system and possibly secondarily in the kidneys. It is then excreted in the urine as unchanged drug (*Drug Facts and Comparisons*, 2002).

Limitations of UFH include the heterogeneity in its size, anticoagulant activity, and pharmacokinetic profile. UFH can range in size from 5000 to 30,000 Da. Agents with higher molecular weights are cleared from the circulation more rapidly than agents with lower molecular weights. UFH is highly bound to plasma proteins and cellular components, including endothelial cells and macrophages, which reduces its therapeutic effect and increases the incidence of immunologic reactions (eg, heparin-induced thrombocytopenia [HIT]). Furthermore, some patients exhibit heparin resistance. This is characterized by no measurable change in anticoagulant effect despite receiving large doses (35,000 U) of heparin daily (Hirsh et al., 1998). UFH also has a nonlinear dose response, so that small changes in dosage can result in large changes in anticoagulant effect. Therefore, UFH is usually restricted to use in the hospital setting because frequent laboratory monitoring is necessary.

Dosage

UFH dosing is based on weight. Initial dosing should be 80 U/kg as an intravenous bolus and then 18 U/kg/h continuous intravenous infusion. UFH effect is monitored by the aPTT. Dosage changes should be made based on aPTT levels monitored every 6 hours until stable and the every 12 hours. For DVT or PE treatment, a therapeutic aPTT of 1.5 to 2.5 times control must be achieved within the first 24 hours of

Table 54.6

Weight-Based Heparin Dosing Nomogram

Activated Partial Thromboplastin Time	Rate Change
Initial dose	80 U/kg bolus, then 18 U/kg/h
<35 (<1.2 × control)	80 U/kg bolus, then increase infusion by 4 U/kg/h
35–45 (1.2–1.5 × control)	40 U/kg/h bolus, then increase infusion by 2 U/kg/h
46–70 (1.5–2.3 × control)	No change
71–90 (2.3–3 × control)	Decrease infusion rate by 2 U/kg/h
>90 (>3 × control)	Hold infusion for 1 h, then decrease infusion rate by 3 U/kg/h

Adapted from Hirsh, J., Raschke, R., et al. (2004). Heparin and low-molecular-weight heparin. *Chest, 126*(suppl. 1), 188S–203S.

therapy to reduce the rate of recurrent thrombotic events and decrease mortality rates. Several dosing nomograms are available to assist clinicians in rapidly attaining a therapeutic aPTT within the first day of therapy. One popular method is the weight-based nomogram (Hirsch et al., 2004) shown in Table 54-6.

Adjusted-dose subcutaneous heparin has been used in patients with limited intravenous access or in those with contraindications to warfarin (eg, pregnancy). Intramuscular injections are not recommended because of the increased risks of bleeding and bruising (Hirsh et al., 1998). UFH in a fixed low dose of 5000 U subcutaneously every 8 to 12 hours is used for VTE prophylaxis and reduces the risk for VTE by 60% to 70%. This regimen may be used in postoperative patients and medical patients with decreased mobility.

Adverse Events

Adverse effects associated with UFH include bleeding, osteoporosis, and thrombocytopenia (see Table 54-2). Less common adverse effects that may occur include hyperlipidemia secondary to the increase in free fatty acid serum levels caused by the induction of lipoprotein lipase, chills, fever, urticaria, and hypersensitivity reactions (*Drug Facts and Comparisons*, 2002). The risk of bleeding increases in patients who have preexisting renal failure, hepatic disease, or cardiovascular disease, who sustained recent trauma or surgery, who have had recent CNS procedures such as surgery or spinal anesthesia, who have a history of or current GI lesions or bleeding, who have a hematologic disorder, and who are using aspirin concurrently. Little is known about the mechanism causing osteoporosis. It is thought that UFH impairs bone deposition and accelerates bone resorption. This is a concern in those requiring long-term treatment with UFH, especially with heparin doses greater than 20,000 U/d administered for more than 3 months or UFH doses less than 20,000 U/d for longer than 12 months. For these patients, it is recommended that baseline bone density should be obtained and calcium supplements considered (Becker et al., 2002). Pregnant patients may receive heparin for the duration of gestation, whereas it is necessary to discontinue oral anticoagulant therapy; they are also at risk for heparin-induced osteoporosis. Thrombocytopenia during heparin therapy may be mild, remain stable, and possibly

reverse itself during therapy. However, platelet counts should be closely monitored during heparin therapy because a drop in platelet count below 150×10^9/L or greater than 50% of baseline necessitates discontinuation of heparin therapy. This may be related to heparin-induced thrombocytopenia (HIT), an antibody-mediated reaction that may cause new venous and arterial thrombosis to occur. A more detailed discussion of HIT and its treatment is presented in Box 54-5.

Low-Molecular-Weight Heparins

Low-molecular-weight heparins (LMWHs) are fragments of UFH, prepared by the depolymerization of porcine heparin. Like UFH, LMWHs produce their major anticoagulant effect by activating antithrombin III, although the LMWH–antithrombin III complex has a weak antithrombin effect, it can inactivate factor Xa. LMWHs are used for prophylaxis of VTE in patients after orthopedic and abdominal surgery and medical patients with decreased mobility or increased risk for VTE and for treatment of DVT/PE. Other uses that will not be discussed in this chapter are in unstable angina and myocardial infarction (Becker et al., 2002). As with UFH, most patients need subsequent treatment with warfarin, depending on the indication for anticoagulation.

Another medication, similar to LMWH and approved only for the prophylaxis of DVT/PE in patients after hip fracture and hip or knee replacement surgery is the pentasaccharide, fondaparinux sodium (Arixtra). It is a 5-saccharide chain that also binds to and activates antithrombin. In studies of patients with these indications, pentasaccharide was more effective than the LMWH, enoxaparin, when given in a daily subcutaneous dose of 2.5 mg. It also had a similar rate of bleeding as compared to enoxaparin. Other advantages of this drug are that there is no interaction with platelets, which conveys no risk for HIT and it is not made from animal products (Becker et al., 2002). However, it is not yet frequently used and is not approved by the Food and Drug Administration (FDA) for use in HIT.

Mechanism of Action

LMWHs preferentially inhibit the activation of factor X but have minimal effects on thrombin (factor II) because of their small size. The average molecular weight of LMWHs ranges from 4000 to 6500 Da with 13 to 22 saccharide units (UFH has a mean molecular weight of 12,000–15,000 Da with 18–50 saccharide units). Only the LMWHs with saccharide chains having 18 or more units can bind to and inhibit thrombin (Becker et al., 2002). UFH has a ratio of anti-Xa to anti-IIa activity of 1:1, and the anti-Xa to anti-IIa activity of LMWHs ranges from 2:1 to 4:1.

LMWH given by the subcutaneous route has a bioavailability greater than 90% of the given dose. In contrast to UFH, LMWH has minimal binding to cells or plasma proteins, which results in the persistence of free drug in the circulation and a longer half-life of activity. The half-lives of LMWHs range from 108 to 252 minutes. Dosing is fixed in prophylaxis but is based on weight for treatment.

As previously noted, the major antithrombotic effect and bleeding effect of LMWHs arise through their ability to

BOX 54–5. HEPARIN-INDUCED THROMBOCYTOPENIA (HIT)

Two types of thrombocytopenia have been associated with heparin, a benign form (type I) and an immune-mediated form (type II), which can cause devastating complications.

Type I HIT

Type I HIT is caused by platelet sequestration, occurs early in therapy, rarely produces platelet counts below 100,000/mm^3, resolves despite continued treatment with heparin, and is considered clinically insignificant.

Type II HIT

Type II HIT occurs after 5 to 15 days of heparin treatment and can cause rapid and dramatic reductions in the platelet count. A platelet count below 100,000/mm^3, often fewer than 50,000/mm^3, or a 50% drop from baseline should alert the practitioner to possible type II HIT. Clinical effects of type II HIT include arterial and venous thrombosis, resulting in DVT, PE, myocardial infraction limb ischemia, and gangrene requiring limb amputation, cerebral thrombosis, and death. Discontinuation of all heparin sources, including heparin flushes and heparin-coated catheters, is required for platelet counts to normalize.

In type II HIT, antibodies directed against the platelet membrane are produced in the presence of heparin. The target antigen is a complex of heparin bound to platelet factor 4 (PF4), which stimulates the release of immunoglobulins (IgGs) and subsequent platelet activation and aggregation. The coagulation cascade is initiated, eventually causing increased platelet consumption and clearance.

Alternatives to Heparin

Low-molecular-weight heparins (LMWHs) are possible alternatives to unfractionated heparin in patients with HIT requiring further anticoagulation therapy. However, cross-sensitivity between LMWHs and unfractionated heparin has been reported in HIT, so LMWHs would not be suitable in such a situation (Howe & Allerman, 1998).

The only recommended agents for treating patients with HIT are the direct thrombin inhibitors (DTIs), lepirudin and argatroban. Lepirudin is a recombinant hirudin product derived from yeast cells. Hirudin is an anticoagulant isolated from the salivary glands of medicinal leeches, used historically to prevent blood clotting. Recombinant technology allowed mass production of hirudin. Unlike heparin, hirudin does not require cofactors for activation (Stringer & Lindenfeld, 1992). Lepirudin (r-hirudin) is a DTI that binds irreversibly to thrombin, thus inactivating the enzyme and preventing further activation of the coagulation cascade.

Lepirudin has anticoagulant activity, with no known interaction with platelets. This product received U.S. Food and Drug Administration approval for anticoagulation in patients with HIT to prevent further thromboembolic complications, based on the results of two trials conducted in Germany (Hoechst Marion Roussel, 1998). These trials evaluated more than 200 patients with HIT. Results showed increases in platelet counts, effective anticoagulation, and reductions in death and the need for limb amputation with lepirudin (Greinacher et al., 1999). An intravenous (IV) bolus of 0.4 mg/kg administered over 15 to 20 seconds is followed by a continuous IV infusion of 0.15 mg/kg, given for 2 to 10 days, or longer, if clinically indicated. The major adverse effect of lepirudin is bleeding, including intracranial hemorrhage. Protamine does not reverse the activity of lepirudin (Hoechst Marion Roussel, 1998). In circumstances where an alternative to heparin is needed, argatroban and lepirudin are reasonable choices (Howe & Allerman, 1998).

Argatroban is a synthetic derivative L-arginine that binds to the thrombin molecule. Although the binding is reversible, there is no known antidote. Argatroban is metabolized predominantly in the liver, with minimal excretion in the urine. As a DTI, argatroban rapidly inhibits both fibrin-bound and freely circulating thrombin and has no cross-reacting with HIT antibodies. The recommended dosing inpatients with HIT is 2 μg/kg/min as a continuous IV infusion adjusted to a target aPTT range of 1.5 to 3.0 times the initial baseline value. A prospective, open-label, historically controlled study evaluated the safety and efficacy of argatroban in over 300 patients with HIT. Two arms were studied: the HIT am, which included those with isolated thrombocytopenia or history of HIT, and the HIT with thrombosis arm. In the HIT arm argatroban significantly reduced the rate of the composite end point of death, amputation, or new thrombosis. When evaluating each end point individually, the rate of new thrombosis was significantly reduced, but death and limb amputation were not. This is because even because even in the presence of a DTI, clot-bound thrombin can continue to activate platelets and generate further thrombus formation. This also explains why argatroban did not significantly reduce the incidence of the composite end point or any of the individual clinical end points compared to controls. Hemorrhage was the most common adverse event associated with argatroban.

---

inactivate factor Xa. UFH is monitored using the aPTT, which primarily reflects anti–activated factor II (IIa) activity, but LMWH has minimal effects on the aPTT. Theoretically, LMWH may be monitored by anti–factor Xa activity, with a target range for treatment regimens of 0.5 to 1.2 U/mL 3 to 4 hours after a subcutaneous dose. Studies have demonstrated that the anti-Xa effect of LMWH is linearly related to the dose administered. Therefore, plasma levels are predictable and anti-Xa activity monitoring is not routinely performed. Monitoring may be considered in selected patients, such as those with renal dysfunction because LMWHs are cleared primarily by the renal route, morbidly obese patients (150 kg) because weight-adjusted dosing has not been evaluated in patients with severe obesity, and pregnant patients because their weight changes, volume shifts occur, and clearance changes as pregnancy progresses (Becker et al., 2002). In addition to the recommendation for monitoring levels in patients with renal dysfunction, dosing adjustments may be necessary when using LMWHs in patients with a creatinine clearance of less than 30 mL/min (Hyers et al, 2001).

Advantages of LMWH over UFH include increased bioavailability secondary to decreased plasma protein binding, a longer half-life, less frequent dosing, and more predictable anticoagulant activity. This profile allows for administration of this medication in the home and may decrease length of hospital stays for patients being treated for DTV/PE or receiving LMWH for prophylaxis.

Three LMWHs are available in the United States, dalteparin (Fragmin), tinzaparin (Innohep), and enoxaparin (Lovenox), and several more are under clinical development (see Table 54-2). A LMWH, ardeparin (Normiflo), was withdrawn by the FDA secondary to safety and effectiveness issues. A heparinoid product, danaparoid, also used in patients for prophylaxis of VTE and the treatment of HIT, is no longer available in the United States because the natural constituents of the drug are no longer readily available, but it is used in the European Union and Canada (Larned et al., 2003).

Dosage

Each LMWH has its own unique dosing regimen because of its unique chemical properties and the relative proportions of anti-Xa to anti-IIa activity (Table 54-7). Because of differences in the manufacturing process, molecular weight, half-life, ratio of anti-Xa to anti-IIa activity, and dose, FDA does not consider these agents therapeutically interchangeable (Hirsh et al., 1998). Enoxaparin at 30 mg every 12 hours or 40 mg daily is currently approved for prophylaxis in medical inpatients and patients after hip, knee, and abdominal surgery. Dalteparin at 2500 U every 12 hours or 5000 U daily is approved for prophylaxis in patients after hip and abdominal surgery. For treatment, current FDA approvals are for enoxaparin at 1 mg/kg every 12 hours or 1.5 mg/kg daily for inpatients with acute DVT with and without PE when administered in conjunction with warfarin and for outpatients with acute DVT without PE when administered in conjunction with warfarin. Tinzaparin at 175 IU/kg daily is FDA approved for inpatient treatment of acute DVT with and without PE when administered in conjunction with warfarin (Becker et al., 2002).

Table 54.7

Pharmacokinetic Profiles of Low–Molecular-Weight Heparins

Product	Trade Name	Molecular Weight (Da)	Half-Life (h)	Anti-Xa/IIa Ratio
dalteparin	Fragmin	5000	3	2.7:1
enoxaparin	Lovenox	4500	4.5	3.8:1
tinzaparin	Innohep	4500	3–4	1.9:1

There are no specific guidelines for dosage adjustments in patients with renal dysfunction although decreased doses should be considered in patients with creatinine clearance of less than 30 mL/min. Howard (2003) describes one study that recommended dosing adjustments that result in an anti-Xa level of 1.0 IU mL. For enoxaparin dosing, it was recommended that dosage be decreased to 0.84 mg/kg twice daily for patients with creatinine clearance of 30 to 60 mL/min and 0.64 mg/kg twice daily for those with creatinine clearance of less than 30 mL/min (Howard, 2003). Another study recommends decreasing enoxaparin dosage to 1 mg/kg once daily for those with a creatinine clearance of 30 mL/min or less (Lovenox package insert, 2002).

Adverse Effects

Adverse effects associated with LMWHs include bleeding, thrombocytopenia, and elevations in liver function test results. Less common effects are injection site reactions, fever, nausea, peripheral edema, wound hematoma, urinary tract infections, and hypochromic anemia. Hemorrhage is the most common complication of LMWH therapy, along with hematoma at the injection or surgical site. The incidence of hemorrhage is similar to or slightly lower than that with use of UFH. The aPTT is not used to monitor therapeutic efficacy, and a patient receiving LMWHs should have periodic CBC and platelet monitoring and hemoccult testing to assess for bleeding. The incidence of thrombocytopenia is much lower than with UFH. Transient, benign thrombocytopenia is seen in approximately 5% of patients treated with LMWH. The immune-mediated thrombocytopenia, HIT, has been reported in fewer than 1% of patients. In patients with active or prior HIT, the thrombocytopenia may be reproduced during the use of LMWH with a reported cross-reactivity in HIT of more than 90% (Spandorfer et al., 2001). Asymptomatic elevations in aspartate aminotransferase and alanine aminotransferase levels have been reported with LMWHs; elevations are reversible with drug discontinuation. As previously described, patients with renal insufficiency may have reduced LMWH elimination. Therefore, careful use is recommended, including dosage reduction or monitoring of anti-Xa concentrations (Hirsh et al., 1998).

Aspirin

Aspirin is the oldest and most frequently used antiplatelet drug. Antiplatelet agents, such as aspirin, decrease platelet aggregation and decrease the formation of arterial thrombi. Aspirin is commonly used in patients for primary prevention of atherosclerotic heart disease to reduce the risk of subsequent myocardial infarction, stroke, and vascular death. It is also used in patients to prevent TIAs and acute ischemic stroke secondary to cerebral vascular disease. Aspirin has also been used as an alternative therapy for patients with atrial fibrillation who are considered poor candidates for anticoagulation and who have no high or moderate risk factors and no clinical or echocardiographic evidence of cardiovascular disease (Patrono et al., 2001). Aspirin use in atherosclerotic heart disease will not be discussed in this chapter.

Mechanism of Action

Aspirin prevents the synthesis of prostaglandin in platelets and other tissues by irreversibly modifying and inhibiting the enzyme cyclooxygenase, which catalyzes the conversion of arachidonic acid to thromboxane A_2, a prostaglandin derivative, which is a potent vasoconstrictor and promoter of platelet aggregation. After discontinuation of aspirin, platelets are impaired for their normal life span of 7 to 10 days because of the irreversible inhibition of cyclooxygenase (Spandorfer et al., 2001). Every 24 hours, 10% of platelets are replaced and 5 to 6 days following aspirin ingestion, approximately 50% of the platelets function normally (Patrono et al., 2001).

Aspirin is rapidly absorbed in the stomach and upper intestine with peak levels occurring 30 to 40 minutes after ingestion. Inhibition of platelet function is evident by 1 hour after ingestion. The half-life of aspirin is 15 to 20 minutes and salicylic acid, to which aspirin is hydrolyzed during absorption, has a half-life of 2 to 3 hours at low doses and may exceed 20 hours at higher doses. Aspirin is eliminated by renal excretion (*Drug Facts and Comparisons*, 2002).

Dosage

The optimal aspirin dosage for thrombotic disorders is still controversial because doses ranging from 30 to 1500 mg/d are effective. Inhibition of platelet aggregation can be shown at doses as low as 20 mg/d given over several days. Maximal inhibition of platelet aggregation occurs at doses of 80 to 100 mg/d. Higher doses of aspirin have other effects such as acetylation of fibrinogen, which results in a diminished capacity for fibrinogen to form fibrin, and the fibrin that is formed is more susceptible to lysis. It is not yet known how these nonplatelet effects of aspirin contribute to its overall antithrombotic properties (Spandorfer et al., 2001). Randomized trials have found lower aspirin doses ranging between 50 and 100 mg/d effective as an antithrombotic agent. The antithrombotic effects of several dosage ranges of aspirin have been compared to untreated control groups with a number of thrombotic vascular disorders. Doses between 50 and 1200 mg/d were effective in transient cerebral ischemia. In acute ischemic stroke, doses of 160 to 300 mg/d were effective in reducing early mortality and stroke recurrence, with a range of 30 to 1300 mg deemed acceptable for stroke prevention (Patrono et al., 2001). The largest trial of antiplatelet agents, the Antiplatelet Trialists' Collaboration, evaluated over 100,000 patients in 145 trials. The study concluded that antiplatelet agents were beneficial in patients with a history of ischemic stroke or TIA and that larger aspirin doses were no more effective than smaller doses. This analysis showed that aspirin doses of 75 to 325 mg/d were as effective as higher doses in secondary prevention in high-risk patients (Spandorfer et al., 2001). However, aspirin doses lower than 300 mg/d produced fewer GI adverse events than doses of 1200 mg/d (Antiplatelet Trialists' Collaboration, 1994). Gastric erosions and hemorrhage can occur even with short courses of aspirin therapy, and enteric-coated preparations do not always prevent GI complications. As a result, the lowest effective aspirin dose should be used (Patrono et al., 1998). Because of its low cost and relatively good safety profile, aspirin is the standard therapy for patients experiencing a first episode of acute, noncardioembolic, ischemic stroke (see Table 54-2). When used for stroke prevention in low-risk patients with atrial fibrillation who have a contraindication to anticoagulation therapy with warfarin, an aspirin dose of 325 mg/d is recommended (Patrono et al., 2001).

A combination product containing 25 mg aspirin and 200 mg extended-release dipyridamole (Aggrenox), administered twice daily, has been approved for preventing recurrent stroke in patients who have experienced a TIA or previous ischemic stroke. Dipyridamole inhibits platelet adhesion, but its full mechanism of action is unknown. A European trial conducted in 6000 patients was the basis for FDA approval of this agent. However, the American College of Chest Physicians consensus guidelines recommend aspirin as the initial choice for a first episode of noncardioembolic ischemic stroke (Albers et al., 1998).

Adverse Effects

The most common adverse effects of aspirin are GI upset, such as nausea, dyspepsia, heartburn, epigastric discomfort, anorexia, and bleeding. These effects are dose related and are more likely to occur at doses greater than 325 mg/d. Although lower doses cause fewer GI symptoms, they still can cause significant GI bleeding (Spandorfer et al., 2001). Aspirin may also potentiate peptic ulcer disease. Chronic therapy may cause persistent iron deficiency anemia. Although modest and unpredictable, aspirin can also cause prolongation of bleeding time and some studies suggest it may increase postoperative bleeding. Other possible adverse effects are leukopenia, thrombocytopenia, purpura, shortened erythrocyte survival time, hives, rashes, angioedema, fever, thirst, and dimness of vision (*Drug Facts and Comparisons*, 2002).

Ticlopidine and Clopidogrel

Ticlopidine and clopidogrel are structurally related antiplatelet agents that differ mechanistically from aspirin. These agents do not affect cyclooxygenase, but prevent platelet aggregation by inhibiting adenosine diphosphate (ADP), a promoter of platelet receptor binding (Patrono et al., 1998).

Ticlopidine is a prodrug that is hepatically metabolized to its active form. The usual dose is 250 mg administered twice daily. The full antiplatelet effect requires 3 to 5 days of oral administration. Although the drug's half-life is 24 to 36 hours, antiplatelet effects persist for up to 10 days after ticlopidine discontinuation, paralleling the platelet life span. The FDA-approved indications for ticlopidine include the secondary prevention of TIAs and ischemic stroke in patients who have had a stroke despite receiving aspirin therapy and coronary artery stenting, although currently clopidogrel is primarily used after coronary stent placement (Patrono et al., 2001). Affecting approximately 2% of patients, neutropenia is the most serious adverse effect of ticlopidine. The greatest risk for neutropenia occurs within the first 3 months of therapy; neutropenia is reversible within 1 to 3 weeks of drug discontinuation. The FDA requires CBC monitoring every 2 weeks for the first 3 months of therapy. Ticlopidine must be discontinued if the absolute neutrophil count (ANC) falls below 1200/mm^3 or if the platelet count drops lower than 80,000/mm^3. Patients need to inform the clinician of any symptoms of neutropenia, such as fever, chills, or sore throat. Due to the risk of life-threatening blood dyscrasias such as neutropenia, agranulocytosis, and thrombotic thrombocytopenic purpura, ticlopidine is reserved for patients who are intolerant or allergic to aspirin or in whom aspirin therapy has failed. Hepatotoxicity is another rare complication of ticlopidine, and baseline liver function tests along with a CBC should be ordered and results reviewed before therapy is initiated. These effects include GI toxicity, rash, and bleeding complications such as ecchymosis, epistaxis, hematuria, conjunctival hemorrhage, GI bleeding, and posttraumatic and preoperative bleeding (see Table 54-2). Adverse effects are relatively common with at least one being reported in more than 50% of patients (*Drug Facts and Comparisons*, 2002).

Structured similarly to ticlopidine, the major advantage of clopidogrel is that neutropenia is not a concern. A dose of 75 mg/d irreversibly inhibits ADP-mediated platelet aggregation (see Table 54-2). Dose-dependent inhibition of platelet aggregation is seen 2 hours after a single oral dose and platelet aggregation and bleeding time return to baseline approximately 5 days after discontinuation of clopidogrel. Absorption is rapid and greater than 50% after oral administration. Clopidogrel is extensively metabolized by the liver. The elimination half-life of the main circulating metabolite is 8 hours with half excreted in urine and half in the feces 5 days after dosing (*Drug Facts and Comparisons,* 2002). This medication received FDA approval with one major study, the CAPRIE (Clopidogrel Versus Aspirin in Patients at Risk of Ischemic Events) trial. A clopidogrel dosage of 75 mg/d was compared with aspirin 325 mg/d in more than 6000 patients. The effects of clopidogrel were similar to those of aspirin in decreasing the risk of stroke, but clopidogrel was superior to aspirin when ischemic stroke, myocardial infarction, and vascular death were considered together. There was no difference between clopidogrel and aspirin in causing neutropenia (CAPRIE Steering Committee, 1996). Current FDA-labeled indications for clopidogrel are prophylaxis against thrombotic events in patients with recent myocardial infarction, recent stroke, and peripheral arterial disease. Clopidogrel is also frequently used for prophylaxis against thrombosis in patients undergoing percutaneous coronary intervention (Micromedex, 2004). It is now recommended that clopidogrel plus aspirin be given prior to coronary intervention and continued for 9 months to a year or longer for patients with coronary artery stents. Currently, an ongoing clinical trial is studying a combination of clopidogrel and aspirin versus warfarin in patients with atrial fibrillation for the prevention of ischemic stroke. Possible adverse effects of clopidogrel, occurring in more than 3% of patients, include flulike symptoms, chest pain, edema, headache, dizziness, dyspepsia, abdominal pain, diarrhea, nausea, arthralgia, purpura, dyspnea, cough, rhinitis, rash, pruritus, depression, and hypercholesterolemia (*Drug Facts and Comparisons*, 2002).

A New Oral Anticoagulant

Since the 1950s, when warfarin was first used in humans, there has been no other comparable oral anticoagulant for the treatment of VTE and VTE prophylaxis. A variety of compounds are currently under development and investigation to be used orally as a long-term anticoagulant. These include inhibitors of factors VIIa, IXa, Xa, and XIIIa, and direct thrombin inhibitors (DTIs; Becker et al., 2001). An agent that is very close to receiving FDA approval and promises to be an effective alternative to warfarin is ximelagatran. This is a DTI being produced and studied by AstraZeneca Pharmaceuticals. It is a prodrug of melagatran. Melagatran inactivates both circulating and clot-bound thrombin by binding to the thrombin active site, thus, inhibiting platelet activation or aggregation and reducing fibrinolysis time (Evans et al., 2004).

Ximelagatran is rapidly absorbed after oral administration and converted to the active form. Maximum concentration is attained approximately 1.6 to 1.9 hours after administration. Melagatran is not metabolized or bound to plasma proteins. It is predominantly cleared via the kidneys with a half-life of 4 to 5 hours, which requires twice-daily dosing.

Selecting the Most Appropriate Agent

In cases of DVT or PE, all patients receive either LMWH or heparin first. Then, drug therapy switches over to oral drug therapy with warfarin. Warfarin is also commonly used in thromboembolism prevention in atrial fibrillation, and native or prosthetic heart valvular disease. For more information, see Table 54-8 and Figure 54-2.

Deep Venous Thrombosis or Pulmonary Embolism

All patients with a diagnostically confirmed DVT of the proximal leg veins or diagnostically confirmed PE should receive a bolus of intravenous UFH followed by a continuous intravenous infusion of UFH, adjusted-dose subcutaneous heparin, or subcutaneous LMWH as initial therapy. A UFH intravenous bolus followed by continuous intravenous infusion UFH therapy or LMWH may also be started before a definitive diagnosis in patients with a high clinical suspicion of UFH and LMWH are used initially as the treatments of choice for DVT or PE because of their rapid anticoagulant effect. However, oral anticoagulation with warfarin is recommended for the remainder of therapy duration (see Box 54-4). Warfarin should be initiated on day 1 after confirmation of DVT/PE and overlapped with UFH or LMWH for approximately 4 to 5 days while warfarin reaches a therapeutic level (Hyers et al., 2001).

Therapy with heparin and warfarin does not dissolve an existing clot but reduces further clot extension and recurrence. A dosage of heparin during initial treatment that prolongs the aPTT to 1.5 to 2.5 times normal is recommended. The target INR for long-term treatment of DVT or PE is a range of 2 to 3, which protects against recurrent events but causes a low incidence of bleeding complications (Hyers et al, 2001). The PIOPED (Prospective Investigation of Pulmonary Embolism Diagnosis) algorithm provides a detailed flow chart for determining therapy for PE (PIOPED Investigators, 1990). The American College of Chest Physicians consensus guidelines also provide algorithms for initial treatment of DVT/PE with both UFH and LMWH and for treatment duration with warfarin.

Table 54.8

Recommended Order of Treatment for Coagulation Disturbances

Order	Agent	Comments
DVT/PE		
Initial therapy	heparin or LMWH	Can now treat with LMWH in the outpatient setting.
Long term	warfarin	Consider patient risk factors for duration of therapy.
Orthopedic Surgery Prophylaxis		
First line	LMWH or warfarin	LMWH is more effective than warfarin but bleeding risk is increased. Duration of warfarin therapy is controversial.
Second line	UFH or IPC	UFH is a more complex option.
Third line	ASA, UFH, dextran	Refer to American College of Chest Physicians Guidelines for more information. Sole therapy with these agents is not recommended.
Prevention of Noncardioembolic Ischemic Stroke		
First line	ASA or clopidogrel	ASA is inexpensive, relatively safe; use clopidogrel in ASA-sensitive patients.
Second line	ASA with dipyridamole or clopidogrel	For patients with ASA allergy
Third line	ticlopidine	Risk of neutropenia
Prevention of Cardioembolic Stroke		
First line	warfarin	For patients with atrial fibrillation, valvular heart disease, prosthetic valve or stroke
Second line	antiplatelet agents	For patients with minor risk conditions
Atrial Fibrillation		
First line	warfarin	Choice is based on patient risk factors.
Second line	ASA	Choice is based on patient risk factors.

ASA, aspirin; IPC, intermittent pneumatic compression; LMWH, low-molecular-weight heparin; UFH, unfractionated heparin.

Several studies have been conducted in an attempt to determine the most appropriate duration of anticoagulation therapy for proximal DVT versus isolated calf DVT and PE. Blanket recommendations have been made and will be discussed here; however, the duration of anticoagulation must always be tailored to the individual patient.

Patient risk factors for recurrent thrombosis influence the duration of oral anticoagulant therapy. Laurent and colleagues (2001) conducted the first controlled trial comparing durations of oral anticoagulant therapy in patients with a first episode of proximal DVT, isolated calf DVT, and PE. The study concludes that 3 or 6 months of therapy for proximal DVT and PE and 6 or 12 weeks for isolated calf DVT produce equivalent outcomes in terms of recurrence in patients, including those with permanent risk factors and idiopathic VTE. However, during the time of this study, several other studies were completed, which found conflicting results. Some argued in favor of shorter therapy (ie, 3 months for first episode VTE) and some were in favor of longer treatment (ie, 6 months up to >1 year). Treatment for isolated calf DVT has been given little attention. The consensus guidelines do offer recommendations for treatment duration, which are currently followed in practice, but further studies are necessary.

A patient with reversible risk factors (ie, surgery, trauma, immobilization, estrogen use, invasive venous catheter) and a first episode of DVT/PE is recommended to be treated for 3 months or more. Those with a first episode of idiopathic VTE are recommended to be treated for 6 months or more. Treatment for 12 months or more is recommended for patients with recurrent idiopathic VTE or a continuing risk factor such as cancer or inherited disorders of coagulation,

such as antithrombin III deficiency and anticardiolipin antibody syndrome (Hyers et al., 2001).

Treatment for symptomatic isolated calf thrombosis is recommended for 6 to 12 weeks or more in addition to follow up with serial noninvasive tests for to 14 days to identify proximal clot extension (Hyers et al., 2001). In practice, unless the thrombosis is confined to a small venous branch for which no anticoagulation treatment is recommended, calf DVTs are treated for at least 3 months.

Traditionally, continuous intravenous infusion UFH was administered in the hospital for DVT or PE. However, several studies using various preparations of LMWHs compared with UFH for treatment of DVT or PE have been conducted. The trial with the most rigorous objective end points compared enoxaparin 1 mg/kg subcutaneously every 12 hours to intravenous continuous infusion UFH in patients with DVT. Bilateral lower extremity venograms and V/Q scans were performed at study entry and 10 days later. A total of 134 patients were evaluated. Of the 67 patients receiving the LMWH enoxaparin, only 1 (1.5%) had a recurrent DVT, compared with 7 of the 67 patients receiving UFH (10.4%). This difference was statistically significant ($P = .002$). No cases of PE occurred in the enoxaparin group, whereas two PEs were documented in the heparin arm of the study (3%). There were no major bleeding events with either treatment (Simmoneau et al., 1993). In the study by Merli and colleagues (2001), 900 patients with symptomatic lower extremity DVT including 287 with confirmed PE in 74 hospitals and 16 countries were studied to compare enoxaparin once or twice daily dosing with intravenous UFH. Equivalent efficacy was seen in the UFH group and

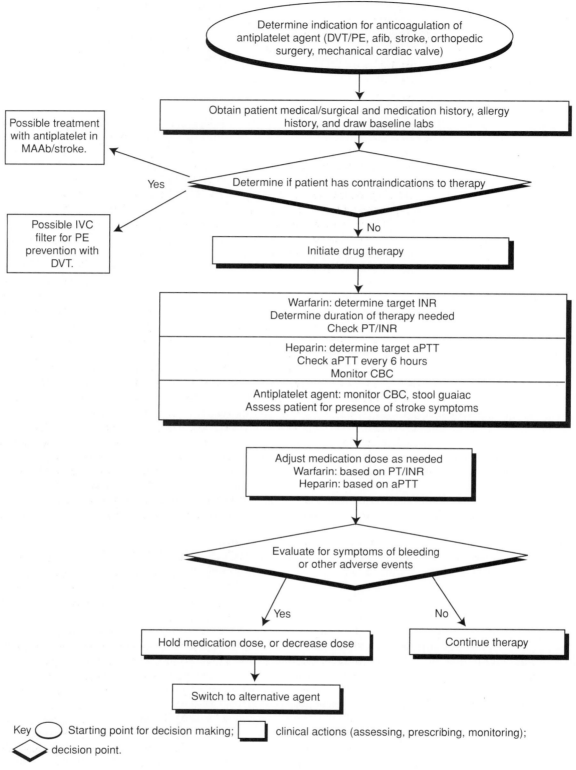

Figure 54–2   Treatment algorithm for coagulation disturbances.

both enoxaparin groups with recurrence found in 4.1% patients receiving UFH, 4.4% of those receiving once daily enoxaparin, and 2.9% of those receiving twice daily dosing. Major hemorrhage occurred in a smaller percentage of the patients in both enoxaparin groups as compared to the UFH

group. Several studies including meta-analyses have shown lower rates of thrombosis recurrence and bleeding with LMWH as compared to UFH (Hyers et al., 2001).

One benefit of LMWH therapy is the potential for treatment outside of the hospital, and at least two studies have documented the use of outpatient subcutaneous LMWH, in place of hospital admission and treatment with intravenous UFH (Koopman et al., 1996; Levine et al., 1996). A total of 253 patients receiving continuous-infusion heparin in the hospital were compared with 247 patients treated with enoxaparin 1 mg/kg actual body weight subcutaneously every 12 hours in the outpatient setting in an open-label study. Thirteen patients (5.3%) receiving enoxaparin had a symptomatic recurrent thromboembolic episode compared with 17 patients (6.7%) receiving heparin. The incidence of major bleeding episodes was similar between the two groups. Patients treated with LMWH were hospitalized for 1.1 days, whereas those in the heparin group were hospitalized for 6.5 days (Levine et al., 1996). The consensus guidelines state that it is estimated that an average of 5 to 6 hospitalization days per patient are saved with the use of outpatient LMWH. This was projected to save approximately $250 million annually in the United States alone. Guidelines for selecting patients appropriate for outpatient therapy have been proposed. These include ensuring the patient is stable, has no severe renal insufficiency, and has low risk of bleeding. Further, appropriate systems for drug administration (oral or subcutaneous), coupled with appropriate access to monitoring, must be ensured (Hyers et al., 2001).

Alternative treatments for VTE are thrombolytic therapy, which is reserved for those with hemodynamically unstable PE or massive ileofemoral thrombosis, and inferior vena caval (IVC) filters. IVC filters are recommended in patients with proximal vein thrombosis or PE or with high risk for these conditions when anticoagulation therapy is contraindicated or has resulted in a complication. IVC filters may also be placed in patients who have suffered recurrent VTE despite adequate anticoagulation, with recurrent embolism or pulmonary hypertension, and with concomitant surgical pulmonary embolectomy or pulmonary thromboendarterectomy (Hyers et al., 2001). There is much controversy over the use of IVC filters and when they are used there is controversy over the need for long-term anticoagulation with an IVC filter because it is thought to be thrombogenic.

Prophylaxis for Deep Venous Thrombosis and Pulmonary Embolism in Patients Undergoing Orthopedic Procedures

Patients undergoing total hip replacement (THR), total knee replacement (TKR), or hip fracture surgery should receive anticoagulation prophylaxis to reduce the high risk of DVT or PE. Several studies have found the prevalence of total DVT at 7 to 14 days after THR, TKR, and hip fracture surgery to be approximately 50% to 60%. The incidence of PE is less certain, but in studies in which a ventilation–perfusion scan was performed, about 7% to 11% of THR and TKR patients had a high probability scan within 7 to 14 days after surgery. It has also been found that total DVT rate is greater in TKR than THR. Overall, the data suggests that asymptomatic VTE is common after orthopedic surgery and, in the absence of prophylaxis, will affect at least half of these patients (Geerts, 2001). Numerous pharmacologic and nonpharmacologic agents have been used in the postoperative setting to decrease the risk of DVT or PE.

First-Line Therapy

For patients undergoing THR or TKR, LMWH is considered more effective than warfarin in preventing VTE, but it does have a higher risk of surgical site bleeding and hematoma. Warfarin therapy with a goal INR range of 2 to 3 is effective as prophylaxis in this group of patients, causes less bleeding risk if monitored properly, and appears to be more cost effective than LMWH in the United States, based on a recent analysis. Therefore, the consensus guidelines recommend that a decision between the use of LMWH and warfarin be made on an institutional level (Geerts, 2001). Currently, for THR, LMWH therapy, started 12 hours before or 12 to 24 hours after surgery, half of the high-risk dose 4 to 6 hours after surgery followed by the high-risk dose the next day, or adjusted dose warfarin started preoperatively or immediately postoperatively is recommended as first-line therapy. For TKR, LMWH or dose-adjusted warfarin is also recommended as first-line therapy. The optimal duration of prophylaxis after THR and TKR is not known. Prophylactic therapy is recommended for at least 7 to 10 days after surgery (Geerts, 2001). However, warfarin is commonly administered for 3 to 6 weeks after surgery. In patients having surgery for hip fracture, LMWH or adjusted-dose warfarin with a goal range of 2 to 3 is recommended as first-line therapy, but the bleeding risk with these agents must be considered.

Second-Line Therapy

Second-line therapy recommended for THR in patients with increased risk of bleeding is the use of adjusted dose UFH started preoperatively, but this is a more complex option and not favored by most surgeons. Additional prophylaxis with intermittent pneumatic compression (IPC) device is thought to improve efficacy, but it must be applied intraoperatively or immediately postoperatively and worn continuously (at least 23 hours a day) until the patient is fully ambulatory. For TKR, UFH is not recommended, but an alternative therapy is the optimal use of IPC devices. For hip fracture surgery, a second-line, alternative treatment is low-dose unfractionated heparin (LDUH) therapy (Geerts, 2001).

Third-Line Therapy

Third-line therapies for prophylaxis after orthopedic surgery include aspirin, LDUH, and dextran because of their decreased effectiveness compared with warfarin or LMWH. Nonpharmacologic measures, such as IPC, provide very effective prophylaxis without the risks of drug therapy (Clagett et al., 1998). Sole therapy with any of the above agents is not recommended by the consensus guidelines (Geerts, 2001).

The most recent consensus guidelines should be consulted for more detailed information. Recommendations for VTE prophylaxis in general, gynecologic, urologic, and neurologic surgeries as well as neurologic trauma and spinal cord injury can be found in the American College of Chest Physicians consensus guidelines for antithrombotic therapy.

Ischemic Stroke

Treatment of Acute Ischemic Stroke

Within 3 hours of symptom onset, tissue plasminogen activator (tPA) or urokinase is recommended for patients who meet eligibility criteria. Within 3 to 6 hours of symptom onset intra-arterial thrombolytic therapy should be offered in selected patients (Albers, Amarenco et al., 2001).

Treatment for acute stroke with antithrombotic agents is to prevent progression of the stroke, prevent recurrence of cerebral thromboembolism, and minimize the occurrence of hemorrhagic transformation. Choosing an antithrombotic agent is difficult because there are different stroke etiologies and subtypes each with different risks. For treatment of acute ischemic stroke in patients not receiving thrombolytic therapy, aspirin 160 to 325 mg/d is recommended and should be started within 48 hours of the onset of stroke. Patients with acute stroke found to be of acute cardioembolic in nature, are progressing, and thought to be a result of ongoing thromboembolism, should be offered early anticoagulation with UFH or LMWH. Early anticoagulation should not be offered if there are potential contraindications such as bleeding. A brain imaging study should be performed prior to initiation of anticoagulation to rule out hemorrhage.

DVT and PE prophylaxis should be instituted after ischemic stroke. For patients with restricted mobility low-dose subcutaneous UFH or LMWH may be used. Patients with intracerebral hematoma may receive low-dose subcutaneous UFH as early as the second day after hemorrhage onset. IPC devices or elastic stockings should be used for patients with contraindications to anticoagulant use.

Prevention of Ischemic Stroke

Noncardioembolic Stroke

First-Line Therapy

For prevention of noncardioembolic ischemic stroke or TIA aspirin 50 to 325 mg/d is recommended because of its low cost, safety profile, and proven effectiveness in several clinical trials with thousands of patients. In several studies aspirin was found to reduce the odds of stroke by approximately 30%. Therefore, aspirin is used as a first-line agent by many practitioners for the prevention of noncardioembolic stroke in high-risk patients. Oral anticoagulants, such as warfarin, are not recommended because they increase the risk for brain hemorrhage and outweigh the possible benefits.

Second-Line Therapy

The combination of aspirin and dipyridamole in comparison to placebo has been found to reduce the risk of stroke in those with prior events by 37% to 38% in two trials. Although aspirin and dipyridamole 25/200 mg twice daily is thought to be more effective than aspirin alone and is an acceptable option as an initial therapy, it is viewed as an alternative treatment to aspirin therapy in the prevention of stroke (Albers, Amarenco et al., 2001).

Clopidogrel 75 mg/d is also acceptable as an option for initial therapy in the prevention of noncardioembolic stroke, but it is regarded as an alternative to aspirin therapy. In the CAPRIE trial, clopidogrel was found to have a risk reduction of about 10% over aspirin for the combined outcomes of stroke, myocardial infarction, and vascular death. There were no major differences between safety profiles and adverse experiences with both clopidogrel and aspirin were minimal. Therefore, clopidogrel should be used as a first-line treatment in patients unable to take aspirin (Albers, Amarenco et al., 2001).

Third-Line Therapy

Ticlodipine seems to be comparable to clopidogrel in the prevention of stroke. However, because it is associated with an approximately 1% risk of severe adverse effects such as neutropenia, it is considered a third line or last choice treatment. Most clinicians have completely abandoned its use because of the associated risks (Albers, Amarenco et al., 2001).

Cardioembolic Stroke

First-Line Therapy

Therapy for prevention of cardioembolic ischemic stroke is oral anticoagulation with warfarin with an INR goal range of 2 to 3 in patients with atrial fibrillation after a recent stroke or TIA as well as for patients with high-risk cardiac conditions such as prosthetic heart valves, valvular heart disease, and coronary artery disease.

Second-Line Therapy

Antiplatelet agents may be offered to patients with minor risk cardiac conditions. There are few data regarding the efficacy of antiplatelet medications in the prevention of cardioembolic stroke. As noted, oral anticoagulants are the treatment of choice, but when there is a contraindication to anticoagulant therapy, antiplatelet agents may be used. If carotid endarterectomy is performed, aspirin 81 to 325 mg/d should be given before and after the procedure (Albers, Amarenco et al., 2001).

Atrial Fibrillation

The risk of thromboembolic stroke in patients with atrial fibrillation who are not receiving anticoagulation is approximately 5%/y, and this risk increases rapidly after the age of 65 (Atrial Fibrillation Investigators, 1994; Laupacis et al., 1998). In the Framingham Heart Study, the risk of stroke in patients with atrial fibrillation rose form 1.5% in those 50 to 59 years of age to 23.5% in those 80 to 89 years old. In patients older than 80 years, atrial fibrillation was the only cardiovascular condition associated with increased risk of stroke.

First-Line Therapy

Six major, well-conducted trials have documented the benefits of warfarin in reducing the risk of stroke in patients with atrial fibrillation. The 5% annual risk of stroke in non–anticoagulated patients was reduced to 1.4% with warfarin, a risk reduction of 68%. Anticoagulation therapy did not significantly increase the incidence of major bleeding events. In contrast, the benefits provided by aspirin alone contributed a 21% risk reduction, much less than the effects provided by warfarin (Laupacis et al., 1998).

The Stroke Prevention in Atrial Fibrillation-II Study results suggested that warfarin is more effective in those older than 75 years as compared to their younger counterparts, but the over 75-year-old age group has a substantial risk of intracerebral bleeds, which negated the benefit of warfarin. However, four other pooled trials did not support these findings. These studies found that most major bleeds occurred at INRs higher than 4 (Kellen, 2004). Therefore, warfarin therapy is not withheld in those over age 75 years. Warfarin versus aspirin therapy is decided based on patient risk factors but is viewed as first-line therapy in patients with any high-risk factor.

The current recommendations for anticoagulation in atrial fibrillation include warfarin with a goal INR range of 2 to 3 for patients with any high-risk factor, such as previous TIA, systemic embolism, stroke, history of hypertension, poor left ventricular function, age 75 years or older, rheumatic mitral valve disease, and prosthetic heart valve or more than one moderate risk factor. Aspirin therapy should be offered to patients with contraindications to warfarin therapy or to those who refuse warfarin therapy. Aspirin in addition to low, fixed-dose warfarin therapy is not recommended.

Second-Line Therapy

Aspirin therapy has shown a 21% to 22% risk reduction in studies as compared to placebo. Warfarin therapy is clearly superior to aspirin in risk reduction for stroke, but it does have a higher risk for hemorrhage. The rate of intracranial hemorrhage, in one primary prevention study, was found to be 1.8% in those older than 75 years treated with warfarin as compared to 0.8% in those treated with aspirin. Therefore the risk intensity for stroke versus that of hemorrhage must be considered when choosing between warfarin and aspirin therapy.

Consensus guidelines suggest that those with only one moderate risk factor, such as age 65 to 75 years, diabetes mellitus, and coronary artery disease with preserved left ventricular function, can receive aspirin 325 mg/d or warfarin with a goal INR range of 2 to 3. Those who are younger than 65 years and with no high or moderate risk factors and no clinical or echocardiographic evidence of cardiovascular disease may receive aspirin 325 mg/d. Table 54-9 summarizes recent recommendations.

Anticoagulation for Elective Cardioversion

Patients with atrial fibrillation undergoing electrical or pharmacologic cardioversion should also receive anticoagulation therapy. The risk of systemic embolization after direct current cardioversion is 5% in patients not receiving anticoagulation compared with 1% in those receiving anticoagulation. Once a thrombus is formed in the heart, 2 to 3 weeks is required for clot organization and adherence to the atrial wall. Therefore, patients with atrial fibrillation should receive warfarin for 3 weeks before cardioversion, which is then continued for 4 or more weeks after the procedure or until normal sinus rhythm has been maintained for 4 or more weeks. Although electrical activity of the atria resumes quickly after successful cardioversion, normal atrial contraction (mechanical activity) may not resume for 3 to 4 weeks, thus requiring continued anticoagulation. Patients may also be offered anticoagulation therapy and then undergo transesophageal echocardiography (TEE) followed by immediate cardioversion if not thrombi are detected.

Prophylaxis Against Systemic Embolism in Patients With Native and Prosthetic Mechanical Heart Valves

The rate of major thrombotic events in patients who have mechanical heart valves and who are not receiving anticoagulation is 8%; anticoagulation therapy decreases this risk by 75% (Carnetiger et al., 1995).

Both the position of the mechanical valve and the type of valve influence the risks for embolism. The prevalence of thromboembolism is higher with a valve in the mitral position than in the aortic position (0.5% versus 0.9% yearly, respectively; Vongpatanasin et al., 1996). The increased risk of embolism with prosthetic mitral valves is attributed to a higher incidence of atrial fibrillation, left atrial enlargement, and damage from rheumatic heart disease. In addition, the risk of thromboembolism is higher in patients with double mechanical valves (ie, aortic and mitral valve replacement) at 1.2% yearly compared with those with only one prosthetic valve.

Regarding the type of valve, caged-ball valves have a higher incidence of major embolism than bileaflet and tilting disk valves. Also, the frequency of thromboembolic events is lower with the second-generation mechanical valves (ie, St. Jude valves) than first-generation valves (ie, Starr-Edwards valves).

The consequences of systemic embolism are more serious than the complications of hemorrhage caused by anticoagulant therapy. Therefore, the guidelines recommend a target INR of 2.5 to 3.5 for tilting disk valve, bileaflet valve in the mitral position, or bileaflet mechanical valve in the aortic position with atrial fibrillation. Warfarin, given to maintain an INR of 2.5 to 3.5, in combination with aspirin, 80 to 100 mg/d, has been proposed as an alternative therapy for patients with mechanical heart valves at increased risk of thromboembolism. These risks include prior stroke, atrial fibrillation, coronary artery disease, enlarged left atrium, left atrial thrombus, double prosthetic valves, and those with caged-ball or caged-disk valves. A low risk of thromboembolic events and bleeding complications has been reported with this combination. Patients who experience systemic embolism despite receiving warfarin at a therapeutic INR between 2.5 and 3.5 can also have aspirin 80 to 100 mg/d added to their regimen. For those with a St. Jude bileaflet aortic valve, CardioMedics bileaflet aortic valve, and

Table 54.9

Risk Stratification for Treating Atrial Fibrillation

Risk Factor Status	Recommendation
No high or moderate risk factors	Aspirin
One moderate risk factor	Aspirin or warfarin
High risk factor	Warfarin with a target INR of 2–3

Medtronic-Hall tilting disk in the aortic position with a normal size left atrium and normal sinus rhythm can be offered warfarin with a goal range of 2 to 3 (Stein et al., 2001).

For bioprosthetic heart valves, either in the mitral or aortic position, oral anticoagulation with warfarin is recommended for the first 3 months after valve insertion with an INR goal range of 2 to 3. On anticoagulation initiation, UFH or LMWH may be used and overlapped with warfarin until the INR is within the therapeutic range for 2 consecutive days. In a patient with a history of a systemic embolism, oral anticoagulation should be continued for 3 to 12 months. In the presence of atrial fibrillation or left atrial thrombus at the time valve implantation, long-term oral anticoagulation is recommended. If the patients have a permanent pacemaker with the bioprosthetic valve, oral anticoagulation is optional. In those in normal sinus rhythm, long-term aspirin therapy at 80 mg/d is recommended (Stein et al., 2001).

In native valvular heart disease, the necessity of anticoagulation depends on the position of the diseased valve and the comorbidities of the patient. Anticoagulation should be offered to those with rheumatic mitral valve disease, mitral stenosis and atrial fibrillation, mitral stenosis in the older patient, an increased left atrium size, left atrium thrombi, or a history of prior embolism. In those with mitral regurgitation, anticoagulation is indicated in the presence of atrial fibrillation, congestive heart failure, cardiac enlargement with a low cardiac output, enlarged left atrium, or a history of a prior embolism. In patients with mitral valve prolapse and a TIA, aspirin is indicated. Warfarin should be instituted only in the case of TIA recurrence. For those who have had a mitral valve repair, the need for anticoagulation is dependent on the type of ring used. No anticoagulation is required for those with a Cosgrove ring, but 3 months of anticoagulation is recommended with the Carpentier ring. Anticoagulation is not indicated in patients with normal sinus rhythm and non–mitral, non–aortic, or non–tricuspid valve disease (Spandorfer et al., 2001).

Special Population Considerations

When considering anticoagulation therapy, special populations are those who pose more difficult issues when it comes to diagnosis and treatment. Those with renal impairment or obesity and pregnant patients are considered special population groups when addressing anticoagulation for various disease states. Obesity and renal impairment were briefly discussed in anticoagulant dosing in the appropriate sections of this chapter. Here we will discuss the special considerations necessary in treating the pregnant patient with VTE or VTE risk.

Pregnancy

Pregnancy is an independent risk factor for VTE. Fatal PE is a common cause of maternal mortality. The increased risk is secondary to changes in both procoagulant and anticoagulant proteins, blood stasis related to decreased venous tone, and obstruction of flow from the gravid uterus, and vascular injury (Spandorfer et al., 2001). In one study, women with known prepregnancy thrombophilia states were found to have an 8-fold risk of VTE. Thrombophilia

also puts women at risk for pregnancy loss and pregnancy complications associated with placental infarction, such as intrauterine growth retardation, preeclampsia, placental abruption, and intrauterine death. Also, women with a history of VTE have an increased risk of recurrence during pregnancy.

Diagnosis of VTE in pregnant women is difficult by clinical evaluation because many nonthrombotic symptoms of pregnancy mimic DVT and PE. In addition, tests used to diagnose DVT can be altered by the compressive effects of the gravid uterus. However, the only way to reduce maternal mortality from VTE is to aggressively investigate symptomatic women with a clinical suspicion of VTE and to offer treatment or prophylaxis to women who are at increased risk for VTE. Treatment and prophylaxis of VTE in pregnancy are based primarily on clinical experience because there are no major clinical studies to support evidence-based practice (Copplestone et al., 2004).

Warfarin is relatively contraindicated in pregnancy because it is a known teratogen and can cause fetal bleeding with the highest risk between 6 an 12 weeks and close to term. In all women of childbearing age who are attempting to be come pregnant or who do become pregnant, warfarin therapy should be discontinued immediately and an alternative agent selected. Heparin is the treatment of choice in pregnant patients requiring anticoagulation therapy, and an extensive body of literature supports the efficacy and safety of heparin. However, heparin is a pregnancy category C medication and some side effects of heparin products may affect the mother, such as osteoporosis, HIT, bleeding, and skin reactions. The LMWHs, which may potentially decrease the risk of osteoporosis and HIT, are an option, and are a pregnancy category B medication. UFH and LMWHs do not cross the placenta and therefore are unlikely to cause hemorrhage or be teratogenic (*Drug Facts and Comparisons*, 2002).

In lactation, warfarin appears in inactive form in breast milk and has not been found to change the PT in nursing infants of women taking warfarin. UFH is not secreted into breast milk. It is not known if LMWHs are secreted into breast milk; however, in practice they are used in nursing mothers when necessary (*Drug Facts and Comparisons*, 2002). Practitioners should review the latest guidelines for assistance in choosing the appropriate treatment for pregnant and nursing mothers.

For prophylaxis in pregnant patients with a prior VTE associated with a transient risk factor, surveillance and postpartum anticoagulation is recommended. Those who have had and idiopathic VTE or a prior VTE and the presence of thrombophilia, but not on long-term anticoagulation, surveillance, mini-dose (5000 IU subcutaneously every 12 hours) or moderate dose (adjusted doses every 12 hours to a target anti-Xa level of 0.1 to 0.3 IU/mL) UFH, or prophylactic LMWH in addition to postpartum anticoagulation is recommended. Pregnant patients with no prior VTE but with confirmed thrombophilia and not on long-term anticoagulation therapy are recommended to be offered surveillance, mini-dose UFH, or prophylactic LMWH in addition to postpartum anticoagulation. When patients have had 2 or more episodes of VTE or are currently on long-term anticoagulation, adjusted-dose UFH, prophylactic LMWH, or adjusted-dose LMWH in addition to long-term postpartum anticoagulation is recommended.

For treatment of VTE in pregnancy, those with an average risk of recurrence should be offered adjusted-dose LMWH throughout pregnancy or an intravenous UFH bolus followed by continuous infusion for 5 or more days and then adjusted-dose UFH until delivery. LMWH and UFH should be discontinued 24 hours before elective induction of labor. Those at very high risk for VTE recurrence (ie, proximal DVT within the prior 2 week period), intravenous UFH, discontinued 4 to 6 hours before expected delivery and anticoagulation for 6 or more weeks postpartum or 3 or more months after VTE occurrence is recommended.

Pregnant women with mechanical cardiac valves pose a special challenge because of the lack of controlled clinical trials, concern regarding the efficacy of subcutaneous heparin and LMWHs in preventing thromboembolic complications, the teratogenic effects of warfarin, and the risks of maternal bleeding. One review of studies including 976 women with 1234 pregnancies found that replacing warfarin with heparin between weeks 6 to 12 of gestation resulted in negligible fetal abnormalities, whereas using warfarin throughout pregnancy caused a 6% risk of fetal defects. Maternal thromboembolic complications were lowest when warfarin was used throughout pregnancy (4% frequency). Complications increased to 9% when warfarin was switched to heparin after the first trimester and further increased to 33% when heparin was used solely. Women experiencing valve thromboses were most often receiving heparin at the time of the event, also raising the concern for heparin efficacy. However, the aPTT values and target aPTTs were not reported in this review. Another limitation of this review was that older mechanical valves with a higher risk of thromboembolism were overrepresented (Chan et al., 2000).

The use of LMWH in pregnant women with mechanical heart valves is supported by data acquired by Ginsberg and colleagues due to the superior pharmacologic properties and lower potential for adverse effects of LMWHs compared with other therapeutic modalities. LMWH use was further supported by a study of 7 pregnant patients treated with LMWH in which there was only one minor bleeding event. Otherwise, the treatment with LMWH appeared to be safe and efficacious.

Consensus guidelines on prophylaxis in pregnant women with mechanical heart valves recommend aggressive adjusted-dose UFH every 12 hours throughout pregnancy to maintain aPTT at 2 times control levels or anti-Xa level maintained at 0.35 to 0.70 IU/mL, adjusted-dose LMWH throughout pregnancy to maintain a 4 hour postinjection anti-Xa level of approximately 1.0 IU/mL, or UFH or LMWH, as just described, until the 13th week of pregnancy and then warfarin until the middle of the third trimester, then restart UFH or LMWH therapy until delivery. Long-term anticoagulation should be resumed postpartum.

Consult the American College of Chest Physicians consensus guidelines for prophylaxis in pregnant women with increased risk for pregnancy loss related to thrombophilia states.

DVT/PE Risk and Airline Travel

Recently, the media has brought to public attention a health risk of long airline flights and DVT and PE development.

This is not a new phenomenon. As we know from Virchow's triad, venous stasis is one of the three components that may lead to blood clotting. The airplane environment, with cramped seating arrangements and discouraged passenger mobility, encourages blood pooling in the lower extremity veins, which may lead to clot formation. Due to several deaths occurring after long airline flights, the connection between the immobility frequently experienced on such fights and the occurrence of DVT/PE has been made and more readily studied and publicized.

The first clue to this issue was in 1940, when an article in *Lancet* documented a marked increase in the monthly incidence of PE among people who spent prolonged periods in cramped quarters in London air-raid shelters. Immobility related to long-distance airline flights and the association with VTE was recognized 14 years later, but did not raise significant concern until two decades later, when in 1977 two British researchers found 8 of 182 patients with a diagnosed PE that developed shortly after prolonged travel in the coach section of an airplane. Since that time, several studies have been conducted and in 2001 researches concluded that airplane travel is a definite risk factor for PE (Ball, 2003).

In addition to the immobility caused by long flights, other environmental factors on aircraft, different from the ground environment, may cause physiologic stresses leading to VTE. These environmental factors include lower barometric pressure that can lead to abdominal distention acting against venous blood return from the lower extremities; decreased partial pressure of oxygen that may lead to increased blood clotting tendencies; and lower humidity (2% as compared to 50% at ground level), which can affect the body fluid content, cause dehydration, hemoconcentration, and clot formation. Cramped seating causes orthostatic stress and the edge of the airplane seat may compress the popliteal vein, both contributing to clot formation. Additional factors include sustained periods of exposure to noise and vibration, turbulence, variable air circulation and lower air quality, temperature changes, disruption of circadian rhythms, and varying exposure to low-level radiation (Ball, 2003).

A recent study by Schwartz and coworkers (2003) looked at 964 passengers returning from long airplane flights and compared them with 1213 controls. Those on anticoagulants or wearing compression stockings were not included. They found 2.8% of the passengers as compared to 1% of the controls had isolated calf muscle venous thrombosis on ultrasound that was not present on baseline testing. All of the passengers had at least one risk factor for VTE. They concluded that fights longer than 8 hours doubles the risk for isolated calf muscle venous thrombosis, which translates into VTE risk.

MONITORING PATIENT RESPONSE

Warfarin

With today's focus on minimizing inpatient costs, shorter hospital lengths of stay are encouraged. However, anticoagulation therapy may not be stabilized before hospital discharge. Enoxaparin subcutaneous injections, when overlapped with warfarin, allow patients to be discharged before a therapeutic INR is achieved. UFH or enoxaparin can be discontinued when the INR is within therapeutic range on two measurements taken 24 or more hours apart. Patients on warfarin therapy, with and without the overlap of UFH or LMWH, need to be evaluated within 3 to 5 days after discharge to avoid increasing the risk of either thromboembolic or bleeding events. The INR is then monitored weekly until a stable INR is reached, which is often defined as two consecutive INRs within the target range measured at least 72 hours apart (Hirsh et al., 1998).

Careful and routine monitoring of the INR is necessary, even in stabilized patients. After the INR is stable for 2 weeks, the interval of laboratory monitoring can be increased to once every 2 weeks, then every 3 weeks (Hirsh et al., 1994). The INR should be checked no less frequently than every 4 weeks because several factors can influence the INR, including diet, alcohol ingestion, physical activity, smoking, use of other medications, changes in patient disease states, and acute illnesses, such as fever and diarrhea (Bussey, 1993; Hirsh et al., 1998). More frequent monitoring is needed if bleeding complications develop or if other factors occur that could potentially interfere with warfarin, such as dietary changes, poor patient compliance, and medication changes (Hirsh et al., 1994).

When unexpected INR results are obtained, several questions should be addressed (Box 54-6). If highly elevated INR results are reported, the practitioner needs to rule out laboratory error and perform the INR test again if necessary before adjusting the warfarin dose. Potentiation of the warfarin effect occurs with exacerbation of congestive heart failure, hepatic disease, fever, hyperthyroidism, and diarrhea. Hepatic dysfunction reduces the synthesis of vitamin K–dependent clotting factors, and hypermetabolic conditions, such as fever or hyperthyroidism, accelerate the clear-ance of vitamin K and vitamin K–dependent clotting factors and lead to increases in the INR (Hirsh et al., 1998). INRs that fluctuate widely without apparent cause should raise the question of therapeutic noncompliance. Instructing patients to bring in all prescription and over-the-counter medications and conducting tablet counts can help determine patient reliability. Identifying trends in the INR, rather than reacting to an individual laboratory result, is also important.

The specimen necessary to obtain an INR value may be retrieved via venipuncture and processed in the laboratory or by fingerstick and processed immediately by a point-of-care (POC) monitor. POC monitors measure a thromboplastin-mediated clotting time that is converted to a PT equivalent by a microprocessor and expressed as a PT and INR. The thromboplastin is impregnated into the testing strips to which a sample of the patient's blood is applied. Samples as small as 10 to 56 µg are required. The ISI and precision of the testing procedure determine the accuracy of the result, but results are typically comparable to that of the laboratory. POC monitors are often used by anticoagulation management services such as Coumadin clinics, which are dedicated to the management of outpatient anticoagulation therapy (Ansell, et al., 2001). Several POC devices are also approved for home use, although they are expensive and only covered under Medicare guidelines for patients with mechanical heart valves. Coaguchek and ProTime are two of the commonly used POC monitors.

Heparin

The aPTT is used to monitor the effect of UFH and is sensitive to thrombin, factor Xa, and factor IXa. A target ratio range of 1.5 to 2.5 (observed aPTT/mean laboratory aPTT) is considered a therapeutic aPTT, which is equivalent to an anti-Xa level of 0.35 to 0.7 IU/mL for most aPTT reagents, and is multiplied by the control aPTT. Blood should be drawn for an aPTT evaluation every 6 hours until the aPTT is stable and within the therapeutic range.

As stated earlier, one of the major advantages of the LMWHs compared with heparin administered by continuous infusion or subcutaneously is that the aPTT does not need to be monitored because LMWHs have a minimal effect on the aPTT. Theoretically, anti-Xa activity can be used to monitor LMWH therapy, but this is not routine and is reserved for morbidly obese patients or those with renal dysfunction and women who are pregnant. Minimal therapeutic anti-Xa levels have not been definitively established. A conservative therapeutic range for twice daily dosing and an anti-Xa level 4 hours after subcutaneous administration is 0.6 to 1.0 IU/mL. For once-daily dosing, the target range 4 hours after dosing is not as clear, but a range of 1.0 to 2.0 IU/mL is deemed reasonable.

Antiplatelet Agents

Unlike the PT/INR with warfarin, the aPTT with heparin, and the anti-Xa level with LMWH, there are no laboratory tests to monitor the therapeutic efficacy of the antiplatelet agents aspirin, clopidogrel, or ticlopidine. Adverse events of these agents, especially bleeding or neutropenia, can be monitored by CBC or guaiac testing to detect blood in the

---

BOX 54–6. QUESTIONS TO ASK WHEN INR RESULTS ARE UNEXPECTED

- Have any warfarin doses been missed in the past 3 to 5 days?
- Have extra warfarin tablets been ingested?
- Is the patient taking a warfarin regimen other than prescribed?
- Is the patient experiencing bleeding problems?
- Is the patient experiencing thromboembolic complications?
- Have any new medications (prescription over-the-counter, herbal) been started, deleted, or changed from the patient's medication regimen?
- Has the patient's underlying condition changed, as in acute congestive heart failure exacerbation, or worsening of renal or hepatic impairment?
- Has the patient had a recent acute febrile or gastrointestinal illness?
- Has thyroid status changed or has a malignancy been diagnosed?

stools. Therapeutic efficacy is most commonly assessed by the absence of new thromboembolic or stroke symptoms.

PATIENT EDUCATION

Patient education regarding anticoagulation therapy should begin at the initiation of therapy. The practitioner should explain the rationale for anticoagulation and the risks and benefits of therapy. Extensive discussion of the potential for drug interactions, the need for frequent laboratory monitoring (Box 54-7), and the importance of stable dietary habits, also is essential for patients receiving warfarin. Patients must be willing to take an active part in treatment.

Patients receiving antiplatelet agents should be taught to recognize the signs and symptoms of bleeding, particularly from the GI tract. Aspirin can cause GI upset, so patients need to be aware of the necessity of taking it with food or meals. Sustained-release aspirin products should not be crushed or chewed because this destroys their delayed-absorption properties. Any large bruises or unusual bleeding should be reported to the practitioner.

Contact sports and dangerous activities, such as motorcycle riding, should be discouraged. Soft-bristled toothbrushes should be used, and electric razors can replace razor blades. Patients engaged in occupations that pose a risk of injury should be instructed to maintain extra caution in the workplace and always wear shoes and gloves as appropriate. Patients should be made aware of signs and symptoms of bleeding such as excessive or unexplained bruising, red or amber urine, and black stools.

Drug Information

Patients on warfarin should know their dosage, tablet size, and tablet color so that they maintain the prescribed regimen and will be able to know if they are given the correct medication from their supplier. Patients should also be cautioned against switching pill brands. Patients should be instructed to inform all health care practitioners (physicians, nurse practitioners, pharmacists, podiatrists, and dentists) that they are receiving anticoagulation therapy. In addition, because the list of potentially interacting substances with warfarin is exhaustive, the practitioner should encourage patients to report any new prescribed or over-the-counter drug, any herbal medicines, or changes in drug dosages. Patients should also be alerted to over-the-counter medications they should avoid, such as NSAIDs. Patients also must be instructed to notify the practitioner of any changes in health status such as fever, diarrhea, viral syndromes, weight changes, and increased fluid retention secondary to congestive heart failure. Patients must also be advised to notify the practitioner monitoring their anticoagulation therapy if they will be having any invasive procedures such as colonoscopy, tooth extraction, and surgery. If this occurs a decision whether or not warfarin will need to be stopped before the procedure, for how long, and if therapy with a shorter acting agent such as LMWH will be needed while the patient is off warfarin. See Box 54-8 for discussion of bridging therapy with LMWH while holding warfarin in preparation for an invasive procedure.

In addition, patients receiving ticlopidine need to be counseled regarding the signs and symptoms of neutropenia (including fever, chills, or sore throat). Those taking both ticlopidine and clopidogrel must be aware of the symptoms of thrombocytopenia (fever, weakness, difficulty speaking, seizures, yellowing of the skin or eyes, dark or bloody urine, or petechiae). Discussing what to do about symptoms of liver dysfunction, such as yellow skin or sclera, dark urine, or light-colored stools, is also recommended.

Patient-Oriented Information Sources

Several types of educational materials are available in several languages (including Spanish) from drug manufacturers, such as Bristol-Myers Squibb Company (1-800-268-6234 or 1-800-COUMADIN). Products include pillboxes, information booklets, audiotapes, videotapes, and Coumadin wallet-sized identification cards. MedicAlert bracelets or pendants are encouraged for patients who need lifelong anticoagulation therapy. The local American Heart Association branch has several pamphlets discussing atrial fibrillation and stroke.

Nutrition

Education concerning food restrictions for patients taking warfarin is essential. Vitamin K_1, the antidote to warfarin, is

---

BOX 54–7. TEACHING ABOUT THERAPEUTIC RANGES FOR ANTICOAGULANT THERAPY

Not only do patients receiving anticoagulant therapy need to know why they are taking medication, they need to know why they must have their blood tested frequently. In taking time to explain the rationale for testing as well as for treatment, the practitioner can help enhance the chances that patients will comply with the therapeutic plan.

INR Goal 2–3
Prophylaxis of venous thrombosis
Treatment of venous thrombosis
Treatment of pulmonary embolism
Prevention of systemic embolism
Atrial fibrillation
Tissue heart valves
Valvular heart disease

INR Goal 2.5–3.5
Mechanical prosthetic heart valves
Hypercoagulable conditions
Antiphospholipid antibodies
Lupus anticoagulant

Adapted from Hirsch, J., Dalen, K. E., Anderson, D. R. et al. (1998). Oral anticoagulants: Mechanism of action, clinical effectiveness, and optimal therapeutic range. *Chest, 114* (Suppl. 5). 44S–69S.

BOX 54–8. MANAGEMENT OF ANTICOAGULATION IN PREPARATION FOR INVASIVE PROCEDURES

When a patient receiving warfarin therapy is scheduled for an invasive diagnostic or treatment procedure, warfarin must be held 4 to 5 days prior to allow the INR to fall to an acceptable level to decrease the risk of bleeding. The type of procedure and the risk of bleeding involved will determine if warfarin therapy must be held. For most dermatologic procedures, such as Moh's surgery, it is not necessary to hold anticoagulation because the risk of bleeding while on anticoagulants is less than the risk of thromboembolic complications when anticoagulation is interrupted. Also, many dental procedures do not require anticoagulation interruption. Routine cleaning, cavity fillings, and root canals can be performed while the patient is receiving therapeutic anticoagulation. Gum scrapping and tooth extractions may require warfarin to be held so that the INR can fall to ≤2.0. Cataract removal, because it is not a very vascular procedure, can also be performed without anticoagulation interruption. Most major surgeries, endoscopic procedures, and urologic procedures require warfarin cessation to reach an INR ≤1.5. The practitioner performing the procedure, regardless of the type of procedure, should always be contacted to discuss the risks of the procedure and to determine the need to interrupt warfarin therapy because each case is individual.

If warfarin cessation is required, the length of interruption required for the INR to fall sufficiently must be determined. For those maintained at an INR of 2 to 3, stopping warfarin 4 to 5 days prior to the procedure should allow the INR to return to near a normal level. For those maintained at an INR of 2.5 to 3.5, stopping warfarin for 5 to 6 days may be required.

Based on the patient's thromboembolic risk, it must then be determined if a fast-acting anticoagulant, such as UFH or LMWH, should be given as a bridge therapy during the period of warfarin cessation. For patients with low risk of thromboembolism, such as patients without VTE for more than 3 months and patients with atrial fibrillation without history of stroke, warfarin may be stopped without the use of UFH or LMWH. Prophylaxis may be given after the procedure, whereas warfarin is restarted if the procedure creates a higher risk of thrombosis. Patients with intermediate risk of VTE should be given low-dose UFH or prophylactic dose LMWH, and high-risk patients, such as those with a recent VTE (>3 months) and those with a mechanical cardiac valve, should be given full-dose UFH or full-dose LMWH starting 1 to 2 days after warfarin is stopped, stopped 24 hours before the procedure, and restarted after the procedure along with warfarin and continued until warfarin is at a therapeutic level. UFH or LMWH should be resumed at the same dose after the procedure while warfarin is resumed and continued until the INR reaches a therapeutic level (Ansell et al., 2001). INR testing should be checked at least every 2 to 3 days to determine if the INR is therapeutic and the UFH or LMWH can be stopped. The risk of bleeding after the procedure with the addition of UFH and LMWH must be discussed with the practitioner performing the procedure and a plan to minimize both the bleeding and thrombotic risk must be arranged.

LMWH is frequently chosen for bridge therapy because it can be administered as an outpatient without frequent monitoring, can be given once or twice a day, and only needs to be held 12 to 24 hours prior to the procedure to decrease the risk of bleeding. When the patient is unable to take LMWH because of a history of HIT, severe renal insufficiency, or cost of the LMWH and no insurance coverage (Lovenox Free Drug program is available for those without insurance coverage who have a qualifying income level; call 888-632-8607), UFH may be used. Frequently the patient must be admitted to the hospital before the procedure for IV UFH because outpatient SC UFH is difficult because monitoring of PTT levels must be performed frequently.

---

naturally found in several plant foods. In contrast, vitamin K_2 is primarily synthesized by normal intestinal flora. The estimated necessary dietary intake of vitamin K_1 is 80 μg/d for men over 25 years old and 65 μg/d for women over 25 years old. In the United States, typical American dietary vitamin K_1 intake is 300 to 500 μg (Suttie, 1992). Excessive amounts of dietary vitamin K_1 may antagonize warfarin's clinical effect and decrease the INR (Pederson et al., 1991). Khan and coworkers (2004) found that for every 100 μg increase in vitamin K_1 intake in the 4 days before an INR measurement, the INR fell by 0.2. In another study, it was found that higher warfarin doses at 5.7 ± 1.7 mg/d was needed by those consuming 250 μg or more vitamin K daily compared to that of 3.5 ± 1.0 mg/d by those consuming less than 250 μg vitamin K daily (Khan et al., 2004). Dark green leafy vegetables (spinach and turnip, collard, and mustard greens), broccoli, Brussels sprouts, and cabbage are the primary sources of vitamin K and contain high amounts, greater than 100 mg/100-g serving. Herbal and green teas may also contain large quantities of vitamin K_1 (1400 mg/100 g), and high levels of vitamin K_1 (50 mg/100 g) are found in soybean and soy products and olive oils, whereas peanut and corn oils contain minimal amounts. Vitamin K is also found in certain plant oils and prepared foods containing these oils, such as baked goods, margarines, and salad dressings. Food preparation with oils rich in vitamin K may also contribute to total vitamin K intake and effect warfarin action (Booth & Centurelli, 1999). The *Coumadin Cookbook* (available from Bristol-Myers Squibb) is a great resource for patients taking warfarin because it provides tips for monitoring and maintaining a consistent vitamin K intake and provides many recipes with a low vitamin K content. Patients should be encouraged to eat a healthy diet, maintain consistency in their choice of foods, and avoid large fluctuations in dietary vitamin K_1 intake. Instructing patients to maintain a consistent intake of vitamin K–containing foods, rather than trying to eliminate all sources of dietary vitamin K_1, is essential (Ferland & Sadowski, 1992). Patients must also be educated on portion sizes and their vitamin K content so that they are not only consistent with the frequency of intake of vitamin K foods, but are also consistent with the number of servings of vitamin K they consume. Fad diets, such as the "cabbage soup" diet, are discouraged and if diets such as the Atkin's diet or low-carbohydrate diets are to be started, the patient must notify the practitioner so that INRs can be more frequently monitored. These diets, when strictly followed, frequently lead to a change in the intake amount of vitamin K foods. Table 54-10 lists examples of vitamin K food content and serving size.

Table 54.10

Vitamin K Content of Selected Foods

Food	Amount of Vitamin K in mg per 100-g Portion
Abalone	23
Asparagus, raw	40
Avocado, raw	40
Broccoli, raw	205
Brussel sprouts, raw	177
Cabbage, raw	145
Canola oil	141
Chinese green tea (dry)	1428
Coleslaw	57
Coriander leaf, cooked	1510
Cucumber peel, raw	360
Endive, raw	231
Green beans, snap	47
Kale, raw	817
Lettuce, raw	210
Margarine, stick*	51
Mayonnaise	81
Mustard greens, raw	170
Nightshade leaf, raw	620
Parsley, raw	540
Purslane, raw	381
Seaweed, purple	1385
Soybean oil	193
Soybeans, raw	47
Spinach leaf, raw	400
Swiss chard, raw	830
Tofu, raw	2
Turnip greens, raw	251
Watercress, raw	250

*1 stick of margarine is equivalent to 113 g.
From Spandorfer, J., Konkle, B. A., & Merli, G. J. (2001). *Management and prevention of thrombosis in primary care*. London: Arnold.

Hidden sources of excess vitamin K include enteral supplements, which can cause resistance to warfarin. Checking the amount of vitamin K in any nutritional supplement is advised because several of these preparations are now marketed directly to patients through the lay press. In addition, many over-the-counter vitamin preparations contain vitamin K, and patients should be counseled to read the label or bring in all medication bottles to the practitioner. Questioning patients regarding any changes in dietary habits may provide clues when the INR varies. Extensive lists of the vitamin K content of common foods are now widely available on the Internet.

Complementary and Alternative Medications

Although there are no complementary or alternative therapies available, newer anticoagulants are on the horizon. The SPORTIF III and V trials evaluated ximelagantran in high-risk patients with atrial fibrillation. The combined results found that a fixed dose of ximelagantran of 36 mg twice daily without coagulation monitoring was not inferior to well-controlled, adjusted-dose warfarin in preventing stroke and systemic embolic events among high-risk patients with atrial fibrillation who did not have impaired renal function. There was also significantly less bleeding events associated with ximelagantran use (Hankey et al., 2004). Ximelagantran has also been studied in orthopedic surgery patients for prevention of VTE. Subcutaneous melagantran followed by oral ximelagantran has been investigated in four European trials and the efficacy of an oral ximelagantran regimen has been evaluated in five U.S. trials (Evans et al., 2004). The EXULT A study found that ximelagantran reduced the risk of VTE following TKR surgery as compared to warfarin. The THRIVE III study looked at prevention of VTE recurrence in patients with a prior history. This study showed that continuing treatment with ximelagantran for 18 months after completion of a standard 6-month course of anticoagulant therapy for VTE reduced the risk of recurrence by 84% versus placebo (Poole, 2003). One adverse event that was found in approximately 6% of study patients was significant excess elevation in liver enzymes, notably alanine aminotransferase. The elevation typically occurred 2 to 6 months after initiation and resolved after cessation of treatment without sequelae (Hankey et al., 2004).

The advantages of ximelagantran in comparison to warfarin are oral administration with a rapid onset of action negating the need for overlap with a heparin product; fixed dosing; no need for anticoagulation monitoring; predictable pharmacokinetic profile, allowing much less food and drug interactions than that with warfarin; and a decreased risk of major bleeding. Disadvantages may be the need for twice-daily dosing, adverse hepatic effects possibly requiring monitoring of liver function for up to 6 months after initiation, the need to evaluate renal function before initiation secondary to renal excretion, and higher cost than warfarin. Overall, it appears that ximelagantran, the first oral DTI, may be a useful and well-accepted alternative to warfarin for those who qualify for use and can afford it.

■ Case Study

D.G. is a 74-year-old woman who arrives at the emergency center complaining of shortness of breath, palpitations, nausea, and vomiting for the past 4 days. Her medical history includes diabetes mellitus, hypertension, congestive heart failure, cataract in the left eye, and degenerative joint disease. She ambulates with a cane and is considered legally blind. The patient's current medications are hydrochlorothiazide 25 mg/d, fosinopril 10 mg/d, metformin 500 mg twice daily, and ibuprofen 800 mg 3 times daily with food.

Vital signs are as follows: blood pressure of 160/95, respiratory rate of 30, and heart rate of 125. ECG shows an irregularly irregular rhythm with a rapid ventricular response. Echocardiography reveals a moderately dilated left atrium, moderately depressed left ventricular systolic function, moderate mitral stenosis, and a thrombus in the apex of the left atrium.

Diagnosis: atrial fibrillation, acute onset

1. List specific goals of treatment for D.G..
2. What dietary and lifestyle changes should be recommended for D.G.?
3. What drug therapy would you prescribe? Why?
4. What are the parameters for monitoring success of the therapy?
5. Describe one or two drug–drug or drug–food interactions for the selected agent.
6. List one or two adverse reactions for the selected agent that would cause you to change therapy.
7. What would be the choice for the second-line therapy?
8. Discuss specific patient education based on the prescribed therapy.
9. What over-the-counter or alternative medications would be appropriate for D.G.?

Bibliography

Starred references are cited in the text.

*Adams, H. P. Jr., Bott, T. G., Crowell, R. M., et al. (1994). Guidelines for the management of patients with acute ischemic stroke. *Stroke, 25,* 1901–1914.

*Albers, G. W., Amarenco, P., Easton, J. D., et al. (2001). Antithrombotic and thrombolytic therapy for ischemic stroke. *Chest, 119* (Suppl. 1), 300S–320S.

*Alpert, J. S., & Dalen, J. E. (1994). Epidemiology and natural history of venous thromboembolism. *Progress in Cardiovascular Disease, 36,* 417–422.

*Albers, G. W., Dalen, J. E., Laupacis, A., et al. (2001). Antithrombotic therapy in atrial fibrillation. *Chest, 119* (Suppl. 1), 194S–206S.

*Albers, G. W., Easton, D., Sacco, R. L., et al. (1998). Antithrombotic and thrombolytic therapy in ischemic stroke. *Chest, 114* (Suppl. 5), 683S–698S.

American Society of Health-System Pharmacists. (1995). ASHP therapeutic position statement on the use of the international normalized ratio system to monitor oral anticoagulant therapy. *American Journal of Health-System Pharmacy, 52,* 529–531.

*Anderson, F. A., & Spencer, F. A. (2003). Risk factors for venous thromboembolism. *Circulation, 107* (23), I9–I16.

*Ansell, J. E. (1993). Oral anticoagulant therapy—50 years later. *Archives of Internal Medicine, 153,* 586–596.

Ansell, J. E., Buttaro, M. L., Voltis, T. O., et al. (1997). Consensus guidelines for coordinated outpatient oral anticoagulant therapy management. *Annals of Pharmacotherapy 31,* 604–615.

*Ansell, J., Hirsh, J., Dalen, J., et al. (2001). Managing oral anticoagulant therapy. *Chest, 119* (Suppl. 1), 22S–38S.

*Antiplatelet Trialists' Collaboration. (1994). Collaborative overview of randomized trial of antiplatelet therapy: I. Prevention of death, myocardial infarction, and stroke by prolonged anti-platelet therapy in various categories of patients. *British Medical Journal, 308,* 81–106.

*Atrial Fibrillation Investigators. (1994). Risk factors for stroke and efficacy of antithrombotic therapy in atrial fibrillation: Analysis of pooled data from five randomized trials. *Archives of Internal Medicine, 154,* 1449–1457.

*Ball, K. (2003). Deep vein thrombosis and airline travel—the deadly duo. *AORN Online, 77* (2), 346–358.

Barr Pharmaceuticals. (1997). Warfarin package insert. Pomona, NY: Author.

Bates, S. M., Greer, I. A., Hirsh, J., & Ginsberg, J. S. (2004). Use of antithrombotic agents during pregnancy: the Seventh ACCP Conference on Antithrombotic and Thrombolytic Therapy. *Chest, 126*(3 Suppl), 627S–644S.

*Beare, P. G., & Myers, J. L. (1994). *Adult health nursing.* St. Louis: Mosby.

*Becker, R. C., Fintel, D. J., & Green, D. (2002). *Antithrombotic therapy.* Caddo, OK: Professional Communications.

*Benet, L. Z., & Goyan, J. E. (1995). Bioequivalence and narrow therapeutic index drugs. *Pharmacotherapy, 15*, 433–440.

*Booth, S. L., & Centurelli, M. A. (1999). Vitamin K: A practical guide to the dietary management of patients on warfarin. *Nutrition Reviews, 57* (9, Pt. I), 288–296.

*Bridgen, M. L., Kay, C., Le, A., et al. (1998). Audit of the frequency and clinical response to excessive anticoagulation in an outpatient population. *American Journal of Hematology, 59*, 22–27.

*Bristol-Myers Squibb Company. (2001). Coumadin tablets package insert. Princeton, NJ: Author.

*Bussey, H. I. (1993). How to monitor the dosage of warfarin. *Heart Disease and Stroke, 23*, 88–92.

Bussey, H. I., Force, R., Bianco, T. M., et al. (1992). Reliance on prothrombin time ratios causes significant errors in anticoagulation therapy. *Archives of Internal Medicine, 152*, 278–282.

*CAPRIE Steering Committee. (1996). A randomized, blinded, trial of clopidogrel versus aspirin in patients at risk of ischemic events (CAPRIE). *Lancet*, 1329–1339.

*Carnetiger, S. C., Rosendaal, F. R., Wintzen, A. R., et al. (1995). Optimal anticoagulant therapy in patients with mechanical heart valves. *New England Journal of Medicine, 333*, 11–17.

*Chan, W. S., Anand, S., & Ginsberg, J. S. (2000). Anticoagulation in pregnant women with mechanical heart valves. *Archives of Internal Medicine, 160*, 191–196.

*Clagett, G. P., Anderson, F. A., Geerts, W., et al. (1998). Prevention of venous thromboembolism. *Chest, 114*(Suppl. 5), 531S–560S.

*Colman, R. W., Marder, V. J., Salzman, E. W., et al. (1994). Overview of hemostasis. In R. W. Colman (Ed.), *Hemostasis and thrombosis: Basic principles and clinical practice* (3rd ed., pp. 3–16). Philadelphia: J. B. Lippincott.

*Crowther, M. A., Donovan, D., Harrison, L., et al. (1998). Low-dose oral vitamin K reliably reverses over-anticoagulation due to warfarin. *Thrombosis and Haemostasis, 79*, 1116–1118.

Dalen, J. E., & Hirsh, J. H. (1998). Fifth ACCP Consensus Conference on Antithrombotic Therapy. *Chest, 114*(Suppl. 5), 429S–769S.

*Diab, F., & Feffer, S. (1994). Hereditary warfarin resistance. *Southern Medical Journal, 87*(3), 407–409.

Diener, H. C., Cunha, L., Forbes, C., et al. (1996). European Stroke Prevention Study 2: Dipyridamole and acetylsalicylic acid in the secondary prevention of stroke. *Journal of the Neurological Sciences, 143*, 1–13.

Drug facts and comparisons. Pocket version, 6th ed. (2002). St. Louis: Facts and Comparisons.

DuPont Pharma. (2000). Coumadin package insert. Wilmington, DE: Author.

*Evans, H. C., Perry, C. M., & Faulds, D. (2004). Ximelagantran/melagantran: A review of its use in the prevention of venous thromboembolism in orthopedic surgery. *Drugs, 64*(6), 649–678.

*Ferland, G., & Sadowski, J. A. (1992). Vitamin K1 (phylloquinone) content of edible oils: Effects of heating and light exposure. *Journal of Agricultural and Food Chemistry, 40*, 1869–1873.

*Fihn, S. D., McDonell, M., Martin, D., et al. (1993). Risk factors for complications of chronic anticoagulation. *Annals of Internal Medicine, 118*, 511–520.

*Geerts, W. H., Heit, J. A., Clagett, G. P., et al. (2001). *Chest, 119* (Suppl. 1), 132S–175S.

*Ginsberg, J. S., & Hirsh, J. (1998). Use of antithrombotic agents during pregnancy. *Chest, 114*(Suppl. 5), 524S–530S.

*Gorski, L. A. (2001). Clinical update: deep vein thrombosis. *Home Healthcare Nurse, 19*(5), 307–310.

*Greinacher, A., Janssens, U., Berg, G., et al. (1999). Lepirudin (recombinant hirudin) for parenteral anticoagulation in patients with heparin-induced thrombocytopenia: Heparin-Associated Thrombocytopenia Study (HAT) investigators. *Circulation, 100*, 587.

Gurwitz, J. H., Avorn, J., Ross-Degnan, D., et al. (1992). Aging and the anticoagulant response to warfarin therapy. *Annals of Internal Medicine, 116*, 901–904.

Haines, S. T., & Bussey, H. I. (1997). Diagnosis of deep vein thrombosis. *American Journal of Health-System Pharmacy, 54*, 66–74.

*Hankey, G. J., Klijn, C. J. M., & Eikelboom, J. W. (2004). Ximelagantran or warfarin for stroke prevention in patients with atria fibrillation. *Stroke, 35*(2), 389–391.

*Harrell, C. C., & Kline, S. S. (1995). Oral vitamin K1: An option to reduce warfarin's activity. *Annals of Pharmacotherapy, 29*, 1229–1232.

*Harrison, L., Johnston, M., Massicotte, M. P., et al. (1997). Comparison of 5 mg and 10 mg loading doses in initiation of warfarin therapy. *Annals of Internal Medicine, 126*, 133–206.

*Hart, R. G., Pearce, L. A., & Koudstaal, P. J. (2004). Transient ischemic attacks in patients with atrial fibrillation: implications for secondary prevention: The European atrial fibrillation trial and stroke prevention in atrial fibrillation III trial. *Stroke, 35*(4), 948–951.

Hirsh, J. (1991). Oral anticoagulant drugs. *New England Journal of Medicine, 324*, 1865–1875.

*Hirsh, J., Dalen, J. E., Anderson, D. R., et al. (2001). Oral anticoagulants: Mechanism of action, clinical effectiveness, and optimal therapeutic range. *Chest, 119*(Suppl. 1), 8S–21S.

Hirsh, J., & Fuster, V. (1994). Guide to anticoagulant therapy. Part 2: Oral anticoagulants. *Circulation, 89*, 1469–1480.

*Hirsh, J., Salzman, E. W., Marder, V. J., et al. (1994). Overview of the thrombotic process and its therapy. In R. W. Colman (Ed.), *Hemostasis and thrombosis: Basic principles and clinical practice* (3rd ed., pp. 1151–1158). Philadelphia: J. B. Lippincott.

*Hirsh, J., Warkentin, T. E., Shaughnessy, S. G., et al. (2001). Heparin and low-molecular-weight heparin. *Chest, 119*(Suppl. 1), 64S–94S.

*Hoechst Marion Roussell. (1998). Refludan package insert. Kansas City, MO: Author.

*Howard, P. A. (2003). Low molecular weight heparins in special populations. *Journal of Infusion Nursing, 26*(5), 304–310.

*Howe, A. M., & Allerman, A. A. (1998). Is immune-mediated heparin-induced thrombocytopenia less common with low-molecular-weight heparins, and should a low-molecular-weight heparin be used in a patient who develops this complication with standard, unfractionated heparin? *Disease Management Clinical Outcomes, 1*(6), 207–210.

*Hull, R. D., Raskob, G. E., Pineo, G. F., et al. (1992). Subcutaneous low-molecular-weight heparin compared with continuous intravenous unfractionated heparin in the treatment of proximal deep venous thrombosis. *New England Journal of Medicine, 325*, 975–982.

*Hyers, T. M., Agnelli, G., Hull, R. D., et al. (2001). Antithrombotic therapy for venous thromboembolic disease. *Chest, 119* (Suppl. 1), 176S–193S.

*Hyers, T., Agnelli, G., Hull, R., et al. (1998). Antithrombotic therapy for venous thromboembolic disease. *Chest, 114*(Suppl. 5), 561S–578S.

*Janetsky, K., & Morreale, A. P. (1997). Probable interaction between warfarin and ginseng. *American Journal of Health-System Pharmacy, 54*, 692–693.

Kannel, W. B., Abbott, R. D., Savage, D. D., et al. (1982). Epidemiologic features of chronic atrial fibrillation: The Framingham Study. *New England Journal of Medicine, 306*, 1018–1022.

*Kellen, J. C. (2004). Implications for nursing care of patients with atrial fibrillation lessons learned from the AFFIRM and RACE studies. *Journal of Cardiovascular Nursing, 19*(2), 128–137.

*Khamashta, M. A., Cuadrado, M. J., Mujic, F., et al. (1995). The management of thrombosis in the antiphospholipid-antibody syndrome. *New England Journal of Medicine, 332*(15), 993–997.

*Khan, T., Wynne, H., Wood, P., et al. (2004). Dietary vitamin K influences intra-individual variability in anticoagulant response to warfarin. *British Journal of Haematology, 124*(3), 348–354.

*Koopman, M. M., Prandoni, P., Piovella, F. O. P. A., et al. (1996). Treatment of venous thrombosis with intravenous unfractionated heparin administered in the hospital as compared with subcutaneously low-molecular-weight heparin administered at home. *New England Journal of Medicine, 333*, 682–687.

*Landefeld, C. S., & Byeth, R. J. (1993). Anticoagulation-related bleeding: Clinical epidemiology, prediction and prevention. *American Journal of Medicine, 95*, 315–328.

*Larned, Z. L., O'Shea, S. I., & Ortel, T. L. (2003). Heparin-induced thrombocytopenia: Clinical presentations and therapeutic management. *Clinical Advances in Hematology & Oncology, 1*(6), 356–364.

*Laupacis, A., Albers, G., Dalen, J., et al. (1998). Antithrombotic therapy in atrial fibrillation. *Chest, 114*(Suppl. 5), 579S–589S.

*Levine, M., Gent, M., Hirsh, J., et al. (1996). A comparison of low-molecular-weight heparin administered primarily at home with unfractionated heparin administered in the hospital for proximal deep vein thrombosis. *New England Journal of Medicine, 334*, 677–681.

Levine, G. N, Kern, M. J., Berger, P. B., et al. (2003). Management of patients undergoing percutaneous coronary revascularization. *Annals of Internal Medicine, 139*(2), 123–136.

*Levine, M., Raskob, G., Landefeld, S., et al. (1998). Hemorrhagic complications of anticoagulant therapy. *Chest, 114*(Suppl. 5), 511S–523S.

Martineau, P., & Tawill, N. (1998). Low-molecular-weight heparins in the treatment of deep-vein thrombosis. *Annals of Pharmacotherapy, 32*, 588–598.

McKenna, R., Cole, E. R., & Vassan, I. (1983). Is warfarin sodium contraindicated in the lactating mother? *Journal of Pediatrics, 103*, 325–327.

Merck and Co. (1997). Mephyton and Aquamephyton package inserts. West Point, PA: Author.

*Micromedex 2004, Micromedex(r) Healthcare Series Vol. 121 Retrieved May 21, 2004, from http://proxy1.lib.tju.edu:2051/mdxcgi/mdxhtml.exe?&tmpl=mdxhome.tm1&SCRNAME=md xhome&CTL=/u01/mdx/mdxcgi/megat.sys

*Morris, B. A., Morrison, R. B., & Yetsko, C. (2002). Venous thromboembolism: prevention & treatment. *RN, 65*(10), 24hf3–24hf9.

Morrison, G. W. (1979). Predicting warfarin requirements. *Lancet, 1*, 829–830.

*Noble, J. (2001). *Textbook of primary care medicine.* St. Louis: Mosby.

*O'Rourke, F., Dean, N., Akhtar, N., et al. (2004). Current and future concepts in stroke prevention. *Canadian Medical Association Journal, 170*(7), 1123–1133.

*Patrono, C., Coller, B., Dalen, J. E., et al. (2001). Platelet-active drugs. *Chest, 119*(Suppl. 1), 39S–63S.

*Patrono, C., Coller, B., Dalen, J. E., et al. (1998). Platelet-active drugs: The relationships among dose, effectiveness, and side effects. *Chest, 114*(Suppl. 5), 470S–488S.

*Pederson, F. M., Hamburg, O., Hess, K., et al. (1991). The effect of dietary vitamin K on warfarin-induced anticoagulation. *Journal of Internal Medicine, 229*, 517–520.

*Pinede, L., Ninet, J., Duhaut, P., et al. (2001). For the Investigators of the Durée Optimale du Traitement AntiVitamines K (DOTAVK) Study. *Circulation, 103*(20), 2453–2460.

*PIOPED Investigators. (1990). Value of the ventilation/perfusion scan in acute pulmonary embolism: Results of the Prospective Investigation of Pulmonary Embolism Diagnosis (PIOPED). *Journal of the American Medical Association, 263*, 2753–2759.

*Poole, R. M. (2003). Ximelagantran reduces risk of VTE. *Inpharma Weekly, 1375*, 9–10.

Raschke, R. A., Beilly, B. M., & Guidry, J. R. (1993). The weight-based heparin dosing nomogram compared with a "standard care" nomogram. *Annals of Internal Medicine, 119*, 874–881.

*Rathbun, S. W., Whitsett, T. L., Vesely, S. K., et al. (2004). Clinical utility of d-dimer in patients with suspected pulmonary embolism and nondiagnostic lung scans or negative CT findings. *Chest, 125* (3), 851–855.

*Salem, D. N., Daudelin, D. H., Levine, H. J., et al. (2001). Antithrombotic therapy in valvular heart disease. *Chest, 119* (Suppl. 1), 207S–219S.

*Salzman, E. W., & Hirsh, J. (1994). The epidemiology, pathogenesis, and natural history of venous thrombosis. In R. W. Colman (Ed.), *Hemostasis and thrombosis: Basic principles and clinical practice* (3rd ed., pp. 3–16). Philadelphia: J. B. Lippincott.

*Schwartz, T., Siegert, G., Oettler, W., et al. (2003). Venous thrombosis after long-haul flights. *Archives of Internal Medicine, 163* (22), 2759–2764.

*Simmoneau, G., Charbonnier, B., Decousus, H., et al. (1993). Subcutaneous low-molecular-weight heparin compared with continuous intravenous unfractionated heparin in the treatment of proximal deep venous thrombosis. *Archives of Internal Medicine, 153*, 1541–1544.

*Spandorfer, J., Konkle, B. A., & Merli, G. J. (2001). *Management and prevention of thrombosis in primary care.* London: Arnold.

*Stein, P. D., Alpert, J. S., Bussey, H. I., et al. (2001). Antithrombotic therapy in patients with mechanical and biological prosthetic heart valves. *Chest, 119*(Suppl. 1), 220S–227S.

Stein, P. D., Alpert, J. S., Dalen, J. E., et al. (1998). Antithrombotic therapy in patients with mechanical and biological prosthetic heart valves. *Chest, 114*(Suppl. 5), 602S–610S.

*Stringer, K. A., & Lindenfeld, J. (1992). Hirudins: Antithrombotic anticoagulants. *Annals of Pharmacotherapy, 26*, 1535–1540.

*Suttie, J. W. (1992). Vitamin K and human nutrition. *Journal of the American Dietetic Association, 92*, 585–590.

*Taylor, J. R., & Wilt, V. M. (1999). Probable antagonism of warfarin by green tea. *Annals of Pharmacotherapy, 33*, 426–428.

*Tyler, V. E. (1996). *The honest herbal* (3rd ed.). Binghamton, NY: Pharmaceutical Products Press.

*Vongpatanasin, W., Hillis, L. D., & Lange, R. A. (1996). Prosthetic heart valves. *New England Journal of Medicine, 335*, 407–416.

Warkentin, T. E., & Kelton, J. G. (1991). Heparin-induced thrombocytopenia. *Progress in Hemostasis and Thrombosis, 10*, 1–34.

Weibert, R. T. (1992). Oral anticoagulant therapy in patients undergoing dental surgery. *Clinical Pharmacokinetics, 11*, 857–864.

Wells, P. S., Holbrook, A. M., Crowther, N. R., et al. (1994). Interactions of warfarin with drugs and food. *Annals of Internal Medicine, 121*, 676–693.

White, R. H., Hong, R., Venook, A. P., et al. (1987). Initiation of warfarin therapy: Comparison of physician dosing with computer-assisted dosing. *Journal of General Internal Medicine, 2*, 141–148.

Wilde, M. I., & Markham, A. (1997). Danaparoid: A review of its pharmacology and clinical use in the management of heparin-induced thrombocytopenia. *Drugs, 54*, 903–924.

55

ANEMIAS

■ KELLY BARRINGER

Anemia is a hidden epidemic in this nation and can have serious consequences if it is left untreated. At least 3.4 million Americans have been diagnosed as anemic and millions more may be undiagnosed or at increased risk of developing anemia. Anemia occurs more frequently among women, African Americans, the elderly, and those with the lowest incomes.

The most common anemia in the United States is hypoproliferative anemia, which includes iron deficiency, chronic kidney disease (CKD), and the inflammation-associated anemia of chronic disease (rheumatoid arthritis, inflammatory bowel disease).

CAUSE

Anemia may develop through blood loss, nutritional deficiency, or malabsorption syndromes, or concurrently with inflammation or malignancy, or be inherited as in sickle cell disease, thalassemia, or hemoglobinopathy. Anemia may also occur from the treatment of diseases such as cancer, HIV/AIDS, or hepatitis C.

PATHOPHYSIOLOGY

Red blood cells (RBCs), also known as erythrocytes, are formed in the marrow of ribs, sternum, clavicle, vertebrae, pelvis, and proximal epiphyses of the humerus and femur. RBCs play a vital role in the support of tissue metabolism by transporting oxygen to and removing carbon dioxide from tissue. To maintain proper tissue oxygenation and sustain a normal acid–base balance, an adequate number of RBCs must be available and they must be a specific shape and size.

The production of RBCs involves a series of maturational steps beginning with a pluripotent cell that differentiates into erythroid precursors. As the cells undergo maturational changes, they lose their nuclei and acquire hemoglobin as a component. The production of RBCs is initiated by the hormone erythropoietin (EPO), which is produced by the kidneys in response to a decrease in tissue oxygen concentration. Decreased tissue oxygen then signals the kidneys to increase production and release EPO. This EPO stimulates the stem cell to differentiate into proerythroblasts; EPO also increases the rate of mitosis and increases the release of reticulocytes from the marrow and induces hemoglobin formation. When hemoglobin synthesis is accelerated, the critical hemoglobin concentration necessary for maturity is reached more rapidly, causing an earlier release of reticulocytes. The appearance of reticulocytes in peripheral circulation indicates that RBC production is being stimulated. The maturation process takes about 1 week. Several days are then required for the reticulocyte to become an erythrocyte. The normal RBC survival time is 120 days. The survival time can be decreased to 18 to 20 days before occurrence of an anemia if the bone marrow functions at maximal capacity. When hemolytic destruction of RBCs exceeds marrow production, anemia will develop, causing the hemoglobin value to decrease.

DIAGNOSTIC CRITERIA

Anemia is a reduction in the number of circulating RBCs (the hemoglobin concentration) or the volume of packed RBCs (hematocrit) in the blood. In adults, anemia is present if the hematocrit is less than 41% (hemoglobin <13.5 g/dL) in men or 37% (hemoglobin <12 g/dL) in women (Table 55-1). Anemias are classified according to their pathophysiologic basis and occur due to decreased production or increased destruction of RBCs (Table 55-2). They are also classified according or cell size using the mean corpuscular volume (MCV). Microcytic anemias are those anemias due to RBCs with a lower than normal size. These include iron deficiency anemia, thalassemia, and anemia of chronic disease. In contrast, macrocytic anemia may be megaloblastic such as folate or vitamin B_{12} deficiency or nonmegaloblastic causes such as myelodysplasia, liver disease, or reticulocytosis.

The signs and symptoms of anemia depend on the rate of development, age, and cardiovascular status of the patient. Rapid onset of anemia is most likely to present with cardiorespiratory symptoms (tachycardia, lightheadedness, breathlessness). Anemia of a chronic nature may present with symptoms including fatigue, weakness, headache, vertigo, faintness, sensitivity to cold, pallor, and loss of skin tone.

Table 55.1

Normal Hematologic Values

Test	Children >2 y	Adults >18 y
Hemoglobin (g/dL)	11.5–15.5	Men 13.5–17.5
		Women 12–16
Hematocrit (%)	34–45	Men 41–53
		Women 36–46
MCV (fL)	75–95	80–100
MCHC (%)	31–37	31–37
MCH (pg/cell)	24–33	26–34
RBC (million/mm³)	3.9–5.2	4.5–5.9
Reticulocyte count, absolute (%)		0.5–1.5
TIBC	250–400	250–400
Ferritin (ng/mL)	7–140	Men 15–200
		Women 12–150
Serum iron (μg/dL)	50–120	Men 50–160
		Women 40–150

MCV, mean corpuscular volume; MCHC, mean corpuscular hemoglobin concentration; MCH, mean corpuscular hemoglobin; TIBC, total iron-binding capacity.

ANEMIAS CAUSED BY INCREASED DESTRUCTION

ACUTE POSTHEMORRHAGIC ANEMIA/CHRONIC BLOOD LOSS

Posthemorrhagic anemia results from massive hemorrhage associated with spontaneous or traumatic rupture or incision of a large blood vessel, erosion of an artery by lesion (peptic ulcer, neoplasm), or failure of normal hemostasis. The sudden loss of one third of blood volume may be fatal, whereas a two-thirds loss of blood volume slowly over 24 hours is without immediate risk.

Diagnostic Criteria

Initial evaluation of anemia includes complete blood count, reticulocyte index, examination of the peripheral blood smear,

Table 55.2

Classification of Anemias by Pathophysiology

Increased destruction
  Blood loss
  Hemolysis
  Sickle cell disease
  G6PD deficiency
  Thrombotic thrombocytopenic purpura
  Hemolytic-uremic syndrome
  Clostridial infection
  Hypersplenism
Decreased production
  Iron deficiency
  Thalassemia
  Anemia of chronic disease
  Aplastic anemia
  Myeloproliferative leukemia

G6PD, glucose-6-phosphate dehydrogenase.

and a stool sample for occult blood. Further studies are indicated based on results from the preliminary evaluation.

During and immediately after hemorrhage, the RBC count, hemoglobin value, and hematocrit may be high due to vasoconstriction. Within a few hours, fluid from tissue enters the circulation resulting in hemodilution causing a drop in the RBC count and hemoglobin value. This result is proportional to the severity of bleeding.

Initiating Therapy

Immediate therapy consists of hemostasis, restoration of blood volume, and treatment of shock. Blood transfusion is the only means of rapidly restoring blood volume.

SICKLE CELL ANEMIA

Sickle cell anemia is an autosomal recessive disorder in which abnormal hemoglobin leads to chronic hemolytic anemia with numerous clinical consequences. It most commonly affects African Americans and, to a lesser extent, Hispanics.

Pathophysiology

Patients with sickle cell disease predominantly make hemoglobin S. Hemoglobin S differs from normal hemoglobin A by the substitution of a single amino acid within one of the two polypeptide chains. Deoxygenation causes RBCs cells to sickle and leads to vaso-occlusion and blockage of microvasculature, which can cause sickle cell crisis. This blockage causes significant damage to the endothelium of the arterial and venous circulation. Crisis occurs when patients are physically stressed (exercise), exposed to high altitude or cold temperatures, or have a high fever or infection. The underlying cause includes hypoxia, dehydration, and acidosis. Sickle cell crises last about a week but may not resolve for several weeks to months. Pain typically occurs in the back, ribs, and limbs. Patients with sickle cell anemia are susceptible to infection, particularly *Streptococcus pneumoniae* and *Haemophilus influenza*, and are prone to gallstones and renal failure. Other complications include chronic leg ulcer, priapism, aseptic necrosis of the humoral and femoral heads, and chronic osteomyelitis. Long-term effects include stroke, heart failure, and death.

Diagnostic Criteria

Examination of a peripheral blood smear for sickling and checking a reticulocyte count can provide supportive data for the diagnosis of sickle cell disease. Hemoglobin electrophoresis or a sickle cell preparation can also be useful in the diagnosis of sickle cell disease. Laboratory findings also show reduced hemoglobin and a RBC count between 2 and 3 million/μL.

For those at risk, techniques such as chorionic biopsy have been used during early gestation (6–8 weeks of pregnancy) to identify sickle cell disease. Genetic counseling and education must also be offered. Risk of the procedure to mother and fetus, risks of false-positive and false-negative results, and the acceptability of therapeutic abortion should also be discussed.

Initiating Drug Therapy

No specific treatment is available for patients with sickle cell anemia. Analgesics, oxygen, and adequate hydration are given for vaso-occlusive episodes. Pneumococcal vaccine is encouraged for preventing pneumococcal infections due to impaired splenic function. Folic acid demands are increased in patients with sickle cell disease because of accelerated erythropoiesis. Therefore, patients are maintained on folic acid supplementation, 1 mg/d, and given transfusions in consultation with a hematologist.

Hydroxyurea

In selected patients, hydroxyurea is used for prophylaxis treatment to reduce the number of crises (acute chest syndrome or >3 crises per year). The effects of hydroxyurea on RBCs include increasing hemoglobin F levels, increasing water content of RBCs, increasing deformability of sickled cells, and altering the adhesion of RBCs to endothelium. Evidence suggests that hydroxyurea reduces the number of chest syndromes and transfusions and may reverse organ dysfunction.

The optimal regimen of hydroxyurea has not been determined. Doses start at 15 mg/kg/d and are increased by 5 mg/kg/d every 2 weeks until marrow suppression is present. The suggested maximum dose is 35 mg/kg/d. The goal of hydroxyurea is to achieve a white blood cell (WBC) count between 5000 and 8000 WBCs/mm^3 and suppression of the granulocyte and reticulocyte counts. Long-term safety of hydroxyurea is uncertain. Hydroxyurea is a cytotoxic agent and has the potential to cause life-threatening cytopenia. This drug should not be used in patients likely to become pregnant or those unwilling or unable to follow instructions regarding treatment. Patients should be monitored for myelotoxicity.

Pain Management

The management of acute painful crisis includes aggressive narcotic analgesia. Morphine 0.1 mg to 0.15 mg/kg every 3 to 4 hours is the drug of choice for severe pain. Meperidine 0.75 to 1.5 mg/kg every 2 to 4 hours may also be use to control severe pain. However, the increased frequency of dosing, coupled with the high rate of addiction, makes this agent less desirable than morphine. Management of mild pain includes acetaminophen, ibuprofen, aspirin, and codeine and oxycodone for moderate pain. Bone pain may respond to oral ketorolac, 30 to 60 mg initially, then 15 to 30 mg every 6 to 8 hours. Bone marrow transplantation has provided a cure in some children (Claster & Vichinsky, 2003).

ANEMIAS CAUSED BY DIMINISHED PRODUCTION OF RED BLOOD CELLS

IRON DEFICIENCY ANEMIA

According to the World Health Organization iron deficiency is the most common anemia (Carley, 2003). Iron deficiency has been implicated as a cause of perinatal complications such as low birth weight and premature delivery in affected mothers. In children, long-term findings include increased susceptibility to infection, poor growth, developmental and behavioral delays, and low mental and motor test scores.

Cause

Iron deficiency is related to insufficient iron intake, inadequate absorption from the gastrointestinal (GI) tract, and increased iron demands; it is exacerbated by chronic intestinal blood loss due to parasitic and malarial infections. Dietary deficiencies result from decreased consumption of animal protein and ascorbic acid as a consequence of chronic alcoholism, food faddism, prolonged illness with anorexia, or poor nutrition (Table 55-3).

Inadequate absorption from the GI tract is usually related to malabsorption syndromes, postgastrectomy, and the presence of certain foods or drugs or unrelenting diarrhea. The prevalence of iron deficiency anemia in the United States is declining as a result of food and formula supplementation. However, it remains of concern in toddlers, adolescents, and women of childbearing age.

Pathophysiology

The predominant use of iron is for the creation of heme groups that are incorporated into hemoglobin and myoglobin. Additionally, iron is involved in the production of cytochromes and other enzymes. Immediately bioavailable, iron is bound in the bloodstream to a specific carrier protein, transferrin. Excess of immediate iron needs are stored in the liver, spleen, and bone marrow as ferritin. Patients with iron deficiency anemia may be asymptomatic or have vague symptoms. Other manifestations include koilonychia (spoon nail), angular stomatitis, glossitis, and pica (eating dirt, paint, clay, ice, or cornstarch).

Diagnostic Criteria

Laboratory findings are critical for the diagnosis. The classic criterion for iron deficiency anemia includes low serum iron and ferritin concentrations and a high total iron-binding capacity (TIBC). In mild iron deficiency, the hemoglobin, hematocrit, and RBC indices remain normal. In the later stages, the hemoglobin and hematocrit levels fall below normal values.

Table 55.3

Causes of Iron Deficiency

Deficient diet
Decreased absorption
Increased requirements
   Pregnancy
   Lactation
Blood loss
   GI
   Menstrual
   Blood donation
Hemoglobinuria
Iron sequestration

A low concentration of ferritin (<0–12 g/L) is the earliest and most sensitive indication of iron deficiency. However, patients with renal or liver disease, malignancies, or infectious or inflammatory processes may have elevated ferritin levels that may not correlate with iron stores in the bone marrow. Transferrin saturation (serum iron divided by TIBC) is also used to assess iron deficiency anemia. Low values (<15%) indicate iron deficiency anemia, although low serum transferrin saturation values may also be present in inflammatory disorders. In this case, TIBC helps to differentiate the diagnosis. A TIBC greater than 400 mcg/dL suggests iron deficiency anemia, whereas values below 200 mcg/dL usually represent inflammatory disease. Free erythrocyte protoporphyrin (FEP) can also be used to distinguish between iron deficiency anemia and thalassemia minor. Iron binds with protoporphyrin to form heme. The serum concentration of protoporphyrin not bound to iron is elevated when iron levels are low. Thus, FEP is elevated in patients with iron deficiency anemia, inflammatory disorders, and lead poisoning. Rarely, a bone marrow examination is performed to assess iron stores.

Initiating Drug Therapy

The treatment of iron deficiency anemia consists of dietary supplementation and iron preparations (Table 55-4). Iron is best absorbed from red meat, fish, and poultry. Plant-based foods are good sources of iron, although they are less easily absorbed. Whole-grain or iron-fortified cereals, breads, and pastas are among the best. Beverages such as tea or milk will reduce the absorption of iron and should be consumed in moderation between meals. Vitamin C (500 mg daily), as well as orange juice, increases the absorption of iron due to the increased stomach acidity. They should be given together and are recommended with meals.

Goals of Drug Therapy

Goals are specific to the patient and include an evaluation of the impact the anemia has on quality of life, activities of daily living, and general well-being. Minimization of the impact chronic iron deficiency anemia has on adequate iron replacement has typically occurred when the serum ferritin level reaches 50 mcg/L and when the hemoglobin and hematocrit have returned to normal levels.

Iron Replacement Therapy

Dosage

Treatment of adult iron deficiency anemia should start with 2 to 3 mg/kg oral elemental iron daily in three divided doses.

Table 55.4

Elemental Iron Content of Various Iron Salts

Iron Salt	% Iron
Ferrous fumarate	33
Ferrous gluconate	11.6
Ferrous sulfate	20
Ferrous sulfate, anhydrous	30

Infants (0–6 mo) should receive 10 to 25 mg/kg/d, also in divided doses. Children 6 months to 2 years old should receive 6 mg/kg/d. Oral iron therapy with soluble ferrous iron salts is the preferred therapy due the improved bioavailability of the ferrous ion. Non–enteric-coated ferrous salts containing ferrous sulfate are the least expensive and provide adequate elemental iron. Typically, a dose of 325 mg ferrous sulfate 3 times daily provides sufficient iron replacement (195 mg elemental iron or about 2.7 mg/kg for a 70-kg adult). Slow-release or sustained-release iron preparations do not dissolve until reaching the small intestines, significantly reducing iron absorption. Iron should be administered daily in divided doses preferably 1 hour before meals.

Time Frame for Response

Therapeutic doses of iron should increase hemoglobin value by 0.7 to 1 g/wk. Reticulocytosis occurs within 7 to 10 days after initiation of iron therapy. Iron therapy should be continued for at least 3 to 6 months. Common causes of treatment failure include noncompliance with therapy, malabsorption, and blood loss equal to the rate of production. Malabsorption can be ruled out by the iron test in which plasma iron levels are determined at half-hour intervals for 2 hours following administration of 50 mg ferrous sulfate. Absorption is satisfactory if iron plasma levels increase by more than 50 ng/dL.

Adverse Events

Adverse reactions to iron are primarily GI difficulties, consisting of discolored feces, anorexia, constipation or diarrhea, nausea, and vomiting. To minimize the GI side effects, iron supplements should be taken with food. However, the impact of this on bioavailability of agents may be as high as a 66% decrease in iron absorption. Changing to a different iron salt or to a controlled-release preparation may also reduce side effects.

Interactions

There is a host of drug–drug interactions with iron preparations. Many antibiotics, such as tetracyclines and fluroquinolones, have a decrease in absorption due to the formation of a chelation product with the ferrous ions. The absorption of iron may be decreased when it is given with products containing aluminum, calcium, or magnesium. This effect may be as much as 30% to 40% reduction in absorption. The theory is that the reduced stomach acidity secondary to the antacid-like properties of products reduces the iron absorption. Similarly, patients taking proton pump inhibitors or H_2-antagonists may also have decreased iron absorption due to the lowered stomach acid. If the patient is taking both medications, space them at least 1 to 2 hours apart. In contrast, acidifying agents such as ascorbic acid (vitamin C) may enhance the absorption of iron-containing salts.

ANEMIA OF CHRONIC RENAL FAILURE

Anemia is a common complication of chronic renal failure. CKD arises as a consequence of diabetes mellitus, hypertension, chronic glomerulonephritis, and polycystic kidney disease. Diabetes and hypertension are the two leading causes of end-stage renal disease according to the U.S. Renal Data System 2001 Annual Data Report. The National Institutes of Health 1993 Consensus Statement of Morbidity and Mortality of Dialysis recommend that patients be referred to nephrologists when serum creatinine levels rise to 1.5 mg/dL for women and 2 mg/dL for men.

Pathophysiology

Patients with chronic renal failure have a decreased EPO production and a decreased RBC life due to a uremic environment. Because of the increased demand for RBC production, patients with chronic renal failure require an increased demand for folic acid. Many patients with chronic renal failure have folic acid deficiency and anemia due to iron loss and blood loss from hemodialysis. Hemodialysis can introduce RBC toxins such as copper, formaldehyde, chlorine, nitrates, and chloramines while removing folic acid (Spivak, 2000).

Initiating Drug Therapy

The National Kidney Foundation's Kidney Disease Outcomes Quality Initiative guidelines recommend that hemoglobin levels be maintained between 11 and 12 g/dL. Studies have shown adverse anemia-related sequelae occur at hemoglobin level less than 11 g/dL. Stable, well-compensated patients may tolerate levels less than 11 g/dL. However, therapy should be considered if hemoglobin levels fall below 9 to 10 g/dL.

Goals of Drug Therapy

The goal of therapy is to elevate or maintain the RBC level (hemoglobin/hematocrit) and to reduce the need for transfusions. Studies suggest that correction of anemia decreases morbidity and reduces hospitalization and mortality among patients with CKD. Benefits of correcting anemia include improvements in quality of life, exercise capacity, cognitive function, and sexual function. Hypertension may develop or worsen in some patients while the hematocrit is increasing. Seizures may occur although the etiology is not well understood.

Epoetin and Darbepoetin

Recombinant EPO (epoetin, Epogen, Procrit) is indicated for the treatment of anemia due to chronic renal failure, zidovudine administration (in HIV-infected patients), and chemotherapy administration. Epoetin is used in patients whose hematocrits are less than 30% to 35%. Other indications include a reduction in blood transfusions in anemic patients undergoing elective, noncardiac, nonvascular surgery. Similarly, darbepoetin is indicated for patients with chronic renal failure and patients receiving chemotherapy.

Mechanism of Action

Epoetin and darbepoetin are recombinant hormones that stimulate the production of RBCs from the erythroid tissues in the bone marrow. Epoetin also stimulates the division and differentiation of erythroid progenitors in bone marrow. Darbepoetin is a longer-acting erythropoietic agent than epoetin (serum half-live of 25 hours versus 8.5 hours).

Dosage

The starting dose of epoetin is 50 to 100 U/kg given subcutaneously or intravenously 3 times a week until the hematocrit approaches 30% to 36% or increases greater than 4 points in a 2-week period. The dosing is the same whether it is given subcutaneously or intravenously. The subcutaneous route provides sustained serum levels compared to the intravenous route.

The recommended starting dose for darbepoetin is 0.45 mcg/kg body weight, administered as a single intravenous or subcutaneous injection once weekly. Dosing is the same whether it is given subcutaneously or intravenously. A target hemoglobin concentration of 12 g/dL should not be exceeded. After initiating therapy, the hemoglobin level should be monitored weekly for at least 4 weeks until the hemoglobin value has stabilized.

All patients receiving erythropoietic stimulation should receive iron supplementation unless iron stores are already in excess. Iron supplementation should be initiated no later than the beginning of treatment and continue throughout the course of therapy. Oral therapy with ferrous sulfate 325 mg once to 3 times daily is adequate. Monitor the patient's hematocrit, blood pressure, clotting times, platelet counts, blood urea nitrogen level, and serum creatinine concentration.

Time Frame for Response

Two to 6 weeks may be required to evaluate the effectiveness or epoetin. If the response is not satisfactory in terms of reduced transfusion requirements or increased hematocrit after 8 weeks of therapy, the dose may be increased up to 300 U/kg 3 times a week. If patients do not respond, it is unlikely that they will respond to higher doses. Maintenance doses are individualized for each patient.

With once-weekly dosing, steady-state serum levels are achieved within 4 weeks with darbepoetin. Dose adjustment should not be increased more frequently than once a month. If the hemoglobin is increasing and approaching 12 g/dL, the dose should be reduced by 25%. If the hemoglobin continues to increase, the dose is withheld temporarily until the hemoglobin begins to stabilize.

Contraindications

Both epoetin and darbepoetin and are contraindicated in patients with uncontrolled hypertension or hypersensitivity to mammalian cell-derived products or human albumin. It is not intended for patients with chronic renal failure who require correction of severe anemia or in patients with iron folate deficiencies or GI bleeding.

Adverse Events

Epoetin and darbepoetin are generally well tolerated. Adverse reactions may include hypertension, headache, seizure, arthralgia, nausea, edema, fatigue, diarrhea, vomiting, chest pain, asthenia, and dizziness. Other adverse reactions include infection, hypertension, hypotension, and myalgia. Serious adverse reactions include vascular access thrombosis, heart failure, sepsis, and cardiac arrhythmia. There are no significant drug interactions.

ANEMIA OF CHRONIC DISEASE

Anemia of chronic disease is a hypoproliferative anemia and is associated with infection, inflammation, and neoplasia (Table 55-5) and accounts for approximately 75% of all cases.

Pathophysiology

Anemia of chronic disease typically occurs despite adequate reticuloendothelial iron stores and is characterized by reduced concentrations of serum iron, transferrin, and TIBC; normal or raised ferritin levels; and high erythrocyte sedimentation rate. EPO production has also been implicated in the pathogenesis. It can mimic or coexist with other types of anemia (Fitzsimons & Brock, 2001). The RBCs are often normochromic and normocytic. In patients with rheumatoid arthritis and Crohn's disease RBCs are similar to the effects of iron deficiency, with hypochromic and microcytic indices.

Diagnostic Criteria

In anemia of chronic disease, the hematocrit rarely falls below 60% of baseline. The MCV is usually normal or slightly reduced. Serum iron values may be unmeasurable, and transferrin saturation may be extremely low. Serum ferritin values should be normal or increased. A serum ferritin value of less than 30 mcg/L suggests coexistent iron deficiency.

Initiating Drug Therapy

Treatment is directed at the underlying cause and at eliminating exacerbating factors such as nutritional deficiencies

---

Table 55.5

Causes of Anemia of Chronic Disease

Common Causes
Chronic infections
  Tuberculosis
  Subacute bacterial endocarditis
  Osteomyelitis
Chronic inflammation
  Rheumatoid arthritis and inflammatory osteoarthritis
  Systemic lupus erythematosus
  Collagen-vascular diseases
  Gout
Malignancies

Less Common Causes
Alcoholic liver disease
Heart failure
Thrombophlebitis
Chronic obstructive lung disease
Ischemic heart disease

---

and marrow-suppressive drugs. Other causes of anemia should be treated before initiating therapy.

Doses of recombinant epoetin are higher than those in renal anemia. Epoetin is administered subcutaneously and doses may vary from 150 to 1500 U/kg/wk.

Goals of Drug Therapy

A good response is likely if, after 2 weeks of therapy, the hemoglobin increases more than 0.5 g/dL. If no response has been observed at 900 U/kg/wk, further escalation is unlikely to be effective. Iron supplements are required to ensure an adequate epoetin response.

THALASSEMIA

The thalassemias are hereditary disorders of hemoglobin synthesis, which are considered among the hypoproliferative anemias. The α-thalassemia syndromes are seen primarily in persons from India and China and are less commonly seen in African Americans. The β-thalassemia syndrome affects primarily persons of Mediterranean origin (Italian, Greek). Every year more than 200,000 babies are born with thalassemia major. They have a life expectancy of less than 30 years and are dependent on blood transfusions. Repeated transfusions result in cirrhosis of the liver, cardiomyopathy, endocrinopathies, and death due to hemosiderosis (Savulescu, 2004).

Pathophysiology

Normal adult hemoglobin is primarily hemoglobin A. Hemoglobin A consists of equal quantities of α- and β-globin chains. Thalassemia is present when a hemoglobinopathy is associated with a decreased production of either the α or β globins or a structurally abnormal globin chain. In α-thalassemia, the production of α-globin chains is controlled by four genes. Mutation of all four genes is incompatible with life (hydrops fetalis). Mutation of only one of the four is considered a silent carrier. Mutations of two of the four genes results in both microcytosis and mild anemia. Mutations of three of the four genes allow excess β chains to form tetramers (hemoglobin H) and results in severe anemia in addition to microcytosis. Physical examination will reveal pallor and splenomegaly. β-Thalassemia is commonly classified by the severity of anemia; many genotypes exist for each phenotype. In β-thalassemia, β-globin chain is controlled by two genes. Mutations of one of two genes results in β-thalassemia trait (β-thalassemia minor). Thalassemia intermedia is associated with dysfunction of both β-globin genes. Clinical severity is intermediate (hemoglobin level of 7–10 g/dL) and patients are usually not dependent on transfusions. Thalassemia major (Cooley anemia) results from mutations of both genes and reveals a majority of hemoglobin F. This results in severe anemia and RBC transfusions are required to sustain life. Clinical problems include growth failure, bony deformities (abnormal facial structure, pathologic fractures), hepatosplenomegaly, jaundice, leg ulcers, and cholelithiasis. As a result of transfusion dependency, iron overload results because of the body's inability to excrete iron from the transfused RBCs. This results in hemochromatosis, heart failure, cirrhosis, and endocrinopathies typically after more than 100 U.

Diagnostic Criteria

α-Thalassemia Trait

Patients with mild anemia have hematocrits between 28% and 40%. The MCV is low despite modest anemia, and the RBC bound is normal or increased. Peripheral blood smear shows microcytic, hypochromia, target cell and acanthocytes (cell with irregularly spaced bulbous projections). The reticulocyte and iron parameters are normal.

Hemoglobin H

Patients have marked hemolytic anemia with a hematocrit between 22% and 32%. The MCV is low. The peripheral blood smear reveals hypochromia, microcytosis, target cells, and poikilocytosis. The reticulocytes count is elevated. A peripheral blood smear demonstrates the presence of hemoglobin.

β-Thalassemia Minor

Patients have modest anemia with a hematocrit between 28% and 40%. The MCV ranges from 55 to 75 fL, and the RBC count is normal or increased. The peripheral blood smear reveals hypochromia, microcytosis, and target cells and basophilic stippling may be present. The reticulocyte count is normal or slightly elevated.

β-Thalassemia Major

Patients have severe anemia and the hematocrit may fall to less than 10%. The peripheral blood smear is bizarre, revealing severe poikilocytosis, hypochromia, microcytosis, target cells, basophilic stippling, and nucleated RBCs.

Initiating Drug Therapy

Patients with mild thalassemia (α-thalassemia trait or β-thalassemia minor) require no treatment. Patients should be identified so that they will not be subjected to repeated evaluation and treatment for iron deficiency. Patients with hemoglobin H should take folate supplements and avoid iron and oxidative drugs such as sulfonamides. Patients with severe thalassemia are maintained on a regular transfusion schedule and receive folate supplementation. Iron chelation therapy with deferoxamine mesylate may be used when transfusions result in tissue iron overload. Deferoxamine is administered by continuous subcutaneous infusion for 10 to 24 h/d. Adverse reactions include local irritation at the injection site, pruritus, hypotension, tachycardia, abdominal discomfort, diarrhea, nausea, and vomiting. Ocular and auditory disturbances may occur and patients should have baseline and annual vision and hearing examinations.

VITAMIN B$_{12}$ DEFICIENCY

Vitamin B$_{12}$ (cyanocobalamin) deficiency, or pernicious anemia, is a disorder of impaired DNA synthesis. Vitamin B$_{12}$ deficiency is considered a macrocytic anemia. There is an increase in incidence with increasing age, suggesting that it is a consequence of gastric epithelial aging. Vitamin B$_{12}$ is essential in maintaining the integrity of the neurologic system.

Table 55.6

Causes of Vitamin B$_{12}$ Deficiency

Dietary deficiency
Decreased production of intrinsic factor
  Pernicious anemia
  Gastrectomy
Helicobacter pylori infection
Fish tapeworm
Pancreatic insufficiency
Surgical resection of ileum
Crohn's disease

Pathophysiology

Vitamin B$_{12}$ deficiency has several causes, including lack of intrinsic factor, inadequate intake, decreased absorption, and inadequate utilization. Other causes include fish tapeworm infestation, *Helicobacter pylori* infection, malignancy, pancreatitis, gluten enteropathy, sprue, and small bowel bacterial overgrowth (Table 55-6). More recently, the increased incidence of obesity and the option of gastric bypass surgery raise greater concerns about vitamin B$_{12}$ deficiency. Vitamin B$_{12}$ is water soluble and obtained by ingestion of meat (beef, pork, organ meat) and dairy products. Its absorption occurs in the terminal ileum and requires intrinsic factor (found in gastric mucosa) for transport across the intestinal mucosa. Ileal absorptive sites may be congenitally absent or destroyed by inflammation or surgical resection. Other causes of decreased absorption include chronic pancreatitis, malabsorption syndromes, and drugs (oral calcium-chelating drugs, aminosalicylic acid, biguanides).

Vitamin B$_{12}$ deficiency can present with gastric mucosal atrophy, neuropsychiatric abnormalities (paranoia, delirium, confusion), and yellow-blue color blindness. GI manifestations include anorexia, intermittent constipation and diarrhea, and poorly localized abdominal pain. An early symptom may be glossitis or weight loss. In the early stages, neurologic symptoms include peripheral loss of position and vibratory sensation in the extremities, weakness, and loss of reflexes. Later stages include spasticity, Babinski responses, and ataxia. Early diagnosis is important because neurologic defects, if left untreated, are irreversible.

Diagnostic Criteria

Serum vitamin B$_{12}$ assay is the most commonly used method for establishing B$_{12}$ deficiency. Normal levels range between 150 and 820 pg/mL. Serum measurement of the MCV is usually elevated above 100 fL. Vitamin B$_{12}$ values below 150 pmol/L in patients with macrocytosis, hypersegmented polymorphonuclear leukocytes, peripheral neuropathy, or dementia is diagnostic of B$_{12}$ deficiency. Mild leukopenia and thrombocytopenia may be present. In patients with a deficiency of intrinsic factor, the Schilling test can confirm a diagnosis.

Initiating Drug Therapy

Pernicious anemia, malabsorption syndromes, or surgical removal of the stomach causes absence of intrinsic factor. Therefore, dietary vitamin B$_{12}$ cannot be absorbed. In this case, therapy consists of parenteral administration of vitamin B_{12}. In the case of inadequate intake, dietary allowance and supplementation can be recommended. The recommended daily requirements of Vitamin B_{12} is 0.3 to 0.5 mcg in infants, 0.7 to 1.4 mcg in children, 2.0 mcg in boys/men and girls/women aged 11 to 51 years, and 2.6 mcg in pregnant and lactating women.

Goals of Drug Therapy

Clinical improvement is evidenced by increased alertness, appetite, and cooperation. Reticulocytosis occurs within 2 to 3 days and peaks within 5 to 8 days. The hematocrit begins to rise within 2 weeks and reaches normal values within 2 months. MCV will increase initially due to increase reticulocytes, then will gradually decrease to normal.

Vitamin B_{12} (cyanocobalamin)

Vitamin B_{12} (cyanocobalamin) 100 mcg daily is given intramuscularly or deep subcutaneously for 6 or 7 days. The same dose is given on alternative days for an additional 7 days, then every 3 to 4 day for another 2 to 3 weeks, then monthly. Vitamin B_{12} therapy must be maintained for life. Oral B_{12} therapy is not usually recommended for pernicious anemia because of insufficient absorption due to lack of intrinsic factor.

FOLATE DEFICIENCY

Pathophysiology

Folic acid is necessary for the production of nucleic proteins, amino acids, purines, and thymine. Humans are unable to synthesize total daily folate requirements and depend on a dietary source. Major sources of folate include fresh vegetables and fruits, yeast, mushrooms, and animal organs such as liver and kidney. The minimum daily requirement is 50 to 100 mcg. Folic acid deficiency results in the development of large functionally immature erythrocytes (megaloblasts). Major causes of folic acid deficiency include inadequate intake, inadequate absorption, inadequate utilization, increased requirement (pregnancy, lactation, infancy, malignancy, increased metabolism), and increased excretion (renal dialysis; Table 55-7). Folic acid deficiency is associated with poor eating habits as seen in the elderly, alcoholics, food faddists, and those who are chronically ill. It is also seen in patients with malabsorption syndromes, Crohn's disease and celiac disease. Several drugs

Table 55.7

Causes of Folate Deficiency

Dietary deficiency
Decreased absorption due to
  Phenytoin
  Sulfasalazine
  Trimethoprim–sulfamethoxazole
Increased requirements
  Chronic hemolytic anemia
  Pregnancy
  Exfoliative skin disease

reported to cause folic acid deficiency include co-trimoxazole, primidone, phenytoin, and phenobarbital.

Symptoms associated with folate deficiency are similar to those in patients with B_{12} deficiency. However, the major difference is the absence of neurologic manifestations.

Diagnostic Criteria

Laboratory assessment of folate status includes a serum folic acid level. Serum folic acid levels less than 4 ng/mL suggest deficiency. A low RBC folate level identifies tissue deficiency; however, the values depend on the laboratory method used. Serum homocysteine measurement provides the best evidence of tissue deficiency. Both methylmalonic acid and homocysteine must be measured because B_{12} uses the same pathway. A normal methylmalonic acid level with an elevated homocysteine level confirms the diagnosis of folate deficiency.

Initiating Drug Therapy

Folic acid 1 mg daily replenishes tissues. Drug such as phenytoin or carbamazepine competitively bind folic acid.

Goals of Drug Therapy

The evaluation of symptomatic improvement is the same as those with B_{12} deficiency.

Folate Replacement

Folic acid is present in most fruits and vegetables (citrus fruits and green leafy vegetables). The recommended dietary allowances for adult men is 0.15 to 0.2 mg and for women, 0.15 to 0.18 mg. Total body stores are approximately 5 mg and supply requirements for up to 2 to 3 months. Folate deficiency is treated by oral replacement therapy. The usual dose of folate is 1 mg daily. Higher doses up to 5 mg daily may be required for folate deficiency due to malabsorption. The duration of therapy depends on the cause of deficiency. Patients with hemolytic anemia or those with malabsorption or chronic malnutrition should receive oral folic acid indefinitely. Side effects include erythema, skin rash, nausea, abdominal distention, altered sleep patterns, irritability, mental depression, confusion, and impaired judgment.

APLASTIC ANEMIA

Aplastic anemia is a condition of bone marrow failure that can be hereditary or arise from injury to or abnormal expression of the stem cell. There are a number of causes of aplastic anemia (Table 55-8). One cause is direct stem cell injury from radiation, chemotherapy, toxins, or pharmacologic agents.

Pathophysiology

Erythrocytes, granulocytes, and platelets, which are normally produced in the bone narrow, decrease to dangerously low levels. The bone marrow becomes hypoplastic with replacement of normal marrow hemopoietic cells by fat

Table 55.8

Causes of Aplastic Anemia

Congenital
Idiopathic/autoimmune
Systemic lupus erythematosus
Chemotherapy
Radiation therapy
Toxins
    Benzene, toluene, insecticides
Drugs
    Chloramphenicol, phenylbutazone, gold salts, sulfonamides, phenytoin,
      tolbutamide
Pregnancy

cells, and pancytopenia develops. This results in bleeding and increased risk of infection. Patients most commonly present with symptoms of anemia (fatigue, dyspnea, weakness) and skin or mucosal hemorrhage or visual disturbance due to retinal hemorrhage (Marsh et al., 2003). Physical examination may reveal signs of pallor, purpura, and petechiae.

Diagnostic Criteria

A complete blood count typically shows pancytopenia. In most cases, the hemoglobin level and neutrophil, reticulocyte, and platelet counts are depressed with a preserved lymphocyte count. The bone marrow aspirate and bone marrow biopsy appear hypocellular with scant amounts of normal hematopoietic progenitors. Magnetic resonance imaging of the vertebrae shows uniform replacement of marrow with fat.

Initiating Drug Therapy

Mild cases of aplastic anemia may be treated with supportive care. RBC transfusions and platelets are given as necessary. Antibiotics are given to treat infections. In severe aplastic anemia (neutrophil count <500/μL, platelet counts <20,000, reticulocytes <1%), the treatment of choice for young adults under age 50, who have an HLA-matched sibling, is allogeneic bone marrow transplantation. For adults over age 50 or those without HLA-matched siblings the preferred treatment is immunosuppression with antithymocyte globulin plus cyclosporine. Androgens, such as oxymetholone, have also been used but care should be taken due to hepatotoxicity.

SPECIAL POPULATION CONSIDERATIONS

Pediatric

Iron deficiency anemia significantly impairs mental and psychomotor development in infants and children. Iron deficiency can be reversed with treatment; however, the reversibility of the mental and psychomotor effects is unclear. Furthermore, iron deficiency increases a child's susceptibility to lead toxicity as lead replaces iron in the absorptive pathway when iron is unavailable.

Young children are at greatest risk of iron deficiency anemia due to rapid growth, increased iron requirements, and lack of iron in the diet. Poverty, abuse, and living in a home with poor household conditions also place children at risk for iron deficiency anemia. Iron deficiency anemia is seen most commonly in children 6 months to 3 years of age. Those at highest risk are low-birth-weight infants after 2 months of age, breast-fed term infants who receive no iron-fortified food or supplemental iron after 4 months of age, and formula-fed term infants who are not consuming iron-fortified formula. During the first months of life, the newborn rapidly uses iron stores due to an accelerated growth rate and increased blood volume. Maternally derived iron stores are generally sufficient for the first 4 to 6 months; however, sustained growth demands an increased iron supply. By the end of the second year of life, the growth rate decreases and accompanying iron needs level off. During adolescence, growth accelerates and iron needs increase. Adolescent girls are at increased risk and need additional iron to compensate for menstrual loss. Patients with iron deficiency who are responding poorly to the usual dietary supplementation regimens should be screened for lead poisoning. Heavy metal poisoning, as with lead and bismuth, is often overlooked.

Geriatric

Anemia should not be accepted as an inevitable consequence of aging. The most common causes of anemia in elderly patients are chronic disease (CKD, infections, malignancies, inflammatory disorders), iron deficiency, and nutritional and metabolic disorders. Anemia resulting from blood loss due to surgery, injury, and GI and genitourinary bleeding is more common in hospitalized patients. Untreated geriatric anemia has been associated with increased mortality, increased prevalence of various comorbid conditions, and decreased function. Low hemoglobin concentration was found to predict early death in nursing home residents in a study by Kikuchi and colleagues (2001). Furthermore, Argyriadou and coworkers (2001) found significant cognitive impairment in those with anemia.

Women

Pregnant women and women who are 4 to 6 weeks postpartum are at increased for anemia. Pregnant women who are iron deficient are at increased risk for a preterm delivery and delivering a low-birth-weight baby. However, two to three times more iron is required in pregnancy and in childhood. In pregnant women who had a previous pregnancy with a fetus or infant with a neural tube defect, the recommended dose is 5 mg daily. Also, women who may become pregnant and have seizure disorders should take folate supplementation.

MONITORING PATIENT RESPONSE

In almost all cases of anemia, evaluation should proceed in an orderly manner and therapy withheld until a specific diagnosis can be made. Patients with significant cardiopulmonary disease, who may be compromised by a decrease oxygen capacity, require immediate correction of anemia. This may require inpatient evaluation and consideration of transfusion therapy when they are experiencing dyspnea, angina, or marked fatigue related to anemia. Once treatment has been initiated, patient response should be evaluated on at least a monthly basis. Once correction has been achieved the need for long-term maintenance can more easily be determined.

PATIENT EDUCATION

Patients need to be told to what extent the anemia accounts for symptoms, what the possible causes are, and what the appropriate workup will be. Patient education and the importance of adherence to therapy are integral to successful management. Because some cases of anemia require the need of medication, the patient needs to be informed about possible side effects and when to report dangerous side effects.

Nutrition

All patients are encouraged to limit the use of alcohol, to avoid tobacco, to exercise, and to consume a diet of meat, poultry, fish, and fresh fruits and vegetables. To prevent deficiency, all patients are encouraged to eat fortified foods (fortified cereals, dairy products) or take supplements as prescribed by their physician. Patients with specific problems, such as pica, may need additional counseling.

Complementary and Alternative Medications

Herbal medicine to supply iron, iodine, and calcium include yellow dock root, Irish moss, and horsetail in equal parts made into a tea. Other herbal medicine for the treatment of iron deficiency include burdock, devil's bit, meadow sweet, mullein leaves, restharrow, salep, silver weed, stinging nettle, strawberry leaves, and toad flax. Patients should be educated that herbs are not regulated by the U.S. Food and Drug Administration and may interact with prescription medications. Patients must also understand that they should report any adverse reactions and stop the herbal medication immediately.

■ Case Study

J.B., an 82-year-old white man, was referred to clinic for evaluation of increasing shortness of breath.

Past medical history

    Pulmonary hypertension

    Hypertension

    Congestive heart failure

    Diabetes mellitus type 2, poor control

    Deep vein thrombosis

    Alcohol abuse

    Chronic obstructive pulmonary disease with respiratory failure

Family history

    Noncontributory

Physical examination

    Height 69 inches, weight 205 lb

    Blood pressure: 138/88

    Pulse 86 bpm, regular

    Lungs clear, neck supple negative for jugular venous distention

    Lower extremities +1 edema

Laboratory findings

    Scr = 1.7 K^+ = 4.2

    BUN = 24 Na^+ = 141

    Hb = 9.8

    Hct = 29.4

Serum ferritin 189 mg/dL

Social history

    Tobacco: 52 pack-years

    Alcohol: distant past

Diagnosis: Anemia of CKD

> 1. List specific goals of treatment for this patient.
>
> 2. What drug therapy would you prescribe? Why?
>
> 3. What are the parameters for monitoring success of the therapy?
>
> 4. Discuss specific patient education based on the prescribed therapy.
>
> 5. List one or two adverse reactions for the selected agent that would cause you to change therapy.
>
> 6. What dietary and lifestyle changes should be recommended for this patient?
>
> 7. What over-the-counter or alternative medications would be appropriate for this patient?
>
> 8. What dietary and lifestyle changes should be recommended for this patient?
>
> 9. Describe one or two drug–drug or drug–food interactions for the selected agent.

Bibliography

Starred references are cited in the text.

Abkowitz., J. (2001). Aplastic anemia: Which treatment? *Annals of Internal Medicine, 135,* 524–526.

Abramson, J., Jurkovitz, C., Vaccarino, V., et al. (2003). Chronic kidney disease, anemia, and incident stroke in a middle-aged, community-based population: The ARIC study. *Kidney International, 64,* 610–615.

Amgen. (2001). ARANESP (darbepoetin alfa) package insert. Thousand Oaks, CA: Amgen.

Angerio, A., & Lee, N. (2003). Sickle cell crisis and endothelin antagonists. *Critical Care Nursing Quarterly, 26,* 225–229.

*Argyriadou S., Vlachonikolis, I., Melisopoulou, H., et al. (2001). In what extent anemia coexists with cognitive impairment in elderly: A cross-sectional study in Greece. *BMC Family Practice, 2*(1), 5.

Blain, H., Hamdan, K., Blain, A., et al. (2002). Aplastic anemia induced by phenytoin: A geriatric case with severe folic acid deficiency. *Journal of the American Geriatrics Society, 50,* 396–397.

Cao, A., & Galanello, R. (2002). Effect of consanguinity on screening for thalassemia. *New England Journal of Medicine, 347,* 1200–1202.

*Carley, A. (2003). Anemia: When is it iron deficiency? *Pediatric Nursing, 29,* 127–133.

*Claster, S., & Vichinsky, E. (2003). Managing sickle cell disease. *British Medical Journal, 327,* 1151–1155.

Cook, L. (2000). A simple case of anemia: Pathophysiology of a common symptom. *Journal of IV Nursing, 23,* 271–281.

*Fitzsimons, E., & Brock, J. (2001). The anaemia of chronic disease: Remains hard to distinguish from iron deficiency anaemia in some cases. *British Medical Journal, 322,* 811–812.

Kaptan, K., Beyan, C., Ugur, A., et al. (2000). *Helicobacter pylori:* Is it a novel causative agent in vitamin B-12 deficiency? *Archives of Internal Medicine, 160,* 1349–1353.

*Kikuchi, M., Inagaki, T., & Sinagawa, N. (2001). Five-year survival of older people with anemia: Variation with hemo- globin concentration. *Journal of American Geriatric Society, 49*(9), 1226–1228.

Looker, A., Cogswell, M., Gunter E. (2002). Iron deficiency— United States, 1999–2000. *Journal of the American Medical Association, 288,* 2114–2116.

*Marsh, J., Ball, W., Darbyshire, P., et al. (2003). Guidelines for the diagnosis and management of acquired aplastic anaemia. *British Journal of Haematology, 123,* 782–801.

Nissenson, A., Goodnough L., & Dubois, R. (2003). Anemia: Not just an innocent bystander? *Archives of Internal Medicine, 163,* 1400–1404.

Platt, O. (2000). Sickle cell anemia as an inflammatory disease. *Journal of Clinical Investigation, 106,* 337–338.

Poskitt, E. (2003). Early history of iron deficiency. *British Journal of Haematology, 122,* 554–562.

Provan, D., & Weatherall, D. (2000). Red cells II: Acquired anaemias and polycythaemia. *Lancet, 355,* 1260–1268.

Robinson, A., & Mladenovic, J. (2001). Lack of clinical utility of folate levels in the evaluation of macrocytosis or anemia. *American Journal of Medicine, 110,* 88–90.

*Savulescu, J. (2004). Thalassaemia major: The murky story of deferiprone. *British Medical Journal, 328,* 358–359.

*Spivak, J. (2000). The blood in systemic disorders. *Lancet, 355,* 1707–1712.

Tefferi, A. (2003). Anemia in adults: A contemporary approach to diagnosis. *Mayo Clinic Proceedings, 78,* 1274–280.

*U.S. Renal Data System. USRDS 2001 Annual Data Report. Bethesda, MD: National Institute of Diabetes and Digestive and Kidney Diseases, National Institutes of Health.

Waddelaw, T. A., & Sproat, T. (2002). Anemias. In J. T. DiPiro (Ed.), *Pharmacotherapy: A pathophysiologic approach* (5th ed., pp. 1729–1745). Stamford, CT: Appleton & Lange.

Weatherall, D. (2000). Red cells I: Inherited anaemias. *Lancet, 355,* 1169–1175.

Yen, P. (2000). Nutritional anemia. *Geriatric Nursing, 21,* 111–112.

Young, N. (2002). Acquired aplastic anemia. *Annals of Internal Medicine, 136,* 534–546.

Visit the Connection web site for the most up-to-date drug information.

ONCOLOGIC DISORDERS

■ EDWARD C. LI

Although cancer is often thought of as a single disease, it is actually a group of diseases that share similar features. Cancer is a result of abnormal cells that do not die and continue to divide and invade nearby or distant organs and tissues, thereby causing problems. Cancer is generally divided into two categories, solid (eg, breast, lung, colorectal, prostate) or hematologic (eg, leukemia, lymphoma, myeloma), and is named according to the site from which the original malignant cell arose.

According to the National Center for Health Statistics, cancer is the second leading cause of death in the United States. In the year 2001, it accounted for 22.9% of total deaths, versus the 29% caused by heart diseases (Jemal et al., 2004). It is estimated that in the year 2004, approximately 1.4 million new cases of cancer will emerge, and 0.6 million people will die from cancer. Also in 2004, cancer of the lung and bronchus will continue to be the leading cause of cancer death in men and women. Breast and prostate cancer attribute approximately one third of the new cases annually in women and men, respectively.

CAUSES

Although the etiology of cancer cannot be attributed to a single source, multiple factors are operative that enable a person to develop the disease. Cancer is essentially a disease of malfunctioning genetic material (ie, DNA), thereby causing excessive and uncontrolled growth of cells, and leading to the development of a tumor. Therefore, it is understandable how cancer can develop if a person has a congenital defect in the genome or if an environmental factor has caused damage to the genetic material. Generally speaking, factors causing cancer are grouped into two major categories: host versus environmental factors.

Host Factors

Host factors are those that occur within the physiology of the patient. These factors can be further divided into three types: hereditary, hormonal, and immunologic impairment. Hereditary factors involve mutated or defected genetic materials that are linked to the development of certain cancers. For example, mutations in the *BRCA1* and *BRCA2* genes (tumor suppressor genes) are commonly seen in patients with a strong family history of hormonal breast cancer. Some studies indicate a relationship between sex hormones and the incidence of prostate and breast cancer. Lastly, a higher incidence of some cancers, such as non-Hodgkin lymphoma and Kaposi sarcoma, in immunocompromised patients offers a strong case that the immune system is a natural defense mechanism against cancer.

Environmental Factors

Environmental factors have also been linked to causing cancer. These are independent of host factors and include exposures to carcinogens, radiation, and infectious agents. Personal lifestyle, such as alcohol and smoking history, are also included in this category. Furthermore, some environmental factors may influence carcinogenesis strongly (such as asbestos exposure and lung cancer), whereas others are simply weak associations. Common chemical carcinogens identified include arsenic, asbestos, benzene, mustard gas, radium, and radon. The radiation beams known to cause cancer include those that are ionizing (x-rays, γ rays, α and β particles) and even ultraviolet light found in sunlight (UVA and UVB). Fortunately, UVA and UVB radiation is unable to penetrate into deeper organs but may cause skin cancer. Currently, radiation produced from cellular or portable telephones is not thought to cause brain cancer, because the type of radiation produced is nonionizing (Frumkin et al., 2001). Furthermore, several retrospective, epidemiologic studies did not detect a higher rate of brain cancer in patients who used cellular telephones. Tobacco use has also been associated with causing cancer, whether it is passive or active use. Although any form of tobacco is harmful, smoking is associated with the highest risk. Lastly, some studies indicate regular alcohol use increases the risk of head/neck, esophageal, and liver cancer.

PATHOPHYSIOLOGY

Exogenous and endogenous factors can contribute to tumor genesis via damage within DNA. These mutations can allow the cancerous cells to proliferate and grow uncontrollably. Normally functioning cells progress through the G_0, G_1, S, G_2, and M phases of the cell cycle during cell division. Mutations in cancerous cells can cause them to divide uncontrollably and provide immortality by preventing cell death. It is through this growth and proliferation that the cancerous cells produce their pathologic effect by invading and damaging local tissue. If left unchecked, these malignant cells may metastasize to different areas of the body and injure other organs.

DIAGNOSTIC CRITERIA

As with other diseases, a comprehensive physical examination and medical history are necessary to evaluate a patient with cancer. Different lifestyle habits or previous medical history may predispose a patient to certain cancers, and these must be considered when making the appropriate diagnosis. Furthermore, the information obtained through the physical examination is important in not only diagnosing the cancer, but also for identifying other constitutional symptoms that must be addressed because of the disease.

Although clinical signs and symptoms are important in discovering cancer, a clear diagnosis cannot be made based on clinical syndromes alone. To establish a correct diagnosis, further workup is required. A biopsy of the mass is normally performed to establish the pathologic features of the cancer. Regional lymph nodes may also be harvested or biopsied to aid with the diagnosis and staging of the disease. In the case of hematologic diseases, such as leukemia or myeloma, a bone marrow biopsy is necessary to evaluate the extent of disease and histologic features of the cancerous cells.

Computed tomography (CT) and positron emission tomography (PET) scans are frequently performed to establish the extent of tumor involvement and monitor for disease progression. Using these tests, clinicians are able to noninvasively evaluate the location, size, and invasion of the tumor. Furthermore, these methods can detect evidence of metastatic disease to other organs.

Different tumors may produce a tumor marker that is measurable in the patient's blood. However, these laboratory values are often used as monitoring parameters for evaluating treatment efficacy over time instead of during the initial diagnosis.

INITIATING DRUG THERAPY

Although chemotherapy is commonly used to treat cancer, it is not the only modality used. Before considering treatment with chemotherapy, it is important to recognize the goals of therapy and apply a treatment strategy that has proven to be efficacious against the specific tumor type. Furthermore, it is important to involve the patient in deciding which treatment option is the best.

Goals of Drug Therapy

Similar to other types of drugs, it is important to weigh the risks versus benefits when initiating therapy with cytotoxic agents. In this case, the goals of using chemotherapy are important to discuss with the patient because of the propensity of these drugs to cause adverse effects. However, it is important to distinguish between response to therapy and the goals of a therapy.

Response to chemotherapy has been standardized according to many different organizations, including the World Health Organization (WHO) and the International Union against Cancer. However, the most commonly used criteria used to evaluate tumor response are the RECIST (Response Evaluation Criteria in Solid Tumors) guidelines developed jointly by the European Organization for Research and Treatment of Cancer (EORTC), the National Cancer Institute of the United States (NCI), and the NCI of Canada Clinical Trials Group. According to these criteria, tumor response to chemotherapy can be reported as complete response (CR), partial response (PR), stable disease (SD), or progressive disease (PD). A CR means no evidence of tumor is left in the patient, whereas a PR means the tumor size has decreased by at least 50%. SD means the tumor did not increase or decrease in size, and PD occurs when tumor size has increased or if new lesions have developed (Therasse et al., 2000). These parameters are different when assessing hematologic malignancies and are based on bone marrow biopsy results. For example, in patients with leukemia, the response is determined by how many leukemia cells remain in the bone marrow after treatment.

To obtain the specific goals of therapy different modalities of treatment may be used. For the most part, the treatment of cancer encompasses a multimodal strategy involving surgery, radiation, chemotherapy, and immunotherapy. The method of chemotherapy administration with respect to each modality is summarized in four strategies:

1. Primary treatment: In this instance, chemotherapy is the only modality used to treat the cancer. This strategy is rarely used because of the superior data available with multimodal therapy. However, it is common to use chemotherapy as the primary treatment of leukemia or lymphoma (ie, liquid tumors) that cannot be treated with surgery because there is no clear mass to remove.
2. Adjuvant therapy: Most of the time when chemotherapy is prescribed, it is used in the adjuvant setting. This strategy involves using either surgery or radiation first to "remove" the primary mass. After a successful procedure, chemotherapy is administered later to eradicate any residual, microscopic disease and prevent further recurrence.
3. Neoadjuvant therapy: In this case, chemotherapy is used before radiation or surgery to shrink the tumor to a more manageable size to allow a better resection. One major reason this strategy is implemented is to decrease the size of an inoperable tumor to a size where operating on the patient would not be as risky.
4. Palliative: This strategy is implemented mostly in patients with advanced or metastatic disease that is impractical to treat with radiation or surgery. The goal is to ultimately prolong survival, decrease symptoms related to the disease, and increase quality of life.

According to the goals of therapy, both the treatment strategy used and the desired response to therapy may vary. For example, a patient may receive primary chemotherapy for an intended cure of disease may hope to obtain a CR, but a patient with metastatic disease may receive palliative chemotherapy in hopes of obtaining a CR, PR, or SD to prolong survival. Generally speaking, treatment of solid tumors diagnosed at earlier stages will attempt for curative therapy with first surgery/radiation with (or without) adjuvant chemotherapy, whereas in more advanced stages (ie, metastatic disease), the goal is palliation of symptoms, increase in quality of life, and prolongation of survival. However, the treatment goals for different cancers differ according to the patient's specific characteristics and treatment protocols.

GENERAL COMMENTS ABOUT CHEMOTHERAPY

Although each chemotherapy agent is different, these groups of agents share certain similarities. For example, all of these agents are considered to be biohazardous. Therefore, special precautions must be in place to ensure proper storage, handling, compounding, and disposal of these drugs. Special procedures must also be followed in case of an accidental spill. Treatment is most often given as a combination of cytotoxic drugs to take advantage of different mechanisms of action to potentially increase efficacy. Furthermore, these combinations have been determined through clinical trials and specific treatment regimens are routinely administered to patients with a specific cancer. For example, the combination doxorubicin/cyclophosphamide is often used for treating breast cancer. This chapter will later discuss the commonly used treatment regimens for selected cancers.

Dosage

Because these agents are toxic and exhibit a narrow therapeutic window (ie, the range of a therapeutic level versus the toxic level is small), the dose of these agents most often must be individualized to each patient. Therefore, the dose to be administered is commonly based on the patient's body surface area (BSA), expressed in square meters (m^2). For example, the dose for doxorubicin given to a patient with breast cancer is 50 mg/m^2. The BSA is calculated through various available algorithms using the patient's height and weight. The BSA for the average patient is 1.73 m^2. Some drugs are exceptions to this rule, and it depends mostly on the individual drug and specific treatment regimen. The specific doses of each agent will not be discussed in this chapter because they vary greatly with each treatment regimen and tumor type. Instead, frequently used chemotherapy regimens will be discussed.

Combinations of agents are typically given in cycles. Each day in a cycle is specifically numbered, and chemotherapy is given on specific days according to the treatment regimen. Once the cycle has ended, it then repeats again, starting with day 1. Depending on the cancer being treated, patients may receive a finite number of cycles or may receive these cycles indefinitely or until disease progression. For instance, with the doxorubicin/cyclophosphamide regimen, both drugs are given on day 1 of each cycle, repeating every 21 days. In this example, day 22 becomes day 1 of the next cycle.

Dose reduction or delays in starting the next cycle may occur depending on the degree of adverse effects seen from the previous cycle of chemotherapy. To receive chemotherapy, patients must meet certain criteria in their complete blood count (white blood cells, hemoglobin/hematocrit, platelets) for each cycle. Sometimes, chemotherapy can be so extremely myelosuppressive that patients do not meet the criteria for receiving chemotherapy for the next cycle. Therefore, the cycle must be delayed until the patient's laboratory values recover to the appropriate level. The doses for the subsequent cycles may be decreased to prevent this treatment delay from happening.

Contraindications, Adverse Events, and Interactions

In general, chemotherapy is cytotoxic and should not be administered to patients who are pregnant or nursing. Most of these agents are pregnancy category D, meaning that although data exist that the drug is harmful to the fetus, under some circumstances it might be appropriate to administer chemotherapy to a pregnant patient, based on risk-versus-benefit assessment. Myelosuppression, alopecia, and nausea/vomiting are commonly seen with most agents, although the severity of these adverse effects may differ. The most common drug interaction seen with all the chemotherapy agents is with live vaccines because of the immunosuppressive nature of these cytotoxic agents. Other drug interactions may occur and are the result of overlapping toxicities or altered pharmacokinetic parameters.

SPECIFIC CLASSES OF AGENTS

Antimetabolites

Antimetabolites are a class of cytotoxic agents that are active in a wide variety of tumor types, such as breast cancer or leukemia. This class of agents has been used for many decades beginning with the introduction of fluorouracil in the 1950s. Despite its antiquity, fluorouracil is still routinely used in practice. Antimetabolites are not commonly given as single agents for the treatment of a particular disease, but are most often given in combination with other agents to help overcome drug-resistant tumors. Antimetabolites ultimately inhibit cell growth and cause cell death by damaging the DNA of the cancerous cells. These drugs achieve this goal by either incorporating into the DNA itself or by inhibiting enzymes that help construct DNA during cell division. Table 56-1 lists the commonly used metabolites and their differences.

The antimetabolites are generally divided into subclasses depending on which building block the drug inhibits. For example, the folate antagonist methotrexate inhibits the enzyme dihydrofolate reductase, preventing the synthesis of thymidylate and purines, basic building blocks of DNA. Pemetrexed not only inhibits dihydrofolate reductase but also three other enzymes involved the formation of DNA building blocks. The purine analogues thioguanine, mercaptopurine, fludarabine, and cladribine (2-CDA) are believed to inhibit ribonucleotide synthesis via structural similarity to purines, allowing them to be incorporated into DNA. Meanwhile, pentostatin inhibits DNA synthesis through an enzymatic process that causes a deficit of building blocks of DNA and RNA. The pyrimidine analogues (cytarabine, gemcitabine, fluorouracil, floxuridine, and capecitabine) similarly to the purine analogues, in that the pyrimidine analogues are similar to the pyrimidine bases. These drugs inhibit DNA synthesis either by incorporating into DNA (fluorouracil, floxuridine, capecitabine) or by inhibiting DNA polymerase (cytarabine, gemcitabine), an enzyme that is crucial in creating the DNA chain from building blocks.

The dosing of antimetabolites varies greatly within of each treatment protocol. For example, the dose of fluorouracil

Table 56.1

Antimetabolites

Generic (Trade) Name(s) and Dosage	Selected Anticancer Activity	Common Dose Range	Selected Adverse Events	Special Considerations
Folate Antagonists				
methotrexate (various)	Breast, head/neck, leukemia, lymphoma, osteosarcoma	Lymphoma: 10–25 mg PO daily for 4–8 d; leukemia: 3.3 mg/m²/d IV	Mucositis, diarrhea, nausea/vomiting, myelosuppression	High doses (>150–12,000 mg/m²) require rescue with leucovorin and serum monitoring; may be given intrathecally
pemetrexed (Alimta)	Mesothelioma	500 mg/m² IV every 21 d	Myelosuppression, rash, fatigue, diarrhea, nausea/vomiting	Vitamin B₁₂ and folate supplementation must be given concurrently.
Purine Analogues				
mercaptopurine, 6-MP (Purinethol)	Leukemia	1.5–2.5 mg/kg/d PO	Myelosuppression, diarrhea, rash, hepatotoxicity	Given orally
thioguanine, 6-TG	Leukemia	2–3 mg/kg/d PO	Myelosuppression, hepatotoxicity, nausea/vomiting	Given orally
cladribine, 2-CDA (Leustatin)	Leukemia	0.09 mg/kg/d IV for 7 d	Myelosuppression, neurotoxicity, nausea, fatigue	Adjust dose for renal or neurotoxicity.
fludarabine (Fludara)	Leukemia, lymphoma	25 mg/m²/d for 5 d, repeat every 4 wk	Myelosuppression, anemia, neurotoxicity (paresthesia, weakness, confusion), nausea/vomiting	Adjust dose for renal or neurotoxicity; do not give with pentostatin—risk of fatal pulmonary toxicity.
pentostatin (Nipent)	Leukemia	4 mg/m² IV every 2 wk	Myelosuppression, neurotoxicity, renal/hepatic toxicity	Do not give with fludarabine—risk of fatal pulmonary toxicity.
Pyrimidine Analogues				
cytarabine, ara-C (Cytosar-U)	Leukemia, lymphoma	100 mg/m²/d or 100 mg/m² every 12 h for 7 d	Myelosuppression, nausea/vomiting, fever, rash mucositis, neurotoxicity (ataxia, somnolence), corneal toxicity	May be given intrathecally; adjust dose for renal/hepatic insufficiency.
fluorouracil, 5-FU (Adrucil)	Breast, colorectal, gastric, head/neck, hepatic, pancreatic	12 mg/kg/d IV for 4 d; other regimens may use up to 1200 mg/m²/d IV	Diarrhea, mucositis, hand–foot syndrome, myelosuppression, photoxicity	Sometimes is given as a continuous infusion up to 4 d; adjust dose for hepatic insufficiency
gemcitabine (Gemzar)	Breast, bladder, lung, pancreatic	1000–1250 mg/m² IV every 1–3 wk	Myelosuppression, rash, fever, fatigue, hepatotoxicity	
capecitabine (Xeloda)	Breast, colorectal, pancreatic	2500 mg/m²/d PO for 14 d	Diarrhea, mucositis, hand–foot syndrome, myelosuppression, thrombocytopenia, phototoxicity	Oral prodrug; it is metabolized into 5-FU inside of tumor cells.
floxuridine (FUDR)	Gastrointestinal, renal cell	0.1–0.6 mg/kg/d	Diarrhea, mucositis, nausea/vomiting, myelosuppression	May be given as an intra-arterial infusion into the hepatic artery to treat liver metastasis.

in the treatment of breast cancer (as part of the cyclophosphamide, methotrexate, fluorouracil regimen) is 600 mg/m² intravenously on days 1 and 8, versus the dose for metastatic colorectal cancer (as part of the FOLFOX regimen), which is 400 mg/m² as an intravenous bolus, then 600 mg/m² intravenously over 22 hours, given on days 1 and 2. A common strategy for dosing methotrexate involves administering a relatively high dose, followed by rescue with leucovorin, the active form of folic acid, to minimize adverse effects such as mucositis. Methotrexate may also be given intrathecally for the treatment of some leukemias. Pemetrexed, another folate antagonist, was recently approved for the treatment of mesothelioma at an intravenous dose of 500 mg/m^2 on day 1 of a 21-day cycle. Administration of vitamin B$_{12}$ and folic acid is necessary to prevent toxicities. The doses of mercaptopurine and thioguanine are relatively more consistent; mercaptopurine usually is given as 1.5 to 2.5 mg/kg/d, whereas thioguanine is given as 2 mg/kg/d for the treatment of leukemia. The doses of the remaining antimetabolites vary according to specific treatment protocols.

Because the mechanism of action of the antimetabolites is to inhibit the building blocks of DNA, its cytotoxic activity depends whether or not the tumor cell is actively synthesizing DNA (eg, in preparation to replicate). Hence, these drugs only work during the synthesis phase (S phase) of the cell cycle and are considered cell cycle-specific cytotoxic agents. It is because of the cell cycle specificity that most of the antimetabolites are given over a longer period of time, as opposed to a single dose. Because it is not known when a patient's tumor cells are in the S phase of cell division, the purpose of multiday dosing is to have a greater chance that an antimetabolite is being administered when these tumor cells do enter the S phase of cell division.

Certain antimetabolites require dose modifications based on the presence and severity of renal or hepatic dysfunction. These agents include (but are not limited to) capecitabine, cytarabine, fludarabine, fluorouracil, methotrexate, and pentostatin. Dose reductions may be clearly stated at times. However, there may be no specific guidelines given for some drugs that may require dose modifications, and it is recommended to "use caution" when administering the drug in these individuals.

Although most of chemotherapy agents in this class are pregnancy category D, methotrexate specifically carries a pregnancy category X label, meaning the drug is contraindicated in patients who are pregnant. Similar to most chemotherapeutic agents, the antimetabolites generally cause myelosuppression, specifically neutropenia, anemia, and thrombocytopenia, and may lead to life-threatening infections or bleeding. Nausea, vomiting, mucositis, diarrhea, and stomatitis are other common adverse effects shared by the antimetabolites. These complications may also be potentially serious, leading to hospitalizations. Specific management of these toxicities from chemotherapy is mentioned later in the chapter. Although many antimetabolites share common adverse effects, the severity of these reactions may differ among agents.

Drug interactions are specific to each antimetabolite and are most often associated with a change in pharmacokinetic parameters. For example, nonsteroidal anti-inflammatory agents (ie, ibuprofen, naproxen) and penicillins may decrease the renal clearance of methotrexate. Therefore, caution should be exercised when concomitantly administering those drugs. Other drug interactions are pharmacodynamic in nature and are seen when two chemotherapeutic agents that have overlapping toxicities are administered together. For example, the combination of pentostatin and fludarabine may result in fatal pulmonary toxicity. Each antimetabolite exhibits different drug interactions, and all medications should be reviewed before they are administered.

Alkylating Agents

Alkylating agents were the first antineoplastic agents to be widely used to treat cancer. After observing that surviving soldiers who were exposed to mustard gas in World War I exhibited low white blood cell counts, a less dangerous analog, mechlorethamine, was developed to treat leukemias and lymphomas. Although newer agents in this class have been developed recently, the alkylating agents remain an important for treating leukemia and lymphoma.

Although there are many different subclasses of alkylating agents, the mechanism of action is essentially the same. Alkylating agents inhibit DNA synthesis by binding to and damaging the DNA itself. Because the damage is so severe, this ultimately results in cell death. Unlike the antimetabolites, alkylating agents are able to damage the DNA of cells in any phase of the cell cycle, although highly actively dividing cells are preferentially selected. Therefore, alkylating agents are considered to be cell cycle nonspecific.

The different types of alkylating agents include the nitrogen mustards (cyclophosphamide, ifosfamide, melphalan, mechlorethamine, chlorambucil), the nitrosoureas (carmustine, lomustine), the platinum analogues (cisplatin, carboplatin, oxaliplatin), and other various agents listed in Table 56-2.

The dosing for each alkylating agent is specific for each treatment regimen and may differ depending on the tumor type that is being treated. For example, cyclophosphamide is used in a wide variety of cancers, and dose may range from 600 mg/m^2 for breast cancer to 1800 mg/m^2 daily for 4 days as a conditioning regimen for stem cell transplantation. However, some doses are relatively consistent for each disease, such as the dose of temozolomide, which is commonly given at 150 mg/m^2 orally daily for 5 consecutive days. Dosing carboplatin differs from other chemotherapy agents, in that the dose is calculated by targeting a specific area under the drug concentration curve (AUC). The target AUC of carboplatin is usually and AUC of 4 to 6, and the actual dose of the drug is calculated using the Calvert equation, which is expressed as: dose of carboplatin (mg) = AUC × (glomerular filtration rate + 25).

The dose-limiting toxicity of most of the alkylating agents is myelosuppression. These agents also cause more nausea and vomiting compared to other classes. The nitrogen mustards cyclophosphamide and ifosfamide can also cause hemorrhagic cystitis because of accumulation of toxic metabolites in the bladder. This can be prevented by giving adequate hydration (to ensure frequent bladder emptying) or by administering mesna, a drug that scavenges the harmful metabolites in the bladder. Busulfan has the tendency to cause seizures, and patients must receive seizure prophylaxis while receiving busulfan. Cisplatin may cause renal toxicity, and all platinum agents may cause peripheral neuropathy. Oxaliplatin may cause patients to become sensitive to cold, causing a painful burning sensation whenever a cold object is touched. Therefore, patients should be instructed to stay away from cold beverages or anything that is cold. This adverse effect usually resolves in a few days.

Topoisomerase Inhibitors

Topoisomerase inhibitors are another class of agents used to treat a wide variety of cancers. They are used in combination with other chemotherapy drugs to treat breast cancer, colorectal cancer, lung cancer, leukemia, lymphoma, or other cancers. Although these drugs are generally further separated into the topoisomerase I and II inhibitors, their mechanism of

Table 56.2

Alkylating Agents

Generic (Trade) Name(s) and Dosage	Selected Anticancer Activity	Common Dose Range	Selected Adverse Events	Special Considerations
Nitrogen Mustards				
cyclophosphamide (Cytoxan)	Breast, leukemia, lymphoma, myeloma, neuroblastoma, ovarian	40–50 mg/kg IV over 2–5 d, 10–15 mg/kg IV every 7–10 d, 3–5 mg/kg twice a wk	Myelosuppression, hemorrhagic cystitis, nausea/vomiting, cardiomyopathy, Stevens–Johnson syndrome	Higher doses may require treatment with mesna to prevent hemorrhagic cystitis.
ifosfamide (Ifex)	Head/neck, lymphoma, sarcoma, testicular	1 g/m²/d for 5 d	Myelosuppression, hemorrhagic cystitis, nausea/vomiting, confusion	Requires treatment with mesna to prevent hemorrhagic cystitis.
melphalan (Alkeran)	Leukemia, myeloma, ovarian	0.15–0.25 mg/kg/d PO daily for 4–7 d; 16 mg/m² IV every 2 wk	Myelosuppression, mucositis, pulmonary fibrosis, hepatitis, secondary malignancies	Decrease dose for renal impairment.
mechlorethamine (Mustargen)	Leukemia, lymphoma	0.4 mg/kg IV each course	Myelosuppression, nausea/vomiting, dermatitis, anemia	Vesicant—avoid extravasation
chlorambucil (Leukeran)	Leukemia, lymphoma	0.1–0.2 mg/kg/d for 3–6 wk, then 2–4 mg/d	Myelosuppression, nausea/vomiting, pneumonitis, rash	Given orally
Nitrosoureas				
carmustine, BCNU (BiCNU)	Brain, lymphoma, myeloma	150–200 mg/m² IV every 6 wk	Myelosuppression, nausea/vomiting, pulmonary toxicity, hepatotoxicity	Available as an implantable wafer for brain tumors
lomustine, CCNU (CeeNU)	Brain, lymphoma	130 mg/m² PO every 6 wk	Myelosuppression, nausea/vomiting, pulmonary toxicity, renal toxicity, neurotoxicity	Given orally
streptozocin (Zanosar)	Carcinoid, pancreatic	500 mg/m²/d IV for 5 d, repeat every 6 wk	Nausea/vomiting, renal toxicity, confusion	Decrease dose for renal impairment.
Alkyl Sulfonates				
busulfan (Myleran)	Leukemia	0.8 mg/kg/dose every 6 h for 16 doses before transplant; 4–8 mg/d for chronic myelogenous leukemia	Myelosuppression, pulmonary toxicity, seizures, hepatic veno-occlusive disease	May require seizure prophylaxis with an antiseizure medication such as phenytoin.
Ethylenimine				
thiotepa (Thioplex)	Bladder, breast, lymphoma, ovarian	0.3–0.4 mg/kg IV every 1–4 wk	Myelosuppression, rash, nausea/vomiting	May be given intravesically into the bladder space to treat bladder cancer
altretamine (Hexalen)	Ovarian	260 mg/m²/d divided into 4 doses for 14–21 d	Myelosuppression, peripheral neuropathy, nausea/vomiting	Given orally
Triazenes				
dacarbazine (DTIC-Dome)	Lymphoma, melanoma, sarcoma	Melanoma: 2–4.5 ng/kg/d for 10 d; lymphoma: 150 mg/m²/d for 5 d	Myelosuppression, nausea/vomiting, hepatotoxicity	Vesicant—avoid extravasation
Imidazotetrazines				
temozolomide (Temodar)	Brain	150 mg/m²/d PO for 5 d	Nausea/vomiting, myelosuppression, fatigue	Given orally—take on an empty stomach to decrease nausea.
Platinum Analogues				
cisplatin (Platinol)	Bladder, esophageal, head/neck, lung, melanoma, ovarian	50–100 mg/m² IV every 3–4 wk	Nausea/vomiting, renal toxicity, myelosuppression, neuropathy, ototoxicity	Usually requires pre- and posthydration to prevent renal toxicity

(continued)

Table 56.2

Alkylating Agents *(Continued)*

Generic (Trade) Name(s) and Dosage	Selected Anticancer Activity	Common Dose Range	Selected Adverse Events	Special Considerations
carboplatin (Paraplatin)	Head/neck, lung, ovarian, testicular	300–360 mg/m^2 IV every 4 wk; or target AUC = 4–6	Myelosuppression, nausea/vomiting, peripheral neuropathy	Dose is based on area under the curve (AUC) using the Calvert formula: Dose = (Target AUC)×(GFR + 25)
oxaliplatin (Eloxatin)	Colorectal	85 mg/m^2 IV every 2 wk	Sensitivity to cold, peripheral neuropathy, myelosuppression, nausea/vomiting, pharyngolaryngeal dysesthesia	Calcium and magnesium are usually given before and after oxaliplatin; patients should be instructed not to drink cold beverages for 2–3 d after infusion.

GFR, glomerular filtration rate.

action is essentially the same. A summary of these agents is listed in Table 56-3.

These drugs exert their cytotoxic effect by binding to topoisomerase, the enzyme responsible for uncoiling the cell's DNA during replication. Although this interaction allows the DNA to be uncoiled for replication, the drug inhibits the re-formation of the DNA double helix, resulting in DNA strand breaks. Although this is the main mechanism of action, some classes of topoisomerase inhibitors exhibit additional mechanisms of cytotoxicity. For example, the anthracyclines (doxorubicin, daunorubicin, idarubicin) and mitoxantrone insert themselves within the DNA bases and cause additional damage. The anthracyclines also generate free radicals that damage the cell's DNA further and contribute to their adverse effect profile.

Although myelosuppression is the major dose-limiting toxicity of all of the topoisomerase inhibitors, other adverse effects are different among subclasses. The camptothecin topoisomerase I inhibitors (irinotecan, topotecan), may cause severe diarrhea. In fact, the diarrhea experienced because of irinotecan can be separated into an early and late phase reaction. The early phase diarrhea can be experienced during or after infusion of the drug, and it is thought to be mediated by the cholinergic pathway. This can be treated by administering atropine. The late diarrhea begins 24 hours after administration and may be treated with loperamide. Nausea and vomiting also occur frequently with these agents.

The anthracyclines also have a unique side effect profile in addition to myelosuppression. As mentioned, oxygen free radicals are generated by the drug and can cause congestive heart failure, especially in patients who have received more than 450 mg/m^2 doxorubicin or daunorubicin in their lifetime. Because of the seriousness of this adverse effect, patients should have their cardiovascular status evaluated through an electrocardiogram or echocardiogram (or both) before beginning therapy with an anthracycline. These drugs are also vesicants if they are extravasated and may discolor bodily fluids.

The epipodophyllotoxins may cause infusion-related reactions, such as hypotension, if they are administered too rapidly. In addition, they frequently cause mucositis and nausea and vomiting. There is also concern for the development of a secondary leukemia, especially with etoposide use.

Antimicrotubules

The antimicrotubule agents are a class of chemotherapy agents derived from natural plant sources. The vinca alkaloids vincristine and vinblastine were isolated from the periwinkle plant. Vinorelbine, however, is a semisynthetic derivative of an alkaloid extracted from the same plant. The taxanes (paclitaxel and docetaxel) owe their origins to the pacific yew tree. Paclitaxel is a naturally occurring compound found and isolated from the bark of the Pacific yew. However, the harvesting of the bark from these trees causes it to die. Therefore, paclitaxel is currently manufactured semisynthetically through derivatives extracted from the European yew needles. Docetaxel is also a semisynthetic product of compounds extracted from the needles of yew trees. These agents are active mostly in solid tumors, with the biggest role in treating breast and lung cancers. However, the vinca alkaloids are also used in treating lymphoma and leukemia. Table 56-4 lists the commonly used antimicrotubule agents.

These agents exert their cytotoxic effects differently than the agents previously discussed in this chapter. Instead of inhibiting DNA formation or causing DNA strand breaks, these agents inhibit mitosis (cell division) by disrupting microtubule function. Because microtubules are most active during the M phase of cell cycle replication, the antimicrotubules have the most cytotoxic effects during this phase and are said to be cell cycle specific.

These agents are given intravenously, and the dosing depends on the specific treatment regimen and tumor type being treated. Caution must be used to prevent accidental administration of a vinca alkaloid intrathecally. The administration of vinca alkaloids intrathecally leads to death or paralysis. Therefore, extra care should be taken so that the vinca alkaloids are not in reach when drugs are given intrathecally. Both paclitaxel and docetaxel require premedications before administration to prevent adverse effects. Patients must be given a steroid, an H$_1$-receptor antagonist (eg, diphenhydramine) and an H$_2$-receptor antagonist (eg, ranitidine, famotidine) to prevent anaphylaxis and hypersensitivity reactions. Patients receiving docetaxel must be premedicated with steroids to prevent fluid retention and hypersensitivity. Dose adjustments are necessary when patients

Table 56.3

Topoisomerase Inhibitors

Generic (Trade) Name(s) and Dosage	Selected Anticancer Activity	Common Dose Range	Selected Adverse Events	Special Considerations
Topoisomerase I Inhibitors—Camptothecins irinotecan (Camptosar)	Colorectal, lung	125 mg/m^2 IV every week for 4 wk	Diarrhea, myelosuppression, nausea/vomiting	May cause acute cholinergic symptoms (sweating, flushing, diarrhea) that can be treated with atropine.
topotecan (Hycamtin)	Leukemia, lung, myeloma, ovarian	1.5 mg/m^2 IV daily for 5 d	Diarrhea, myelosuppression, nausea/vomiting	
Topoisomerase II Inhibitors—Anthracyclines doxorubicin (Adriamycin)	Bladder, breast, endometrial, gastric, leukemia, lymphoma, ovarian, sarcoma	40–45 mg/m^2 IV every 21–28 d	Myelosuppression, cardiotoxicity, nausea/vomiting, vesicant	Lifetime doses ≥450 mg/m^2 increase the risk for heart failure; anthracyclines are red in color and may discolor body fluids.
daunorubicin (Cerubidine) idarubicin (Idamycin)	Leukemia, lymphoma	12 mg/m^2 IV daily for 3 d	Myelosuppression, cardiotoxicity, mucositis, hepatotoxicity, nausea/vomiting, vesicant	Lifetime doses ≥150 mg/m^2 increase the risk for heart failure; anthracyclines are red in color and may discolor body fluids.
epirubicin (Ellence)	Breast	100–120 mg/m^2 IV on d 1 and 8	Myelosuppression, cardiotoxicity, mucositis, nausea/vomiting, secondary leukemia, vesicant	Lifetime doses ≥900 mg/m^2 increase the risk for heart failure; anthracyclines are red in color and may discolor body fluids.
Topoisomerase II Inhibitors—Epipodophyllotoxins etoposide, VP-16 (VePesid)	Lung, testicular, stem cell mobilization for autologous stem cell transplantation	35–100 mg/m^2 IV daily for 4–5 d; oral dose is twice the IV dose	Myelosuppression, Stevens–Johnson syndrome, diarrhea, mucositis, nausea/vomiting, secondary leukemia	Rapid infusions may cause hypotension; etoposide is also available orally.
teniposide (Vumon)	Lung, leukemia	165 mg/m^2 IV twice weekly for 8–9 doses; 250 mg IV weekly for 4–8 doses	Myelosuppression, diarrhea, mucositis, nausea/vomiting, neurotoxicity, hypersensitivity	Rapid infusions may cause hypotension.
Topoisomerase II Inhibitors—Miscellaneous mitoxantrone (Novantrone)	Leukemia, prostate	Leukemia: 12 mg/m^2 IV daily for 3 d; prostate: 12–14 mg/m^2 IV every 21 d	Myelosuppression, mucositis, diarrhea, nausea/vomiting, cardiotoxicity, hepatotoxicity, secondary leukemia	Lifetime doses ≥100 mg/m^2 increase the risk for heart failure; mitoxantrone is blue in color and may discolor body fluids.

have hepatic dysfunction. The dose of vinca alkaloids should be decreased by 50% for bilirubin levels of 1.5 to 3.0 mg/dL and should not be given if the value is any higher. Docetaxel should also not be given if the bilirubin is greater than the upper limit of normal. Paclitaxel, however, can be used cautiously, but a dose reduction may be necessary.

In general, the dose-limiting toxicity of the antimicrotubules is the development of peripheral neuropathy. Patients may experience a tingling and numbness in their extremities that may warrant discontinuation or dose reduction of the offending drug. The vinca alkaloids may cause constipation and are vesicant drugs. The taxanes are myelosuppressive and therefore blood counts need to be monitored after administration. These agents also cause nausea and vomiting, but to a lesser degree than the antimetabolites or alkylating agents.

Caution must be exercised when administering these agents with other drugs that affect drug metabolism through liver enzymes. Most of the antimicrotubules are cleared through the liver, and drug concentrations in the body may be affected by coadministering other drugs that affect these liver enzymes. Some examples include cyclosporine, tacrolimus,

Table 56.4

Antimicrotubules

Generic (Trade) Name(s) and Dosage	Selected Anticancer Activity	Common Dose Range	Selected Adverse Events	Special Considerations
Vinca Alkaloids				
vincristine (Oncovin)	Leukemia, lung, lymphoma, myeloma, sarcoma	1–2 mg/m^2 IV every wk; max of 2 mg/dose	Peripheral neuropathy, constipation, vesicant	Fatal if given intrathecally
vinorelbine (Navelbine)	Breast, cervical, lung	25–30 mg/m^2 IV every wk	Peripheral neuropathy, constipation, vesicant	Fatal if given intrathecally
vinblastine (Velban)	Bladder, lymphoma, melanoma, prostate, testicular	Adults: 3.7 mg/m^2 as a single dose; increase dose by 1.8 mg/m^2 every wk until toxicity or a maximum dose of 18.5 mg/m^2 weekly	Hypertension, myelosuppression, peripheral neuropathy, constipation, vesicant	Fatal if given intrathecally
Taxanes				
paclitaxel (Taxol)	Breast, lung, ovarian,	135–175 mg/m^2 IV every 3 wk	Anaphylaxis, myelosuppression, bradycardia, hypotension, peripheral neuropathy, nausea/vomiting	Patients must be premedicated with a steroid, an H$_1$-receptor antagonist (eg, diphenhydramine), and an H$_2$-receptor antagonist (eg, ranitidine).
docetaxel (Taxotere)	Bladder, breast, gastric, lung, prostate	60–100 mg/m^2 IV every 3 wk	Peripheral neuropathy, fluid retention, myelosuppression, diarrhea, nausea/vomiting	Premedicate with steroids to decrease incidence of fluid retention.

erythromycin, carbamazepine, phenytoin, phenobarbital, fluconazole, ketoconazole, itraconazole, and warfarin.

Antitumor Antibiotics and Enzymes

The antitumor antibiotics are a relatively older class of agents and are less commonly used in clinical practice today than the agents discussed previously. Table 56-5 lists the agents in this class. The enzymes L-asparaginase and pegaspargase are used exclusively in treating leukemia. Mitomycin C is thought to produce its cytotoxic effects via a similar mechanism as the alkylating agents, resulting in DNA strand breaks. Bleomycin also cleaves DNA strands, but through the formation of oxygen free radicals. Dactinomycin is incorporated into DNA, which results in the inhibition of RNA and protein synthesis. The enzyme L-asparaginase and its modified form, pegaspargase, exhibit their antitumor effects by destroying the amino acid asparagine. This amino acid is necessary for protein synthesis in leukemia cells and the destruction ultimately leads to cell death.

Each antitumor antibiotic exhibits a unique side effect profile. Mitomycin C and dactinomycin both cause myelosuppression, whereas bleomycin does not. Mucositis, nausea, and vomiting are common with all three agents, but are relatively mild compared to agents previously discussed. Bleomycin also causes pulmonary toxicity, which may start as an interstitial pneumonitis and may progress to pulmonary fibrosis. Although this adverse effect may occur in any patient, the incidence is higher in patients who have received more than 450 U in their lifetime.

The major toxicities of the enzymes L-asparaginase and pegaspargase are hypersensitivity reactions, and a skin test using L-asparaginase before administering the dose may be performed to detect patients who may experience this reaction. In patients who have documented hypersensitivity to L-asparaginase, the modified formulation may be used because it is less likely to induce a reaction. Other adverse effects of these enzymes include nausea, hepatotoxicity, and coagulopathy.

Hormonal Agents

The hormonal antineoplastic agents do not have the same cytotoxic effects as the agents previously described; they are not considered biohazardous agents and therefore do not require the same special handling precautions as mentioned before. Nonetheless, they are of major importance in treating the hormone-sensitive tumors, breast and prostate cancer. Table 56-6 lists and compares these agents.

In contrast to being cytotoxic agents, the hormonal agents are cytostatic, meaning they prevent the growth of the tumor instead of causing cell death. The antiestrogens (tamoxifen, toremifene, fulvestrant) act by blocking the receptor that allows estrogen to stimulate the growth of breast cancer cells. In contrast, the aromatase inhibitors (anastrazole, letrozole, exemestane, aminoglutethimide) act by decreasing the levels of estrogen in the body and preventing the hormone from stimulating breast cancer cell growth. The antiandrogens (bicalutamide, flutamide, nilutamide) act similarly to the antiestrogens but instead block a receptor that enables testosterone from stimulating prostate cancer growth. The administration of luteinizing hormone-releasing hormone (LHRH) agonists (goserelin, leuprolide, triptorelin) ultimately results in the suppression of testosterone, preventing it from stimulating the growth of prostate cancer cells.

Table 56.5

Antitumor Antibiotics and Enzymes

Generic (Trade) Name(s) and Dosage	Selected Anticancer Activity	Common Dose Range	Selected Adverse Events	Special Considerations
Antitumor Antibiotics				
bleomycin (Blenoxane)	Lymphoma, testicular	10–20 U/m² once-twice weekly	Pulmonary fibrosis, pneumonitis, dermal reactions (hyperpigmentation, rash, hyperkeratosis)	Pulmonary fibrosis is dose dependent and therefore the dose should not exceed 400 U.
mitomycin C (Mutamycin)	Bladder, gastric, hepatocellular, pancreatic	20 mg/m² IV every 6–8 wk	Myelosuppression, hemolytic uremic syndrome, nephrotoxicity, vesicant	Can be given intra-arterially as part of chemoembolization for hepatic lesions.
dactinomycin (Cosmegen)	Sarcoma, trophoblastic neoplasia, Wilms tumor	12–15 μg/kg IV daily for 5 d	Myelosuppression, diarrhea, acne, erythema, nausea/vomiting, vesicant	
Enzymes				
L-asparaginase (Elspar)	Leukemia	6,000 U/m² IM days 4, 7, 10, 13, 16, 19, 22, 25, and 28; or 1000 U/kg/d for 10 d	Hypersensitivity, weakness, fatigue, coagulopathy, skin rash, urticaria, hepatotoxicity	A skin test is recommended before administration to test for hypersensitivity reactions.
pegaspargase (Oncaspar)	Leukemia	2500 U/m² IM every 14 d	Hypersensitivity, coagulopathy, weakness, fatigue, hepatotoxicity	Pegaspargase is a modified version of L-asparaginase; its half-life is longer and therefore it can be administered less frequently.

Most of the antiestrogens, antiandrogens, and aromatase inhibitors are taken orally every day, except for fulvestrant, which is given as two consecutive intramuscular injections every month. The LHRH agonists leuprolide and triptorelin are given as intramuscular injections every 1 to 4 months, whereas goserelin is given as a subcutaneous injection every 1 to 3 months, depending on the dose.

Almost all of these agents are contraindicated in pregnancy because of the harmful effects to the fetus. Adverse effects include hot flashes and nausea. The antiestrogens increase a patient's risk for endometrial cancer; the aromatase inhibitors can cause osteoporosis and bone pain. Both antiestrogens and aromatase inhibitors increase the risk for thrombosis. The antiandrogens and LHRH agonists both can cause gynecomastia, but hepatotoxicity is a problem with the antiandrogens.

Antibodies

Antitumor antibodies are a relatively new class of anticancer agents that are both structurally and mechanistically different than traditional cytotoxic agents. Fundamentally, these agents act by binding to a specific receptor on tumor cells or other another substrate, leading to either direct cell death or inhibition of tumor proliferation. These antibodies are synthesized synthetically by using DNA recombinant technology, resulting in a humanized antibody that acts against a specific target. Table 56-7 lists the antibodies used to treat cancer and the specific targets of those drugs.

The most common adverse effect related to all of the monoclonal antibodies are hypersensitivity and infusion related reactions, usually manifested in hypotension and is related to the rate of infusion. Specifically, trastuzumab may cause heart failure, bevacizumab may cause hypertension and bleeding, and cetuximab may cause an acneiform rash.

Gemtuzumab ozogamicin is a combination antibody and antitumor antibiotic. The gemtuzumab antibody specifically targets the CD33 receptors on leukemia cells and delivers a cytotoxic agent directly to the malignant cell. The agents gemtuzumab ozogamicin, ibritumomab tiuxetan, and tositumomab have a more severe side effect profile because these antibodies facilitate the delivery of cytotoxic agents to the tumor cells. Adverse effects associated with this drug include myelosuppression and hepatotoxicity. Ibritumomab tiuxetan and tositumomab are radiolabeled antibodies that deliver radioisotopes to lymphoma cells that express the CD20 receptor. These agents may cause myelosuppression, chills, fatigue, and nausea. However, there is a risk for developing hypothyroidism and exposing others to radiation when being treated with tositumomab.

Targeted Therapy

Targeted therapy is a term used to describe the newest class of agents developed to fight cancer. In general, these agents are small molecules designed to inhibit a specific receptor overexpressed in a specific cancer and induce cell death. For example, the drug imatinib (Gleevec) is designed to inhibit the BCR-ABL tyrosine kinase pathway found in chronic leukemia cells. Furthermore, gefitinib (Iressa) is another small molecule designed to inhibit the epidermal growth factor receptor tyrosine kinase pathway. It is currently being used to treat lung cancer but is being investigated for activity in other cancers. Currently, multiple targeted therapy

Table 56.6

Hormonal Agents

Generic (Trade) Name(s) and Dosage	Selected Adverse Events	Common Dose Range	Contraindications	Special Considerations
Antiestrogens				
tamoxifen (Nolvadex)	Hot flashes, nausea, DVT/PE, cataracts, endometrial cancer	20–40 mg/d PO	Pregnancy, history of PE/DVT (relative contraindication)	Most commonly used to prevent breast cancer recurrence in the adjuvant setting; usual length of therapy is 5 y; also used to treat metastatic breast cancer.
toremifene (Fareston)	Hot flashes, nausea, DVT/PE, cataracts, endometrial cancer	60 mg PO daily	Pregnancy	Indicated for patients with metastatic breast cancer; continue therapy until disease progression.
fulvestrant (Faslodex)	Hot flashes, nausea, abdominal pain, injection site pain, anemia	250 mcg IM monthly	Pregnancy	For the treatment of metastatic breast cancer in patients who are estrogen receptor positive
Aromatase inhibitors				
anastrozole (Arimidex)	Hot flashes, nausea, bone pain; osteoporosis, DVT/PE	1 mg PO daily	Pregnancy	Can be used to prevent breast cancer recurrence in the adjuvant setting or to treat metastatic breast cancer.
letrozole (Femara)	Hot flashes, nausea, bone pain; osteoporosis, DVT/PE	2.5 mg PO daily	Pregnancy	New data suggest using letrozole after 5 y of tamoxifen may decrease incidence of breast cancer recurrence.
exemestane (Aromasin)	Hot flashes, nausea, bone pain; osteoporosis, DVT/PE	25 mg PO daily after meals		Used for the treatment of metastatic breast cancer after failing tamoxifen
aminoglutethimide (Cytadren)	Rash/adrenal insufficiency (administer with hydrocortisone to decrease incidence); nausea, dizziness, hypotension, pancytopenia	250 mg PO bid for 2 wk, then increase to 250 mg PO qid		First-generation aromatase inhibitor; must give with hydrocortisone (60 mg PO qhs, 20 mg PO qam and q 2pm for 2 wk, then 20 mg PO qhs, 10 mg PO qam and q 2pm).
Antiandrogens				
bicalutamide (Casodex)	Gynecomastia, nausea, hot flashes, anemia, hepatotoxicity	50 mg PO daily	Women, pregnancy	Most commonly given with a LHRH agonist
flutamide (Eulixin)	Gynecomastia, nausea, hot flashes, anemia, leukopenia, thrombocytopenia, hepatotoxicity	250 mg PO q8h	Pregnancy, severe hepatic impairment	Most commonly given with a LHRH agonist for B2C or D2 prostate cancer
nilutamide (Nilandron)	Gynecomastia, nausea, hot flashes, anemia, hepatotoxicity, blurred/impaired vision, interstitial pneumonitis	300 mg PO daily (as one dose or 3 divided doses) for 1 mo, then 150 mg daily thereafter	Hepatic impairment, respiratory insufficiency	Used in combination with orchiectomy or LHRH agonist; may give 100 mg PO every 8 h as monotherapy
Luteinizing Hormone-Releasing Hormone (LHRH) Agonists				
leuprolide (Lupron)	Hot flashes, gynecomastia, bone pain, nausea/vomiting, edema, thrombosis, impotence	7.5 mg IM monthly, *or* 22.5 mg IM every 3 mo, *or* 30 mg IM every 4 mo	Pregnancy	Also available as an implantable device for the palliative treatment of prostate cancer
goserelin (Zoladex)	Hot flashes, gynecomastia, bone pain, impotence, thrombosis	3.6 mg SC every 28 d *or* 10.8 mg SC every 3 mo	Pregnancy	Indicated for neoadjuvant therapy in stage B2-C prostate cancer
triptorelin (Trelstar)	Hot flashes, gynecomastia, bone pain, impotence, thrombosis	3.75 mg IM monthly	Pregnancy	

DVT, deep view thrombosis; PE, pulmonary embolism.

Table 56.7

Antibodies

Generic (Trade) Name(s) and Dosage	Selected Anticancer Activity	Common Dose Range	Selected Adverse Events	Special Considerations
rituximab (Rituxan)	Lymphoma, leukemia	375 mg/m^2 IV every wk for 4–8 doses	Hypersensitivity, infusion related reactions, cardiac toxicity, fever	Specifically targets the CD20 receptor on B cells.
trastuzumab (Herceptin)	Breast	4 mg/kg IV for 1 dose, then 2 mg/kg IV weekly	Cardiomyopathy, infusion-related reactions	Specifically targets the HER2/neu receptor in breast cancer
bevacizumab (Avastin)	Colorectal	5 mg/kg IV every 2 wk	Hypertension, bleeding, infusion related reactions, thrombosis	Specifically targets vascular endothelia growth factor (VEGF); it is the first anti-angiogenesis drug to be FDA approved
cetuximab (Erbitux)	Colorectal	400 mg/m^2 IV for 1 dose, then 250 mg/m^2 IV every wk	Infusion-related reactions, acneiform rash, asthenia	Specifically targets the epidermal growth factor receptor (EGFR).
gemtuzumab ozogamicin (Mylotarg)	Acute myeloid leukemia	9 mg/m^2 IV every 2 wk for 2 doses	Infusion-related reactions (dyspnea, hypotension, anaphylaxis), myelosuppression, hepatotoxicity	The gemtuzumab component specifically targets the CD33 receptor on leukemia cells while an attached cytotoxic agent causes cell death
ibritumomab tiuxetan (Zevalin)	Non-Hodgkin lymphoma	In-111 ibritumomab tiuxetan 5 mCi for 1 dose, then Y-90 ibritumomab tiuxetan 0.4 mCi/kg (max = 32 mCi) 7–9 d later; all doses given within 4 h after rituximab 250 mg/m^2 IV	Myelosuppression, secondary malignancies, asthenia, fever, chills	A monoclonal antibody component targets the CD20 receptors and facilitates delivery of a radioisotope to lymphoma cells to induce apoptosis.
tositumomab (Bexxar)	Non-Hodgkin lymphoma	450 mg tositumomab IV followed by iodine I-131 tositumomab; repeat 6–7 d later	Myelosuppression, secondary malignancies, asthenia, hypothyroidism, fever, chills, risk of radiation exposure to others	A monoclonal antibody component targets the CD20 receptors and facilitates delivery of a radioisotope to lymphoma cells to induce apoptosis.

agents are being investigated for a wide variety of tumor types. Because these are agents are small molecules that bind to a specific receptor on tumor cells, these agents are not biohazardous and are not subject to the same precautions as chemotherapy.

These agents represent the future of treating oncologic disorders. Instead of administering a highly cytotoxic agent that destroys normal, healthy host cells in addition to the harmful tumor cells, the targeted therapy agents are able to specifically target the receptors located in the malignant cell. Therefore, these agents are generally well tolerated compared with conventional chemotherapy. Furthermore, these agents are administered orally. However, much research still needs to be completed before it is known how to most effectively use these agents for treating cancer.

Selecting the Most Appropriate Chemotherapy Regimens

Chemotherapy is often used in combination with surgery or radiation therapy or both, depending on the specific tumor type and stage of disease. Combination chemotherapy is often used to take advantage of different mechanisms of action to

overcome drug resistance. The following section describes the most commonly used regimens to treat the most commonly treated cancers.

Breast Cancer

In the treatment of breast cancer, chemotherapy is primarily used in the adjuvant setting, after surgery or radiation is performed. Adjuvant therapy is given to eradicate any residual micrometastatic disease and usually consists of doxorubicin/cyclophosphamide (4 cycles), fluorouracil/doxorubicin/cyclophosphamide (6 cycles), or cyclophosphamide/methotrexate/fluorouracil (6 cycles). Table 56-8 presents the specifics regarding each treatment regimen. After adjuvant therapy is administered, patients with hormone-dependent tumors may have therapy initiated with tamoxifen or an aromatase inhibitor for a duration of 5 years. The purpose of this therapy is to prevent breast cancer recurrence.

If breast cancer has recurred or is metastatic, the primary treatment option for those tumors that are hormone dependent is a hormonal antineoplastic agent. Otherwise, treatment with chemotherapy is indicated in patients with non–hormone-dependent tumors and those in whom all hormonal

Table 56.8

Common Breast Cancer Regimens*

Chemotherapy Agents	Dose/Regimen	Cycle
doxorubicin (*Adriamycin*)	60 mg/m² IV on d 1	21 d
*c*yclophosphamide	600 mg/m² IV on d 1	
*f*luorouracil	500 mg/m² IV on d 1	21 d
doxorubicin (*Adriamycin*)	50 mg/m² IV on d 1	
*c*yclophosphamide	500 mg/m² IV on d 1	
*c*yclophosphamide	100 mg/m² PO on d 1–14	28 d
*m*ethotrexate	40 mg/m² IV on d 1 and 8	
*f*luorouracil	600 mg/m² IV on d 1 and 8	
*c*yclophosphamide	600 mg/m² IV on d 1	28 d
*m*ethotrexate	40 mg/m² IV on d 1	
*f*luorouracil	600 mg/m² IV on d 1	
doxorubicin (*Adriamycin*)	50 mg/m² IV on d 1	21 d
paclitaxel	220 mg/m² IV on d 2	
capecitabine (*Xeloda*)	1250 mg/m² PO bid on d 1–14	21 d
docetaxel (*Taxotere*)	75 mg/m² on d 21	
paclitaxel	175 mg/m² IV on d 1	21 d
paclitaxel	135 mg/m² IV on d 1	28 d
vinorelbine	30 mg/m² IV on d 1 and 8	
trastuzumab	4 mg/kg IV loading dose over 90 min then 2 mg/kg IV over 30 min	Every 7 d
gemcitabine	725 mg/m² IV on d 1, 8, and 15	28 d
vinorelbine	30 mg/m² IV	7 d

*Italicized letters provide common acronyms for regimens.

therapy has failed. Examples of some chemotherapy regimens used in this setting include FAC and CMF. However, regimens containing paclitaxel, docetaxel, and vinorelbine have been used. Furthermore, patients who overexpress the HER2/neu oncogene may benefit from therapy with the monoclonal antibody, trastuzumab (Herceptin).

Prostate Cancer

The role of chemotherapy in treating prostate cancer is minimal. Early stage prostate cancer is typically treated by watchful waiting, prostatectomy, or radiation. However, patients who present with more advanced disease may receive radiation/prostatectomy plus hormonal therapy using LHRH agonists or antiandrogens (or both) in the primary treatment or neoadjuvant setting. Those with metastatic disease are typically treated with LHRH agonists alone, antiandrogens alone, or LHRH agonists plus antiandrogens, depending on response. Patients who have disease recurrence despite appropriate treatment with hormonal therapy (ie, hormone-refractory disease) may be candidates for systemic chemotherapy. However, these therapies historically produce low response rates of approximately 4% to 9% (Oh & Kantoff, 1998). However, chemotherapy may still be used to treat patients who have exhausted all other therapeutic options. Some chemotherapy options include mitoxantrone plus steroids, estramustine plus vinblastine/paclitaxel/docetaxel/etoposide, and doxorubicin plus ketoconazole. Figure 56-1 depicts the algorithm for treating metastatic prostate cancer.

Lung Cancer

Chemotherapy plays an important role in patients with non–small-cell lung cancer (NSCLC) who present with

advanced disease (stages III-IV) or in patients with inoperable, less advanced disease. Often chemotherapy is combined with radiation to produce the best outcomes. Small-cell lung cancer is a chemosensitive disease; it is treated with chemoradiation for limited stage disease and chemotherapy alone for extensive disease. Table 56-9 lists the chemotherapy regimens commonly used in treating lung cancer. Combination regimens are usually used as first-line therapy, whereas single agent regimens are commonly seen in patients who have progressive disease. Combination regimens usually include a platinum agent (cisplatin, carboplatin), a taxane (paclitaxel, docetaxel), or gemcitabine (Schiller et al., 2002). The single-agent regimens used are docetaxel, gemcitabine, and vinorelbine. Currently,

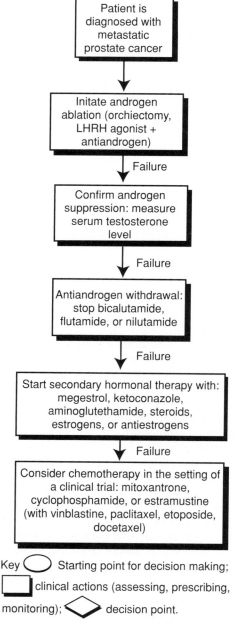

Figure 56-1 Algorithm for treatment of prostate cancer. (Adapted from Oh, W.K., & Kantoff, P.W. [1998]. Management of hormone refractory prostate cancer: Current standards and future prospects. *Journal of Urology, 160,* 1220–1229.)

Table 56.9

Common Lung Cancer Regimens

Chemotherapy Agents	Dose/Regimen	Cycle
Non–Small-Cell Lung Cancer		
cisplatin	75 mg/m² IV on d 1	21 d
paclitaxel	135 mg/m² IV over 24 h on d 1	
cisplatin	100 mg/m² on d 1	28 d
gemcitabine	1000 mg/m² on d 1, 8, and 15	
cisplatin	75 mg/m² on d 1	21 d
docetaxel	75 mg/m² on d 1	
carboplatin	AUC 6 mg/mL/min on d 1	21 d
paclitaxel	225 mg/m² over 3 h on d 1	
etoposide	100–120 mg/m²/d on d 1–3	21 d
carboplatin	300–325 mg/m² IV on d 1	
gemcitabine	1200 mg/m² IV on d 1 and 8	21 d
vinorelbine	30 mg/m² IV on d 1 and 8	
docetaxel	75 mg/m² IV over 1 h on d 1	21 d
gemcitabine	1000 mg/m² IV on d 1, 8 and 15	28 d
vinorelbine	30 mg/m² IV	Every 7 d
Small-Cell Lung Cancer		
etoposide	80 mg/m²/d IV on d 1–3	21 d
cisplatin	80 mg/m² IV on d 1 (or 27 mg/m²/d IV d 1–5)	
cyclophosphamide	1000 mg/m² IV on d 1	21 d
doxorubicin	45 mg/m² IV on d 1	
vincristine	1.5 mg/m² IV on d 1	

gefitinib (Iressa) at a dose of 250 mg by mouth daily is approved by the Food and Drug Administration (FDA) for third-line treatment of NSCLC in patients who have failed prior chemotherapy with a platinum agent and docetaxel.

Colorectal Cancer

Surgery is the main treatment of choice for patients who present with colon cancer. Those who present with rectal cancer will receive surgery plus radiation. Chemotherapy plays a role in colorectal cancer when a patient presents with stage III or IV disease; it is given in the adjuvant setting for stage III cancers and as palliative therapy for stage IV disease. The chemotherapy regimens used are the same for both colon and rectal cancer. Table 56-10 lists the commonly used chemotherapy regimens.

Fluorouracil and leucovorin have long been used to treat colorectal cancer. Leucovorin is not a chemotherapy agent, but in this case is used synergistically in combination with fluorouracil to increase the cytotoxicity. Irinotecan and oxaliplatin are relatively new agents and were approved by the FDA in 1996 and 2002, respectively. They are combined with fluorouracil and leucovorin for the treatment of metastatic colorectal cancer. In early 2004, two new agents, bevacizumab and cetuximab, were also approved by the FDA for this disease. Capecitabine is considered an oral formulation of fluorouracil and is sometimes given in place of fluorouracil/leucovorin.

Leukemias and Lymphomas

Leukemias and lymphomas are two different types of cancers that are sensitive to chemotherapy. In fact, chemotherapy represents the main treatment modality because of the systemic nature of these diseases. Acute leukemias are typically induced into remission (ie, induction therapy), then are further treated with consolidation therapy to prevent disease relapse. Patients with acute lymphoblastic leukemia (ALL) will receive maintenance therapy after consolidation to further decrease their risk of relapse. Typical chemotherapy agents used for treating ALL include cytarabine, anthracyclines, and mitoxantrone. Etoposide is sometimes added into treatment regimens. The treatment of ALL follows a complicated treatment regimen and includes agents such as anthracyclines, vincristine, corticosteroids, asparaginase, methotrexate, and cyclophosphamide in the induction and consolidation phases. Maintenance therapy is achieved by using mercaptopurine, corticosteroids, vincristine, and methotrexate administered regularly for 2 to 3 years.

Different treatment regimens are used to treat different type of lymphomas. A common regimen for treating aggressive non-Hodgkin lymphoma is the CHOP regimen (cyclophosphamide, doxorubicin, vincristine, and prednisone). Sometimes, rituximab is added to this regimen if the tumor cells express the CD20 antigen. Indolent, low-grade lymphomas may be treated with fludarabine, either as a single agent or in combination with other agents.

Special Considerations

There are certain patient specific parameters that must be considered when starting chemotherapy. Patients with renal and hepatic dysfunction may be at an increased risk for toxicity if certain chemotherapy agents are administered. For example, the anthracyclines (doxorubicin, daunorubicin, idarubicin), taxanes (docetaxel, paclitaxel), vinca alkaloids (vincristine, vinblastine, vinorelbine), etoposide, imatinib, and thiotepa are cleared from the body via the liver. Therefore,

Table 56.10

Common Colorectal Cancer Regimens

Chemotherapy Agents	Dose/Regimen	Cycle
fluorouracil (5-FU)	600 mg/m² IV on d 1, 8, 15, 22, 29, and 35	8 wk
leucovorin	500 mg/m² on d 1, 8, 15, 22, 29, and 35	
irinotecan	100–125 mg/m² IV on d 1, 8, 15, and 22	6 wk
fluorouracil (5-FU)	600 mg/m² IV on d 1, 8, 15, and 22	
leucovorin	500 mg/m² on d 1, 8, 15, and 22	
oxaliplatin	85 mg/m² IV on d 1	14 d
fluorouracil (5-FU)	400 mg/m² IV bolus, then 600 mg/m² via continuous IV infusion over 22 hs], given on d 1 and 2	
leucovorin	200 mg/m² IV before 5-FU bolus on d 1 and 2	
capecitabine	1250 mg/m² PO bid on d 1–14 (may be substituted for 5-FU/leucovorin in above regimens)	21 d
bevacizumab	5 mg/kg IV every 2 weeks (should be added to the above irinotecan or oxaliplatin regimens)	Every 2 wk
cetuximab	400 mg/m² IV × 1 dose, then 250 mg/m² IV weekly	Weekly

caution must be exercised when administering these agents to patients who have underlying hepatic dysfunction; doses may need to be adjusted. With some agents, the drug should be omitted from the regimen if the hepatic dysfunction is too severe.

Drugs that are eliminated renally include the platinums (cisplatin, carboplatin), cyclophosphamide, ifosfamide, bleomycin, fludarabine, methotrexate, etoposide, and topotecan. Similarly to hepatic dysfunction, caution should be exercised when administering these agents to patients with renal dysfunction, and they may be omitted or the dosage decreased depending on the degree of dysfunction.

MONITORING PATIENT RESPONSE

Goals of therapy and response criteria have been previously discussed in this chapter. Monitoring for a patient's response may incorporate the use of imaging studies and laboratory values (such as specific tumor markers), along with a standard physical examination and review of systems performed by the practitioner. Solid tumors are generally monitored for response through the use of CT or PET scans; practitioners will assess these imaging studies at regular intervals to monitor the change in size of each tumor. Some cancer will also produce "tumor markers" that are measurable in the bloodstream. Examples include the prostate-specific antigen (PSA) for prostate cancer and carcinoembryonic antigen (CEA) for pancreatic and colorectal cancer. These values may also be assessed at regular intervals to measure the trend. Hematologic malignancies are different in that bone marrow biopsies are performed at regular intervals to assess whether there is residual disease present. The patient's overall clinical status is also important to assess. Review of factors such as nausea, vomiting, appetite, fatigue, and pain should be evaluated regularly to assess whether there is an improvement in these parameters.

MANAGING COMPLICATIONS OF CHEMOTHERAPY

Because of the cytotoxic nature of chemotherapy, many complications may occur after administration of these agents. These include, but are not limited to, febrile neutropenia, nausea/vomiting, mucositis, diarrhea, and extravasation. Although some of these complications are serious and can often be fatal, they can be managed if they are identified early.

Febrile Neutropenia

Febrile neutropenia is a common complication associated with myelosuppressive chemotherapy. It is defined as having a temperature of 38.3°C (or ≥38°C for 1 hour) and having or anticipating a neutrophil count of 500 cells/mm^3 or less (Hughes et al., 2002). Although approximately one half of these patients are actually infected, they should all should seek medical attention immediately because of the high mortality rates.

There are two strategies for managing febrile neutropenia: treatment and prevention. Once a patient becomes febrile while neutropenic, broad-spectrum antibiotics should be administered to adequately cover both gram-positive and gram-negative bacteria such as *Staphylococcus* species, *Pseudomonas aeruginosa*, and *Escherichia coli*. Such agents include cefepime, imipenem, piperacillin/tazobactam, or ceftazidime. Generally speaking, higher doses of these broad-spectrum antibiotics are necessary to cover the appropriate suspected organisms. Cefepime should be given intravenously as 2 g every 8 hours; imipenem 500 mg is given every 6 hours, piperacillin/tazobactam can be given as 4.5 g intravenously every 6 hours or 3.375 g intravenously every 4 hours, and ceftazidime 2 g every 8 hours. These doses assume normal renal function and should be adjusted accordingly. An aminoglycoside (gentamicin, tobramycin, amikacin) may also be added to the regimen in patients who are expected to have prolonged neutropenia or those who are clinically unstable. If a patient has a compromised vascular access device or is hemodynamically unstable, additional gram-positive coverage with vancomycin (1 g every 12 hours for normal renal function) may be required. Patients are continued on antibiotics and monitored closely until the fever resolves and the neutrophil count recovers. Those who are persistently febrile and neutropenic despite being given the broad-spectrum antibiotics may require additional antifungal therapy, especially against the *Aspergillus* species. Common agents used for this purpose include amphotericin B and voriconazole.

The use of colony-stimulating factors (filgrastim, pegfilgrastim, sargramostim) has not been proven to decrease the mortality of febrile neutropenia once a patient has been admitted into the hospital and is actively being treated for this complication. However, it has been shown to decrease the time that these patients are neutropenic. Therefore, it is recommended that colony-stimulating factors not be used in all patients who are already experiencing febrile neutropenia. Instead, select patients with additional complications and poor prognostic factors are possible candidates (Ozer et al., 2000).

The role of colony-stimulating factors lies in the prevention of febrile neutropenia. These agents are routinely given to patients who have had a history of febrile neutropenia, have had a cycle delayed because of neutropenia, or are receiving a chemotherapy regimen that is likely to cause febrile neutropenia in 40% or more of patients (Ozer et al., 2000). The dose for this indication is 5 mg/kg for filgrastim (usually rounded to a 360- or 480-mg dose) and 250 mg/m^2 for sargramostim given subcutaneously once daily starting 24 hours after chemotherapy ends and continuing until the absolute neutrophile count (ANC) is 10,000 cells/mm^3 or higher. Pegfilgrastim is given as a single 6-mg subcutaneous dose 24 hours after chemotherapy ends and should not be given if chemotherapy is to be given within the next 14 days.

Chemotherapy-Induced Nausea and Vomiting

Nausea and vomiting are adverse effects commonly associated with chemotherapy. Despite advances in medicine, approximately one half of patients vomit within 5 to 6 days after receiving chemotherapy (Gralla et al., 1999). Therefore, it is important to properly identify patients at higher risk and properly administer the correct antiemetic agents to prevent or treat nausea and vomiting.

Table 56.11

Emetogenic Levels of Cancer Chemotherapeutic Agents

LEVEL 1	LEVEL 2	LEVEL 4
(<10% Frequency)	(10%–30% Frequency)	(60%–90% Frequency)
androgens	asparaginase	carboplatin
bleomycin	cytarabine (<1 g/m^2)	carmustine (<250 mg/m^2)
busulfan (oral, <4 mg/kg/d)	docetaxel	cisplatin (<50 mg/m^2)
capecitabine	doxorubicin (<20 mg/m^2)	cyclophosphamide (>750 mg/m^2 to ≤ 1500
chlorambucil (oral)	etoposide	mg/m^2)
cladribine	fluorouracil (<1000 mg/m^2)	cytarabine (>1 g/m^2)
corticosteroids	gemcitabine	dactinomycin (>1.5 mg/m^2)
fludarabine	methotrexate (>50 mg/m^2; <250 mg/m^2)	doxorubicin (>60 mg/m^2)
hydroxyurea	mitomycin	irinotecan
interferon	paclitaxel	melphalan (IV)
melphalan (oral)	temozolomide	methotrexate (>1000 mg/m^2)
mercaptopurine	teniposide	mitoxantrone (>15 mg/m^2)
methotrexate (≤ 50 mg/m^2)	thiotepa	oxaliplatin
rituximab	topotecan	procarbazine (oral)
thioguanine		
trastuzumab	LEVEL 3	LEVEL 5
tretinoin	(30%–60% Frequency)	(>90% Frequency)
vinblastine	aldesleukin	carmustine (>250 mg/m^2)
vincristine	cyclophosphamide (IV, <750 mg/m^2)	cisplatin (≥ 50 mg/m^2)
vinorelbine	dactinomycin (≤ 1.5 mg/m^2)	cyclophosphamide (>1500 mg/m^2)
	doxorubicin hydrochloride (20–60 mg/m^2)	dacarbazine (≥ 500 mg/m^2)
	epirubicin hydrochloride (≤ 90 mg/m^2)	lomustine (>60 mg/m^2)
	idarubicin	mechlorethamine
	ifosfamide	pentostatin
	methenamine (oral)	streptozocin
	methotrexate (250–1000 mg/m^2)	
	mitoxantrone (≤ 15 mg/m^2)	

The most highly emetogenic agent in the combination should be identified, and the contribution of other agents should be considered by using the following rules: (1) **level 1** and **level 2** agents do not contribute to the emetogenicity of a given regimen; (2) adding a **level 3** or **level 4** agent increases the emetogenicity of the combination by one level per agent. The dose, route and schedule of administration, concomitant therapies, and patient's prior emetic history influence the emetic potential of any individual drug (adapted from Hesketh et al., 1997).

Risk factors for developing chemotherapy-induced nausea or vomiting include female gender, younger age, history of motion/morning sickness, poor performance status, and previous vomiting due to chemotherapy. Patients with increased alcohol consumption have a lower risk of vomiting due to chemotherapy. Specific chemotherapy agents and regimens are stratified into five different levels depending on the probability to cause vomiting if there is no prophylaxis. Level 5 emetogenicity is the highest level available, with a probability of 90% or more of patients vomiting if not adequately premedicated with antiemetics. Examples of agents in their respective level of emetogenicity are listed in Table 56-11.

Nausea and vomiting can further be divided into three categories: acute, delayed, and anticipatory. Acute nausea/vomiting occurs within the first 24 hours after chemotherapy. Any vomiting for up to 5 days afterward is considered delayed nausea/vomiting. Anticipatory nausea/vomiting occurs before chemotherapy is administered and is usually associated with a poor response to a previous cycle (see Chapter 28).

The treatment of chemotherapy-induced nausea and vomiting is divided into prevention and treatment. Prevention starts with premedications before the chemotherapy is administered; typically a corticosteroid (usually dexamethasone) is given 30 minutes before chemotherapy. A serotonin antagonist such as dolasetron, granisetron, or ondansetron is added if patients are receiving a moderately or highly emetogenic regimen (ie, levels 3–5). A benzodiazepine such as lorazepam may also be considered at this time if the patient is experiencing anticipatory nausea/vomiting. For the prevention of delayed nausea/vomiting, patients should continue to take dexamethasone for 5 days total if they received a level 4-5 emetogenic regimen. They should also continue to receive a serotonin antagonist daily for 3 days total. For patients receiving highly emetogenic chemotherapy containing cisplatin, aprepitant (Emend) should be given before chemotherapy in addition to the dexamethasone and serotonin antagonist on day 1, but should be given in place of a serotonin antagonist on days 2 and 3. The most commonly used agents for breakthrough nausea or vomiting are prochlorperazine, promethazine, and haloperidol, taken as needed.

Oral Mucositis

Oral mucositis is a common and severe adverse effect of chemotherapy. It is often associated with significant morbidity, such as infection, narcotic use, and hospital stay. Oral mucositis is also associated with increased 100-day mortality in recipients of stem cell transplants (Rubenstein et al., 2004). It is a common dose-limiting side effect of most chemotherapy agents, but occurs most commonly in patients receiving fluorouracil or high-dose chemotherapy (eg, melphalan or cyclophosphamide for stem cell transplantation).

Many options are available for the prevention of oral mucositis, but therapy often begins with good oral hygiene to decrease associated complications. To prevent oral mucositis, oral cryotherapy (with ice chips) has been useful when administering fluorouracil. Once mucositis has occurred, little can be done to reduce its duration. Instead, treatment is usually palliative. Topical preparations that include ingredients such as viscous lidocaine, magnesium hydroxide, aluminum hydroxide, and diphenhydramine may have some benefit in reducing the pain from mucositis. Rinsing with saline and bicarbonate preparations may also have benefit. Systemic opioids have also been effective in treating pain associated with oral mucositis.

Diarrhea

Chemotherapy may induce diarrhea by damaging the intestinal mucosa, thereby leading to decreased absorption and increased secretion of fluids in the gastrointestinal tract. The most common causative agents include irinotecan and fluorouracil, but it can also occur with most other chemotherapy agents, especially those used to treat colorectal cancer (Saltz, 2003). The diarrhea experienced by patients may range from a mild, increase of daily stools to a life-threatening state that requires hospitalization for hemodynamic support. Therefore, it is important to identify and treat chemotherapy-induced diarrhea.

Management of chemotherapy-induced diarrhea includes adequate hydration with clear liquids that contain sugars or electrolytes. Diet can be modified once diarrhea is experienced. Patients should avoid milk (because of induced lactose intolerance) and spicy, fried, or greasy foods. Instead, a diet consisting of easily digestible foods such as bananas, rice, applesauce, and toast (ie, the BRAT diet) has been recommended. Drugs that can be used to manage diarrhea include loperamide and diphenoxylate/atropine. Loperamide is given at a different dosing schedule than what is generally recommended; 4 mg should be given at the onset of diarrhea, then 2 mg should be given every 2 hours (or 4 mg every 4 hours if during bedtime) until the diarrhea stops. Octreotide at doses of 100 to 500 mcg 3 times daily may be used for more severe cases that require patient hospitalization.

Extravasation

Extravasation occurs when the chemotherapy has infiltrated the tissue surrounding the vascular access during administration. This usually occurs with peripheral access devices and seldom occurs when patients have central catheters. Although this may be a problem with all intravenously administered chemotherapy agents, those that are able to cause local tissue necrosis (ie, vesicants) are especially problematic. These agents include the anthracylines, vinca alkaloids, and mechlorethamine. Other agents may be irritants if extravasated but do not directly cause local tissue damage. Patients may complain of pain, burning, itching, or tingling if extravasation does occur.

When administering vesicant agents, care must be used to prevent extravasation. When available, central access catheters should be used to administer these agents. However, they can be administered peripherally if given with free-flowing intravenous fluids over a couple of minutes. Blood return should periodically be checked during administration. If extravasation does occur, the infusion should be stopped, as much drug as possible should be aspirated, and cold compresses can be applied if the agent the extravasated was an anthracycline, versus warm compresses for vinca alkaloids. Dimethyl sulfoxide (for anthracyclines) or thiosulfate (for mechlorethamine) may also be applied, but few data are available to support its regular use.

PATIENT EDUCATION

When patients are receiving chemotherapy, they must be educated regarding these agents because of the severe and often life-threatening side effects of these drugs. Patients may often be asked to sign a consent form stating they have been well informed of the toxicities of the specific agents they are receiving. Patients should also be notified of the common complications associated with chemotherapy, especially febrile neutropenia, so they are able to quickly recognize the symptoms and seek medical attention immediately. Patients should also be told of the realistic goals of the chemotherapy, whether it is for palliative treatment or curative intent. This should allow the patient to adequately judge the risks versus benefits of receiving chemotherapy.

■ Case Study

T.G. is a 62-year-old man with a history of diffuse large B-cell lymphoma, diagnosed approximately 6 months ago. He presents to the clinic today for his fourth cycle (of 8) of R-CHOP, which is rituximab 375 mg/m^2 on day 1, cyclophosphamide 750 mg/m^2 on day 1, doxorubicin 50 mg/m^2 on day 1, vincristine 1.4 mg/m^2 (2 mg max) on day 1, and prednisone 40 mg/m^2/d on days 1 to 5. Initially, he presented with painful cervical lymphadenopathy, chills, night sweats, and fatigue. These symptoms have improved since starting chemotherapy, but he has recently been complaining of painful tingling and burning in his feet. He was recently treated with antibiotics in the hospital for an episode of febrile neutropenia that lasted 7 days and caused a delay in starting this cycle.

➤ 1. List at least two major adverse effects of each of the chemotherapy agents T.G. is receiving.

➤ 2. What level of emetogenicity is the chemotherapy regimen T.G. is receiving, and what agents should T.G. receive before chemotherapy?

➤ 3. Should T.G. receive prophylaxis therapy with a colony-stimulating factor to prevent febrile neutropenia? Why or why not?

➤ 4. What agent in T.G.'s chemotherapy regimen is likely causing the neuropathy?

➤ 5. What concerns must be addressed when administering doxorubicin?

Bibliography

*Starred references are cited in the text.

Adams, V. R., & Bence, A. K. (2003). Guide for the administration and use of cancer chemotherapeutic agents 2003. *Oncology Special Edition, 6,* 123–138.

*Adams, V. R., Sheehan, J. B., Holdsworth, M. T. (2003). Guide to cancer chemotherapy regimens 2003. *Oncology Special Edition, 6,* 139–154.

*Frumkin, H., Jacobson, A., Gansler, T., et al. (2001). Cellular phones and risk of brain tumors. *CA Cancer Journal for Clinicians, 51,* 137–141.

*Gralla, R. J., Osoba, D., Kris, M. G., et al. (1999). Recommendations for the use of antiemetics: Evidence-based, clinical practice guidelines. *Journal of Clinical Oncology, 17,* 2971–2994.

*Hesketh, P. J., Kris, M. G., Grunberg, S. M., et al. (1997). Proposal for the classifying the acute emetogenicity of cancer chemotherapy. *Journal of Clinical Oncology, 15,* 103–109.

*Hughes, W. T., Armstrong, D., Bodey, G. P., et al. (2002). 2002 Guidelines for the use of antimicrobial agents in neutropenic patients with cancer. *Clinical Infectious Diseases, 34,* 730–751.

*Jemal, A., Tiwari, R. C., Murray T., et al. (2004). Cancer statistics, 2004. *CA Cancer Journal for Clinicians, 54,* 8–29.

*Oh, W. K., & Kantoff, P. W. (1998). Management of hormone refractory prostate cancer: Current standards and future prospects. *Journal of Urology, 160,* 1220–1229.

*Ozer, H., Armitage, J. O., Bennett, C. L., et al. (2000). 2000 Update of recommendations for the use of hematopoietic colony-stimulating factors: Evidence-based, clinical practice guidelines. *Journal of Clinical Oncology, 18,* 3558–3585.

*Rubenstein, E. B., Peterson, D. E., Schubert, M., et al. (2004). Clinical practice guidelines for the prevention and treatment of cancer chemotherapy-induced oral and gastrointestinal mucositis. *Cancer, 100*(9 Suppl), 2026–2046.

*Saltz, L. B. (2003). Understanding and managing chemotherapy-induced diarrhea. *Journal of Supportive Oncology, 1,* 35–46.

*Schiller, J. H., Harrington, D., Belani, C. P., et al. (2002). Comparison of four chemotherapy regimens for advanced non-small cell lung cancer. *New England Journal of Medicine, 346,* 92–98.

*Therasse, P., Arbuck, S. G., Eisenhauer, E. A., et al. (2000). New guidelines to evaluate the response to treatment in solid tumors. *Journal of the National Cancer Institute, 92,* 205–216.

Visit the Connection web site for the most up-to-date drug information.

XIII

Pharmacotherapy in Health Promotion

57

IMMUNIZATIONS

■ CATHERINE KIRBY AND VIRGINIA P. ARCANGELO

Although the tendency is to place the primary focus of immunization efforts on infants and preschool children, immunization prophylaxis is important for all age groups— infants through older adults. This is particularly true when the potential loss of time from work, additional cost of health care, the possible need for additional caretakers, and potential side effects are considered. The dollar amount of these effects may be monumental. Relocation, change in job status or field of employment, travel, assumption of care- taker responsibilities, and the like may also place a person into a different risk category, requiring a review of immu- nization status. The challenge faced by practitioners is to develop a system that facilitates review of immunization sta- tus at all health care visits so that no opportunity is missed to update immunizations for those who are not adequately vaccinated and thus inadequately protected against prevent- able diseases.

Immunization prophylaxis offers an opportunity to prevent disease, improve clinical outcomes for those at high risk, and realize significant savings to the person in terms of cost, time, and resources. The plan to eradicate transmissible communi- cable diseases by the year 2000 and the reduced number of reported cases of communicable diseases have had a signifi- cant impact on preventing communicable diseases, reducing preventable complications, and improving clinical outcomes. In the United States, immunization has sharply curtailed or practically eliminated diphtheria, measles, mumps, pertussis, congenital and acquired rubella, tetanus, and *Haemophilus influenzae* type B disease. However, because these diseases persist in the United States and other countries, immunization prophylaxis needs to be continued. Recommendations for immunization prophylaxis come from multiple sources, including:

Advisory Committee on Immunization Practices (ACIP)
American Academy of Pediatrics (AAP)
American Academy of Family Physicians
Canadian Task Force on the Periodic Health Examination
U.S. Preventive Task Force and the Centers for Disease
    Control and Prevention

The Centers for Disease Control and Prevention (CDC) is responsible for providing vaccine management, technical assistance, information, epidemiology, and assessment. In January of each year, the immunization schedule is reviewed and revised as indicated.

CHARACTERISTICS OF IMMUNIZATIONS

Many infectious diseases can be prevented by immunopro- phylaxis, which is accomplished either through active or passive immunization. Active immunization involves giving a person either live or attenuated (live but killed; inactivated) vaccine to stimulate the development of immune system defenses against future natural exposure.

Active immunization involves administration of all or part of a microorganism or a modified product of that microor- ganism (eg, toxoid, a purified antigen, or an antigen pro- duced by genetic engineering) to evoke an immune response that mimics the response of the body to natural infection but that usually presents little or no risk to the recipient. Protec- tion may be afforded for a limited time or for a lifetime. If protection is for a limited time, the vaccine must be read- ministered at specified intervals.

Passive immunization is used for those people who have already been exposed or who have the potential to be exposed to certain infectious agents. Passive immunization involves the administration of a preformed antibody when the recipient has a congenitally acquired defect or immun- odeficiency, when exposure is likely to result in high-risk complications, or when time does not permit adequate pro- tection by active immunization (eg, immunizations against rabies or hepatitis B). In addition, passive immunity can be used therapeutically during active disease states to help sup- press the effects of a toxin or the inflammatory response.

VACCINES

Vaccines are the pharmacologic substances used to provide or boost immunity to disease. The major constituents of vaccines include active immunizing antigens (toxoid, live virus, or killed bacteria), suspending fluid, preservatives, stabilizers, antibiotics, and adjuvants. The differences depend on the manufacturer, and the person prescribing or administering the vaccine should check the package insert for the active and inert ingredients for each product. Potential allergic reactions may result from one or more of the preservatives, stabilizers,

Table 57.1

Vaccines Licensed in the United States and Their Routes of Administration

Vaccine[*]	Type	Route[†]
Adenovirus[‡]	Live virus	Oral
Anthrax[§]	Inactivated bacteria	SC
BCG	Live bacteria	ID (preferred) or SC
Cholera	Inactivated bacteria	SC, IM, or ID
DTP	Toxoids and inactivated bacteria	IM
DTaP	Toxoids and inactivated bacterial components	IM
Hepatitis A	Inactivated viral antigen	IM
Hepatitis B	Inactivated viral antigen	IM
Hib conjugates	Polysaccharide–protein conjugate	IM
Reconstituted with DTP	Polysaccharide–protein conjugate with toxoids and inactivated bacteria	IM
Reconstituted with DTaP	Polysaccharide–protein conjugate with toxoids and inactivated bacterial components	IM
Hib conjugate (PRP-OMP)-hepatitis B	Polysaccharide–protein conjugate with inactivated virus	IM
Influenza	Inactivated virus (whole virus), viral components	IM
Japanese encephalitis	Inactivated virus	SC
Lyme disease	Inactivated protein	IM
Measles	Live virus	SC
Meningococcal	Polysaccharide	SC
MMR	Live viruses	SC
Measles—rubella	Live viruses	SC
Mumps	Live viruses	SC
Pertussis[§]	Inactivated bacteria	IM
Plague	Inactivated bacteria	IM
Pneumococcal	Polysaccharide	IM or SC
Poliovirus:		
OPV	Live virus	Oral
IPV	Inactivated virus	SC
Rabies	Inactivated virus	IM or ID[‖]
Rubella	Live virus	SC
Tetanus	Toxoid	IM
Diphtheria-tetanus (dT, DT)	Toxoids	IM
Typhoid		
Parenteral	Inactivated bacteria	SC
Parenteral	Capsular polysaccharide	SC (boosters may be ID)
Oral	Live bacteria	Oral
Varicella	Live virus	SC
Yellow fever	Live virus	SC

[*]Vaccine abbreviations: BCG, bacillus Calmette-Guerin vaccine; DTP, diphtheria and tetanus toxoids and pertussis vaccine, adsorbed; DTaP, diphtheria and tetanus toxoids and acellular pertussis vaccine, adsorbed; Hib, *Haemophilus influenzae* type b vaccine; MMR, live measles–mumps–rubella viruses vaccine; OPV, oral poliovirus vaccine; IPV, inactivated poliovirus vaccine; dT, tetanus and diphtheria toxoid (for children ≥7 y and adults); DT, diphtheria and tetanus toxoids (for children <7 y).
[†]Route abbreviations: SC, subcutaneous; ID, intradermal; IM, intramuscular.
[‡]Available only to U.S. Armed Forces.
[§]Distributed by BioPort Corp., Lansing, MI.
[‖]Human diploid cell rabies vaccine for intradermal use is different in constitution and potency from the intramuscular vaccine; it should be used for pre-exposure immunization only. Rabies vaccine adsorbed (RVA and RabAvert) should not be used intradermally.
From cdc.gov/nip. Accessed on 4/21/05.

adjuvants, or antibiotics in the vaccine, and the recipient's sensitivity to one or more of the additives should be anticipated as a hypersensitivity. Current vaccines licensed in the United States are identified in Table 57-1.

RECOMMENDED CHILDHOOD AND ADOLESCENT IMMUNIZATION SCHEDULE

The recommended childhood immunization schedule for the United States is listed in Table 57-2. Table 57-3 presents the recommended immunizations for children who have not been immunized in the first year of life.

Recommendations for hepatitis B; diphtheria, tetanus, and pertussis (DTaP); *H. influenzae* type B disease; poliomyelitis; measles, mumps, and rubella (MMR); and varicella are included for birth to 16 years of age. Combination vaccines

are available that assist in reducing the number of injections a child must receive at any one time. In addition, recommended acceptable ranges for administration provide some flexibility regarding the number of injections administered at any one time as recommendations for catch-up vaccinations. A consideration for flexible scheduling should include parental or guardian compliance with appointments as well as office follow-up methods used for those patients who do not keep scheduled appointments for immunizations.

Special Circumstances

Preterm infants and children who are immunocompromised, infected with human immunodeficiency virus (HIV), lack a spleen, or have a personal or family history of seizures require special consideration when immunization prophylaxis is reviewed and administered.

Table 57.2

Recommended Childhood Immunization Schedule—United States, January–December 2000

Vaccines* are listed under the routinely recommended ages. Bars indicate range of acceptable ages for immunization. Catch-up immunization should be done during any visit when feasible. Shaded blocks indicate vaccines to be assessed and given if necessary during the early adolescent visit.

Catch-up Vaccination

Range of Acceptable Ages for Vaccination

Vaccine	Birth	1 mo	2 mo	4 mo	6 mo	12 mo	15 mo	18 mo	4–6 y	11–12 y	14–16 y
Hepatitis B[†]		Hep B-1									
			Hep B-2			Hep B-3				Hep B[‡]	
Diphtheria, tetanus, pertussis[‡]			DTaP	DTaP	DTaP		DTaP		DTaP	Td	
H. influenzae type b[§]			Hib	Hib	Hib	Hib					
Polio[l]			IPV[l]	IPV		IPV[l]			IPV[l]		
Measles, mumps, rubella[¶]						MMR			MMR[¶]	MMR[¶]	
Varicella**						Var				Var**	
Hepatitis A[††]								24 mo–12 y Hep A—in selected areas			

On October 22, 1999, the Advisory Committee on Immunization Practices (ACIP) recommended that Rotashield (RRV-TV), the only U.S.-licensed rotavirus vaccine, no longer be used in the United States (*MMWR*, Volume 48, Number 43, Nov. 5, 1999). Parents should be reassured that their children who received rotavirus vaccine before July are not at increased risk for intussusception now.

*This schedule indicates the recommended ages for routine administration of currently licensed childhood vaccines as of 11/1/99. Additional vaccines may be licensed and recommended during the year. Licensed combination vaccines may be used whenever any components of the combination are indicated and its other components are not contraindicated. Providers should consult the manufacturers' package inserts for detailed recommendations.

†*Infants born to hepatitis B surface antigen (HBsAg)-negative mothers* should receive the 1st dose of hepatitis B (Hep B) vaccine by age 2 months. The 2nd dose should be at least one month after the 1st dose. The 3rd dose should be administered at least 4 months after the 1st dose and at least 2 months after the 2nd dose, but not before 6 months of age for infants.
Infants born to HBsAg-positive mothers should receive hepatitis B vaccine and 0.5 mL hepatitis B immune globulin (HBIG) within 12 hours of birth at separate sites. The 2nd dose is recommended at 1 month of age and the 3rd dose at 6 months of age.
Infants born to mothers whose HBsAg status is unknown should receive hepatitis B vaccine within 12 hours of birth. Maternal blood should be drawn at the time of delivery to determine the mother's HBsAg status; if the HBsAg test is positive, the infant should receive HBIG as soon as possible (no later than 1 week of age).
All children and adolescents (through 18 years of age) who have not been immunized against hepatitis B may begin the series during any visit. Special efforts should be made to immunize children who were born in or whose parents were born in areas of the world with moderate or high endemicity of hepatitis B virus infection.

‡The 4th dose of DTaP (diphtheria and tetanus toxoids and acellular pertussis vaccine) may be administered as early as 12 months of age, provided 6 months have elapsed since the 3rd dose and the child is unlikely to return at age 15–18 months. Td (tetanus and diphtheria toxoids) is recommended at 11–12 years of age if at least 5 years have elapsed since the last dose of DTP, DTaP, or DT. Subsequent routine Td boosters are recommended every 10 years.

§Three *Haemophilus influenzae* type b (Hib) conjugate vaccines are licensed for infant use. If PRP-OMP (PedvaxHIB or ComVax [Merck]) is administered at 2 and 4 months of age, a dose at 6 months is not required. Because clinical studies in infants have demonstrated that using some combination products may induce a lower immune response to the Hib vaccine component, DTaP/Hib combination products should not be used for primary immunization in infants at 2, 4, or 6 months of age, unless FDA-approved for these ages.

lTo eliminate the risk of vaccine-associated paralytic polio (VAPP), an all-IPV schedule is now recommended for routine childhood polio vaccination in the United States. All children should receive four doses of IPV at 2 months, 4 months, 6–18 months, and 4–6 years. OPV (if available) may be used only for the following special circumstances:
1. Mass vaccination campaigns to control outbreaks of paralytic polio.
2. Unvaccinated children who will be traveling in <4 weeks to areas where polio is endemic or epidemic.
3. Children of parents who do not accept the recommended number of vaccine injections. These children may receive OPV only for the third or fourth dose or both; in this situation, health care providers should administer OPV only after discussing the risk for VAPP with parents or caregivers.
4. During the transition to an all-IPV schedule, recommendations for the use of remaining OPV supplies in physicians' offices and clinics have been issued by the American Academy of Pediatrics (see *Pediatrics,* December 1999).

¶The 2nd dose of measles, mumps, and rubella (MMR) vaccine is recommended routinely at 4–6 years of age but may be administered during any visit, provided at least 4 weeks have elapsed since receipt of the 1st dose and that both doses are administered beginning at or after 12 months of age. Those who have not previously received the second dose should complete the schedule by the 11–12-year-old visit.

**Varicella (Var) vaccine is recommended at any visit on or after the first birthday for susceptible children, that is, those who lack a reliable history of chickenpox (as judged by a health care provider) and who have not been immunized. Susceptible persons 13 years of age or older should receive 2 doses, given at least 4 weeks apart.

††Hepatitis A (Hep A) is shaded to indicate its recommended use in selected states and/or regions; consult your local public health authority. (Also see *MMWR* Oct. 01, 1999;48[RR12]; 1–37).

From Centers for Disease Control and Prevention. (2000). Recommended childhood immunization schedule—United States, 2000. Recommendations of the Advisory Committee on Immunization Practices. *Morbidity and Mortality Weekly Report.*

Table 57.3

Recommended Immunization Schedules for Children Not Immunized in the First Year of Life*

Recommended Time/Age	Immunization(s)[†,‡,§]	Comments
Younger Than 7 y		
First visit	DTaP, Hib,[†] HBV, MMR	If indicated, tuberculin testing may be done at same visit. If child is 5 y of age or older, Hib is not indicated in most circumstances.
Interval after first visit		
1 mo (4 wk)	DTaP, IPV, HBV, Var[§]	The second dose of IVP may be given if accelerated poliomyelitis vaccination is necessary, such as for travelers to areas where polio is endemic.
2 mo	DTaP, Hib,[†] IPV	Second dose of Hib is indicated only if the first dose was received when younger than 15 mo.
≥8 mo	DTaP, HBV, IPV	IPV and HBV are not given if the third doses were given earlier.
Age 4–6 y (at or before school entry)	DTaP, IPV, MMR[⊥]	DTaP is not necessary if the fourth dose was given after the fourth birthday; IPV is not necessary if the third dose was given after the fourth birthday.
Age 11–12 y	See Recommended Childhood Immunization Schedule for United States, January 2000.	
Age 7–12 y		
First visit	HBV, MMR, dT, IPV	IPV also may be given 1 mo after the first visit if accelerated poliomyelitis vaccination is necessary.
Interval after first visit		
2 mo (8 wk)	HBV, MMR, Var,[§] dT, IPV	
8–14 mo	HBV,[¶] dT, IPV	IPV is not given if the third dose was given earlier.
Age 11–12 y	See Recommended Childhood Immunization Schedule for United States, January 2000	

*Table is not completely consistent with all package inserts. For products used, also consult manufacturer's package insert for instructions on storage, handling, dosage, and administration. Biologics prepared by different manufacturers may vary, and package inserts of the same manufacturer may change. Therefore, the physician should be aware of the contents of the current package insert.

Vaccine abbreviations: HBV indicates hepatitis B virus vaccine; Var, varicella vaccine; DTaP, diphtheria and tetanus toxoids and acellular pertussis vaccine; Hib, *Haemophilus influenzae* type b conjugate vaccine; IPV, inactivated poliovirus vaccine; MMR, live measles–mumps–rubella vaccine; dT, adult tetanus toxoid (full dose) and diphtheria toxoid (reduced dose), for children ≥7 years and adults.

[†]If all needed vaccines cannot be administered simultaneously, priority should be given to protecting the child against those diseases that pose the greatest immediate risk. In the United States, these diseases for children younger than 2 years usually are measles and *Haemophilus influenzae* type b inflection; for children older than 7 years, they are measles, mumps, and rubella. Before 13 years of age, immunity against hepatitis B and varicella should be ensured.

DTaP, HBV, Hib, MMR, and Var can be given simultaneously at separate sites if failure of the patient to return for future immunizations is a concern.

For further information on pertussis and poliomyelitis immunization, see the respective chapters (Pertussis, p. 435, and Poliovirus Infections, p. 465).

[‡]See *Haemophilus influenzae* Infections, p. 262, and Table 3.11 (p. 268).

[§]Varicella vaccine can be administered to susceptible children any time after 12 months of age. Unvaccinated children who lack a reliable history of chicken pox should be vaccinated before their 13th birthday.

[⊥]Minimum interval between doses of MMR is 1 month (4 weeks).

[¶]HBV may be given earlier in a 0-, 2-, and 4-month schedule.

Source: cdc.gov/nip. Accessed on 4/21/05.

Preterm Infants

Preterm infants born to mothers who are negative for the hepatitis B surface antigen (HBsAg) should have hepatitis B immunization delayed until they weigh at least 2 kg or they are about to be discharged from the hospital. At the chronologic age of 2 months (including those infants still hospitalized), the infant should be given the immunizations routinely scheduled for that age. Note that inactivated poliovirus is the preferred vaccine because of the possible transmission of poliomyelitis (Pickering, 2003).

Preterm infants who are born to mothers who test positive for HBsAg should receive hepatitis B immune globulin within 12 hours of birth and concurrent hepatitis B vaccine (in the appropriate dose per package insert) at a different site. If the maternal HBsAg status is unknown, the vaccine should be given in accordance with the protocol for a mother who tests positive for HBsAg (Pickering, 2003). In addition, preterm infants who have chronic respiratory disease should receive the influenza vaccine annually in the fall beginning at age 6 months.

Immunosuppressed Children

Children who are immunosuppressed or immunodeficient are at risk for actually contracting the disease or experiencing serious adverse effects from live-bacteria or live-virus vaccines. Live vaccines are therefore contraindicated. In general, experience with vaccine administration to an immunosuppressed or immunodeficient child is limited. Efficacy is suboptimal because their ability to develop immunogenicity to a specific agent is altered owing to a depressed immune system.

Theoretical considerations are the only guide because experiential data are lacking or adverse consequences have not been reported.

Children with a deficiency in antibody-synthesizing capacity cannot respond to vaccines. These children should receive regular doses of immune globulin, usually intravenous immune globulin, that provide passive protection against many infectious diseases. Specific immune globulins (eg, varicella-zoster immune globulin) are available for postexposure prophylaxis for some infections. An exception appears to be the judicious use of live-virus varicella vaccine in children with acute lymphocytic leukemia in remission, in whom the risk of natural varicella outweighs the risk from the attenuated vaccine virus. This vaccine may be obtained from the manufacturer on a compassionate use protocol for patients between 12 months and 17 years of age who have acute lymphocytic leukemia in remission for at least 1 year.

Children With Transplants

Transplant recipients (eg, bone marrow transplant recipients) should also be viewed in a special light. Some experts elect to reimmunize all children without serologic evaluation, and others, because of the limited amount of data, recommend that immunization protocols be developed for these children in conjunction with experts in the fields of infectious disease and immunology. Information about the use of live-virus vaccines in organ transplant recipients is also limited. Only inactivated poliovirus vaccine should be given to transplant recipients and their household contacts.

Children Taking Corticosteroids

Children receiving corticosteroids also need careful consideration and thorough review of their medical history, including a review of the underlying disease, the specific dose and schedule of corticosteroids prescribed, and current immunization status, which includes an evaluation of risk factors relative to infectious disease. In general, children who have a disease (which suppresses the immune response) and who are receiving either systemic or locally administered corticosteroids (which also suppress the immune response) should not be given live-virus vaccines except in special circumstances. The guidelines for administering a live-virus vaccine to patients receiving corticosteroid therapy are based on the dosage in relation to the child's weight in kilograms and the duration of corticosteroid therapy. The following treatments do not contraindicate administration:

1. Topical therapy or local injections of corticosteroids
2. Physiologic maintenance doses of corticosteroids
3. Low or moderate dosage of systemic corticosteroids (<2 mg/kg/d of prednisone [Deltasone] or its equivalent or <20 mg/d or on alternate days if the child weighs >10 kg)

Special consideration should be given if high-dose corticosteroids are prescribed. Administration of high-dose corticosteroids (≥2 mg/kg/d of prednisone or its equivalent or ≥20 mg/d if the child weighs >10 kg) given daily or on alternate days for 14 days or less preempts administration of live-virus vaccines until the treatment is discontinued. Some experts recommend delaying immunization until 2 weeks after discontinuation of therapy.

Patients who receive high doses of systemic corticosteroids—daily or on alternate days for 14 days or more—should not receive live-virus vaccines until steroid therapy has been discontinued for at least 1 month. In addition, if clinical or laboratory evidence of systemic immunosuppression results from prolonged application, live-virus vaccines should not be administered until corticosteroid therapy has been discontinued for at least 1 month.

Children With Seizures

Infants and children with a personal or family history of seizures are at increased risk for having a convulsion after receiving either pertussis (as DTaP) or measles (as MMR) vaccine. Seizures are usually brief, self-limited, and generalized and occur in conjunction with fever (Pickering, 2003). However, in the case of DTaP vaccine administered during infancy, administration may coincide with or hasten the inevitable recognition of a seizure-related disorder, such as infantile spasms or epilepsy. This causes confusion about the role of the pertussis vaccine, and in this instance, pertussis immunization should be deferred until a progressive neurologic disorder is excluded or the cause of the seizure diagnosed.

Measles immunization, however, is usually given at an age when the cause and nature of the seizure activity have been established. Therefore, measles immunization should not be deferred in children with a history of one or more seizures.

Adolescents

Adolescents continue to be adversely affected by vaccine-preventable disease, including varicella, hepatitis B, measles, and rubella. In November 1996, the CDC issued recommendations for immunizing adolescents. Recommendations for adolescents at 11 and 12 years of age aim to improve the vaccine coverage and to establish routine visits to health care providers. These strategies reflect the recommendations of the ACIP, AAP, American Academy of Family Physicians, and American Medical Association. In addition to providing an opportunity for administering needed vaccines, such as hepatitis B, varicella, second dose of MMR, and tetanus and diphtheria booster, this visit provides an opportunity to render other recommended preventive services, including health behavior guidance; screening for biomedical, behavioral, and emotional conditions; and delivery of other health services. For more information, see Table 57-4.

IMMUNIZATION RECOMMENDATIONS FOR ADULTS

Immunization prophylaxis is as important for adults as it is for children. However, the practice of routinely reviewing and updating the vaccination status of adults remains an issue. Obstacles that affect adult vaccination rates include:

1. The practitioner's limited knowledge of specific recommendations
2. The patient's reluctance or refusal to be vaccinated
3. Liability and reimbursement issues

Table 57.4

Adolescent Vaccine-Specific Recommendations

Vaccine	Recommendations and Comments
Hepatitis B	Vaccinate adolescents 11–12 y of age who have not been previously vaccinated with 3-dose series of hepatitis B. In addition, those >12 y who are at increased risk for HBV infection should be vaccinated. Ensure completion of the series through a systematic approach for scheduling appointments and follow-up if missed.
MMR (second dose)	Administer the second dose of MMR to adolescents who have not received 2 doses of MMR at 12 mo of age or older.
Tetanus (Td) booster	Administer a booster dose of Td vaccine to adolescents at ages 11–12 or 14–16 y if they have received the primary series of vaccinations and if no dose has been received during the past 5 y. All subsequent doses (in the absence of tetanus prone injury) should be administered at 10-y intervals.
Varicella	Administer varicella virus vaccine to adolescents ages 11–12 y who do not have a reliable history of chickenpox and who have not been vaccinated with varicella virus vaccine.
Influenza	Administer annually to adolescents who, because of an underlying medical condition, are at risk for complications associated with influenza. Also, vaccinate adolescents who have close contact with people at high risk for complications associated with influenza.
Pneumococcal	Administer to adolescents who have chronic illnesses associated with increased risk for pneumococcal disease or its complications. Use adolescents' visits to providers to ensure that the vaccine has been administered to people for whom it is indicated.
Hepatitis A	Administer to unvaccinated adolescents who fall into the following categories: • Plan to travel or work in a country that has high or intermediate endemicity of hepatitis A virus (HAV) infection • Reside in a community that has a high rate of HAV infections and periodic outbreaks of hepatitis A • Are administered clotting factors • Have any of the following conditions or risk behaviors: chronic liver disease, use of illegal injecting/noninjection drugs, or if they are males who have sex with males.

From Centers for Disease Control and Prevention. (1996). Immunization of adolescents: Recommendations of Advisory Committee on Immunization Practices (ACIP), American Academy of Pediatrics, American Academy of Family Physicians and the American Medical Assoc. *Morbidity and Mortality Weekly Report 45*(RR-l3), 1–16.

As a result, many adults continue to be affected adversely by vaccine-preventable diseases such as varicella, hepatitis B, measles, and rubella. The ACIP and the CDC recommend that an overall review of vaccine status should be completed on all adults at 50 years of age. Table 57-5 summarizes risk factors and recommendations for adult immunizations.

DISEASE-SPECIFIC VACCINE RECOMMENDATIONS

Pneumococcal Vaccine 23-Valent

Pneumococcal infection causes an estimated 40,000 deaths annually in the United States, accounting for more deaths than any other vaccine-preventable bacterial disease. *Streptococcus pneumoniae* colonizes the upper respiratory tract and can cause disseminated invasive infections, including bacteremia and meningitis, pneumonia and other lower respiratory tract infections, and upper respiratory tract infections, including otitis media and sinusitis. The pneumococcal vaccine protects against invasive bacteremic disease, although existing data suggest that it is less effective in protecting against other types of pneumococcal infections.

In April 1997, the ACIP recommended that pneumococcal vaccine be used more extensively, particularly for identified high-risk populations (Table 57-6 and Box 57-1). Two available vaccines include 23 purified capsular polysaccharide antigens of *S. pneumoniae*. These replaced the earlier 14-valent vaccines in 1983. Revaccination should be considered for those people who previously received the 14-valent vaccine and who are at high risk for fatal infection. If an elderly patient's vaccination status is unknown, he or she should receive one dose of the vaccine. There are no data to support revaccination beyond two doses.

Response to Vaccine

Antibodies develop within 2 to 3 weeks in healthy young adults; immune responses are not consistent among all 23 serotypes in the vaccine. Antibody concentrations and responses to individual antigens tend to be lower in the following populations:

• The elderly
• People with alcoholic cirrhosis, chronic obstructive pulmonary disease, type 1 diabetes mellitus, Hodgkin's disease
• People with chronic renal failure requiring dialysis, renal transplantation, nephrotic syndrome
• People with acquired immunodeficiency syndrome, HIV infection

Special Circumstances

Antibody response is diminished or absent in people who are immunocompromised or who have leukemia, lymphoma, or multiple myeloma. The antibody levels to most pneumococcal vaccine antigens remain elevated for at least 5 years in healthy adults.

A more rapid decline (within 3–5 years) occurs in certain children who have undergone splenectomy after trauma and in those who have sickle cell disease. Antibody concentrations also decline after 5 to 10 years in elderly people, those who have undergone splenectomy, patients with renal disease requiring dialysis, and people who have received transplants. A lower antibody response or rapid decline in antibody levels is also noted in patients with Hodgkin's disease and multiple myeloma. At least 2 weeks should elapse between immunization and the initiation of chemotherapy or immunosuppressive therapy.

Table 57.5

Summary of Recommendations for Adult Immunization

Vaccine Name and Route	For Whom it Is Recommended	Schedule
Influenza ("flu shot") Give IM	• Adults age 50 y or older • People 6 mo to 65 y of age with medical problems such as heart disease, lung disease, diabetes, renal dysfunction, hemoglobinopathies, immunosuppression, and/or those living in chronic care facilities • People (≥6 mo of age) working or living with at-risk people • All health care workers and those who provide key community services • Healthy pregnant women who will be in their 2nd or 3rd trimesters during the influenza season • Pregnant women who have underlying medical conditions should be vaccinated before the flu season, regardless of the stage of pregnancy. • Anyone who wishes to reduce the likelihood of becoming ill with influenza • Travelers to areas where influenza activity exists	• Given every year • October through November is the optimal time to receive an annual flu shot to maximize protection, but the vaccine may be given at any time during the influenza season (typically December through March) or at other times when the risk of influenza exists. • May be given with all other vaccines but at a separate site
Pneumococcal Give IM or SC	• Adults age 65 or older • People 2–65 y old who have chronic illness or other risk factors	• Routinely given as a one-time dose; administer if previous vaccination history is unknown. • One-time revaccination is recommended 5 y later for people at highest risk of fatal pneumococcal infection or rapid antibody loss (eg, renal disease) and for people ≥65 y if the 1st dose was given prior to age 65 and ≥5 y have elapsed since previous dose. • May be given with all other vaccines but at a separate site
Hepatitis B (Hep-B) Give IM; brands may be used interchangeably.	• High-risk adults, including household contacts and sex partners of HBsAg-positive people; users of illicit injectable drugs; heterosexuals with more than one sex partner in 6 mo; men who have sex with men; people with recently diagnosed STDs; patients in hemodialysis units and patients with renal disease that may result in dialysis; recipients of certain blood products; health care workers and public safety workers who are exposed to blood; clients and staff of institutions for the developmentally disabled; inmates of long-term correctional facilities, and certain international travelers. *Note:* Prior serologic testing may be recommended depending on the specific level of risk and/or likelihood of previous exposure • All adolescents *Note:* In 1997, the NIH Consensus Development Conference, a panel of national experts, recommended that hepatitis B vaccination be given to all persons infected with hepatitis C virus. *Ed. note: Do serologic screening for people who have emigrated from endemic areas. When HBsAg-positive people are identified, offer them appropriate disease management. In addition, screen their household members and intimate contacts and, if found susceptible, vaccinate.*	• Three doses are needed on a 0, 1, 6 mo schedule. • Alternative timing options for vaccination include: 0, 2, 4 mo 0, 1, 4 mo • There must be 4 wk between doses #1 and #2, and 8 wk between doses #2 and #3. Overall there must be at least 4 mo between doses #1 and #3. • **Schedule for those who have fallen behind:** If the series is delayed between doses, do not start the series over. Continue from where you left off. • May be given with all other vaccines but at a separate site.
Hepatitis A (Hep-A) Give IM; brands may be used interchangeably.	• People who travel outside of the U.S. (except for Northern and Western Europe, New Zealand, Australia, Canada, and Japan) • People with chronic liver disease, including people with hepatitis C virus infection; people with hepatitis B who have chronic liver disease; illicit drug users; men who have sex with men; people with clotting factor disorders; people who work with hepatitis A virus in experimental lab settings (this does not refer to routine medical laboratories); and food handlers where health authorities or private employers determine vaccination to be cost-effective *Note:* Prevaccination testing is likely to be cost effective for people >40 y of age as well as for younger people in certain groups with a high prevalence of hepatitis A virus infection.	• Two doses are needed. • The minimum interval between dose #1 and #2 is 6 mo. • If dose #2 is delayed, do not repeat dose #1. Just give dose #2. • May be given with all other vaccines but at a separate site.
dT (tetanus, diphtheria) Give IM	• All adolescents and adults • After the primary series has been completed, a booster dose is recommended every 10 y. Make sure patients have received a primary series of 3 doses. • A booster dose as early as 5 y later may be needed for the purpose of wound management, so consult ACIP recommendations.	• Booster dose every 10 y after completion of the primary series of 3 doses • **For those who have fallen behind:** The primary series is 3 doses: • Give dose #2 four weeks after #1. • #3 is given 6–12 mo after #2. • May be given with all other vaccines but at a separate site

(continued)

Table 57.5

Summary of Recommendations for Adult Immunization (*Continued*)

Vaccine Name and Route	For Whom it Is Recommended	Schedule
MMR (measles, mumps, rubella) Give SC	• Adults born in 1957 or later who are ≥18 y of age (including those born outside the U.S.) should receive at least one dose of MMR if there is no serologic proof of immunity or documentation of a dose given on or after 1st birthday • Adults in high-risk groups, such as health care workers, students entering colleges and other post–high school educational institutions, and international travelers should receive a total of two doses • All women of childbearing age (ie, adolescent girls and premenopausal adult women) who do not have acceptable evidence of rubella immunity or vaccination *Note:* Adults born before 1957 are usually considered immune, but proof of immunity may be desirable for health care workers.	• One or 2 doses are needed. • If dose #2 is recommended, give it no sooner than 4 wk after dose #1. • May be given with all other vaccines but at a separate site • If varicella vaccine and MMR are both needed and are not administered on the same day, space them at least 4 wk apart.
Varicella (Var; "chickenpox shot") Give SC	• All susceptible adults and adolescents should be vaccinated. Make special efforts to vaccinate susceptible people who have close contact with people at high risk for serious complications (eg, health care workers and family contacts of immunocompromised people) and susceptible people who are at high risk of exposure (eg, teachers of young children, day care employees, residents and staff in institutional settings such as colleges and correctional institutions, military personnel, adolescents and adults living with children, nonpregnant women of childbearing age, and international travelers who do not have evidence of immunity) *Note:* People with reliable histories of chickenpox (such as self- or parental report of disease) can be assumed to be immune. For adults who have no reliable history, serologic testing may be cost effective because most adults with a negative or uncertain history of varicella are immune.	• Two doses are needed. • Dose #2 is given 4–8 wk after dose #1. • May be given with all other vaccines but at a separate site • If varicella vaccine and MMR are both needed and are not administered on the same day, space them at least 4 wk apart. • If the second dose is delayed, do not repeat dose #1. Just give dose #2.
Polio (IPV) Give IM or SC	• Not routinely recommended for people 18 y of age and older *Note:* Adults living in the U.S. who never received or completed a primary series of polio vaccine need not be vaccinated unless they intend to travel to areas where exposure to wild-type virus is likely. Previously vaccinated adults should receive one booster dose if traveling to polio endemic areas.	• Refer to ACIP recommendations regarding unique situations, schedules, and dosing information. • May be given with all other vaccines but at a separate site
Lyme disease Give IM	• Consider for people 15–70 y of age who reside, work, or recreate in areas of high or moderate risk and who engage in activities that result in frequent or prolonged exposure to tick-infested habitat. • People with a history of previous uncomplicated Lyme disease who are at continued high risk for Lyme disease (See description in the first bullet.) • See ACIP statement for a definition of high and moderate risk.	• Three doses are needed. Give at intervals of 0, 1, and 12 mo. Schedule dose #1 (given in y 1) and dose #3 (given in y 2) to be given several weeks before tick season. See ACIP statement for details. • Safety of administering Lyme disease vaccine with other vaccines has not been established. • ACIP says if it must be administered concurrently with other vaccines, give it at a separate site.

HBsAg, hepatitis B surface antigen.

From the Advisory Committee on Immunization Practices (ACIP) by the Immunization Action Coalition with review by ad hoc team—August 1999.

Note: For specific ACIP immunization recommendations refer to the full statements that are published in the *MMWR.* To obtain a complete set of ACIP statements, call (800) 232-2522, or to access individual statements, visit CDC's web site: www.cdc.gov/nip/publications/ACIP-list.htm

This table will be revised approximately once a year because of the changing nature of national immunization recommendations. Check our web site (www.immunize.org) to make sure you have the most current copy.

Revaccination is recommended once for patients who are 2 years of age or older, who are at highest risk for serious pneumococcal infection, and who are likely to have a rapid decline in antibody levels provided that 5 years have elapsed since receiving the first dose of vaccine.

Pneumococcal Conjugate Vaccine

In June 2000, the U.S. Food and Drug Administration licensed a heptavalent pneumococcal conjugate vaccine, PCV7 (Prevnar). This vaccine is recommended for universal use in children 23 months of age and younger. The number of doses for the primary series varies with the age of the child at the first dose (Table 57-7).

Children 24 to 59 months of age who are at high risk for invasive pneumococcal infection and who have not been previously immunized should also receive 23-valent vaccine to expand the serotype coverage. Indications for children 24 months of age and older who are considered to be at moderate or low risk remain under investigation because current data are insufficient to recommend routine administration (Table 57-8).

Influenza Vaccine

Influenza and pneumonia are the sixth leading cause of death in the United States and fifth in older adults. Fatalities from influenza begin to rise in midlife and are highest in

Table 57.6

Recommendations for the Use of Pneumococcal Vaccine

Groups for Which Vaccination Is Recommended	Strength of Recommendation*	Revaccination†
Immunocompetent People‡		
People aged ≥65 y	A	Second dose of vaccine if patient received vaccine ≥5 y previously and was age <65 y at the time of vaccination
People aged 2–64 y with chronic cardiovascular disease,§ chronic pulmonary disease, or diabetes mellitus	A	Not recommended
People aged 2–64 y with alcoholism, chronic liver disease,¶ or cerebrospinal fluid leaks	B	Not recommended
People aged 2–64 y with functional or anatomic asplenia**	A	If patient is aged >10 y: single revaccination ≥5 y after previous dose. If patient is aged ≤10 y: consider revaccination 3 y after previous dose
People aged 2–64 y living in special environments or social settings††	C	Not recommended
Immunocompromised People		
Immunocompromised people aged ≥2 y, including those with HIV infection, leukemia, lymphoma, Hodgkin's disease, multiple myeloma, generalized malignancy, chronic renal failure, or nephrotic syndrome; those receiving immunosuppressive chemotherapy (including corticosteroids); and those who have received an organ or bone marrow transplant	C	Single revaccination if ≥5 y have elapsed since receipt of first dose. If patient is aged ≤10 y: consider revaccination 3 y after previous dose

*The following categories reflect the strength of evidence supporting the recommendations for vaccination:
  A = Strong epidemiologic evidence and substantial clinical benefit support the recommendation for vaccine use.
  B = Moderate evidence supports the recommendation for vaccine use.
  C = Effectiveness of vaccination is not proven, but the high risk for disease and the potential benefits and safety of the vaccine justify vaccination.
†Strength of evidence for all revaccination recommendations is "C."
‡If earlier vaccination status is unknown, patients in this group should be administered pneumococcal vaccine.
§Including congestive heart failure and cardiomyopathies.
\Including chronic obstructive pulmonary disease and emphysema.
¶Including cirrhosis.
**Including sickle cell disease and splenectomy.
††Including Alaskan Natives and certain American Indian populations.
From Centers for Disease Control and Prevention. (1997). Prevention of Pneumococcal disease: Recommendation of Advisory Committee on Immunization Practices (ACIP). *Morbidity and Mortality Weekly Report, 46*(RR-8), 1–24.

BOX 57-1. CHILDREN AT HIGH OR MODERATE RISK OF INVASIVE PNEUMOCOCCAL INFECTION

High Risk (attack rate of invasive pneumococcal disease > 150/100,000 cases/y)
- Sickle cell disease, congenital or acquired asplenia, or splenic dysfunction
- Infection with human immunodeficiency virus

Presumed High Risk (attack rate not calculated)
- Congenital immune deficiency: some B- (humoral) or T-lymphocyte deficiencies, complement deficiencies (particularly C1, C2, C3, and C4 deficiencies), or phagocytic disorders (excluding chronic granulomatous disease)
- Chronic cardiac disease (particularly cyanotic congenital heart disease and cardiac failure)
- Chronic pulmonary disease (including asthma treated with high-dose oral corticosteroid therapy)
- Cerebrospinal fluid leaks

- Chronic renal insufficiency, including nephrotic syndrome
- Diseases associated with immunosuppressive therapy or radiation therapy (including malignant neoplasms, leukemias, lymphomas, and Hodgkin's disease) and solid organ transplantation*
- Diabetes mellitus

Moderate Risk (attack rate of invasive pneumococcal disease > 20 cases/100,000/y)
- All children 24–35 mo of age
- Children 36–59 mo of age attending out-of-home care
- Children 36–59 mo of age who are of Native American, Alaskan Native, or African American descent

*Guidelines for the use of pneumococcal vaccines for children who have received bone marrow transplants are currently undergoing revision (CDC, personal communication).

Table 57.7

AAP Recommended Schedule of Doses for Heptavalent Pneumococcal Conjugate Vaccine (PCV7), Including Primary Series and Catch-up Immunizations, in Previously Unvaccinated Children

Age at First Dose	Primary Series	Booster Dose*
2–6 mo	3 doses, 6–8 wk apart	1 dose at 12–15 mo of age
7–11 mo	2 doses, 6–8 wk apart	1 dose at 12–15 mo of age
12–23 mo	2 doses, 6–8 wk apart	
≥24 mo†	1 dose	

*Booster doses to be given at least 6 to 8 wk after the final dose of the primary series.
†The AAP is not recommending *universal* immunization of low- and moderate-risk children in this age group at this time.

persons with chronic disease. Measures available to reduce the incidence of influenza include immunoprophylaxis with inactivated (killed virus) vaccine and chemoprophylaxis. Before the influenza season gets under way, vaccination of people at risk and those likely to transmit influenza to at-risk populations is the most effective measure. The vaccine is associated with a decrease in influenza-related respiratory illness in all age groups, decreased hospitalization and death in people at high risk, decreased incidence of otitis media in children, and decreased work and school absenteeism.

Two types of influenza vaccine are available—inactivated virus and live attenuated vaccine (in the form of nasal spray). The live virus is recommended for those 5 to 49 years old and is contraindicated in patients who are immunocompromised and require a protected environment, health care workers, and household members who are in close contact with the immunocompromised individual. If a live virus is given, the patient should not have contact with those who are immunocompromised for 7 days.

Groups at Risk

People at increased risk for influenza-related complications include:

1. Those 50 years of age or older
2. Children aged 6 to 23 months

3. Adults and children with pulmonary disease, including asthma
4. Adults and children who have required regular medical follow-up or hospitalization during the preceding year because of chronic metabolic diseases (including diabetes mellitus), renal dysfunction, hemoglobinopathies, or immunosuppression (including immunosuppression caused by medications or HIV infection)
5. Children and teenagers on long-term aspirin therapy who might be at risk for development of Reye syndrome after influenza
6. Women in the second or third trimester of pregnancy during the influenza season
7. Persons who live with or care for persons at high risk, including health care workers and household contacts (including children birth to 23 months)

Transmission of Influenza

Just as immunizing people in groups at high risk for flu and its complications is important, so too is immunizing those who are most likely to transmit the disease. Groups that can transmit influenza to people at high risk include health care workers (in hospital and outpatient settings and in emergency response service), employees of nursing homes and chronic care facilities who have contact with patients or residents, employees of assisted living and other residences for people in high-risk groups, providers of home care to people at high risk (eg, visiting nurses, volunteers), household contacts of high-risk individuals, and providers of essential community services. Additional populations for consideration include people with HIV infection, breast-feeding mothers, people traveling to foreign countries, students or other people in institutional settings, and the general populace who want to reduce the likelihood of contracting influenza.

The dose for all age groups is outlined in Table 57-9.

The optimal time for an organized influenza vaccination campaign in the United States is October through mid-November. However, the vaccine can be given as early as September so as not to miss an opportunity for vaccination. Antibody development after vaccination in healthy adults can take as long as 2 weeks and as long as 6 weeks in children—or 2 weeks after the second dose.

Table 57.8

AAP Recommendations for Pneumococcal Immunization With Heptavalent Pneumococcal Conjugate Vaccine (PCV7) or 23-Valent Pneumococcal Polysaccharide (23PS) Vaccines for Children at High Risk* for Pneumococcal Disease

Age	Previous Doses	Recommendations
≤23 mo	None	PCV7
24–59 mo	4 doses of PCV7	1 dose of 23PS at 24 mo, at least 6–8 wk after last dose of PCV7
		1 dose of 23PS, 3–5 y after the first dose of 23PS
24–59 mo	1–3 doses of PCV7	1 dose of PCV7
		1 dose of 23PS, 6–8 wk after the last dose of PCV7
		1 dose of 23PS, 3–5 y after the first dose of 23PS
24–59 mo	1 dose of 23PS	2 doses of PCV7, 6–8 wk apart, beginning at least 6–8 wk after last dose of 23PS
		1 dose of 23PS, 3–5 y after the first dose of 23PS
24–59 mo	None	2 doses of PCV7, 6–8 wk apart
		1 dose of 23PS, 6–8 wk after the last dose of PCV7
		1 dose of 23PS, 3–5 y after the first dose of 23PS

*Children at high risk are those with sickle cell disease, asplenia, or splenic dysfunction, and those with HIV infection.

Table 57.9

Influenza Vaccine* Dosage, by Age Group—United States, 2000–2001 Season

Age Group	Product	Dosage	No. of Doses	Route
6–35 mo	Split virus only	0.25 mL	1 or 2*	IM
3–8 y	Split virus only	0.50 mL	1 or 2*	IM
9–12 y	Split virus only	0.50 mL	1	IM
>12 y	Whole or split virus	0.50 mL	1	IM

*Two doses administered at least 1 mo apart are recommended for children <9 y of age who are receiving the vaccine for the first time.
From Centers for Disease Control and Prevention. (2000). Prevention and control of influenza: Recommendations of Advisory Committee of Immunization Practices (ACIP). *Morbidity and Mortality Weekly Report, 49*(RR-3), 1–38.

Chemoprophylaxis with antiviral agents, amantadine (Symmetrel), rimantadine (Flumadine), zanamivir (Relenza), and oseltamivir (Tamiflu) can also be helpful. When administered within 48 hours of the onset of illness, they can reduce the severity and shorten the duration of illness in otherwise healthy people. In November 2000, the FDA also approved oseltamivir (Tamiflu) for use in the prevention of influenza in adults and children 13 years and older. For more information, see Table 57-10.

Prevention of Meningococcal Disease

Approximately 3000 cases of meningococcal diseases occur in the United States each year, with a fatality rate of 10% despite antibiotic therapy early in the illness. During 1991 to 1998, the highest rate occurred among infants younger than 12 months of age. Mortality rates for people 18 to 23 years of age were higher than those for the general population.

In June 2000, the ACIP recommended that the following high-risk groups be considered for meningococcal vaccine:

- People with terminal complement component deficiencies and those who have anatomic or functional asplenia
- Research, industrial, and clinical laboratory personnel who are exposed routinely to *Neisseria meningitidis* in solutions that may be in aerosol form

- Travelers with prolonged contact with the local population in countries where *N. meningitidis* is epidemic or hyperendemic

In addition, in an effort to educate students and parents about the risk of disease and the vaccine, the ACIP issued the following recommendations regarding the use of meningococcal polysaccharide vaccines for college students:

- Providers of medical care to incoming and current college freshmen, particularly those who plan to or already live in dormitories and residence halls, should, during routine medical care, inform these students and their parents about meningococcal disease and the benefits of vaccination. ACIP does not recommend that the level of increased risk among freshmen warrants any specific changes in living situations for freshmen.
- College freshmen who want to reduce their risk for meningococcal disease should either be administered vaccine or directed to a site where vaccine is available.
- The risk for meningococcal disease among non-freshman college students is similar to that for the general population. However, the vaccine is safe and efficacious and, therefore, can be provided to non-freshman undergraduates who want to reduce their risk for meningococcal disease.

Table 57.10

Recommended Daily Dose for Anti-influenza Treatment and Prophylaxis

Antiviral Agent	Age Group (y)			
	1–9	10–13	14–64	≥65
amantadine (Symmetrel)				
Treatment	5 mg/kg/d up to 150 mg in 2 divided doses	100 mg bid	100 mg bid	≤100 mg/d
Prophylaxis	5 mg/kg/d up to 150 mg in 2 divided doses	100 mg bid	100 mg bid	≤100 mg/d
rimantadine (Flumadine)				
Treatment	NA	NA	100 mg bid	100 or 200 mg/d
Prophylaxis	5 mg/kg/d up to 150 mg in 2 divided doses	100 mg bid	100 mg bid	100 or 200 mg/d
zanamivir (Relenza)				
Treatment	NA	10 mg bid	10 mg bid	10 mg bid
Prophylaxis	NA	NA	NA	NA
oseltamivir (Tamiflu)				
Treatment	NA	NA	75 mg bid	75 mg bid
Prophylaxis	NA	NA	NA	NA

NA, not applicable.
From Centers for Disease Control and Prevention. (2000). Prevention and control of influenza: Recommendations of Advisory Committee on Immunization Practices (ACIP). *Morbidity and Mortality Weekly Report, 49*(RR-3), 1–38.

- Colleges should inform incoming or current freshmen, particularly those who plan to live or already live in dormitories or residence halls, about the meningococcal disease and the availability of a safe and effective vaccine.
- College students who are at higher risk for meningococcal disease because of an underlying immunodeficiency or who are traveling to areas where *N. meningitidis* is epidemic or hyperendemic should be vaccinated.
- College students who are employed as research, industrial, and clinical laboratory personnel who are exposed routinely to *N. meningitidis* in solutions that may be in aerosol form should be considered for vaccination.

ADVERSE EVENTS ASSOCIATED WITH VACCINES

Risks of vaccination vary from inconvenient to severe and life-threatening. Common vaccine side effects (eg, fever and local irritation to DTaP vaccine) are usually mild to moderate in severity and without permanent consequences. However, serious side effects and adverse reactions are possible, although the occurrence of an adverse event does not prove causation by the vaccine (ie, the adverse event may be caused by factors other than the vaccine).

Reporting of adverse events is important because it may provide clues to unanticipated adverse reactions. It is important to interview the patient or guardian regarding any side effects after past immunizations. Any unexpected, reported, and observed event that required medical attention soon after the administration should be described in detail in the patient's medical record and reported using the Vaccine Adverse Events Reporting System (VAERS).

The VAERS is a result of the National Childhood Injury Act of 1986, which made provisions for health care providers to report occurrences of certain adverse events and to maintain permanent immunization records. Pertinent information to be reported includes a detailed description of the event (signs and symptoms reported and observed) and the time from administration of vaccine to presentation of signs and symptoms.

Pertinent patient history information should be noted regarding any existing physician-diagnosed allergies, medical conditions, and birth defects as well as any illness at the time of vaccine administration. In addition, information about the vaccine must be included. Documentation should identify the type of vaccine, the manufacturer, lot number, site and route of administration, and any previous doses received.

Staff from VAERS contact the provider (reporter) for follow-up of the patient's condition at 60 days and at 1 year after the initial reporting of adverse events. Box 57-2 contains the VAERS form.

CONTRAINDICATIONS TO VACCINATIONS

The primary contraindications to vaccine administration are acute febrile illness, allergy to a vaccine component, or history of hypersensitivity/anaphylactic reaction to vaccine constituents. Table 57-11 includes a detailed listing of contraindications by vaccine. The four main types of hypersensitivity reactions include:

1. Allergic reactions to egg-related antigens (eg, MMR, yellow fever)
2. Mercury sensitivity in some recipients of vaccines or immune globulin
3. Antibiotic-induced allergic reactions (eg, inactivated or oral poliovirus vaccine—trace streptomycin, neomycin, and polymyxin B; MMR, including single or combined with varicella—trace neomycin)
4. Hypersensitivity to other vaccine components, including the infectious agent

Acute febrile illness suggesting a moderate to severe illness is sufficient reason to defer vaccination until the person recovers. Guidelines in this instance are based on the provider's assessment of the illness and the vaccines scheduled for administration.

The rationale for withholding vaccination in moderate to severe illness, with or without fever, is that evolving signs and symptoms associated with the illness may be difficult to distinguish from the reaction to the vaccine. Minor illness (minor respiratory, gastrointestinal, or other illness) and low-grade fevers are not contraindications to immunization. The benefit of the immunization at the recommended age, regardless of the presence of mild illness, outweighs the risk of vaccine failure (Pickering, 2003).

Pregnancy is an additional contraindication to the administration of live-virus vaccines. In some cases, immunization of immunodeficient and immunosuppressed children is contraindicated (see the preceding discussions on immunocompromised children).

PATIENT AND PROVIDER EDUCATION AND ISSUES

Patient and health care provider/practitioner education, updates on immunization protocols, and established office systems with designated areas of responsibility are significant factors in improving immunization rates. Office routines and systems should incorporate pediatric immunization standards (Box 57-3) and facilitate use of all possible opportunities to review and update the immunization status of each patient. Tickler systems, chart reminders, and flow sheets that identify needed immunizations clearly and visibly are useful adjuncts to patient care.

A team approach to staff involvement also helps to enhance vaccination rates. Support staff should be aware of immunization needs when scheduling return or preventive visits as well as visits for illness or minor health problems. Visual reminders on the patient's chart or visit-encounter form can be used to alert the practitioner to review specific vaccine needs or requests. Box 57-4 presents recommendations related to the immunization schedule, and Box 57-5 offers answers to frequently asked questions about immunization.

Vaccines should be stored in the office in sufficient amounts to meet the needs of the patients. Staff should have specific assignments to monitor stock levels, lot numbers, and expiration dates. Vaccines should be stored according to the manufacturer's recommendations with a back-up system to identify times when power outages may have affected vaccines, particularly during nonbusiness hours. Methods can range from plugging in a digital clock in the same outlet to

BOX 57-2. VACCINE ADVERSE EVENT REPORTING SYSTEM FORM

VACCINE ADVERSE EVENT REPORTING SYSTEM
24 Hour Toll-Free Information 1-800-822-7967
P.O. Box 1100, Rockville, MD 20849-1100
PATIENT IDENTITY KEPT CONFIDENTIAL

For CDC/FDA Use Only

VAERS Number _____

Date Received _____

Patient Name:

Last   First   M.I.

Address

_____

_____

_____

City   State   Zip

Telephone no. (____) _____

Vaccine administered by (Name):

_____

Responsible
Physician _____

Facility Name/Address

_____

_____

_____

City   State   Zip

Telephone no. (____) _____

Form completed by (Name):

_____

Relation   ☐ Vaccine Provider ☐ Patient/Parent
to Patient ☐ Manufacturer   ☐ Other

Address (if different from patient or provider)

_____

_____

_____

City   State   Zip

Telephone no. (____) _____

| 1. State | 2. County where administered | 3. Date of birth ___/___/___ mm dd yy | 4. Patient age | 5. Sex ☐ M ☐ F | 6. Date form completed ___/___/___ mm dd yy |

7. Describe adverse events(s) (symptoms, signs, time course) and treatment, if any

8. Check all appropriate:
☐ Patient died   (date ___/___/___ mm dd yy)
☐ Life threatening illness
☐ Required emergency room/doctor visit
☐ Required hospitalization (____ days)
☐ Resulted in prolongation of hospitalization
☐ Resulted in permanent disability
☐ None of the above

9. Patient recovered ☐ YES ☐ NO ☐ UNKNOWN

10. Date of vaccination   11. Adverse event onset
___/___/___ mm dd yy   ___/___/___ mm dd yy
Time _____ AM/PM   Time _____ AM/PM

12. Relevant diagnostic tests / laboratory data

13. Enter all vaccines given on date listed in no. 10

	Vaccine (type)	Manufacturer	Lot number	Route/Site	No. Previous Doses
a.					
b.					
c.					
d.					

14. Any other vaccinations within 4 weeks prior to the date listed in no. 10

	Vaccine (type)	Manufacturer	Lot number	Route/Site	No. Previous doses	Date given
a.						
b.						

15. Vaccinated at:
☐ Private doctor's office/hospital   ☐ Military clinic/hospital
☐ Public health clinic/hospital   ☐ Other/unknown

16. Vaccine purchased with:
☐ Private funds ☐ Military funds
☐ Public funds   ☐ Other/unknown

17. Other medications

18. Illness at time of vaccination (specify)

19. Pre-existing physician-diagnosed allergies, birth defects, medical conditions (specify)

20. Have you reported this adverse event previously?
☐ NO   ☐ To health department
☐ To doctor   ☐ To manufacturer

Only for children 5 and under

22. Birth weight
_____ lb. _____ oz.

23. No. of brothers and sisters

21. Adverse event following prior vaccination (check all applicable, specify)

	Adverse Event	Onset Age	Type Vaccine	Dose no. in series
☐ In patient				
☐ In brother or sister				

Only for reports submitted by manufacturer/immunization project

24. Mfr./ imm. proj. report no.

25. Date received by Mfr./imm. proj.

26. 15 day report?
☐ Yes ☐ No

27. Report type
☐ Initial ☐ Follow-Up

Health care providers and manufacturers are required by law (42 USC 300ss-25) to report reactions to vaccines listed in the Table of Reportable Events Following Immunization. Reports for reactions to other vaccines are voluntary except when required as a condition of immunization grant awards.

Form VAERS-1(poa)

---

use of alarm systems on the freezer or refrigerator. An inexpensive method of detecting a power outage uses a cup of ice with a penny or other coin placed on top of the ice. The length of a power outage may be judged by how far the coin sinks in the previously completely frozen ice. If power outages occur, the pharmaceutical manufacturer should be contacted for information about vaccine use, revised expiration dates, or unusable vaccine. Staff members should not automatically assume that vaccine should be discarded.

A central log book, maintained by date and time and including lot numbers and expiration dates of the vaccines, is recommended. Used with patient schedule information and chart documentation, the log book helps identify patients should a pharmaceutical company notify the office

Table 57.11

Guide to Contraindications and Precautions to Immunizations, January 2000

Vaccine	True Contraindications and Precautions	Not True (Vaccines May Be Given)
General for all vaccines (DTaP/DTP[c] IPV, OPV, MMR, Hib, HBV, Var)	Anaphylactic reaction to a vaccine contraindicates further doses of that vaccine. Anaphylactic reaction to a vaccine constituent contraindicates the use of vaccines containing that substance. Moderate or severe illnesses with or without a fever	Mild to moderate local reaction (soreness, redness, swelling) after a dose of an injectable antigen Low-grade or moderate fever after a prior vaccine dose Mild acute illness with or without low-grade fever Current antimicrobial therapy Convalescent phase of illnesses Prematurity (same dosage and indications as for normal, full-term infants) Recent exposure to an infectious disease History of penicillin or other nonspecific allergies or fact that relatives have such allergies Pregnancy of mother or household contact Unvaccinated household contact
DTaP/DTP[c]	Encephalopathy within 7 d of administration of previous dose of DTaP/DTP Precautions:[1] Fever of ≥40.5°C (104.8°F) within 48 h after vaccination with a prior dose of DTaP/DTP Collapse or shock-like state (hypotonic–hyporesponsive episode) within 48 h of receiving a prior dose of DTaP/DTP Seizures within 3 d of receiving a prior dose of DTaP/DTP[d] Persistent, inconsolable crying lasting 3 h, within 48 h of receiving a prior dose of DTaP/DTP Guillain-Barré syndrome (GBS) within 6 wk after a dose[e]	Family history of seizures[d] Family history of sudden infant death syndrome Family history of an adverse event after DTaP/DTP administration
IPV	Anaphylactic reaction to neomycin or streptomycin Precaution: pregnancy	
OPV[f,g]	Infection with HIV or a household contact with HIV Known altered immunodeficiency (hematologic and solid tumors; congenital immunodeficiency; and long-term immunosuppressive therapy) Immunodeficient household contact Precaution: pregnancy	Breast-feeding Current antimicrobial therapy Mild diarrhea
MMR[j]	Anaphylactic reactions to neomycin Pregnancy Known altered immunodeficiency (hematologic and solid tumors; congenital immunodeficiency; severe HIV infection and long-term immunosuppressive therapy) Anaphylactic reaction to gelatin Precautions: Recent (within 3–11 mo, depending on product and dose) immune globulin administration[h] Thrombocytopenia or history of thrombocytopenic purpura[h,i]	Tuberculosis or positive PPD Simultaneous tuberculin skin testing[j] Breast-feeding Pregnancy of mother of recipient Immunodeficient family member or household contact Infection with HIV Nonanaphylactic reactions to eggs or neomycin
HIB	None	
Hepatitis B	Anaphylactic reaction to baker's yeast	
Varicella	Pregnancy Anaphylactic reaction to neomycin and to gelatin Infection with HIV Known altered immunodeficiency (hematologic and solid tumors; congenital immunodeficiency; and long-term immunosuppressive therapy) Precautions: Recent IG administration Family history of immunodeficiency	Pregnancy Immunodeficiency in a household contact Household contact with HIV Pregnancy in the mother of the recipient

[a]DTaP, diphtheria and tetanus toxoids and acellular pertussis; DTP, diptheria and tetanus toxoids and pertussis; IVP, inactivated polio virus; OPV, oral polio virus; MMR, measles–memps–rubella; HIB, *Haemophilus influenzae* type b; HBV, hepatitis B virus; var, varicella; PPD, purified protein derivative (tuberculin); PPD, purified protein derivative.
These guidelines, originally issued in the 1993 have been updated to give current recommendations as of 2000 (based on information available as of December 1999).
Note: This information is based on the recommendations of the Advisory Committee on Immunization Practices (ACIP) and the Committee on Infectious Diseases of the American Academy of Pediatrics (AAP). Sometimes these recommendations vary from those in the manufacturers' product label. For more detailed information, providers should consult the published recommendations of the ACIP, AAP, and the manufacturer's package inserts.
[b]The events or conditions listed as precautions, although not contraindications, should be carefully reviewed. The benefits and risks of administering a specific vaccine to an individual under the circumstances should be considered. If the risks are believed to outweigh the benefits, the immunization should be withheld; if the benefits are believed to outweigh the risks (eg, during an outbreak of foreign travel), immunization should be given. Whether and when to administer DTaP (or DTP) to children with proven or suspected underlying neurologic disorders should be decided on an individual basis.
[c]DTP is no longer recommended in the United States.
[d]Acetaminophen given before administering DTaP (or DTP) and thereafter every 4 h for 24 h should be considered for children with a personal or a family history (ie, siblings, parents) of seizures.
[e]The decision to give additional doses of DTaP (or DTP) should be based on consideration of the benefit of further vaccination vs. the risk of recurrence of GBS. For example, completion of the primary series in children is justified.
[f]A theoretical risk exists that the administration of multiple live virus vaccines within 30 d (4 wk) of one another if not given on the same day will result in suboptimal immune response. No data substantiate this risk, however.
[g]OPV is no longer recommended for routine use in the United States.
[h]An anaphylactic reaction to egg injection formerly was considered a contraindication unless skin testing and, if indicated, desensitization had been performed. However, skin testing is no longer recommended (as of 1997).
[i]The decision to vaccinate should be based on consideration of the benefits of immunity to measles, mumps, and rubella vs. the risk of recurrence of exacerbation of thrombocytopenia after vaccination, or from natural infections of measles or rubella. In most instances, the benefits of vaccination will be much greater than the potential risks and justify giving MMR, particularly in view of the even greater risk of thrombocytopenia after measles and rubella. However, if a prior episode of thrombocytopenia occurred in close temporal proximity to vaccination, not giving a subsequent dose may be prudent.
[j]Measles vaccination may temporarily suppress tuberculin reactivity. MMR vaccine may be given after, or on the same day as, TB testing. If MMR has been given recently, postpone the TB test until 4–6 wk after administration of MMR. If giving MMR simultaneously with tuberculin skin test, use the Mantoux test and not multiple puncture tests, because the latter require confirmation of positive, which would have to be postponed 4–6 wk.
[k]Varicella vaccine should not be given to a member of a household with a family history of immunodeficiency until the immune status of the recipient and other children in the family is documented.
From cdc.gov/nip. Accessed on 4/21/05.

BOX 57-3. STANDARDS FOR PEDIATRIC IMMUNIZATION PRACTICES

Standard 1. Immunization services are readily available.

Standard 2. No barriers or unnecessary prerequisites to the receipt of vaccines exist.

Standard 3. Immunization services are available free or for a minimal fee.

Standard 4. Providers use all clinical encounters to screen and, when indicated, immunize children.

Standard 5. Providers educate parents and guardians about immunization in general terms.

Standard 6. Providers question parents or guardians about contraindications and, before immunizing a child, inform them in specific terms about the risks and benefits of the immunizations their child is to receive.

Standard 7. Providers follow only true contraindications.

Standard 8. Providers administer simultaneously all vaccine doses for which a child is eligible at the time of each visit.

Standard 9. Providers use accurate and complete recording procedures.

Standard 10. Providers co-schedule immunization appointments in conjunction with appointments for other child health services.

Standard 11. Providers report adverse events after immunization promptly, accurately, and completely.

Standard 12. Providers operate a tracking system.

Standard 13. Providers adhere to appropriate procedures for vaccine management.

Standard 14. Providers conduct semiannual audits to assess immunization coverage levels and to review immunization records in the patient populations they serve.

Standard 15. Providers maintain up-to-date, easily retrievable medical protocols at all locations where vaccines are administered.

Standard 16. Providers operate with patient-oriented and community-based approaches.

Standard 17. Vaccines are administered by properly trained individuals.

Standard 18. Providers receive ongoing education and training on current immunization recommendations.

From Centers for Disease Control and Prevention. (1993). Standard for pediatric immunization practices: Recommended by National Vaccine Advisory Committee (ACIP). *Morbidity and Mortality Weekly Report, 42* (RR-5), 1–13.

BOX 57–4. IMMUNIZATION SCHEDULE TIPS

Restarting Vaccine Series

With the exception of oral typhoid vaccine, it never is necessary to restart a vaccine series because the interval has been prolonged—although every effort should be made to adhere to the recommended schedule.

Vaccines Given Too Soon

These will not be accepted at school entry and revaccination will be recommended.

Lack of Written Vaccination Record

An attempt should be made to verify vaccination status. If no record can be verified, the child should be considered unimmunized and should be revaccinated as appropriate for age.

Hepatitis B

In the case of an *interrupted* or *incomplete* series, resume the series; do not repeat or restart. Dose should be appropriate in accord with the manufacturer's instructions.

The *third dose* should be given at least 2 mo after the second dose and at least 4 mo after the first dose, but not before 6 mo of age.

PPD/MMR

PPD can be done before or at the same time as the measles vaccine is administered. Give PPD 4 to 6 wk after measles vaccine, if measles is given first, because measles can reduce the reactivity of PPD. This reduction in reactivity is due to mild suppression of cell-mediated immunity, which can lead to false-negative test results.

DtaP

The fourth dose can be given if a child is ≥12 mo of age and 6 mo have elapsed since DTaP dose 3 (especially if the child is unlikely to return at 15 to 18 mo of age). The fifth dose should be given at 4 to 6 y. Children should not receive more than six doses of diphtheria or tetanus-containing toxoid before their seventh birthday. No pertussis-containing vaccines are licensed for use in people ≥7 y of age.

HIB

No HIB vaccine should be given to infants younger than 6 wk of age and is not recommended after age 5 y. Minimum age for last HIB is 12 mo, if at least 2 mo have passed since the previous dose. DTaP/HIB combination products should not be used for primary series (2, 4, 6 mo of age).

Varicella

Dosage for people 12 mo and older: Single 0.5-mL dose subcutaneously suffices for protection 12 mo to 12 y. People 13 y of age and older should receive two 0.5-mL doses at least 4 wk apart.

BOX 57–5. QUESTIONS AND ANSWERS ABOUT IMMUNIZATION

Q. How long should the vaccination needle be?

A. Subcutaneous injections for children and adults: ⅝ to ¾ in., 23- to 25-gauge needle.

Intramuscular injections for infants and children: minimum needle length of ⅞ in. for anterolateral thigh and minimum of ⅝ in. for deltoid injection; for adults: 1 to 1½ in. needle (Humiston & Atkinson, 1998).

Q. What are the immunization recommendations for children of parents or household residents who were never vaccinated for polio?

A. If the unvaccinated or inadequately vaccinated person resides in the household, an all-IVP schedule is recommended for the child. Parents and household contacts may receive IVP too.

Q. Which HIB vaccines are the best?

A. Different manufacturers' products are considered interchangable for the primary series and the booster. However, no HIB vaccine is recommended for infants younger than 6 wk of age. If it is given, it may make the child incapable of responding to subsequent doses.

Q. Are there special recommendations if someone in the family or household has an immune system problem?

A. Yes. The person receiving a polio vaccine should receive only IPV (not OPV because the virus is shed in the stool for up to 6 wk). Other live vaccines and all inactivated vaccines may be given as usual.

Q. What are some special concerns related to pregnancy?

A. There are no contraindications to immunization of a household member if another household member is pregnant. However, if a woman in the household wants to become pregnant and also wants to be vaccinated, she should wait to become pregnant at least 1 mo after receiving mumps, measles, varicella and 3 mo after receiving rubella.

Q. What happens if someone has an extra vaccination?

A. Extra doses of live vaccine do not appear to have adverse consequences and they may boost immunity. Extra doses of inactivated vaccines can induce very high antibody titers. If these people are revaccinated, large local inflammatory reactions may ensue.

Q. Is it harmful to receive vaccines simultaneously?

A. No evidence exists that simultaneous administration of vaccines reduces vaccine effectiveness or increases adverse events.

Q. What are the implications of an error, such as previous administration of a vaccine at the wrong site, in a wrong dose, by a wrong route?

A. Unfortunately, they do not count. Only full doses in acceptable sites should be counted. Revaccinate according to age. The exception to the rule is live vaccines (MMR, varicella), which are recommended to be administered subcutaneously—intramuscular administration of these vaccines is not likely to decrease immunogenicity. *Note:* Reducing or dividing doses of any vaccine including those to preterm or low–birth-weight infants is not indicated.

Q. What is the recommended way to administer multiple injections to infants?

A. The recommended approach is to place the vaccine most likely to cause a local adverse reaction (eg, DTP) in one leg and the two less reactive in different sites in the other leg.

Q. How effective is the varicella vaccine?

A. Effectiveness is 70% to 90% protection against infection with 95% protection against severe disease. Protection persists at least 7 to 10 y. The risk of transmission appears low but somewhat higher if the vaccinee develops a varicella-like rash after vaccination. Recommend that vaccinees avoid contact with immunocompromised people when the rash is present.

Q. Why is the MMR vaccine given twice?

A. The second dose is given because 2% to 5% of people do not develop immunity after the first dose, and 95% of the people who did not respond to the first dose respond to the second.

Note: Birth before 1957 is generally considered evidence of rubella immunity; laboratory evidence of immunity is recommended. Combined MMR vaccine is the drug of choice if vaccination is needed.

Q. What is the standard dosing schedule for hepatitis B vaccine?

A. There is no standard dose. That is why it is so important to read the package insert for hepatitis B vaccine carefully. The formulations vary and the appropriate microgram dose must be selected.

Q. What should be done if the patient spits out the dose of OPV?

A. There is no definite rule regarding how much can be spit out before repeating the dose. If in the judgment of the person administering the vaccine a substantial amount was spit out, regurgitated, or vomited, another dose can be administered within 5 to 10 min at the same visit. If the repeated dose is not retained, neither dose should be counted. OPV should be readministered at the next visit (Humiston & Atkinson, 1998).

of a vaccine recall or a need to reimmunize patients receiving a specific lot of vaccine.

In addition, practice decisions need to be made regarding immunization screening processes to be used for all populations. A focus on adolescent and adult populations as well as infants and children is critical. Current recommendations include routine screening at 11 and 12, and at 50 years of age. An interim process for high-risk people in combination with aforementioned recommended screenings provides the best mechanism for implementing a comprehensive immunization program.

Several Web sites provide vaccine information: www.aap.org, www.cdc.gov/nip, www.cdc.gov/nvpo, www.immunizationinfo.org.

■ Case Study 1

J.V. is a 45-year-old woman, married with no children. She presents on October 10 for a follow-up visit for type 2 diabetes mellitus diagnosed 2 months ago. Her history is significant for the following:

- Type 2 diabetes mellitus controlled with diet and exercise
- Recent graduation from a physical therapy program and working in a pediatric hospital
- Immunization status: routine childhood immunizations received with the exception of varicella and hepatitis B. She does not recall having chickenpox. Her last tetanus shot was 11 years ago.
1. In assessing and treating J.V., what is your plan to update her immunizations?
2. What factors would you consider most important and why?
3. Which vaccines would be a priority and why?

■ Case Study 2

L.L. is a 10-month-old Hispanic boy who presents in November for the first time. He has not had any contact with the health care system since he was 2 months old. He lives in a house with 7 immigrants and poor sanitation. The only immunizations that he has had are hepatitis B (2 shots), 1 HIB, 1 DTaP, 1 IPV, and 1 Prevnar.

1. What immunizations would you administer at this visit?
2. When would you schedule his next visit and what immunizations would you give at that visit?

Bibliography

*Starred references are cited in the text.

Advisory Committee on Immunization Practices. (2004). Prevention and control of influenza. *Morbidity and Mortality Weekly Report, 53*(RR 6), 1–40.

American Academy of Pediatrics, Committee on Infectious Diseases. (1999a). Poliomyelitis prevention: Revised recommendations for use of inactivated and live oral poliovirus vaccines. *Pediatrics, 103,* 171–172.

*Centers for Disease Control and Prevention. (2004). Notice to readers—Childhood immunization schedule—United States-July-December 2004. *Morbidity and Mortality Weekly Report, 53.*

Centers for Disease Control and Prevention. (2000). Prevention of pneumococcal disease among infants and young children: Recommendations of the Advisory Committee on Immunization Practices (ACIP). *Morbidity and Mortality Weekly Report, 49*(RR-9), 1–35.

Centers for Disease Control and Prevention. (2000a). Prevention and control of influenza: Recommendations of Advisory Committee on Immunization Practices (ACIP). *Morbidity and Mortality Weekly Report, 53*(RR-61).

*Centers for Disease Control and Prevention (2003). Notice to readers—Recommended adult immunization schedule—United States 2003–2004. *Morbidity and Mortality Weekly Report, 52*(40), 965.

Centers for Disease Control and Prevention. (2000b). Prevention and control of meningococcal disease. Meningococcal disease and college students: Recommendations of the Advisory Committee on Immunization Practices (ACIP). *Morbidity and Mortality Weekly Report, 49*(RR-7), 1–20.

*Pickering, L. (Ed.). (2003). *The 2003 red book: Report of the Committee on Infectious Diseases* (26th ed.). Elk Grove Village, IL: American Academy of Pediatrics.

Wu, J. J. (2004). Vaccines and immunotherapy for prevention of infectious diseases having cutaneous manifestations. *Journal of American Academy of Dermatology, 50*(4), 495–528.

Zimmerman, R. K. (1999). Should rotavirus vaccine be recommended for universal use? An affirmative view. *Journal of Family Practice, 48*(2), 146–147.

Zimmerman, R. K. (2001). Pneumococcal conjugate vaccine for young children. *American Family Physician, 63*(10), 1991–1998.

Visit the Connection web site for the most up-to-date drug information.

SMOKING CESSATION

■ JESSICA O'HARA AND JEEGISHA R. PATEL

Cigarette smoking is a chronic condition that leads to significant morbidity and mortality. Smoking is the most preventable cause of death in our society (American Cancer Society [ACS], 2004).

In 2000, about 4.9 million smoking-related, premature deaths occurred throughout the world (ACS, 2004). In the United States, tobacco use is responsible for nearly 1 in 5 deaths per year (Centers of Disease Control [CDC], 2002a). Cigarette smoking kills an estimated 264,000 men and 178,000 women in the United States each year (CDC, 2004a). Smoking accounts for at least 30% of all cancer deaths and 87% of lung cancer deaths (ACS, 2004).

Lung cancer mortality rates are about 22 times higher for current male smokers and 12 times higher for current female smokers compared with lifelong nonsmokers (ACS, 2004). Smoking is associated with increased risk for cancers of the mouth, pharynx, larynx, esophagus, pancreas, uterine, cervix, kidney, and bladder. In addition to the variety of cancers, smoking is a major cause of heart disease, cerebrovascular disease, chronic bronchitis, and emphysema, and is associated with gastric ulcers (ACS, 2004).

Smoking causes approximately $157.7 billion in annual health-related economic costs, including adult medical-related productivity costs, adult medical expenditures, and medical expenditures for newborns (CDC, 2002a). According to the CDC, nationwide medical care costs attributable to smoking have been estimated to be more than $50 billion annually (CDC, 2004b). In addition, they estimate the value of lost earnings and loss of productivity to be at least another $47 billion a year (CDC, 2004b).

An estimated 46.2 million adults in the United States smoke cigarettes (ACS, 2004). According to the ACS (2004a), men were more likely to smoke (25.2%) than women (20.2%). Cigarette smoking was highest among American Indians and Alaska natives (32.7%) and lowest among Asian Americans (12.4%) (CDC, 2004a). Cigarette smoking among adults aged 18 and older declined 40% between 1965 and 2000, from 42% to 22% (CDC, 2004a). Smoking prevalence among adults decreased by an average of 1% per year from 1993 to 2000 (CDC, 2004a). Current smoking among U.S. high school students increased significantly from 28% in 1991 to 36% in 1997 (CDC, 2002b). It has been estimated that approximately 3000 children and adolescents become addicted to nicotine each day (Fiore et al., 2000). And

although 70% of smokers report that they would like to quit, only 2% to 3% actually reach this goal each year (CDC, 2004b). The Agency for Health Care Policy and Research (AHCPR) recommends that all health care professionals, including physicians, pharmacists, nurses, and others, ask about and document their patients' smoking status (Fiore et al., 2000). The 2000 guidelines urge clinicians to treat tobacco use disorder as a chronic disease similar in many respects to other diseases such as hypertension, diabetes mellitus, and hyperlipidemia and to provide patients with appropriate advice and pharmacotherapy (Fiore et al., 2000).

PATHOPHYSIOLOGY

Nicotine is the addictive substance in cigarette smoke. It is absorbed and distributed to most tissues of the body, where it binds with nicotinic receptors and produces its physiologic effects on the heart, brain, and other organ systems. Nicotine is a ganglion receptor agonist whose pharmacologic effects are highly dependent on dose (McEvoy, 2001). These effects include central and peripheral nervous system stimulation and depression, respiratory stimulation, skeletal muscle relaxation, catecholamine release by the adrenal medulla, peripheral vasoconstriction, and increased blood pressure, heart rate, CO, and O_2 consumption (McEvoy, 2001). Activation of nicotine receptors in the brain produces relaxation or arousal, increases attention, improves learning and problem-solving skills, and decreases stress and tension (Rennard & Daughton, 2000).

A common endocrine and metabolic effect of nicotine is weight loss. Smokers tend to weigh between 2.7 and 4.5 kg less than nonsmokers (McEvoy, 2001). Additional endocrine effects include increased risk of osteoporosis and earlier menopause (McEvoy, 2001). Finally, smoking alters the liver's metabolic effects by inducing hepatic (cytochrome P450) enzymes. This action is related to the increased metabolism of certain medications such as theophylline and acetaminophen.

DIAGNOSTIC CRITERIA

Chronic nicotine ingestion may lead to physical and physiologic dependence and tolerance to some of its pharmacologic effects. Nicotine dependence disorder has been defined as a form of substance abuse that can lead to clinically important impairment of distress (American Psychiatric Association [APA], 1994). The key features required for the diagnosis of nicotine dependence are continued use despite wanting to quit, prior attempts at quitting, persistent use in face of physical illness, tolerance, and presence of withdrawal symptoms (Prochazka, 2000). Box 58-1 identifies the APA criteria for nicotine dependence (and withdrawal). Another clinical assessment tool for nicotine dependence is the Fagerstrom Test for Nicotine Dependence (Mallin, 2002). This test places significant importance on "time to the first cigarette of the day" (Heatherton et al., 1991). Nicotine has a relatively short half-life and smokers may experience significant discomfort on waking unless they quickly have their first cigarette (Mallin, 2002). However, only the number of cigarettes smoked per day has been shown to correlate with the degree of nicotine dependence. Therefore, the use of the Fagerstrom test is recommended (Box 58.2), in addition to the APA criteria for diagnosis of nicotine dependence among smokers.

Patients who are addicted to nicotine may experience withdrawal symptoms. Onset of these symptoms usually occurs within 24 hours and may last for days or weeks or longer (Rennard & Daughton, 2000). Nicotine withdrawal is associated with a well-described syndrome characterized by irritability, awakening from sleep, bradycardia, anxiety, impaired concentration, impaired reaction time, restlessness, drowsiness, confusion, hunger, and weight gain (Rennard & Daughton, 2000). Tobacco status should be asked about and documented for all patients at every visit. The AHCPR recommends that tobacco use status be adopted as the "5th vital sign" along with blood pressure, temperature, pulse, and respiration rates (Fiore et al., 2000).

INITIATING DRUG THERAPY

The AHCPR guidelines recommend that all clinicians aggressively motivate and assist their smoking patients to quit (Fiore et al., 2000). Analysis of the updated guidelines suggests that a wide variety of clinicians can effectively implement these strategies and those interventions as brief as 3 minutes can increase cessation rate significantly (Fiore et al., 2000). The panel reminds clinicians that effective treatment of tobacco dependence now exists and that every patient should receive at least minimal treatment every time he or she visits a clinician. The first step in this process, identification and assessment of tobacco use status, separates patients into 3 treatment categories:

1. Patients who use tobacco and are willing to quit should be treated using the 5 As: Ask, Advise, Assess, Assist, and Arrange (Fig. 58-1).

BOX 58–1. APA CRITERIA FOR DEPENDENCE AND WITHDRAWAL

Dependence
Nicotine dependence is a maladaptive pattern of substance use, leading to clinically important impairment or distress, as manifested by three or more of the following at any time in a 12-month period:

1. Tolerance occurs, as defined by either of the following: a need for markedly increased amounts of the substance to achieve intoxication or the desired effect, or a markedly diminished effect with continued use of the same amount of the substance.
2. Withdrawal occurs, as manifested by either of the following: the characteristic withdrawal syndrome for the substance, or the taking of the same (or a closely related) substance to relieve or avoid withdrawal symptoms.
3. The substance is often taken in larger amounts or for a longer period than was intended.
4. There is a persistent desire or unsuccessful efforts to cut down or control substance abuse.
5. A great deal of time is spent in activities necessary to obtain the substance (eg, visiting multiple doctors or driving long distances), use the substance (eg, chain smoking), or recover from its effects.
6. Important social, occupational, or recreational activities are given up or reduced because of substance abuse.
7. The substance use is continued despite the knowledge that there is a persistent or recurrent physical or psychological problem likely to have been caused or exacerbated by the substance (eg, current cocaine use despite the recognition of cocaine-induced depression, or continued drinking despite the recognition that an ulcer was made worse by alcohol consumption).

Withdrawal
Withdrawal symptoms may be initiated and characterized by the following:

1. Daily use of nicotine for at least several weeks.
2. Abrupt cessation of nicotine use, or reduction in the amount of nicotine used, followed within 24 h by four or more of the following:
   a. Dysphoric or depressed mood
   b. Insomnia
   c. Irritability, frustration, or anger
   d. Anxiety
   e. Difficulty concentrating
   f. Restlessness
   g. Decreased heart rate
   h. Increased appetite or weight gain
3. The symptoms cause clinically significant distress or impairment in social, occupational, or other important areas of functioning.
4. The symptoms are not due to a general medical condition and are not better accounted for by another mental disorder.

BOX 58–2. FAGERSTOM TOLERANCE TEST FOR NICOTINE DEPENDENCE

Write the number of the answer that is most applicable on the line to the left of the question.

_____1. How soon after you awake do you smoke your first cigarette?
0. After 30 min
1. Within 30 min

_____2. Do you find it difficult to refrain from smoking in places where it is forbidden such as the library, theater, or doctor's office?
0. No
1. Yes

_____3. Which of all the cigarettes you smoke in a day is the most satisfying?
0. Any other than the first one in the morning
1. The first one in the morning

_____4. How many cigarettes a day do you smoke?
0. 1–15
1. 16–25
2. >26

_____5. Do you smoke more during the morning than during the rest of the day?
0. No
1. Yes.

_____6. Do you smoke when you are so ill that you are in bed most of the day?
0. No
1. Yes

_____7. Does the brand you smoke have low, medium, or high nicotine content?
0. Low
1. Medium
2. High

_____8. How often do you inhale the smoke from your cigarette?
0. Never
1. Sometimes
2. Always

Scoring Instructions: Add you up your responses to all the items. Total scores should range from 0 to 11, where 7 or greater suggests physical dependence to nicotine.

TOTAL SCORE: _____

Heatherton, T. F. Kozlowski, L. T., Frecker, R. C., et al. (1991). The Fagerstrom Test for Nicotine Dependence: A revision of the Fagerstrom Tolerance Questionnaire. _British Journal of Addictions, 86,_ 1119–1127.

2. Patients who use tobacco but are unwilling to quit at this time should be treated with the 5 Rs of motivational interventions: Relevance, Risks, Reward, Roadblocks, and Repetition (Fig. 58-2).

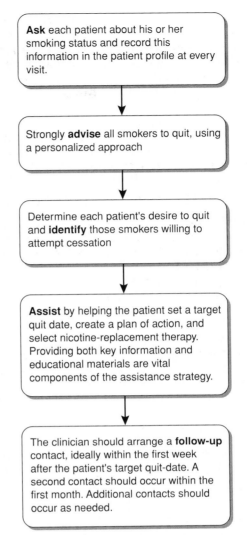

Ask each patient about his or her smoking status and record this information in the patient profile at every visit.

↓

Strongly **advise** all smokers to quit, using a personalized approach

↓

Determine each patient's desire to quit and **identify** those smokers willing to attempt cessation

↓

Assist by helping the patient set a target quit date, create a plan of action, and select nicotine-replacement therapy. Providing both key information and educational materials are vital components of the assistance strategy.

↓

The clinician should arrange a **follow-up** contact, ideally within the first week after the patient's target quit-date. A second contact should occur within the first month. Additional contacts should occur as needed.

Figure 58–1   AHCPR model strategies for smoking cessation. (From Agency for Health Care Policy and Research. _Helping smokers quit._ AHCPR Publication No. 96-0693. Rockville, MD: Author.)

3. Patients who have quit using tobacco recently should be provided relapse-prevention treatment. Clinicians should reinforce the patient's decision to quit, review the benefits of quitting, and assist the patient in resolving any residual problems arising from quitting (Fiore et al., 2000).

Once the diagnosis of nicotine dependence is made, the next step is to assess the patient's readiness to change (Mallin, 2002). The five-step transtheoretical model of stages of change (SOC) is useful for assessing the patient's readiness to quit. The SOC model identifies smoking behavior change as a process involving movement through a series of five motivational stages (Mallin, 2002):

- Stage 1—Precontemplation: the patient has no intention to quit.
- Stage 2—Contemplation: a smoker is interested in quitting but has no definite plans.
- Stage 3—Preparation: the smoker in this stage is planning to quit within the next month and has made a failed attempt to quit during the previous year.

Relevance

Encourage the patient to indicate why quitting is personally relevant, being as specific as possible. Motivational information has the greatest impact if it is relevant to a patient's disease status or risk, family or social situation (e.g., having children in the home), health concerns, age, gender, and other important patient characteristics (e.g., prior quitting experience, personal barriers to cessation).

Risks

The clinician should ask the patient to identify potential negative consequences of tobacco use. The clinician may suggest and highlight those that seem most relevant to the patient. The clinician should emphasize that smoking low-tar/low-nicotine cigarettes or use of other forms of tobacco (e.g., smokeless tobacco, cigars, and pipes) will not eliminate these risks.

Rewards

The clinician should ask the patient to identify potential benefits of stopping tobacco use. The clinician may suggest and highlight those that seem most relevant to the patient. Examples of rewards include improved health, food will taste better, improved sense of smell, save money, feel better about yourself, home, car, clothing, breath will smell better, can stop worrying about quitting, and perform better in physical activities.

Roadblocks

The clinician should ask the patient to identify barriers or impediments to quitting and note elements of treatment (problem solving, pharmacotherapy) that could address barriers. Typical barriers might include withdrawal symptoms, fear of failure, weight gain, lack of support, depression and enjoyment of tobacco.

Repetition

The motivational intervention should be repeated every time an unmotivated patient visits the clinic setting. Tobacco users who have failed in previous quit attempts should be told that most people make repeated quit attempts before they are successful.

Figure 58–2   Tobacco users unwilling to quit: The "5 R's." (AHCPR. [2000]. A clinical practice guideline for treatment use and dependence: A US Public Health Service report. *JAMA, 283*[24] 3244–3254.)

- Stage 4—Action: the smoker makes a serious effort to quit by modifying his or her behavior and environment. During this stage, the patient has abstained anywhere from 1 day to 6 months. After 6 months of abstinence, the patient enters the final stage.
- Stage 5—Maintenance

The first step in any cessation program should be to target a quitting date with the patient. This date should be identified; otherwise the patient may never actually make the attempt to stop smoking. In addition, picking a definite date provides the patient with an obtainable goal and avoids overwhelming the patient with the thought of having to change an entire lifestyle.

Nonpharmacologic approaches to smoking cessation consist of various individual and group behavioral interventions, including self-management, group counseling and support, nicotine fading, and aversion techniques (APA, 1996). Behavioral therapy is based on the theory that learning processes operate in the development, maintenance, and cessation of smoking (APA, 1996). The core feature of behavioral therapies is to educate the patient about the benefits of smoking cessation. When used alone, these interventions have low success rates because they do not satiate cravings or prevent withdrawal symptoms. However, patients who are highly motivated or who smoke only a few cigarettes a day may benefit the most from these approaches. The APA recommends using multicomponent behavioral therapy as first-line treatment (APA, 1996).

Self-Management

Self-management techniques are commonly used to make patients more aware of their smoking habits and cues. By becoming more familiar with the environment and events that precede smoking a cigarette, patients may be able to interrupt these patterns by avoiding certain situations. If a relapse occurs, the patient should determine what may have triggered the failed attempt and eliminate those factors. Some nondrug methods to enhance smoking cessation and prevent relapse include getting rid of ashtrays, drinking lots of water and breathing deeply between sips, avoiding places with smoke-filled air, making a dental appointment to get teeth cleaned, exercising, calling on friends or family for support and encouragement, eating a balanced diet, and avoiding the routine that causes craving a cigarette (ie, drinking coffee every morning with a cigarette; Mallin, 2002).

Group Counseling and Support

The AHCPR expert panel emphasized that there is a strong dose-response relationship between the intensity of tobacco dependence counseling and its effectiveness. Treatments involving person-to-person contact (via individual, group, or proactive telephone counseling) are consistently effective and their effectiveness increases with treatment intensity. Three types of counseling and behavioral therapies were especially effective and should be used with all patients who are attempting tobacco cessation:

- Provision of practical counseling (problem-solving/skills training)
- Provision of social support as part of treatment (intra-treatment social support)
- Help in securing social support outside treatment (extra-treatment social support)

Group counseling programs help to educate the patient on the risks and benefits of smoking cessation. In addition, the patient is presented with strategies to cope with and avoid situations that may lead to relapse. Finally, a social support structure provides the patient with continuous encouragement and reinforcement. These programs are intended to keep the patient motivated to quit smoking

Nicotine Fading

Nicotine fading consists of a slow decrease in the intake of nicotine. This can be accomplished by decreasing the number of puffs taken or the number of cigarettes smoked per day or by switching to a brand of cigarettes that contains less nicotine. However, the success rate of this technique is limited because the patient can compensate by inhaling more deeply or for longer periods.

Aversion Therapy

Finally, aversion techniques have been used to make smoking less desirable to the patient. The first method, satiation, requires the patient to smoke double or triple the usual amount in a short time. In the second method, rapid smoking, the patient must inhale rapidly every 6 to 8 seconds until the cigarette is finished or the patient is nauseated. The use of these methods is limited because of possible health problems and compliance issues.

A health care professional who merely advises his or her patient to quit smoking is providing at least minimal assistance in the efforts.

Goals of Drug Therapy

All patients attempting to quit should be encouraged to use effective pharmacotherapies for smoking cessation. Long-term smoking cessation pharmacotherapy should be considered as a strategy to reduce the likelihood of relapse (Doering, 2002). As with other chronic diseases, the most effective treatment of tobacco dependence requires the use of multiple modalities (Fiore et al., 2000). According to the AHCPR guidelines, clinicians should encourage all patients initiating a quit attempt to use one or a combination of efficacious pharmacotherapies, although pharmacotherapy use requires special consideration in some patient groups (ie, those with medical contraindications, those smoking fewer than 10 cigarettes a day, pregnant/breast-feeding women,

and adolescent smokers; Doering, 2002). Long-term abstinence is the ultimate goal of treatment of nicotine dependence. Initial goals include moving smokers from not contemplating smoking cessation to contemplating, and to attempting to quit or quitting for a short period of time.

Drug therapy known as *nicotine replacement therapy* (NRT) aims to control nicotine levels in the bloodstream so that withdrawal does not occur while the patient is adjusting to life without cigarette smoking. The goal of therapy is to maintain the cessation of smoking for a period that allows the patient to develop preventive strategies to avoid relapse.

The primary mechanism of action by which NRT enhances smoking cessation is to obtain plasma levels of nicotine that can relieve or prevent withdrawal symptoms (Okuyemi et al., 2000). The pharmacokinetic effects underlie the concept of nicotine replacement as an aid to smoking cessation, providing that steady-state levels of nicotine can prevent a smoker from experiencing intense withdrawal while not providing the reinforcing peaks achieved from smoking (Le Houezec, 2003). Smokers can, therefore, achieve abstinence by dealing with the various behavioral aspects of smoking. Once abstinence is achieved, the smoker can taper of the nicotine by gradual reduction (Le Houezec, 2003).

One benefit of NRT includes not exposing the smoker to the carcinogens and other toxins in cigarette smoke. NRT is approved by the U.S. Food and Drug Administration (FDA) as an aid to smoking cessation for the relief of nicotine withdrawal symptoms when used as part of a comprehensive behavioral program. The guideline panel identifies six first-line medications (bupropion SR, nicotine gum, nicotine inhaler, nicotine nasal spray, nicotine patch, and nicotine lozenge) (Table 58-1). Two second-line medications (clonidine and nortriptyline) are also identified for smoking cessation but are not approved by the FDA. The gum and patch are recommended as initial therapy by the APA and AHCPR guidelines. The AHCPR found in research studies that the abstinence rate with the gum and patch was 1.4 to 2 times that of placebo at 12 months after therapy. In addition, the APA guidelines reported that the quit rates for the gum and patch were increased by 1.6 to 2.4 compared with psychological therapy alone. The use of the inhaler, nasal spray, and lozenge requires further evidence and therefore should be reserved as alternatives (Table 58-2). It is important that the patient stops smoking completely before initiating treatment, regardless of which formulation is used.

Transdermal Patches

Although both the gum and patch are recommended as initial therapy, the AHCPR guidelines recommend that the patch be routinely used in clinical practice (Fiore et al., 2000). The recommendation is based on the finding that the patch has fewer compliance problems and requires less patient education on the use of the product compared with the gum. Currently, three NRT patch formulations are marketed and all available over the counter (see Table 58-1): Habitrol, Nicoderm CQ, and Nicotrol. Patch brands differ in rate control mechanisms, starting dose, and weaning regimen (Okuyemi et al., 2001).

The Habitrol and Nicoderm CQ patches are available as 21-mg (6–8 weeks), 14-mg (2–4 weeks), and 7-mg (2–4 weeks) regimens. In general, if patients smoke more than

Table 58.1

Overview of Selected Agents Used in Smoking Cessation

Generic (Trade) Name and Dosage	Selected Adverse Events	Contraindications	Special Considerations
Nicotine Products			
nicotine patch (Nicotrol) 15 mg patch qd for 6 wk	Cutaneous irritation, GI disturbances, dizziness, headaches	Those who continue to smoke, chew tobacco, or use other nicotine products	Patch worn for only 16 h/d Available without a prescription Not indicated for people smoking fewer than 10 cigarettes per day
nicotine patch (Habitrol, others) ≥10 cigarettes/d: 21 mg for 6 wk, then 14 mg for 2–4 wk, then 7 mg for 2–4 wk <10 cigarettes/d: 14 mg for 6 wk, then 7 mg for 2–4 wk	Same as above	None noted	Patch worn for 24 h/d
nicotine patch (Nicoderm CQ) ≥10 cigarettes/d: 21 mg for 6 wk, then 14 mg for 2 wk, then 7 mg for 2 wk <10 cigarettes/d: 14 mg for 6 wk, then 7 mg for 2 wk	Same as above	Same as above	Same as above
nicotine polacrilex gum (Nicorette) Start: 2 mg q1–2h wk 1–6 2 mg q2–4h wk 7–9 2 mg q4–8h wk 10–12 Range: 1–24 pieces per day See text for use of 4-mg dose	Sore throat, hiccups, undesirable taste,	Dentures, temporomandibular joint disease, dizziness	Gum should be chewed until patient feels a tingling sensation, then "parked" between cheek and gum. Repeat chewing every 15–30 min.
nicotine nasal spray (Nicotrol NS) Start: 1–2 sprays in each nasal hourly (one spray = 0.5 mg) Range: 1–40 sprays per day	Nasal irritation, sore throat, dizziness, headache	Hypersensitivity to preservatives Rhinitis, sinusitis	No more than 5 sprays per hour
nicotine inhaler (Nicotrol inhaler) Start: 6 cartridges per day; self-titrated to avoid withdrawal Range: 6–16 cartridges per day	Throat irritation, dizziness, headache, cough	Hypersensitivity to menthol	A minimum of 6 cartridges must be used for 3–6 wk. Do not use for >6 mo.
nicotine lozenge (Commit) First cigarette within 30 min of waking: 4 mg First cigarette >30 min after waking: 2 mg One lozenge every 1–2 h for first 6 wk, then one every 2–4 h for wk 7–9, and one lozenge every 4–8 h for wk 10–12.	Hiccups, dyspepsia, dry mouth, and irritation/soreness of the mouth	Those who continue to smoke, chew tobacco, or use other nicotine products.	Lozenge should be placed in mouth and allowed to dissolve for about 20–30 min. Do not swallow or chew the lozenge. Occasionally move the lozenge from one side of the mouth to other until completely dissolved.
Non-nicotine Products bupropion (Zyban) Start: 150 mg PO qd for 3 d, then increase to 150 mg PO bid for 7–12 wk Range: 150–300 mg/d	Headache, dry mouth, insomnia	History of seizures during the second week of therapy	Patient must set a target quit date.

10 cigarettes per day, they should start with the highest dose. After approximately 1 to 2 months, patients switch to progressively lower-dose patches until they are effectively weaned off the patch. The Nicotrol patch is a single-dose patch of 15 mg and is intended for daytime use only as a 16-hour patch. Treatment for patients using the patch is recommended for 6 weeks.

The Habitrol patch may be left on for 24 hours and applied at the same time each day; however, the Nicotrol patch must be removed before going to sleep to avoid sleep disturbances. A new patch should then be applied on waking. Nicoderm CQ may be left on for 16 or 24 hours. Patients requiring a cigarette on awakening would benefit from the 24-hour patch. Only one patch should be applied at a time.

The most common side effects of the transdermal patches include a mild skin reaction with pruritus and erythema (Okuyemi et al., 2001). The skin reactions are usually mild and self-limiting, resolving within 24 hours of removing the

Table 58.2

Recommended Order of Treatment for Smoking Cessation

Order	Agents	Comments
First line	Nicotine gum or patch	The patch leads to fewer compliance problems, less patient education time and greater ease of use.
		It is recommended that the patch be used routinely in clinical practice unless contraindicated or the patient has failed the patch or prefers gum.
Second line	Nicotine nasal spray, inhaler, buproprion, or lozenge	These products are the newest smoking cessation therapies and therefore data are limited. They should be reserved for patients who fail first-line therapy.
		Product selection is patient specific and dependent on the reason for failure of first-line therapy.
Third line	Combination therapy	Useful combinations include the patch plus the gum, the patch plus the nasal spray, and the patch plus bupropion.

patch. Rotating application sites or wearing a 16-hour patch decreases the incidence of these events. Less common, sleep disturbances have been reported with the 24-hour patches (Okuyemi et al., 2001). When this occurs, it is difficult to distinguish if it is a result of the patch or nicotine withdrawal. The transdermal patches are contraindicated for patients with systemic eczema, unstable angina, or pregnancy and within 1 month of a myocardial infraction (Okuyemi et al., 2001).

The initial patch should be applied immediately on awakening on the patient's targeted quit date. The application site should be clean and dry before applying the patch. The patient should press the patch onto a hairless portion of the upper outer arms or upper chest and hold it for approximately 10 seconds. To decrease irritation that may occur with the patches, the patient should rotate application sites with each new patch. It is common to experience mild tingling, itching, or burning sensations for the first minute after application. If these symptoms persist for more than 4 days, however, the prescriber should be notified and an alternative method should be used.

If the patch gets wet or if it falls off, a new patch should be applied to a different site, and then removed at the original time the first patch would have been removed. Proper disposal of the patch is important. After the patch is removed, it should be placed in the wrapper from the newly applied patch and discarded responsibly—out of the reach of children and pets.

It is important to advise patients not to use the patch if they use other nicotine-containing products or continue to smoke or chew tobacco unless informed by their physician. Instruct patients not to smoke even if they are not wearing the patch. Nicotine in the skin will be entering the bloodstream for several hours after the patch is removed.

Nicotine Gum

Nicotine polacrilex gum (Nicorette) was the first NRT to be approved and is now available without a prescription. The initial dose is one 2-mg piece of gum. The patient should chew the gum slowly until he or she senses a peppery taste or tingling. Then the gum should be "parked" between the cheek and the gingiva to increase absorption. This cycle should be repeated with the same piece of gum approximately every minute for 15 to 30 minutes. The gum is more effective if used on a fixed schedule as opposed to an "as-needed" basis (APA, 1996). Therefore, the patient should be advised to chew one piece of gum every 1 to 2 hours. A 4-

mg dose is also available and may be used as the initial dose in the following:

- Patients with a history of severe withdrawal symptoms
- Patients who smoke more than 20 cigarettes per day
- Patients who smoke immediately on awakening
- Patients for whom the 2-mg gum failed
- Patients who request it

The initial duration of therapy is 6 weeks regardless of what strength is used. Over the next 6 weeks, the patient should be slowly weaned off the gum to avoid withdrawal symptoms. The maximum dose is 24 pieces per day for the 2-mg dose and 12 pieces per day for the 4-mg dose (see Table 58-1).

The patient should be advised not to smoke while using the gum. In addition, food and fluid should not be taken for at least 15 minutes before and after chewing the gum because certain foods (eg, coffee, tea, carbonated beverages) cause the saliva to become more acidic and therefore decrease the absorption of the gum. Patients should dispose of the gum and wrapper properly to avoid ingestion by small children and pets.

Common adverse effects of nicotine gum use include jaw muscle aches and fatigue, oral sores, hiccups, belching, throat irritation, and nausea. Some of these events (ie, hiccups, throat irritation, nausea) result from rapid chewing, leading to excessive nicotine release and absorption. Patient education on the proper use of the gum decreases the incidence of these events.

Nicotine Nasal Spray

The nicotine nasal spray is a prescription product and is marketed under the brand name Nicotrol NS. Because of limited data, a high side effect profile, and increased risk for dependence, this formulation should be reserved for patients who have failed to quit smoking by using the gum or patch or who are highly dependent smokers who require nicotine replacement at a quicker rate than the gum and patch can provide (Silagy et al., 2002).

The recommended initial dosage of the nasal spray is one or two 0.5-mg doses in each nostril per hour (one spray contain 0.5 mg nicotine). The dosage may be increased as needed to prevent withdrawal symptoms. The maximum dose is 5 sprays per hour or 40 sprays per day. After the initial 6 to 8 weeks of treatment, the dosage should be slowly tapered over the next 4 to 6 weeks. Using the nasal spray for longer than 6 months is not recommended because there is no greater efficacy and it increases the risk for dependence.

Before administering the first dose, the patient must prime the pump. This is accomplished by pumping the medication into a tissue 6 to 8 times until a fine spray appears. If the spray is not used for 24 hours or more, the pump must be primed again. Once the pump is ready for use, the patient must follow the manufacturer's directions. For a summary, see Box 58-3. The difference between the nicotine nasal spray and other nasal sprays is that the patient must remember not to sniff or inhale while administering Nicotrol NS. If the spray comes in contact with the mouth, eyes, or skin, the patient should rinse the area immediately with cold water to prevent toxicity. The patient must be aware that it takes approximately 1 week to adjust to the side effects.

Common side effects of the nicotine nasal spray include throat irritation, rhinitis, sneezing, coughing, and watery eyes. These events can occur in more than 75% of patients. The nicotine inhaler is associated with dyspepsia, throat or mouth irritation, oral burning, rhinitis, and cough after inhalation.

Nicotine Inhaler

In 1998, the nicotine inhaler became available as a prescription drug for smoking cessation. The inhaler is thought to improve smoking cessation through two mechanisms. When it is used, it mimics the hand-to-mouth ritual that occurs when smoking a cigarette and it produces a sensation of inhaled smoke on the back of the throat. However, because of the limited evidence, the inhaler should be reserved for patients who have failed initial treatment with other products (see Table 58-1).

BOX 58–3. HOW TO USE A NICOTROL INHALER

STEP 1: Blow your nose to make sure it is clear.
STEP 2: Tilt your head back slightly and insert bottle tip into nostril as far as it is comfortable.
STEP 3: Breathe in through your mouth and hold your breath.
STEP 4: Press on the bottom of the bottle with your thumb to release one spray. Breathe out through your mouth. Do not sniff or inhale through your nose and do not swallow while spraying. If your nose runs after releasing the spray, gently sniff to keep the spray in your nose. Wait 2–3 min before blowing your nose.
STEP 5: If you are to use one spray in each nostril, repeat steps 2–4 for the other nostril.
STEP 6: Wipe bottle tip and replace the cap.

The inhaler consists of a mouthpiece and a cartridge. These two separate pieces are pressed together to break the seal on the cartridge. Once the seal is broken, the nicotine-filled air is inhaled into the mouth as a cigarette would be inhaled. The best results have been found when the patient takes shallow, frequent puffs over 20 minutes. Once a cartridge is opened, it is good only for 1 day.

The recommended dose is 6 to 16 cartridges per day. A minimum of six cartridges must be used for at least 3 to 6 weeks and continued for 3 months. The dose should then be tapered over the next 6 to 12 weeks. Use of the Nicotrol Inhaler should not exceed 6 months. Like the nasal spray, the inhaler must be used for 1 week before the patient adjusts to the side effects. Finally, because the cartridges contain high concentrations of nicotine, they should be stored and disposed of in a place that cannot be accessed by children and pets.

Nicotine Lozenge

The newest formulation of NRT is the nicotine lozenge (Commit), which was approved by the FDA in October 2002 and is available over the counter without a prescription. The nicotine lozenge is available in 2-mg and 4-mg strength tables. One study found that treatment with the nicotine lozenge results in significantly greater 28-day abstinence at 6 weeks for the 2-mg (46.0% versus 29.7%; $P<.001$) and the 4-mg lozenges compared with placebo (48.7% versus 20.8%; $P<.001$; Shiffman et al., 2004). Similar treatments were maintained for a full year. Use of more lozenges also resulted in reducing cravings and withdrawal (Shiffman et al., 2004).

The nicotine lozenge helps control cravings by delivering craving-fighting medicine quickly. The lozenge uses a unique method for smokers to determine their degree of physical dependence on nicotine. This indicator is called time to first cigarette (TTFC). With TTFC, those who smoke their first cigarette within 30 minutes of waking are directed to use the 4-mg strength, whereas those who smoke their first cigarette after 30 minutes of waking are directed to use the 2-mg strength (Shiffman et al., 2002). It is recommended that during the first 6 weeks, an individual should take one lozenge every 1 to 2 hours, for at least 9 a day. This dosage is then reduced to one lozenge every 2 to 4 hours in weeks 7 to 9, and every 4 to 8 hours in weeks 10 to 12. The recommended length of treatment of therapy for the nicotine lozenge is 12 weeks.

The patient should be advised not to eat or drink for 15 minutes before using the nicotine lozenge. The lozenge should be placed in the mouth and sucked on for 20 to 30 minutes to allow the lozenge to slowly dissolve. The lozenge should not be swallowed or chewed. The patient will feel a warm or tingly sensation. Occasionally, the lozenge should be moved from one side of the mouth to the other until it is completely dissolved. Only one lozenge should be used at a time and patients should not use more than 5 lozenges in 6 hours or more than 20/d.

The most common side effects of the nicotine lozenge are hiccups, dyspepsia, dry mouth, and irritation/soreness in the mouth and throat (Glover et al., 2002). These effects mainly occurred in patients who chewed or swallowed the lozenge. Patient education on how to properly administer the lozenge can help decrease these incidences. Finally, because the lozenge looks similar to hard candy, it should be stored and disposed properly to avoid access to children.

Nonnicotine Therapies: Bupropion

Several nonnicotine products have been tested for smoking cessation, but the FDA has approved only one. Bupropion is the first nonnicotine product approved for smoking cessation. The drug has been commonly used as an antidepressant under the brand name Wellbutrin SR. It is available by prescription as an aid to smoking cessation under the brand name Zyban SR. The exact mechanism of action is unknown; however, it is believed to be related to dopaminergic or noradrenergic properties. In a randomized double-blind, placebo-controlled trial (Dale et al., 2001), 27% of patients who received the active drug were abstinent at 6 months, compared with 16% of patients taking placebo ($P < .001$).

The initial dose of Zyban SR is 150 mg/d for 3 days to decrease the incidence of insomnia. After 3 days, the dose can be increased to 150 mg twice a day for 7 to 12 weeks. Dosages higher than 300 mg/d are not recommended because of the increased risk of seizures. Unlike NRT, Zyban SR therapy should be initiated while the patient is still smoking because the drug takes approximately 1 week to reach steady-state plasma concentrations. The patient should set a target quit date during week 2 of therapy. If the patient has not made significant improvements by week 7 of treatment, the attempt is unlikely to be successful and the medication should be discontinued. Tapering the dose is not required when stopping the medication.

The most common side effects of Zyban SR are dry mouth and insomnia. Other adverse events that can occur include nervousness or difficulty concentrating, rash, and constipation. Seizures have also occurred but are very rare (Dale et al., 2001).

It is important that patients taking Zyban SR participate in behavioral therapy programs that include counseling both during and after therapy. Patients need to be informed not to use Wellbutrin or Wellbutrin SR while taking Zyban SR because these medications all contain bupropion. In addition, monoamine oxidase inhibitors should not be used during or within 14 days of Zyban SR treatment. The interaction between these agents increases bupropion toxicity (ie, seizures, psychotic changes).

Second-Line Agents: Clonidine and Nortriptyline

Two second-line nonnicotine products are also available to aid in smoking cessation but are not approved by the FDA for smoking cessation. These two products are clonidine and nortriptyline, which are both available only with a prescription. Clonidine therapy has been examined for use in treatment of nicotine addiction because of its availability to reduce withdrawal symptoms in people addicted to narcotics or alcohol (Jones et al., 2000). Clonidine therapy is usually started 3 to 7 days before the quit date. Oral clonidine can be given 0.05 mg/d initially, and the dosage can then be adjusted upward as tolerated to 0.15 to 0.75 mg/d administered in divided doses (Fiore et al., 2000). Alternatively, the clonidine transdermal patch can be used at a dosage of 0.1 to 0.2 mg/d. Duration of therapy is for 3 to 10 weeks. Those

with rebound hypertension should not use clonidine. Common side effects include dry mouth, drowsiness, dizziness, and sedation (Anderson et al., 2002).

Nortriptyline is another second-line nonnicotine agent that has been effective and well tolerated for the treatment of addiction to smoking (Da Costa et al., 2002). Nortriptyline dosage ranges from 75 to 100 mg/d and duration for 12 weeks. It is contraindicated in those with risk of arrhythmias. Common side effects include sedation and dry mouth (Da Costa et al., 2002).

The AHCPR guidelines recommend the use of these two products as second-line therapy because they are not FDA approved for the treatment of nicotine dependence and withdrawal.

Combination Drug Therapy

Although all the drugs discussed above have only been approved as single pharmacologic agents, combined treatment may be appropriate for smokers who are unable to quit with monotherapy. Three combinations of nicotine replacement have shown to be safe and effective in smoking cessation (Okuyemi et al., 2000).

A double-blind, placebo-controlled trial concluded that the addition of the gum to the patch significantly increases quit rates from 23% to 34% at 12 weeks and from 15% to 28% at 24 weeks, respectively (Kornitzer et al., 1995). Side effects were not significantly increased by combined use of the patch and gum. Another study also reported higher quit rates when the patch is combined with the nasal spray than with the patch alone (51% versus 35% at 6 weeks and 37% versus 25% at 3 months for the combination of patch and spray and patch alone, respectively; Blondal et al., 1999). Combination treatment should be considered for smokers with significant craving or withdrawal symptoms despite adequate doses of single agents and should be continued for 3 to 6 months (Okuyemi et al., 2000).

The third combination is the use of the transdermal patch and bupropion. A double-blind, placebo-controlled study compared sustained-release bupropion, a nicotine patch, and both for smoking cessation in 732 smokers. Abstinence rates at 12 months were 35.5% in the combination (bupropion plus nicotine patch) group compared with 30.3% for the nicotine patch alone and 15.6% for the placebo and pill group (Jorenby et al., 1999). They concluded that abstinence rates were significantly higher with bupropion in combination with nicotine patch than with the patch alone. These findings suggest that bupropion may be used in combination with the nicotine patch in patients without contraindications to either drug when necessary (Okuyemi et al., 2000). Patients should be started on bupropion 150 mg/d for 3 days, then 150 mg twice daily for 1 to 2 weeks prior to quit date. Transdermal nicotine patch therapy should be added starting on the quit date and treatment continued for 3 to 6 months (Okuyemi et al., 2000).

Selecting the Most Appropriate Agent

Which therapeutic agent is most effective depends on the patient and the patient's smoking history, among other factors. For a review of the recommended order of treatment and the clinical guidelines for prescribing pharmacotherapy

Table 58.3

Clinical Guidelines for Prescribing Pharmacotherapy for Smoking Cessation

Who should receive pharmacotherapy for smoking cessation?	All smokers trying to quit, except in the presence of special circumstances. Special consideration should be given before using pharmacotherapy with selected populations: those with medical contraindications, those smoking fewer than 10 cigarettes/d, pregnant/breastfeeding women, and adolescent smokers.
What are the first-line pharmacotherapies recommended?	All five of the FDA-approved pharmacotherapies for smoking cessation are recommended, including bupropion SR, nicotine gum, nicotine inhaler, nicotine nasal spray, and the nicotine patch.
What factors should a clinician consider when choosing among the five first-line pharmacotherapies?	Because of the lack of sufficient data to rank-order these five medications, choice of a specific first-line pharmacotherapy must be guided by factors such as clinician familiarity with the medications, contraindications for selected patients, patient preference, previous patient experience with a specific pharmacotherapy (positive or negative), and patient characteristics (eg, history of depression, concerns about weight gain).
Are pharmacotherapeutic treatments appropriate for lighter smokers (eg, 10–15 cigarettes/d)?	If pharmacotherapy is used with lighter smokers, clinicians should consider reducing the dose of first-line nicotine replacement therapy (NRT) pharmacotherapies. No adjustments are necessary when using bupropion SR.
What second-line pharmacotherapies are recommended?	Clonidine and nortriptyline.
When should second-line agents be used for treating tobacco dependence?	Consider prescribing second-line agents for patients unable to use first-line medications because of contraindications or for patients for whom first-line medications are not helpful. Monitor patients for the known side effects of second-line agents.
Which pharmacotherapies should be considered with patients particularly concerned about weight gain?	Bupropion SR and nicotine replacement therapies, in particular nicotine gum, have been shown to delay, but not prevent, weight gain.
Are there pharmacotherapies that should be especially considered in patients with a history of depression?	Bupropion SR and nortriptyline appear to be effective with this population.
Should nicotine replacement therapies be avoided in patients with a history of cardiovascular disease?	No. The nicotine patch in particular is safe and has been shown not to cause adverse cardiovascular effects.
May tobacco dependence pharmacotherapies be used long-term (eg, 6 mo or more)?	Yes. This approach may be helpful with smokers who report persistent withdrawal symptoms during the course of pharmacotherapy or who desire long-term therapy. A minority of individuals who successfully quit smoking use ad libitum NRT medications (gum, nasal spray, inhaler) long term. The use of these medications long term does not present a known health risk. Additionally, the FDA has approved the use of bupropion SR for a long-term maintenance indication.
May pharmacotherapies ever be combined?	Yes. There is evidence that combining the nicotine patch with either nicotine gum or nicotine nasal spray increases long-term abstinence rates over those produced by a single form of NRT.

AHCRP. (2000). *A clinical practice guideline for treating tobacco use and dependence.* A U.S. Public Health Service Report. *Journal of the American Medical Association,* *283*(24), 3244–3254 (reprinted).

according to the AHCPR guidelines for smoking cessation, see Tables 58-2 and 58-3 and Figure 58-3.

Special Population Considerations

Female patients should be monitored for pregnancy because NRT can harm the fetus. The nicotine gum is pregnancy category C and the patches, nasal spray, inhaler, and lozenge are category D (positive evidence of risk). Zyban SR is category B (no adequate, well-controlled studies in pregnant women). These medications should be reserved for patients in whom nonpharmacologic therapy has not worked or those experiencing severe withdrawal symptoms. In pregnant patients, the benefits of using smoking cessation medications should outweigh the risks of smoking.

Nicotine replacement therapy should be used with caution in those patients with cardiovascular disease because it can cause tachydysrhythmia and worsen angina. However, the risks are small compared with the cardiovascular effects of smoking. Nicotine concentrations are higher and delivered more rapidly from cigarettes compared with NRT products.

MONITORING PATIENT RESPONSE

Smoking status must be monitored in all patients. As mentioned, patients starting NRT must stop smoking completely before initiating treatment to avoid nicotine toxicity. Common signs of nicotine toxicity include nausea, vomiting, diarrhea, hypersalivation, abdominal pain, perspiration, dizziness, headache, hearing and visual disturbances, confusion, and weakness. On the other hand, patients beginning treatment with Zyban SR must set a quit date after the medication has been taken for 1 to 2 weeks.

A follow-up telephone call from the practitioner should occur approximately 2 to 4 days after the patient's scheduled quit date. If the patient is aware of the future call, compliance may be improved. In addition, the follow-up call may help detect ineffective use or adverse events early in the course of treatment. Additional follow-up contacts should occur as needed. If the patient has been successful at the time of the call, the clinician should offer congratulations and additional support. However, if the patient has relapsed, it is important to reassure the patient that it is not indicative of ultimate failure. Many smokers attempt to quit several times before achieving their goal. The reasons for failure should be identified and eliminated for the next attempt and the patient should be encouraged to try again.

Duration of therapy must be monitored to evaluate if tolerance or physical dependence occurs to NRT. Dependence is most common with the nicotine nasal spray because of its rapid delivery of nicotine. Proper dosage titration and weaning schedule should be monitored as well to prevent withdrawal symptoms from occurring.

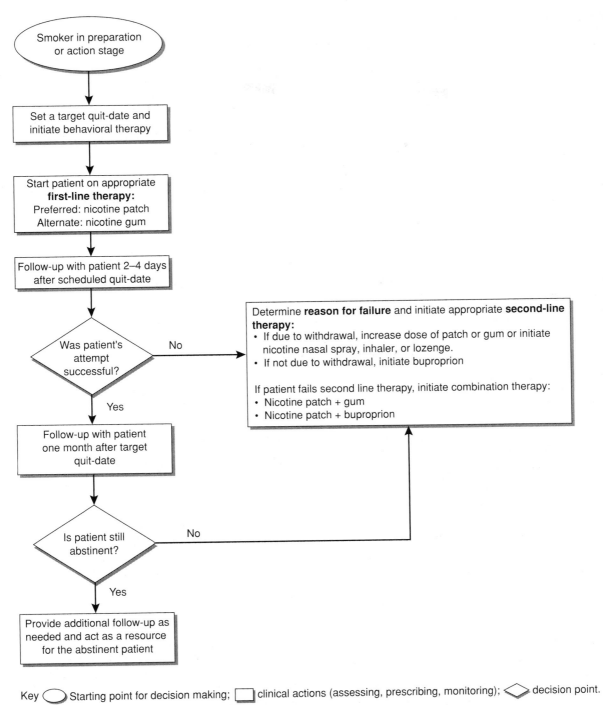

Figure 58–3   Treatment algorithm for smoking cessation.

PATIENT EDUCATION

The occurrence of adverse events with any medication has a definite correlation with patient compliance. Therefore, it is important that both the practitioner and patient be aware of the common side effects that may occur when using smoking cessation products. In addition, the patient needs to be informed that tolerance to the adverse effects associated with NRT usually occurs.

Weight gain is a common outcome of smoking cessation and many patients are hesitant to quit for this reason. Approximately 2 to 3 kg is gained over the first year after cessation (Anderson et al., 2001). The mechanism for this is thought to be a slowing of metabolism. As mentioned earlier, the average smoker weighs 2.7 to 4.5 kg less than the average nonsmoker (McEvoy, 2001). Therefore, with the cessation of smoking, the average former smoker should weigh approximately the same as the average nonsmoker.

Patients must be informed that weight gain is possible but not significant. In addition, the health risk is small compared with continued smoking. The increase in weight can be dealt with after the patient has achieved complete abstinence. If weight gain is a major deterrent to treatment, nicotine gum may be used because it may delay the weight gain.

Furthermore, patient counseling on the proper use of nicotine products including dose and administration can improve efficacy and safety of the medications. Although the important role of pharmacotherapy is addressed, it should be recognized that a sustained reduction in smoking prevalence will require social desirability of limiting access to cigarettes and increasing availability as well as use of effective cessation intervention (Anderson et al., 2001). Finally, as the effort to promote smoking cessation interventions is sustained, increase in quit rates will be expected as well as an ultimate decrease in smoking-related morbidity and mortality among both children and adults.

■ Case Study

A.P., a 46-year-old white man, has been smoking 1.5 packs of cigarettes per day for the last 28 years. He has a very stressful job as executive of a large marketing company. A.P. and his coworkers frequently go to "happy hour" at the local bar after a long day at work. When he is at home, A.P. has a sedentary lifestyle that consists of lounging by the pool or watching television. He tried to quit smoking "cold turkey" 2 years ago and remained abstinent for approximately 1 year, but has never tried any pharmacologic smoking cessation aids. During his previous attempt to quit, he became very anxious, irritable, and depressed and had trouble sleeping and concentrating at work. He has a medical history of hypertension for the last 10 years and he has not complied with the therapeutic regimen. His family has been encouraging him to stop smoking for years. He is currently at the doctor's office for his blood pressure check-up and inquires about smoking cessation options.

1. What symptoms experienced by this patient during his previous attempt to quit smoking are consistent with physical dependence to nicotine?

2. What motivational level (stage of change) is this patient in?

3. When A.P. reaches the action stage, what pharmacologic options are available for him?

4. Which smoking cessation aid would you recommend starting in this patient? Why?

5. What adverse events could you see with the product that you chose in the previous question?

6. What are some nondrug methods that may enhance smoking cessation in this patient?

Bibliography

Starred references are cited in the text.

*Agency for Health Care Policy and Research. (2000). A clinical practice guideline for treating tobacco use and dependence. A U.S. Public Health Service report. *Journal of the American Medical Association, 283*(24), 3244–3254.

*American Cancer Society. (2004). *Cancer facts and figures*. Atlanta, GA: Author.

*American Psychiatric Association. (1994). *Diagnostic and statistical manual of mental disorders* (4th ed.). Washington, DC: Author.

*American Psychiatric Association. (1996). Practice guideline for the treatment of patients with nicotine dependence. *American Journal of Psychiatry, 153*(Suppl. 10), 1–31.

*Anderson, J. E., Jorenby, D. E., Scott, W. J., et al. (2002). Treating tobacco use and dependence; and evidence based clinical practice guideline for tobacco cessation. *Chest, 121*(3), 932–941.

*Blondal, T., Gudmundsson, L. J., Olafsdottir, I., et al. (1999). Nicotine nasal spray with nicotine patch for smoking cessation: Randomized trial with six year follow up. *British Medical Journal, 318*, 285–289.

*Centers for Disease Control and Prevention. (2002a). Annual smoking-attributable mortality, years of potential life, list and economic costs-United States, 1995–1999. *Morbidity and Mortality Weekly Report, 51*(14), 300–303.

*Centers for Disease Control and Prevention. (2002b). Trends in cigarette smoking among high school students—United States, 1991–2001. *Morbidity and Mortality Weekly Report, 51*, 409–412.

*Centers for Disease Control and Prevention. (2004a). State-specific prevalence of current cigarette smoking among adults—United States, 2002. *Morbidity and Mortality Weekly Report Highlights, 50* (53), 1277–1280.

*Centers for Disease Control and Prevention. (2004b). Health effects of cigarette smoking. Fact Sheet. Accessed: April 1, 2004 at www.cdc.gov.

*Da Costa, C. L., Younes, R. N., & Lourenco, M. T. (2002). Stopping smoking: A prospective, randomized, double-blind study comparing nortriptyline to placebo. *Chest, 122*, 403–408.

*Dale, L. C., Glover, E. D., Sachs, D. P., et al. (2001). Bupropion for smoking cessation. *Chest, 119*, 1357–1364.

*Doering, P. L. (2002). Substance-related disorders: Alcohol, nicotine, and caffeine. In J. T. Dipiro (Ed.). *Pharmacotherapy: A pathophysiologic approach* (5th ed.). New York: McGraw-Hill.

*Fiore, M. C., Bailey, W. C., Cohen, S. J., et al. (2000). *Treating tobacco use and dependence: Clinical practice guidelines.* Rockville, MD: U.S. Department of Health and Human Services, Public Health Service, Agency for Health Care Policy and Research.

*Glover, E. D., Glover, P. N., Franzon, M., et al. (2002). A comparison of a nicotine sublingual tablet and placebo for smoking cessation. *Nicotine Tobacco Research, 4,* 441–450.

Gold, P. B., Rubey, R. N., & Harvey, R. T. (2002). Naturalistic, self-assignment comparative trial of bupropion SR, a nicotine patch, or both for smoking cessation treatment in primary care. *American Journal of Addictions, 11*(4), 315–331.

*Heatherton, T. F., Kozlowski, L. T., Frecker, R. C., et al. (1991). The Fagerstrom Test for Nicotine Dependence: A revision of the Fagerstrom Tolerance Questionnaire. *British Journal of Addictions, 86,* 1119–1127.

Hurt, R. D., Sachs, D. P. L., Glover, E. D., et al. (1997). A comparison of sustained-release buproprion and placebo for smoking cessation. *New England Journal of Medicine, 337,* 1195–1202.

*Jones, J. M., Lewis, M. L., & Stembridge, N. Y. (2000). Counseling against cigarette smoking. *US Pharmacist, 23*(2).

*Jorenby, D. E., Leischow, S. J., Nides, M. A., et al. (1999). A controlled trial of sustained release buproprion, a nicotine patch, or both for smoking cessation. *New England Journal of Medicine, 340,* 685–691.

*Kornitzer, M., Boutsen, M., Thijs J., et al. (1995). Combined use of nicotine patch and gum in smoking cessation: a placebo controlled clinical. *Preventive Medicine, 24,* 41–47.

*Le Houezec, J. (2003). Nicotine pharmacokinetics in nicotine addiction and nicotine replacement: A review. *International Journal of Tuberculosis and Lung Disease, 7*(9), 809–810.

*Mallin, R. (2002). Smoking cessation integration of behavioral and drug therapies. *American Family Physician, 65*(16), 1107–1114.

*McEvoy GE, Ed. (2001). *Miscellaneous Autonomic Drugs 12:92.* AHFS Drug Information. Bethesda, MD: American Society of Health-System Pharmacists.

McRobbie, H., & Hayek, P. (2001). Nicotine replacement therapy in patients with cardiovascular disease: Guidelines for health professionals. *Addiction, 96,* 1547–1551.

*Okuyemi, K. S., Ahluwalia, J. S., & Harris, K. J. (2000). Pharmacotherapy of smoking cessation. *Archives of Family Medicine, 9,* 270–281.

*Okuyemi, K. S., Ahluwalia, J. S., & Wadland, W. C. (2001). The evaluation and treatment of tobacco use disorder. *Journal of Family Practice, 50*(11), 987–997.

Patterson, F., Jepson, C., Kaufmann V., et al. (2003). Predictors if attendance in a randomized clinical trial of nicotine replacement therapy with behavioral counseling. *Drug and Alcohol Dependence, 72,* 123–131.

*Prochazka, A. V. (2000). New development in smoking cessation. *Chest, 117,* 169S–175S.

*Rennard, S. I., & Daughton, D. M. (2000). Smoking cessation. *Chest, 117,* 360S–364S.

*Shiffman, S., Dresler, C. M., Hajek, P., et al. (2002). Efficacy of a nicotine lozenge for smoking cessation. *Archives of Internal Medicine, 162*(22), 2632–2633.

*Shiffman, S., Dresler, C. M., Rohay, J. M., et al. (2004). Successful treatment with a nicotine lozenge of smokers with prior failure in pharmacological therapy. *Addiction, 99*(1), 83–92

*Silagy, C., Lancaster, T., Stead, L., et al. (2002). Nicotine replacement therapy for smoking cessation. *The Cochrane Library,* Volume (Issue 4). Accessed April 2004 at www.cochrane.org.

Wallstrom, M., Nilsson, F., & Hirsch, J. M. (2000). A randomized, double-blind, placebo controlled clinical evaluation of a nicotine sublingual tablet in smoking cessation. *Addiction, 95*(8), 1161–1171.

Wilson, K., Gibson, N., William, A., et al. (2000). Effects of smoking cessation on mortality after myocardial infarction: meta-analysis of cohort studies. *Archives of Internal Medicine, 160,* 2939–2944.

Visit the Connection web site for the most up-to-date drug information.

59

MENOPAUSE AND HORMONE REPLACEMENT THERAPY

■ VIRGINIA P. ARCANGELO

Menopause is the permanent cessation of menstruation resulting from loss of ovarian function. It is an endocrinopathy resulting from failure of the ovary to produce estrogen. Menopause is not an acute condition but rather a gradual transition from perimenopause to menopause and finally postmenopause. The perimenopause, that period from the first changes in ovarian function (which can be identified only in the laboratory) to final menstruation, can range from 2 to 8 years.

Every day about 5000 women enter menopause. The age of menopause in America has not changed significantly during the 20th century, but life expectancy has significantly increased. American women today can expect to live beyond 80 years of age. The median age of menopause in the United States is between 49 and 51 years, with a range of 41 to 59 years, so the average life expectancy of a woman reaching menopause is approximately 30 more years. Factors that contribute to menopause at an earlier than average age include a history of irregular menses before the perimenopause, African American heritage, cigarette smoking, and weight reduction diets. Approximately 4% of women undergo a nonsurgical menopause before 40 years of age (U.S. Preventive Services Task Forces, 2002).

The increased incidence of chronic disease in postmenopausal women appears to be influenced by decreased levels of estrogen or progesterone. The probability of developing coronary heart disease is 46%, stroke 20%, hip fracture 15%, breast cancer 10%, colorectal cancer 6%, and endometrial cancer 2.6%. Postmenopausal women have a 1.4- to 3-fold increased risk for Alzheimer's disease over men.

PHYSIOLOGY

Menopause involves an age-related loss of ovarian function and a resulting decrease in estrogen secretion by the ovarian follicular unit. The ovary produces 17-β-estradiol, the major circulating estrogen. At birth, approximately 1 to 2 million ovarian follicles are present. By 45 years of age, the number drops to approximately 10,000.

At middle perimenopause, the woman herself notices changes in her menstrual pattern. The menstrual pattern can change in one or all of three different ways as a result of unstable maturation of ovarian follicles. The time span from the first day of one menstrual period to the first day of the next may increase, the amount of blood lost and the number of days of bleeding may increase or decrease, or menstrual cycles may become anovulatory.

Amenorrhea in menopause results from the remaining follicles becoming resistant to the effect of follicle-stimulating hormone (FSH). The ovaries begin with a large number of follicles that atrophy during the reproductive years at a steady rate until there are too few to produce significant amounts of estradiol. During the perimenopause, estradiol and progesterone production declines. The reduction in hormone levels reduces the negative-feedback loop of the hypothalamic-pituitary system, which leads to a rise in FSH levels.

Estrogen has an impact on many body tissues and systems: bone, teeth, brain, eyes, vasomotor, heart, colon, and urogenital. Ovarian failure causes changes in many organ systems, but the changes are subtle and usually not distressing to women. The most noticeable change is amenorrhea. This is the change in reproductive function that all women experience. After 1 year of amenorrhea, women are considered postmenopausal.

Morbidity in the older woman seems to result from decreased hormone production. There is an unfavorable alteration in lipid profile and in the endothelium and vasoreactivity, predisposing postmenopausal women to cardiovascular disease, which increases in incidence after menopause because of increasing serum lipid levels. Coronary heart disease develops in approximately half of postmenopausal women; 30% die as a result and 20% have a stroke.

Most women seek treatment for menopausal symptoms such as vasomotor symptoms, insomnia, and mood changes. Approximately 85% of women experience vasomotor responses in the form of hot flashes or flushes, which are transient sensations ranging from warmth to intense heat that can last from 30 seconds to several minutes. Hot flashes are not linked to decreasing estrogen levels; rather, they are thought to be caused by gonadotropin-releasing factors that affect the autonomic nervous system, which leads to vasomotor instability. They are the most annoying consequences of menopause for many women. They can disrupt sleep. In addition, women experience vaginal atrophy and vaginal dryness, which can be very bothersome for sexually active women.

There is atrophy of the genitourinary system as a result of menopause. The vagina, vulva, urethra, and bladder have a large number of estrogen receptors. As estrogen levels decrease, there is the potential for urinary and sexual dysfunction. The vulva loses collagen, adipose tissue, and the ability to retain water. There is a shortening and narrowing of the vagina; the walls become thin and pale and elasticity decreases. Vaginal secretions decrease, thereby decreasing vaginal lubrication. The urethra may become irritated as well.

Osteoporosis, a progressive decrease in bone mass leading to potential fractures, is common. Approximately 1.3 million osteoporosis-related fractures are estimated to occur yearly in postmenopausal women.

INITIATING DRUG THERAPY

The treatment of menopause has a long and interesting history; bloodletting, purgatives, and powdered ass penis have all been tried to relieve the symptoms of menopause (Utian, 1997). Today, an increasing number of women are using behavioral changes and herbs to manage menopausal symptoms. Women who reduce intake of refined carbohydrates, caffeine, and alcohol report a reduction in hot flashes. Wearing only cotton clothing and maintaining low environmental temperatures makes many women more comfortable during hot flashes.

The phytoestrogens, those estrogens obtained from food, are being marketed in oral form under the trade name of Promensil. Phytoestrogens are also found in a number of common foods (Box 59-1). Phytoestrogens appear to block estrogen stimulation of the breast and uterus, but they must be used for 4 to 6 weeks, before improvement is noticed.

Women are also turning to other herbs for managing menopause (Table 59-1) such as soy or black cohash.

Estrogen decreases the frequency of night sweats and periods of wakefulness during the night, reduces sleep latency (time between going to bed and falling asleep), and improves sleep in postmenopausal women with sleeping difficulty.

About 1 year after menopause, a woman often experiences vulvovaginal symptoms, including vaginal dryness, itching, and burning. These symptoms increase in intensity the further a woman is from menopause. There is a loss of collagen and adipose tissue in the vulva, loss of the protective covering of the clitoral glans, and thinning and loss of elasticity of the vaginal surface. In the Women's Health Initiative (WHI) HOPE (Health, Osteoporosis, Progestin, Estrogen) study, women taking conjugated equine estrogen (CEE) or CEE with medroxyprogesterone acetate (MPA) at all doses had a significant increase in vaginal cells (Utian et al., 2001).

Women with low levels of estrogen are more likely to report sexual problems from vaginal dryness, pain, and burning during intercourse. Hormone therapy can reverse these symptoms. Shifren and colleagues (2000) reported that women aged 31 to 56 who had undergone oophorectomy and hysterectomy and reported sexual dysfunction had improvements in overall sexual function with the use of CEE plus transdermal testosterone.

An increase in irregularity of periods and symptoms of hypoestrogenism signal perimenopause. Treatment of perimenopause reflects a consideration of waning but still present fertility, and contraception must be considered. A combination hormone contraceptive has the dual advantage of alleviating hypoestrogenic symptoms and providing contraception.

Studies of Hormone Replacement

Until recently, hormone replacement therapy (HRT) was the gold standard for menopause therapy and prevention of osteoporosis. It was believed that HRT had cardioprotective effects. Recent studies have changed prescribing patterns for postmenopausal women.

The use of hormone therapy for menopausal symptoms was the standard approach until the results of the WHI were released in 2002. The purpose of the WHI was to study interventions for preventing and controlling common chronic conditions in postmenopausal women. In the early 1990s, randomized controlled studies had proven the efficacy of hormone therapy for relieving hot flashes and vaginal atrophy and for improving bone mineral density (BMD) and lipid levels. However, the only data about clinical outcomes for fractures, dementia, and cardiovascular disease came from observational studies.

WHI was to be an 8- to 10-year study with an observational component of 93,700 women and a randomized controlled component with 68,000 women. The randomized part

---

BOX 59–1. FOOD SOURCES OF PHYTOESTROGENS

Soybeans and soy products
Cashews
Peanuts
Oats
Corn
Wheat
Apples
Almonds

Table 59.1

Herbal Treatment of Menopausal Symptoms

Menopausal Symptom	Herbal Treatment	Usual Dose	Adverse Events and Contraindications
Hot flashes	Black cohosh (Cimicifuga)	40–200 mg/d; not to be taken for >6 mo	Not to be used during pregnancy Potential side effects: GI disturbances, hypotension
	Isoflavins (soy)	20–40 mg/d	Flatulence
	Vitamin E	400 U/d	
Mood swings	St. John's wort (Hypericum)	300 mg tid	Do not take with any antidepressant. May cause sun sensitivity

had 3 arms—hormone therapy (estrogen alone, estrogen plus progestin, and placebo), a low-fat diet, and calcium plus vitamin D. The estrogen used was continuous-combined CEE 0.625 mg daily and 2.5 mg MPA mg daily. The estrogen plus progestin arm was stopped early (after about 5.2 years). This group also had increased risk of coronary events, stroke, pulmonary embolism, and invasive breast cancer. The thought is that because there was an increased incidence of invasive breast cancer, HRT promotes the growth of existing breast cancer rather than causing cancer. There was a reduced risk of colorectal cancer and hip fractures. Many of the risks appeared in year 1 (coronary and venous thromboembolic events) and year 2 (stroke). It was determined based on the data that the risk–benefit profile of estrogen plus progestin was such that its use for primary prevention of chronic conditions was not validated and it should not be prescribed to prevent chronic conditions.

Quality of life (QOL) data have been reported for the estrogen plus progestin arm of WHI. Approximately 16,600 women completed surveys at baseline and year 1. About 1500 women completed surveys at year 3. At year 1 there was statistically significant improvement in sleep disturbance, physical functioning, and bodily pain as compared with placebo group. However, the differences were so small that there is a question about clinical significance. There was no significant difference at year 3. In women reporting moderate to severe vasomotor symptoms, those taking estrogen plus progestin had significant improvement in the severity of hot flashes and night sweats.

In the HOPE study, healthy postmenopausal women aged 40 to 65 were randomly assigned to treatment with CEE alone (0.625, 0.45, or 0.3 mg daily), CEE plus MPA (0.625/2.5, 0.45/2.5, 0.45/1.5 or 0.3/1.5 mg daily), or placebo. Over 13 cycles, women in all active treatment groups had a significant reduction in vasomotor symptoms. In women taking CEE alone, benefit increased with increased dosage. In women taking CEE plus MPA, the benefit was comparable with all doses.

The Heart and Estrogen/Progestin Replacement Study trials (HERS) were conducted to determine if estrogen and progestin therapy alters the risk of coronary heart disease events in postmenopausal women. The drugs were CEE and MPA and placebo. There were more coronary heart disease events in the first year but fewer in years 4 and 5. In HERS there was an increase in deep vein thromboembolism and pulmonary embolism and biliary tract surgery. There was no cardiac protection in women with previously diagnosed coronary heart disease.

The Postmenopausal Estrogen/Progestin Interventions (PEPI) trial studied healthy women aged 45 to 64. They were randomly assigned to treatment with different hormone regimens (CEE, cyclic CEE plus MPA, continuous CEE plus MPA, or cyclic CEE plus micronized progesterone). The women in the placebo group lost BMD at the spine and hip. Women who took hormone therapy gained BMD in the spine and hip.

In a recent meta-analysis of observational studies, postmenopausal women who used HRT at any time were found to have an incidence of dementia of 34% less than never-users. An analysis of 3 prospective studies in different cohorts of women showed that those who used HRT had a reduced risk of Alzheimer's disease (AD) from 41% to 60% (LeBlanc et al., 2001). In the Cache County study, an observational study of dementia in healthy older adults showed

that current users who had been using HRT for more than 10 years had a nonsignificant reduction in risk of AD but those who had started use within the past 3 years or 3 to 10 years had nonsignificant increase in the risk of AD compared with never-users (Zandi et al., 2002). In the HERS population, women who had used CEE plus MPA for a mean of 4.2 years did not perform better on tests of cognition than women who had used placebo (Grady et al., 2002). The WHI Memory Study (WHIMS) showed that estrogen plus progestin increased the risk for probable dementia in women 65 or older and did not prevent mild cognitive impairment in these women (Rapp et al., 2003).

Because only oral CEE 0.625 mg and MPA 2.5 mg were studied, it is not possible to generalize response to other forms of estrogen or progestin, other routes of administration, or other doses.

Studies of Nonhormonal Therapy for Hot Flashes

There has been an evaluation of nonhormonal therapy for hot flashes because of the controversy about HRT. Anecdotal improvement was seen in hot flashes in women using agents that inhibit neuronal uptake of serotonin. Relief was found with fluoxetine (Prozac, Sarafem), venlafaxine (Effexor), and paroxetine (Paxil) (Loprinzi et al., 1998). Based on these observations, clinical trials were conducted with venlafaxine and paroxetine. In the venlafaxine pilot, 12.5 mg twice a day was used. There was an approximately 50% decrease in hot flashes. A pilot study using paroxetine 20 mg showed a reduction in hot flashes of about 65% (Stearns et al., 2000).

Further study was done with venlafaxine (extended release) at doses of 37.5 mg, 75 mg, and 150 mg. This was a 4-arm double-blind placebo-controlled study. There was a 37% reduction in hot flashes with 37.5 mg compared to a 61% reduction with 75 and 150 mg. There was improvement in libido and QOL scores in the venlafaxine groups (Loprinzi et al., 2000).

A placebo-controlled crossover study with fluoxetine 20 mg was conducted. There was a 50% decrease of hot flashes with fluoxetine (Loprinzi et al., 2002).

Pilot studies have shown that gabapentin (Neurontin) in low doses can alleviate hot flashes (Guttuso, 2000). Further studies have to be conducted.

Recommendations on Use of HRT

The U.S. Preventive Services Task Force (2002) recommends against the routine use of estrogen and progestin for prevention of chronic conditions in postmenopausal women. HRT has benefits and harms. The benefits are the increase in BMD, decrease in the risk of fracture, and decrease in the incidence of colorectal cancer. The harms are increased risks for breast cancer, venous thromboembolism, coronary heart disease, stroke, and cholecystitis.

Both the American College of Obstetrics and Gynecology (ACOG) and the North American Menopause Society (NAMS) recommend against the use of HRT for primary or secondary prevention of cardiovascular disease. They caution against the use of HRT to prevent osteoporosis; other therapies should be used. The use of HRT is acceptable for control of menopausal symptoms but not for prolonged use. At each visit a risk–benefit analysis is done by the patient and provider and the decision to continue therapy is made based on that discussion.

The decision to prescribe HRT should be a joint one between the provider and the patient. When discussing HRT, the women must be informed of the risks. Many women choose pharmacotherapy to relieve the symptoms of menopause. In prescribing HRT, a complete and thoughtful history and physical examination are conducted. The standard family and personal history should be augmented with questions about the woman's gynecologic history, menopausal symptoms, and attitudes toward menopause and her goals in using HRT.

The routine physical examination should also include the patient's measured height, a gynecologic examination, and clinical breast examination. Investigative studies should include a pregnancy test, mammogram, and Papanicolaou (Pap) smear. Conditions that predispose women to increased risk of endometrial cancer include a lifelong history of irregular menses, polycystic ovary disease, or a recent history of irregular menses occurring closer than 21 days apart or menses lasting longer than 10 days. These women should have an endometrial biopsy before beginning HRT.

Low-dose oral contraceptives can be used to prevent and control symptoms until the patient reaches menopause and to ensure prevention of conception because these women are still fertile. To check if the patient taking oral contraceptives is menopausal, FSH levels can be determined on the last hormone-free day. Oral contraceptives are contraindicated in smokers older than 35 years of age. Oral contraceptives are discussed in Chapter 60.

If the choice is to use HRT, therapy should be individualized. Individual needs should be assessed and menopausal symptoms evaluated.

All continuous HRT regimens can cause breakthrough bleeding. About 30% of all women who are recently menopausal have some breakthrough bleeding; this decreases with women who are more than 3 years postmenopausal. Amenorrhea usually occurs within 1 year of initiating therapy.

Data from the WHI shows that short-term use of combined estrogen and progestin increases the incidence of breast cancer and abnormal mammograms. Those women in the study taking HRT were diagnosed at a more advanced stage of breast cancer. The risk is increased less than 1 per 100 women over baseline.

The use of HRT is recommended for the prevention of postmenopausal osteoporosis, treatment of moderate to severe vasomotor symptoms, and treatment of moderate to severe vulvar and vaginal atrophy.

Goals of Drug Therapy

The goal of hormone therapy is treatment of menopausal symptoms. It is no longer to prevent long-term chronic conditions, especially heart disease. HRT generally refers to treatment with estrogen and progestin used in women with an intact uterus and ERT refers to treatment with estrogen alone, used in women who have no uterus.

Estrogen

In the postmenopausal woman, short-term estrogen therapy is the choice for treating symptoms such as hot flashes, vaginal dryness, and sleep disturbances. It is not to be used for prevention of coronary heart disease. The therapy should be a

short as possible. Therapy for 1 to 4 years seems to outweigh the risks, but therapy for longer than 4 years is questionable.

No other method provides such consistent and complete relief of menopausal symptoms as HRT. Use the lowest possible dose. Doses as low as 0.3 mg have been shown to provide effective relief from hot flashes and vaginal discomfort. Transdermal doses of estradiol as low as 12.5 μg have been effective.

It is recommended that HRT be prescribed at lower doses. Postmenopausal women using CEE alone had a significantly reduced risk of first coronary events when compared with nonusers. Women using a higher dose had a significantly higher risk of stroke but women using the lower dose did not. A different preparation of estrogen can be used such as 17-β-estradiol, ethinyl estradiol, or esterified estrogen.

HRT comes in nonoral forms. These forms seem to better mimic the release of hormones as the ovaries would produce if they were still functional. There are transdermal options with steady-state pharmacokinetics and less hepatic metabolism. There is not an increase in C-reactive protein seen with these as with oral therapy. Vaginal rings containing estrogen are another option.

Dosage

For the management of moderate to severe vasomotor symptoms, the dose for CEE, esterified estrogen, and estropipate is 0.3 to 0.625 mg/d, with 0.3 the recommended dose. The 17-β-estradiol oral dose is recommended at 0.25 to 0.5 mg and the 17-β-estradiol patch 0.025 mg/d. Estrogen can be taken continuously or on a cyclic schedule with 1 week off per month. The lowest dose that controls symptoms is recommended. It does takes longer to achieve maximal benefit with low dose.

Local products for vaginal symptoms include vaginal estradiol ring (Estring 0.0075 mg/d) and estradiol acetate (Femring 0.05 and 0.10 mg/d). The rings are inserted every 3 months. Additionally there are vaginal topical preparations and 17-β-estradiol suppositories (Vagifem 0.025) and cream (Estrace vaginal cream, 2–4 gm/d for 1–2 weeks, then 1–2 g/d for 1–2 weeks, then 1 g 1–3 times weekly), and CEE (Premarin vaginal cream 0.5–2 g daily for 3 weeks on and 1 week off). Dienestrol (Ortho Dinestrol Vaginal Cream 1–2 applicatorsful/d for 1–2 weeks, then half the dose for 1–2 weeks, then 1 applicatorful 1–3 times weekly) is another vaginal cream available. Local products have the lowest systemic absorption.

Adverse Events

To avoid serious adverse events, the practitioner does not prescribe HRT/ERT if it is absolutely contraindicated (Box 59-2 lists the absolute and relative contraindications).

Adverse events include intolerance to contact lenses from steepening of corneal curvature, headache, depression, gallbladder disease, nausea, vomiting, abdominal cramps, increased blood pressure, thromboembolic disease, breakthrough bleeding, edema, breast cancer, and breast tenderness.

The results of the WHI showed that for every 10,000 women taking HRT for 1 year, there was an increase of 8 strokes, 7 cases of coronary heart disease, 8 more invasive breast cancers, and 8 additional pulmonary embolisms. There was a decreased incidence of 6 colorectal cancers and 5 fewer hip fractures.

BOX 59–2. WHEN HRT IS CONTRAINDICATED

Absolute Contraindications
- Known or suspected breast cancer
- Known or suspected endometrial cancer
- Undiagnosed genital bleeding
- Acute liver disease
- Active thromboembolic disease or history of thromboembolic disease
- Known or suspected pregnancy

Relative Contraindications
- Chronic liver dysfunction
- Uncontrolled or poorly controlled hypertension
- Acute intermittent porphyria

Interactions

Drug interactions with CEE include increased effects of corticosteroids and decreased levels of estrogen with barbiturates, phenytoin (Dilantin), and rifampin (Rifadin). Patients taking phenytoin excrete estrogen more quickly. There can be increases in thyroxine and serum triglyceride levels. An increased dose is needed in smokers because only half the serum level achieved in nonsmokers is reached. Alcohol increases the circulating levels of estrogen.

Progestin

Progesterone is secreted by the corpus luteum. It acts on the endometrium to change proliferative endometrial tissue to secretory tissue. Progesterone is given as a part of HRT to women with an intact uterus. It decreases the risk of estrogen-induced irregular bleeding, endometrial hyperplasia, and carcinoma. It is not needed in women without a uterus.

Progestins may increase the risk of breast cancer above that with estrogen alone. However, women who have a uterus must take progestogens to protect against endometrial cancer and hyperplasia. The progestogens tend to attenuate the positive cardiovascular effects of estrogen. This shows a need to use the lowest possible dose of progestin other than MPA. Some are more metabolically inert (micronized progesterone, trimegestone, drospirenone).

The PEPI trial showed that CEE with cyclic micronized progesterone had the best lipid profile of any of the combined regimens. Micronized progesterone and norethindrone acetate (NETA) have better side effect profiles than MPA.

The progesterone studied in the WHI study was medroxyprogesterone. Micronized progesterone showed the best lipid profile in the PEPI trial, so it may be the best preparation to use. Another option is norethindione acetate.

Dosage

The recommended daily dose is 0.5 to 5 mg for a woman with an intact uterus. The lowest dose is recommended. One study showed NETA doses as low as 0.1 mg were effective in providing endometrial protection when combined with oral 17-β-estradiol 1.0 mg. The standard dose of NETA is 0.5 mg (Kurman et al., 2000).

Contraindications

Thrombophlebitis, hepatic disease, breast cancer, undiagnosed vaginal bleeding, pregnancy, and lactation contraindicate progesterone use. Cautious use is recommended with epilepsy, migraine, asthma, and cardiac or renal dysfunction.

Adverse Events

Adverse events include bloating, abdominal cramping, edema, irritability, weight gain, headache, breakthrough bleeding, breast tenderness, and acne.

Combination Products

Products that combine estrogen and progestin provide ease of administration and include CEE/MPA, estradiol/norgestimate, and ethinyl estradiol/NETA.

Testosterone

The slight decrease in testosterone production that accompanies menopause can cause a significant decrease or complete loss of libido in some women. For these women, testosterone can be added to HRT in doses of 1.25 to 2.5 mg methyltestosterone. The adverse events of testosterone in these doses are hirsutism, voice change, and a decrease in the high-density lipoprotein cholesterol level. Long-term use is associated with the risk of hepatocellular neoplasm, increased edema, and possible elevation of cholesterol level. The only indication for treatment is severe vasomotor disturbances and decreased libido.

The most frequent treatment choice is either Estratest, which is 1.25 mg esterified estrogen and 2.5 mg methyltestosterone, or Estratest H.S., which is 0.625 mg esterified estrogen and 1.25 mg methyltestosterone. Estratest H.S. may be used safely as long as lipid levels are normal. Estratest, with its 1.25 mg esterified estrogen, is a high dose of estrogen and should be used only for short periods. Topical testosterone, which has recently received a great deal of attention in the lay press, is not commercially available in the United States.

Nonhormonal Therapy

The most effective alternatives to HRT for the relief of vasomotor symptoms are the selective serotonin reuptake inhibitors (SSRIs), venlafaxine (Effexor) and paroxetine (Paxil). They have been shown to significantly reduce hot flashes in randomized trials, with venlafaxine 75 mg and paroxetine 20 mg or paroxetine CR 12.5 mg and 25 mg having the greatest effect.

Venlafaxine (Effexor), extended release, is the best studied nonhormonal therapy for hot flashes. It is recommended that therapy start at 37.5 mg/d for 1 week. If hot flashes are controlled at that dose, then it is maintained. If they are not controlled, the dose should be increased to 75 mg/d. Also recommended is paroxetine (Paxil) 12.5 to 25 mg daily. Results are usually seen in 1 to 2 weeks.

Selecting the Most Appropriate Agent

For women who have had a hysterectomy, the only component needed for HRT is estrogen. The patient needs to decide which estrogen delivery method—transdermal, vaginal, or oral—is desirable for her. Transdermal estrogen is easy to use, which increases compliance. Some women, however, find the concept of a transdermal patch aesthetically unpleasing and they may select an oral estrogen. Both dosage forms have the same effect of reducing hot flashes and preventing osteoporosis. Oral agents have a greater impact on lipid levels. The oral and transdermal products are discussed in Table 59-2.

Estrogen must be combined with progestin to prevent endometrial hyperplasia and the possibility of endometrial carcinoma in a woman with an intact uterus. Currently, the only progestin approved by the U.S. Food and Drug Administration (FDA) for oral HRT is MPA.

The woman who has not had a hysterectomy must also select a delivery method for HRT—oral, transdermal, or vaginal—and must also decide if she wants to use cyclic, continuous, or continuous combined HRT.

Progestin exposure should be minimized. Women using HRT who receive MPA 5 or 10 mg every 3 months have only slightly higher rates of hyperplasia (1.5%) (Doren, 2000). In one study, women on lower-dose estrogen, CEE 0.3 mg daily plus MPA 10 mg daily for 14 days every 6 months, the rate of endometrial hyperplasia was only 1.6% (Ettinger et al., 2001), suggesting that quarterly or biyearly progestin schedules are almost as effective as monthly or continuous regimens at preventing endometrial hyperplasia, although more study needs to be done.

Short-term use is recommended. Risk of breast cancer does not substantially increase until after 5 years and most women's menopausal symptoms abate within 5 years after onset of menopause.

For women with vasomotor symptoms with contraindications to HRT, or who choose not to use HRT, venlafaxine and paroxetine are recommended.

Administration Options

Oral therapy is the most popular, but therapy is available in transdermal and vaginal preparations as well. Transdermal estrogen is recommended if it is desirable to avoid the first-pass phenomenon in women who have liver disease or who are prone to gallbladder disease. Vaginal preparations are used to relieve genitourinary symptoms associated with menopause.

First-Line Therapy

For a woman with an intact uterus, the most popular regimen is continuous combined oral therapy. Continuous use of estrogen and progestin prevents withdrawal bleeding.

Second-Line Therapy

If the woman cannot tolerate oral estrogen because of intolerance to pills or gastrointestinal (GI) upset, or compliance issues, transdermal or vaginal preparations are recommended. The transdermal and vaginal routes, which bypass the liver, are also preferred for women who smoke or who have a history of gallbladder disease, fibrocystic breast disease, thrombophlebitis, elevated triglyceride levels, migraines, or hypertension. Additionally, nonhormonal therapy, such as SSRIs, can be used.

Third-Line Therapy

If vasomotor symptoms are intolerable, estrogen doses can be increased to the next higher dose. If the woman experiences decreased libido, methyltestosterone can be added at a dose of 1.2 to 2.5 mg/d. If this therapy is used, the practitioner must monitor liver function and electrolyte levels every 3 to 6 months. See Table 59-3 and Figure 59-1 to review the order of therapy.

MONITORING PATIENT RESPONSE

The patient should be seen 2 months after starting therapy and then in 6 months to check response to therapy, blood pressure, and side effects. After that, annual visits are required.

The health status of a woman on HRT must be evaluated annually. The woman should have an annual clinical breast examination and mammogram if she is older than 40 years of age. Annually, the patient's medical history should be reviewed for the past year, including questions about vaginal bleeding. Any woman on continuous combined HRT who has vaginal bleeding beyond the first year of treatment should be evaluated with an endometrial biopsy. The physical examination should include:

- Height measurement to screen for osteoporosis
- Weight measurement to screen for obesity
- Blood pressure evaluation to screen for cardiovascular disease
- Clinical breast examination and review of procedures for breast self-examination
- Full pelvic examination, including Pap smear

Prescriptions for HRT should not be renewed without a full annual history and physical. Encouraging new HRT users to call the practitioner at the end of 3 months of therapy helps the patient to discuss any concerns or problems with HRT.

At each visit, the risks and benefits of HRT must be discussed and documented. At that time it should be a mutual decision whether to continue or stop the therapy.

Discontinuing HRT should be done gradually. It may be done in several ways. The patient may begin to skip more days between doses or the dose may be decreased at 4- to 6-week intervals.

More than 75% of women discontinue HRT in less than 1 year because of undesirable side effects. Another influence is that the woman may not feel any different when taking the medication. Education is an important aspect of prescribing HRT.

PATIENT EDUCATION

Drug Information

Several options are available for the postmenopausal woman with vasomotor symptoms. If she decides to begin HRT, the decision must be an informed decision. To make an informed decision, the patient must be provided with detailed information on the risks and benefits of therapy and other options available. It is also important to understand the side effects and that there may be monthly bleeding. Key teaching points include:

- The patient must be aware that it may be 4 weeks or more before symptoms disappear.

Table 59.2

Overview of Selected Agents Used to Treat Menopausal Symptoms

Generic (Trade) Name and Dosage	Side Effects	Contraindications	Special Considerations
Oral Hormone Replacement			
Conjugated equine estrogen (CEE) (Premarin) Usual daily dose 0.3–0.65 mg Doses available: 0.3, 0.45 and 0.625 mg	Nauses, vomiting, breakthrough bleeding, edema, weight changes, swollen/tender breasts, hypertension, depression, hair loss, changes in libido	Estrogen-dependent neoplasia Thrombophlebitis or thromboembolic disorder Pregnancy Undiagnosed vaginal bleeding	May cause GI upset, so take with food.
estradiol (Estrace) 1 mg/d	Same as above	Same as above	Same as above
Combination products			
CEE and MPA (Prempro) Doses 0.5/1.5, 0.4/1.5, 0.625/2.5, 0.625/5 mg	Same as above	Same as above	Same as above
ethinyl estradiol & norethindine acetate (NETA)			
Femhrt 1/5 5 mcg/1 ng	Same as above	Same as above	Same as above
estradiol (NETA) 1 mg/0.5 ng	Same as above	Same as above	Same as above
(Estratest) esterified estrogen 1.25 mg and methyltestosterone 2.5 mg (Estratest H.S.) esterified estrogen 0.625 mg and methyltestosterone 1.25 mg Taken daily for 3 wk then 1 wk off	Liver function changes, nausea, breakthrough bleeding, edema, weight gain, hypertension, depression, intolerance to contact lenses, changes in libido, virilization, jaundice, gallbladder disease	Breast or endometrial cancer, undiagnosed genital bleeding, thromboembolic disease, pregnancy, lactation	Report any adverse events immediately. May take at bedtime to prevent nausea.
Progesters			
medroxyprogesterone (Amen, Curretab, Cycrin, Provera) 2.5–10 mg either daily or cyclic	Vision changes, migraine, porphyria, depression, insomnia, jaundice, nausea, thrombophlebitis, pulmonary embolism, increased blood pressure, breakthrough bleeding, breast tenderness, rash, hirsutism, increased weight, decreased glucose tolerance	Thrombophlebitis, hepatic disease, breast cancer, undiagnosed vaginal bleeding, pregnancy, lactation Caution in epilepsy, migraine, asthma, cardiac dysfunction	Report any adverse events immediately. May take at bedtime to prevent nausea.
norethindione acetate (NETA) Aygestin dose 2.5–10 mg/d	Same as above	Same as above	Same as above
Transdermal Hormone Replacement			
estradiol (Alora, Estraderm, Vivelle) Change transdermal patch twice a week Alora—0.05, 0.075, 0.1 mg/d Vivelle—0.0375, 0.05, 0.075, 0.1 mg/d	Irritation at application site, headache, breakthrough bleeding, nausea, abdominal cramps,	Undiagnosed abnormal vaginal bleeding, thromboembolic disorder, pregnancy, breast or estrogen-dependent tumor	Apply to clean, dry area on lower abdomen, hips, or buttocks (not breast or waistline). Rotate application sites. Use 3 wk on and 1 wk off in patient with intact uterus; continuous in patient without uterus.
estradiol (Climara)—0.025, 0.0375, 0.05, 0.075, 0.1 Change transdermal patch once a week 0.05, 0.075, 0.1 mg/d	Same as above	Same as above	Same as above
estradiol and NETA (CombiPatch) Change transdermal patch twice a week (0.05 mg estradiol and 0.14 mg norethindrone, 0.05 mg estradiol and 0.25 mg norethindrone)	Same as above	Same as above	Apply to clean, dry area on lower abdomen, hips or buttocks (not breast or waistline). Combination therapy
Vaginal Hormones			
estradiol 0.01% (Estrace Vaginal Cream) Initially 2–4 g/d for 1–2 wk, then 1–2 g/d for 1–2 wk; maintenance dose: 1 g, 1–3 times a week (3 wk on and 1 wk off)	Uterine bleeding, vaginal candidiasis	Breast or estrogen-dependent cancer, thrombophlebitis, undiagnosed genital bleeding, pregnancy, lactation, impaired liver function	Need to take progestin if uterus present.
Estring (vaginal ring) 0.0015/d ring into vagina; replaced every 90 d Femring 0.05, 0.1/d	Headache, leukorrhea, back pain, urinary tract infection, vaginitis, vaginal pain, abdominal pain, bacterial growth	Same as above	Remove while treating vaginitis. Reevaluate every 3–6 mo.
Premarin vaginal cream 0.625 mg/g 0.5–2 g/d	Nausea, vomiting, breakthrough bleeding, edema, weight changes, swollen/tender breasts, hypertension, depression, hair loss, changes in libido	Same as above	Therapeutic regimen consists of 3 wk on therapy and 1 wk off

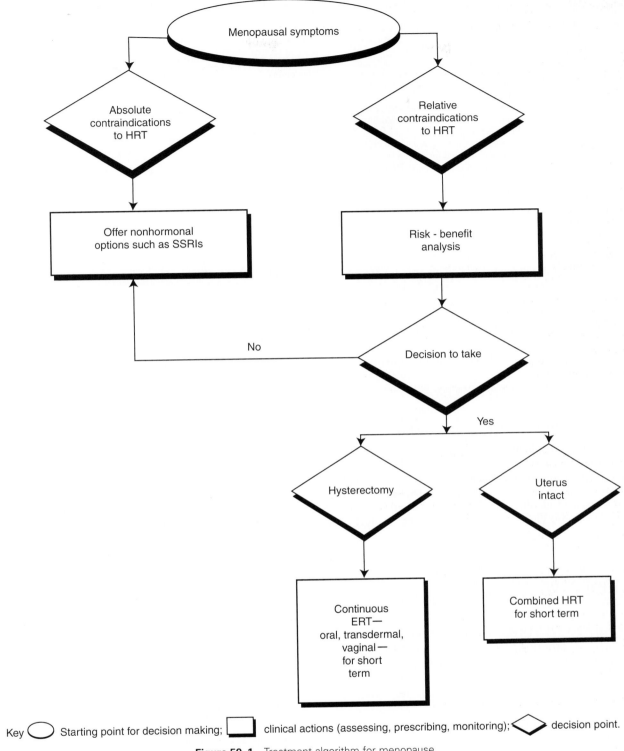

Figure 59–1 Treatment algorithm for menopause.

- HRT can be taken with food or at bedtime to prevent nausea.
- The patient should be taught how to perform a monthly breast self-examination.
- The patient should be familiar with danger signs of adverse events—abnormal vaginal bleeding, pain in the calf or chest, shortness of breath, coughing blood, severe headache, jaundice, breast lump, and vision changes. These should be reported immediately to the health care provider.

Assess the presence and severity of menopausal symptoms and how they impair the patient's QOL. Discuss all reasonable treatment options and prescribe HRT at the lowest dose for the shortest period of time.

When using hormonal products for the treatment of symptoms of vulvar and vaginal atrophy, use topical preparations.

Perform an annual risk–benefit assessment.

If discontinuing HRT, taper it. Reduce the estrogen component and maintain the progestin component. Taper for at

Table 59.3

Recommended Order of Therapy

Order	Agents	Comments
First line	HRT/ERT short-term for treatment of menopausal symptoms at the lowest therapeutic dose for the shortest period of time. Therapy can be oral, transdermal, or vaginal. Combination therapy must be used for a woman with an intact uterus.	At each visit the risk/benefits must be discussed and a mutual dicision made whether to continue therapy.
Second line	If vasomotor symptoms are not controlled, higher estrogen doses can be used for a short period of time.	
Third line	If there is contraindication to HRT/ERT or if the decision is made not to use this therapy, consider SSRIs for treatment relief or alternative therapies. If the women experience decreased libido, testosterone can be added at a dose of 1.2–2.5 mg of methyltestosterone.	It testosterone is used, liver function and electrolytes must be monitored every 3–6 mo.

least 4 weeks. If the patient develops vasomotor symptoms, return to the previous dose and continue therapy.

Patient information sources for menopause include:

Harvard Women's Health Watch: www.health.harvard.edu/newsletters

The National Council for Reliable Health Information: www.ncrhi.org/main.htm

The North American Menopause Society: www.menopause.org

Nutritional and Lifestyle Changes

The woman in menopause who is symptomatic needs to be instructed to wear loose, cotton clothing. Environmental adjustments may be helpful, such as keeping the temperature lower. A reduction in the intake of caffeine, simple carbohydrates, and alcohol also helps. She should go to bed just to sleep and have sex. If she is unable to sleep, she should leave the bed and read or do some other activity that is relaxing.

Complementary and Alternative Medicine

A randomized trial of vitamin E showed that the treatment group had one less daily hot flash (Barton et al., 1998). Some clinical trials have shown improvement of hot flashes with soy and black cohash and some have shown no improvement (Faure et al., 2002; Quella et al., 2000).

Soy, chickpeas, and other legumes contain isoflavins, which exhibit estrogenic properties. They can provide some symptom relief, although their effectiveness in menopause is still being investigated.

Black cohash is also used to treat menopause. It purportedly induces vaginal maturation and improves hot flashes. However, no long-term scientific data are available currently.

■ Case Study

E.P., a 51-year-old Asian woman who is 68 inches tall and weighs 130 pounds, presents complaining of amenorrhea for the past 8 months. She wakes up at least 5 times a night with hot flashes and experiences them at least 10 times a day. She is very uncomfortable and sleep deprived. At the visit a Pap smear is done and a mammogram is negative. Her FSH level is 32 IU/mL. She has no family history of breast cancer, but her mother has osteoporosis.

1. List specific goals for treatment of E.P.

2. What drug therapy would you prescribe? Why? For how long?

3. What are the parameters for monitoring success of the therapy?

4. Discuss patient education and counseling necessary in this situation.

5. List two adverse reactions of the prescribed therapy.

6. What would be the choice for second-line therapy if E.P. could not tolerate the treatment of choice and symptoms were still present?

> → 7. What alternative therapy may be suggested?
>
> → 8. What dietary and lifestyle modifications should be made?
>
> → 9. Describe contraindications to HRT.

Bibliography

Starred references are cited in the text.

*Barton, D., Loprinzi, C., Quela, S., et al. (1998). Prospective evaluation of vitamin E for hot flashes in breast cancer survivors. *Journal of Clinical Oncology, 16,* 495–500.

*Doren, M. (2000). Hormonal replacement regimens and bleeding. *Maturitas, 34,* S17–S23.

*Ettinger, B., Pressmen, A., & VanGessel, A. (2001). Low-dosage esterified estrogens opposed by progestin at 6 month intervals. *Obstetrics and Gynecology, 98,* 205–211.

*Faure, E., Chantre, P., & Mares, P. (2002). Effects of a standardized soy extract on hot flushes: A multicenter, double-blind randomized, placebo-controlled study. *Menopause, 9,* 329– 334.

Gold, E. B., Sternfield, B., Kelsey, J. L., et al (2000). Relationship of demographic and lifestyle factors to symptoms in a multi-racial/ethnic population of women 40 to 55 years of age. *American Journal of Epidemiology, 152,* 463–473.

Grady, D. (2003). Postmenopausal hormones—Therapy for symptoms only. *New England Journal of Medicine, 348,* 1835–1837.

*Grady, D., Yaffe, K., Kristof, M., et al. (2002). Effects of postmenopausal function on cognitive function: The Heart and Estrogen/progestin Replacement Study, *American Journal of Medicine, 113.* 543–548.

Grodstein, F., Newcomb, P. A., & Stampfer, M. J. (1999). Postmenopausal hormone therapy and risk of colorectal cancer: A review and meta-analysis. *American Journal of Medicine, 106,* 574–582.

*Guttosa, T. J. (2000). Gabapentin's effect on hot flashes and hypothermia. *Neurology, 54,* 2161–2163.

Hackley, B., & Rousseau, M. E. (2004). Managing menopausal symptoms after the Women's Health Initiative. *Journal of Midwifery Women's Health, 49*(2), 87–95.

*Kurman, R. J., Felix, J. C., Archer, D. F., et al. (2002). Norethindrone acetate and estradiol-induced endometrial hyperplasia. *Obstetrics and Gynecology, 96,* 373–379.

*LeBlanc, E. S., Janowsky, J., Chan, B. K., et al. (2001), Hormone replacement therapy and cognition: Systematic review and meta-analysis. *Journal of the American Medical Association, 285,* 1489–1499.

*Loprinzi, C. L., Kugler, J. W., Sloan, J. A., et al. (200). Venlafaxine in management of hot flashes in survivors of breast cancer: A randomized controlled trial. *Lancet, 356,* 2059–2063.

*Loprinzi, C. L., Pisansky, T. M., Fonseca, R., et al. (1998). Pilot evaluation of venlafaxine hydrochloride in the therapy of hot flashes in cancer survivors. *Journal of Clinical Oncology, 16,* 2377–2381.

*Loprinzi, C. L., Sloan, J. A., Perez, E. A., et al. (2002). Phase III evaluation of fluoxetine for treatment of hot flashes. *Journal of Clinical Oncology. 20,* 1578–1583.

Mattox, J., & Shulman, L. (2001). Combined oral hormone replacement therapy formulations. *American Journal of Obstetrics and Gynecology, 185,* S38–S46.

Mulnard, R. A., Cotman, C. W., Kawas, C., et al. (2000). Estrogen replacement therapy for treatment of mild to moderate Alzheimer's disease: A randomized controlled trial: Alzheimer's Disease Cooperative Study. *Journal of the American Medical Association, 283,* 1007–1015.

*Quella, S. K., Loprinzi, C. L., Barton, D. L., et al. (2000). Evaluation of soy phytoestrogens for the treatment of hot flashes in breast cancer survivors. A North Central Cancer Treatment Group Trial. *Journal of Clinical Oncology, 18,* 1068–1074.

*Rapp, S. R., Espeland, M. A., Shumaker, S. A., et al. (2003). Effect of estrogen plus progestin on global cognitive function in postmenopausal women. The Women's Health Initiative Memory Study: A randomized controlled trial. *Journal of the American Medical Association, 289,* 2663–2672.

Rousseau, M. E. (2002). Hormone replacement therapy: Short-term versus long-term use. *Journal of Midwifery Women' Health, 47,* 461–470.

*Shifren, J. L., Braunstein, G. D., Simon, J. A., et al. (2000). Transdermal testosterone treatment in women with impaired sexual function after oophorectomy. *New England Journal of Medicine, 343,* 682–688.

Shumaker, S. A., Legault, C., Rapp, S. R., et al. (2003). Estrogen plus progestin and in incidence of dementia and mild cognitive impairment in postmenopausal women. The Women's Health Initiative Memory Study: A randomized controlled trial. *Journal of the American Medical Association, 289,* 2651–2662.

*Stearns, V., Isaacs, C., Rowland, J., et al. (2000). A pilot trial assessing the efficacy of paroxetine hydrochloride (Paxil) in controlling hot flashes in breast cancer survivors. *Annals of Oncology, 11,* 17–22.

Torgerson, D. J., & Bell-Seyer, S. E. (2001). Hormone replacement therapy and the prevention of nonvertebral fractures: A meta-analysis of randomized trials. *Journal of the American Medical Association, 285,* 2891–2897.

*U.S. Preventive Services Task Force. (2002). Postmenopausal hormone replacement therapy for primary prevention of chronic conditions: Recommendations and rationale. *Annals of Internal Medicine, 137*(10), 834–839.

*Utian, W. H. (1997). Menopause: A modern perspective from a controversial history. *Maturitas, 26*(2), 73–82.

*Utian, W. H., Shoupe, D., Bochman, G., et al (2001). Relief of vasomotor symptoms and vaginal atrophy with lower doses of conjugated equine estrogen and medroxyprogesterone acetate. *Fertility Sterility, 75,* 1065–1079.

Writing Group for the PEPI Trial. (1995). Effects of estrogen or estrogen/progestin on heart disease risk factors in post menopausal women. *Journal of the American Medical Association, 273,* 199–208.

Writing Group for the Women's Health Initiative. (2002). Risks and benefits of estrogen plus progestin in healthy postmenopausal women. *Journal of the American Medical Association, 288,* 321–333.

*Zandi, P. P., Carlson, M. C., Plassman, B. L., et al (2002). Hormone replacement therapy and incidence of Alzheimer's disease in older women: The Cache County Study. *Journal of the American Medical Association, 288,* 2123–2129.

Visit the Connection web site for the most up-to-date drug information.

CONTRACEPTION

■ ELENA M. UMLAND AND VIRGINIA P. ARCANGELO

Contraception is the inhibition of pregnancy by a process, device, or method. The U.S. Food and Drug Administration (FDA) first approved oral contraception (OC), the use of hormones to prevent pregnancy, in the 1960s, and the last law prohibiting its use in the United States was overturned in 1973 (Speroff & Darney, 2000). Regardless of the type used, one of contraception's major benefits is its potential impact on the rate of unplanned pregnancies. Current estimates are that approximately half of all pregnancies in the United States are unintended. Of these, more than half of all pregnant women choose elective abortions, which translates into 25% of all pregnancies being terminated (Speroff & Darney, 2000). Unintended pregnancies that continue, including both unwanted and mistimed pregnancies, are positively associated with late-entry prenatal care, low birth weight, child abuse or neglect, and behavioral problems in children (Moos et al., 1997). The importance of this high rate of unintended pregnancy and the effects of its related consequences have been illustrated in the *Healthy People 2010* objectives (National Institutes of Health, 1999). This initiative suggests a reduction in unintended pregnancies from 49% to 30% by the year 2010. One way that this decrease may be achieved is through the increased awareness of contraception and the various available options.

Over the past 25 years, the widespread use of contraception in health care in the United States has expanded opportunities for women. Its use has allowed women to take on roles beyond (or in addition to) motherhood. Contraception has increased women's ability to decide when pregnancy and subsequent child-rearing will occur.

Data from 1995 illustrated that 93% of women in the United States between the ages of 15 and 44 years used some form of contraception. Box 60-1 illustrates the contraceptive methods of choice among 60% of women aged 15 to 44 years who used contraception. Studies have shown that age and desire for future pregnancy greatly influence a woman's method of choice. Reversible forms of contraception are the regimens of choice among women between 15 and 24 years of age as well as among women who have never been married and those who are planning future pregnancies. Oral, transdermal, and vaginal hormonal contraception are a first choice because return of fertility after discontinuing use is expected. At 48 months after discontinuing this regimen, 82% of patients 30 to 34 years of age have given

birth. Among women 25 to 29 years of age, the pregnancy rate is 92% at the same time after discontinuation (Speroff & Darney, 2000).

PHYSIOLOGY

A woman's ability to reproduce begins after she has completed the developmental stage of puberty. The average age of the onset of puberty is 11.2 years, whereas the length of time for the completion of this process is 4 years. Menarche, the last step in the pubertal process, is when menses commences. The average age for menarche is 12.7 years.

The cause or trigger for the onset of puberty is not completely understood. It is thought that a decreased sensitivity of the hypothalamus and pituitary glands to already circulating sex hormones results in an increased production of luteinizing hormone (LH) and follicle-stimulating hormone (FSH). Increased LH and FSH further stimulate the gonadal response of increased secretion of estrogen, progesterone, and testosterone. LH subsequently surges, inciting the release of ova. In the absence of fertilization, menses ensues.

A woman's menstrual cycle can be described in terms of either the follicular or luteal phase. In addition, in each of these phases, endometrial, ovarian, and pituitary hormone-secreting changes occur. These two major phases and the physiologic changes occurring in each are illustrated in Figure 60-1.

The endometrial changes can be subdivided. Menstruation, occurring on days 1 to 4 of the menstrual cycle, is the shedding of the endometrial lining. The next three phases are the proliferative phase (day 4 or 5 through ovulation), the secretory phase (immediately after ovulation), and the implantation phase (approximately days 21–27). During these phases, the endometrial lining is prepared for implantation of a fertilized ovum. In the event that an ovum does not implant, the next phase, endometrial breakdown, begins once again.

Relative to the ovarian changes that occur during the menstrual cycle, three major subdivisions can be identified: the follicular, ovulatory, and luteal phases. During the follicular phase, a dominant follicle is produced that will be released and await possible fertilization. The regulatory hormone largely responsible for this portion of the ovarian phase of the menstrual cycle is FSH. FSH stimulates the conversion of androgens to estrogen in the granulosa cells of the ovaries. Stimulation by FSH contributes to the development of a dominant follicle that produces further estrogen. The overall increase in estrogen production stimulates development of the glandular epithelium of the uterine lining, increases cervical mucous production and reduces the viscosity of this mucus, and increases vaginal pH.

Opposing the normal negative feedback mode of the menstrual cycle, in which high concentrations of estrogen inhibit the release of FSH and LH, the eventual peak in estrogen in this late follicular phase stimulates a surge in LH. The LH surge is subsequently responsible for the final maturation, release, and rupture of the dominant follicle. Follicular rupture and ovulation occur approximately 24 to 36 hours after the beginning of the LH surge and encompass the ovulatory phase of the menstrual cycle.

After the ovulatory phase, the luteal phase of the menstrual cycle enables the implantation of a fertilized ovum and maintenance of the uterine lining. The corpus luteum that remains after the follicle ruptures, releasing the ovum, secretes progesterone and 17-β-estradiol. The secretion of these hormones increases the secretory activity of the endometrial glands. Cervical mucus also increases in viscosity. In the event that pregnancy occurs, the life of the corpus luteum is extended to continue production of these hormones. In the absence of pregnancy, the corpus luteum dies, estrogen and progesterone levels decline, and menstruation occurs.

INITIATING DRUG THERAPY

Given the normal menstrual cycle, pregnancy can be inhibited by preventing fertilization, manipulating hormones of the menstrual cycle such that ovulation never occurs, or interfering with implantation. Contraceptive options may be nonpharmacologic or pharmacologic. Table 60-1 identifies these options and the failure rates of each.

Nonpharmacologic options include periodic abstinence, barrier devices, and intrauterine devices (IUDs) and systems. Periodic abstinence, which means avoiding sexual intercourse during the period of maximum fertility, includes several assumptions. First, the viability of sperm in the female reproductive tract is 2 to 7 days. Second, the life span of the ovum is 1 to 3 days. It is assumed, therefore, that the period of maximum fertility occurs in the 5 days before ovulation and ends on the day of ovulation. Prediction of

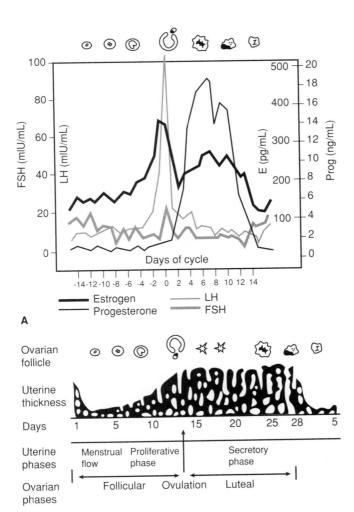

Figure 60–1 Comparison of the phases of the reproductive cycle. **A.** Plasma hormone concentrations in the normal female reproductive cycle. **B.** Ovarian events and uterine changes during the menstrual cycle. (From Bullock, B. A. & Henze, R. L. [2000]. *Focus on pathophysiology.* Philadelphia: Lippincott Williams & Wilkins, p. 1100.)

Table 60.1

Contraceptive Options and Rates of Failure

Contraceptive Method	Failure Rates*
Cervical cap	9%–32%
Combination oral contraceptive pills	0.3%–8%
Condom and spermicides	2%–21%
Depot medroxyprogesterone acetate	0.3%–3%
Diaphragm and spermicides	6%–18%
Intrauterine device	0.6%–2%
Mirena	0.5%–3%
Orthoevra patch	0.3%
Periodic abstinence	1%–25%
Progesterone mini pills	0.5%–3%
Sterilization	0.1%–0.4%

*Ranges may vary depending on typical or perfect use.

ovulation is important in recognizing the dates to avoid sexual intercourse. Several methods may be incorporated into the periodic abstinence method to identify better the time of ovulation. Examples include the use of ovulation predictor kits, monitoring of basal body temperature, and testing of cervical mucus. The increase in progesterone concentration just before the LH surge is accompanied by a 0.4°F to 0.8°F increase in basal body temperature. The woman measures her body temperature orally with a basal thermometer just before arising from bed daily. She also may observe cervical mucus as a guide to predicting ovulation. Midcycle cervical mucus, just before ovulation, is clear, thin, and stringy. Peak mucous production occurs on the day of ovulation. After this, the mucus becomes sticky and wet. Intercourse, with a low presumed risk of pregnancy, is permitted beginning on the fourth day of this sticky, wet mucus.

Other nonpharmacologic options for the prevention of pregnancy include the use of barrier devices such as condoms, diaphragms, and cervical caps. These options vary not only in their efficacy rates but in their abilities to prevent sexually transmitted diseases (STDs). The male latex condom helps to prevent the spread of human papilloma virus and many other STDs. It is the only contraceptive option clinically proven to prevent the spread of the human immunodeficiency virus (HIV). The female condom has been shown to act as a barrier to most STDs; however, limitations include its cost of approximately $2.50 per condom. More important, despite the positive laboratory data, clinical data showing that its use protects against the spread of HIV are lacking.

The diaphragm and cervical cap are both devices that require fitting by a health care provider. The woman can insert a diaphragm up to 6 hours before intercourse and must leave it in place for at least 6 hours (but no more than 24 hours) after intercourse. The diaphragm has been shown to reduce the risk of cervical gonorrhea, pelvic inflammatory disease (PID), and tubal infertility secondary to STDs. It is not, however, effective against HIV infection, and urinary tract infections are twice as common in diaphragm users compared with nonusers. Comparably, the cervical cap may be left in place for a total of 48 hours. It must remain in place, however, for at least 8 hours after sexual intercourse. Like the diaphragm, it has not been shown to afford any protection against HIV infection.

The third major type of nonpharmacologic contraception is the IUD. Although its mechanism of action is not clearly understood, it is thought to prevent pregnancy through production of a "spermicidal intrauterine environment." The intrauterine environment is rendered unreceptive to sperm or the implantation of a fertilized ovum should fertilization occur. Commonly used IUDs include the Lippes Loop and the copper IUD. Progesterone-implanted intrauterine systems have also begun to be used. In addition to the proposed mechanism of the IUD, the continued release of progesterone contributes to the contraceptive action of this device through production of viscous cervical mucus, which further impedes the sperm's ability to reach the ovum.

Goals of Drug Therapy

In addition to, or in place of, the nonpharmacologic contraceptive options available, pharmacologic options do exist.

The primary mechanism by which these agents prevent pregnancy is through manipulation of the normal menstrual cycle, effects on cervical mucus, or both. Estrogen plus progesterone or progesterone alone is used to interfere with the process of ovulation, conception, or both. Optimal contraception features, as defined by the World Health Organization include:

- Safe
- Effective
- Convenient
- Maintain regular bleeding episodes
- Rapidly reversible

Combined (Estrogen and Progestin) Oral, Transdermal, and Vaginal Contraceptives

The combination contraceptive agents contain estrogen, usually in the form of ethinyl estradiol or mestranol. Doses of estrogen range from 20 to 35 mg; 98% of all prescribed OCs contain less than 35 mg estrogen, and even OCs with as little as 20 mg estrogen are considered effective. Pills with low estrogen content are considered safer than higher-dose OCs for certain patients, including perimenopausal women, those with a family history of heart disease, and smokers younger than age 35 (although women who take OCs and smoke remain at an increased risk of myocardial infarction and stroke due to OC-associated changes in coagulation factors). Progesterone is in the form of desogestrel, ethynodiol diacetate, levonorgestrel, norethindrone, norethindrone acetate, norgestimate, or norgestrel. A synthetic progesterone (drospirenone [DRSP]) is also available. It has antiandrogenic and antimineralocorticoid properties. It is associated with less water retention than other progesterones, less negative emotional affect, and less appetite increase after 6 months of use.

In any combination, the doses used today are substantially lower than the doses used when OCs were first approved in the 1960s. From the 1960s through the mid-1970s, the average estrogen dose declined from 150 mg/d to 35 mg/d. Likewise, the mean progesterone dose was reduced from 10 mg/d to 0.5 to 1 mg/d. The reasons for these large dosage reductions included increased knowledge regarding their efficacy in preventing pregnancy. In addition, many of the side effects observed with these agents were related to high doses. The dose reductions are beneficial, therefore, from the standpoints of both efficacy and toxicity.

The mechanism of action of combination contraceptive agents is the suppression of the pituitary gonadotropins FSH and LH by the continued high concentrations of circulating estrogen and progesterone. The suppression of LH, primarily by the progesterone component, inhibits the LH surge that is responsible for ovulation. Progesterone also exerts its influence through its effects on increasing cervical mucous viscosity, thus impairing sperm transport. FSH suppression, largely through estrogen's influence, prevents the selection and emergence of a dominant follicle. Therefore, the combination of estrogen and progesterone inhibits selection of a dominant follicle and ovulation.

In addition to their influence on the reproductive cycle, the hormones used in OC pills (OCPs) exert other actions. All forms of progesterone exhibit some estrogenic, androgenic, or anabolic activity. For example, highly androgenic forms of progesterone affect lipid and carbohydrate metabolism and promote the appearance of acne, weight gain, and hirsutism. As such, practitioners should consider the various progesterone formulations relative to their androgenic effects when choosing an OCP regimen. The least androgenic forms include the newer, third-generation progesterones, desogestrel and norgestimate. In addition to their relative lack of androgenic side effects, they are also more potent than the other progesterones, norethindrone, norethindrone acetate, ethynodiol diacetate, and norgestrel. Knowledge of the differences in the progesterone formulations becomes important when managing (or prospectively avoiding) certain side effects of the OCPs.

Many options exist when choosing an OC regimen for a patient. In general, the combination OCPs are divided into monophasic (Alesse, Brevicon, Demulen, Yasmin, others), biphasic (Jenest-28, others), and triphasic (Ortho-Novum 7/7/7, Ortho Tri-Cyclen, others) combinations. Tables 60-2 and 60-3 list the available formulations. Monophasic combinations provide a set amount of estrogen and progesterone daily for 21 days. Placebo or nothing is given on days 22 to 28, the days during which a woman menstruates. The monophasic combinations may be useful in managing adverse effects

Table 60.2

Monophasic Contraception

Brand Name	Hormonal Components
Alesse	20 µg EE, 0.1 mg levonorgestrel
Brevicon	35 µg EE, 0.5 mg norethindrone
Demulen	50 µg EE, 1.0 mg ethynodiol diacetate
Demulen 1/35	35 µg EE, 1.0 mg ethynodiol diacetate
Desogen	30 µg EE, 0.15 mg desogestrel
Levlen	30 µg EE, 0.15 mg levonorgestrel
Loestrin 1/20	20 µg EE, 1.0 mg norethindrone acetate
Loestrin 1.5/30	30 µg EE, 1.5 mg norethindrone acetate
Lo-Ovral	30 µg EE, 0.3 mg norgestrel
Mircette	20 µg EE, 0.15 mg desogestrel days 1–21; 10 µg EE days 24–28
Modicon	35 µg EE, 0.5 mg norethindrone
NEE 0.5/35	35 µg EE, 0.5 mg norethindrone
NEE 1/35	35 µg EE, 1 mg norethindrone
Nelova 0.5/35	35 µg EE, 0.5 mg norethindrone
Nelova 1/35	35 µg EE, 1 mg norethindrone
Nordette	30 µg EE, 0.15 mg levonorgestrel
Norethin 1/50M	50 µg EE, 1 mg norethindrone
Norethin 1/35E	35 µg EE, 1 mg norethindrone
Norinyl 1 + 50	50 µg mestranol, 1 mg norethindrone
Norinyl 1 + 35	35 µg EE, 1 mg norethindrone
Norlestrin 2.5/50	50 µg EE, 2.5 mg norethindrone acetate
Ortho-Cept	30 µg EE, 0.15 mg desogestrel
Ortho-Cyclen	35 µg EE, 0.25 mg norgestimate
Ortho-Novum 1/35	35 µg EE, 1 mg norethindrone
Ortho-Novum 1/50	50 µg EE, 1 mg norethindrone
Ovcon 35	35 µg EE, 0.4 mg norethindrone
Ovcon 50	50 µg EE, 1 mg norethindrone
Ovral	50 µg EE, 0.5 mg norgestrel
Seasonale	30 µg EE, 0.15 mg levonorgestrel
Yasmin	30 µg EE, 3 mg drospirenone

EE, ethinyl estradiol.

Table 60.3

Biphasic and Triphasic Oral Contraceptive Pills

Brand Name	Hormonal Components
Biphasic Oral Contraceptive Pills	
Jenest-28	35/35 µg EE, 0.5/1 mg norethindrone
NEE 10/11	35/35 µg EE, 0.5/1 mg norethindrone
Ortho-Novum 10/11	35/35 µg EE, 0.5/1 mg norethindrone
Triphasic Oral Contraceptive Pills	
Estrostep	20/30/35 µg EE, 1 mg norethindrone acetate
Ortho-Novum 7/7/7	35/35/35 µg EE, 0.5/0.75/1 mg norethindrone
Ortho Tri-Cyclen	35/35/35 µg EE, 0.18/0.215/0.25 mg norgestimate
Tri-Levlen	30/40/30 µg EE, 0.05/0.075/0.125 mg levonorgestrel
Tri-Norinyl	35/35/35 µg EE, 0.5/1/0.5 mg norethindrone
Triphasil	30/40/30 µg EE, 0.05/0.075/0.125 mg levonorgestrel

EE, ethinyl estradiol.
Adapted from Kaunits, A. M., & Ory, H. (1997). Dialogues in contraception. *Dialogues, 5*(4), 1–20.

such as break-through vaginal bleeding. Also, women who are sensitive to fluctuations in hormone levels that occur with the biphasic and triphasic OCPs may respond more positively to the monophasic formulations.

A variation to the traditional monophasic OCP has been introduced. This formulation provides a constant amount of estrogen and progesterone daily on days 1 to 21. The woman takes placebo tablets on days 22 to 23. On days 24 to 28, a lower dose of estrogen alone is given. The rationale for providing estrogen on days 24 to 28 is to help manage problems in women who may have exhibited symptoms of estrogen deficiency during the traditional week-long placebo period. This includes, for example, women who experience rebound headaches in the absence of estrogen during days 22 to 28.

The biphasic and triphasic OCP combinations were developed to mimic more closely the normal fluctuations in hormones experienced during the menstrual cycle. Changes in the estrogen or progesterone components occur every 7 to 10 days in these products. The phasic OCPs have not been shown to have any proven advantages in efficacy over the monophasic products. The major difference between the biphasic and triphasic regimens and the monophasic regimens is the net amount of progesterone delivered per cycle. The biphasic and triphasic regimens contain, in general, less progesterone (see Tables 60-2 and 60-3). Therefore, for women experiencing progesterone-related side effects, changing to a regimen containing lower doses of a product with less androgenic effects may be most beneficial.

Seasonale is an extended-cycle birth control pill. It is a 91-day regimen (84 active pills and 7 placebo pills). This reduces menses from 10 to just 4 a year. It works just like a traditional 28-day OC but extends the cycle. There may be a higher incidence of break-through bleeding during early cycles.

When initiating therapy for patients, a contraceptive regimen is started relative to the woman's menstrual cycle. One can either initiate a day 1 start or a Sunday start regimen. Women who follow a day 1 start regimen begin the contraceptive agent on the first day of their period, regardless of the day of the week. Likewise, women who follow Sunday start regimens begin the OCP pack on the Sunday directly after the onset of menses. This means that the woman will not menstruate on a weekend, which is desirable to many patients. OCP packs are produced with the Sunday start regimen in mind. In the event that a patient is a day 1 start, the pharmacist places a special label on the pack noting the beginning day of the pack and the end. The situation in which the day 1 versus Sunday start becomes an issue is relative to missed doses, which is discussed later in the chapter.

A new form of contraception is the transdermal patch. This is a combination hormonal contraception that releases 150 mcg norelgestromin and 20 mcg ethinyl estradiol a day. The patch can be applied to the abdomen, buttocks, upper outer arm, or upper torso on clean, dry, healthy skin free of lotions. The patient can bathe, shower, or swim while wearing the patch. A new patch is applied each week, worn for 7 days, and removed and replaced with a new patch. During the fourth week no patch is worn. The first patch should be applied on the first day of menses and a new one on the same day the next week. Detachment has been shown in only 5% of cases, but if it becomes loose or falls off, it must be replaced with a new patch. If the patch is off for more than 24 hours, a new cycle is started and backup methods of birth control used for the next 7 days.

The most frequent complaint from users of the patch is reactions at the application site. Women who weigh more than 198 pounds may experience a higher failure rate and should use a different form of contraception.

Combination contraceptive vaginal rings are also available. The NuvaRing is a flexible transparent device inserted into the vagina by the patient. It releases 15 mcg ethinyl estradiol and 120 mcg etonogestrel daily. It is removed after 3 weeks for 1 week and a new ring is inserted. Lower hormonal doses are required with the vaginal ring because there is no hepatic or gastrointestinal interference. It can remain in place during bathing, swimming, and intercourse.

It has been shown that there is a mean of 5.88 cycles for conception following discontinuation of combined hormonal contraception (Stenchever et al., 2001).

Progestin-Only Hormonal Contraceptives

Progesterone alone to prevent pregnancy may be used in the dosage formulations of oral tablets, intramuscular injections, or subdermal implants. Regardless of the formulation, they are the hormonal contraceptive options of choice in women who cannot take or cannot tolerate estrogen-containing formulations. For example, the progesterone-only formulations are beneficial in women who are breast-feeding their infants. In ease of administration, compliance, and efficacy, however, the formulations vary greatly.

The progesterone-only contraceptive pill (Micronor, others), commonly referred to as the *mini-pill*, contains a very low dose of progesterone. Table 60-4 lists the available

Table 60.4

Progesterone-Only Oral Contraceptive Pills

Brand Name	Hormonal Component
Micronor	0.35 mg norethindrone
Nor-QD	0.35 mg norethindrone
Ovrette	0.075 mg norgestrel

formulations and active components of each. The mini-pills do not consistently suppress the pituitary gonadotropins LH and FSH. Their primary effect is exerted through changing the endometrial and cervical mucous environments. The time from dosing to changes in the cervical mucus is 2 to 4 hours. The impermeability of the mucus declines 22 hours after the dose. Therefore, to help ensure maximum efficacy, it is imperative that the woman take the pill at exactly the same time daily. Recommendations are that if the dose is more than 3 hours late, the woman should use a backup form of contraception. When beginning the mini-pill, the woman should start on the first day of menses and use backup contraception for the first 7 days. The woman takes the mini-pill daily without a placebo week, as is exercised with the combination OCPs.

The FDA approved the use of intramuscularly injected medroxyprogesterone acetate (depo MPA) in 1992. The dose of depo MPA used suppresses ovulation in addition to affecting cervical mucus. Depo MPA is dosed every 13 weeks and is a good choice for women for whom daily compliance with a combination or progesterone-only OCP is an issue. When beginning depo MPA, recommendations are that it be given within the first 5 days of the onset of menses. It can be given to women postpartum and to those who are breast-feeding. Subsequent doses must be given no later than 13 weeks from the prior dose to ensure efficacy. If a woman presents later than 13 weeks for her next injection, the provider needs to determine that the patient is not pregnant before administering the drug.

In addition to the positive compliance effects of this dosage formulation, women wishing future pregnancy also frequently prefer depo MPA. On discontinuation of depo MPA, 70% of women conceive within the first year and 90% within 24 months. Limitations to the use of depo MPA include the occurrence of menstrual changes in most women and episodes of unpredictable bleeding lasting more than 7 days. The latter problem occurs more commonly in the first few months of therapy.

The Intrauterine System

Another form of contraception is intrauterine systems (IUSs). One is Mirena, which is inserted by the clinician into the patient's uterine cavity to prevent pregnancy. It contains levonorgestrel, which is released at 20 mg/d into the uterine lining; it thickens the cervical mucus, suppresses ovarian function, and inhibits sperm movement. It also thins the uterine lining, making it an unfavorable environment for implantation. The IUS is approved for as long as 5 years of continuous use. Because the IUS contains no estrogen component, it is appropriate for women in whom estrogen is contraindicated. The IUS may also be an effective treatment for women with dysmenorrhea, menorrhagia, and anemia and may serve as an effective transition from contraception to hormone replacement therapy. Little maintenance is required. The patient must check the string after each menstrual period to ensure that it is still in place. For women who choose to become pregnant, the device can be removed by the clinician at any time; no waiting period is required before conception, and IUS use is not associated with a decline in fertility. This system has been shown to lessen dysmenorrhea and bleeding.

Also available is the standard copper-containing IUD, but greater dysmenorrhea and bleeding are associated with this system.

Emergency Contraception

In addition to the traditional prospective form of preventive contraception, the use of combination OCPs also has been studied in preventing pregnancy after coitus has occurred. The FDA has approved the Yuzpe regimen, 100 mg ethinyl estradiol plus 1 mg norgestrel or 0.5 mg levonorgestrel within 72 hours of unprotected intercourse, to be repeated in 12 hours, as emergency contraception. Box 60-2 illustrates formulations used in emergency contraception. Providers must be aware of the formulation prescribed, such that the dosage strength equals that which has been approved. Monophasic regimens are recommended. If a biphasic or triphasic regimen is chosen, however, the patient must be aware of which tablets and how many she needs to take. Also, practitioners must stress the importance of not using the placebo tablets.

Although the exact mechanism of action of emergency contraception is not clear, several mechanisms have been proposed. These include inhibition or delay of ovulation, alteration of the endometrium, interference with implantation of the fertilized egg, and interference with tubal transport of sperm or egg.

Common side effects include nausea and vomiting. Recommendations are that if the patient vomits within 4 hours of the dose, she should repeat the dose.

Another regimen studied as emergency contraception is the progestin-only regimen. This regimen uses 0.75 mg levonorgestrel within 72 hours of unprotected intercourse, followed by the same dose 12 hours later. In a clinical trial comparing its use with the Yuzpe regimen, the progestin-only group exhibited a pregnancy rate of 1.1% compared with 3.2% in the Yuzpe group. In addition, the levonorgestrel-only regimen resulted in significantly lower rates of nausea, vomiting, dizziness, and fatigue.

Regardless of the regimen chosen, a woman should menstruate within 21 days. If she does not, the clinician should instruct her to follow up with her provider to determine whether pregnancy has occurred. In addition, the practitioner should take this opportunity to discuss other forms of contraception so that emergency contraception does not become the woman's routine method of pregnancy prevention.

Nausea and vomiting are the most common adverse effects after treatment with the Yuzpe regimen. Other common adverse effects include fatigue, breast tenderness, headache, abdominal pain, and dizziness. Levonorgestrel alone is better tolerated than the Yuzpe regimen. According the American College of Obstetricians and Gynecologists and the World Health Organization, there are no absolute medical contraindications to the use of emergency contraception with the exception of pregnancy. The daily dose of steroidal hormones provided in these products is high; however, they are taken for only a short time, and thus, the contraindications cited for cyclical combination OCPs are not thought to apply. There is no evidence of increased risk or confirmed safety in women who have contraindications to daily use of OCs.

Drug Interactions

Any agent that increases gastrointestinal motility or causes diarrhea may reduce the plasma concentration of ethinyl estradiol by decreasing its absorption. Agents, such as ascorbic acid, that inhibit sulfation of ethinyl estradiol in the gastrointestinal tract may increase the bioavailability of ethinyl estradiol and lead to an increase in estrogenic adverse effects.

Ethinyl estradiol is metabolized by the cytochrome P450 (CYP) 3A4 enzyme pathway. Drugs known to induce CYP3A4 (phenytoin, primidone, barbiturates, carbamazepine, ethosuximide, topiramate, methsuximide, rifampin, and griseofulvin) can lead to decreased plasma ethinyl estradiol levels and may cause failure of emergency contraception. Reports suggest that the enterohepatic circulation of ethinyl estradiol is decreased in women taking antibiotics, which may lead to a decrease in systemic concentrations of ethinyl estradiol. Ethinyl estradiol may interfere with the metabolism of other compounds. It can inhibit microsomal enzymes, which may slow the metabolism of other drugs (ie, analgesic anti-inflammatory drugs such as antipyrine, antidepressant agents, theophylline, and ethanol), increasing their plasma and tissue concentrations and increasing the risk of adverse effects. There is a potential interaction between warfarin and levonorgestrel given as an emergency contraceptive. The proposed mechanism is the displacement of warfarin by levonorgestrel from the FIS binding site of human alpha$_1$-acid glycoprotein, the main transport protein for drugs in the plasma. This potential interaction should be considered so that the patient's

---

BOX 60–2. FORMULATIONS FOR EMERGENCY CONTRACEPTION

- Alesse   5 tablets followed by 5 tablets 12 h later
- Levlen   4 tablets followed by 4 tablets 12 h later
- Lo-Ovral   4 tablets followed by 4 tablets 12 h later
- Nordette   4 tablets followed by 4 tablets 12 h later
- Tri-Levlen   4 tablets followed by 4 tablets 12 h later
- Triphasil   4 tablets followed by 4 tablets 12 h later
- Ovral   2 tablets followed by 2 tablets 12 h later
- Preven   Specially packaged for emergency contraception; pregnancy test included; 2 tablets followed by 2 tablets 12 h later (ethinyl estradiol and levonorgestrel)
- Plan B   Specially packaged for emergency contraception; 1 tablet followed by 1 tablet 12 h later (levonorgestrel alone)

Table 60.5

Treatment Order for Available Hormonal Contraceptive Agents

Clinical Scenario	Therapeutic Options

Women with acne, hirsutism, obesity, controlled hypertension or history of pregnancy-related hypertension, hypercholesterolemia, smoker younger than 30 y,* family history of heart disease, depression, family history of breast or ovarian cancer, benign breast disease, diabetes mellitus, dysmenorrhea, abnormal menstrual cycles, persistent anovulation, concurrently taking antiepileptic medication†	First line:
	  30–35 µg ethinyl estradiol daily + progesterone with low androgenic potential (norgestimate or desogestrel or monophasic norethindrone 0.4–0.5 mg daily)
	Second line:
	  30–35 µg ethinyl estradiol daily + levonorgestrel triphasic or norethindrone 1 mg monophasic or triphasic or norethindrone acetate 1 mg or ethynodiol diacetate 1 mg or levonorgestrel 0.1 mg

New-start patients, adolescents, perimenopausal women, postpartum, nonlactating women	

Endometriosis	First line:
	  Monophasic continuous therapy: 30–35 µg ethinyl estradiol + progesterone with medium to high androgenic potential
	Second line:
	  Monophasic continuous therapy: 30–35 µg ethinyl estradiol + norgestrel 0.3 mg or norethindrone acetate 1.5–2.5 mg or levonorgestrel 0.15 mg

Postpartum, lactating	Progesterone-only mini-pill
Noncompliance	Depot medroxyprogesterone acetate or levonorgestrel subdermal implants
Break-through bleeding—first half of cycle	Change to combination pill with higher estrogen content in first half of cycle
Break-through bleeding—second half of cycle	Change to combination pill with higher progestin content in second half of cycle

*Recommended dose of ethinyl estradiol <50 µg/d.

†Recommended dose of ethinyl estradiol = 50 µg/d secondary to drug interaction of increased metabolism or use of progesterone-only product.

Adapted from Kaunitz, A. M., & Ory, H. (1997). Dialogues in contraception. *Dialogues, 5*(4), 1–20; and Darney, P. D. (1997). OC practice guidelines: Minimizing side effects. *International Journal of Fertility, 42*(Suppl. 1), 158–169.

international normalized ratio levels can be monitored because the Yuzpe regimen for emergency contraception generally would not be recommended in women with a history of deep vein thrombosis who are receiving anticoagulant therapy.

Selecting the Most Appropriate Agent

With the wide variety of forms of hormonal contraception, many questions exist about which agent should be used first and for whom. Table 60-5 addresses some of these issues and is provided as a guide to the prescription of hormonal contraception.

MONITORING PATIENT RESPONSE

Therapeutic drug monitoring of hormonal contraception includes, primarily, monitoring for adverse effects and preventing complications from their use. Before using any of the hormonal regimens, all sexually active patients should receive a gynecologic examination with Papanicolaou smear to observe cervical cytology. They also should have a thorough physical examination before beginning use, including information such as blood pressure and weight. A lipid panel, including baseline total cholesterol, high-density lipoprotein cholesterol, and triglyceride levels may be especially important in women with other risk factors for heart disease. Identification of blood glucose control before and after initiating hormonal contraception is important in women with diabetes mellitus.

In addition to the initial workup and physical examination, it is also important to maintain a high index of suspicion for adverse effects associated with the use of either the estrogen or progesterone components, or both, in women receiving hormonal contraception. It is estimated that 25%

to 50% of women discontinue hormonal contraception within the first 12 months of use because of physical side effects. Therefore, it is important to look for these side effects and know how to manage them. Box 60-3 identifies side effects related to excess estrogen and progesterone.

Side effects due to insufficient estrogen and progesterone, such as break-through bleeding, also may occur. In the first half of the menstrual cycle, break-through bleeding is likely due to insufficient estrogen; in the second half of the cycle, it is likely due to insufficient progesterone. Therefore, practitioners can simplify management by adding supplemental estrogen or progesterone when appropriate or changing to a new regimen with higher estrogen or progesterone as necessary.

PATIENT EDUCATION

Poor outcomes secondary to the use of hormonal contraception may include treatment failures, potentially life-threatening side effects, or side effects beyond those commonly expected, as noted in Box 60-3. Treatment failures frequently are related to compliance with the regimen. In the case of combination OCs, guidelines exist that explain what to do in the event of a missed pill (or pills) to help ensure continued contraceptive efficacy. Table 60-6 illustrates these guidelines. Another cause of treatment failure includes drug interactions that may affect the efficacy of the hormonal contraceptive. Agents proven to reduce circulating estrogen concentrations, therefore affecting efficacy, include rifampin (Rifadin), phenytoin (Dilantin), and carbamazepine (Tegretol). Recommendations to reduce the risk of treatment failure relative to these agents include the use of higher daily doses of estrogen (50 mg ethinyl estradiol) or use of progesterone-only options.

BOX 60–3. CAUSES OF SIDE EFFECTS OF HORMONE CONTRACEPTION

Too Much Estrogen
Heavy bleeding
Cystic breasts
Breast enlargement
Breast tenderness
Dysmenorrhea
Bloating
Premenstrual edema
Gastrointestinal symptoms
Premenstrual headache
Premenstrual irritability
Cervical extrophy

Too Little Estrogen
Bleeding (spotting) early in cycle
Too-light bleeding
Bleeding throughout the cycle
Amenorrhea

Too Much Progestin
Increased appetite
Candidiasis
Depression
Fatigue
Cervicitis

Too Little Progestin
Bleeding fewer days
Bleeding (spotting) late in cycle
Heavy bleeding
Delayed-withdrawal bleeding
Bloating
Dysmenorrhea
Premenstrual edema
Gastrointestinal symptoms
Premenstrual headache
Premenstrual irritability

BOX 60–4. ABSOLUTE CONTRAINDICATIONS TO THE USE OF COMBINATION ORAL CONTRACEPTIVE PILLS

- Thrombophlebitis, thromboembolic disorders, cerebral vascular disease, coronary occlusion*
- Markedly impaired liver function
- Breast cancer (known or suspected)
- Abnormal vaginal bleeding in the absence of a diagnosed cause
- Pregnancy
- Smokers older than age 35 y

*Includes a past history or other situations that may put the patient at risk for development of these conditions.

Patients can best avoid life-threatening side effects of the hormonal contraceptives, especially combination OCs, if they follow the contraindications to their use. Box 60-4 identifies absolute contraindications to the use of combination OCs. In addition, the acronym *ACHES* is useful in teaching patients about the potential severe side effects that may occur with the use of OCPs. Clinicians should instruct patients to call their primary care provider if any of the following occur:

- Severe **A**bdominal pain (indicative of gallbladder disease)
- **C**hest pain (potentially related to pulmonary embolism or myocardial infarction)
- **H**eadache (relative to stroke, hypertension, or migraine)
- **E**ye problems (relative to stroke or hypertension)
- **S**evere leg pain (indicative of deep vein thrombosis)

It is crucial to relay this information to the patient. Early recognition and treatment of these adverse events saves lives.

The increased risk of certain types of cancer has been linked to the use of hormonal contraception, especially combination OCPs. Data from 1995 illustrate that, per 100,000 users of combination OCPs, 151 cases of breast cancer, 125 cases of cervical cancer, and 41 cases of liver cancer could be attributed to their use (Schesselman, 1995). Clinicians should consider these increased risks when deciding on an initial contraceptive regimen for a patient.

Table 60.6

Guidelines for Missed Pills

Number of Missed Pills	Recommended Action
One pill	Take missed pill as soon as possible and resume schedule; back-up method of contraception is not necessary.
Two pills during wk 1 or 2	Take two pills daily for 2 d; then finish pack; it is unlikely that a back-up method of contraception is needed, but it is advised for 7 d.
Two pills during wk 3*	Take daily pill until Sunday, then start a new pack; use back-up method of contraception immediately and for 7 d.
Three or more missed pills*	Take daily pill until Sunday, then start a new pack; use back-up method of contraception immediately and for 7 d.

*If a day 1 start—start a new pack and use back-up method of contraception immediately and for 7 d.
From Speroff, L., & Darney, P. (2000). *A clinical guide for contraception* (3rd ed.). Philadelphia: Lippincott Williams & Wilkins.

BOX 60–5. NONCONTRACEPTIVE BENEFITS OF COMBINED ORAL CONTRACEPTIVES

- Decreased iron deficiency anemia
- Decreased dysmenorrhea
- Decreased dysfunctional uterine bleeding
- Decreased incidence of ovarian cysts
- Improvement in acne
- Decreased incidence of pelvic inflammatory disease
- Decreased risk of osteoporosis
- Decreased incidence of endometrial cancer
- Decreased risk of benign breast disease

Many women are unaware of the health risks and side effects of the various forms of hormonal contraception. Likewise, 25% of women are unaware that the use of combination contraceptive agents imparts benefits in addition to the prevention of pregnancy. Some of these benefits include a 50% to 60% reduction in ovarian cancer risk with 5 years of use. This benefit persists for up to 10 or more years after discontinuation. In addition, 50% to 60% reductions in PID risk and 30% to 50% reductions in the occurrence of menstrual disorders have been observed with combination agents.

Another benefit of OCPs is their use in other indications. For example, 60% to 94% of women with endometriosis who are treated with daily monophasic contraceptive agents for 6 to 9 months experience symptomatic improvement. After treatment, a 5% to 10% annual recurrence rate of the disease is noted. Benefits of contraceptive agents are listed in Box 60-5.

Several Web sites contain patient information on contraception: www.contraception.net, www.contraceptiononline.org, and www.plannedparenthood.org.

■ Case Study

J.L., a 27-year-old account executive, presents to the Family Medicine office for her annual checkup with her primary care provider. She has no significant past medical history. Her medications include calcium carbonate 500 mg orally twice a day and a multivitamin daily. She exercises regularly. Her family history is significant for cardiovascular disease (her father had a myocardial infarction [MI] at 54 years of age and died of a further MI at 63 years of age). She notes that she has been dating her current partner for approximately 5 months. She is interested in a reliable form of contraception. After discussing the various contraceptive options, she decides that an OC would best fit her needs.

1. Before prescribing an OCP regimen, what tests or examinations would you like to perform?

2. Identify three different OCP regimens that could be chosen for J.L. Note their differences and why you chose them.

3. Identify the potential side effects that need to be relayed to J.L. Note especially those effects for which J.L. should seek immediate medical care.

Bibliography

*Starred references are cited in the text.

Bullock, B. A., & Henze, R. L. (2000). *Focus on Pathophysiology.* Philadelphia: Lippincott Williams & Wilkins.

Burkman, R. T. (1989). Noncontraceptive benefits of oral contraceptives. *International Journal of Fertility, 34,* 50–55.

*Darney, P. D. (1997). OC practice guidelines: Minimizing side effects. *International Journal of Fertility, 42*(Suppl. 1), 158–169.

Davidson, M. R. (2003). Contraception update. *Clinical Reviews 13*(6), 52–59.

Handbook of Adolescent Medicine. (2003). *Adolescent Medicine, 14*(2), 309–335.

Hatcher, R. A., Trussel, J., Stewart, F., et al. (2004). *Contraceptive technology* (18th ed.). New York: Ardent Media.

Hatcher, R. A., Zieman, M., Cwiak, C., et al. (2004). *Managing contraception.* New York: Ardent Media.

Herndon, E. J., & Zieman, M. (2004). New contraceptive options. *American Family Physician 69*(4), 853–860.

*Kunitiz, A. M., & Ory H. (1997). Dialogues in contraception. *Dialogues 5*(4), 1–20.

Kaunitz, A. M. (1994). Long-acting injectable contraception with depot medroxyprogesterone acetate. *American Journal of Obstetrics and Gynecology, 170,* 1543–1549.

Levine, D. W., & Hillard, P. J. A. (1998). The menstrual cycle and abnormal uterine bleeding. In L. A. Wallis, et al. (Eds.) *Textbook of women's health* (p. 602). Philadelphia: Lippincott-Raven.

*Moss, M. K., Peterson, R., Meadows, K., et al. (1997). Pregnant women's perspectives on intendedness of pregnancy. *Women's Health Issues, 7,* 385–392.

*Schesselman, J. J. (1995). Net effects of oral contraceptive use on the risk of cancer in women in the United States. *Obstetrics and Gynecology 85,* 793–801.

*Speroff, L., & Darney, P. (2000). *A clinical guide for contraception* (3rd ed.). Philadelphia: Lippincott Williams & Wilkins.

*Stenchever, M. A., Droegemuller, W., Herbst, A. L., et al. (2001). *Comprehensive Gynecology* (4th ed.). St. Louis: Mosby.

Task Force on Postovulatory Methods of Fertility Regulation. (1998). Randomised controlled trial of levonorgestrel versus the Yuzpe regimen of combined oral contraceptives for emergency contraception. *Lancet, 352,* 428–433.

*U.S. Department of Health and Human Services. (2001). *Healthy people 2010.* McLean, VA: International Medical Publishing.

Weismiller, D. G. (2004). Emergency contraception. *American Family Physician 70*(4), 707–714.

Visit the Connection web site for the most up-to-date drug information.

WEIGHT LOSS

JESSICA O'HARA, ANDREW M. PETERSON, AND EILEEN GLEASON DONNELLY

Obesity has reached epidemic proportions, affecting more than 300 million people worldwide (World Health Organization [WHO], 2003). It is the second leading cause of preventable death in the United States, accounting for approximately 300,000 deaths per year (U.S. Department of Health and Human Services [DHHS], 2001). According to the most recent survey from the National Health and Nutrition Examination Survey (NHANES) for 1999 to 2000, 64.5% of U.S. adults are overweight (body mass index [BMI] exceeds 25) and 30.5% are obese, with a BMI exceeding 30 (Flegal et al., 2002).

The prevalence of overweight adults has risen dramatically since the early 1980s, with the potential for the entire U.S. adult population to be overweight within a few generations (Hill, 1998). This alarming increase has also affected the nation's youth, with 15.5% of U.S. children and adolescents aged 12 to 19 years old, 15.3% aged 6 through 11 years old, and 10% aged 2 through 5 years old being overweight, according to NHANES 1999–2000. This is compared with 10.5%, 11.3%, and 7.2%, respectively, in 1988–1994 (NHANES III; Ogden et al., 2002). Women and minorities have a higher proportion of obesity among the general population.

CAUSES

Researchers attribute the rise in obesity to caloric imbalances. During the 1980s, the effects of modernization combined with an unprecedented abundance of cheap, energy-dense food produced a population that ate more while becoming increasingly sedentary (Taubes, 1998). Xavier Pi-Sunyer, a Columbia University obesity researcher and National Institutes of Health (NIH) Obesity Task Force chairperson, stated "Food is probably cheaper and more available than it ever has been in history." Coupled with the increased food supply is the transformation of our society from a primarily labor-intensive work force during the agricultural age to a more sedate work force during the industrial and information ages. In other words, researchers theorize that Americans have been getting fatter in the last decades of the 20th century because of too much food and too little activity.

Researchers link obesity to the development of chronic debilitating disease states such as heart disease, type 2 diabetes mellitus, and cancer. Because of these links, the WHO and

health officials, such as former U.S. Surgeon General C. Everett Coop, have declared obesity a global epidemic (James et al., 2001; Wickelgren, 1998). These leading health officials claim that obesity is not only hurting the individuals involved but draining the economy as well. In the United States, the NIH claims that overweight/obese people are costing citizens more than $50 billion annually in direct health care costs with an additional $30 billion spent on weight loss products and services (NIH, 1998). Therefore, obesity accounts for over 5% of annual health care costs in the United States.

Genetic Factors

Obesity tends to run in families, suggesting that it may have a genetic cause. However, family members share not only the genes but the diet and lifestyle habits that may contribute to obesity. Separating these lifestyle factors from genetic factors is difficult. Still, growing evidence points to heredity as a strong determinant of obesity.

Environmental Factors

Although genetics may play a role in the development of obesity, the WHO Consultation on Obesity concluded that behavioral and environmental factors are primarily responsible for the dramatic increase in obesity during the past two decades (Racette et al., 2003). Environment includes lifestyle behaviors, such as what a person eats and how active he or she is. Americans tend toward high-fat diets, often putting taste and convenience ahead of nutritional content when choosing meals. Most Americans also do not get enough exercise. Since 1980, weights in the United States have been increasing at an alarming rate. The NHANES III showed that the prevalence of obesity had increased from 14.5% in 1980 to 22.5% of the population in 1994 (Taubes, 1998). The most recent NHANES (1999–2000) reports that this prevalence has increased to 30.5% (Flegal et al., 2002).

Psychological Factors

Psychological factors may also influence eating habits. Many people eat in response to negative emotions such as boredom, sadness, anger, and anxiety. Studies in the 1970s found that overeaters may be treating themselves for depression. The key is the chemical serotonin, which is produced by ingestion of starch and which regulates mood. Overeaters may be scrambling to boost their serotonin levels and also their moods.

Other Causes

Some illnesses can cause obesity. These include hypothyroidism, Cushing syndrome, depression, and some neurologic problems. Certain drugs, such as steroids and some antidepressants, may cause excessive weight gain.

PATHOPHYSIOLOGY

Obesity is not a disorder of body weight regulation. Obese people can regulate their weight appropriately, but that regulation is centered at an elevated homeostatic set point. After adolescence, body weight is usually highly stable, increasing slowly by approximately half a pound yearly over the course of a lifetime. Research studies performed on twins and adopted siblings show that genetic factors strongly influence the homeostatic set point of individuals.

Weigle (1990) suggests that body weight is set at the point of balance between various feedback loops regulating adipose mass. The genetic influence could be mediated by circulating factors or factors that regulate satiety. People with a high set point have lower amounts of these factors and thus have to gain relatively more adipose tissue before appetite and energy expenditure balance. The theory is that it is an extraordinarily difficult feat to cure obesity by dietary energy restriction. Most patients who lose weight through dieting regain that weight, indicating that the weight-regulating system is very strong. "Only persons with incredibly strong will power or the ability to tolerate physical discomfort are likely to be successful in this attempt to defeat a homeostatic mechanism . . . " (Weigle, 1990).

When calorie intake exceeds energy expenditure over the long term, the excess energy is stored as fat. Everyone needs a certain amount of stored body fat for energy, heat insulation, shock absorption, and other functions. As a rule, women have more fat than men. Problems arise when men have more than 25% body fat and women more than 30%.

Body fat distribution is an important health consideration that has been widely overlooked by health care practitioners in terms of risk factors for obesity. Many recent research data suggest that it is not only how much fat a person has but also its distribution in the body that affects the risk for disease associated with that fat.

Women typically collect fat in the lower part of the trunk (hips and buttocks), giving their body a pear shape. Men usually build up fat in the upper trunk and intra-abdominal regions, giving them more of an apple shape. Excess body fat, particularly when distributed in the intra-abdominal region, increases the risk of hypertension, coronary artery disease, type 2 diabetes, gallbladder disease, sleep apnea, gout, and certain types of cancer (National Institute of Diabetes and Digestive and Kidney Disease [NIDDK], 2000).

Diagnostic Criteria

The standard for body fat measurement is densitometry, which determines the density of a body submersed in water.

However, the cost and technical requirements limit its usefulness in the clinical setting. The following paragraphs describe measurements more commonly used in clinical practice.

Weight-for-Height Tables

Weight-for-height tables usually have a range of acceptable weights for a person of a given height. A problem with using weight-for-height tables is that clinicians disagree about which is the best table to use. Many versions are available, and all cite different weight ranges. Some tables take a person's frame size, age, and sex into account; others do not. A limitation of all weight-for-height tables is that they do not distinguish excess fat from muscle (Table 61-1).

Body Mass Index

The BMI is the measurement of choice for clinicians and researchers studying obesity. Besides its simplicity, which eases use in clinical practice, associations have been demonstrated between BMI and adiposity, disease risk, and mortality (NIDDK, 2000; Racette et al., 2003). In general, when BMI exceeds 25, morbidity and mortality rise proportionally (Sheperd, 2003).

The BMI takes into account both a person's height and weight (BMI = kg/m^2). In Table 61-2, the mathematics and metric conversions have already been done. To use the table, find the appropriate height in the left-hand column and then move across the row to the given weight. The number at the

Table 61.1

Height and Weight Table

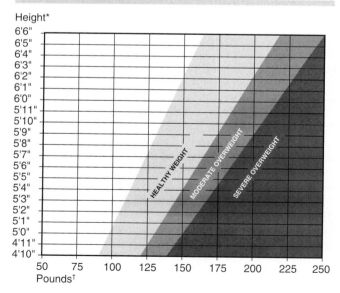

* Without shoes.

† Without clothes. The higher weights apply to people with more muscle and bone, such as many men.

Source: Report of the Dietary Guidelines Advisory Committee on the Dietary Guidelines for Americans, 1995, pages 23–24.

From *Understanding adult obesity*. National Institute of Diabetes and Digestive and Kidney Diseases on-line publication.

Table 61.2

Body Mass Index Conversion Chart*

Body Mass Index (kg/m²)	19	20	21	22	23	24	25	26	27	28	29	30	35	40
Height (in.)						**Body Weight (lbs)**								
58	91	96	100	105	110	115	119	124	129	134	138	143	167	191
59	94	99	104	109	114	119	124	128	133	138	143	148	173	198
60	97	102	107	112	118	123	128	133	138	143	148	153	179	204
61	100	106	111	116	122	127	132	137	143	148	153	158	185	211
62	104	109	115	120	126	131	136	142	147	153	158	164	191	218
63	107	113	118	124	130	135	141	146	152	158	163	169	197	225
64	110	116	122	128	134	140	145	151	157	163	169	174	204	232
65	114	120	126	132	138	144	150	156	162	168	174	180	210	240
66	118	124	130	136	142	148	155	161	167	173	179	186	216	247
67	121	127	134	140	146	153	159	166	172	178	185	191	223	255
68	125	131	138	144	151	158	164	171	177	184	190	197	230	262
69	128	135	142	149	155	162	169	176	182	189	196	203	236	270
70	132	137	146	153	160	167	174	181	188	195	202	207	243	278
71	136	143	150	157	165	172	179	186	193	200	208	215	250	286
72	140	147	154	162	169	177	184	191	199	206	213	221	258	294
73	144	151	159	166	174	182	189	197	204	212	219	227	265	302
74	148	155	163	171	179	186	194	202	210	218	225	233	272	311
75	152	160	168	176	184	192	200	208	216	224	232	240	279	319
76	156	164	172	180	189	197	205	213	221	230	238	246	287	328

*Each entry gives the body weight in pounds for a person of a given height and body mass index. Pounds have been rounded off. To use the table, find the appropriate height in the left-hand column. Move across the row to a given weight. The number at the top of the column is the body mass index for the height and weight.
From *Understanding adult obesity*. National Institute of Diabetes and Digestive and Kidney Diseases on-line publication.

top of the column is the BMI for that height and weight. Table 61-3 gives the current guidelines for classification of obesity based on BMI. Similar to the weight-for-height tables, a limitation of BMI is that it does not distinguish excess fat from muscle. Therefore, some muscular people may be mistakenly classified as obese using BMI alone. In addition, it does not take body fat distribution into account, which is an independent predictor of health risk (NIH, 1998).

Waist Circumference

Clinicians are concerned over where fat is located in the body. People whose fat is concentrated mostly in the abdomen are more likely to have many of the health problems associated with obesity. Waist circumference is a marker of abdominal fat and a good predictor of disease risk. Waist circumference is found my measuring the circumference around the waist at the level of the iliac crest (just above the hip bone). A waist circumference exceeding 40 inches (102 cm) in men and 35 inches (88 cm) in women signifies increased health risk in those who have a BMI of 25 to 34.9.

Waist-to-Hip Ratio

Because upper body obesity carries greater risks, patients with central obesity, particularly younger patients, should be targeted for weight reduction. Similar to waist circumference, waist-to-hip ratio is a good indicator of who is at risk based on body fat distribution. However, recent guidelines state that the measurement of waist-to-hip ratio provides no advantage over waist circumference alone (NIH, 2000).

To find someone's waist-to-hip ratio, measure the waist at its narrowest point, and then measure the hips at the widest point. Divide the waist measurement by the hip measurement. Women with waist-to-hip ratio exceeding 0.85 or men with waist-to-hip ratios over 1.0 are at the greatest risk for disease associated with obesity.

INITIATING DRUG THERAPY

Experts generally agree that people who are 20% or more overweight, especially the severely obese, can gain significant health benefits from weight loss. Many obesity experts believe that people who are less than 20% above their healthy weight should try to lose weight if they have any of the following risk factors:

- Family history of certain chronic diseases
- Preexisting medical conditions
- High waist-to-hip ratio

Table 61.3

Classification of Obesity by Body Mass Index (BMI)

	BMI (kg/m²)
Underweight	<18.5
Normal	18.5–24.9
Overweight	25.0–29.9
Obesity, class	
I	30.0–34.9
II	35.0–39.9
III (extreme)	≥40

People with close relatives who have had heart disease or diabetes are more likely to have these problems if they are obese. High blood pressure, high cholesterol levels, or elevated glucose levels are all warning signs of some obesity-associated diseases. Finally, people whose weight is concentrated around their abdomen may be at greater risk for heart disease, diabetes, or cancer than people of the same weight whose fat is concentrated in the thighs and buttocks.

There are no "magic cures" for obesity. The most successful strategies include calorie reduction, increased physical activity, and behavior therapy designed to improve eating and physical activity habits (Nonas, 1998). Many guidelines advise physicians to have their patients try lifestyle therapy for at least 6 months before embarking on physician-prescribed drug therapy. Weight-loss drugs approved by the U.S. Food and Drug Administration (FDA) for long-term use may be tried as part of a comprehensive weight-loss program that includes dietary therapy and physical activity in carefully selected patients (BMI >30 without additional risk factors, BMI >27 if the patient has other risk factors including type 2 diabetes, high blood pressure, dyslipidemia, coronary artery disease, or sleep apnea) who had been unable to lose weight or maintain weight loss with nondrug therapies (Table 61-4).

Table 61.4

Overview of Agents Prescribed to Suppress Appetite

Generic (Trade) Name and Dosage	Selected Adverse Events	Contraindications	Special Considerations
amphetamine sulfate (Amphetamine, others) Start: 5–10 mg ac Range: 5–30 mg Long acting: 10–15 mg every morning	Palpitations, tachycardia, CNS stimulation, dry mouth	MAOIs, hyperthyroidism, glaucoma, symptomatic cardiovascular disease or moderate–severe hypertension Safety in people <3 y not established	Schedule 2 drug Do not crush or chew sustained release dosage form
dextroamphetamine (Dexedrine, Oxydess) Start: 5–10 mg ac Range: 5–30 mg Long acting: 5–15 mg every morning	Same as above	Same as above, but safety in people <12 y not established	Same as above
methamphetamine (Desoxyn) Start: 5 mg ac Range: 20–25 mg/d Long acting: 10–15 mg every morning	Palpitations, tachycardia, CNS stimulation, dry mouth	Same as above	Same as above
diethylpropion (Tenuate, Tenuate dospan) Start: 25 mg ac or 75 mg qd (long acting) Range: 75 mg/d	Same as above	Same as above	Schedule 4 drug
phendimetrazine (Bontril, Prelu-2, others) Start: 35 mg bid, 1 h before meals Range: 35–105 mg qd Long acting: 105 mg every morning before breakfast	Palpitations, tachycardia, CNS stimulation, dry mouth	MAOIs, hyperthyroidism, glaucoma, symptomatic cardiovascular disease or moderate–severe hypertension Safety in people <12 y not established	Schedule 3 drug
phentermine (Adipex-P, Fastin, Ionamin) *phentermine:* 8 mg tid (30 min before breakfast) *Adipex-P:* 37.5 mg qd (2 h after breakfast) *Ionamin:* 15 mg qd (before breakfast or 10–14 h before bedtime)	Headache, insomnia, nervousness, CNS stimulation	Same as above	Ionamin is a resin complex. This resin complex reaches peak plasma concentrations in 8 h.
sibutramine (Meridia) Start: 10 mg qd Range: 5–15 mg qd	Constipation, dry mouth, insomnia, headache	MAOIs, selective serotonin reuptake inhibitors, sumatriptan, dextromethorphan, cardiovascular disease or moderate–severe hypertension, safety in people <16 y not established	Metabolized by cytochrome P450 3A4 subsystem, schedule 4
orlistat (Xenical) 120 mg tid with meals	Oily spotting, flatus with discharge, fecal urgency, fatty/oily stool	Chronic malabsorption syndrome or cholestasis Safety in people <12 y not established	May decrease absorption of fat-soluable vitamins (A, D, E, K)

MAOI, monoamine oxidase inhibitor.

BOX 61–1. ALTERNATIVE WEIGHT-LOSS THERAPIES

Stimulant Herbs: Coffee and Chinese Ephedra (200 mg and 20 mg tid)

Coffee contains the stimulant caffeine. Chinese ephedra contains the stimulants ephedrine and pseudoephedrine. Both ephedrine and caffeine increase the basal metabolic rate. They also seem to depress appetite. Caffeine has a mild antidepressant and diuretic effect. Despite their availability over the counter, these two stimulant herbs are not very popular for diet therapy because large doses must be taken, often with unpleasant side effects: insomnia, irritability, jitters, and elevated blood pressure.

Diuretic Herbs

Herbs with diuretic properties—buchu, celery seed, dandelion, juniper, parsley, and uva ursi—are used as a short-term strategy. In this way, diuretics can help people lose several pounds of "water weight." But the body senses the increased water loss diuretics cause and reacts with increased thirst to replace lost fluids. If diuretics continue to be ingested, the body eventually adjusts and retains water despite them. Herbal diuretics do not play a major role in permanent weight control.

Psyllium

Psyllium is the seed of the plantain plant. It is rich in a spongy fiber called *mucilage*. When psyllium comes in contact with water, its mucilage absorbs the fluid and expands substantially. In the stomach, psyllium expansion can produce feelings of fullness. Psyllium seed is sold in bulk in health food stores and herb shops. It is also available in a familiar product, the bulk-forming laxative Metamucil.

Hot, Spicy Herbs

Red pepper and mustard (1 teaspoon with each meal) are two herbs that give hot foods their heat and that increase the basal metabolic rate. As the basal metabolic rate increases, calories burn faster and weight decreases more rapidly. Another weight-loss benefit of hot spices is associated with thirst. Hot herbs stimulate thirst, so the person drinks more liquids, filling up on water instead of food, which also contributes to weight loss.

Goals of Drug Therapy

Goals of therapy are to reduce body weight and maintain a lower body weight for the long-term (NIH, 2000). A modest weight loss of 5% to 10% can lead to beneficial effects on cardiovascular risk factors associated with obesity including improvements in glycemia, blood pressure, and plasma lipid profiles. Recent studies have also shown that modest weight loss may help prevent or delay the appearance of type 2 diabetes and hypertension (Vidal, 2002). Data also suggest that voluntary modest weight loss is associated wit a 25% reduction in total mortality in patients with type 2 diabetes (Williamson et al., 2000). Proper food choices and regular aerobic exercise are preferable ways of attaining this weight loss as opposed to calorie restriction. When body weight drops below the set point by exercise, energy expenditure appears to adapt to the new weight, unlike weight loss by calorie restriction, which elicits strong counter-regulatory mechanisms (Weigle, 1990).

The 2000 guidelines published by the NIH (NIH, 2000) suggest that an initial weight loss goal of 10% over 6 months is reasonable. This should be accomplished through a reduction of caloric intake by 500 to 1000 kcal/d, resulting in a rate of loss 1 to 2 lb/wk (0.45-0.9 kg/wk).

Eating behavior, like mood and personality, is thought to be the result of a mixture of neurotransmitters in the brain. Pharmaceutical approaches to weight loss may be more effective than attempts at behavioral therapy, just as antidepressants have been found in general to be more effective for treating clinical depression than psychotherapy. Amphetamines were once a popular prescription drug for weight con-

trol; however, one of the many complaints associated with their use was that all the weight that had been lost during drug therapy was regained after the drug was discontinued. Americans spent at least $467 million on prescription drugs in 1996 and another $32 million on over-the-counter diet aids such as pills and herbal therapies (Wickelgren, 1998) (Box 61-1).

Obesity must be treated as a chronic medical condition in the same way that hypertension is a chronic medical condition (Fig. 61-1). Seen in this light, weight gain after drug discontinuation is no different from rising blood pressure after the discontinuation of antihypertensive medication. The pharmaceutical industry is very much aware of the marketing potential of a pill that would help combat the lifelong challenge of obesity. Much research time and money have been put into the development of such a pill during the 1990s. Lifelong drug therapy for obesity and the drug risk factors involved are factors that have yet to be addressed by researchers, whose studies have been over the short term (24 months being the longest). At present, drug therapy is used during the weight-loss phase of treatment, with drug safety beyond 2 years of total treatment not yet established. Therefore, it is critical not only to lose weight, but also to maintain the weight loss through changes in lifestyle and dietary habits.

Over-the-Counter Agent: Phenylpropanolamine

For years, phenylpropanolamine (Dexatrim, others) has been recommended for use as an over-the-counter weight-loss product. However, in October 2000, the FDA's Nonprescription Drug Advisory Committee issued a statement relating phenylpropanolamine to hemorrhagic strokes. As such, the FDA no longer considers phenylpropanolamine safe, and therefore, it is no longer available in the U.S market.

Anorexiants

Amphetamine and nonamphetamine agents are used to treat obesity. The nonamphetamine derivatives are considered anorexiants. Other terms for these nonamphetamine agents include *anorectics* or *anorexigenics*. These agents (see Table 61-4) include benzphetamine, diethylpropion (Tenuate), mazindol (Sanorex), phenmetrazine, phendimetrazine (Bontril), and phentermine (Adipex-P). These agents are considered adjuncts to dietary restriction and an exercise program for weight loss. The effects of these agents are often short lived because tolerance may develop to the anorexigenic effect after a few weeks.

In 1992, an article on the long-term effects of a combination of anorexiants and amphetamine-like drugs on weight loss was published (Weintraub et al., 1992). This article started the "fen-phen" craze of the 1990s. Citing 121 patients

losing some 30 pounds each, the study touted the benefits of the combination of products. Each component, fenfluramine and phentermine (hence "fen-phen"), was an FDA-approved drug for treating obesity. However, because of reports of valvular heart disease (Connolly et al., 1997) and primary pulmonary hypertension (Dillon et al., 1997), fenfluramine and its dextrorotary congener, dexfenfluramine (Redux), have been voluntarily withdrawn from the market.

Mechanism of Action

The mechanism of action of anorexiants is not well established. One theory is that they stimulate the satiety center in the hypothalamic and limbic regions of the brain, possibly inducing appetite suppression. However, this has not been conclusively proven, and an alternative theory is that central nervous system (CNS) stimulation results in weight loss (McEvoy, 1999). Diethylpropion and phentermine are adrenergic agents, whereas fenfluramine is dopaminergic. Mazindol acts on both adrenergic and dopaminergic pathways (Hebel, 1999).

The absorption of these drugs is not affected by food, and the primary route of elimination is renal. The drugs are

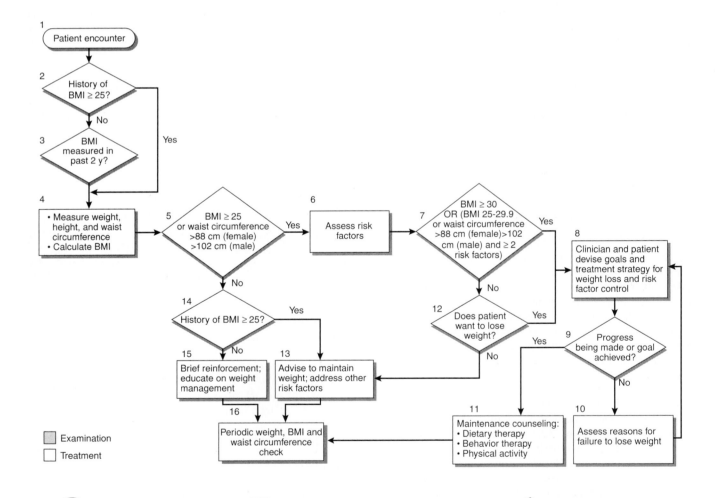

Figure 61–1   Treatment algorithm for obesity. (From the National Heart, Lung and Blood institute. [2000]. *The Practical guide: Identification, evaluation and treatment of overweight and obesity in adults* [publication No. 00–4084] Washington, DC: National Institutes of Health.]

considered short-acting agents, with half-lives ranging from 1.9 to 9.8 hours. For this reason, these agents are often dosed 3 times daily, and are also formulated in extended-release forms for once-daily dosing. The dosing varies by individual response, but it is recommended to start at the lowest dose and increase based on weight loss and tolerance of adverse events.

Contraindications

All of these agents have a potential for abuse, and as such are classified as Schedule III (C-III) drugs. Caution should be used when prescribing these agents in patients with a history of substance abuse.

Because they lead to increased levels of norepinephrine and dopamine, these agents are contraindicated in patients taking monoamine oxidase inhibitors (MAOIs). The combination may cause an increased pressor effect, resulting in hypertensive crisis.

Adverse Events

Adverse events include CNS stimulation such as insomnia, tremor, and headache. Overstimulation may result in an impairment of ability to perform activities requiring mental alertness (eg, driving or operating heavy machinery). Occasionally, urinary frequency, blurred vision, and changes in libido may occur.

Other adverse effects include dry mouth and nausea as well as cardiovascular effects such as increases in blood pressure and tachycardia. For this reason, blood pressure and heart rate should be monitored on a biweekly or monthly basis, and even more frequently in patients with preexisting hypertension. Caution should also be used when these agents are prescribed for patients with diabetes. The decrease in caloric intake may decrease a patient's blood glucose level, requiring adjustment of insulin or oral hypoglycemic agents.

Serotonin and Norepinephrine Reuptake Inhibitor: Sibutramine

Another type of anorexiant is sibutramine (Meridia). Sibutramine inhibits both serotonin and norepinephrine reuptake, slowing the dissipation of the brain's existing serotonin. This is the first weight loss drug to be classified as a serotonin and norepinephrine reuptake inhibitor. It causes weight loss in laboratory rats by altering both food intake and metabolic rate. Sibutramine controls food intake for 24 hours by enhancing a feeling of satiety. It also appears to induce thermogenesis in rats, resulting in increased oxygen consumption. Studies have shown that sibutramine decreases the amount of centrally deposited fat, which, as noted, is associated with adverse health outcomes. Sibutramine therapy also results in decreased levels of triglycerides, low-density lipoprotein (LDL), and total cholesterol, as well as increased high-density lipoprotein cholesterol levels. Also, sibutramine seems to improve glucose utilization. Weight loss with sibutramine appears to be related to dose and is influenced by the intensity of the behavioral component of therapy. Ultimate efficacy of the medication can be predicted if the patient has lost 4 pounds after 4 weeks of therapy.

The STORM (Sibutramine Trial of Obesity Reduction and Maintenance) trial evaluated the effects of sibutramine on weight maintenance after an initial period of weight loss. Patients (n=605) with BMIs between 30 and 45 received sibutramine 10 mg/d for 6 months along with a low-calorie diet (600 kcal/d deficit). Patients who lost at least 5% of initial body weight after the 6 months were randomized to receive sibutramine 10 to 20 mg/d or placebo for 18 months. Of these patients, 42% and 50%, respectively, did not complete the study. Among completers, 43% of the sibutramine group and 16% of the placebo group maintained at least 80% of their weight loss after 2 years (James et al., 2000).

Dosage

The recommended starting dose of sibutramine is 10 mg once daily. If the patient gains weight while on therapy, the dose may be increased to 15 mg/d. If the patient has problems tolerating the medication, the dose may be decreased to 5 mg/d.

Contraindications/Precautions

Sibutramine is contraindicated in patients taking MAOIs. It should not be used in patients with a major eating disorder or poorly controlled hypertension. The drug should also be avoided in patients with a history of coronary artery disease, congestive heart failure, arrhythmia, stroke, or severe renal or hepatic disease. Sibutramine should be used with caution in patients with narrow-angle glaucoma or a history of seizures. Sibutramine is not indicated in patients younger than 16 years of age.

Adverse Events

Although sibutramine is classified as Schedule IV, there is no evidence of abuse potential with this medication. The adverse events most frequently reported by patients receiving sibutramine therapy were dry mouth, headache, constipation, decreased appetite, and insomnia. These events are generally mild and transient. Due to its mechanism of action, sibutramine can lead to increases in blood pressure (average of 1–3 mm Hg) and pulse rate (average of 4–6 bpm).

Antidepressants

Some antidepressant medications have been studied as appetite suppressants. These medications are FDA approved for the treatment of depression, and their use in weight loss is an "off-label" use. Fluoxetine (Prozac) is a selective serotonin reuptake inhibitor that has the unexpected side effect of weight loss. It is not clear how it aids in weight loss; it may limit appetite, or it may increase the basal metabolic rate. Because some people overeat when depressed, it may reduce food consumption secondary to depression. Studies of the antidepressants usually have found that patients lost moderate amounts of weight for up to 6 months. However, most studies indicate patients who lost weight while taking antidepressants tended to regain weight while they were still on drug therapy.

The choice of one agent over another has not been well studied in controlled trials. The choice can be influenced by the formulary of the patient's health maintenance organization or the cost to the patient. Each agent may help curb a patient's appetite, but, as noted earlier, these agents are used only as adjuncts to therapy.

Medications Affecting Fat Absorption or Metabolism: Orlistat

Orlistat (Xenical) differs from previously available weight-loss medications in that it works nonsystemically, acting locally in the gastrointestinal (GI) tract. Orlistat is a GI lipase inhibitor that facilitates weight loss by lowering absorption of dietary fat, on average by 30%. In research, orlistat users saw small, but significant drops in their total cholesterol, LDL, blood pressure, and blood sugar and insulin levels. Absorption of vitamins A, D, and E and β-carotene also was impaired.

In a randomized trial evaluating the long-term effects of orlistat, Davidson and colleagues (1999) compared the effects of dietary intervention coupled with orlistat versus dieting for a 2-year period. The researchers randomized patients with a BMI of 30 to 43 to orlistat 120 mg 3 times daily versus placebo. The results showed that patients taking orlistat had an average 3-kg greater weight loss than those taking placebo after 1 year. Nearly 35% of patients removed from orlistat therapy after the first year regained the weight by the end of the second year, compared with 60% in the placebo group (Davidson et al., 1999). Although the difference in weight loss between placebo and orlistat is small (3 kg = 6.6 lb), the sustained weight loss after drug discontinuation is remarkable. Two trials conducted in Europe showed similar results (Hollander, 2003). These studies showed that the best predictor for efficacy was a weight loss of greater than 5% initial body weight after 3 months of therapy.

The addition of orlistat to lifestyle therapy reduced the incidence of type 2 diabetes by 37% in patients with impaired glucose tolerance in a 4-year, randomized, double-blind study conducted in Sweden. In patients who already have type 2 diabetes, the addition of orlistat to current diabetes therapy (sulfonylureas, metformin, or insulin) resulted in significantly greater weight loss than the placebo group. The decrease in HbA_{1c} was also greater in the orlistat group (Hollander, 2003).

Dosage

Orlistat should be administered at a dose of 120 mg 3 times a day, during or up to 1 hour after a meal containing fat. The meal should contain less than 30% fat, and orlistat should not be taken with a meal containing no fat. The maximum daily dose is 360 mg/d. A primary concern with the use of orlistat is the potential for decreased absorption of the fat-soluble vitamins, A, D, E, and K. Multivitamins should be taken by all patients taking orlistat and these should be separated from the orlistat by 2 or more hours to ensure vitamin absorption.

Contraindications/Precautions

Orlistat is contraindicated in patients with chronic malabsorption syndrome or cholestasis. In addition, orlistat is not indicated in patients younger than 12 years of age.

Adverse Events

There are no systemic side effects of orlistat due to its lack of absorption. The primary side effects of orlistat include diarrhea, fatty stools, and flatulence. Patients should be advised of this because the fatty stools may appear as an oily leakage, particularly after flatus, and may cause embarrassment. Nausea and abdominal pain may also occur. GI effects associated with orlistat worsen with the more fat the dieters eat. However, data suggest that concomitant administration of natural fiber (psyllium mucilloid) may significantly reduce the self-reported frequency and severity of GI side effects associated with orlistat (Cavaliere et al., 2001). Caution should be used in patients taking oral warfarin (Coumadin) because orlistat may inhibit the absorption of vitamin K, resulting in an increased international normalized ratio.

Amphetamines

These agents are not widely used in the treatment of obesity primarily because of their high risk of abuse. As schedule II (C-II) agents, there are often restrictions on the amount and duration of therapy, and some states even prohibit these drugs from being prescribed for weight loss. Nonetheless, they have been and may continue to be used for weight-loss purpose, although they remain a last line of therapy for the obese patient.

The three forms of amphetamines are amphetamine, methamphetamine (Desoxyn), and dextroamphetamine (Dexedrine). Although each agent exerts similar effects, their potency varies, and therefore the dosing for each varies.

Mechanism of Action

The amphetamines cause an increase in the release of norepinephrine from central noradrenergic neurons and possibly a release of dopamine from the mesolimbic system at higher doses. Similar to the anorexiants, the mechanism of action for weight loss appears to be exerted at the hypothalamic feeding center.

These agents are completely absorbed when administered orally and are widely distributed throughout the body. The plasma half-life varies from approximately 7 hours to more than 30 hours, depending on the urinary alkalinization. At an acidic pH, the half-life is short because these agents are protonated in the acidic urine and are not reabsorbed. For every 1-unit increase in pH, the half-life increases by approximately 7 hours (McEvoy, 1999) because of an increase in urinary reabsorption.

Dosage

As a result of the short half-life of these agents, several long-acting dosage forms are available. The dosing of these agents is 5 to 10 mg 30 minutes to 1 hour before meals, and the last dose should be administered more than 6 hours before bedtime to minimize the side effect of insomnia. Because amphetamines display tachyphylaxis, tolerance may occur early on in therapy.

When they are used to treat obesity, these agents should be used at the lowest effective dose with intermittent courses of therapy. The dosage should not exceed 30 mg amphetamine sulfate or 15 mg of the long-acting form of methamphetamine or dextroamphetamine. A 3- to 6-week course of therapy followed by an "off" period of half the treatment time (eg, 4 weeks of drug therapy followed by 2 weeks off, then 4 weeks on) is recommended.

Selecting the Most Appropriate Agent

The selection of the most appropriate agent for treating an obese patient depends on a number of factors. Previous use of anorexiants or other weight-loss agents is essential to determine which agent the patient considers to be effective. In addition, the clinician must assess the abuse or dependency potential of the patient because of the controlled nature of the approved prescription agents. The side effect profile must be considered, particularly in patients with hypertension, dysrhythmia, or stroke.

All pharmacotherapeutic treatment should be anchored with appropriate dietary restrictions and counseling as well as physical activity. The decreases in caloric intake and the increases in caloric expenditure associated with these behaviors are essential to the effective weight reduction associated with medications. It is important to keep in mind that the amount of weight loss obtained will vary with each individual, but it appears to be no more than 10% of initial weight no matter which agent is selected (Weigle, 2003).

First-Line Therapy

The agents for first-line therapy include sibutramine and orlistat. Both of these agents have FDA approval for long-term maintenance of weight loss and should be considered for first-line therapy. However, patients with a history of hypertension, coronary artery disease, congestive heart failure, dysrhythmias, or stroke should not use sibutramine. Therefore, orlistat may be a reasonable first choice in these patients.

Second-Line Therapy

If sibutramine was chosen as first-line therapy, then orlistat should be considered a second-line agent, and vice versa. Agents that can be purchased without a prescription usually are not recommended for long-term weight loss because of the lack of efficacy data and the potential side effects.

Third-Line Therapy

No single agent is considered a third-line therapy, but surgery is often considered in patients with a BMI of 40 or higher in whom dietary, physical, and pharmaceutical therapies have failed, or in those with a BMI of 35 or higher with obesity-related comorbidities.

Combination Therapy

The combination of drugs with different mechanisms of action may provide additive or synergistic effects. However, data suggests that adding orlistat to sibutramine therapy produces no additional weight loss than sibutramine alone (Wadden et al., 2000).

Special Population Considerations

Smokers

Smoking in itself is a risk factor for cardiovascular disease. The additional burden of obesity places the obese smoker in a much higher risk category for long-term cardiovascular effects. Coupled with this is the increase in metabolism induced by smoking. The obese patient, who then quits smoking, runs the risk of gaining weight or thwarting efforts at weight loss. Special attention should be paid to this category of patient. A much greater level of attention should be paid to the lifestyle changes these patients need to make, and a continued reinforcement of the need for abstinence from smoking versus weight loss should be emphasized.

Ethnicity

There appears to be no specific relationship between ethnicity and response to drug therapy for weight loss. However, dietary changes and lifestyle changes, when offered, must be offered within the patient's cultural context.

Socioeconomic Status

Although obesity is a chronic disease with many adverse health consequences, it is a physical disability that is intensely stigmatized in our society. Many people, including some health care professionals, do not view obesity as a condition that deserves medical intervention or sympathy. Studies have shown a striking inverse relationship between obesity and socioeconomic status in the developed world, particularly among women (Gortmaker et al., 1993). A research study performed by Gortmaker and colleagues found that being overweight during adolescence has a particularly detrimental effect on socioeconomic achievement. They studied the relationship between being overweight and education attainment, marital status, household income, and self-esteem in 10,039 randomly selected people aged 16 to 24 years in 1981.

To assess the social consequences of obesity, the investigators compared disability from obesity with that associated with other forms of chronic illness. Seven years later, the overweight women were less educated, less likely to have been married, and had lower household incomes and 10% higher rates of household poverty than women who had not been overweight, independent of baseline socioeconomic status and aptitude test scores (Gortmaker et al., 1993). Similar trends were also found among men, but the relationship was weaker. It has been said that obesity is due to low socioeconomic status, yet the results of this study indicate that the inverse is also true: low socioeconomic status is influenced by obesity (Gortmaker et al., 1993).

MONITORING PATIENT RESPONSE

One of the most painful aspects of obesity may be the emotional suffering it causes. American society places great emphasis on physical appearance, often equating attractiveness with slimness, especially in women. The messages, intended or not, make overweight people feel unattractive. Therefore, obese individuals may suffer from social stigmatization, discrimination, and low self-esteem, which may also lead to depression. The social stigma of being obese has created a $40-billion-a-year weight-loss industry that preys on Americans' desire to be thin, with weight-loss treatments, such as diets and dietary foods, that are clearly ineffective, counterproductive, and associated with adverse effects.

Certain drugs that are used to treat psychosis, depression, and epilepsy can cause marked weight gain (Weigle, 2003). This may lead to decreased patient compliance with therapy or increased risk of adverse health outcomes. Newer drugs that treat these conditions are available, which cause less weight gain or even weight loss. Therefore, the patient's medication history should be monitored and adjusted as needed.

The patient should be monitored for weight loss, decreases in BMI, and changes in waist-to-hip ratios. In addition, patients taking anorexiants or amphetamines should have their blood pressure monitored at least monthly, if not biweekly. Weight loss should not be faster than 1 to 2 lb/wk over a sustained period, usually 6 or more months. During this period, empiric evidence (NIH, 1998) suggests that frequent visits to a health care practitioner, with reinforcement of dietary and lifestyle changes, improve weight loss and maintenance of weight loss.

PATIENT EDUCATION

Patients should be educated that obesity is more than just a cosmetic problem. It is a health hazard. Someone who is 40% overweight is twice as likely to die prematurely as an average-weight person. This effect is seen after 10 to 30 years of being obese. Research evidence indicates that a sedentary lifestyle confers an even greater risk than being overweight (Wickelgren, 1998).

Dieting as a way of weight loss is not only ineffective but risky. Severely energy-restricted or unbalanced diets are linked to deficiency syndromes, gallstones, dysrhythmias, and sudden cardiac death. Even balanced diets lead to chronic fatigue, impaired concentration, cold intolerance, mood changes, and malaise as weight drops below the set point. Cycles of dietary deprivation followed by refeeding ("yo-yo" dieting) may contribute to hypertension, congestive heart failure, and peripheral edema. Yo-yo dieting may enhance metabolic efficiency, thus promoting weight gain. It may also lead to low self-esteem as the dieter fails either to lose weight or maintain a weight loss (Weigle, 1990).

Patients should be educated on the fact that obesity has been linked to several serious medical conditions, such as diabetes, heart disease, high blood pressure, and stroke. It is also associated with higher rates of certain types of cancer. Obese men are more likely than nonobese men to die from cancer of the colon, rectum, and prostate. Obese women are more likely than nonobese women to die from cancer of the gallbladder, breast, uterus, cervix, and ovaries.

For more information regarding overweight or obesity, practitioners and patients should contact the following organizations or visit their Web sites. The Web site addresses listed below will direct people to the obesity section of the organization's Web site.

American Obesity Association
   1250 24th Street, NW
   Suite 300
   Washington, DC 20037
   202-776-7711
   www.obesity.org
Division of Nutrition and Physical Activity, National Center
   for Chronic Disease Prevention and Health Promotion,
   Centers for Disease Control and Prevention
   4770 Buford Highway, NE, MS/K-24
   Atlanta GA 30341-3717
   770 488-5820
   www.cdc.gov/nccdphp/dnpa/obesity/
National Institutes of Health
   9000 Rockville Pike
   Bethesda, Maryland 20892
   301-496-4000
   http://health.nih.gov/result.asp/476
WHO Regional Office for the Americas
   525, 23rd Street, NW
   Washington, DC 20037
   202-974-3000
   www.who.int/health_topics/obesity/en/
The Surgeon General
   Office of the Surgeon General
   5600 Fishers Lane
   Room 18-66
   Rockville, MD 20857
   www.surgeongeneral.gov/topics/obesity/

■ Case Study

A.P. is a 34-year-old woman who comes into your clinic looking for a medication to help her lose weight. She states that she has tried several times to lose weight but seems to gain it back within months after stopping her dieting. She tried fen-phen a few years ago with some success, but stopped the drug therapy when she heard about the heart problems. She informs you that she has had a follow-up test and that there were no problems found with her heart.

Your workup reveals a normal, young, well-developed woman in no acute distress. She is 66 inches tall and weighs 179 lb. She has no abnormal laboratory values, including a cholesterol level of 187 mg/dL. Her blood pressure is somewhat elevated at 138/87. She has no other pertinent medical history, no allergies to medications, and she takes only birth control pills. She does not smoke or drink alcohol. She works as a secretary in an office. She has a BMI of 29.

Diagnosis: obesity

1. What would be a good weight goal for A.P.? What BMI?

2. What dietary and lifestyle changes should be recommended to A.P.?

3. What drug therapy would you prescribe? Why?

4. What would you monitor for and how often would you monitor these parameters?

5. Describe one or two drug–drug or drug–food interactions for the selected agent.

6. What patient education would you provide based on the prescribed therapy?

7. Describe one or two adverse reactions for the selected agent that would cause you to change therapy.

8. If one of these occurred, what would be the choice for the second-line therapy?

9. What over-the-counter or alternative medications would be appropriate for this patient?

Bibliography

Starred references are cited in the text.

Campfield, L. A., Smith, F. J., & Burn, P. (1998). Strategies and potential molecular targets for obesity treatment. *Science, 280,* 1383–1387.

Camuzzie, A. C., & Allison, D. B. (1998). The search for human obesity genes. *Science, 280,* 1374–1377.

Carek, P. J., et al. (1997). Management of obesity: Medical treatment options. *American Family Physician, 55*(2), 551–558, 561–562.

*Cavaliere, H., Floriano, I., & Medeiros-Neto, G. (2001). Gastrointestinal side effects of orlistat may be prevented by concomitant prescription of natural fibers (psyllium mucilloid). *International Journal of Obesity Related Metabolic Disorders, 25,* 1095–1099.

*Connolly, H. M., Crary, J. L., McGoon, M. D., et al. (1997). Valvular heart disease associated with fenfluramine-phentermine (Fen-phen). *New England Journal of Medicine, 337,* 581–588.

*Davidson, M. H., Hauptman, J., DiGirolamo, M., et al. (1999). Weight control and risk factor reduction in obese subjects treated for 2 years with orlistat: A randomized controlled trial. *Journal of the American Medical Association, 281,* 235–242.

*Dillon, K. A., Putnam, K. G., & Avorn, J. L. (1997). Death from irreversible pulmonary hypertension associated with short-term use of fenfluramine and phentermine (Letter). *Journal of the American Medical Association, 278,* 132.

Duke, J. (1997). *The green pharmacy.* Emmaus, PA: Rodale Press.

Expert Panel on the Identification, Evaluation, and Treatment of Overweight and Obesity in Adults. (1998). Executive summary of the clinical guidelines on the identification, evaluation, and treatment of overweight and obesity in adults. *Archives of Internal Medicine, 158,* 1855–1867.

*Flegal, K. M., Carroll, M. D., Ogden, C. L., et al. (2002). Prevalence and trends in obesity among U.S. adults 1999–2000. *Journal of the American Medical Association, 288,* 1723–1727.

*Gortmaker, S. L, et al. (1993). Social and economic consequences of overweight in adolescence and young adulthood. *New England Journal of Medicine, 329,* 1008–1012.

*Hebel, S. K. (Ed.). (1999). Anorexiants. *Drug facts and comparisons.* St. Louis: Facts and Comparisons.

*Hill, J. O. (1998). Environmental contributions to the obesity epidemic. *Science, 280,* 1371–1373.

*Hollander, P. (2003). Orlistat in the treatment of obesity. *Primary Care in Clinical and Office Practice, 30,* 427–440.

*James, P. T., Leach, R. , Kalamara, F., et al. (2001). The worldwide obesity epidemic. *Obesity Research, 9*(Suppl 5), S228–S233.

*James, W. P., Astrup, A., Finer, N., et al., for the STORM study group. (2000). Effect of sibutramine on weight maintenance after weight loss: A randomized trial. Sibutramine Trial of Obesity Reduction and Maintenance. *Lancet, 356,* 2119–2125.

Kiberstis, P. A., & Marx, J. (1998). Regulation of body weight. *Science, 280,* 1363.

*McEvoy, G. K. (Ed.). (1999). *AHFS drug information 99.* Bethesda, MD: American Society of Health-System Pharmacists.

*National Institute of Diabetes and Digestive and Kidney Diseases. (2000). Overweight, obesity, and health risk. *Archives of Internal Medicine, 160,* 898–904.

*National Institutes of Health. (1998). *Clinical Guidelines on the identification, evaluation, and treatment of overweight and obesity in adults.* (NIH Publication No. 98-4083). Bethesda, MD: Author. Available at http://www.nhlbi.nih.gov/guidelines/obesity/ob_home.htm. Accessed March 2, 2004.

*National Institutes of Health. (2000). *The practical guide: Identification, evaluation and treatment of overweight and obesity in adults.* (NIH Publication No. 00-4084). Bethesda, MD: Author. Available at http://www.nhlbi.nih.gov/guidelines/obesity/prctgd_c.pdf. Accessed March 1, 2004.

National Institutes of Health. (2001). *Understanding adult obesity* (NIH Publication No. 01-3680). Bethesda, MD: Author. Available at http://www. niddk.nih.gov/health/nutrit/pubs/unders.htm #tables. Accessed March 1, 2004.

National Institutes of Health. (2003a). *Prescription medications for the treatment of obesity* (NIH Publication No. 97-4191). Bethesda, MD: Author. Available at http://www.niddk.nih.gov/health/nutrit/pubs/presmeds.htm. Accessed March 2, 2004.

National Institutes of Health. (2003b). *Do you know the health risks of being overweight?* (NIH Publication No. 03-4098). Bethesda, MD: Author. Available at http://www.niddk.nih.gov/health/nutrit/pubs/health.htm. Accessed March 2, 2004.

*Nonas, C. A. (1998). A model for chronic care of obesity through dietary treatment. *Journal of the American Dietetic Association, 98*(Suppl. 2), S16–S22.

*Ogden, C. L., Flegal, K. M., Carroll, M. D., et al. (2002). Prevalence and trends in overweight among U.S. children and adolescents

1999–2000. *Journal of the American Medical Association, 288,* 1728–1732.

*Racette, S. B., Deusinger, S. S., & Deusinger, R. H. (2003). Obesity: Overweight prevalence, etiology, and treatment. *Physical Therapy, 83,* 276–288.

*Sheperd, T. M. (2003). Effective management of obesity. *Journal of Family Practice, 52,* 34–42.

*Taubes, G. (1998). As obesity rates rise, experts struggle to explain why. *Science, 280,* 1367–1368.

*U.S. Department of Health and Human Services. (2001). *The Surgeon General's call to action to prevent and decrease overweight and obesity.* Rockville, MD. Available at http://www.surgeongeneral.gov/topics/obesity/calltoaction/factsheet03.pdf. Accessed March 1, 2004.

*Vidal, J. (2002). Updated review on the benefits of weight loss. *International Journal of Obesity, 26*(Suppl 4), S25–S28.

*Wadden, T. A., Berkowitz, R. I., Womble, L. G., et al. (2000). Effects of sibutramine plus orlistat in obese women following 1 year of treatment by sibutramine alone: A placebo-controlled trial. *Obesity Research, 8,* 431–437.

*Weigle, D. S. (1990). Human obesity: Exploding the myths. *Western Journal of Medicine, 153,* 421–428.

*Weigle, D. S. (2003). Pharmacological therapy of obesity: Past, present, and future. *Journal of Clinical Endocrinology and Metabolism, 88,* 2462–2469.

*Wickelgren, I. (1998). Obesity: How big a problem? *Science, 280,* 1364–1367.

*Weintraub, M., et al. (1992). Long-term weight control: National Heart, Lung, and Blood Institute–funded multi-modal intervention study—Conclusions. *Clinical Pharmacology and Therapeutics, 51,* 642–646.

*Williamson, D. F., Thompson, T. J., Thun, M., et al. (2000). Intentional weight loss and mortality among overweight individuals with diabetes. *Diabetes Care, 23,* 1499–1504.

*World Health Organization. (2003). *Obesity and overweight: Fact sheet.* Available at: http://www.who.int/hpr/NPH/docs/gs_obesity.pdf. Accessed March 1, 2004.

Yaes, R. J. (1993). Futility and avoidance: Medical professionals in the treatment of obesity. *Journal of the American Medical Association, 270,* 1423.

Visit the Connection web site for the most up-to-date drug information.

XIV

Integrative Approach to Patient Care

62

THE ECONOMICS OF PHARMACOTHERAPEUTICS

■ SAMIR K. MISTRY AND JOSHUA J. SPOONER

As little as 100 years ago, health insurance in the United States was scarce. Although President George Washington signed a law establishing prepaid health care in 1798, health insurance plans were slow to develop. Traditionally, patients paid health care providers and hospitals directly for their services on a fee-for-service basis. This system worked well for patients in times of good health; however, a serious injury or illness could leave the patient facing financial ruin.

ORIGINS OF MANAGED CARE

Modern health insurance's origins can be traced to 1929, when the Baylor University Hospital in Dallas began to offer 1500 school teachers up to 21 days of hospital care a year for $6 per person (Starr, 1982). Other groups also entered into agreement to prepay for Baylor's services. Shortly thereafter, several other Dallas-area hospitals followed suit and offered similar plans. Other early health insurance plans included the Kaiser Health Plans (early to mid-1930s) and the Group Health Association in Washington, DC (1937). As the country slid into the Depression and hospital revenues plummeted by 75% per patient, hospitals began to rely on insurance payments for a greater proportion of their operating budget (Starr, 1982).

Most health plans offered indemnity insurance (also known as fee-for-service insurance), in which patients paid for health care expenses out of their own pockets and then requested reimbursement from the insurer (often 80%). Unfortunately, indemnity insurance did little to control health care expenditures because physicians and hospitals received payments proportional to the volume of services they provided. Health care costs escalated further during the 1960s because of increased labor costs, increased use of specialists, unnecessary procedures, and the cost of care for the poor and uninsured (Navarro & Cahill, 1999).

Concerned with the rising cost of providing health care, insurance providers sought a way to slow the increases in expenditures. After extensive lobbying and negotiations in Congress, President Richard Nixon signed the federal Health Maintenance Organization (HMO) Act into law on December 29, 1973. This act encouraged the growth of managed care by providing grants and loans to develop HMOs, overturned restrictive state laws regulating health providers, defined a basic package of services that HMOs were required to offer, and established procedures by which HMOs could become federally qualified. The act also provided other support for the expansion of HMOs.

Because HMOs could be cost effective without reducing the quality of care, they were an attractive health insurance alternative for employers. The rate of enrollment in HMOs grew rapidly during the 1980s and 1990s and rivaled preferred provider organizations (PPOs) as the leading source of health insurance in the United States in the late 1990s (Hoechst Marion Roussel, 1998) before undergoing a decline in enrollment in the next decade (Kaiser Family Foundation, 2003). The federal government encouraged Medicare recipients to enroll in HMOs to manage the health care costs of beneficiaries; HMOs were reimbursed on a prospective basis by the government. The states soon followed suit, offering HMO-based options to Medicaid recipients.

The goal of this chapter is to provide a brief review of pharmacoeconomics, educate the reader about the methods used by managed care organizations (MCOs) to manage health care expenditures, explain how these methods are developed and implemented, and review how MCOs evaluate the practices of contracted providers. Understanding the rationale, benefits, and limitations associated with MCOs can be a factor in helping practitioners select appropriate drug therapy for their patients.

OVERVIEW OF PHARMACOECONOMICS

One of the most important aspects of managed care pharmacy involves the MCOs' emphasis on economics in the decision-making process. *Pharmacoeconomics* is the description and analysis of the costs of drug therapy to health care systems and society (Bootman et al., 1996). Because they evaluate both cost and human data, studies on pharmacoeconomics are important tools for MCOs in making drug therapy decisions. To provide an overview, some different pharmacoeconomic study designs are described in the following sections.

Cost–Benefit Analysis

A cost–benefit analysis is used to determine the overall cost of a particular intervention or protocol by evaluating all pertinent data and converting the data to a monetary end point (eg, U.S. dollars or E.U. Euros). Most often, this type of analysis is used to compare two different programs that also have different units for end points because the data can then be converted to one common unit (usually the dollar). The limitation to this analysis involves the evaluation of "intangible" end points or data that cannot be equated to a monetary value.

Cost Minimization Analysis

A cost minimization analysis evaluates the cost of two or more interventions with equivalent components or end points and determines which intervention is least costly. The most appropriate use for such analyses involves situations in which every aspect of compared interventions is identical except the cost of the intervention. Because efficacy and safety are identical, the cost of each intervention becomes the differential outcome. The outcomes of these analyses are also expressed in a monetary end point.

Cost-Effectiveness Analysis

A cost-effectiveness analysis may help determine the best program or intervention, where the desired outcome is a combination of both a monetary end point and a nonmonetary end point relative to an improvement in health (eg, life expectancy, blood glucose measurements). An example of this would be dollars per life-year saved.

Cost–Utility Analysis

A cost–utility analysis, which is closely related to a cost-effectiveness analysis, measures data in terms of quality of life. Quality of life is an assessment of a patient's well-being and social functioning, which can assist practitioners in determining a patient's response to drug therapy (Bootman et al., 1996). Along with traditional clinical results (eg, laboratory values, blood pressure, serum glucose level), a cost–utility analysis provides a more complete evaluation of a patient's progress and compares the cost of an intervention or program in terms of more intangible end points, rather than dollars. These analyses predominantly use quality-adjusted life-years (QALYs) gained as a major outcome. The QALY is symbolic of healthy years of life and is the unit of measurement that encompasses outcomes (eg, morbidity and mortality) in preferential sequence. This method has been very successful in evaluating various procedures compared with drug therapy in which a patient's quality of life is the chosen outcome (Bootman et al., 1996).

Pharmacoeconomic research compares cost and consequence with respect to pharmaceutical products and their impact on individuals, the health care system, and society. Such parameters are seldom analyzed in most studies.

FORMULARIES AND PHARMACY AND THERAPEUTICS COMMITTEES

An evaluation of American health expenditures identified $1.55 trillion in total health care spending in 2002; this was a 9.3% increase in expenditures over the previous year (Levit et al., 2004). Of this $1.55 trillion in health expendi-

tures, $162.4 billion (10.5%) was spent on prescription drugs. Although this represents a small portion of overall health care expenditures, it has been identified by many MCOs as a target for intervention due to large annual increases in prescription drug spending. Prescription drug spending increased 15.3% in 2002, close to the 16.4% and 15.9% increases seen in 2000 and 2001 (Levit et al., 2004).

Formularies

One of the most effective methods by which an MCO can improve the quality of care provided to patients and slow the increasing costs of providing a prescription benefit is by using a formulary (Troy, 1999). A medication formulary is simply a list of medications approved for use within a HMO, third-party payer, or pharmacy benefit manager (Navarro & Cahill, 1999). Formularies are usually organized by therapeutic area and medication class, with the formulary status and reimbursement category listed for each medication.

Formularies encourage the use of medications considered to be safer, more clinically effective, or more cost effective than other medications. When an MCO wants to limit the use of a drug for a specific reason (cost, safety, efficacy, or therapeutic class), a formulary allows the flexibility to implement such restrictions or limitations.

Evolution of Formularies

The use of formularies and formulary systems can be traced back to 1925, when the physicians and pharmacists of Syracuse University Hospital collaborated to establish a formulary system to monitor drug use and reduce therapeutic duplication (the unnecessary use of two or more medications to treat the same condition) in its drug therapy program (Sonnedecker, 1976). By the 1960s, formularies were being implemented in hospitals throughout the country with the guidance of the *American Hospital Formulary Service*, a prominent set of formulary development materials published by the American Society of Hospital Pharmacists. Following the HMO Act of 1973, many HMOs adopted the hospital formulary to monitor medication use. Formularies were initially used by managed care as an inventory control mechanism for staff-model HMOs (Dillon, 1999), but they evolved into effective tools for monitoring and regulating medication utilization for all types of MCOs. By 2003, 71% of managed care plans were using formularies (Kaiser Family Foundation, 2003).

Structure of Formularies

Although the format of a formulary differs from plan to plan, it usually contains the same fundamental information. Arranged by therapeutic class, most formularies list the name of the drug, its brand/generic status, an estimate of the drug's relative cost, and its formulary status and patient co-payment level. An example of a formulary is shown in Table 62-1. A "formulary medication" is a drug that is covered (reimbursed) by the health plan; formulary medications can be subdivided into different groups such as preferred and nonpreferred agents. "Preferred" agents are drugs that the health plan would prefer the practitioner to prescribe, either due to efficacy, safety, or cost issues. "Nonpreferred" drugs

Table 62.1

Example of a Formulary

Drug Class X Drug Name	Brand/Generic	Relative Cost	Formulary Status/Co-pay Tier
Drug A	Generic	$	First tier / $5.00
Drug B	Generic	$	First tier / $5.00
Drug C	Generic	$$	First tier / $5.00
Drug D	Brand	$$$$	Second tier / $15.00
Drug E	Brand	$$$$	Second tier / $15.00
Drug F	Brand	$$$$$	Second tier / $15.00
Drug G	Brand	$$$$	Third tier / $35.00
Drug H	Brand	$$$$$$	Third tier / $35.00
Drug I	Brand	$$$$$$$$	Prior authorization required / $35.00
Drug J	Generic	$	Nonformulary
Drug K	Brand	$$$$$	Nonformulary

are not the preferred agents of the health plan, but will nonetheless be covered by the plan. "Nonformulary medications" are drugs that are not on the formulary; health plans generally do not cover nonformulary medications or require specific documentation (eg, prior authorization) by a prescriber before being covered by the plan.

Most formularies can be divided into two specific groups: closed formularies and open formularies. Closed formularies (also knows as *restrictive* formularies) limit clinicians to prescribing from a small list of preferred agents (Troy, 1999). Rigid formulary systems were used by health plans and pharmacy benefit managers through the 1990s (Navarro, 1998). Open formularies usually do not involve a preferred group of agents, allowing the prescriber a greater selection of medications to choose from. Although some limitations exist in open formularies, providers usually can override restrictions with less effort than within a closed formulary. Both open and closed formularies are viewed as two extremes. Between the extremes are formularies that vary in their restrictiveness or openness.

Impact of Formularies on Patients

The price that consumers pay for prescriptions varies from plan to plan. Patients are commonly required to pay a portion of the cost of the prescription, also known as the co-payment, or "co-pay." Co-pay amounts can differ due to many variables: the product's formulary status, the brand/generic status of the product, the quantity of medication dispensed, the days' supply of medication (number of days worth of medication) dispensed, and the pharmacy used to fill/refill the prescription.

Most co-pays are set to cover up to a 1-month supply of medication (28–34 days of therapy, depending on the health plan). Thus, a patient who received a prescription for a 5-day course of therapy with rofecoxib for dental pain would likely have the same co-payment as a patient who received a prescription for a 30-day course of therapy of rofecoxib for arthritis.

Some plans may allow patients to get more than a 1-month supply of medication at a time for a maintenance medication (a medication that is taken at a stable dose for long periods of time, such as antihypertensives and antihyperlipidemics). For maintenance medications, most health plans allow patients to receive a 90-day supply of medication once the

dose has been stabilized. Health plans usually charge patients three co-pays for a 90-day supply (three 1-month supply co-pays). For example, if a patient paid a $10 co-pay for a 1-month supply, then the 90-day supply would cost $30. Health plans often offer reduced co-payments as an enticement for patients to order their maintenance medications from a mail-order pharmacy service; a 90-day supply of medication might only cost a patient one or two co-payments instead of three.

In the rigid formulary systems in the 1990s, a two-tiered prescription co-payment system was used by most health plans and PBMs; the lower co-payment tier was used for generic medications, whereas the higher co-payment tier was used for formulary brand name medications. Nonformulary medications were rarely covered by health plans or PBMs without prior approval; if granted, the prescription would fall into the higher co-payment tier. Nonformulary medications that were not approved by the health plan were not covered; either the patient paid the full retail price for the prescription, or the prescription was switched to a formulary agent by the prescribing physician.

Fueled by increasing prescription costs (Kaiser Family Foundation, 2001) and charges of restrictions of care (Flanagan, 2002; Horn et al., 1998; Talley, 1997), health plans and PBMs have begun to abandon the two-tiered formulary system in favor of three- and four-tiered systems (PBM News, 2001). Within these formulary systems, the first two tiers are set up the same as the previous two-tiered system, with the first (lowest) tier co-payment reserved for generic products and the second tier co-payment reserved for preferred brand name products. Agents in the third tier are the nonpreferred brand name products; the co-payment is substantially higher than the second tier co-payment. Some plans have added a fourth tier to their formulary for lifestyle drugs (impotence medications, wrinkle creams, hair restoration medications, etc.) with the highest prescription co-payments (PBM News, 2001). Three- and four-tiered formularies have introduced value considerations to patients: Do they value a specific third-tier product enough to pay the higher co-payment or will a second-tier product (with a lower co-payment) be suitable for their needs? The multiple-tiered co-payment has been proven to successfully move patients to products in the first and second tiers of the formulary without restricting access to prescription products (Fairman et al., 2003).

Functions of Formularies

Formularies have been used to promote the safe, effective, and cost-effective use of medications. Formularies can promote the use of generic medications, help to avoid the overuse or inappropriate use of certain medications (such as antibiotics), prevent the use of medications that may be harmful to certain patient populations (such as sedative/hypnotics in the elderly) or contraindicated in others (such as isotretinoin during pregnancy), and limit the use of medications with a high abuse potential (such as benzodiazepines and narcotic analgesics). Through generic substitution requirements, quantity/age/gender limits, or more specific regulations, MCOs can set up their formularies to promote a evidence-based and cost-effective approach to drug therapy.

Generic Substitution

A highly effective method of reducing the cost of the pharmacy benefit is generic substitution. Generic substitution is the process of dispensing an appropriate generic equivalent of a prescribed brand name drug. Prescribing generic products can reduce the cost of providing prescription medications for patients by 10% to 15% without reducing the quality of care (Friedman & Hanchak, 1999). Generic substitution has been supported by cost minimization analyses; as the brand and generic agents are considered identical in composition and activity, cost becomes the contributing factor for an agent's selection.

As noted in Chapter 1, a generic drug is considered equal, or bioequivalent, to a brand name drug and must undergo stringent testing and comply with specific criteria established by the U.S. Food and Drug Administration (FDA). The FDA has set certain therapeutic equivalence evaluation codes to show the relative bioequivalence of generic agents to the brand name drugs (U.S. Food and Drug Administration, 2004). There are two basic rating codes: A and B. The "A" rating indicates that the drug is considered therapeutically equivalent to other pharmaceutically equivalent products. The "B" rating indicates that the agent is not therapeutically equivalent to other pharmaceutically equivalent agents. Both A- and B-rated drugs are further differentiated based on dosage form. An "AB" rating states that the product's bioequivalence problems have been resolved, and evidence exists supporting the bioequivalence to pharmaceutically equivalent agents.

An example of generic substitution is dispensing the diuretic furosemide when the prescriber writes the prescription for Lasix, and the prescriber has not indicated that the brand name product is medically necessary. In such a situation, the pharmacist is filling the prescription with an FDA-approved, bioequivalent form of the brand name drug. Some insurance plans may allow the patient or physician to request the brand name agent, but this often results in a higher co-payment for the patient (Gross, 1998). The increase in co-payment may be as large as the difference in cost to the health plan between the brand and generic agents.

To maximize generic substitution, plans may use restrictive strategies such as "dispense as written" (DAW) blocks. A DAW code describes the rationale for the drug's selection and is entered into the prescription claim by the pharmacist before it is transmitted to the health plan for adjudication.

There are DAW codes for "substitution permissible" (DAW 0), "dispense as written" (DAW 1), "patient requests brand" (DAW 2), as well as other choices to provide a rationale for the chosen agent. A health plan can require that the patient receive an acceptable generic substitution for a brand name product unless a suitable DAW code has been entered. A DAW code of 7 is used for products with a narrow therapeutic index. Due to the risk of disrupting the level of drug in the patient's blood, drugs with a narrow therapeutic index do not have to be automatically substituted for an equivalent generic agent. A DAW of 7 informs the health plan that either the physician, pharmacist, or patient has elected to continue use of the brand name product. Drugs in this category include warfarin (Coumadin) and digoxin (Lanoxin).

Therapeutic Interchange

Therapeutic interchange is defined as the procedure of dispensing prescribed medications that are chemically different but deemed therapeutically similar to the medication prescribed (American Society of Consultant Pharmacists [ASCP], 2003). In general, therapeutic interchange involves the substitution of drugs that are different chemical compounds but are considered to exert the same therapeutic effect and have similar toxicity and side effect profiles (eg, nonsedating antihistamines: substitution of fexofenadine [Allegra] for desloratadine [Clarinex]). The use of therapeutic interchange has increased significantly because of a large influx of new medications that do not offer any therapeutic advantages over existing therapies but are priced lower than established products. These medications are commonly known as "me too" drugs. The angiotensin II receptor blockers (ARBs) offer the best example of "me too" drugs. In 2004, a total of 7 ARBs were on the market, with very little difference between them except price.

Pharmaceutical manufacturers offer rebates to health plans to compete for preferred status on formularies, which lowers the prescription benefit cost. Controversies tend to arise when discounts are used to exchange one drug over another when the drugs are in different classes. If a therapeutic interchange involves two drugs of the same therapeutic class, it can be considered an example of therapeutic minimization because the only difference between the two agents is cost (assuming that the safety/efficacy data for the two agents are equal).

Therapeutic interchange is used for reasons other than controlling costs, including promoting the use of agents associated with fewer drug–drug interactions (eg, substitution of fluconazole [Diflucan] for ketoconazole [Nizoral]), or of agents with a more convenient dosing schedule (eg, once-daily enalapril [Vasotec] instead of 2- to 3-times daily captopril [Capoten]). These interventions may prevent unnecessary drug–drug interactions or enhance medication compliance, which could, in turn, decrease overall health care costs and improve patient care.

In the retail pharmacy setting, therapeutic interchange must be verified and accepted by the prescribing practitioner. In the institutional setting, therapeutic interchange does not necessarily require a prescriber's approval if the institution's pharmacy and therapeutics (P&T) committee approves the specific interchange protocol (Chase et al., 1998). The American Medical Association (AMA) endorses the practice of therapeutic interchange in settings that have an organized medical staff and a functioning P&T committee (AMA, 1994).

Prior Authorization

Prior authorization refers to a preapproval process that health plans may require for certain prescriptions before they will cover it (Feldman et al., 1999). The primary purpose of a prior authorization process is to control the use of and prevent the overuse of nonpreferred medications or nonformulary medications. Prior to the recent move by health plans toward increasingly open formularies with three and four tiers of co-payments, health plans would require prior authorizations for most nonformulary drugs, expensive drugs, newly approved drugs, and drugs with less expensive alternatives (Dillon, 1999). Over 75% of commercial health plans used prior authorization programs in 2002 (Takeda Pharmaceuticals, 2003), and prior authorization is used by a majority of the states in their Medicaid programs (National Conference of State Legislatures [NCSL], 2004).

The criteria for approval of each drug undergoing the prior approval process will depend on the drug, the patient, the disease state involved, and the prescribing practitioner. Some prior authorizations may require a diagnosis along with pertinent laboratory values, whereas others may require a patient to fail therapy with certain drugs that are indicated to treat the same disease as the restricted agent. Other criteria may include patient demographics, such as age or gender limits, or prescriber limits, where only specific specialty types are allowed to prescribe for certain medications (eg, only allowing dermatologists to prescribe isotretinoin).

The usual chain of events involving prior authorization starts with a patient presenting a pharmacist with a prescription for a newly prescribed medication. The pharmacist, after submitting a claim and having it rejected, learns that the medication requires prior authorization (often from a message sent with the rejected claim). The pharmacist or patient then contacts the prescriber, tells the prescriber that the medication prescribed requires prior authorization, and requests that the prescriber contact the MCO to explain why the patient requires that medication. Prescribers can decide to either contact the MCO and pursue prior authorization, or they may choose not to pursue prior authorization and select an alternative agent. MCOs often accept prior authorization requests from practitioners by mail, fax, or telephone. Completing the prior authorization process may result in the drug's approval for use in that patient, or the MCO may again reject the claim and offer a list of alternative medications that are covered by the plan.

If the prescriber knows that the drug requires prior authorization, the necessary paperwork can be completed to have the drug approved for the patient before the patient enters the pharmacy. Problems arise when the patient and prescriber are unaware of which agents on the MCO's formulary require prior authorization. This confuses many patients, possibly leading them to think that the prescriber ordered the wrong medication or the pharmacist made an error in filling the prescription (Lisi, 1997).

MCOs have increased their efforts to prospectively review prescriptions requiring prior authorization during the claim adjudication process (Takeda Pharmaceuticals, 2003). When a pharmacy sends a claim for a prior authorization drug to the PBM for adjudication, the PBM can review the patient's prescription claim history and the claim itself to determine if the prior authorization criteria have been met. This step can decrease the number of rejected prescription claims and minimize the time and efforts of prescribers, pharmacists, and patients in obtaining prior authorizations. When initiated effectively by informing practitioners of the drug's status and the preapproval process, prior authorization can become a very efficient mechanism for controlling costs and drug use.

Medical Necessity

Some MCOs use the term *medical necessity* interchangeably with *prior authorization*. In most settings, a drug considered a medical necessity is a nonformulary drug that is usually extremely expensive and that may have less expensive alternatives or is indicated only for rare disorders (Glassman et al., 1997; Roy-Byrne et al., 1998). Some MCOs make medical necessity drugs available only after failure of drug therapy with a drug requiring prior authorization. MCOs carefully evaluate drugs before classifying them as medical necessity drugs, knowing that the drugs will be restricted if they are covered. Like the criteria for medications requiring prior authorization, the criteria for coverage vary from drug to drug.

PHARMACY AND THERAPEUTICS COMMITTEE

Structure and Function

A P&T committee is a group that meets periodically to review and revise the MCO's formulary. The committee is composed primarily of physicians and may include nurse practitioners, physicians' assistants, administrators, and pharmacists. The physicians on the committee often comprise a diverse group from various fields of practice, with general practitioners and several specialty types (eg, neurology, cardiology, psychiatry, gastroenterology) represented. The committee is a well-balanced mix of practitioners who can view health care policies from different perspectives and provide sound recommendations.

Formulary Management

The main responsibilities of a P&T committee are to revise the formulary, create and implement medication policies, and provide education for practitioners. Formulary reviews include evaluating new medications for formulary consideration, periodic drug class reviews, and utilization analyses. A major goal of the P&T committee is to provide cost-effective, clinically safe, and effective therapy. Frequent formulary revisions are needed for several reasons: pharmaceutical manufacturers are introducing new agents more rapidly than ever before, the addition and deletion of agents must reflect the current standards of health care practice (Navarro & Cahill, 1999), and the results of clinical studies can potentially change guidelines for disease management.

The inclusion and exclusion of new agents is a time-intensive process for P&T committees because each new

BOX 62-1. CRITERIA NEEDED FOR A NEW AGENT TO BE ADDED TO A FORMULARY

1. Source of supply and reliability of manufacturer and distributor
2. Pharmacologic considerations (drug class, adverse effect profile, mechanism of action, therapeutic indications, drug–drug interactions, similarity to existing drugs, clinical advantages)
3. Unlabeled uses and their appropriateness
4. Bioavailability data
5. Pharmacokinetic data
6. Dosage ranges by route and age
7. Risks versus benefits regarding clinical efficacy and safety of a particular drug relative to other drugs with the same indication
8. Patient risk factors relative to contraindications, warnings, and precautions
9. Special monitoring or drug administration requirements
10. Pharmacoeconomic data
11. Cost comparisons against other drugs available to treat the same medical condition(s)

(Adapted from Dillon, M. J. [1999]. Drug formulary management. In R. P. Navarro [Ed.], *Managed care pharmacy practice* (pp. 145–165). Gaithersburg, MD: Aspen Publishers.)

agent must meet certain criteria before it can be placed on a formulary as a preferred product (Box 62-1). The committees usually evaluate peer-reviewed journal articles and the FDA-approved product labeling for the new agent. The committee must consider the issue of bias when evaluating results provided by any literature provided by the pharmaceutical manufacturer. Literature that includes data comparing the new agent with an agent currently used to treat the same disorder is useful for comparing one drug with another. If the new agent meets enough of the criteria, the P&T committee then recommends addition of the agent to the formulary. A P&T committee can add the drug to the formulary unconditionally or may recommend implementation of certain restrictions on the coverage (prior authorization, quantity limitations, step therapy) of the new agent to allow its inclusion in the formulary.

Because of the increase in prescription drug spending by health plans, cost now plays a more significant role in formulary status, although cost should be considered only after safety and efficacy data are evaluated. To promote a drug's addition to a formulary, pharmaceutical manufacturers may offer discounts to MCOs as incentives.

Development of Practice Guidelines or Treatment Algorithms

Another responsibility of a P&T committee is to develop or approve potential practice guidelines or treatment algorithms for the MCO. Guidelines provide useful recommendations for practitioners treating various diseases. They may be based on current consensus practice guidelines, or they may be developed by the P&T committee using current clinical data. A main purpose of guidelines or algorithms is to provide a standard of therapy to minimize variations in disease management (Dillon, 1999).

ENSURING FORMULARY AND PRACTICE GUIDELINE COMPLIANCE

One of the reasons MCOs develop formularies and practice guidelines is to help lower the cost of the prescription drug benefit. Unfortunately, merely printing and distributing formularies and algorithms often is not enough to alter prescribing practices. Patients and pharmacists may also be wary of the formulary system, failing to understand both its necessity and usefulness. Educational programs, including seminars, newsletters, provider (pharmacy and physician) communications, and one-on-one meetings, are useful tools to improve formulary compliance but do not ensure it. Thus, MCOs have developed a variety of payment and reimbursement strategies to improve compliance. The following sections describe the ways that MCOs evaluate formulary and treatment guideline compliance and how MCOs use different levels of payments to improve compliance.

Prescriber Incentives for Compliance

MCOs can monitor compliance to the formulary and treatment guidelines with a variety of tools. Many MCOs use the level of peer compliance to determine the amount of a prescriber's or practice's year-end incentives. Prescribers can be eligible for a bonus incentives if they meet specific criteria established by the MCO or if their compliance is superior to that of their peers.

Some MCOs may tie a portion of a provider's compensation to the level of compliance. If a practitioner fails to follow practice guidelines closely and inexplicably high prescription costs result, an MCO may withhold a portion of the provider's compensation. In a capitated plan, the provider receives a fixed, predetermined, per-member payment by the MCO to provide services for members, regardless of how much or how frequently a member uses service. Providers can reap financial reward if they can provide services at a cost lower than their level of payment. On the other hand, they are responsible for all costs if expenses should rise above their level of payment. Approximately 60% of MCOs offer a capitated plan (Dalzell, 2003). However, the percentage of health plans that capitate pharmacy benefit utilization continues to decrease; in 2000, fewer than 2% of health plans used a capitated pharmacy benefit (Greene, 2002).

Evaluating Compliance: Percentage Formulary Compliance

The simplest way for an MCO to evaluate formulary compliance is to determine the prescriber's percentage of prescriptions for generic and branded formulary products. Although this method is useful for determining formulary compliance (eg, the use of generic and branded formulary angiotensin-converting enzyme [ACE] inhibitors compared with nonformulary branded ACE inhibitors), it does not evaluate the quality of prescribing. Just because a formulary agent is prescribed does not make the prescription appropriate. It may be more important to determine if the prescriber is following practice guidelines. A prescriber who prescribes a formulary agent but is not following treatment guidelines has the same percentage formulary compliance as a prescriber who uses a different and potentially less expensive or more appropriate formulary medication by following treatment guidelines. Also, prescribers who use medically necessary or appropriate but nonformulary drugs are penalized in this system. This becomes an issue if a patient is unresponsive, allergic, or intolerant to the formulary agent. Many MCOs have initiated programs to evaluate the quality of physician prescribing by implementing physician profiling programs, where clinicians evaluate questionable prescribing with the physicians.

Because of the aforementioned limitations with percentage formulary compliance, MCOs also use another tool to evaluate compliance, the per-member–per-month (PMPM) reports.

Health Care Trend Reporting

When analyzing health care trends for any MCO, many variables are reviewed and factored in to evaluate and justify the trends during any particular year. The PMPM reports are a unit of measure related to each enrollee for each month. When used to evaluate prescribing practices, average PMPM prescription costs are determined for each provider. Theoretically, prescribers who adhere to formulary and practice guidelines achieve lower PMPM prescription costs than their peers who do not. This is not a foolproof method to evaluate compliance because a small number of patients requiring expensive therapy (eg, chemotherapy) can substantially increase a prescriber's PMPM. More frequently, MCOs use PMPMs to evaluate prescription costs for a specific disease. An example of a disease-specific PMPM report appears in Table 62-2. Although prescriber A is responsible for the highest dollar expenditure on antihyperlipidemics, his PMPM prescription cost is close to the average of the prescriber's peers. On the other hand, despite prescriber C's low overall dollar expenditure on lipid agents, his PMPM prescription cost is the highest.

Another factor that is considered in evaluating health care trends is drug cost. Monitoring the rate of increase in drug cost has become a significant factor in overall health care spending. As the prices of prescription medications increase, MCOs are adjusting their overall plan designs to compensate for that increase. These adjustments may include changes to preferred and nonpreferred products on drug formularies, implementation of prior authorization and step therapy programs for expensive products, increases in member co-payments, or increases in member premiums.

Improving Formulary Compliance

MCOs have a unique opportunity to improve formulary and practice guideline compliance by providing financial incentives to other people (beside clinicians) who participate in dispensing medication to the patient: the dispenser (pharmacist) and the recipient (patient). These financial incentives include bonuses, differential reimbursement rates, and different levels of prescription co-payment.

Pharmacist Reimbursement

An MCO can influence pharmacists as a secondary step in limiting the use of nonformulary medications. As a part of the contracting process, MCOs may impose requirements on pharmacies if the pharmacy wishes to serve members of the plan. MCOs can require that pharmacies dispense generic products when available, unless the physician requires the prescription to be DAW or the medication (eg, digoxin [Lanoxin], warfarin [Coumadin]) has a narrow therapeutic index. Many states already require automatic generic substitution when applicable. To reduce wasted or unused medication, MCOs often impose a limit on the amount of medication that a pharmacist can dispense—usually no more than 1 month's worth at a time for medications to treat chronic illnesses (hypertension or diabetes mellitus) or a shorter duration for medications such as antibiotics.

Pharmacies that are successful in increasing formulary compliance or reducing member pharmacy costs may be eligible for bonuses or they may receive a higher reimbursement rate. Alternatively, pharmacies that fail to meet the requirements of the contract may receive a lower reimbursement rate or have their contract terminated altogether. MCOs frequently audit the claims of pharmacies with a higher-than-average number of DAW orders to ensure that the prescriber requires the brand name drug.

Patient Prescription Co-payment

The impact of prescription co-payment on patients was reviewed earlier in this chapter. In summary, as formularies have progressively become more open, health plans have responded by using differential co-payments in an effort to encourage patients to use lower-cost generic or preferred brand products. Patients who are hesitant to pay a high prescription co-payment when lower priced alternatives are available frequently ask their physician to prescribe the product with the lower co-payment; the physician will often comply with the patient's request if they believe the change can be made without adversely affecting the outcome of care.

CURRENT ISSUES IN MANAGED CARE

One of the largest challenges to face managed care recently has been the financial impact of high-cost injectable drugs

---

Table 62.2

Per-Member–Per-Month (PMPM) Prescription Costs for Patients Receiving Antihyperlipidemic Therapy

Prescriber	Number of Member Months	Lipid Prescription Costs ($)	PMPM Prescription Costs ($)
A	561	45,183	80.54
B	240	18,818	78.41
C	285	25,639	89.96
D	496	36,248	73.08
E	357	30,780	86.22
F	489	40,223	82.31

products. Many MCOs have contracted with companies that make specialty injectable drugs to manage the distribution of these agents. These companies provide a cost-effective distribution center for injectable medications. This has unfortunately removed the ability of many physicians to bill injectable drugs through the medical benefit and forced them to seek reimbursement through the specialty injectable companies.

A new factor to enter the managed care landscape is the movement of prescription products to over-the-counter (OTC) status. The most recent products include nonsedating antihistamines (Claritin), proton pump inhibitors (Prilosec OTC), and H_2-receptor blockers (Pepcid, Zantac, Axid, and Tagamet). This has provided MCOs the opportunity to implement cost-effective strategies to decrease the cost of the prescription medications within the previously mentioned therapy classes. Many MCOs have implemented third-tier co-payments for all prescription drugs in therapy classes that have an OTC available (Reed, 2003). Other MCOs have implemented step therapy programs, which require a trial of an OTC product prior to reimbursement of the prescription products. The movement of prescription products to OTC status also increases patient convenience because products that previously required prescriptions from a physician are now available without a prescription. Questions remain about the safety of allowing patients to diagnose and treat conditions without the direct supervision of physicians.

In the late 1990s, a backlash against MCOs—particularly HMOs—began. Critics argue that MCOs focus more on cost containment than quality improvement and that further compromises in quality are in the future (Talley, 1997). Patients have begun suing MCOs for denial of services or failure to reimburse for treatment. Congress, in turn, is examining ways to restructure these organizations to be more consumer friendly. The merits of a health care consumer's bill of rights have been discussed.

One cause of discontent among health care purchasers is the cost of insurance premiums, which began to rise at a rate greater than that of inflation starting in the mid-1990s. The average family premium cost over $9000 in 2003 (Kaiser Family Foundation, 2003). Some of this price increase can be attributed to increasing expenditures for medications. The increase in expenditures for prescription drugs is the effect of three factors: rising use, rising prices, and the increased availability of novel medications. The influence of direct-to-consumer advertising, manufacturer pricing policies, and the increase in the number of "me too" drugs on the rising cost of health care continues to be debated. This much remains clear: if prescription drug spending continues to increase as projected (Heffler et al., 2004), MCOs will have to modify the extent to which they cover prescription drugs.

Despite its critics and shortcomings, managed care is likely to grow and remain the leading manner of financing and delivering health care in the United States. Through more effective communication and cooperation, practitioners and MCOs may some day resolve their conflicting issues. It is imperative for practitioners and MCOs to understand each other's role in health care. Although practitioners and MCOs have quite different responsibilities in health care, both groups share a common goal: the delivery of high-quality care to patients.

Bibliography

Starred references are cited in the text.

Academy of Managed Care Pharmacy. (2000). *A format for the submission of clinical and economic evaluation data in support of formulary consideration by managed health care systems in the United States.* Alexandria, VA: Academy of Managed Care Pharmacy.

*American Medical Association. (1994). AMA policy on drug formularies and therapeutic interchange in inpatient and ambulatory patient care settings. *American Journal of Hospital Pharmacy, 51,* 1808–1810.

*American Society of Consultant Pharmacists. (2003). *Guidelines for implementing therapeutic interchange in long-term care.* Public Policy Guidelines: www.ascp.com/public/pr/guidelines/therapeutic.shtml.

*Bootman, J. L., Townsend, R. J., & McGhan, W. F. (1996). Introduction to pharmacoeconomics. In J. L. Bootman, R .J. Townsend, & W. F. McGhan (Eds.), *Principles of pharmacoeconomics* (2nd ed., pp. 4–19). Cincinnati, OH: Harvey Whitney Books.

Campbell, G., & Sprague, K. L. (2001). The state of drug decision-making: Report on a survey of P&T committee structure and practices. *Formulary, 36,* 644–655.

*Chase, S. L., Peterson, A. M., & Wardell, C. J. (1998). Therapeutic-interchange program for oral histamine H_2-receptor antagonists. *American Journal of Hospital Pharmacy, 55,* 1382–1386.

*Dalzell, M. (2003). Has capitation weathered the storm? *Managed Care,* July 2002, 18–26.

*Dillon, M. J. (1999). Drug formulary management. In R. P. Navarro (Ed.), *Managed care pharmacy practice* (pp. 145–165). Gaithersburg, MD: Aspen Publishers.

*Fairman, K. A., Motheral, B. R., & Henderson, R. R. (2003). Retrospective, long-term follow-up study of the effect of a three-tier prescription drug co-payment system on pharmaceutical and other medical utilization and costs. *Clinical Therapeutics, 25,* 3147–3161.

*Feldman, S., Fleischer, A., & Chen, G. J. (1999). Is prior authorization of topical tretinoin for acne cost effective? *American Journal of Managed Care, 5,* 457–463.

Fins, J. J. (1998). Drug benefits in managed care: Seeking ethical guidance from the formulary? *Journal of the American Geriatrics Society, 46,* 346–350.

*Flanagan, J. (2002). *HMO light and tight plan will restrict access to care and provide fewer patient protections.* The Foundation for Taxpayer and Consumer Rights. www.consumerwatchdog.org/healthcare/pr/pr002772.php3. Accessed March 4, 2004.

*Friedman, Y. M., & Hanchak, N. A. (1999). Pharmacy program performance measurement. In R. P. Navarro (Ed.), *Managed care pharmacy practice* (pp. 199–220). Gaithersburg MD: Aspen Publishers.

Fullerton D. S., & Atherly D. S. (2004). Formularies, therapeutics, and outcomes: New opportunities. *Medical Care. 42*(4 Suppl.), 39–44.

*Glassman, P., Jacobson, P., & Asch, S. (1997). Medical necessity and defined coverage benefits in the Oregon health plan. *American Journal of Public Health, 87,* 1053–1058.

*Greene, J. (2002). The road back to capitation? *Healthplan Magazine.* [On-line] http://www.aahp.org/Content/NavigationMenu/Inside_AAHP/Healthplan_Magazine/The_Road_Back_to_Capitation_.htm. Accessed September 7, 2004.

*Gross, D. J. (1998). Prescription drug formularies in managed care: Concerns for the elderly population. *Clinical Therapeutics, 20,* 1277–1291.

*Heffler, S., Smith, S., Keehan, S., et al. (2004). Health spending projections through 2013. *Health Affairs, 4,* W79–W93.

*Hoechst Marion Roussel. (1998). *The managed care digest series 1998.* Kansas City, MO: Author.

*Horn, S. D., Sharkey, P. D., & Phillips-Harris, C. (1998). Formulary limitations and the elderly: Results from the Managed Care Outcomes Project. *American Journal of Managed Care, 4,* 1105–1113.

*Kaiser Family Foundation. (2001). *Employer health benefits 2001 annual survey.* (Publication No. 3138.). Menlo Park, CA: Author.

*Kaiser Family Foundation. (2003). *Employer health benefits 2003 annual survey.* (Publication No. 3369). Menlo Park, CA: Author.

Keech, M. (2001). Using health outcomes data to inform decision-making. *Pharmacoeconomics, 19,* 27–31.

*Levit, K., Smith, C., Cowan, C., et al. (2004). Health spending rebound continues in 2002. *Health Affairs, 23,* 147–159.

*Lisi, D. (1997). Ethical issues for pharmacists in managed care. *American Journal of Health-System Pharmacy, 54,* 1041–1045.

Luce, B. R., Lyles, A. C., & Rentz, A. M. (1996). The view from managed care pharmacy. *Health Affairs, 15,* 168–176.

Lyles, A., & Palumbo, F. B. (1999). The effect of managed care on prescription drug costs and benefits. *Pharmacoeconomics, 15*(2), 129–140.

Marion Merell Dow, Inc. (1993). *Managed care digest, HMO edition.* Kansas City, MO: Author.

Monane, M., Nagle, B., & Kelly, M. (1998). Pharmacotherapy: Strategies to control drug costs in managed care. *Geriatrics, 53*(9), 53–63.

*National Conference of State Legislatures. (2004). *Pharmacy cost containment strategies.* http://www.ncsl.org/programs/health/forum/cost/strat6.htm. Denver, CO: Author.

*Navarro, R. (Ed.). (1998). *Pharmacy benefit report: Trends and forecasts.* East Hanover, NJ: Novartis Pharmaceuticals.

*Navarro, R. P., & Cahill, J. A. (1999). The U.S. health care system and the development of managed care. In R. P. Navarro (Ed.), *Managed care pharmacy practice* (pp. 3–28). Gaithersburg, MD: Aspen Publishers.

*PBM News. (2001, Fall). *Use of multiple-tier plan designs continue to increase.* (On-line). Available: http://www.pbmi.com/pbmnews/V6N4_plandesigns.html.

Penna, P. M. (2002). AMCP format for formulary submissions: Who is using them, who will be evaluating them, and what regulatory concerns do they raise? International Society for Pharmacoeconomics and Outcomes Research Seventh International Meeting, Arlington, VA.

*Reed, C. (2003). *Rx reimbursement brief: Claritin OTC status triggers series of changes.* (On-line) *PBM News.* http://www.pbmi.com/pb,news/V8N1_claritin.html.

*Roy-Byrne, P., Russo, J., Rabin, L., et al. (1998). A brief medical necessity scale for mental disorders: Reliability, validity, and clinical utility. *Journal of Behavioral Health Services and Research, 25,* 412–424.

Smith, S., Freeland, M., Heffler, S., et al. (1998). The next ten years of health spending: What does the future hold? *Health Affairs, 17*(5), 128–140.

*Sonnedecker, G. (1976). *Kremer's and Urdang's history of pharmacy.* Madison, WI: American Institute of the History of Pharmacy.

*Starr, P. (1982). *The social transformation of American medicine.* New York: Basic Books.

Sweet, B. T., Wilson, M. W., Waugh, W. J., et al. (2002). Building the outcomes-based formulary. *Disease Management and Health Outcomes, 10,* 525–530.

*Takeda Pharmaceuticals. (2003). *The prescription drug benefit cost and plan design survey report* (Publication MC01-0049-3). Lincolnshire, IL: Takeda Pharmaceuticals North America.

*Talley, C. R. (1997). Managed care backlash. *American Journal of Health-System Pharmacy, 54,* 1049.

*Troy, T. (1999). Defining your firm's formulary. *Managed Healthcare, 25–37.*

*U.S. Food and Drug Administration. (2004). *Approved drug products with therapeutic equivalence evaluations* (24th ed.). Rockville, MD: United States Department of Health and Human Services.

Visit the Connection web site for the most up-to-date drug information.

INTEGRATIVE APPROACHES TO PHARMACOTHERAPY—A LOOK AT COMPLEX CASES

■ VIRGINIA P. ARCANGELO AND ANDREW M. PETERSON

The cases presented in each of the chapters on disorders were designed to help the learner think through the process of evaluating the drug therapy needed for a patient. The cases were simple ones, typically involving a single problem related to the disorders discussed in that chapter. This chapter, however, uses cases involving patients with multiple problems, which forces the learner to assess the problems and prioritize them. When faced with multiple problems in a single patient, the practitioner then must decide among a variety of treatment options. This level of complexity is reflective of real-life situations and requires a systematic approach to the patient to manage the complexities.

THE COMPLEXITY OF PATIENTS

The reality of life is that patients are complex individuals with multiple competing issues and priorities. Patients have economic, social, emotional, and cultural issues that affect their medical conditions.

Medications are expensive, with the 2003 average prescription price for a branded medication being $83.66 and generic medication $30.58 (National Association of Chain Drug Stores [NACDS], 2004). Nearly two thirds of elderly patients use medications on a daily basis with an average of 8 prescription medications per person in the elderly (Chrischilles et al., 1992). The monthly cost alone could range from $240 to $640, clearly prohibitive for some patients without a prescription drug coverage plan. The selection, then, of treatment options must consider the cost of the treatment, because if patients cannot afford the treatment they will not follow the plan.

In addition, the social and emotional impact of a diagnosis must be considered. Patients requiring insulin injections to maintain adequate blood sugar levels need assistance in making the lifestyle change necessary to incorporate the injections as well as the monitoring into their daily routine. The emotional reminder of "illness associated with chronic medication-taking behavior" must be addressed at the initial and subsequent visits. Lastly, culturally accepted treatment options are important considerations; injectable medications containing human blood products (eg, albumin) may not be acceptable to patients who are of the Jehovah's Witness faith. In another vein, Asian cultures view illness as an inevitable consequence of life and, as a result, may not seek care or may refuse treatment.

GENERAL OVERVIEW OF METHODS FOR ASSESSING PATIENTS AND DRUG THERAPY

One of the more common methods for organizing medical information is the problem-oriented medical record (POMR). Each of the patient's medical problems is identified and prioritized in order of importance. The order of the problems depends on the acuity and severity of the situation. Typically, the most severe and acute problems are listed first, followed by the chronic conditions, and then problems requiring preventive measures (eg, smoking cessation).

In addition to the prioritized problem list, the POMR system uses the "SOAP" note technique for organizing information associated with each problem. The acronym SOAP stands for (S)ubjective, (O)bjective, (A)ssessment and (P)lan. The subjective and objective components are the data that support the identification of the prioritized problem. The subjective data refer to information provided by the patient (or other individual), which cannot be independently verified. The objective data often are laboratory data or health assessments (eg, blood pressures) performed or observed by the practitioner.

The information needed in this part of the SOAP note includes the chief complaint (CC), history of the present illness (HPI), past medical history, family and social history, medication history, and the results of the review of systems, and physical examination and laboratory results. This data collection is key in the assessment of the patient.

The assessment section of the SOAP note integrates the subjective and objective information and is where the practitioner delineates the potential diagnosis related to the problem. The rationale for the diagnosis should be included as well as an indication of the severity and acuity of the problem. The last portion of the note is the therapeutic plan. In this section, the practitioner may include additional diagnostic tests necessary to confirm or rule out the suspected diagnosis. This diagnostic plan may also include referral to other practitioners as necessary. The other portion of the plan section should include information about changes in therapeutic plans such as adding/deleting drug therapy, identifying desired outcomes, and monitoring parameters.

Anticipating Problems

One of the key elements to a good practitioner is the ability to plan for unintended consequences. A patient may become noncompliant with a medication due to an adverse event and not report the event or the noncompliance to you, before your next scheduled visit. The result is the patient foregoes treatment for an identified problem for an unknown period of time. When confronted, the patient will admit to the noncompliance but indicate that he did not "want to bother you" with the problem. Upfront discussions regarding the potential consequences (adverse reactions, noncompliance) will help reduce the frequency of these types of encounters. As a practitioner, you should always consider what you will do if your patient has a drug reaction, takes an interacting drug, or even stops taking the drug.

Other Information Needed Before Prescribing

When taking a medication history, the practitioner needs to assess specific information related to drug therapy. An inventory of patient-reported allergies is vital to a good medication history. These allergies include an assessment of the drug allergies. A patient may report a symptom as an allergy, but the clinician must assess the validity of the report. For example, a patient may report abdominal discomfort as an allergy to erythromycin but in reality, the reported symptom is an adverse effect of the drug. This type of report is not a true allergy and would not preclude the patient from receiving that drug or a related drug. However, the practitioner must consider the impact the symptom has on the patient's willingness to take a prescribed medication. If the patient was prescribed a medication that would cause distress, the patient is less likely to take it.

Food allergies are also important to assess. Reports of allergies to shellfish or other iodine-containing foods are important to know when prescribing medications such as intravenous contrast dyes.

Further, within this section of the patient history, the practitioner must not only assess prescription medication use, but also obtain a good history of nonprescription and complementary and alternative medication use. In 2002, 19% of adults used natural products as part of their personal treatment plan. The most commonly used products were echinacea (40.3%), ginseng (24.1%), and gingko biloba (21.1%; Barnes et al., 2004). The potential for drug–drug and drug–disease interactions with these, and other agents, exists and must be considered as part of the treatment plan.

Questions

As noted earlier, each disorder chapter had a simple case with a series of questions designed to help you work through the pharmacotherapeutic approach to the patient. These nine questions are indicative of a thought process that should be followed when developing the pharmacotherapeutic aspect of the care plan. The following real-life cases are more complex than those in the disorder chapters and are designed to help the learner integrate the treatment plan for patients with multiple disorders. We use the same nine questions, in varying forms, to exemplify the thought process. The answers provided may not be the only "right" answers. Other choices of drug therapy may clearly be available or as time progresses, we may learn that there are better choices due to new drug development and new research on existing drugs. We encourage you to use this process to help you think through the problem, not just come up with an answer.

CASES

■ Case 1: Diabetes/Lipids/HTN/CAD with Microalbuminuria

J.S. is a 52-year-old white man who is an accountant who was diagnosed with type 2 diabetes mellitus 5 years ago. The disease has been controlled with diet. He also has osteoarthritis of his right knee and a strong family history of coronary artery disease (CAD). He comes to the office complaining of frequent urination, blurry vision, and fatigue. He leads a very sedentary life. He does walk his dog for 10 minutes every night but that is the only exercise he gets. He does not regularly check his blood sugar.

Weight 250 lb

Height 70 in.

BP 142/88

Pulse 72

Current medications: naproxen 500 mg bid, as needed

Labs values:

   Glucose 260 mg/dL

   HgbA$_{1c}$ 8.9%

   Total cholesterol 250 mg/dL

     LDL 140 mg/dL

     HDL 30 mg/dL

     Triglycerides 280 mg/dL

   Creatinine 1.0 mg/dL

   BUN 14 mg/dL

   AST 15

   ALT 20

   Urine microalbumin +

Issues: J.S. has type 2 diabetes mellitus. In addition, he is obese, has hyperlipidemia, hypertension, and microalbuminuria. All of these factors must be considered in determining which medications are appropriate for J.S.

List Specific Goals for Treatment for J.S.

One of the primary goals for J.S. is to lower his risk for developing complications associated with metabolic syndrome. These include microvascular complications such as retinopathy, neuropathy, nephropathy, and the macrovascular complications of heart attack, stroke, and death. Preventing these are the long-term goals. The intermediate goals for J.S. are as follows:

Maintaining fasting blood glucose at <120 mg/dL
Maintaining HgbA$_{1c}$ at <7%
Preventing complications of diabetes mellitus
Prevention of cardiovascular morbidity and mortality by reducing blood pressure to <120/80
Reducing total cholesterol to <200 mg/dL
Reducing low-density lipoprotein to <70 mg/dL

What Drug Therapy Would You Prescribe? Why?

J.S.'s profile indicates metabolic syndrome. Appropriate medications for him would include biguanides and thiazolidinediones because they decrease peripheral insulin resistance. Either one is appropriate because his renal function (creatinine) and liver function are within normal levels. Pioglitazone (Actos) is an appropriate choice because it has been demonstrated to increase high-density lipoprotein (HDL).

Blood pressure control is also an issue with J.S. It is recommended that in the diabetic patient angiotensin-converting enzyme (ACE) inhibitors or angiotensin receptor blockers (ARBs) be used to protect kidney function. The addition of either of these agents is appropriate.

Hyperlipidemia is also a problem with J.S.. His total cholesterol should be under 200 mg/dL with his LDL less than 70 mg/dL. His HDL should be more than 40 mg/dL. A statin should be started at the lowest therapeutic dose.

What Are the Parameters for Monitoring Success of the Therapy?

Success of therapy for diabetes mellitus is determined by measurement of HgbA$_{1c}$ every 3 months. If the HgbA$_{1c}$ level does not show a downward progression or is not below 7%, the dosage of the drug should be increased or if J.S. is at the maximum dose, a second and sometimes a third drug is added. Liver function tests should be done every 2 months for the first year of therapy with pioglitazone and periodically afterward because of the potential for hepatotoxicity.

Success of therapy for hypertension is measured by blood pressure readings. Ideally, blood pressure for a diabetic patient should be under 120/80. Lipid therapy is monitored by repeat lipid profiles in 4 to 6 weeks with liver function tests performed to make sure that the statin has not caused a rise of aspartate aminotransferase (AST) or alanine aminotransferase (ALT). This is also an important measurement for the pioglitazone.

Discuss Specific Patient Education Based on the Prescribed Therapy

Patient education includes teaching the signs and symptoms of hypoglycemia, dietary modifications for lowering blood sugar and cholesterol. Consideration should be given to having J.S. see a dietitian to review specific changes in his diet to meet the therapeutic lifestyle changes needed to maximize drug therapy efficacy.

Additional discussion should focus on the potential side effects of these agents. If J.S. experiences muscle aches and pains, he should seek attention to rule out rhabdomyolysis secondary to the statin. Similarly, ACE-inhibitor cough, while not life-threatening, is a common side effect and J.S. should monitor for it.

List One or Two Adverse Reactions for the Selected Agent that Would Cause You to Change Therapy

If J.S. is taking an ACE inhibitor and developed a cough, it would be appropriate to switch to an ARB.

If myalgias occur, this could be a side effect of the statin and sometimes lowering the dose or switching to another statin may rectify this. Additionally, creatine kinase (CK) should be measured to see if it is increases. Patients may experience myalgias, however, without increased CK. If the symptoms persist on another statin, ezetimibe (Zetia) may be considered.

Pioglitazone may cause edema. If this occurs, J.S. can be switched to metformin.

What Would Be the Choice for Second-Line Therapy?

If J.S.'s blood glucose is not controlled or his HgbA$_{1c}$ is above 7%, an insulin secreatagogue can be added to the therapy.

If his blood pressure is not at an appropriate level, a second antihypertensive agent may be added. A diuretic is often very effective in combination with other drug therapy.

If lipids have not reached therapeutic levels, exetimibe can be added to the current statin for further reduction.

What Over-the-Counter or Alternative Medications Would Be Appropriate for J.S.?

Aspirin 81 mg daily is recommended for prophylaxis of heart attack or stroke. Higher doses than this can slightly increase the risk of a peptic ulcer and offer little additional benefit. Fish oil is recommended for hyperlipidemia. Cinnamon has been investigated for lowering blood sugar levels in patients with diabetes.

What Lifestyle Changes Would You Recommend to J.S.?

J.S. needs to reduce his weight. This can be accomplished by dietary changes and increased exercise. If he has a high sodium intake, reducing this to 100 mEq or less daily can help to reduce his blood pressure. J.S. is encouraged to follow a low-fat diet to reduce his cholesterol and reduce his risk for a major cardiac event. Fat intake should be restricted to 25% to 35% of total calories.

Describe One or Two Drug–Drug or Drug–Food Interactions for the Selected Agent

Pioglitazone can interact with decongestants, which decrease its hypoglycemic efficacy.

There may be a decreased antihypertensive effect with nonsteroidal anti-inflammatory drugs (NSAIDs) and antihypertensive agents so blood pressure must be carefully be monitored. Some statins have an interaction with grapefruit. Grapefruit can increase the 3-hydroxy-3-methylglutaryl-coenzyme A (HMG CoA) inhibitor levels. St. John's wort can decrease statin levels.

■ Case 2: Elderly/Statin/Warfarin Comes Down With an Infection

M.T. is a 66-year-old woman with a chief complaint of generalized feeling poor and a 24-hour history of dysuria, urinary frequency, and urgency. She has had recent sexual activity. She has a 1-year history of atrial fibrillation. She is also has type 2 diabetes and hypercholesterolemia. She had a hysterectomy 3 years ago.

Her medications include: simvastatin, 40 mg qd; diltiazem extended release, 180 mg bid; sotalol, 80 mg bid; warfarin, 7.5 mg qd; metformin, 850 mg bid; calcium carbonate, 1000 mg qd.

Most recent pertinent labs:

INR 2.2   Creatinine 1.3 mg/dL

All others WNL

Physical exam—unremarkable except for urinalysis: WBC 10–15 cells/hpf, RBCs, 1–5 cells/hpf, bacteria 2–5/hpf, nitrite negative

Allergies: NKDA

Diagnosis: Acute uncomplicated urinary tract infection (UTI)

What Specific Goals Do You Have for M.T.'s Current Condition?

The goals of treatment for M.T. include eradication of the urinary bacteria and a return to a normal urinary habit.

What Drug Therapy Would You Prescribe? Why?

A variety of drug choices are available for M.T. Antibiotic therapy is the mainstay of treatment because UTIs are typically bacterial in nature. One of the most common organisms causing an uncomplicated UTI is *Escherichia coli*. The first-line therapy for treating this type organism in a UTI is typically sulfamethoxazole–trimethoprim (Bactrim). This agent concentrates well in the urine and has good activity against *E. coli*. Often, a single-day or a 3-day treatment regimen of double-strength sulfamethoxazole–trimethoprim is sufficient to eradicate the organism. However, in patients with diabetes, single-dose treatment is not recommended. There are some reports of an increasing resistance to this agent, which may be endemic to a geographical region (Butler et al., 2001).

In the case of M.T., however, sulfamethoxazole–trimethoprim may not be the best first choice. Due to her atrial fibrillation, she is receiving warfarin as venous thromboembolism (VTE) prophylaxis. The drug–drug interaction between warfarin and sulfamethoxazole–trimethoprim can lead to increased international normalized ratios (INRs). Although her INR is 2.2 (within the desired range of 2–3), the protein binding displacement of warfarin caused by the sulfamethoxazole component can lead to unacceptable changes in the coagulation factors. This would place M.T. at risk for a minor or a major bleed, particularly if she were to inadvertently injure herself through a fall. Instead, she would be a candidate for a fluoroquinolone antibiotic such as levofloxacin or ciprofloxacin. For purposes of further discussion, M.T. will be prescribed levofloxacin.

Consideration should be given to the appropriate dose of levofloxacin. For uncomplicated UTIs, the dose is typically 250 mg orally daily for 3 days. Typically, a fluoroquinolone dose adjustment should be made for patients with renal dysfunction (estimated creatinine clearance [CrCl] <50 mL/min). However, because the drug concentrates well in the urine, and the dose is low to begin with, the adjustment is not necessary for UTIs until the CrCl is 20 mL/min or less.

What Are the Parameters for Monitoring Success of the Drug Therapy?

The primary parameter would be a resolution of the symptoms. M.T. should return to a normal urinary habit within 48 to 72 hours after initiation of antibiotic treatment. A repeat urinalysis after treatment ends would confirm bacterial eradication, but often is unnecessary if symptoms resolve. If the symptoms do not resolve, then a urine culture is indicated.

Discuss Specific Patient Education Based on the Prescribed Therapy

The patient should be educated on the need for taking levofloxacin for the entire 3 days even if the symptoms begin to resolve. Information regarding increasing water/fluid intake should also be part of the patient education process.

Describe One or Two Drug–Drug or Drug–Food Interactions for Levofloxacin

The patient should also be advised not to take the levofloxacin with chelating agents such as iron supplements, magnesium- or aluminum-containing antacids, or zinc products. If M.T. needs to take one or more of these, then the levofloxacin should be taken 2 hours before or after the agent.

Further, quinolones have been reported to enhance the effects of warfarin anticoagulation when administered concomitantly. No specific dosage adjustments are needed with either medication, but the INR should be monitored closely to prevent bleeding complications.

List One or Two Adverse Reactions for the Levofloxacin That Would Cause You to Change Therapy

Many side effects can be associated with quinolone antibiotics. Common ones include gastrointestinal (GI), neurologic, and cardiac disturbances. The GI effects such as vomiting and diarrhea put her at risk for dehydration, worsening her metabolic state. The neurologic effects such as seizures, delirium, and abnormal coordination put her at risk for falls and the development of a major bleed.

What Would Be the Choice for the Second-Line Therapy?

An alternative agent, besides sulfamethoxazole–trimethoprim, is nitrofurantoin 50 mg 4 times a day for 7 days. Nitrofurantoin is typically less effective than the other two agents when treating UTIs. Further, the lack of tissue penetration may predispose the patient to a recurrent UTI. It is recommended that urinary cultures be taken 3 days after completion of the 7-day course of therapy to document bacteria eradication.

What Over-the-Counter or Alternative Medications Would Be Appropriate for M.T.?

There are no over-the-counter of complementary/alternative medications appropriate to treat M.T.'s infection. The practitioner should discourage the use of these types of medications, particularly those that may interact with her warfarin.

What Dietary and Lifestyle Changes Should Be Recommended for M.T.?

M.T. should be encouraged to drink plenty of water, particularly while taking the antibiotic. The water helps to flush the bacteria out of the system. Also, M.T. should be encouraged to urinate when she has the urge; she should not hold back on urination because this may increase the bacterial growth. Also, M.T. should be sure to urinate after sexual activity to prevent future UTIs.

■ Case 3: Postmenopausal/Hypothyroid/Osteoporosis

L.L. is a 56-year-old white woman who has not menstruated for 1 year. She is waking up at night with hot flashes, and, consequently is tired all of the time. During the day she has 8 to 10 hot flashes and is very uncomfortable. She wants to do something about the hot flashes. Her gynecologic exam and Pap smear are normal and you order a dual-energy x-ray absorptiometry (DEXA) scan.

PMH: Hypothyroidism

Medications: Vitamin C 1000 mg daily

Synthroid 112 μg daily

Ibuprofen as needed for back pain

Multivitamin daily

Weight 115 lbs

Height 5'6" (she was 5'8" 2 years ago)

BP 118/76

DEXA scan: t score of –2.6 left hip and –2.0 lumbar spine

TSH 7.4

Issues: L.L. is postmenopausal and is symptomatic for hot flashes. She also has osteoporosis. Another area of concern is poor control of hypothyroidism.

List Specific Goals for Treatment for L.L.

For L.L., there are two types of outcomes desired: humanistic and clinical. The humanistic outcomes relate to the quality of life. In the short run, this would mean a reduction in the menopausal symptoms for L.L. and an improvement in the symptoms related to poor thyroid control. In the long run, the clinical goal would be to prevent the development of fractures. L.L.'s DEXA scan results shows that she is at risk for fractures, and if she continues on this course, the risk will only increase. Therefore, goals of therapy include:

- Reduction of menopausal symptoms
- Prevention of fracture
- Maintenance of thyroid function at normal levels

What Drug Therapy Would You Prescribe? Why?

L.L. should be prescribed a low-dose combination of hormone therapy including estrogen and progesterone because she has an intact uterus. A dose of 0.3 mg estrogen and 1.5 mg progesterone is acceptable. She should be kept on this therapy for the shortest possible time just for relief of menopausal symptoms.

Alendronate (Fosamax) 70 mg is a suitable choice for osteoporosis. It is given once a week.

L.L.'s Synthroid dose must be increased because she is still hypothyroid. An increase to 125 μg will be made.

What Are the Parameters for Monitoring Success of the Therapy?

Patient history of menopausal symptom relief is the key to determining if hormone therapy is successful. L.L. should return in 2 months to check response to hormone replacement therapy (HRT) and blood pressure. It is recommended that L.L. stay on HRT for the shortest possible time to prevent cardiac events.

L.L.'s thyroid-stimulating hormone (TSH) level should be rechecked in 6 to 8 weeks. If it is within normal levels, the dose of Synthroid should remain at 125 μg. TSH should be monitored in 6 months and then yearly if it is stable.

A DEXA scan should be repeated every 2 years to ensure effectiveness of therapy. There should be little to no change in the DEXA scan results during therapy with alendronate. Compliance should also be checked.

Discuss Specific Patient Education Based on the Prescribed Therapy

L.L. must be told that it may take at least 4 weeks of HRT before she notices a significant change in menopausal symptoms. It is important that she be taught the correct method for performing a monthly breast self-exam and to report any palpable masses. Any abnormal vaginal bleeding is to be reported immediately.

Thyroid medications should be taken 1 hour before or 4 hours after any other medications, especially calcium and iron supplements. It needs to be stressed that L.L. will require life-long thyroid replacement.

Alendronate must be taken at least 30 minutes before any other food or liquid (except what is used to take the medicine). L.L. should remain in a sitting or standing position for at least 30 minutes after ingestion to prevent damage to the esophagus.

List One or Two Adverse Reactions for the Selected Agent That Would Cause You to Change Therapy

Adverse reactions of HRT include GI upset and elevated blood pressure. Adverse reactions of Synthroid include palpitations and nervousness. If this occurs, the TSH level needs to be checked because it indicates too high a dose of Synthroid. An adverse event associated with alendronate is severe GI upset.

What Would Be the Choice for Second-Line Therapy?

Use of a transdermal hormone patch can reduce menopausal symptoms and many side effects. If the patch does not contain progesterone, supplemental progesterone must be given to prevent uterine hyperplasia.

Calcitonin would be a second-line therapy for osteoporosis for L.L. A selective estrogen receptor modulator (SERM) would not be appropriate with HRT because the combination increases the risk of clots.

What Over-the-Counter or Alternative Medications Would Be Appropriate for L.L.?

Black cohash can be used in place of HRT with some relief of symptoms. Calcium at a dose of 1500 mg with 400 U vitamin D is recommended for postmenopausal women in addition to the alendronate but should be taken at least 2 hours after the alendronate because it can interfere with absorption.

What Lifestyle Changes Would You Recommend to L.L.?

L.L. should wear cool clothing to diminish the hot flashes. Weight-bearing exercises are important in the patient with osteoporosis because they build bone mass.

Describe One or Two Drug–Drug or Drug–Food Interactions for the Selected Agent

Synthroid absorption is decreased if given with calcium products and should be taken 1 hour before or 4 hours after calcium. Antacids can decrease absorption of alendronate.

■ Case 4: Asthma/ADHD/Allergies With Exacerbation of Allergy

N.J. is an 11-year-old boy with a 5-year history of attention deficit hyperactivity disorder (ADHD) and a 7-year history of asthma. He also experiences perennial allergic rhinitis. N.J.'s mother is bringing him into your office due to an exacerbation of this allergy. The symptoms he presents with include increased cough and runny nose, sneezing. He has no other medical history. The following is his current list of medications.

Concerta 36 mg every morning

Albuterol inhaler, 2 puffs as needed (uses 1–2 times a day)

Singulair 5 mg PO daily

Zyrtec 5 mg PO daily

List Specific Goals of Treatment for N.J.

The obvious goal is to decrease the coughing and other allergic symptoms. However, it is not clear if the cough is a secondary manifestation of the uncontrolled asthma or as a result of the rhinorrhea associated with the allergies. Therefore, an additional goal would be to improve the asthma control. Specific goals related to asthma would be a decrease in the frequency of use of the albuterol inhaler.

What Drug Therapy Would Be Appropriate for N.J.? Why?

For the treatment of the allergies, consider adding on a short course of diphenhydramine 25 mg orally every 6 hours to the already existing cetirizine. Watch for the potential oversedation due to the combination of antihistamines. There should be relief of the runny nose, and if secondary to the rhinorrhea, there should also be a decrease in the cough within 24 to 48 hours.

As for the asthma, the National Asthma Education and Prevention Program (NAEPP) update of 2002 recommends that all persons with persistent asthma be prescribed an inhaled corticosteroid controller. N.J.'s moderate persistent asthma should also be treated with a long-acting β_2 agonist such as salmeterol. A good product to consider would be the combination product, Advair Diskus. This product contains both fluticasone and salmeterol in three different dosage strengths (100/50, 250/50, and 500/50 per inhalation). The fluticasone dose increases (100 mg, 250 mg, and 500 mg), whereas the salmeterol component remains constant. An appropriate starting dose for N.J. is one inhalation of the 100/50 Advair Diskus twice daily. Improvement in the asthma symptoms should be seen within a week of constant therapy.

The data on the combination of a leukotriene inhibitor to an inhaled corticosteroid, with or without a long-acting β agonist, show that there is little additive benefit in patients with moderate asthma. Therefore, the leukotriene inhibitor should be discontinued while the inhaled corticosteroid and long-acting β agonist are added.

What are the Parameters for Monitoring Success of the Therapy?

For the allergies, a reduction in the rhinorrhea, and if appropriate, a decrease in the cough would be good clinical markers of success. For the asthma, the primary indicator would be a decreased use of the short-acting β agonist as well as improved lung function such as improved peak flow readings.

Discuss Specific Patient Education Based on the Prescribed Therapy

An investigation of the potential changes in the household or other environmental changes should be part of the workup. Discussion with the mother and child regarding triggers is a key to preventing these exacerbations.

Also, specific education regarding the appropriate way of using the Advair Diskus is needed. The Web site, www.advair.com, is a good source of information regarding appropriate use of the product.

Finally, the patient needs to be educated about the use of this agent as a long-term controller and not a symptom reliever. Advair is not intended to relieve acute symptoms of asthma and use of it in this manner could result in excessive β₂-agonist activity and a worsening of asthma.

List One or Two Adverse Reactions for the Selected Agent That Would Cause You to Change Therapy

Several cardiovascular effects may warrant changing therapy in patient's taking salmeterol. These include palpitations, chest pain, and tachycardia. If these occur, the clinician should be notified immediately and alternative therapy should be considered. When considering alternative therapy, a thorough review of the use of short-acting β₂ agonists must also be considered because these will also produce similar

symptoms. Further, an increasing need for short-acting β₂ agonists or a perceived lack of benefit of short-acting β₂ agonists may be a sign of seriously worsening asthma and the patient should notify the clinician immediately.

What Would be the Choice for the Second-Line Therapy for Treating N.J.?

Budesonide, triamcinolone, and beclomethasone are acceptable alternatives to the fluticasone present in the Advair. Dose equivalency and the frequency of administration are considerations. Typically, the dosing administration should be kept to twice daily, because 3 or 4 times daily may lead to noncompliance.

An alternative to the salmeterol is another long-acting β₂ agonist, formoterol fumarate (Foradil Aerolizer). This agent is a dry-powder capsule that is administered via an aerolizer twice daily. The patient must be educated on using the capsule/aerolizer product properly and told that the capsule is not to be swallowed.

There are advantages to the two distinct medications. The dose of the inhaled corticosteroid can be tailored without consideration of too much or too little long-acting β₂ agonist. Also, the β₂ agonist can be administered independently of the inhaled corticosteroid in cases like exercise-induced asthma. However, the two separate products increase the risk of noncompliance.

What Over-the-Counter or Alternative Medications Would be Appropriate for N.J.?

For treating the rhinorrhea, diphenhydramine is an over-the-counter antihistamine. Other antihistamines are also available over the counter, but do not have the same anticholinergic or H₁-antagonistic properties and are less likely to be of value to N.J.

What Dietary and Lifestyle Changes Should be Recommended for N.J.?

Avoidance of allergen triggers should be considered one of the primary lifestyle changes. Removal of carpets from the bedroom, keeping pets out of rooms in which N.J. spends time, and washing sheets/linens in hot water weekly are some of the strategies for reducing environmental allergens. Exposure to second-hand smoke should also be minimized.

■ Case 5: Depression/GERD

M.M. is a 60-year-old African American man who presents with a 3-month history of lack of sleep because he awakens every 2 hours and cannot get back to sleep. He lacks desire to do anything that he previously enjoyed, has an increased appetite, and does not want to leave his house. It is an effort for him to go to work every morning. Additionally, he says that when he eats anything, he gets burning in his stomach and esophagus and is awakened at night with indigestion.

Social history: Married for 35 years to the same woman. Two grown children. His 15- year-old dog died 3 months ago. He took the dog everywhere with him. He smokes 1/2 pack of cigarettes a day.

BP 126/80

P 76

Weight 204 lb

Height 67 in.

Rest of physical exam WNL

Labs:

TSH 3.4

PSA 0.6

Cholesterol 212 mg/dL

LDL 128 mg/dL

HDL 40 mg/dL

Issues: M.M. has the symptoms of depression. Insomnia is an issue. He also has the symptoms of new-onset gastroesophageal reflux disease (GERD).

List Specific Goals for Treatment for M.M.

The goals of therapy for M.M. relate to quality of life as well as clinical goals. Relieving the depressive symptoms should help M.M. enjoy life and feel better, but the time frame for response is 4 to 6 weeks, provided the initial therapy works. This should be discussed with M.M. as therapy is initiated. A depression scale, such as the Hamilton Depression Scale (HAM-D), might be given to determine a baseline level of depression and as a means of monitoring progress as treatment continues. A specific goal might be a 50% decrease or better from the baseline HAM-D score.

However, relief of indigestion and providing adequate sleep are more immediate goals that should be achievable within the first week of therapy. Progress on these short-term goals is likely to help M.M. continue with the therapy for relieving the long-term problem of depression. Therefore, specific goals are:

• Relief of symptoms of depression
• Provision of adequate sleep
• Relief from indigestion

What Drug Therapy Would You Prescribe for M.M.? Why?

Paroxetine is a good choice because it promotes better sleep. It is best to give this agent in the evening due to the slight sedative effects. If another agent is on formulary at a substantially lower cost, such as sertraline, it can be prescribed and taken in the morning. Ambien might be prescribed concomitantly with sertraline to aid in inducing sleep.

A proton pump inhibitor (PPI) would be a reasonable choice for relief of his GERD now, but because this is new-onset GERD, he should be referred for an endoscopy.

What are the Parameters for Monitoring Success of the Therapy?

Follow-up history is the best way to monitor therapy for depression. Readministration of a depression scale with an improved score would indicate successful therapy. Also indication of 8 hours of sleep a night demonstrates successful therapy. Patient-reported frequency and severity of GERD episodes is a good tool to determine success of therapy for GERD. This would be in addition to any structural changes that might have been identified in the baseline endoscopy. If indicated from the baseline tests, a follow-up endoscopy might be indicated.

Discuss Specific Patient Education Based on the Prescribed Therapy

The overall premise is the promotion of "good sleep habits," which include setting a routine bedtime, instituting regular exercise habits, using the bed for sleeping only, and getting in bed only when ready for sleep. Occasional completion of a sleep log is an important tool for the clinician to evaluate the effectiveness of therapy.

Lifestyle changes are as important as drug therapy in managing GERD. Discussion with the patient and family should cover the following important dietary changes: avoidance of excess alcohol and food intake; decreased amounts of chocolate and spicy, fried, or fatty foods eaten; and avoidance of the recumbent position for at least 3 hours after meals. Because these recommended changes involve many activities or foods that are pleasurable for the patient, they should be eliminated gradually—one at a time. A nutritionist can be consulted to help the patient learn to choose and prepare less problematic foods.

Additional measures include teaching the patient to elevate the head of the bed approximately 4 to 6 inches (using blocks); to avoid tight, restrictive clothing; and to lose weight if necessary. Smoking cessation is another goal of patient education.

List an Adverse Reaction for the Selected Agents That Would Cause You to Change Therapy

If M.M. complains of decreased libido from the paroxetine, then consideration should be given to lowering the dose or changing to a non–selective serotonin receptor inhibitor therapy. This is particularly important if it becomes upsetting to him because he and his wife have a very satisfying sexual relationship.

What Would Be the Choice for Second-Line Therapy?

Lowering the dose of paroxetine might help with the side effects. However, if this is not possible, bupropion is an appropriate choice for second-line therapy for the depression, particularly as it relates to the sexual side effects.

What Over-the-Counter or Alternative Medications Would be Appropriate for M.M.?

Some patients, especially those with delayed sleep phase insomnia, may benefit from the administration of exogenous melatonin; however, further study is necessary.

Peppermint is used by some for the treatment of GERD. It relaxes the sphincter of Oddi by reducing calcium influx and stimulates bile flow in animals by the choleretic action of its flavonoid components. The menthol has a direct spasmolytic effect on smooth muscle of the digestive tract.

What Lifestyle Changes Would you Recommend to M.M.?

Lifestyle modifications are essential for the patient with GERD. Although drug therapy will help reduce the level of acid in the stomach and promote healing, lifestyle changes will aid in preventing the symptoms from returning. These lifestyle changes include dietary changes, such as avoiding irritating foods like caffeine, alcohol, and spicy foods. Further, refraining from eating at least 3 hours before bedtime and elevating the head of the bed by at least 6 inches will help reduce nighttime symptoms. Weight loss will also reduce the frequency of GERD symptoms. Lastly, smoking cessation will reduce the frequency of GERD.

The overall premise is the promotion of "good sleep habits," which include setting a routine bedtime, instituting regular exercise habits, using the bed for sleeping only, and getting in bed only when ready for sleep. Occasional completion of a sleep log is an important tool for the clinician to evaluate the effectiveness of therapy.

Describe One or Two Drug–Drug or Drug–Food Interactions for the Selected Agents

Paroxetine is an inhibitor of the CYP 2D6 system and might increase the serum concentrations of cough suppressants such as dextromethorphan and codeine, so care must be taken when using these agents during the cough/cold season. The PPIs, omeprazole, lansoprazole, and pantoprazole, are inhibitors of the CYP2C19 system and would increase levels of drugs such as diazepam, phenytoin, or amitriptyline.

CONCLUSION

These are a few examples of the decision-making process in prescribing medications. Most patients do not present with just one diagnosis and are taking several medications and these factors must be considered in deciding on the best pharmacologic approaches. The intent of these examples is to help the reader understand *possible* solutions to some common problems. Not all the problems are addressed fully, nor would they be in real-life. The complexity of patients requires the practitioner to begin to judge which problems should be addressed first and with what therapy. As the relationship between the practitioner and the patient continues, other problems can be addressed.

Bibliography

Starred references are cited in the text.

*Barnes, P. M., Powell-Griner, E., McFinn, K., et al. (2004). Complementary and alternative medication use among adults; United States, 2002. *Advance Data from Vital and Health Statistics.* 343.

*Butler, K. H., Reed, K. C., & Bosker, G. (2004). New diagnostic modalities, alterations in drug resistance patterns, and current antimicrobial treatment guidelines for the hospital and outpatient setting. Part I: Diagnosis, evaluation, and principles of antibiotic selection. Clinical Consensus Reports. http://www.ahcpub.com/ahc_root_html/ccr/uti_pt1.html. Accessed September 25, 2004.

*Chrischilles, E. A., Foley, D. J., Wallace, R. B., et al. (1992). Use of medications by persons 65 and over: Data from the established populations for epidemiologic studies of the elderly. *Journal of Gerontology, 47,* M137–144.

*National Association of Chain Drug Stores. (2004). National association of chain drug stores. http://www.nacds.org/wmspage.cfm?parm1=507. Accessed September 25, 2004.

Visit the Connection web site for the most up-to-date drug information.

INDEX

■ *Note:* Page numbers followed by "f" denote figures; those followed by "t" denote tables; and those followed by "b" denote boxes.